Kistner's Gynecology *and* Women's Health

Kistner's Gynecology and Women's Health

Seventh Edition

Kenneth J. Ryan, M.D.

Kate Macy Ladd Professor Emeritus of Obstetrics, Gynecology, and Reproductive Biology
Brigham and Women's Hospital
Harvard Medical School
Boston, Massachusetts

Ross S. Berkowitz, M.D.

William H. Baker Professor of Gynecology
Director of Gynecology and Gynecologic Oncology
Department of Obstetrics and Gynecology
Brigham and Women's Hospital
Harvard Medical School
Boston, Massachusetts

Robert L. Barbieri, M.D.

Kate Macy Ladd Professor of Obstetrics, Gynecology and Reproductive Biology
Harvard Medical School
Chairman, Department of Obstetrics and Gynecology
Brigham and Women's Hospital
Boston, Massachusetts

Andrea Dunaif, M.D.

Chief, Division of Women's Health
Department of Medicine and of Obstetrics and Gynecology
Brigham and Women's Hospital
Boston, Massachusetts

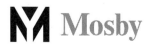

St. Louis Baltimore Boston Carlsbad Chicago Minneapolis New York Philadelphia Portland
London Milan Sydney Tokyo Toronto

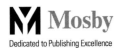
Mosby
Dedicated to Publishing Excellence

Editor-In-Chief: Sally Schrefer
Editor: Geoff Greenwood
Developmental Editor: Rebecca Gruliow
Project Manager: Deborah L. Vogel
Designer: Bill Drone

SEVENTH EDITION

Composition by Graphic World, Inc.
Printing/binding by Maple-Vail Book Mfg. Group

Mosby, Inc.
11830 Westline Industrial Drive
St. Louis, Missouri 63146

Library of Congress Cataloging-in-Publication Data

Kistner's gynecology and women's health / [edited by] Kenneth J. Ryan
 . . . [et al.] —7th ed.
       p.   cm.
    Rev. ed. of: Kistner's gynecology / [edited by] Kenneth J. Ryan,
Ross S. Berkowitz, Robert L. Barbieri. 6th ed. c1995.
    Includes bibliographical references and index.
    ISBN 0-323-00201-3
    1. Gynecology. 2. Women—Health and hygiene. I. Ryan, Kenneth J.
II. Kistner, Robert W. (Robert William), Gynecology.   III. Kistner's gynecology.
IV. Ryan, Kenneth J.   V. Kistner, Robert W. (Robert William), Gynecology.
VI. Kistner's gynecology.   VII. Title: Gynecology and women's
health.   VIII. Title: Gynecology and women's health.
    [DNLM: 1. Genital Diseases, Female.   2. Genital Neoplasms, Female.
3. Women's Health.   4. Genital Diseases, Female.   5. Genital
Neoplasms, Female.   6. Women's Health.   WP 140 K61 1999 / WP 140
K61 1999]
RG101.G923 1999
618.1—dc21
DNLM/DLC
for Library of Congress   99–24042
                                                                CIP

99 00 01 02 03 / 9 8 7 6 5 4 3 2 1

Contributors

David W. Bates, M.D.
Division of General Medicine
Department of Medicine
Brigham and Women's Hospital
Boston, Massachusetts

Joan M. Bengtson, M.D.
Department of Obstetrics and Gynecology
HCHP-Brigham and Women's Hospital
Boston, Massachusetts

Katherine T. Chen, M.D.
Obstetrics and Gynecology
Brigham and Women's Hospital
Boston, Massachusetts

Sarah Feldman, M.D.
Division of Gynecologic Oncology
Brigham and Women's Hospital
Boston, Massachusetts

Janis H. Fox, M.D.
Center for Reproductive Medicine
Department of Obstetrics and Gynecology
Brigham and Women's Hospital
Boston, Massachusetts

Elizabeth S. Ginsburg, M.D.
Center for Reproductive Medicine
Department of Obstetrics and Gynecology
Brigham and Women's Hospital
Boston, Massachusetts

Donald P. Goldstein, M.D.
Division of Gynecologic Oncology
Brigham and Women's Hospital
Boston, Massachusetts

Marie-Andrée Harvey, M.D.
Division of Urogynecology
Department of Obstetrics and Gynecology
Brigham and Women's Hospital
Boston, Massachusetts

Joseph A. Hill, M.D.
Chief, Division of Reproductive Medicine
Department of Obstetrics and Gynecology
Brigham and Women's Hospital
Boston, Massachusetts

Mark D. Hornstein, M.D.
Center for Reproductive Medicine
Department of Obstetrics and Gynecology
Brigham and Women's Hospital
Boston, Massachusetts

Helen H. Kim, M.D.
Center for Reproductive Medicine
Department of Obstetrics and Gynecology
Brigham and Women's Hospital
Boston, Massachusetts

Susan Caruso Klock, Ph.D.
Reproductive Endocrinology
Department of Obstetrics and Gynecology
Northwestern University Medical School
Chicago, Illinois

Marc R. Laufer, M.D.
Center for Reproductive Medicine
Department of Obstetrics and Gynecology
Brigham and Women's Hospital
Boston, Massachusetts

Karen L. Miller, M.D.
Department of Medicine and Gerontology
Brigham and Women's Hospital
Boston, Massachusetts

Michael G. Muto, M.D.
Division of Gynecologic Oncology
Brigham and Women's Hospital
Boston, Massachusetts

Rapin Osathanondh, M.D.
Family Planning Service
Department of Obstetrics and Gynecology
Brigham and Women's Hospital
Boston, Massachusetts

Mitchell S. Rein, M.D.
Chief, Department of Obstetrics and Gynecology
Salem Hospital/North Shore Medical Center
Salem, Massachusetts

Neil M. Resnick, M.D.
Department of Medicine and Gerontology
Brigham and Women's Hospital
Boston, Massachusetts

Laurel W. Rice, M.D.
Department of Obstetrics and Gynecology
University of Virginia Health Sciences Center
Charlottesville, Virginia

Ellen E. Sheets, M.D.
Division of Gynecologic Oncology
Brigham and Women's Hospital
Boston, Massachusetts

Barbara L. Smith, M.D.
Director, Comprehensive Breast Health Center
Department of Surgery
Massachusetts General Hospital
Boston, Massachusetts

Elizabeth A. Stewart, M.D.
Center for Reproductive Medicine
Department of Obstetrics and Gynecology
Brigham and Women's Hospital
Boston, Massachusetts

Ann E. Taylor, M.D.
Reproductive Endocrine Unit
Department of Medicine
Massachusetts General Hospital
Boston, Massachusetts

Ruth E. Tuomala, M.D.
Maternal-Fetal Medicine
Department of Obstetrics and Gynecology
Brigham and Women's Hospital
Boston, Massachusetts

Eboo Versi, M.D.
Director, Division of Urogynecology
Department of Obstetrics and Gynecology
Brigham and Women's Hospital
Boston, Massachusetts

Brian W. Walsh, M.D.
Center for Reproductive Medicine
Department of Obstetrics and Gynecology
Brigham and Women's Hospital
Boston, Massachusetts

Louise Wilkins-Haug, M.D., Ph.D.
Director, Antenatal Diagnostic Center
Department of Obstetrics and Gynecology
Brigham and Women's Hospital
Boston, Massachusetts

Preface to Seventh Edition

For the Seventh Edition of this text, the title has been changed to *Kistner's Gynecology and Women's Health* (from *Kistner's Gynecology*) to recognize the broad scope and expanded interest in the field of women's health care. Although over the past 35 years, previous editions of Kistner have appealed largely to students, trainees, and practitioners in gynecology, this new edition should be useful not only for gynecologists but for internists, family practitioners, and women's health specialists who are devoting more of their time and effort to women's medical issues. The authors for this textbook are appropriately drawn from the ranks of internists, as well as gynecologists, with two of them trained in both fields.

We have added a fourth editor, the distinguished endocrinologist, Andrea Dunaif, M.D., who in 1997 became Chief of the newly established Division of Women's Health in the Department of Medicine and of Obstetrics and Gynecology at the Brigham and Women's Hospital and Harvard Medical School. Dr. Dunaif joined Dr. Ann Taylor in providing a new chapter for this edition on "Polycystic Ovary and Hyperandrogenism." Other new chapter subjects include David Bates' "Evidence-Based Gynecology" and "Geriatric Gynecology and Aging" by Karen Miller, Eboo Versi, and Neil Resnick.

Kistner's Principles and Practice of Gynecology was first published in 1964, and since then each new edition has been a standard text in the field. The book was a distillation of the teaching and practice of gynecology at the Free Hospital for Women, which was founded in 1875, and a continuation of prior texts by Dr. William Graves, the first Professor of Gynecology at Harvard Medical School. It was at the Free Hospital that John Rock collaborated with Celso Garcia and others at the Worcester Foundation in the development of the birth control pill in the 1950s. Robert W. Kistner (1917-1990) started at the Free Hospital for Women in 1952 and became an Associate Clinical Professor of Obstetrics and Gynecology in 1984. He was a very skilled and popular gynecological surgeon, endocrinologist, and teacher who distilled his knowledge of the field into this text. As the field expanded he engaged the help of colleagues for subsequent editions. The current editors are pleased to be able to carry on the tradition. We wish to express our appreciation to all of the contributors for this Seventh Edition, for their scholarship and hard work, and to acknowledge our debt to authors of prior editions that provide the foundation for the current effort. Finally we wish to recognize the able assistance of Susan Holman, Ph.D., who as manuscript coordinator had a central role in the preparation of the book with help in editing, communicating with authors and the publishers, and smooth processing of manuscripts.

Kenneth J. Ryan

Ross S. Berkowitz

Robert L. Barbieri

Andrea Dunaif

Preface to First Edition

This work is designed both as a textbook and as a general reference book of gynecology to meet the needs of undergraduate medical students, young practitioners of gynecology, and specialists in this field. The format of each chapter is similar, the purpose being to provide a uniform and organized approach to the understanding of multiple disease processes of each organ of the female genital tract. Thus, in each chapter the embryology, anatomy, and histology are correlated with specific malformations. Morphologic variations are correlated with physiologic alterations. Recent advances in the diagnosis and therapy of infectious processes are described in detail. Particular emphasis has been given to the relationship of premalignant to malignant neoplasms, and methods for the prophylaxis of certain tumors are suggested. Because of the importance and increasing incidence of endometriosis a separate chapter on this disease is included. Particular emphasis has been placed on hormonal therapy, and details of management outlined.

Because of my interest in the practical endocrinologic aspects of gynecology, a chapter is devoted to steroid therapy. In this chapter an attempt is made to obviate many of the difficulties of administration associated with the new synthetic preparations. I have included (1) a brief resume of basic steroid chemistry, (2) a summation of the pharmacology and physiology of androgen, estrogens, and progesterone, together with a similar discussion of the synthetic progestins, and (3) a discussion of proved and proposed indications for the use of these steroids, with specific contraindications and optimum dosage.

The observations and opinions expressed in this text summarize the sum and substance of the teaching and practice at the Free Hospital for Women during the past 15 years. This hospital was opened on November 2, 1875, and has been in continuous operation since that time. It is the only remaining specialty hospital in the United States whose primary objective is the diagnosis and treatment of medical and surgical diseases of the female.

The Free Hospital for Women became internationally known because of *The Textbook of Gynecology* written by Dr. William P. Graves, formerly Professor of Gynecology at Harvard Medical School. Although the fourth and last edition of Graves' textbook appeared in 1928, since that time a multiplicity of original and important contributions has been published by the members of the staff. Outstanding among these have been the innumerable works of Drs. George and Olive Smith concerning the measurement and metabolism of ovarian steroids and gonadotropic hormones during the menstrual cycle, the period of conception, and subsequent pregnancy. During the years 1938 through 1957 Drs. John Rock and Arthur T. Hertig accomplished their monumental studies on the earliest stages of human growth following fertilization. From 1928 through 1958 Dr. Rock directed intensive study and research projects relating to the etiologic factors in infertility. The pathogenesis of carcinoma in situ of the cervix and its relationship to invasive carcinoma have undergone thorough investigation and evaluation by Drs. Paul Younge, Arthur T. Hertig, and Donald G. MacKay. During the past seven years the synthetic progestational agents have been subjected to extensive clinical investigation in specific gynecologic disorders such as endometriosis and endometrial carcinoma.

In preparing a work of this type, material must be gathered not only from the author's personal experience but to a still greater extent from the work of others. I have, therefore, attempted to include the important observations of numerous authors who have published data concerning the clinical material at the Free Hospital for Women. From the great number of publications consulted there have been several to which I have had frequent recourse, both for new material and for corroboration of personal observations. I must, therefore, express a general acknowledgment of indebtedness to Drs. George and Olive Smith, Arthur T. Hertig, Christopher J. Duncan, Paul A. Younge, Donald G. MacKay, and John Rock. I have also drawn on the writings of the late Joe V. Meigs and Langdon Parsons, both former residents at the Free Hospital for Women. In writing the sections on the relationship of endocrinology to gynecology I have received the greatest assistance from the excellent works, *Endocrine and Metabolic Aspects of Gynecology* by Joseph Rogerts, *Human Endocrinology* by Herbert S. Kupperman, and *The Endocrinology of Reproduction,* edited by Joseph T. Velardo. The reader is referred to these publications for additional and specific details.

I am indebted to Mrs. Edith Tagrin for the excellent illustrations and to Mr. Leo Goodman and Dr. Robert Ehrmann for the photomicrographs. Dr. Arthur T. Hertig and

Dr. Hazel M. Gore have also kindly given their excellent photomicrographs previously published in *Tumors of the Female Sex Organs,* published by the Armed Forces Institute of Pathology. The student is advised to refer to these fascicles for a complete survey of the pathology of tumors of the female genital tract.

I also wish to acknowledge a deep indebtedness to the tireless fingers and indefatigable efforts of my secretaries, Mrs. Ann Gregory Metzger, Mrs. Constance M. Rakoske, Mrs. Linda Angelico, and Mrs. Rachel Markiewicz. Valuable assistance has been given to me by the Administrator of the Free Hospital for Women, Miss Lillian Grahn. Finally, the courtesies of the staff of Year Book Medical Publishers have made the final preparation of this manuscript a pleasant task.

Robert W. Kistner

Acknowledgments

The Seventh Edition of *Kistner's Gynecology,* now titled *Kistner's Gynecology and Women's Health,* has developed and grown from the legacy and scholarly contributions of the earlier editions. The first few editions were primarily the work of Robert Kistner, M.D., who was later joined by other invited participants who contributed to the book. Some of the authors of the previous editions have not written for the Seventh Edition and we wish to acknowledge that material from prior editions and authors may have been carried forward to this work in terms of content, figures, organizational structure, and concepts. We wish to express appreciation and indebtedness to the following authors from the Sixth Edition:

Beryl R. Benacerraf, M.D. - Pelvic Ultrasonography

Daniel W. Cramer, M.D. - Biostatistics and Epidemiology

Andrew J. Friedman, M.D. - Uterine Corpus

Howard M. Goodman, M.D. - Cervix

R. Ian Hardy, M.D., Ph.D. - Infertility Treatment

Isaac Schiff, M.D. - Infertile Couple

Frederick H. Sillman, M.D. - Vulva

John Yeh, M.D. - Fallopian Tube and Ectopic Pregnancy

Contents

Detailed Contents

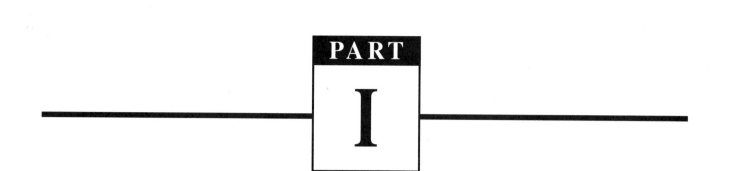

PART

I

GYNECOLOGY OVERVIEW

1

Evidence-Based Gynecology

DAVID W. BATES

KEY ISSUES

1. Evidence-based medicine represents a new paradigm.
2. Practicing medicine in this way requires developing skills for evaluating the primary literature and using those skills on a regular basis when confronted with clinical dilemmas.
3. Such skills are essential for keeping up with changes in medical knowledge.
4. Practicing evidence-based medicine may not only optimize outcomes for patients, it may be immensely rewarding for the provider.

Traditionally, clinicians learned how to practice medicine and to choose interventions by using various approaches—consulting experienced colleagues, searching through textbooks, listening to expert panels, and heeding their own experiences. However, no physician has a sufficiently large practice to make epidemiologically sound judgments, and our feelings about treatments tend to be colored by recent, and particularly by bad, experiences. Thus, the science of clinical investigation has grown up, and many have begun to advocate that clinicians make choices about therapy and diagnosis and make recommendations for prognosis based on the available evidence.

This concept is referred to as evidence-based medicine (Evidence-Based Medicine Working Group, 1992). When using an evidence-based approach, practitioners make decisions by reviewing the available evidence about a given therapy or situation instead of simply asking a colleague about it. This demands that a set of skills be developed so one can learn how to evaluate different types of studies and become facile at performing literature searches. Fortunately, there are now guides about how to do this effectively. This approach can be applied to all areas of medicine, not only gynecology. However, many within gynecology have called for

the profession to make this change (Frigoletto, 1997; Olive and Pritts, 1997; Peipert and Bracken, 1997; Zinberg, 1997).

THE OLD PARADIGM

Guyatt et al (1993) argue that this difference is sufficiently profound to be considered a paradigm shift (Evidence-Based Medicine Working Group, 1992) or a new way of viewing the world. They describe the old paradigm as based on several precepts:

1. Unsystematic observations from clinical experience are a valid way of building and maintaining one's knowledge about patient prognosis, the value of diagnostic tests, and the efficacy of treatment.
2. The study and understanding of the basic mechanisms of disease and of pathophysiologic principles are a sufficient guide for clinical practice.
3. A combination of thorough, traditional medical training and common sense is sufficient to allow one to evaluate new tests and treatments.
4. Content expertise and clinical experience are a sufficient base from which to generate valid guidelines for clinical practice (Evidence-Based Medicine Working Group, 1992).

THE NEW PARADIGM

Guyatt et al (1993) also present the assumptions of the new paradigm:

1. Clinical experience and the development of clinical instincts (particularly with respect to diagnosis) are crucial and necessary elements in becoming a competent physician. Many aspects of clinical practice cannot, or will not, ever be adequately tested. Clinical experience and its lessons are particularly important in these situations. At the same time, systematic attempts to record observations in a reproducible and unbiased fashion markedly

increase the confidence one can have in knowledge about patient prognosis, the value of diagnostic tests, and the efficacy of treatment. In the absence of systematic observation, one must be cautious in the interpretation of information derived from clinical experience and intuition, for it may at times be misleading.

2. The study and understanding of basic mechanisms of disease are necessary but insufficient guides for clinical practice. The rationales for diagnosis and treatment, which follow from basic pathophysiologic principles, may in fact be incorrect, leading to inaccurate predictions about the performance of diagnostic tests and the efficacy of treatments.

3. Understanding certain rules of evidence is necessary to interpret correctly the literature on causation, prognosis, diagnostic tests, and treatment strategy (Evidence-Based Medicine Working Group, 1992).

"KEEPING UP" WITH THE LITERATURE

The task of keeping up with current evidence is increasingly daunting. However, knowing what information is new and should result in a change in practice is important. The traditional track record for adopting even effective new therapies suggests that substantial delays are common; for example, it took physicians on average 3 years to change their practices after the publication of guidelines on a variety of topics (Grilli and Lomas, 1994).

This explosion in knowledge must be juxtaposed with the limited time most clinicians have for its assimilation, yet it is critical that they develop an efficient process to assimilate knowledge. Sackett (1997) has pointed out that a major criticism of evidence-based medicine is that no one has time to practice it. In fact, though few data are available, the best evidence suggests that most practicing physicians devote no more than 30 to 60 minutes a week to reading the literature (Sackett, 1997). What can be done with so little time? If the clinician has to travel to the evidence, the answer is almost nothing. Just getting to the library and back can take 30 minutes. However, if the evidence comes to the clinician, the outlook is much better (Sackett, 1997). Sackett suggests that clinicians should have access to many sources, among them *Best Evidence* (available on CD or floppy disk; call 800-523-1546, extension 2600, or contact on the World Wide Web at www.acponline.org), a compilation of pre-screened evidence (the abstracts) and clinical expertise (the commentaries) that also includes the first volume of *Evidence-Based Medicine* and the *ACP Journal Club*. One approach for finding articles is to subscribe to one or more of the services that look for important information, such as *Journal Watch* (cost is $98; contact on the World Wide Web at www.jwatch.org). Clinicians trained in evidence-based techniques survey the key journals (more than most physicians can read on their own) and write brief summaries of the articles. A clinician who finds something useful can then obtain the full text of the article.

In general, there are three ways to identify new information (Sackett, 1981): to find it through general reading, to find it by conducting a specific literature search, or to have someone else give it to you. Regarding general reading, it would be impossible to keep up with everything. Nonetheless, it probably does make sense to scan a few key journals on a regular basis and read the articles that are of interest.

However, scanning journals is insufficient; performing literature searches and evaluations when confronted with a clinical question is fundamental to practicing evidence-based medicine. This implies several things, namely, ready access to the tools for a computerized literature search, the skill to perform such a search, and the critical judgment to evaluate the articles identified. Among the tools that allow searches of medical databases are Medline (including PubMed), Ovid, and Paperchase. PubMed's advantage is that it is free, and it is available on the World Wide Web (www.ncbi.nlm.nih.gov/PubMed). One drawback of PubMed, however, is that, unlike Paperchase, it will not allow searches or terms to be merged. After a little practice with any of these tools, it is usually possible to find the best evidence about a specific condition in a few minutes.

Another key factor is learning how to scan a journal or evidence summary; this must be done ruthlessly, given time constraints. Sackett (1981) has described one approach (Box 1-1). First, read the title. If it is not interesting, stop. Second, read the authors' names. Third, read the conclusions and decide whether they would be of interest if they were true. Fourth, read the methods and decide whether they are valid. Using this approach, reading the *New England Journal of Medicine* can often be accomplished in less than 30 seconds if there are no articles of interest that week. A corollary of this is that the "throw-away" journals are best avoided because time is too precious.

ASKING A CLINICAL QUESTION

Here is a scenario. Shortly after completing your residency, you see a 23-year-old patient who has had dysuria for 2 days. She has no other medical condition, and she is sexually active but takes oral contraceptives. She has not had fever or chills, but she has had five previous urinary tract infections in the past several years. A urine dipstick is positive for 4+ leukocyte esterase. When you suggest a 7-day course of trimethoprim-sulfamethoxazole, which everyone used where you trained, she tells you that her former gynecologist told her that a 3-day course was as effective and that she regularly would get a yeast infection with a 7-day course. You give her the 3-day course but resolve to evaluate the literature.

That afternoon, a quick search reveals a number of relevant papers (Greenwood and Slack, 1986; Inter-Nordic Urinary Tract Infection Study Group, 1988; Iravani et al, 1995; Saginur and Nicolle, 1992). Investigators in two recent randomized trials suggest that 3-day therapy is more effective than single-dose therapy (Iravani et al, 1995; Saginur and Nicolle, 1992). The consensus concerning a 7- to 14-day

BOX 1-1
**GUIDES FOR SELECTING ARTICLES MOST
LIKELY TO PROVIDE VALID RESULTS**

Primary Studies
Therapy

- Was the assignment of patients to treatments randomized?
- Were all patients who entered the trial properly accounted for and attributed at its conclusion?

Diagnosis

- Was there an independent, blind comparison with a reference standard?
- Did the patient sample include an appropriate spectrum of the sort of patients to whom the diagnostic test will be applied in clinical practice?

Harm

- Were there clearly identified comparison groups that were similar in the important determinants of outcome (other than the one of interest)?
- Were outcomes and exposures measured similarly in the groups compared?

Prognosis

- Was there a representative patient sample at a well-defined point in the course of the disease?
- Was follow-up sufficiently long and complete?

Integrative Studies
Overview

- Did the review address a clearly focused question?
- Were the criteria used to select articles for inclusion appropriate?*

Practice Guidelines

- Were the options and outcomes clearly specified?
- Did the guideline use an explicit process to identify, select, and combine evidence?*

Decision Analysis

- Did the analysis faithfully model a clinically important decision?
- Was valid evidence used to develop the baseline probabilities and utilities?*

Economic Analysis

- Were two or more clearly described alternatives compared?
- Were the expected consequences of each alternative based on valid evidence?*

From Oxman AD, Sackett DL, Guyatt GH: Users' guides to the medical literature. I. How to get started. *JAMA* 1993; 270:2093-2095.

*Each of these guidelines makes an implicit or an explicit reference to the investigators' need to evaluate the validity of the studies reviewed to produce an integrative article. The validity criteria used to make this evaluation depend on the area addressed (therapy, diagnosis, prognosis, or harm), and they are presented in the part of the box dealing with primary articles.

course versus a 3-day course was reached in the late 1980s (Greenwood and Slack, 1986; Inter-Nordic Urinary Tract Infection Study Group, 1988). Three days proved as effective and resulted in fewer side effects in some trials. You decide to change the length of therapy you suggest for patients with this condition.

OVERVIEW OF MAIN TYPES OF STUDIES

Articles that prove to be of value generally are designed to assess therapy, diagnosis, harm, or prognosis, and a small number of domain-specific guides can be used to evaluate whether articles from each domain are likely to give valid results (Box 1-1) (Oxman et al, 1993). Another way to classify clinical studies is as cross-sectional studies, case-control studies, cohort studies, and randomized controlled trials. Among the four main study types—cross-sectional, case-control, cohort, and randomized trials—the strength of the evidence increases from first to last, but so does the expense. Thus, we will never have randomized trial information about everything, and we must realize that much useful information can be drawn from less rigorous study designs. Integrative studies are of increasing importance; main categories are overviews, practice guidelines, decision analyses, and economic analyses (see Box 1-1). One widely used evaluation scheme for ranking the strength of evidence is that used by the U.S. Preventive Services Task Force (Box 1-2).

Therapy and Prevention

Perhaps the largest quantity of data concerns therapy. For drugs especially to be adopted, they must be proven effective in randomized, controlled trials, and trials are becoming

BOX 1-2
**EVALUATION SYSTEM OF THE U.S. PREVENTIVE
SERVICES TASK FORCE**

Quality of Evidence

- I. Evidence obtained from at least one properly randomized controlled trial.
- II-1. Evidence obtained from well-designed controlled trials that were not randomized.
- II-2. Evidence obtained from well-designed cohort or case-control analytic studies, preferably from more than one center or one research group.
- II-3. Evidence obtained from multiple time series with or without the intervention. Dramatic results in uncontrolled experiments (such as the results of the introduction of penicillin treatment in the 1940s) could also be regarded as this type of evidence.
- III. Opinions of respected authorities, based on clinical experience; descriptive studies and case reports or reports of expert committees.

From U.S. Preventive Services Task Force: *Guide to clinical preventive services,* ed 2, Baltimore, 1996, Williams & Wilkins.

6 PART I   Gynecology Overview

BOX 1-3
GUIDES FOR SELECTING ARTICLES ABOUT THERAPY

Are the Results of the Study Valid?
Primary Guides
- Was the assignment of patients to treatments randomized?
- Were all patients who entered the trial properly accounted for and attributed at its conclusion?
- Was follow-up complete?
- Were patients analyzed in the groups to which they were randomized?

Secondary Guides
- Were patients, health workers, and study personnel "blind" to treatment?
- Were the groups similar at the start of the trial?
- Aside from the experimental intervention, were the groups treated equally?

What Were the Results?
- How large was the treatment effect?
- How precise was the estimate of the treatment effect?

Will the Results Help Me in Caring for My Patients?
- Can the results be applied to my patient care?
- Were all clinically important outcomes considered?
- Are the likely treatment benefits worth the potential harms and costs?

From Guyatt GH, Sackett DL, Cook DJ: Users' guides to the medical literature. II. How to use an article about therapy or prevention. A. Are the results of the study valid? *JAMA* 1993; 270:2598-2601.

---

common for procedures as well. A series of questions can be asked when evaluating such a study (Box 1-3) (Guyatt et al, 1993).

The most important validity checks are whether treatment was randomized, whether patients who entered the trial were accounted for at the conclusion, whether follow-up was complete, and whether patients were analyzed in the groups to which they were randomized. Randomized trials have become the standard for evaluating the effectiveness of a therapy, in part because 30% to 40% of patients respond positively to a placebo. If more than 10% of patients are lost to follow-up, this can significantly bias the findings, particularly if the treatment is sufficiently noxious that it causes patients to drop out. Analyzing by assignment of randomized group refers to whether the analysis was conducted on an "intention-to-treat" basis. For example, if the study concerns a surgical therapy and only patients undergoing the therapy are included, but 20% of those patients choose not to undergo surgery, that 20% could be the group most likely to do poorly. Excluding them would bias the results in favor of the therapy.

If the results are valid, the next steps are to assess the size and then the precision of the estimated treatment effect. Size

is important because results can be statistically significant without being clinically significant and vice versa. For example, in a satisfaction scale measuring a large population, a new drug could show an improvement of four points, which is highly statistically significant. However, this may or may not be clinically significant. On the other hand, a small study of a new cancer therapy may be associated with a 15% mortality rate, whereas a conventional cancer therapy may be associated with a 20% mortality rate ($p = 0.15$). Although this is not statistically significant, clinically it is very important. Precision is important, too, because if the confidence intervals around the 15% mortality rate are 3% to 45%, the situation is very different than if they are 10% to 23%.

Tests to determine whether the results will help care for your patients are also important. The first thing to consider is whether the study population is sufficiently similar to your own to generalize to this group. This is a real issue because most papers are written at referral centers. Disease prevalence and treatment outcomes may be substantially different in those centers than they are in different regions of the country and different parts of the world. Next to consider is whether all clinically important outcomes were considered. If a study indicates a large reduction in length of stay but does not address patient satisfaction, it would be suspect. In addition, it is important to assess whether a treatment's benefits are worth the potential harms or costs. If treatment improves a patient's survival but causes severe disfiguration or is extremely costly, it may not be worthwhile.

Therapy

You see in your office a 39-year-old woman who weighs 360 pounds and is 5-feet, 5-inches tall. She has large fibroids in her uterus, experiences substantial pain with her menstrual periods, and wants to have a hysterectomy. You concur. However, you are concerned about the likelihood of postoperative infection and want to do everything you can to minimize the risk of this. When you bring up this case in your group's weekly conference, the senior clinician, who trained in England, states emphatically that drains in obese patients raise the probability of infection and should be avoided. Another member of your group, who trained on the west coast of the United States, says that although she cannot remember the citation, she learned during her residency that drains could reduce the probability of infection under some circumstances. One of the residents says that during a recent meeting, there was an abstract presentation on a trial showing that drains decreased the likelihood of infection. They all hold strong opinions on the issue. During your residency, you were taught not to use drains, but you decide to evaluate the evidence.

In a quick PubMed search from your office, using the query "surgical drains in obese patients," you find a randomized, controlled trial in which 197 obese patients undergoing gynecologic surgery were randomized either to receive or not to receive a drain (Gallup et al, 1996). The assignment was randomized, follow-up was complete, and an intention-to-treat analysis was performed. The complication rate was 20% (22/109) among the group receiving a drain and 31% (27/88) among the group without a drain ($p = 0.09$). Although this result does not meet the threshold of 0.05, the difference in these complication rates appears meaningful to you. Evaluating other important outcomes, you find that wound breakdowns occurred in 7 of 109 (6.4%) patients with drains and 10 of 88 (11.4%) without drains ($p = 0.2$). You also find two earlier studies, one a larger retrospective study of 14,854 wounds of all types suggesting that the probability of wound infection doubles if a drain is present (National Academy of Sciences, 1964). Findings of the other study were similar (Public Health Laboratory Service, 1960). You have your assistant retrieve full-text versions of the three studies. When you review them, you find that in the latter two studies, drain placement was not randomized and was at the discretion of the surgeon. It seems to you that surgeons will place drains more often if they think infection is likely. Thus, you place more weight on the randomized trial, though you would like to see a larger, confirmatory study. You present the information at the group's quality conference the following week.

Diagnosis

The key issues for evaluating studies of diagnostic tests are whether there was an independent, blind comparison with a reference standard and whether the sample included an appropriate spectrum of patients (Box 1-4) (Jaeschke et al, 1994). The first is the more important; if a reference or "gold standard" is available, the test should be compared to it, and those performing the results should be blinded to the patient's clinical characteristics. This is essential for tests with results that are ambiguous and that involve interpretation, such as mammography. In one large study of mammography, radiologists agreed on only 78% of diagnoses (Elmore et al, 1994). When a new test is evaluated, it should be studied in a group similar to those in which it will be used clinically. For example, if a test for a new type of arthritis is under evaluation, the comparison group should be other adults with rheumatic disease or vague joint complaints, not healthy medical students.

A 54-year-old woman comes to your office with postmenopausal bleeding. Her menstrual periods stopped 4 years ago. She works as a medical secretary and is worried she may have uterine cancer. She has recently read in a magazine that cancer is sometimes missed by endometrial biopsy and that ultrasonography may be a better test. Although you have heard several abstract presentations at national meetings about new radiologic studies for the evaluation of postmenopausal bleeding, your practice standard has been to perform endometrial biopsies to look for endometrial cancer. You perform the biopsy in your office but resolve to review the literature and get back to your patient about it.

You perform a literature search on uterine hemorrhage and ultrasonography and find several articles, notably one from Dubinsky et al (1997), which you read in detail. This group performed a prospective study of transvaginal sonography with endometrial biopsy in 329 consecutive women

---

BOX 1-4
EVALUATING AND APPLYING DIAGNOSTIC TEST STUDY RESULTS

Are the Results of the Study Valid?
Primary Guides

- Was there an independent, blind comparison with a reference standard?
- Did the patient sample include an appropriate spectrum of patients to whom the diagnostic test will be applied in clinical practice?

Secondary Guides

- Did the results of the test influence the decision to perform the reference standard?
- Were the methods for performing the test described in sufficient detail to permit replication?

What Were the Results?

- Are likelihood ratios for the test results or data necessary for their calculation provided?

Will the Results Help Me in Caring for My Patients?

- Will the reproducibility of the test result and its interpretation be satisfactory in my setting?
- Are the results applicable to my patient?
- Will the results change my management?
- Will patients be better off as a result of the test?

From Jaeschke R, Guyatt G, Sackett DL: Users' guides to the medical literature. III. How to use an article about a diagnostic test. A. Are the results of the study valid? *JAMA* 1994; 271:389-391.

---

who underwent endometrial biopsy. The reference standard was pathology on specimens obtained during surgery, but it is difficult from the article to determine how many patients actually underwent a surgical procedure; 94 underwent myomectomy or hysterectomy. Of the 329 women who underwent endometrial biopsy, results were negative in 302. Among 259 patients who underwent transvaginal ultrasonography, 65 had endometrial thickening. Among these patients, 8 had carcinoma (positive predictive value of 12%). Endometrial biopsy detected only 33% of the malignancies, whereas ultrasonography detected at least 67%, though not all patients whose ultrasound was positive had biopsy specimens taken.

You find this report provocative and are disturbed by the low sensitivity of endometrial biopsy, and decide to continue to follow this issue in the literature. You elect not to change your practice yet because you would like to see confirmation of these results from other sites with more patients undergoing the reference standard procedure. You also want to know the relative costs of the procedures, the yield in terms of identifying other pelvic diseases, and the fate of patients whose carcinoma is missed on the initial biopsy (because if they all come to attention soon and undergo curative hysterectomy, the low initial sensitivity is not as great a concern).

Harm

To assess harm, determine whether there was a clearly identified comparison group, or groups, similar to the study group with respect to the outcome measured, whether outcomes and exposures were measured similarly in the groups, and whether follow-up was sufficiently long (Box 1-5) (Levine et al, 1994).

A 52-year-old woman comes to your office. Her menstrual periods decreased in frequency in the past 2 years, and 6 months ago they stopped. She would like to begin hormonal replacement therapy, but she has a strong family history of heart disease. Her total cholesterol serum is 273 mg/dl with a low-density lipoprotein of 155 mg/dl and a high-density lipoprotein (HDL) of 35 mg/dl; her internist plans to begin therapy for this. Because she has an intact uterus, her risk for endometrial cancer is too high to use unopposed estrogen. You are concerned that adding a progestational agent will negate the cardiovascular benefits of the estrogen, and you want to offer her the best available therapy for her cardiac risk profile.

A PubMed search finds the Postmenopausal Estrogen/Progestin Interventions (PEPI) trial (Writing Group for the PEPI Trial, 1995), in which 875 women 45 to 64 years of age, who had no known contraindications to hormone replacement therapy, were randomized to one of five groups administered different regimens. The follow-up period lasted only 3 years. Primary outcomes were results of clinical tests, including HDL-C, rather than cardiovascular outcomes. The group in which the greatest improvement in HDL-C occurred was that given conjugated equine estrogen alone (not an option in your patient) and conjugated equine estrogen plus cyclic micronized progesterone, 200 mg/day for 12 days per month. There were significant increases in the HDL-C levels for both groups (to 0.14 mmol/L for the group receiving estrogen alone and to 0.11 mmol/L for the group receiving micronized progesterone). No adverse effects on systolic blood pressure or insulin level were found. Although you would prefer to see long-term data on the association between progestins and myocardial infarction, you elect to use the above regimen with micronized progesterone.

Prognosis

The key differentiating issues regarding prognosis are whether study patients were identified at similar points in the disease course and whether the results will be useful for

---

BOX 1-5
GUIDES FOR SELECTING ARTICLES ABOUT HARM

Are the Results of the Study Valid?
Primary Guides

- Were there clearly identified comparison groups that were similar with respect to important determinants of outcome, other than the one of interest?
- Were the outcomes and exposures measured in the same way in the groups compared?
- Was follow-up sufficiently long and complete?

Secondary Guides

- Is the temporal relationship correct?
- Is there a dose-response gradient?

What Are the Results?

- How strong is the association between exposure and outcome?
- How precise is the estimate of the risk?

Will the Results Help Me in Caring for My Patients?

- Are the results applicable to my practice?
- What is the magnitude of the risk?
- Should I attempt to stop the exposure?

From Levine M, Walter S, Lee H: Users' guides to the medical literature. IV. How to use an article about harm. *JAMA* 1994; 271:1615-1619.

BOX 1-6
GUIDES FOR SELECTING ARTICLES ABOUT PROGNOSIS

Are the Results of the Study Valid?
Primary Guides

- Were there representative and well-defined samples of patients at a similar point in the course of the disease?
- Was follow-up sufficiently long and complete?

Secondary Guides

- Were objective and unbiased outcome criteria used?
- Was there adjustment for important prognostic factors?

What Are the Results?

- How large is the likelihood of the outcome event(s) in a specified time?
- How precise are the estimates of likelihood?

Will the Results Help Me in Caring for My Patients?

- Were the study patients similar to my own?
- Will the results lead directly to selecting or avoiding therapy?
- Are the results useful for reassuring or counseling patients?

From Laupacis A, Wells G, Richardson WS: Users' guides to the medical literature. V. How to use an article about prognosis. *JAMA* 1994; 272:234-237.

reassuring or counseling other patients (Box 1-6) (Laupacis et al, 1994). For instance, if a genetic test can determine that a patient will have a severely debilitating illness late in life but no therapy is available, some patients may find the information useful whereas others may not.

A 24-year-old woman comes to you in tears after her partner has been told he has genital herpes and that he must have contracted it from her. He is angry with her and wants to know why she did not tell him she had herpes. She has had no previous lesions that she is aware of, though she has had three prior partners. Although their relationship is over, she has several questions. Did she give him the infection? If so, is there anything she can do to prevent giving it to others? You know that genital herpes can be asymptomatic, and you tell her that she may have given it to him without knowing it. However, you are vague about the likelihood that she indeed did give him the infection and what she can do about it in the future.

Later that afternoon, you perform a quick Medline search and find a study that sheds some light on this. Langenberg et al (1989) compare a group of 28 women with potentially asymptomatic genital herpes simplex with a group of 67 patients from a gynecology clinic. Of the 28 women with suspected asymptomatic infection, 14 were referred because they were thought to have transmitted genital herpes simplex virus to a sex partner. After counseling about the clinical symptoms of genital herpes and a 5-month follow-up, symptomatic genital herpes developed in 40% of the women and was documented on a repeat visit. They could now be counseled to avoid sex during these episodes. Although this group came from a referral clinic and the women were predominantly black and unmarried, it seems to you that the results are valid. Your patient badly wants more information about what is likely to happen to her and what she should do differently in the future. You call her and relay this information, including what to look for. She is grateful. Six weeks later, a vulval lesion develops that is culture positive for herpes simplex. You refer her to your nurse practitioner for additional counseling.

Overviews

Overviews are increasingly common in the medical literature (Oxman et al, 1994). Key questions include whether the overview addressed a focused question and whether the inclusion criteria were appropriate. Whether meta-analyses agree with the results of large clinical trials is particularly important. In one recent study evaluating this question, investigators found that 35% of the time, the outcomes of 12 large trials were not predicted accurately in published meta-analyses (LeLorier et al, 1997). Hence, though meta-analyses are useful tools, their results often differ from those of large randomized trials on the same subject.

Your clinic's quality group is meeting to evaluate its approach to routine care after abortion. The infection rate after induced abortion is 14%, and the group is trying to decide how this can be improved. Some members use prophylactic antibiotics for all patients, whereas others use them only for selected patients. Group members cite randomized trials with differing results, each supporting their positions (Heisterberg, 1987; Heisterberg and Gnarpe, 1988; Levallois and Rioux, 1988). You volunteer to conduct a literature search and to report back to the group the following month so that a consensus can be reached.

Your search reveals a meta-analysis on this topic in which the authors identify 12 randomized, controlled trials and combine the results using a fixed-effects model (Sawaya et al, 1996). They address a specific question, and the inclusion criteria seem reasonable. The results are striking: the overall summary relative risk for genital tract infection after abortion in women receiving antibiotic therapy rather than placebo was 0.58 (95% confidence interval, 0.47 to 0.71), and this held even for women in groups at low risk. Based on these data, your group decides to begin routine prophylaxis for all women undergoing this procedure.

Practice Guidelines

Criteria for evaluating a practice guideline include whether all important options and outcomes are clearly specified, whether a reasonable process is used to combine evidence, whether the recommendations are practical and clinically relevant, and determining the impact of uncertainty associated with the evidence (Hayward et al, 1995).

A new patient, a 41-year-old woman, comes to see you. She wonders whether she should have a mammogram. She has read that several organizations make different recommendations, and she cannot understand why. You explain that some of the evidence is conflicting, and you decide to review the guidelines because this is an issue that comes up daily in your practice and you want to remain current and to understand the underlying data supporting the recommendations.

Many well-designed studies show reductions in breast cancer mortality rates for women 50 to 69 years of age. However, the 1996 U.S. Preventive Services Task Force Report concludes that the evidence is insufficient to support screening women from 40 to 50 years of age (Frame et al, 1997) because no study has shown that screening women younger than 50 results in a reduced mortality rate. One meta-analysis of eight trials suggested that screening can reduce mortality rates by 23% (Smart et al, 1995), but it excluded the Canadian National Breast Screening Study from the analysis for a number of reasons, one of which was that the follow-up was not yet sufficiently long. However, another meta-analysis of 13 studies, published the same year, found no reduction in the mortality rates of 40- to 49-year-old women (Kerlikowske et al, 1995). Moreover, this area has become so highly politicized that even the Senate has become involved (Fletcher, 1997). You conclude that the jury is still out and that you will explain to your patients that uncertainty remains about this question and that although you will not recommend routine mammography for this age group, you will offer it to women who want it or appear to be at high risk.

Decision Analyses

In evaluating a clinical decision analysis, you must determine whether important strategies and outcomes were covered; whether probabilities were assigned in a reasonable fashion; how strong the evidence about them is; whether utilities—the values patients place on different health states—were used in a reasonable way; whether uncertainty was considered; whether, in the baseline analysis, one strategy is dominant; and whether uncertainty could change the result (Richardson and Detsky, 1995).

A 45-year-old woman comes to see you for a routine visit. She has an intact uterus, has been married for 22 years, and has had no other relationships. She has no gynecologic complaints, had 17 consecutive normal Papanicolaou smears, and asks you why she must continue to have one every year. She has read that one every 3 years is now reasonable for patients who have had multiple normal smears, and she asks why the recommendation was changed. You do know that the other practitioners in your group obtain them every 3 years, but you are unsure how that interval was determined so you decide to review the primary literature.

A Medline search on the terms "Pap smear and frequency" identifies a mathematical model published by Eddy (Eddy, 1987) evaluating the costs and benefits of performing Pap smears at varying intervals. These data show that compared with annual screening, screening every 2, 3, 5, and 10 years retains 99%, 97%, 89%, and 69% of the effectiveness of annual screening for reducing the frequency of invasive cancer. The supporting data from the British Columbia screening program seem reasonably solid. One shortcoming, however, is that a full, formal sensitivity analysis, in which all parameters to which the model is sensitive were varied to determine whether the conclusions could be altered, was not performed. In spite of this, the analyses performed suggest that it is unlikely the basic conclusion—that screening every third year is nearly as effective as annual screening—will change. You feel more comfortable discussing this issue with patients and explaining the rationale for the policy change.

Economic Analyses

In evaluating an economic analysis, some key issues are whether the analysis provides a full comparison of strategies, whether costs and outcomes have been properly obtained, what the incremental costs and outcomes of strategies are, whether these differ by subgroup, and whether the results are affected by uncertainty (Drummond et al, 1997).

You are the director of an infertility group and you are trying to decide how many cycles of therapy to offer patients routinely. You know the chances of success decrease with the number of cycles and depend on risk factors. However, it has been difficult to isolate the costs of continuing, and you have seen a few successes, even with large numbers of cycles. This is especially critical to you now because your largest patient group is now capitated, and you are about to sign a contract that will make you subcapitated across the network; hence, you will receive one sum no matter how much service you provide. You want to give couples considering in vitro fertilization a reasonable chance for a successful outcome, but it must be at a reasonable cost. You remember an article about the cost effectiveness of in vitro fertilization but not all the details.

A quick PubMed search turns up the article, a cost-effectiveness analysis on the cost of a successful delivery with in vitro fertilization (Neumann et al, 1994). Because of their good chance for success, couples with a diagnosis of tubal disease have lower costs, ranging from $50,000 per delivery for the first cycle to $72,727 for the sixth. On the other hand, in couples in whom the woman is older than 40 and the diagnosis is male-factor infertility, the cost is $160,000 for the first cycle and $800,000 for the sixth. The estimates of costs and outcomes seem reasonable, and the results appear robust in a sensitivity analysis. The subgroup differences are large. Your group uses these data to plan a budget. Although you decide to give every infertile couple access to in vitro fertilization and not to use maximization of the number of deliveries as the sole criterion, your group decides to limit the number of cycles offered and to provide fewer cycles for couples with low chances of conceiving.

CONCLUSIONS

Developing an evidence-based approach to practice requires some effort, and though it is challenging, it is also rewarding. Because decisions are made on the basis of interpretation of evidence, this approach is more intellectually stimulating than listening to experts. Nonetheless, it quickly becomes clear to anyone using this approach how thin our knowledge base is; expert opinion will be useful for the forseeable future. An evidence-based approach moves the practitioner closer to the goal of implementing therapy when it is likely to benefit the patient and avoiding it when it is not. Such skills are particularly important with the increased penetration of managed care, which places a premium not on doing everything possible, as was the case with the fee-for-service arrangement, but on doing what works.

REFERENCES

Drummond MF, Richardson WS, O'Brien BJ, et al: Users' guides to the medical literature. XIII. How to use an article on economic analysis of clinical practice. A. Are the results of the study valid? Evidence-Based Medicine Working Group. *JAMA* 1997; 277:1552-1557.

Dubinsky TJ, Parvey HR, Maklad N: The role of transvaginal sonography and endometrial biopsy in the evaluation of peri- and postmenopausal bleeding. *AJR* 1997; 169:145-149.

Eddy DM: The frequency of cervical cancer screening. Comparison of a mathematical model with empirical data. *Cancer* 1987; 60:1117-1122.

Elmore JG, Wells CK, Lee CH: Variability in radiologists' interpretations of mammograms. *N Engl J Med* 1994; 331:1493-1499.

Evidence-Based Medicine Working Group: Evidence-based medicine. A new approach to teaching the practice of medicine. *JAMA* 1992; 268:2420-2425.

Fletcher SW: Whither scientific deliberation in health policy recommendations? Alice in the Wonderland of breast-cancer screening. *N Engl J Med* 1997; 336:1180-1183.

Frame PS, Berg AO, Woolf S: U.S. Preventive Services Task Force: Highlights of the 1996 report. *Am Fam Physician* 1997; 55:567-576, 581-582.

Frigoletto FD: CPR: Can we be resuscitated? *Obstet Gynecol* 1997; 89:1-4.

Gallup DC, Gallup DG, Nolan TE, et al: Use of a subcutaneous closed drainage system and antibiotics in obese gynecologic patients. *Am J Obstet Gynecol* 1996; 175:358-361.

Greenwood D, Slack R: Short-course treatment of urinary tract infection. *Chemioterapia* 1986; 5:244-248.

Grilli R, Lomas J: Evaluating the message: The relationship between compliance rate and the subject of a practice guideline. *Med Care* 1994; 32:202-213.

Guyatt GH, Sackett DL, Cook DJ: Users' guides to the medical literature. II. How to use an article about therapy or prevention. A. Are the results of the study valid? *JAMA* 1993; 270:2598-2601.

Hayward RS, Wilson MC, Tunis SR, et al: Users' guides to the medical literature. VIII. How to use clinical practice guidelines. A. Are the recommendations valid? *JAMA* 1995; 274:570-574.

Heisterberg L: Prophylactic antibiotics in women with a history of pelvic inflammatory disease undergoing first-trimester abortion. *Acta Obstet Gynecol Scand* 1987; 66:15-18.

Heisterberg L, Gnarpe H: Preventive lymecycline therapy in women with a history of pelvic inflammatory disease undergoing first-trimester abortion: A clinical, controlled trial. *Eur J Obstet Gynecol Reprod Biol* 1988; 28:241-247.

Inter-Nordic Urinary Tract Infection Study Group: Double-blind comparison of 3-day versus 7-day treatment with norfloxacin in symptomatic urinary tract infections. *Scand J Infect Dis* 1988; 20:619-624.

Iravani A, Tice AD, McCarty J: Short-course ciprofloxacin treatment of acute uncomplicated urinary tract infection in women. The minimum effective dose. The Urinary Tract Infection Study Group. *Arch Intern Med* 1995; 155:485-494.

Jaeschke R, Guyatt G, Sackett DL: Users' guides to the medical literature. III. How to use an article about a diagnostic test. A. Are the results of the study valid? *JAMA* 1994; 271:389-391.

Kerlikowske K, Grady D, Rubin SM: Efficacy of screening mammography. A meta-analysis. *JAMA* 1995; 273:149-154.

Langenberg A, Benedetti J, Jenkins J, et al: Development of clinically recognizable genital lesions among women previously identified as having "asymptomatic" herpes simplex virus type 2 infection. *Ann Intern Med* 1989; 110:882-887.

Laupacis A, Wells G, Richardson WS: Users' guides to the medical literature. V. How to use an article about prognosis. *JAMA* 1994; 272:234-237.

LeLorier J, Gregoire G, Benhaddad A: Discrepancies between meta-analyses and subsequent large randomized, controlled trials. *N Engl J Med* 1997; 337:536-542.

Levallois P, Rioux JE: Prophylactic antibiotics for suction curettage abortion: Results of a clinical controlled trial. *Am J Obstet Gynecol* 1988; 158:100-105.

Levine M, Walter S, Lee H: Users' guides to the medical literature. IV. How to use an article about harm. *JAMA* 1994; 271:1615-1619.

National Academy of Sciences, National Research Council: Postoperative wound infections: The influence of ultraviolet irradiation of the operating room and various other factors. *Ann Surg* 1964; 160(suppl):1-132.

Neumann PJ, Gharib SD, Weinstein MC: The cost of a successful delivery with in vitro fertilization. *N Engl J Med* 1994; 331:239-243.

Olive DL, Pritts EA: What is evidence-based medicine? *J Am Assoc Gynecol Laparosc* 1997; 4:615-621.

Oxman AD, Cook DJ, Guyatt GH: Users' guides to the medical literature. VI. How to use an overview. *JAMA* 1994; 272:1367-1371.

Oxman AD, Sackett DL, Guyatt GH: Users' guides to the medical literature. I. How to get started. *JAMA* 1993; 270:2093-2095.

Peipert JF, Bracken MB: Systematic reviews of medical evidence: The use of meta-analysis in obstetrics and gynecology. *Obstet Gynecol* 1997; 89:628-633.

Public Health Laboratory Service: Incidence of surgical wound infection in England and Wales. *Lancet* 1960; 2:659-663.

Richardson WS, Detsky AS: Users' guides to the medical literature. VII. How to use a clinical decision analysis. A. Are the results of the study valid? *JAMA* 1995; 273:1292-1295.

Sackett DL: How to read clinical journals: I. Why to read them and how to start reading them critically. *Can Med Assoc J* 1981; 124:555-558.

Sackett DL: . . .So little time, and. . . . *Evidence-Based Medicine* 1997; March/April:39.

Saginur R, Nicolle LE: Single-dose compared with 3-day norfloxacin treatment of uncomplicated urinary tract infection in women. Canadian Infectious Diseases Society Clinical Trials Study Group. *Arch Intern Med* 1992; 152:1233-1237.

Sawaya GF, Grady D, Kerlikowske K: Antibiotics at the time of induced abortion: The case for universal prophylaxis based on a meta-analysis. *Obstet Gynecol* 1996; 87: 884-890.

Smart CR, Hendrick RE, Rutledge JH: Benefit of mammography screening in women ages 40 to 49 years. Current evidence from randomized controlled trials. *Cancer* 1995; 75: 1619-1626.

U.S. Preventive Services Task Force: *Guide to clinical preventive services*, ed 2, Baltimore, 1996, Williams & Wilkins.

Writing Group for the PEPI Trial: Effects of estrogen or estrogen/progestin regimens on heart disease risk factors in postmenopausal women. The postmenopausal estrogen/progestin interventions (PEPI) trial. *JAMA* 1995; 273:199-208.

Zinberg S: Guest editorial: Evidence-based practice guidelines: A current perspective. *Obstet Gynecol Surv* 1997; 52:265-266.

2

Medical Ethics and Risk Management

KENNETH J. RYAN

KEY ISSUES

1. The starting point for medical ethics and medical risk management is reflected by the wisdom of Dr. Francis Weld Peabody: "The secret of the care of the patient is in caring for the patient."

2. In ethical deliberation, it is not necessary to rely on a single moral theory founded either on rules, rights, or obligations, or on the consequences of choices made. Ethical judgment, in practice, is usually based on some combination of the anticipated means and ends (consequences) of our actions, and no single theory completely captures this process in applied medical ethics.

3. The principles most applicable to ethical choice in medicine include respect for human beings (caring for the patient), beneficence and nonmaleficence (helping and not harming), and justice (fairness in the selection and treatment of patients).

4. Ethical considerations are integral to the practice of gynecology. They involve the competency and skill with which this form of medicine is practiced, the nature of the physician-patient interaction, and the value choice options in such issues as assisted reproduction, abortion, women's issues, and terminal care.

5. An evaluation of risk management experience with malpractice claims illustrates the importance of communication with patients, of the documentation and adequacy of the informed consent process, and of postoperative care.

MORAL THEORIES AND PRINCIPLES

Buttressed by the Hippocratic oath, medical ethics has always been considered an integral part of medicine. Its application, though, is largely dependent on the character of the physician and on societal and cultural traditions. In their comments on doctors and on the limitations of medical care, Plato and Montaigne considered it advantageous for physicians to experience the illnesses they would treat (Frame, 1965). In the twentieth century, the writings of physicians about their personal experiences with disease have provided inspiration and guidance to succeeding generations of doctors. As Montaigne put it: "He should catch the pox if he wants to know how to treat it. Truly, I should trust such a man" (Frame, 1965). When Francis Weld Peabody, a physician and physiologist, delivered his now famous 1926 Harvard lecture, "The Care of the Patient," he already knew he had cancer and had less than 1 year to live (Scannell, 1986). At the end of his presentation, based on his own experience with a fatal disease, Peabody gave this eloquent definition of good doctoring: "One of the essential qualities of the clinician is interest in humanity, for the secret of the care of the patient is in caring for the patient" (Peabody, 1927). Few would argue that this is the best place to start; however, challenged as we are by the post–World War II emphasis on individual autonomy and patient rights and by the advances of modern technology, the complexity of medical ethics now requires something more.

Theories

In the evolution of the teaching of medical ethics during the past 20 years, two major theories of modern moral philosophy have been advanced as the ultimate justification for applying ethics in the care of patients. These are Kantian deontology (rule-based morality) and utilitarianism (outcome-based morality). Trying to make moral choices within either a rule-based or an outcome-based system proves too rigid. Common experience is that we often appeal to means and ends (rules and outcomes) and that no single viewpoint is always appropriate. There is no neat, simple theory or principle that substitutes for experience and judgment. Sometimes we must break so-called moral rules to prevent serious injustice or harm; more often, we have to invoke rules to protect against unfair or harmful outcomes. Other useful theories applicable to medical ethics have been proposed. They are based on such concepts as justice, rights, and virtues, but no theory can encompass all ethical concerns, and none should be expected to (Larmore, 1987).

Principles

Principles have been invoked as second-order guides to ethical behavior, but, as do the theories that supersede them, they require judgment in application and have no fixed hierarchical order. Principles can conflict with one another because what is best for the patient medically (beneficence) may not be what the patient accepts (autonomy). In the 1970s, the U.S. Congress asked members of one of its commissions, formed to investigate human subject research abuse, to define the principles that should underlie the conduct of research and the practice of medicine supported by the government. The response was published in *The Belmont Report*, named for the meeting site of the commission deliberations (The National Commission, 1978). Since then, ethical principles have been used widely as guides in applied ethical deliberation, but they require judgment in their application. The principles of *The Belmont Report* are "respect for persons, beneficence and justice." *Respect for persons* encompasses Peabody's "interest in humanity," the Kantian injunction to treat people as ends and not means, and the modern concept to honor individual rights and autonomy. It is more fundamental than simply respecting autonomy, and it accommodates the need for protection for those with diminished autonomy. In practice, respect for persons is expressed in obtaining and adhering to the informed consent of patients and in ensuring that their autonomous choices are informed, or at least questioned, when they seem not to be in the patient's interest. *Beneficence* involves benefiting and not harming the patient, thus encompassing the often-cited separate principle of nonmaleficence. It is expressed by a careful analysis of the risks and benefits inherent in medical choices, and it harks back to the Hippocratic ideal of benefiting, or at least not harming, the patient. In the current social and legal climates of the supremacy of patient rights and patient autonomy, it is considered wrong from a legal, and a moral, perspective for physicians to provide care, no matter how beneficial, if the patient does not agree to it. The tradition of paternalism in medicine has given way to respect for autonomy. This can be frustrating to a physician because at times a patient's choice is not in the patient's best medical interests. *Justice* is the principle that pays tribute to the philosopher John Rawls' monumental work, *A Theory of Justice* (Rawls, 1971). It is concerned with fairness in the selection and treatment of research subjects and patients. Because not everyone in the United States has health insurance and there is no comprehensive health care program for the entire population, the concept of justice becomes important. It should be a critical, if not an overriding, principle in dis-

---

BOX 2-1
PRINCIPLES OF MEDICAL ETHICS

- Respect for Persons, as manifested by obtaining informed consent and providing counsel, honoring the patient's autonomous choices, and protecting patients with diminished autonomy.
- Beneficence, as manifested by evaluating risks of benefits and harms and by trying to maximize benefits and reduce harms.
- Justice, as manifested by fairness in providing access to health care services.

---

cussions of Medicare and Medicaid, affordability and portability of health insurance, and universal health coverage. It is also an appropriate economic consideration in discussions of where and how physicians are educated and who should reap the benefits of their training (Box 2-1).

ETHICS AND THE PRACTICE OF GYNECOLOGY
Making Moral Judgments and Resolving Conflict

From the foregoing discussion of theories and principles, it should be clear that making wise ethical choices requires judgment and experience. Ethical reasoning cannot be grounded in an appeal to one theory or principle, especially when conflicts exist and there is no one correct choice but a range of morally defensible options (Larmore, 1987). In approaching ethical problems, it is important to assemble all relevant facts about the patient's medical and social situation, to specify the ethical issues in question, and to identify comparable or analogous situations or case studies and their resolutions. One can then explore possible options and expected outcomes for congruence with the requirements of conventional ethical rules and principles. It is also helpful to review the arguments made in the past for or against a given course of action in comparable cases, to discuss cases with colleagues, and, when appropriate, to seek consultation with an ethics committee.

Ethics, Science, and Competency in Medicine

Medicine is increasingly dependent on a scientific understanding of disease causation and treatment. The introduction of evidence-based medicine (Chapter 1) highlights the ethical obligation of physicians to know and use the scientific literature for the optimal diagnosis and treatment of their patients. Continued medical education has become a necessity, and the competence and skill of the physician have ethical dimensions. In the credentialing process of the surgical disciplines, competence has been increasingly challenged, especially when new techniques, such as laparoscopic surgery or micromanipulation, are introduced or when continued competence depends on an adequate case-load for the maintenance of surgical skills (Byington, 1997).

Doctor-Patient Relationship

One major focus of ethics in medical practice has been the so-called doctor-patient relationship. The American Medical Association expects physicians to provide competence, honesty, compassion, and respect for human dignity in patient care (Mappes and Zembaty, 1991). In 1973, the American Hospital Association formulated a *Patient's Bill of Rights* that stresses considerate and respectful patient care; complete disclosure of information on the patient's medical status; and sufficient disclosure of information to the patient when informed consent is sought for a diagnostic test, procedure, treatment, or alternative. It also calls for the physician to obtain patient consent for any involvement in teaching and research activities. Although they are increasingly difficult to maintain with the electronic flow of information and insurance requirements, the patient's privacy and confidentiality should be protected.

Ethical and Political Issues in Reproductive Care

No issues in ethics have been more controversial and far-ranging than those involving medical procedures and treatments that either prevent, interrupt, or enable human pregnancy through special, "unnatural" means. These include contraception, abortion, and assisted-reproductive technologies. Because they all "interfere" with or artificially enhance the natural process of begetting a child, in or out of wedlock, the processes have run afoul of religious and social traditions. It is hard to imagine now, but there was a Connecticut law that made the sale or use of birth control devices or counseling in birth control illegal. This was overturned in 1965 by the U.S. Supreme Court decision in *Griswold v. Connecticut* that established a right to privacy in such matters. In 1972, the Supreme Court decision in *Eisenstadt v. Baird* established the right of unmarried persons to have access to contraceptives for their own use, which invalidated a Massachusetts law that interfered with such access (Garrow, 1994). The conservative religious view is best represented by the Vatican's *Instruction on Respect for Human Life in Its Origin and on the Dignity of Procreation,* which describes as illicit any interference with natural procreation through coitus between married couples. It rejects all forms of contraception, and it rejects abortion at any time during pregnancy. Assisted-reproductive technologies, such as in vitro fertilization, gamete freezing, artificial insemination, surrogate pregnancy, and other manipulations of the gametes, are similarly denounced as contrary to nature and contrary to the traditional religious belief that a child should be conceived by a married couple through natural means. Initially, the chief objections to assisted reproduction concerned the safety of the child. This has been largely overcome as the result of more than 20 years of experience that has demonstrated the procedure to be as safe for the offspring as normal procreation. However, the in vitro fertilization process

and its attendant research include the discarding of embryos not used for pregnancy. Religious, ethical, and cultural objections remain because of this loss of embryos. Other objections have been raised about the adverse effects on marriage, the child, and the family, but the effects of assisted reproduction, whether positive or negative, are difficult to study or prove. Arguments about what is natural have abated because much of what modern medicine achieves is the protection of people from the misfortunes inflicted by nature. In any case, people desperate to have children will use almost any means medicine makes available.

Objections to providing contraceptives for minors and unmarried persons have largely dissipated with changes in the law and in public attitudes. The more urgent concerns are that at least half the pregnancies among American women and girls are unplanned and that half of those end in abortion. For some, the ethical issue is that contraceptives are not used responsibly, and for others, the ethical issue is that unmarried persons, especially adolescents, engage in inappropriate sexual activity. Public policy suffers when attempts are made to overcome one of these problems at the expense of the other. For example, it is easier and less expensive to provide access to contraception than it is to provide sex education. The fact is that both should be addressed.

Assisted-Reproductive Technologies: Social Uses, Ovum Donation, Surrogacy, Postmenopausal and Posthumous Pregnancy, and Cloning

Although at first only married, infertile couples used assisted-reproductive technologies, these technologies are now sought by single heterosexuals and homosexuals for whom conventional infertility is not even a problem. This raises questions about the legitimacy of such requests for medical resources, about the wisdom of intentional single parenting, and about the suitability of homosexual couples as rearing parents. Although these issues provoke much controversy, there is a counterargument about the current sad state of society and families with normal reproduction that ends in rampant incidences of divorce, child abuse, deadbeat parents, and general family breakdown. Single parenting has become a way of life because of the high divorce rate, and many states allow homosexual couples to adopt children. The use of a surrogate to carry a pregnancy to term has in some instances involved a sister or a mother who bears a child for a sibling or a daughter who has no uterus or who for medical reasons cannot bear the child herself. In other instances, a surrogate is hired to carry a child to term and is paid a fee for her time and service, with the belief that the child is not being bought or sold (which is illegal). This has been controversial. Sometimes a surrogate has refused to give up a child, and claims have been made of the exploitation of poor or psychologically unstable women. Surrogacy is illegal in many countries, and in some states surrogacy contracts cannot be enforced. A surrogate can be impregnated through artificial insemination, which makes her both a biologic and a gestating mother. An embryo can be transferred so that the surrogate has no genetic relationship to the child. In the latter instances, courts have been less apt to side with the surrogate if she tries to void the contract and keep the child.

The technology has gone beyond the simple in vitro fertilization of the gametes of married couples to donations of ova, sperm, and spare embryos. Because ovum donation is more involved than sperm collection and because it involves donor risk and financial inducement (Ryan, 1996), it has received special scrutiny. Collecting oocytes from aborted fetuses for in vitro maturation and for later donation has been particularly controversial not only because of the involvement of aborted fetuses but also because of the very impersonal nature of the process and the possible effects on the offspring (Ethics Committee, 1997).

Ovum donation and assisted reproduction have been used to overcome the infertility of premature menopause. Few concerns have been voiced about this, but it has also been used in women in their sixties after the natural menopause. The arguments for and against helping older, postmenopausal women become pregnant include whether it is in the best interests of the woman and the child given the medical risks of pregnancy in older women, the shorter life expectancy of the older mother, and the unnaturalness of it. Some people feel it is acceptable because it gives women gender equality with men, who can beget children at advanced ages (Ethics Committee, 1997).

Posthumous reproduction has become possible now that gametes can be collected and stored for later use if one of the parents dies. Through in vitro fertilization, a surrogate can carry the pregnancy if the biologic mother dies or the biologic mother can still become pregnant if her husband dies. If a woman has cancer, gametes can be collected before radiation therapy or chemotherapy to protect them for later reproduction, or they can be used posthumously if she does not survive. Similarly, sperm can be collected if a man has a terminal illness. Embryos can be created and frozen while both parents are alive and implanted posthumously after the death of one or both of them. The most critical issues are the adequate consent of both prospective biological and rearing parents and the well-being of the child or children so conceived, including adequate arrangements for their upbringing (Ethics Committee, 1997).

Cloning is the latest reproductive technology to arouse major ethical concerns. It was reported in 1997 that cloning had been accomplished in sheep. The possibility that it might be tried in humans made everyone sit up and take notice. This cloning involved transferring the genetic material from a differentiated adult somatic cell to a fertilized egg from which the nucleus had been removed. The egg was stimulated to develop. Then it was transferred to a surrogate ewe for gestation and birth. The biologic parent in this case is the adult from which the somatic cell was taken, and the offspring is a genetic copy or clone of that adult. The issues raised when in vitro fertilization was first reported resur-

faced about cloning. It was unnatural, it was unsafe (actually, more than 200 attempts resulted in many deformed embryos before the first and only success), and it would not be in the best interests of the offspring. Most people felt it should not be tried in humans until its safety could be established. Others felt it should never be tried because it was so far out of sync with nature and our concept of reproduction. Others felt the psychologic burden of being a clone (that is, an identical "twin" born many years later) would be insurmountable. At first, it was imagined that only an idiosyncratic, narcissistic millionaire would want to make this attempt at immortalization, but other applications could be considered if this were the only reproductive method available for a threatened human species that could not reproduce sexually. Potential uses have included trying to develop cell lines or organ sources for transplantation needs. Although some limited applications may seem morally acceptable, the controversy over the method remains, and its safety is a major obstacle to even contemplating its application in humans any time soon (National Bioethics Advisory Committee, 1997).

Abortion

It seems as if modern medical ethics developed out of the chaotic social and political fights over abortion in the 1960s. Just before *Roe v. Wade,* the U.S. Supreme Court decision of 1973 that established abortion as a constitutional right, there had been a mounting sympathy for women who sought abortions. Before that time, abortion was condemned publicly but tolerated privately. It was easily available to the wealthy but restricted and dangerous for the poor. A major cause of maternal death was infection or bleeding resulting from illegal abortions. Another impetus to legalizing abortion was that prenatal diagnosis became available through amniocentesis in the 1960s, and many parents did not want knowingly to carry a seriously deformed child to term. A rubella epidemic during the same period created an intense demand for pregnancy termination by parents who feared severely crippling defects in their infants. It was at this time that model laws were being developed to allow abortion under strict criteria: the life or health of the mother was endangered, the pregnancy was the result of rape or incest, or the child would have severe genetic defects. The *Roe v. Wade* decision preempted such laws and made abortion available with no restrictions, at least in the first trimester. There has been an intense battle for the moral high ground on this issue. Those who feel that the life of the fetus is sacred from conception (pro-life) pit themselves against those who feel a woman should have a right to control how her body is used and to choose whether to continue a pregnancy and become a mother (pro-choice). The middle ground holds that the fetus gains in moral status as it develops and that there is less concern about abortion early in pregnancy. The middle-ground perspective contends that restrictions are justified in the second trimester, especially after viability is reached. All these positions have been defended as ethical. Not everyone regards the fertilized egg to be the moral equivalent of a full-term infant. At the extremes, there is no accommodation for the other side's deeply held ethical convictions (Ryan, 1992). Now the focus is on how social harmony and civility can be maintained rather than how to change the opponent's moral views. Arguments, fought mostly at the periphery of abortion, are about destructive operations in late pregnancy (partial-birth abortion), parental consent before abortions in adolescents, and adequate or required counseling for everyone seeking abortion. In the years after the *Roe v. Wade* decision, other Supreme Court decisions have modified the law and reflected public concerns. In 1989, in *Webster v. Reproductive Health Services,* the Supreme Court established a state's right to impose some regulations on abortion, such as a requirement to test for viability. In the 1992 *Planned Parenthood of Southeastern Pennsylvania v. Casey* judgment, however, the Court insisted that in the process of regulation, a state could not put an "undue" burden on a woman's right to abortion (Butler and Walbert, 1992; Garrow, 1994). The ethical strife surrounding abortion points out the inadequacy of moral theory and principles to deal with complex issues such as this concerning the conflicting interests of women, the unborn fetus, and a pluralistic society. Violence against abortion clinics and personnel, progressing even to the murder of physicians who perform abortions, reveals the extremes to which fervent ethical advocacy can lead.

In 1995 in the United States, more than 1.2 million abortions were performed, primarily on single women (80%) older than 25 years (47%). The incidence at age 19 or younger was 20%, and at ages 20 to 24 it was 33%. Of those who had abortions, 60% were white (Leonard, 1997). In public opinion polls, the majority still supports abortions in early pregnancy but feel restrictions are needed as pregnancy advances (Goldberg and Elder, 1998).

Pain, Terminal Care, Assisted Suicide, Euthanasia

Physicians in general do a poor job in pain relief, especially when it comes to cancer pain. This is both an ethical and a medical problem. Pain can be relieved in more than 90% of patients with cancer through relatively simple means (Jacox, Carr, and Payne, 1994). Undertreatment for pain is largely the result of inadequate training of physicians. It is especially important to overcome the negative feelings of physicians and patients about the use of drugs for pain relief and the overblown fears of addiction to prescription drugs. In any case, relief of intractable pain is not the only basis of requests for assisted suicide or euthanasia from patients who are terminally ill. In most instances, requests for assisted suicide and euthanasia have to do with feelings of hopelessness and depression and are not always associated with terminal illness (Emanuel, 1997).

Whether to maintain life when all hope for recovery seems gone was challenged in 1989 in the Nancy Cruzan case. The Missouri Supreme Court found that Ms. Cruzan's parents should not remove life support by denying the use of a feeding tube for their daughter, who was in a persistent vegetative state because of injuries suffered in a car crash. The Court decided that, unless she had given formal instructions before the accident about removing life support, the state could keep Nancy Cruzan alive out of respect for the sanctity of life. The Supreme Court concurred and did establish that a person has the right to make such a request for removal of support by way of an advance directive or a living will that must be honored if they subsequently become incapacitated (Pence, 1995). This removal of life support (respirator, antibiotics, or food and fluid) is often termed passive euthanasia to distinguish it from active euthanasia, which involves the administration of drugs to cause death rather than letting "nature take its course." Philosophers, and occasionally the courts, have denied a material or a moral difference between passive and active euthanasia (omission versus commission) because in each "death is the intended outcome." There is, however, an emotional feeling of culpability and finality of action in active euthanasia that challenges the belief that they are the same.

There has always been a strong presumption that a physician's obligation is to try to maintain life and not to engage in euthanasia, but this was before the advent of modern life support systems that can keep brain-dead persons "alive." The intrusiveness of modern intensive care and the options for total body radiation and bone marrow transplantation in, for example, patients with cancer, offer opportunities for medical treatment that not everyone wants to endure. A physician's duty is no longer as clear as it once was, and patient and family involvement have become more important (Beauchamp, 1997). There have been many stories of excessive care in futile cases, engendering the sense that patients and their families have lost control. Some still believe that life should be maintained at all costs. The situation has been likened to the moral issues and arguments about abortion 25 years earlier. Physician-assisted suicide and active euthanasia are illegal in most states, but they are more widely practiced and condoned than publicly acknowledged. In Oregon, a law was first passed in 1994 permitting physician-assisted suicide, but it was challenged in the courts for 3 years. The legislature then asked for a referendum, and, in November 1997, 60% of the voters affirmed the Death with Dignity Act to allow a terminally ill patient to obtain a lethal dose of drugs from a physician (Knight-Ridder Service, 1998). The first death under the new law, of an 80-year-old woman with terminal breast cancer, took place 4 months later (Egan, 1998). In the states of Washington and New York, laws were passed against physician-assisted suicide that were then overturned by federal courts in those districts, only to be reaffirmed by the U.S. Supreme Court in a 9-0 decision that there is no constitutional right to physician-assisted suicide (Greenhouse, 1997). On the other hand, 51% of the public believes that physician-assisted suicide ought to be legal (Rosenbaum, 1997).

In defense of physician-assisted suicide was a "philosopher's brief" that was sent to the Supreme Court as it was considering the case (Dworkin, 1997). The argument concerned privacy and stated that if patients have the right to refuse care, they should have the right to determine when to die. This is the passive-active euthanasia argument in a different form. The arguments against physician involvement in assisted suicide and euthanasia are that they could lead to abuse and that, in the absence of adequate health insurance, they are economic and social forms of coercion. In Holland, where euthanasia is widely practiced but not legally sanctioned, there have been reports of euthanasia in patients who were not terminally ill and in patients who did not give their consent (Emanuel, 1997).

If physician-assisted suicide becomes the norm, it is feared that people with serious illness would feel they have to defend why they should not give up and die. To others, it would impair the physician-patient relationship and the constancy of medicine in the defense of life. It is believed that morphine is used in patients who are terminally ill not only to relieve pain but to hasten or cause death and that this is a nonsanctioned form of euthanasia. An important aspect of care is to discuss such matters with patients ahead of time and to have them draw up living wills or advanced directives so they and their families can express their preferences and maintain their sense of control and dignity.

Discouraging conclusions to a study of the treatment of terminally ill patients in prestigious teaching hospitals are that physicians do not know their patients' wishes regarding resuscitation and that they are not effective in dealing with their patients' pain and discomfort. When an intervention was tried to overcome these deficiencies, it did not work. Even though physicians were given detailed and accurate prognostic assistance on when to expect death, trained nurses were used to facilitate communication between patients, families, and staff, and physicians had written instructions on their patients' desires, it did not change practice. There was no significant effect, compared with results seen in a control group, on length of time in intensive care, in a coma, or on a machine before death or pain relief (Support Principal Investigators, 1995).

It is clear that the physicians and the public are ambivalent about physician-assisted suicide and euthanasia, yet no one is satisfied with the way terminal illness and chronic disease are handled. For the present, more effective pain relief and advanced directives from patients are clear ethical imperatives. The rights of patients to forgo medical care and futile therapy at the end of life and their preferences for hospice care should be observed. With such measures, the apparent pressure for euthanasia or physician-assisted suicide may decrease enough to provide time for society to work out how it wants to deal with these issues.

HYPOTHETICAL CASE STUDIES

1. A 33-year-old nulliparous patient is referred to you with a large intramural fibroid tumor, heavy irregular bleeding, anemia, and a desire to preserve her fertility. During the course of history taking, the patient identifies herself as a long-standing Jehovah's Witness, which precludes her from accepting a blood transfusion or even prebanking her own blood. Your usual treatment plan is iron therapy, preoperative use of a gonadotrophin-releasing hormone agonist, and myomectomy. Occasionally, you have obtained court orders to transfuse blood to Jehovah's Witnesses, and you are uneasy about promising the patient now that you will not give her a blood transfusion if she bleeds massively during surgery. You have never allowed a patient to exsanguinate when life could be saved by a blood transfusion.

Commentary: This case illustrates the conflict between an autonomous patient's desire for surgery on the condition that she not be made to undergo a blood transfusion and the physician's sense of moral obligation not to let a patient die when a blood transfusion could prevent death and not to have conditions placed on his or her ability to provide appropriate medical care. In such cases it is important to understand the strength and basis of the patient's convictions and to be certain that the patient understands the risks involved. The surgeon should also understand the depth of his or her own convictions and be aware of the changes in public attitudes and in the courts that favor respecting the patient's wishes in such matters. The surgeon's options are to provide surgery and promise to not transfuse or to refer the patient to another surgeon. The option of performing surgery and then a transfusion, if necessary, with or without a court order, would be considered unethical because it would violate the patient's religious beliefs and autonomous choice. This course of action is generally not available, even in emergencies, because of new institutional and legal rules against such practices.

2. A 24-year-old married nulliparous woman is referred to you for infertility services. It has already been determined that she has no identifiable problems with reproductive function, but her husband has azoospermia. The patient requests artificial insemination, but rather than using an anonymous donor's sperm from a sperm bank, she requests use of her brother-in-law's sperm. Her sister and brother-in-law already have two children of their own. The patient's husband and brother-in-law agree to the procedure, but the brother-in-law feels it would be demeaning to be tested for acquired immunodeficiency syndrome and other sexually transmitted diseases.

Commentary: This case is typical of a wide variety of requests for assisted reproduction. The arrangements are socially provocative, and the moral issues are subtle. Some physicians may feel artificial insemination is wrong in all cases. It is important to be certain that the patient's sister, husband, and brother-in-law have no reservations about the proposal and that all are made aware of the possible implications for their future relationships and for the children conceived in such a manner. Fertility programs should include counseling for infertile couples and gamete donors so they can review all the concerns about such arrangements. Although the brother-in-law may object to standard procedures for sperm processing, the physician would be ill advised to forego standard safety procedures under any circumstances.

RISK MANAGEMENT

The purpose of risk management is to achieve a reduction in medical malpractice claims, usually by reviewing previous cases and by identifying patient care and surgical practices that should be changed or improved to reduce complications, bad outcomes, and patient dissatisfaction. The process has a strong affinity to the "ethical" practice of medicine in that each stresses the value of a good doctor-patient relationship, adequate informed consent, and appropriate surgical skills, experience, and competence.

Changes in the practice of the specialty have created new problems that can reduce patient satisfaction and create a sense of abandonment. Surgery is performed either on the day of admission or on an ambulatory basis, thus reducing the opportunity for immediate preoperative evaluation and consultation that once occurred as part of a hospital admission. Similarly, postoperative stays are shortened or nonexistent, and opportunities for counseling for postoperative care and physical surveillance are necessarily curtailed. The rise in laparoscopic surgery has occasioned a corresponding increase in claims associated with complications and questions about the competence and skill of the operators. This highlights the need for adequate training and credentialing for novel procedures and equipment. Major factors in malpractice claims include delays in diagnosis, especially with breast cancer; improper techniques that result in complications; and improper or unnecessary surgery (Box 2-2). Adequate defense of the level of care comes best from adequate records completed in a timely fashion covering the preoperative evaluation, counseling, and informed consent process; a complete operative note; and documentation of postoperative care (Byington, 1997).

Informed Consent

At one time, informed consent was ridiculed as impossible to obtain because of the information gap between patients and their physicians. It was also considered ineffective as a defense in malpractice cases, largely because the consent process and form were perfunctory. These attitudes can no longer be considered correct. Patients are better informed than ever about medical matters because of reports in newspapers, magazines, newsletters, and television. It is unnecessary to detail for them the minutiae of therapy or the structure of drugs as long as they are provided with enough information to make a fully informed choice. This includes the types of treatment and the probable benefits and risks. Patients want to know about common complications and about serious or catastrophic ones, even if they are rare. They want to know about the therapeutic experience of the

---

**BOX 2-2
MAJOR ALLEGATIONS IN MALPRACTICE CLAIMS INVOLVING GYNECOLOGISTS, 1987 TO 1996***

Categories	Percentage of Total
Hysterectomy-related injuries	20
Laparoscopic complications	12
Failure to diagnose (including breast cancer)	11
Negligence in surgery	10
Abortion-related issues	9
Failed sterilization	7
Consent issues	6
Medication injuries	5
Retained foreign body	4

*Data courtesy of Harvard Risk Management Foundation.

**BOX 2-3
COMPONENTS OF THE INFORMED CONSENT PROCESS**

- Provide information and education about the patient's diagnosis and range of therapies, the risks and benefits of each therapeutic option, and the expected outcome of no therapy and of each therapeutic intervention. Provide information a reasonable patient would want to make an informed choice.
- Provide information at the appropriate level of comprehension, including language translation if needed, to ensure that the patient understands the options.
- Ascertain that the patient is making the choice freely, without intimidation or coercion.
- Establish that the patient does not have limited understanding and is acting independently based on the information given.
- Obtain a signed consent form, and record the process in the patient's file.

---

physician and the institution. It is important not to misrepresent your level of experience and technical skill. Patients want to know about alternative therapies and the effects of no therapy at all. Some patients may convey to you that they trust you and prefer not to know details, but such attitudes may change if there are postoperative complications. You cannot force patients to listen to material they clearly do not want to hear, but it should be made available to them, and any refusal should be documented. The legal and moral emphases on the patient's right to make an autonomous choice strengthen the value of well-documented, informed consent in the courts because they undercut the excuse of not knowing or not being informed. The material has to be provided to the patient in language and descriptive detail appropriate to the patient's need, including translation to the patient's native language if necessary. Educational materials to supplement the informed consent process also should be provided. It is necessary to establish that the patient is free to choose without coercion any alternative presented to her. It must also be established that the patient has no limitations to understand and to act on the information given (Box 2-3). It is wise to allow the patient sufficient time to respond to the information, preferably by taking the informed consent and educational documents home and thinking about them for a few days. It is unwise to obtain consent for an elective procedure just before anesthesia is given, and a signed consent form obtained by a resident physician, nurse, or employee rather than by the surgeon is more likely to be questioned. Not only should the physician obtain a signed informed consent document, the informed consent process should be outlined in the patient's chart (Keyes, 1997).

CONCLUSION

The complexities of medical ethics may seem daunting. I am heartened by a quote from Thomas Nagel in his book, *The View from Nowhere*, in which he discusses ethical theory: "Common sense doesn't have the last word in ethics or anywhere else, but it has, as J.L. Austin said about ordinary language, the first word: it should be examined before it is discarded" (Nagel, 1986).

REFERENCES

Beauchamp TL: Justifying physician assisted deaths. In LaFollette H, editor: *Ethics in practice,* Cambridge, Mass, 1997, Blackwell Scientific.

Butler JD, Walbert DF: Abortion, medicine and the law. In *Facts on file,* New York, 1992, Facts on File.

Byington M: Commentary: plus ca change: forum. *Harvard Risk Found* 1997; 18:1.

Dworkin RD et al: Assisted suicide: The philosopher's brief. *New York Review of Books,* 1997: March 27, 41-47.

Egan T: First death under an assisted suicide law, *The New York Times,* p A14, March 26, 1998.

Emanuel E: The painful truth about euthanasia, *The Wall Street Journal,* p A16, Jan 7, 1997.

Ethics Committee of the American Society of Reproductive Medicine: Ethical considerations of assisted reproductive technologies. *Fertility sterility* 1997; 67(suppl 2):2S-9S.

Frame DM: *The complete essays of Montaigne,* Stanford, 1965, Stanford University Press.

Garrow DJ: *Liberty and sexuality,* New York, 1994, Macmillan.

Goldberg C, Elder J: Public still backs abortion, but wants limits, poll says, *The New York Times,* p 1, Jan 16, 1998.

Greenhouse L: Court 9-0 upholds state laws prohibiting assisted suicide, *The New York Times,* p 1, June 27, 1997.

Jacox A, Carr DB, Payne R: New clinical practice guidelines for the management of pain in patients with cancer. *N Engl J Med* 1994; 330:651-655.

Keyes C: The evolution of informed consent for health care treatment: forum. *Harvard Risk Management Found* 1997; 18:14-15.

Knight-Ridder Service: In Oregon, legal doctor-assisted suicide may face federal obstacles, *Boston Globe,* p A13, April 12, 1998.

Laramore CE: *Patterns of moral complexity,* Cambridge, 1987, Cambridge University Press.

Leonard M: Abortion, 25 years after Roe v Wade, *Boston Globe,* p F1, Dec 14, 1997.

Mappes TA, Zembaty JS: *Biomedical ethics,* ed 3, New York, 1991, McGraw-Hill.

Nagel T: *The view from nowhere.* New York: Oxford University Press, 1986.

National Bioethics Advisory Commission: *Report and recommendations: cloning human beings,* Rockville, Md, 1997.

National Commission for the Protection of Human Subjects: *The Belmont Report,* DHEW Pub No (OS) 78-0012, Washington, DC, 1978, US Government Printing Office.

Peabody FW: The care of the patient. *JAMA* 1927; 88:877-882.

Pence G: *Classic cases in medical ethics,* New York, 1995, McGraw-Hill.

Rosenbaum DE: Americans want a right to die, *The New York Times,* p 3, June 8, 1997.

Ryan KJ: Abortion or motherhood: Madness and suicide. *Am J Obstet Gynecol,* 1992; 166: 1029-1036.

Ryan KJ: Ethical and legal implications. In Adashi EY, Rock JA, Rosenwaks Z, editors: *Reproductive endocrinology, surgery and technology.* Philadelphia, 1996, Lippincott-Raven.

Scannell GJ: The care of the patient. *Harvard Medical Alumni Bulletin,* Winter 1986-87; 45-49.

The Support Principal Investigators: A controlled trial to improve care for seriously ill hospitalized patients. *JAMA* 1995; 274:1591-1598.

PART II

THE REPRODUCTIVE SYSTEM AND DISEASE

3

The Menstrual Cycle

ROBERT L. BARBIERI

KENNETH J. RYAN

KEY ISSUES

1. The menstrual cycle is dependent on the integrated actions of the hypothalamus, pituitary gland, ovarian follicle, and endometrium.
2. Like a metronome, the hypothalamus sets the beat for the menstrual cycle by the pulsatile release of gonadotropin-releasing hormone (GnRH). GnRH pulses occur every 1 to 1.5 hours in the follicular phase and every 2 to 4 hours in the luteal phase of the cycle.
3. Pulsatile GnRH secretion stimulates the pituitary gland to secrete luteinizing hormone (LH) and follicle-stimulating hormone (FSH). The pituitary gland translates the tempo set by the hypothalamus to a signal, LH and FSH secretions, that can be understood by the ovarian follicle.
4. In the ovarian follicle, LH stimulates theca cells to produce androstenedione, and FSH stimulates granulosa cells to convert the androstenedione produced by the theca to estradiol. After ovulation, the follicle is transformed into the corpus luteum, which, stimulated by LH or human chorionic gonadotropin (hCG), secretes progesterone. Progesterone prepares the endometrium for implantation of the conceptus.
5. Estradiol stimulates the endometrium to proliferate. Estradiol plus progesterone cause the endometrium to become differentiated to a secretory epithelium. During the midluteal phase of the cycle, when progesterone production is at its peak, the secretory endometrium is optimally prepared for the implantation of a preembryo.

There are two views of the menstrual cycle: the clinical view of cyclic bleeding and the theoretical/physiologic view of the mechanisms underlying the integration of the menstrual cycle. In this chapter, an attempt will be made to develop both perspectives.

The idealized menstrual cycle lasts 28 days, with ovulation occurring at approximately day 14. The first day of menses is considered to be the first day of a new menstrual cycle. At the level of the endometrium, the menstrual cycle consists of four main phases: (1) the menses; (2) the proliferative phase; (3) the ovulatory phase, when the proliferative endometrium is transformed into a secretory endometrium; and (4) the secretory phase, when the endometrium is prepared for the implantation of the embryo (Fig. 3-1). The proliferative endometrium is characterized by a high rate of cell division in the endometrial glands, whereas the secretory endometrium is characterized by a low rate of cell division in the glands. The secretory epithelium fills the luminal spaces with carbohydrates and proteins essential to implantation of the embryo.

At the level of the ovary, the menstrual cycle can be characterized by two main phases. The first half of the cycle is the follicular phase. The second half of the cycle is the luteal phase. Corresponding to the endometrial phases of menses and proliferation is the ovarian follicular phase. *Follicle* is derived from the Greek and denotes a fluid-filled bag or sack. During the middle and late follicular phases of the cycle, the ovary is dominated by a fluid-filled cyst that contains the maturing oocyte. Corresponding to the endometrial secretory phase of the cycle is the ovarian luteal phase. *Luteal* is Latin and means "yellow body." Before and after ovulation, the follicle is transformed into the corpus luteum, which is yellow-orange because of the high concentration of cholesterol esters and other lipids.

CYCLE LENGTH

Menstruation is the cyclic uterine bleeding experienced by most women of reproductive age. Normal menstruation represents the cyclic shedding of the uterine secretory

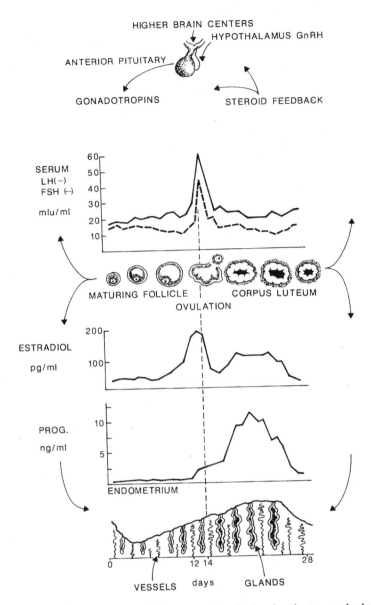

Fig. 3-1. Diagrammatic representation of the menstrual cycle showing the temporal relationships of the pituitary secretion of the gonadotropins follicle-stimulating hormone *(FSH)* and luteinizing hormone *(LH)* with ovarian follicular estradiol production and of luteal progesterone and estradiol production. In addition, the progressive response of the endometrium to the sequential change in steroids is portrayed.

endometrium because of a decline in estradiol and progesterone production caused by the regressing corpus luteum.

The clinician routinely asks each woman about the regularity of the menstrual interval, the length of menses, and the volume of menstrual flow. Treloar et al (1967) reported on the menstrual interval and its regularity in white women who attended the University of Minnesota (Table 3-1). Data were collected prospectively for 30 years, and approximately 275,000 cycles were available for analysis. In this study, the mean age of menarche is approximately 13 years, and the mean age of menopause is approximately 52 years of age. Menstrual cycle lengths are most regular in women between 20 and 40 years of age, and the average length is 28 days. However, the median normal cycle length declined

from 29 days at age 20 to 27 days at age 40. This decrease in cycle length is caused by a decrease of 2 days in the length of the follicular phase of the cycle. Findings of a recently completed study of the menstrual cycles of 1000 women replicate the earlier results (Belsey and Pinol, 1997).

The association of menstruation with the lunar cycle is a romantic notion. Although the lunar cycle is precisely 28 days long, the menstrual cycle of most women does not repeat itself like clockwork throughout their reproductive lives. Menstrual cycle length demonstrates significant variability in the 5 years after menarche and the 5 years before menopause. In the study by Treloar et al (1967), in the 5 years after menarche, cycle length ranges from 22 to 45 days. In the 5 years before menopause, the cycle length

Table 3-1   Median and 5% Upper and Lower Bounds on Menstrual Interval in Days from 275,947 Menstrual Cycles

Chronologic Age (Years)	Menstrual Interval (Days)		
	5% Lower Bound	Median	5% Upper Bound
17	22	28	40
25	23	28	37
33	22	27	34
41	22	26	32
49	15	27	>80

Modified from Treloar AE et al: Variation of human menstrual cycle through reproductive life. *Int J Fert* 12: 77-126, 1967.

ranges from 15 to 55 days. In general, polymenorrhea is present if the cycle length is shorter than 22 days, and oligomenorrhea is present if the cycle length is longer than 35 days.

A working knowledge of menstrual cycle length is especially important for couples who practice the rhythm method of contraception. Because of the ability of the cervical mucus to act as a long-term reservoir for sperm, this method is most effective when a couple refrains from sexual intercourse from the first day of menses until 2 days after the completion of ovulation; by then, the oocyte is no longer capable of fertilization or normal embryo development (Wilcox et al, 1995).

Age at menarche and length of menstrual cycle are important modulators of disease risk. For example, in a prospective study of menstrual cycle characteristics and risk for fracture in menopause, Cooper and Sandler (1997) observe that late menarche (after age 14) is associated with a threefold increase in the risk for wrist fracture. Cycle lengths longer than 31 days are associated with a twofold increase in wrist fractures. Similar correlations between late menarche, or oligomenorrhea, and an increase in hip and vertebral fracture is also reported. Late menarche is associated with a decreased risk for breast cancer, endometriosis, and uterine leiomyomata. In general, late menarche and long cycle intervals are associated with a decreased risk for estrogen-dependent disease. Conversely, early menarche and short cycle intervals are associated with an increased risk for estrogen-dependent disease. Similarly, late age at menopause is associated with an increased risk for estrogen-dependent diseases such as breast cancer (Kelsey et al, 1993).

MENSTRUAL FLOW

Menstrual bleeding occurs only in higher apes and humans; most mammals do not slough the lining of the uterus at the end of each nonfertile cycle. This striking difference in the reproductive process is probably related to the evolution of viviparity and the unique placentation of primates. Although there are no menstrual periods in other mammals, some do have cyclic bleeding at the time of ovulation and sexual receptivity. This is typically seen in the domestic dog.

The average duration of menstruation is between 3 and 7 days. Menstruation that is shorter (hypomenorrhea) or longer (hypermenorrhea) than this range is abnormal. The amount of blood loss is generally 80 mL or less. When menstrual blood loss exceeds 80 mL, there is a good correlation with anemia (hemoglobin concentration less than 120 g/L). Because trying to determine the extent of menstrual blood loss by patient estimates is difficult, checking for anemia is one practical way to monitor the extent of menstrual flow.

INTEGRATION OF THE MENSTRUAL CYCLE

The important structural and functional components of the female reproductive system are the hypothalamus, which controls the pulsatile release of gonadotropin-releasing hormone (GnRH); the pituitary gland, which controls the pulsatile release of luteinizing hormone (LH) and follicle-stimulating hormone (FSH); the ovaries, which control follicular development, with cyclic secretion of estradiol, progesterone, inhibins, and gamete maturation; and the uterus, which controls cyclic endometrial growth and shedding (Figs. 3-1 and 3-2). An overview of the interaction of these units will be provided.

The Hypothalamus

The hypothalamus is bounded at its anterior border by the optic chiasm and extends caudad to the mammillary bodies. The dorsal portion of the hypothalamus constitutes the floor of the third ventricle and its lateral walls. The base of the hypothalamus, or infundibulum, contains the infundibular stalk and the hypothalamic-hypophyseal portal vascular system perfusing the pituitary gland (Fig. 3-3). The hypothalamus contains approximately 10,000 GnRH neurons that drive the menstrual cycle by secreting GnRH in a pulsatile manner. The embryonic precursors of the GnRH neurons develop in the olfactory bulb and migrate to the arcuate and preoptic nuclei. Improper development of the olfactory bulb at an early stage of embryogenesis can result in both anosmia and amenorrhea because of the absence of the GnRH neurons (Kallman syndrome). The main function of the GnRH neurons is to receive neural signals from the brain and to transform these neural signals into an endocrine output, the pulsatile release of GnRH. The arcuate nucleus is a neuroendocrine transducer that converts an electrical signal (neuron) to an endocrine signal. To determine the appropriate pulse frequency and amplitude of GnRH secretion, the hypothalamus monitors numerous environmental cues, including body composition, stress, nutritional status, and emotion. From a teleologic perspective, it is inefficient to ovulate and reproduce if the environment is hostile to the nurturing of a newborn.

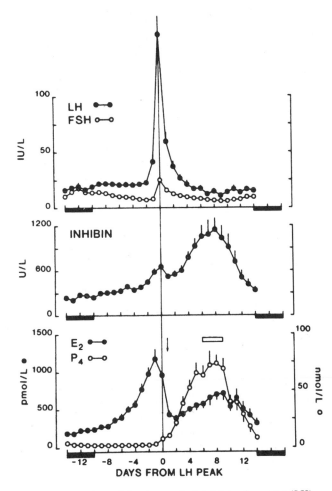

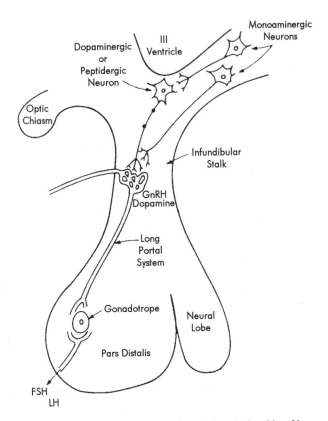

Fig. 3-3. Diagrammatic representation of the relationship of hypothalamic neurons to hypophyseal portal blood vessels that have privileged access to pituitary gonadotropes. (From Ryan KJ: The endocrine pattern and control of the ovulatory cycle. In Insler V, Lunenfeld B, editors: *Infertility: Male and female,* New York, 1986, Churchill Livingstone.)

Fig. 3-2. Overview of the changes in luteinizing hormone *(LH),* follicle-stimulating hormone *(FSH),* total inhibin estradiol, and progesterone throughout the menstrual cycle. (From Roseff SJ, Bangah ML, Kettel LM, et al: Dynamic changes in circulating inhibin levels during the luteal-follicular transition of the human menstrual cycle. *J Clin Endocrinol Metab* 1989; 69:1033.)

GnRH is a decapeptide with a short half-life (5 minutes). The short half-life of GnRH results from the rapid degradation of the peptide by tissue and plasma endopeptidases, which cleave the 6-7 and 9-10 peptide bonds. GnRH is secreted in a pulsatile fashion, and information is contained in the pulse interval and the pulse amplitude. The release of GnRH in neurosecretory bursts and the short half-life of GnRH ensures that each pulse is sharp and crisp. During the follicular phase of the cycle, GnRH pulses are characterized by high frequency, every 60 to 90 minutes, and low amplitude. During the luteal phase of the cycle, GnRH pulses are characterized by low frequency, every 120 to 240 minutes, and high amplitude.

In classic experiments on the rhesus monkey, Knobil (1980) demonstrated that if the arcuate nucleus is destroyed (loss of GnRH), the pituitary gland can no longer secrete gonadotropins and amenorrhea ensues. Exogenous administration of hourly pulses of GnRH can restart the system. If GnRH was administered with abnormally long interpulse intervals, normal menstrual cycles were not reestablished.

Knobil has since identified an electrical pulse-generating signal in the hypothalamus that stimulates the release of GnRH from the arcuate nucleus. These experiments demonstrate the primacy of GnRH in driving menstrual cyclicity.

Early investigators hypothesized that if GnRH was given as a continuous infusion, superovulation could be achieved. Surprisingly, continuous infusion of GnRH resulted in the cessation of gonadotropin secretion and amenorrhea. This unexpected finding has been exploited by the creation of GnRH agonist analogues with a long half-life. These GnRH agonist analogues suppress gonadotropin secretion and cause the cessation of ovarian estradiol secretion and amenorrhea. These GnRH agonist analogues are approved for the treatment of estrogen-dependent diseases such as endometriosis (Chapter 19) and uterine leiomyomata (Chapter 7) and the treatment of gonadotropin-dependent precocious puberty.

The factors that control GnRH secretion are not fully delineated, but steroid hormones and neurotransmitters influence the pulse frequency and amplitude of GnRH secretion. The administration of estradiol plus progesterone causes a decrease in GnRH pulse frequency. From a physiologic perspective, this means that in the luteal phase of the cycle, GnRH pulse frequency will be low and there will be no stimulus to develop a new follicle. This effect is the key to the efficacy of most combination estrogen-progestin contraceptives. By suppressing GnRH secretion and LH and FSH secretion, combination estrogen-progestin contraceptives block gonadotropin secretion and prevent the development of a competent ovarian follicle, thereby blocking ovulation. Norepinephrine and endogenous opioid peptides are neurotransmitters that regulate GnRH secretion. Norepinephrine appears to be the principal neurotransmitter that stimulates GnRH secretion, and endogenous opioid peptides appear to suppress GnRH secretion. The link between opioids and GnRH secretion may be one mechanism by which stress suppresses GnRH secretion.

Abnormalities in GnRH Pulse Frequency Are Associated with Menstrual Dysfunction

In the monkey, abnormalities in menstrual function can be induced by experimental manipulations that decrease or increase GnRH pulse frequency. In the human, decreased GnRH pulse frequency is associated with oligomenorrhea or amenorrhea, and increased GnRH pulse frequency is associated with the polycystic ovary syndrome. Because GnRH is not present in high concentrations in the peripheral circulation, LH pulses are measured as proxies for GnRH pulses. Khoury et al (1987) measured LH pulses in 14 women with amenorrhea and in 25 women with normal ovulation. The ovulating women had LH pulses every 90 minutes. The anovulatory women had LH pulses every 480 minutes. Administration of the opioid antagonist naloxone increased LH pulse frequency to one pulse every 140 minutes. This study suggests that low GnRH pulse frequency contributes to the development of amenorrhea in some women. This study also suggests that hypothalamic opioid activity may contribute to the low GnRH pulse frequency observed in amenorrheic women.

Polycystic ovary syndrome (PCOS) is characterized by irregular menses, oligoovulation or anovulation, and hyperandrogenism. In many women with PCOS, GnRH pulse frequency is significantly increased. Waldstreicher et al (1988) measured LH pulse frequency in 12 women with PCOS and in 21 ovulating women during the follicular phase. In women with normal ovulatory cycles, the mean LH interpulse interval was 90 minutes in the early follicular phase. In women with PCOS, the mean LH interpulse interval was 60 minutes. The LH pulse frequency correlated positively with circulating estradiol. This study suggests that elevated GnRH pulse frequency may contribute to the development of PCOS.

Pituitary Gland: Major Link Between Brain and Ovary

The pituitary gland, with its pulsatile secretion of gonadotropins, is the major link between the brain and ovarian function. During embryonic development, the anterior lobe of the pituitary gland is derived from a pinching off of a portion of the oral cavity, whereas the posterior lobe of the pituitary gland is an extension of the neural tissue linked to the hypothalamus. The two lobes come into apposition to form

the definitive adenohypophysis attached to the median eminence by the infundibular stalk. The adult pituitary weighs 0.5 g and measures $10 \times 13 \times 6$ mm. The anterior pituitary comprises three fourths of the total gland. The gland sits in the sphenoid bone in a cavity known as the *sella turcica,* and it is separated from the cranial cavity by the dura mater, which the pituitary stalk and the blood vessels penetrate. The anterior pituitary is comprised of a range of cell types, each type specific for one or more of the pituitary hormones. It is thought that one cell type is specific for both LH and FSH (gonadotropes) and that another is specific for prolactin (lactotrope) (Pelletier et al, 1978).

The pituitary gonadotropes receive signals from the hypothalamus in the form of pulsatile GnRH secretion. In response, the pituitary synthesizes and secretes FSH and LH in pulses that match the GnRH signal. The secretion of gonadotropins by the pituitary is also modulated by the negative feedback of steroid hormones, especially ovarian estradiol, which keeps FSH and LH levels in the 10 to 20 mIU/mL range during most of the cycle. At menopause or after oophorectomy, when estradiol is no longer secreted, gonadotropins are released from negative feedback control and rise to more than 50 mIU/mL. Gonadotropins are glycoproteins, each composed of two subunits associated by noncovalent bonds and designated α and β. In common with thyroid-stimulating hormone (TSH) and human chorionic gonadotropin (hCG), FSH and LH each contain the same α subunit containing 89 amino acids. It is the β subunit that is different for each of these four hormones and that confers their biologic and immunologic specificity (Parsons and Pierce, 1981).

Ovarian Development

During embryonic development, primitive germ cells migrate from the yolk sac to the mesonephric ridge, where the definitive ovary develops. The primitive germ cells, or oogonia, divide by mitosis and increase their numbers to several million until about 6 months of intrauterine development, when mitotic division stops. Starting at 8 to 13 weeks of gestation, oogonia continually enter meiosis until they all are converted to oocytes, which are arrested in the dictyate stage. The process is completed by 6 months after birth. Oocytes remain arrested in the meiotic prophase until stimulated to resume meiosis during the LH surge of each ovulatory cycle. The number of oocytes continually declines during life. At puberty, only 300,000 oocytes remain, of which only a few hundred will be ovulated in a woman's lifetime.

The primordial follicle represents the earliest stage of follicular development. The primordial follicle consists of the oocyte surrounded by a basal lamina and a few spindle-shaped (pregranulosa) cells. The primordial follicle develops into a primary follicle, when the oocyte is surrounded by cuboidal granulosa cells. In the primary follicle, cuboidal granulosa cells secrete glycoproteins that surround the oocyte in a shell called the *zona pellucida*. These developmental steps can occur in the absence of gonadotropin stimulation. The primary follicle becomes a secondary follicle when the granulosa cells divide and develop into multiple layers surrounding the oocyte. It is at this point that follicles are recruited for each ovarian cycle during active reproductive life (Dorrington and Armstrong, 1979).

Follicular Development

Resting follicles are recruited into a cohort of active follicles, only one of which will be destined to ovulate; the remainder undergo atresia. Each follicle begins as an oocyte surrounded by a layer of granulosa cells, which is surrounded by a band of modified fibroblast-like cells called *theca interna*. Both FSH and LH are necessary for the secondary follicle to fully develop. LH stimulates the thecal cells to divide and produce androgens, which can be converted to estrogens by the granulosa cells. FSH stimulates the granulosa cells to divide and to increase the enzymes necessary to convert thecal androgens to estradiol (aromatization). Granulosa cell numbers increase dramatically to approximately 50 million in the dominant follicle. The follicle increases in volume by forming a fluid-filled cavity, or antrum, of approximately 5 mL, and its diameter increases some 400-fold to 2.5 cm. The follicle destined to ovulate can be identified by the following characteristics: it has FSH in its antral fluid; it has the optimal number of granulosa cells for its size; and it produces estradiol in preference to androgens.

In general, the follicles destined for atresia have not captured enough FSH to complete maturation. They have fewer granulosa cells and more androgen than estrogen in their follicular fluid. High androgen concentrations in the follicular fluid are associated with atresia (McNatty et al, 1979). Oocytes derived from the mature, healthy follicle will resume meiosis more often than oocytes derived from follicles destined for atresia.

The follicular development of the dominant follicle thus creates an environment in which the oocyte matures and is ready to resume meiosis. Enough estradiol is secreted from its granulosa cells to trigger the LH surge of the pituitary by positive feedback, which will cause the follicle to ovulate when it is "ripe." The estradiol produced by the same follicle induces endometrial proliferation, which prepares the uterus for implantation. It has been demonstrated that if the ripe follicle is destroyed, the estradiol level drops quickly; the FSH level rises in response to a transient release from negative feedback, and it takes 2 weeks for another follicle to develop to the same stage. In other words, the 2-week timing of the follicular phase of the cycle depends on the ability of the ovary to respond. The "clock" is in the ovary, even though it depends on the hypothalamus and the pituitary to make it run (DiZerga and Hodgen, 1981).

Follicular Microenvironment

An important feature of the ovarian follicle is that granulosa cells and oocytes are separated from the systemic circulation by a basement membrane. All proteins entering the follicle must pass through the basement membrane and granulosa cells. This feature allows each follicle to develop a unique microenvironment. Two adjacent follicles may have markedly different microenvironments. Many studies suggest that follicles that create a microenvironment rich in FSH and estradiol are the follicles most likely to grow rapidly, gain dominance, and ovulate. This is not surprising because both FSH and estradiol are potent stimulators of granulosa cell mitosis. Follicles that contain low concentrations of FSH and estradiol grow poorly and undergo atresia (follicular demise). The factors that regulate the development of the microenvironment have not been fully delineated. However, follicles that capture a large percentage of total ovarian blood flow appear to be at an advantage in the race to produce a microenvironment rich in FSH. Although each follicle is exposed to the same circulating concentration of FSH, the follicle with the greatest total blood flow receives the largest flux of FSH.

Selection and Dominance

At the beginning of the follicular phase of the cycle (day 1 of menses), there are approximately four antral follicles measuring approximately 4 mm in diameter in the ovaries. By day 12 of the cycle, only *one* large antral follicle measuring approximately 20 mm in diameter remains. The process by which the four small antral follicles are winnowed to one large, preovulatory antral follicle is called the process of selection. The mechanisms underlying the process of selection have not been fully characterized. However, the status of the follicular microenvironment is probably crucial to the process of selection. The small antral follicle that is able to create a microenvironment optimally conducive to growth will achieve dominance and go on to ovulate.

On day 4 of the follicular phase, no single follicle has achieved dominance. A dominant follicle emerges by day 8 of the cycle. Once a dominant follicle is established, no new large antral follicles can appear until that dominant structure undergoes atresia at the end of the luteal phase. The dominant follicle prevents the growth of other new structures by steroid (estrogen, progesterone) and protein (inhibin, follicle-regulatory protein) secretions that feedback to inhibit FSH secretion. Surgical removal of the dominant follicle is followed by the growth of a new cohort of small antral follicles that compete to become dominant. The processes of selection and dominance help ensure that, on the average, only one egg is ovulated each cycle. For mother and fetus, singleton gestation is clearly associated with better outcomes than is multiple gestation.

Ovulation

The timing of ovulation is determined by the dominant ovarian follicle. When the dominant ovarian follicle produces enough estrogen to sustain a circulating estradiol concentration in the range of 300 pg/mL for 48 hours, the hypothalamic pituitary unit responds by secreting a surge of gonadotropins (Fig. 3-4). The gonadotropin surge is characterized by an increase in LH pulse frequency (implying an increase in GnRH pulse frequency) and amplitude, resulting in a marked increase in serum LH. Before the LH surge, estradiol concentrations rise rapidly with a doubling time in the range of 60 hours. The mean duration of the LH surge is approximately 48 hours, with an ascending limb of 14 hours, a plateau of 14 hours, and a descending limb of approximately 20 hours. The gonadotropin surge is characterized by modest increases in serum FSH.

The LH surge stimulates four events in the ovary that result in ovulation: (1) an increase in intrafollicular proteolytic enzymes (plasmin), which destroys the basement membrane of the follicle and allows follicular rupture; (2) luteinization of the granulosa cells and theca, which results in increased progesterone production; (3) resumption of meiosis in the oocyte, which prepares it for fertilization; and (4) an influx of blood vessels into the follicle, which prepares it to be-

come a corpus luteum. Granulosa cells and theca contribute to the total mass of the corpus luteum. The beginning of the LH surge *precedes* ovulation by approximately 35 to 44 hours. The temporal relationship between the LH surge and ovulation is used to great advantage in in vitro fertilization programs. During most of them, oocyte harvesting is scheduled for 34 to 36 hours after the administration of exogenous hCG gonadotropin. This allows the eggs to mature fully before they are harvested, but it prevents their ovulation in the peritoneal cavity.

Luteal Phase of the Cycle

The events of the follicular phase are controlled by the estradiol secreted from the dominant follicle. The events of the luteal phase are controlled by progesterone, secreted by the corpus luteum. After ovulation, the follicle collapses and undergoes reorganization. There is an ingrowth of thecal cells and blood vessels, and the granulosa cells luteinize. Granulosa cells then increase in size and develop the characteristic morphologic changes of luteinzation. Lutein cells develop receptors on their surfaces to bind and internalize serum cholesterol bound to low-density lipoprotein (LDL) cholesterol. This cholesterol becomes a major precursor for the production of the increased amounts of progesterone now synthesized by the corpus luteum. This progesterone induces a secretory change in the estrogen-primed endometrium to prepare it for pregnancy. Estradiol is also produced by the corpus luteum, and the production of both steroid hormones is dependent on continued stimulation by pituitary LH. If pregnancy occurs, the corpus luteum will be stimulated by hCG from the conceptus. This will extend the life span of the corpus luteum until the placenta can assume its endocrine function at approximately 7 to 8 weeks of pregnancy. If pregnancy does not occur, the corpus luteum regresses (Fig. 3-5). The lowered level of steroid hormones and inhibins induces the pituitary gland to increase gonadotropin secretion, and a new cycle of follicular recruitment begins. The lowered steroid hormone levels also cause collapse of the endometrial vasculature, and menstruation results. Why the corpus luteum regresses in the primate at the end of each nonfertile cycle is not completely understood. In many animals, prostaglandin produced by the uterus in response to progesterone reaches the corpus luteum and causes luteolysis in a form of negative feedback. In these animals, simple hysterectomy will prolong the life of the corpus luteum. It is thought that in the primate, prostaglandin produced locally in the corpus luteum causes its own destruction.

Ovarian Compartments

It should be apparent from the foregoing description of ovarian function during the menstrual cycle that the ovary is a dynamic organ with cyclic changes in morphology and hormone secretion. The ovary can be thought of in terms of three major compartments—the follicles, the corpora lutea, and the stroma. The follicular compartment contains all the

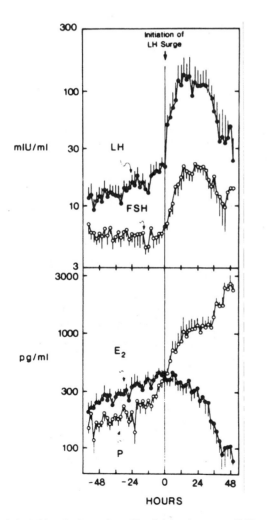

Fig. 3-4. Midcycle dynamics of luteinizing hormone *(LH),* follicle-stimulating hormone *(FSH),* estradiol, and progesterone. (From Hoff JD, Quigley ME, Yen SSC: Hormonal dynamics at midcycle: A reevaluation. *J Clin Endocrinol Metab* 1983; 57:792.)

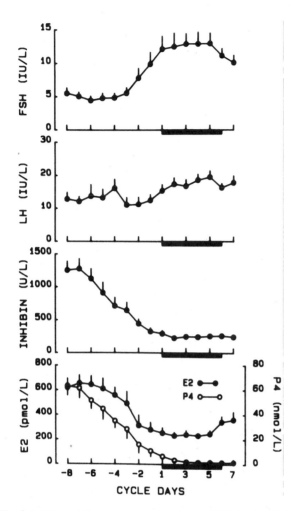

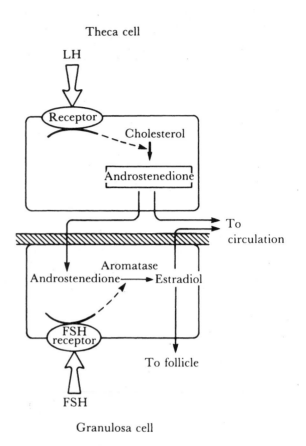

Fig. 3-5. Mean daily serum concentrations of follicle-stimulating hormone *(FSH),* luteinizing hormone *(LH),* total inhibin, estradiol, and progesterone during the spontaneous luteal-follicular transition in 12 women. (From Roseff SJ, Bangah ML, Kettel LM, et al: Dynamic changes in circulating inhibin levels during the luteal-follicular transition of the human menstrual cycle. *J Clin Endocrinol Metab* 1989; 69:1033. Copyright © The Endocrine Society.)

Fig. 3-6. Diagram of the relationship between granulosa cells and thecal cells of the follicle. Note the transport of luteinizing hormone *(LH)*–stimulated thecal androstenedione to follicle-stimulating hormone *(FSH)*–stimulated granulosa cell for dramatization to estradiol. (From Ryan KJ: The endocrine pattern and control of the ovulatory cycle. In Insler V, Lunenfeld B, editors: *Infertility: Male and female,* New York, 1986, Churchill Livingstone.)

primordial and primary follicles that are hormonally and structurally quiescent until they are recruited by pituitary FSH and LH into the cohort of growing follicles for a given cycle. The follicular compartment also includes the growing follicles that are actively secreting hormones. From the pool of growing follicles, the dominant follicle will be selected for ovulation, and the others will regress. The estradiol secreted from the ovary during the early follicular phase of the cycle is derived predominantly from the cohort of developing follicles. The dominant follicle, however, provides the bulk of the estradiol. After the LH surge, estradiol production declines rapidly. Ovarian steroid production is next dominated by the corpus luteum, in turn derived from the ruptured follicle. This compartment makes progesterone and estradiol until it regresses. Follicles and corpora lutea in various stages of development are distributed in the stromal compartment of the ovary, which consists of largely dense

fibroblast-like cells. The stroma itself produces androgens that become the dominant secretory product of the ovary whenever follicles or corpora lutea are not functional and LH concentrations are elevated. This can occur in anovulatory states, such as PCOS, and after menopause when follicles and oocytes are depleted (Ryan and Smith, 1965; Savard et al, 1965).

Two-Cell Theory

The concept of ovarian compartments evolved from studies on isolated follicles, corpora lutea, and stroma studied in vitro. From such studies it was discovered that thecal cells had LH receptors and could make androstenedione and testosterone. Granulosa cells, on the other hand, had FSH receptors and, when stimulated with FSH, responded by increasing their ability to metabolize androgens to estrogens. This explained the need for both LH and FSH for follicular development (Ryan and Petro, 1966). A theory evolved that the theca, in response to LH, makes androgens, which diffuse to the granulosa cells. Under the effect of FSH, the androgen is converted to estrogen (Fig. 3-6).

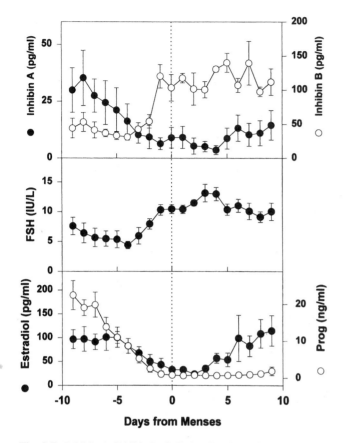

Fig. 3-7. Inhibin A, inhibin B, follicle-stimulating hormone *(FSH)*, estradiol, and progesterone concentrations in the luteal-follicular transition of women with normal menstrual cycles. (From Welt CK, Martin KA, Taylor AE, et al: Frequency modulation of follicle-stimulating hormone (FSH) during the luteal-follicular transition: Evidence for FSH control of inhibin B in normal women. *J Clin Endocrinol Metab* 1997; 82:2645-2652.) Copyright © The Endocrine Society.)

Ovarian Regulatory Proteins

As noted earlier, estradiol secreted by the ovary is carried in the circulation to the pituitary gland, where it inhibits FSH secretion. The ovarian granulosa cells also secrete inhibin A and inhibin B (Fig. 3-7). These proteins travel in the circulation to the pituitary gland, where they markedly inhibit FSH secretion. Inhibins are dimeric proteins that consist of an α subunit with a disulfide linkage to either a β-A subunit (inhibin A) or a β-B subunit (inhibin B). In the follicular phase of the menstrual cycle, the small developing follicles predominantly secrete inhibin B. In the preovulatory and luteal phases of the cycle, the granulosa cells in the large dominant follicle and the luteinized granulosa cells in the corpus luteum predominantly secrete inhibin A (Fig. 3-7). The feedback of the inhibins on pituitary FSH secretion is critical to development of a single dominant follicle. Paradoxically, homodimers of the subunit of inhibin, such as activin A (β-A/β-A) or activin B (β-B/β-B) are capable of stimulating gonadotropin secretion (Tsonis and Sharpe, 1986). Follistatin, unrelated to inhibin or activin, is a protein that is present in follicular fluid and can suppress pituitary FSH

secretion by binding and inactivating activin (Nakamura et al, 1990).

The development of the dominant follicle is critically dependent on the pituitary hormones FSH and LH. Growth factors such as the insulin-like growth factors (IGF) can modulate the action of FSH and LH by amplifying (or attenuating) their stimulatory signals. IGF-I is produced in granulosa cells from healthy follicles and can stimulate the expression of IGF-I receptors on granulosa cells. IGF-I acts synergistically with FSH to stimulate cyclic adenosine monophosphate, estradiol, and progesterone production in granulosa cells. In turn, FSH and estradiol increase the amount of granulosa cell IGF-I receptors, and estradiol increases the amount of IGF-I synthesized by granulosa cells (Giudice, 1991; Zhou and Bondy, 1993).

The ovary is capable of producing most of the IGF-binding proteins (IGFBPs). IGFBPs bind IGF and most often act as IGF antagonists. For example, in the porcine ovary, IGFBP-3 is capable of blocking the ability of FSH to stimulate estradiol and progesterone secretion in granulosa cells, probably by binding and inactivating IGF-I (51). These observations suggest that some forms of IGFBP may be FSH antagonists. The release of the IGFBPs in the rat ovary is highly regulated. IGFBP-2 and IGFBP-6 are released in the theca. IGFBP-3 is released in the corpora lutea during luteolysis. IGFBP-4 and IGFBP-5 are released from some atretic granulosa cells (Erickson et al, 1991; Erickson et al, 1992).

Steroid Structure

The cyclopentanophenanthrene-ring structure is the basic carbon skeleton for all steroid hormones. The carbon skeleton consists of a five-carbon cyclopentane ring conjoined to a phenanthrene molecule, which is itself made up of three six-carbon rings configured as shown in Figure 3-8. Carbons are shared where each of the rings meet, so that carbons 5, 10, 8, 9, 13, and 14 are common to adjoining rings. The rings are designated A, B, C, and D. The numbering of the carbons of the skeleton is important for indicating where hydroxyl groups, side chains, and other additions are added to the rings to define specific hormones. The numbering allows precise designation of the steroid structure and should be kept in mind to distinguish among the hormones, which are all closely related. Because the ring systems are relatively planar and rigid, stereoisomers that must be distinguished also occur. In general, molecules or atoms that extend in space above the plane of the ring are designated β, and those below the plane are designated α.

There are three physiologically important steroid nuclei: estrane (18 carbon atoms), androstane (19 carbon atoms), and pregnane (21 carbon atoms) (Fig. 3-8). All the important gonadal steroids are derivatives of these three steroid nuclei. Specific suffixes and symbols are used to indicate changes in these basic structures. For example, when the C-4 and C-5 carbon bonds are unsaturated and a double bond is present, the suffix "ene" replaces the "ane" ending. If a keto (=O)

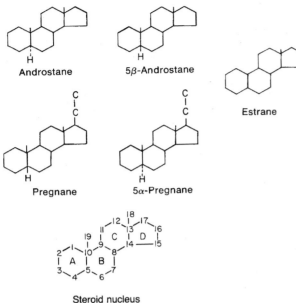

Androstane   5β-Androstane

Estrane

Pregnane   5α-Pregnane

Steroid nucleus
(Cyclopentanophenanthrene)

Fig. 3-8. Structural formula showing the basic steroid nucleus with appropriate numbering of the carbon atoms. Basic C-18 steroid estrane, C-19 steroids, androstane, 5β-androstane, and basic C-21 steroids pregnane and 5α-pregnane are illustrated.

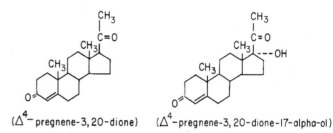

(Δ^4− pregnene-3, 20-dione)   (Δ^4−pregnene-3, 20-dione-17-alpha-ol)

Fig. 3-9. Structural formulas. **A,** Progesterone. **B,** 17α-hydroxyprogesterone.

The Core Reactions

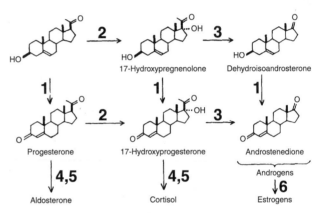

Fig. 3-10. The ovary, the testis, and the adrenal produce six common core steroids. The core Δ^5 steroids are pregnenolone, 17α-hydroxypregnenolone, and dehydroepiandrosterone. The core Δ^4 steroids are progesterone, 17α-hydroxyprogesterone, and androstenedione. The core steroids are the important precursors for the production of all gonadal steroids, glucocorticoids, and mineralocorticoids. Progesterone is an important gonadal steroid and is the precursor for all mineralocorticoids. 17α-hydroxyprogesterone is the precursor for all glucocorticoids. Androstenedione is the precursor for the androgens and estrogens. Enzyme 1 is 3β-hydroxysteroid-dehydrogenase-isomerase; enzyme 2 is 17α-hydroxylase; enzyme 3 is 17, 20-lyase; enzyme 4 is 21-hydroxylase; enzyme 5 is 11β-hydroxylase; and enzyme 6 is aromatase.

group is substituted for two hydrogens, the suffix "one" is used together with the number of the carbon to which it is attached. The 4-ene-3-one grouping is present in many biologically active steroids (testosterone, progesterone, cortisol). If a hydroxy (OH) group is substituted for a hydrogen, the suffix "ol" is used.

In Figure 3-9 the structural formula for progesterone is shown. Progesterone is a derivative of the C-21 compound pregnane. Because there is a double bond in ring A, the term *pregnane* is changed to *pregnene*. The position of the double bond (between carbon atoms 4 and 5) is designated as Δ-4. Two ketone groups are present, one on the carbon 3 and another on the carbon 20 atom—hence, 3, 20-dione (meaning two ketone groups). Therefore, the systematic name for progesterone is Δ-4 pregnene-3, 20-dione. Figure 3-9 also shows the structure and systematic name for 17-hydroxyprogesterone. Note that the OH group at the C-17 position is below the plane of the carbon ring and is designated 17-α-ol.

Biochemistry of Steroid Biosynthesis

The quantitatively important sources of steroid production are the ovaries, the testes, and the adrenals. Each of these glands makes hormones that are unique to that gland. For example, the ovary secretes large amounts of estradiol. The testis secretes large amounts of testosterone. The adrenal gland is responsible for the production of cortisol and aldosterone. In addition to these unique steroid products, each gland can produce some common "core" steroids, such as progesterone, 17-hydroxyprogesterone, and androstenedione (Fig. 3-10). These core steroids are the important pre-

cursors for the production of all gonadal steroids, glucocorticoids, and mineralocorticoids. A discussion of the biosynthesis of these core steroids follows.

Cholesterol is the parent steroid from which all gonadal steroids, glucocorticoids, and mineralocorticoids are derived. Classical concepts of steroidogenesis state that steroid-producing glands, such as the ovaries, synthesize cholesterol from acetate and then use the cholesterol to produce progestins, estrogens, and androgens. However, recent evidence suggests that plasma cholesterol is the precursor for some adrenal and ovarian steroid hormones. In the circulation, cholesterol is carried in lipoprotein packages that consist of a core of hydrophobic cholesterol and cholesterol esters surrounded by a shell of amphoteric phospholipids and apoproteins. The LDL and the high-density lipoproteins (HDL) contain most of the cholesterol present in the circulation. Adrenal and ovarian cells responsible for steroido-

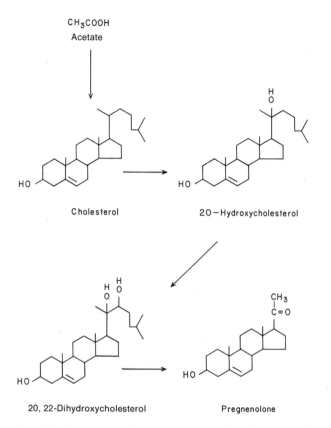

Fig. 3-11. Conversion of acetate to pregnenolone through cholesterol, 20-hydroxycholesterol, and 20, 22-dihydroxycholesterol.

genesis have membrane receptors for the LDL lipoprotein package. Circulating LDL binds to these receptors and becomes incorporated into the cell by a process of endocytosis. Cholesterol from the LDL is released for use by the cell by the action of lysosomal enzymes.

Once cholesterol is released from the lipoprotein package, it must be transported to the mitochondria, where it binds to the cholesterol cleavage enzyme and is metabolized to pregnenolone (Fig. 3-11). Pregnenolone is then metabolized to the other core steroids (progesterone, 17α-hydroxyprogesterone, and androstenedione) by three enzyme systems (Fig. 3-10). In turn, progesterone can be secreted or metabolized to the important mineralocorticoid aldosterone, 17α-hydroxyprogesterone can be secreted or metabolized to the important glucocorticoid cortisol, and androstenedione can be secreted or metabolized to the gonadal steroids testosterone and estradiol (Fig. 3-12).

There are only three types of reactions that steroids undergo: (1) removal or addition of hydrogen, as in the conversion of pregnenolone to progesterone (3β-hydroxysteroid dehydrogenase); (2) hydroxylation (addition of OH), as occurs in the conversion of progesterone to 17α-hydroxyprogesterone [17α-hydroxylase]; and (3) conjugation reactions, such as sulfoconjugates and glucuroconjugates.

The conversion of cholesterol (C-26) to progesterone (C-21), to androstenedione (C-19), and finally to estradiol (C-18), requires the sequential removal of different carbon

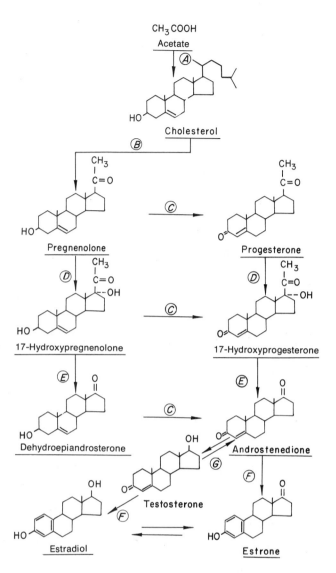

Fig. 3-12. Possible metabolic pathways for the ovarian biogenesis of estrogens. Letters above arrows denote the following metabolic pathways and the enzyme systems involved: **A,** formation of the sterol nucleus; **B,** cleavage of cholesterol side chain with formation of C-21 steroid; **C,** isomerase reaction with changing of double bond from C-5 to C-4, and dehydrogenation at C-3: 3β-ol dehydrogenases; **D,** 17α-hydroxylation (introduction of hydroxy radical in a position on C-17); **E,** cleavage of side chain, converting C-21 to C-19 steroids; **F,** aromatization (introduction of double bonds to *ring A* with conversion of C-19 to C-18 steroids); **G,** 17β-ol dehydrogenase reactions (reversible) (conversion of hydroxy radical in position β on C-17 to ketone group or vice versa). (From Smith OW, Ryan KJ: Estrogen in the human ovary. *Am J Obstet Gynecol* 1962; 84:141.)

side chains. These cleavage reactions are accomplished by multiple hydroxylations (mono-oxygenations) of neighboring carbon bonds. This produces a highly unstable intermediate compound that reaches a lower energy state by separation of the carbon side chain from the parent steroid nucleus. For example, in the conversion of cholesterol to pregnenolone, multiple hydroxylations occur at the C-20 and C-22 carbon bond that results in a breakdown of the parent compound to pregnenolone and the isocaproic aldehyde side chain (Fig. 3-11). Cholesterol cleavage enzyme 17, 20-lyase, and aromatase involve cleavage of the carbon side chains from the parent molecule (Figs. 3-10 to 3-12).

Steroid hormones are produced in the gonads and adrenals and are secreted into the circulation. There they are transported to peripheral tissues, where additional chemical transformations can occur. In the liver, multiple hydroxylation, hydration, and conjugation reactions occur that lead to a loss of steroid activity. However, in some peripheral tissues, potent steroid agonists can be locally produced from weak precursors. For example, the weak androgen androstenedione can be converted in fat tissue to the important estrogen estrone by the enzyme aromatase. In the pilosebaceous unit, the weak androgen androstenedione can be converted to the potent androgen dihydrotestosterone. This *peripheral conversion* is of utmost importance in such disease states as polycystic ovarian disease and endometrial hyperplasia. Another important peripheral conversion is that of androstenedione to the potent androgen testosterone. In normal women, 50% of circulating testosterone arises from the peripheral conversion of androstenedione derived from the ovary and the adrenal.

Steroid Pathways in the Ovarian Follicle and Corpus Luteum

Steroid biosynthetic pathways were defined for the human ovarian follicle based on enzymatic studies of tissue in vitro and on studies of isolated and recombined granulosa and thecal cells (Ryan et al, 1968). The pathway involves the steps just described. The 2-carbon acetate molecule can be converted to the 27-carbon cholesterol molecule by a series of complex reactions. There is then a loss of part of the cholesterol side chain to form the 21-carbon pregnenolone. Pregnenolone is converted to progesterone. Pregnenolone and progesterone are converted to form 19-carbon androgens, which are then transformed to 18-carbon estrogens. Although theca and granulosa cells can carry out all these steps, the theca is most facile in taking acetate to androgens, and the granulosa cells are most facile in the aromatization step to form estrogens from androgens. In the corpus luteum, a new form of steroid production takes place. The acetate-to-cholesterol steps are bypassed, and the cell uses preformed cholesterol obtained from the bloodstream to make progesterone. This probably accounts, in part, for the jump in progesterone production in the transition from the follicle to the corpus luteum. To sequester cholesterol, the luteal cells develop receptors that can bind LDL cholesterol for internalization and processing (Tureck and Strauss, 1982).

Interconversion of Androgens and Estrogens

A unique feature of estrogen production is that all estrogens are derived from androgens. In women, androstenedione is converted to estrone by the enzyme aromatase. Aromatase activity is significant in the ovarian granulosa cell and the placenta. Adipose tissue and other peripheral tissue contain small quantities of aromatase that account for the conversion of androstenedione to estrone in menopausal women. Estrone is converted to estradiol by the type 1 17β-hydroxysteroid dehydrogenase. Type 1 17β-hydroxysteroid dehydrogenase is present at high levels in the granulosa cell and placenta. Type 1 17β-hydroxysteroid dehydrogenase cannot efficiently convert androstenedione to testosterone. This limits the amount of testosterone, a potent androgen synthesized in the granulosa cell and placenta. The type 3 17β-hydroxysteroid dehydrogenase, present in the testis, can efficiently convert androstenedione to testosterone. Interestingly, the ovarian Sertoli-Leydig cell tumors express high levels of the type 3 17β-hydroxysteroid dehydrogenase and can efficiently convert androstenedione to testosterone (Barbieri and Gao, 1997).

Endometrium
Estrogen and Progesterone Effects on the Endometrium

The purpose of the menstrual cycle is to generate a single oocyte for fertilization and to prepare the endometrium for implantation. Estradiol stimulates proliferation, gland formation, and vascular growth in the endometrium. It increases the endometrial production of its own intracellular receptors, which augments its response, and the production of progesterone receptors. It is highly likely that estrogen does not directly cause mitosis in the endometrium. It achieves this secondarily through regulatory proteins such as those described for the ovary.

Spotting at the time of ovulation may represent an endometrial response to the sharp drop in the estrogen level just before the corpus luteum forms and before progesterone can continue to develop the cells. After ovulation the endometrium is ready to respond to progesterone because progesterone receptors were developed by estradiol in the early phase of the cycle. Progesterone causes gland development and decidualization of the stromal cells and the development of further spiraling and tortuosity of the underlying vasculature. This is a suitable lining for implantation and placentation if pregnancy occurs. In the sterile cycle, progesterone and estrogen production by the corpus luteum declines as a result of luteolysis, and menstrual bleeding ensues, with the collapsing of blood vessels and the sloughing of the endometrium. This is true menstrual bleeding of a well-developed secretory endometrium after progesterone withdrawal, which is generally more orderly in duration and amount than withdrawal bleeding from estrogen alone. This is the basis for treating anovulatory bleeding with progesterone.

Dating the Endometrium

Specific changes occurring in the stromal and the glandular elements of the endometrium during the menstrual cycle have been of interest to the pathologist and the clinician. By close scrutiny of these changes, it has been possible to date the endometrium (within a range of approximately 48 hours), particularly in the postovulatory phase of the cycle. This correlation between the date of the cycle and the

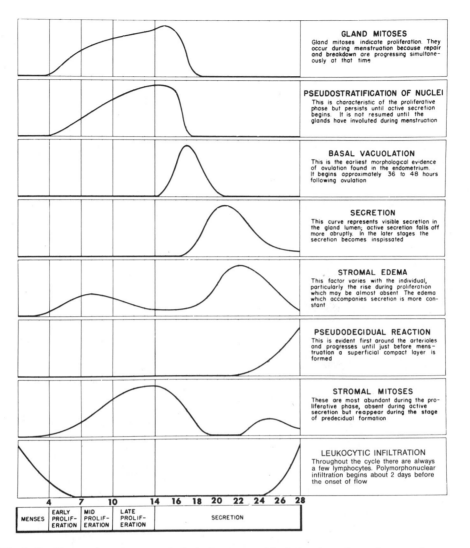

Fig. 3-13. Changes in various morphologic features used in dating the endometrium; graphs correlate with their appearance and disappearance during the menstrual cycle. (From Noyes RW, Hertig AT, Rock J: Dating the endometrial biopsy. *Fertil Steril* 1950; 1:3.)

histologic appearance of the endometrium has particular importance in the study of the infertile patient. For simplicity, a 28-day cycle with ovulation on the 14th day will be described. The first day of the menstrual period will be considered the first day of the cycle; the menstrual flow lasts 4 to 7 days. The *proliferative phase* of the cycle begins at the termination of the *menstrual phase.* The postovulatory phase, or *secretory phase,* of this cycle extends from day 14 to day 28. It should be remembered that the changes to be described occur only in the functional layers of the endometrium and not in the basal layer or in the lower uterine segment. Biopsies of endometrial specimens, therefore, have significance only if an adequate amount of functional endometrium is obtained. It is recognized that all parts of the endometrium do not undergo simultaneous change. Tissue responsiveness varies, depending on the blood supply, adjacent leiomyomata, and so forth. In the normal cycle, however, an approximation of dating within 48 hours is often of considerable help.

Proliferative Phase. Under the stimulation of estrogen, the endometrium gradually rebuilds its substance. The early proliferative phase extends from day 4 through day 7, the middle proliferative phase extends from day 8 through day 10, and the late proliferative phase lasts from day 11 until the time of ovulation on day 14 (Fig. 3-13). Discussion of the histologic characteristics of each phase follows (Noyes et al, 1950).

Early proliferative phase (Fig. 3-14). The glands of the endometrium are short and narrow. With mitotic activity, some glands remaining from the menstrual phase may show secretory exhaustion. The surface epithelium regenerates between the opening of the glands. The stroma is compact and has few mitoses. Stellate or spindle-shaped cells contain little cytoplasm and large nuclei.

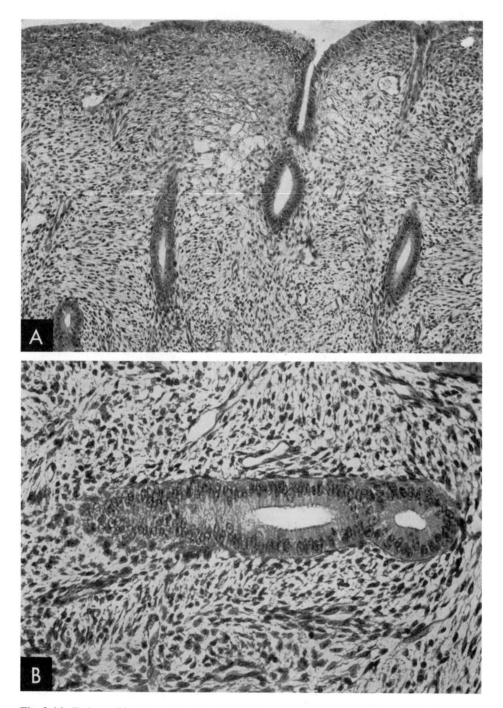

Fig. 3-14. Early proliferative endometrium. **A,** Surface epithelium thin; glands sparse, narrow, and straight (×150). **B,** Few mitoses in glands and stroma; little pseudostratification of gland nuclei (×400). (From Noyes RW, Hertig AT, Rock J: Dating the endometrial biopsy. *Fertil Steril* 1950; 1:3.)

Middle proliferative phase (Fig. 3-15). The glands are longer and have a slightly curved effect. There is early pseudostratification of the nuclei that appear superimposed in layers, but all cells are attached at the same level. The stroma has edema of variable degrees. There are numerous mitotic figures. Scanty cytoplasm and edema give a "naked nucleus" effect. The surface epithelium is covered with columnar epithelium.

Late proliferative phase (Fig. 3-16). The glands are tortuous as a result of active growth. There are numerous mitoses and pseudostratification of the nuclei. The stroma is dense and has an active growth pattern and numerous mitoses.

Secretory Phase. Changes after ovulation result from the effects of estrogen and progesterone on an endometrium previously stimulated or "primed" with estro-

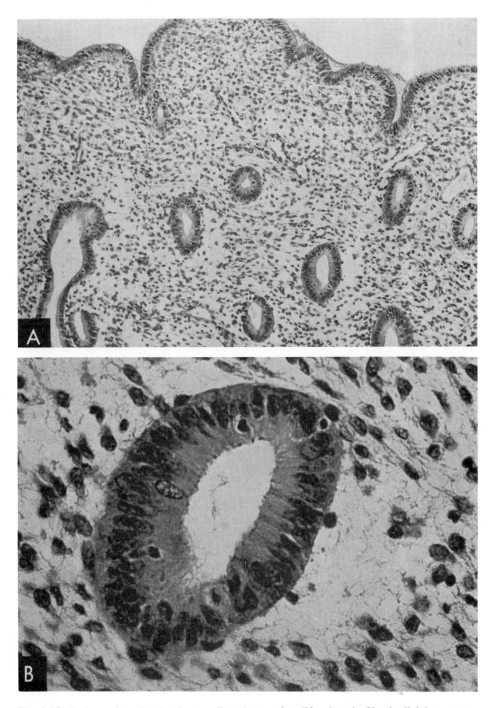

Fig. 3-15. Endometrium showing intermediate degree of proliferation. **A,** Glands slightly tortuous; tall columnar surface epithelium. Extracellular fluid is not always as marked as in this section (×150). **B,** Glands show numerous mitoses with pseudostratification becoming marked. Note the "naked nucleus" type of stromal cell with fine anastomosing processes (×400).

gen. As previously mentioned, this phase lasts approximately 14 days; the first 7 days are characterized by typical changes in the glandular epithelium. During the last 7 days, specific stromal changes occur that may be used for dating purposes.

Day 15. Except for occasional vacuoles below the nuclei of the glands, day 15 shows essentially a late proliferative pattern.

Day 16. It is the last day of pseudostratification. Basal vacuoles are seen in most of the glands, and there are mitoses in the glands and stroma.

Day 17 (Fig. 3-17). The characteristic pattern of subnuclear glycogen vacuoles is evident, and there is homogeneous cytoplasm above the nuclei of the glands. The position of the nuclei is regular. There is a loss of pseudostratification of cells and an increase in diameter and tortuosity. It is

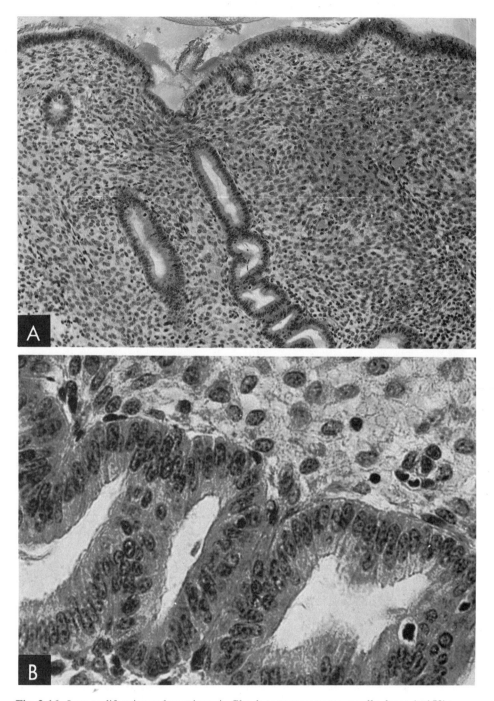

Fig. 3-16. Late proliferative endometrium. **A,** Glands tortuous; stroma usually dense (×150). **B,** Epithelial nuclei pseudostratified and oval (×400). (From Noyes RW, Hertig AT, Rock J: Dating the endometrial biopsy. *Fertil Steril* 1950; 1:3.)

rare for mitotic figures to appear in the glands and the stroma.

Day 18. Subnuclear vacuoles appear smaller as the nuclei move back toward the base of the cell. Secretion of glycogen into the lumen of the gland begins; there are no mitoses.

Day 19. Few subnuclear vacuoles are seen. It resembles the day 16 pattern except for the secretion in the lumen of the gland and the absence of pseudostratification and mitoses.

Day 20 (Fig. 3-18). Occasionally there are subnuclear vacuoles. Acidophilic secretion is prominent in the gland lumen.

Day 21. Beginning stromal effects are evident. Stroma cells have dark, dense nuclei with filamentous cytoplasm. Stromal edema is beginning.

Day 22. Day 22 is the maximum point of stromal edema. Thin-walled spiral arterioles may be seen. Secretion in the gland lumen is active but is subsiding and undergoing inspissation.

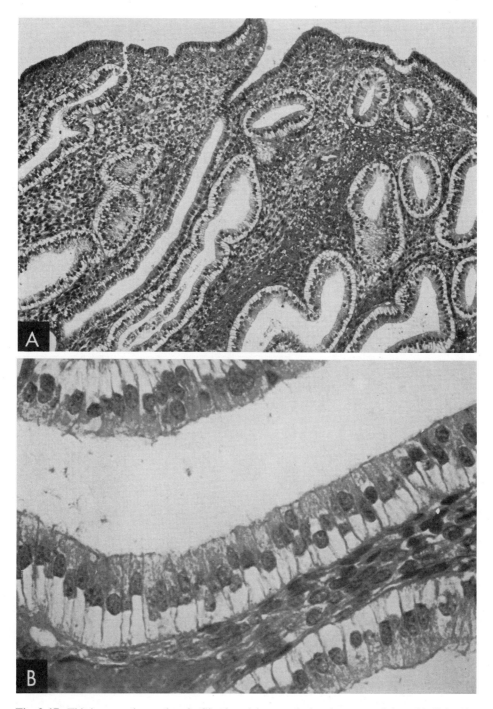

Fig. 3-17. Third postovulatory day. **A,** Gland nuclei are pushed to the center of the epithelial cells with cytoplasm above and vacuoles below them (×150). **B,** Gland mitoses rare; pseudostratification decreasing (×400). (From Noyes RW, Hertig AT, Rock J: Dating the endometrial biopsy. *Fertil Steril* 1950; 1:3.)

Day 23. The edema of stroma persists, but a condensation of the stroma around the spiral arterioles is also characteristic. This is caused by enlargement of the stromal nuclei, with a concomitant increase in the cytoplasm, and it is called the *predecidual change.*

Day 24 (Fig. 3-19). Predecidual collections surrounding arterioles are marked. There are active stromal mitoses, but stromal edema is lessening. The endometrium is now beginning to undergo involution unless it is maintained by pregnancy.

Day 25 (Fig. 3-20). The predecidua is forming beneath the surface epithelium, and there is some edema around the arterioles. Lymphocytic infiltration of the stroma is beginning.

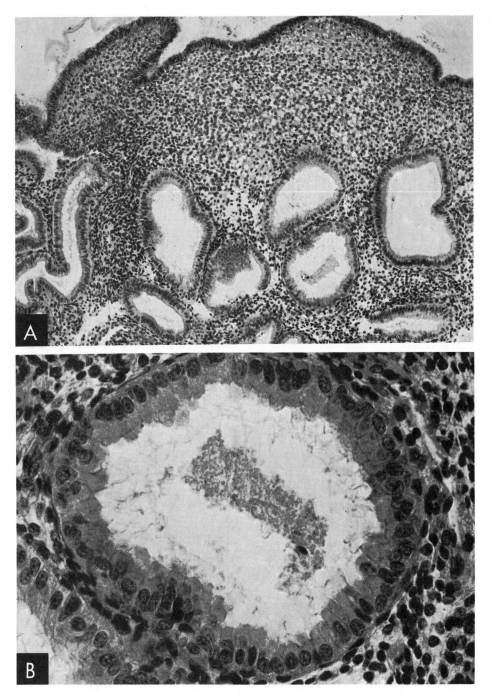

Fig. 3-18. Sixth postovulatory day, corresponding to the beginning of implantation in the fertile cycle. **A,** Secretion in gland lumen at peak; beginning of accumulation of extravascular fluid in stroma (×150). **B,** Subnuclear vacuoles rare; nuclei round and basally located (×400). (From Noyes RW, Hertig AT, Rock J: Dating the endometrial biopsy. *Fertil Steril* 1950; 1:3.)

Day 26. A gradual increase in predecidua is seen throughout the stroma, and there is an infiltration by polymorphonuclear leukocytes.

Day 27. The predecidua is prominent around the blood vessels and under the surface epithelium. There is marked infiltration by polymorphonuclear leukocytes.

Day 28. Focal necrosis of the predecidua is beginning, and there are small areas of stromal hemorrhage. Stromal

cells are clumped together. There is extensive polymorphonuclear leukocytic infiltration. Tortuous glands appear to have undergone secretory "exhaustion."

Certain changes in the glands and stroma may indicate physiologic changes occurring in the endometrium. Thus, *gland mitoses* indicate active proliferation and growth and may be found from day 3 or 4 until day 16 or 17 of the cycle. *Pseudostratification* of the gland nuclei begins after the

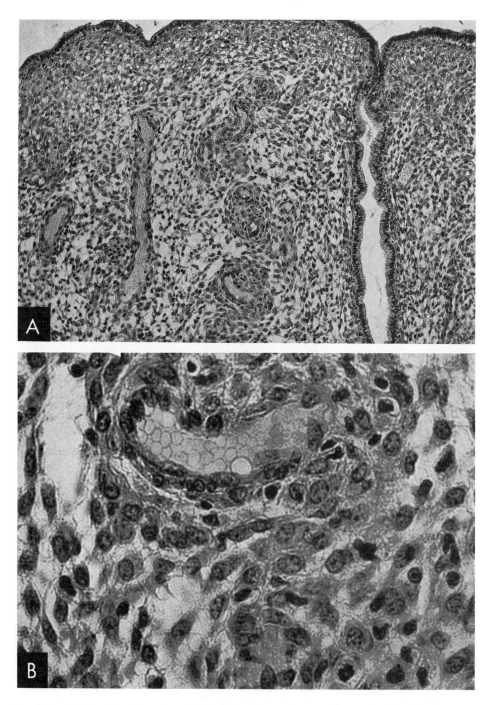

Fig. 3-19. Tenth postovulatory day. **A,** Spiral arterioles and surrounding predecidua still more prominent; extracellular fluid subsiding (×150). **B,** Thickening of periarteriolar predecidual cuff, stromal mitosis evident (×400). (From Noyes RW, Hertig AT, Rock J: Dating the endometrial biopsy. *Fertil Steril* 1950; 1:3.)

postmenstrual revolution and usually disappears by day 17. It is an indication of proliferative glandular growth; its appearance is caused by crowding of the nuclei when the gland is sectioned transversely. *Basal vacuolation* is the earliest morphologic evidence of ovulation that is discernible in the endometrium. Although one vacuole may be seen occasionally in the absence of progesterone, basal vacuoles are usually identified between day 15 and day 19. The glycogen is

pushed into the gland lumen at approximately day 19 or 20. The characteristic lining up of the nuclei above the vacuoles is best seen on day 17, and it is an excellent indication of recent ovulation.

The secretory function of the glands is evident from day 18 until day 22 by the appearance of loose, feathery material in the lumina. If the blastocyst implants itself on the surface of the endometrium approximately 6 days after ovulation,

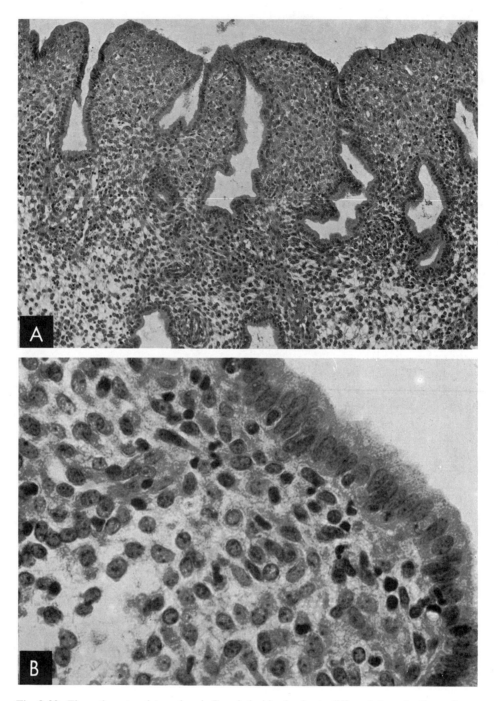

Fig. 3-20. Eleventh postovulatory day. **A,** Pseudodecidua begins to differentiate under the surface epithelium. Stroma of the stratum spongiosum still contains extracellular fluid, except in areas near a spiral arteriole (×150). **B,** Round-cell infiltration accompanies predecidual differentiation. Stromal cells swell to become predecidual (×400). (From Noyes RW, Hertig AT, Rock J: Dating the endometrial biopsy. *Fertil Steril* 1950; 1:3.)

morphology and function are well correlated. Days 20 to 22 are critical from the standpoint of nutrient material. The *edema* of the stroma, most striking between days 22 and 23, may represent an effort by the endometrium to simplify the implantation process by lessening tissue resistance. Periarterial *predecidual reaction* is evident, beginning at approximately days 23 and 24, and may represent a protective mechanism against premature vascular disruption. The predecidua is looked on as providing a supporting framework for newly developed blood vessels to aid in their increased load should pregnancy supervene. These changes in morphologic features are graphically summarized in Figure 3-13.

CLINICAL PEARLS: INTEGRATION OF THE MENSTRUAL CYCLE

The hypothalamus is the conductor that sets the tempo for the menstrual cycle. When the hypothalamus is simultaneously exposed to estrogen and progesterone, GnRH pulse generation is suppressed. Suppression of GnRH pulse generation results in the suppression of pituitary LH and FSH secretion and in the cessation of ovarian follicular development and ovulation. Combined estrogen-progestin contraceptives are effective in suppressing fertility by their actions on the hypothalamus to suppress GnRH and on the pituitary to suppress LH and FSH secretion. Combined estrogen-progestin contraceptives are often prescribed as 21 active pills, followed by 7 days off medication. During the 7 days off medication, hypothalamic GnRH secretion and pituitary LH and FSH secretion increase. If the first pill in a new contraceptive pack is not started on time, the GnRH and LH and FSH secretion can stimulate the development of a dominant follicle that can be ovulated. This makes the first pill of the new contraceptive pack the most important of all the pills. It is important to start the first pill of a new cycle on time to maximize the contraceptive efficacy of oral contraceptives.

More complete suppression of GnRH secretion can be achieved by avoiding the 7 days off medication and prescribing combined estrogen-progestin agents in a continuous fashion. In disease states such as PCOS, in which GnRH pulse generation is abnormally high, suppression of GnRH with continuous combined estrogen-progestin may have clinical importance (Ruchhoft et al, 1996). Continuous administration of oral contraceptives may better suppress GnRH, LH, FSH, and ovarian androgens and may result in better control of hirsutism and acne.

Many women with oligomenorrhea have elevated levels of free testosterone but no clinical evidence of hirsutism or acne. In one study, Allen et al (1997) report that among women with no hirsutism and cycle lengths between 35 and 45 days, most have normal circulating androgens (free testosterone, testosterone, androstenedione, and dehydroepiandrosterone sulfate). However, among women without hirsutism and with cycle lengths greater than 45 days, 40% had at least one elevated circulating androgen (Allen et al, 1997).

Although women with PCOS have elevated LH levels, it is difficult to separate precisely the overlap of LH in women with normal ovulatory cycles and in those with PCOS. This problem results partly from the fact that LH concentrations are dependent on body mass index (BMI). Women with high BMI have lower LH levels (Bohlke et al, 1998) (Fig. 3-21). Because many women with PCOS are obese, their LH levels are similar to those seen in lean women with normal cycles but higher than those seen in obese women with normal cycles. If the LH is adjusted for BMI, the LH concentration of women with PCOS is higher than that seen in women with normal cycles in 95% of cases (Morales et al, 1996; Hoffman et al, 1996).

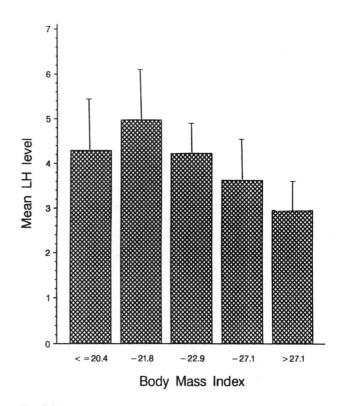

Fig. 3-21. Relationship between body mass index and luteinizing hormone *(LH)* in women with normal menstrual cycles. In obese women, the normal range for LH is lower than that observed in women of normal body mass. (From Bohlke K, Cramer DW, Barbieri RL: The relation of luteinizing hormone levels to body mass index in premenopausal women. *Fertil Steril* 1998; 69: 500-504.)

The endometrium requires exposure to estrogen and then to progesterone to prepare for implantation. Exposure of the endometrium to high concentrations of a synthetic progestin before the proliferative-secretory transition is complete can force the endometrium to advance in its maturation, disrupting its proper preparation for implantation. This physiologic feature is used for postcoital contraception. Women in whom barrier contraception fails (such as when a condom ruptures) or who have been sexually assaulted can be prescribed 100 μg ethinyl estradiol and 1 mg norgestrel immediately, with a repeat dose in 12 hours, to minimize the chance of pregnancy. Norgestrel advances endometrial maturation so that it is out of phase and not conducive to supporting implantation. The failure rate of postcoital contraception is approximately 1%. Human chorionic gonadotropin should be assayed before therapy, and therapy must be instituted within 72 hours of exposure.

In the absence of estrogen stimulation, the endometrium is quiescent and amenorrhea is the rule. For women with severe uterine bleeding in association with medical problems, such as a coagulopathy or severe thrombocytopenia, suppression of estrogen with a GnRH agonist analogue will typically result in amenorrhea and a reduction in transfusion requirements. A less effective alternative is to use estrogen-progestin combination pills in the hope that the progestin component of the pill will keep endometrial growth to a minimum.

Many women have noticed that some diseases seem to be exacerbated at the time of menses. However, the association between a medical condition and menses is often difficult to document. A number of investigators have demonstrated that there is an association between the exacerbation of asthma and the onset of menses in some women. For example, Chandler et al (1997) report that women with asthma have a significant decrease in forced expiratory volume in 1 second (FEV_{-1}) at the time of menses. The administration of exogenous estradiol improved asthma symptom scores and returned FEV_{-1} to normal.

AMENORRHEA
Primary Amenorrhea

Primary amenorrhea is present when the first menses has not appeared by the time a girl is 16 years of age. Primary amenorrhea usually is caused by a genetic or a congenital defect and often is associated with disorders of puberty. Girls who reach 14 years of age and have not had breast development should undergo the same evaluation used for girls with primary amenorrhea.

In a large case series, it was found that the most common causes of primary amenorrhea are gonadal dysgenesis resulting from chromosomal abnormalities, such as 45 X, 45 X/46 XX, and 46 XY (45% of cases); physiologic delay of puberty (20% of cases); müllerian agenesis (15% of cases); transverse vaginal septum or imperforate hymen (5% of cases); absence of hypothalamic GnRH production, such as Kallman syndrome (5% of cases); anorexia nervosa (2% of cases); and hypopituitarism (2% of cases). Less common causes of primary amenorrhea are hyperprolactinemia, hypothyroidism, pituitary tumors, Cushing disease, and craniopharyngioma (1% of cases).

Primary amenorrhea is evaluated efficiently by focusing on the presence or absence of breast development, the presence or absence of the uterus and cervix, and the FSH level. If the FSH level is elevated and there is no breast development, the most likely diagnosis is gonadal dysgenesis. If the FSH is elevated, a karyotype must be obtained to search for a 46 XY karyotype. Gonadal dysgenesis in association with a 46 XY karyotype is associated with a high peripubertal risk for gonadoblastoma and dysgerminoma. In these circumstances, surgical removal of the gonads is necessary. If pelvic ultrasonography shows that the uterus is absent, the probable diagnosis is müllerian agenesis.

Secondary Amenorrhea

Secondary amenorrhea is present when a woman who has been menstruating has not had a period for more than three cycle intervals, or 6 months. A common cause of secondary amenorrhea is pregnancy, and this possibility can be excluded by measuring the circulating hCG. After excluding pregnancy, the most common causes of secondary amenorrhea are hypothalamic dysfunction (35% of cases); pituitary disease (19% of cases); ovarian failure (10% of cases); polycystic ovary disease (30% of cases); and uterine disease (5% of cases). Less common causes of secondary amenorrhea (1% of cases) include adrenal hyperplasia, hypothyroidism, ovarian tumors, and adrenal tumors (Table 3-2, Fig. 3-22).

Secondary amenorrhea caused by hypothalamic dysfunction is usually associated with decreases in GnRH pulse frequency and amplitude caused by low body mass, low body fat, poor nutrition, stress, strenuous exercise, or combinations of all the above. Women with normal cycles who undertake conditioning exercise often have menstrual abnormalities. Those of normal body mass whose lives include stress or poor nutrition can experience anovulation and menstrual abnormalities. A less common cause of secondary amenorrhea is infiltrative diseases of the hypothalamus (lymphoma, histiocytosis). Hypothyroidism occasionally appears as secondary amenorrhea, probably because of changes in GnRH production.

The single most common cause of secondary amenorrhea of pituitary origin is hyperprolactinemia resulting from a prolactinoma (18% of cases). Other pituitary causes of secondary amenorrhea include empty sella syndrome, Sheehan syndrome, and Cushing disease (1% of cases).

Prolactinomas

Many pituitary tumors are monoclonal, indicating that a somatic mutation in a single progenitor cell is the cause of the tumor formation. In one study, 100% of growth hormone (GH)–producing tumors and 75% of adrenocorticotropic hormone–producing tumors were demonstrated to be monoclonal (Herman et al, 1990). In GH-secreting tumors, mutations in the gene that codes for the Gs protein have been reported in 10 of 25 tumors, resulting in the production of a mutant Gs protein that is constituitively activated (Landis and Harsh, 1990). Genetic mutations are the primary cause of pituitary tumors. Factors that change during the reproductive years (for example, estradiol, progesterone, dopamine) are secondary modulators of tumor phenotype. In general, pituitary tumors are benign and slow growing. The discussion below, derived from numerous reviews and previous publications (Barbieri, 1998), focuses on the treatment and evaluation of prolactinomas.

In the initial evaluation of a suspected prolactinoma, it is important to measure circulating prolactin, thyroxine, thyroid hormone–binding globulin uptake, thyrotropin (TSH), and serum IGF-I. A structural study of the hypothalamus and pituitary is useful, and computerized evaluation of the visual fields is necessary if compression of the optic chiasm is suspected. This evaluation excludes occult hypothyroidism (thyroxine, TSH) and acromegaly (IGF-I) as causes of hyperprolactinemia.

Table 3-2 Common Causes of Secondary Amenorrhea (Excluding Pregnancy) and Relative Frequencies

Organ	Cause	Relative Frequency (%)
Hypothalamus	Abnormalities of height/weight and nutrition	15
	Exercise	10
	Stress	10
	Infiltrative disease (craniopharyngioma, sarcoidosis, histiocytosis)	<1
Pituitary	Prolactin-secreting pituitary tumor	18
	Empty sella syndrome	1
	Sheehan syndrome	<1
	ACTH-secreting pituitary tumors (Cushing disease)	<1
Ovary	Premature ovarian failure	10
	Polycystic ovarian disease	30
Uterus	Asherman syndrome	5
Other	Late-onset adrenal hyperplasia	<1
	Hypothyroidism or hyperthyroidism	<1
	Ovarian tumors	<1

ACTH, Adrenocorticotropic hormone.

Women with significant hyperprolactinemia are usually anovulatory and require treatment to ovulate and become pregnant. If a woman with hyperprolactinemia does not want to become pregnant, treatment with estrogen–progestin combinations will reduce the risk for osteoporosis and regulate the menstrual cycle. In women with microprolactinomas, treatment with estrogen–progestin combinations appears to be safe and is associated with few tumor complications, including tumor growth (Corenblum and Donovan, 1993).

For infertile women with significant hyperprolactinemia, treatment is usually required to induce ovulation and achieve pregnancy. Controversy continues as to whether surgery or dopamine agonist treatment is better as a first-line therapy for the infertile woman with hyperprolactinemia; many authorities support the concept that dopamine agonist therapy is better (Thorner, 1997).

The four goals for the treatment of a prolactinoma are to suppress prolactin and induce ovulation, to decrease tumor size, to preserve pituitary reserve, and to prevent recurrence (Barbieri and Ryan, 1983). Treatment with a dopamine agonist is effective in achieving the first three. For example, bromocriptine can normalize prolactin levels, establish regular ovulation, decrease tumor size, and preserve pituitary reserve (McGregor et al, 1979; Molitch et al, 1985). A disadvantage of dopamine agonist treatment is that it is ineffective in preventing tumor recurrence once treatment

is discontinued. Four dopamine agonists—bromocriptine, pergolide, quinagolide, and cabergoline—are effective in the treatment of hyperprolactinemia. Cabergoline is administered once a week and may be more efficacious than bromocriptine in the treatment of microadenomas (Webster et al, 1994). Little information is available concerning the effects of pergolide, quinagolide, and cabergoline on pregnancy. In contrast, substantial experience has accumulated that bromocriptine is safe to use during pregnancy and results in no significant increase in recognizable malformations. In women who conceive using bromocriptine, the rate of congenital abnormalities is no higher than it is in a control group (Raymond et al, 1985). The most common problems with bromocriptine therapy are the side effects of nausea, vomiting, and postural hypotension. These can be minimized by starting treatment at 0.625 mg/day (one quarter of a tablet) and increasing to the target dosage over the course of a few weeks. In some patients, dosages as low as 2.5 mg/day (one tablet) are effective. Prolactin levels can be checked every month for the first 3 months, then every 3 months until the prolactin level returns to normal.

Pituitary tumors are commonly classified by size as microadenomas (<10 mm in diameter) or macroadenomas (>10 mm in diameter). Macroadenomas are sometimes associated with extrasellar extension, local invasion, or compression of the optic chiasm. During pregnancy the clinical manifestations of microadenomas and macroadenomas are

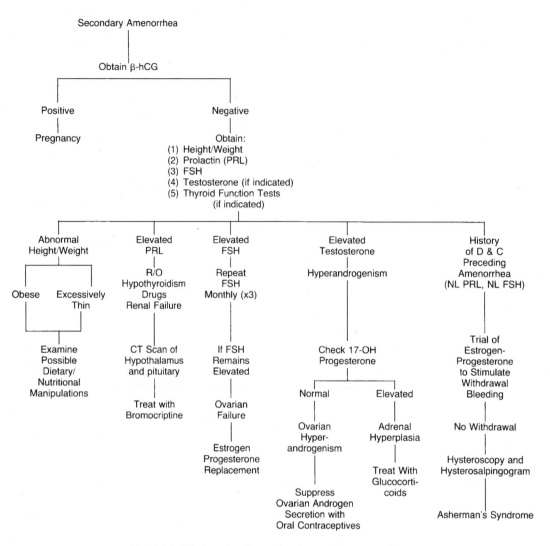

Fig. 3-22. Work-up for diagnosis of secondary amenorrhea.

significantly different from one another. In pregnant women, microadenomas generally are benign, show no evidence of pituitary secretory function loss, and carry a low risk for neurologic complications. For example, of 215 women with microprolactinomas who became pregnant, changes in visual fields, polytomograms, or neurologic signs occurred in less than 1%. Headaches developed in approximately 5% (Barbieri, 1994).

Most women with microprolactinomas have no neurosurgical complications during pregnancy. Bromocriptine can be administered to those in whom neurologic symptoms, such as headache or cranial nerve dysfunction, do develop. Occasionally, neurosurgical intervention is required during pregnancy because of marked tumor enlargement and neurologic sequelae.

In contrast, pituitary insufficiency and neurosurgical complications are common in pregnant women with macroadenomas. Testing for panhypopituitarism should be conducted before dopamine agonist treatment is instituted in women with macroprolactinoma. A study of 60 pregnant

women with macroadenomas (Bergh et al, 1978) revealed that changes in visual fields, polytomograms, or neurologic signs developed in approximately 20%. One approach to treatment for women with macroprolactinomas is to discontinue bromocriptine therapy when they become pregnant and to resume it if symptoms or signs of increasing tumor volume occur. An alternative plan is to continue bromocriptine treatment throughout pregnancy (Konopka et al, 1983; Holmgren et al, 1986).

For infertile women with prolactinomas, some authorities recommend surgical treatment before attempts at pregnancy to reduce the need for dopamine agonist treatment and to decrease the incidence of neurologic complications during pregnancy (Wilson, 1997). However, microsurgical resection of a prolactinoma can result in death (0.3% of patients) or in serious morbidity, such as a cerebrospinal fluid leak (0.4% of patients). Surgery is successful in producing a long-term cure in only 60% of patients. Breast-feeding does not worsen the clinical course of prolactinomas and can be encouraged (Molitch, 1985).

Empty Sella Syndrome

The roof of the pituitary gland (the diaphragm sella) is perforated by the pituitary stalk, which connects the hypothalamic median eminence to the pituitary. If the perforation in the diaphragm sella is excessively large, the pia mater and accompanying cerebrospinal fluid can herniate into the pituitary fossa. Herniation of this fluid, which is under reasonably high pressure, can produce compression atrophy of the pituitary gland that results in hypopituitarism and amenorrhea. The empty sella syndrome can be documented by high-resolution magnetic resonance imaging or computed tomography of the pituitary. Therapy is directed to the specific replacement of documented hormonal abnormalities.

Sheehan Syndrome

Sheehan syndrome is the onset of hypothalamic and pituitary dysfunction after severe obstetric hemorrhage and maternal hypotension at delivery. During pregnancy the pituitary volume increases by approximately 100%. The increase in pituitary size and the low-flow, low-pressure nature of the portal circulation may make the pituitary and parts of the hypothalamus susceptible to ischemia brought on by obstetric hemorrhage and hypotension. In developing countries, the risk for obstetric hemorrhage resulting in significant hypotension is much greater than it is in the developed world. Consequently, the majority of cases of Sheehan syndrome occur in developing countries. World wide, Sheehan syndrome is the most common cause of hypopituitarism.

In Sheehan syndrome, every imaginable pattern of pituitary hormone deficiency can be observed. Growth hormone and prolactin deficiencies are the usual manifestations. In a study of 10 African women with Sheehan syndrome, Jialal et al (1984) reported the pituitary hormone response to a combination intravenous insulin (0.1 U/kg), TRH (200 μg), and GnRH (100 μg) challenge test. The pattern of pituitary hormone response revealed the following loss of secretory reserve: 100% of the women had prolactin and GH deficiencies, 90% had cortisol deficiency, 80% had TSH deficiency, 70% had LH deficiency, and 40% had FSH deficiency. These pituitary abnormalities cause failure of lactation, failure of hair growth over areas shaved for delivery, poor wound healing after cesarean section, and muscle weakness.

The best single test to diagnose Sheehan syndrome is to administer TRH 100 μg intravenously and to take prolactin measurements at 0 and 30 minutes. The ratio of prolactin at 30 minutes to prolactin before the TRH injection (time 0) should be >3 (Barbieri et al, 1985). If the ratio is subnormal, the patient should undergo a complete evaluation for panhypopituitarism.

Loss of anterior pituitary hormone reserve is the most common indicator of Sheehan syndrome. Mild hypothalamic and posterior pituitary dysfunction occur frequently in women with Sheehan syndrome. Sheehan and Whitehead (1965) reported that at autopsy, 90% of women with postpartum hypopituitarism demonstrated "atrophy and scarring" of the neurohypophysis. Whitehead (1965) performed detailed studies on the hypothalamus of 13 patients and observed atrophy of the supraoptic and paraventricular nuclei. Clinical studies demonstrate that most women with Sheehan syndrome have mild defects in vasopressin secretion and maximal urinary concentration capability (Bakiri et al, 1984; Bakiri and Benmiloud, 1984).

Ovarian Causes of Secondary Amenorrhea

Ovarian failure (10% of patients) and polycystic ovary syndrome (30% of patients) can cause secondary amenorrhea. Women with PCOS often have hirsutism or acne. PCOS is reviewed in Chapter 15.

Loss of all ovarian follicles results in the cessation of normal ovarian cyclicity (ovarian failure). Ovarian failure before age 40 is termed premature ovarian failure. Loss of all ovarian follicles results in a marked increase in the serum FSH level secondary to a loss of both estrogen and inhibin-feedback inhibition of FSH. Therefore, ovarian failure is most accurately diagnosed after measuring a patient's serum FSH level. In women with complete ovarian failure, the FSH level will usually be greater than 25 mIU/mL. In women with incipient ovarian failure, the FSH levels can fluctuate markedly between 15 and 25 mIU/mL. Measurements of FSH and estradiol levels during menses for 3 months will often assist the physician in gauging the permanency of the ovarian failure.

One cause of premature ovarian failure is genetic abnormality in the sex chromosomes. Although most of these patients have ovarian failure before puberty, some will have a few years of normal menstrual function and then cease to menstruate. Therefore, any woman with ovarian failure before age 30 should be screened for chromosomal abnormalities by karyotyping or by polymerase chain reaction screening for Y-chromosome elements.

Ovarian failure can also be the result of autoimmune processes. Antiovarian antibodies and ovarian failure can develop in women with polyglandular autoimmune endocrine disease (hypoparathyroidism, Addison disease, hypothyroidism, diabetes mellitus). One of the best-studied examples of autoimmune ovarian failure occurs in women with myasthenia gravis. Myasthenia gravis produces anti-acetylcholine receptor antibodies, which results in neuromotor abnormalities, and anti-FSH receptor antibodies, which results in accelerated loss of developing follicles. This accelerated follicular destruction leads to premature ovarian failure.

Ovarian failure can be caused by chemotherapy (especially alkylating agents such as cyclophosphamide), radiotherapy (as little as 500 cGy to the ovaries), wedge biopsy of the ovaries, and infections (Koyama, 1977).

There is no specific therapy for ovarian failure. Women with premature ovarian failure are at a high risk for osteoporosis and cardiovascular disease caused by hypoestrogenism; estrogen replacement therapy should be offered unless specific contraindications exist. Advances in assisted-reproduction technologies have made it possible for women with ovarian failure to become pregnant through a procedure using donor eggs and in vitro fertilization. A donor egg is fertilized with sperm from the partner of the woman with ovarian failure, who is treated with estrogen and progesterone to prime the uterus to receive the developing embryo. The availability and success of donor egg programs suggest that in young women, a conservative approach should be taken toward the removal of a normal uterus at the time of oophorectomy for an adnexal abnormality. For a full discussion of the benefits of hormone replacement therapy, see Chapter 21.

Uterine Causes

Asherman Syndrome. Asherman syndrome is the presence of intrauterine scar tissue that interferes with normal endometrial growth and shedding. In women with this condition, intrauterine scar tissue usually develops after vigorous curettage of the infected endometrium early in the pregnancy. The patient's history is an important clue to the presence of Asherman syndrome. A commonly used endocrine manipulation to test for its presence is to prescribe 2.5 mg conjugated estrogens daily for 35 days and medroxyprogesterone for the last 10 of those days (days 26 to 35). If there is no withdrawal bleed after such a challenge, it strongly suggests the presence of Asherman syndrome. The diagnosis can be confirmed by a radiologic test (hysterosalpingogram) or by direct visualization of the scar tissue (hysteroscopy).

The typical treatment of Asherman syndrome involves surgical lysis of the intrauterine adhesions (with hysteroscopy), followed by long-term stimulation of the endometrium with estrogen. In some women who become pregnant after therapy for Asherman syndrome, placentation defects such as placenta accreta develop.

Laboratory Evaluation of Secondary Amenorrhea

The goal of laboratory evaluation for secondary amenorrhea is to ensure that no serious disease process, such as hypothalamic or pituitary tumor or premature ovarian failure, is causing it. The initial step in this process is to exclude the possibility of pregnancy. At times this can be accomplished through patient history and physical examination, but a measurement of the serum or urine hCG level is a more sensitive and specific method of ruling out pregnancy. Serum prolactin and FSH levels are usually measured in women with amenorrhea. An elevated serum prolactin level can have multiple causes (pregnancy, tumor, pituitary tumor, hypothyroidism, renal failure, psychoactive drugs), each of which requires additional evaluation. An elevated FSH level suggests the presence of ovarian failure. Some authorities recommend a progestin withdrawal test to diagnose ovarian failure. In the authors' opinion, the sensitivity (less than 50%) and specificity (less than 50%) of the progestin withdrawal test for the diagnosis of ovarian failure are poor, and it is not recommended for this purpose (Rebar and Connolly, 1990).

Two tools that may be of value in the diagnosis of secondary amenorrhea are serum testosterone and thyroid function tests. Occasionally, women with ovarian androgen overproduction have amenorrhea. Usually signs such as hirsutism and acne point to this diagnosis. Oligomenorrhea or amenorrhea sometimes develop in women with hypothyroidism or hyperthyroidism. A good screening tool for thyroid disease is a plasma TSH test because it screens for hyperthyroidism and hypothyroidism.

Although the progestin withdrawal test is of little value in diagnosing ovarian failure, it can be of value in evaluating hypothalamic-pituitary function among patients with secondary amenorrhea. The test consists of administering progestin and monitoring uterine bleeding in the week after the progestin challenge. Before administration of the test, pregnancy must be excluded. Progestin can be administered orally (medroxyprogesterone acetate, 10 mg/day for 5 days) or parenterally (100 mg progesterone in oil). Bleeding in the week after the progestin challenge is a sign that significant endogenous estrogen production is present and, hence, that the uterus is normal. Absence of bleeding in the week after the progestin challenge suggests very low endogenous estrogen production or Asherman syndrome. Low endogenous estrogen production is usually caused by severe hypothalamic-pituitary dysfunction with little GnRH, LH, or FSH output. Women with amenorrhea and abnormal progestin withdrawal test results must be evaluated carefully and followed up closely. Occasionally, they may have large hypothalamic or pituitary tumors that are endocrinologically silent, so many clinicians suggest they undergo structural study of the hypothalamus and pituitary.

ABNORMAL AND EXCESSIVE UTERINE BLEEDING

Abnormal uterine bleeding is one of the most common clinical problems in gynecology. Uterine bleeding is abnormal if the bleeding pattern is *irregular*. This is defined as polymenorrhea (less than 22 days between cycles); oligomenorrhea (more than 35 days between cycles); hypermenorrhea or abnormal *duration* (more than 7 days of bleeding); or menorrhagia or abnormal *amount* (more than 80 mL blood loss during menses). Menometrorrhagia is an all-encompassing term used to describe irregular or excessive bleeding, or both, during menstruation or between menstrual cycles.

Abnormal uterine bleeding can have myriad causes, among them pregnancy (including spontaneous abortion, ectopic pregnancy, gestational trophoblastic disease); tumors of the uterus (benign and malignant); infection (endometritis); hormonal abnormalities (anovulation and estrogen therapy); intrauterine foreign bodies (intrauterine device); and coagulopathies (Box 3-1). The differential diagnosis of abnormal uterine bleeding is complex, but a systematic approach to the patient with uterine bleeding usually results in the diagnosis of a treatable disease process.

The endometrium is a remarkably dynamic tissue. During the follicular phase of the menstrual cycle, under the stimulation of estrogen, the endometrium grows from 0.5 to 3.5 mm in thickness. Histologically, this growth is marked by many *mitoses* in the endometrial glands (proliferative phase). During the luteal phase of the menstrual cycle, the production of large amounts (25 mg/day) of progesterone by the corpus luteum causes the endometrium to stop growing and to differentiate in preparation for the implantation of an embryo (secretory phase). At the end of the menstrual cycle, the programmed demise of the corpus luteum results in the withdrawal of progesterone and estrogen and the sloughing of the endometrium with menstrual bleeding.

The initiation and termination of normal menstrual bleeding requires the orderly interaction of hormonal and structural events. The luteal-phase endometrium consists of three zones: basalis, stratum spongiosum, and stratum compactum. The inferior-most zone is the basalis, which connects the base of the endometrium to the myometrium. The basalis is the source of endometrial regeneration after menstrual sloughing. The stratum spongiosum is the middle zone of the endometrium. In the luteal phase, the stratum spongiosum is the largest zone and represents 50% of total endometrial thickness. The most impressive histologic feature of the stratum spongiosum is the presence of spiral or coiled arteries. These spiral arteries are vasoactive. Just before the onset of menstruation, decreases in estrogen and progesterone levels and increases in prostaglandin levels cause the spiral arteries to undergo intense vasoconstriction. The vasospasm in the spiral arteries causes ischemia in the upper zones of the endometrium and initiates menstrual sloughing of the endometrium. The superficial layer of the endometrium is the stratum compactum. The strata spongiosum and compactum comprise the "functional" zones of the endometrium, which participate in the cyclic process of menstruation.

The mechanisms by which pregnancy or tumors of the uterus cause abnormal uterine bleeding are easily understood. Implantation of the embryo involves invasion of the trophoblast into the endometrium and parasitization of the maternal blood supply. If the pregnancy degenerates, the maternal blood supply becomes directly exposed to the uterine cavity and bleeding ensues. Tumors of the uterus can cause abnormal bleeding by disrupting the normally continuous endometrial surface. Discontinuity in the endometrial surface results in bleeding. Endometritis produces abnormal uterine bleeding by disrupting the continuity of endometrial glands and blood vessels. The first step in the normal process of clotting is the formation of a platelet plug. Any disease that interferes with the formation of a platelet plug (von Willebrand disease or thrombocytopenia) can have as a symptom abnormal uterine bleeding. The hormonal abnormality that is the most common cause of abnormal uterine bleeding is anovulation. Long-term exposure of the endometrium to estrogen, without the stabilizing effects of progesterone, produces a fragile endometrial surface that is prone to bleeding.

BOX 3-1
DIFFERENTIAL DIAGNOSIS OF ABNORMAL UTERINE BLEEDING

I. Pregnancy
 • Spontaneous abortion
 • Ectopic pregnancy
 • Gestational trophoblastic disease
II. Tumors of the uterus
 • Benign
  1. Cervical polyps
  2. Endometrial polyps
  3. Fibroids
 • Malignant
  4. Cervical cancer
  5. Endometrial cancer
  6. Fallopian tube cancer
III. Infection
 • Endometritis
 • Cervicitis
IV. Hormonal abnormalities
 • Endogenous (anovulation, dysfunctional uterine bleeding)
 • Exogenous (hormone administration, e.g., estrogen)
V. Intrauterine foreign body (e.g., intrauterine device)
VI. Coagulopathies
 • Platelet disorders
 • Clotting factor abnormalities

Diagnostic Evaluation

History taking should record the temporal pattern, the duration, and the amount of bleeding. Patients should be asked about contraceptive and sexual practices and the use of hormonal medication. If the patient has had bleeding during previous surgery and a family history of abnormal bleeding, this requires discussion. The main focus of the physical examination is to determine intravascular volume status (orthostatic hypotension, tachycardia). Careful pelvic examination assesses whether the bleeding is vaginal or uterine, provides a thorough evaluation of uterine size, and indicates whether the uterus is enlarged, irregular, or tender. Examination of the skin for ecchymoses or petechiae may provide evidence of underlying coagulopathy.

Laboratory evaluation of abnormal uterine bleeding should include a complete blood cell (CBC) count, a Papanicolaou smear, a sensitive blood pregnancy test (b-hCG), and a biopsy specimen from the endometrium, if necessary. The CBC provides evidence for the diagnosis of anemia or thrombocytopenia. The Papanicolaou smear provides evidence for the presence of cervical cancer and, in some instances, endometrial cancer. A normal β-hCG test result rules out pregnancy. The endometrial biopsy specimen provides for a direct evaluation of endometrial histology (endometrial cancer, hyperplasia, endometritis). Results of these four tests, combined with a complete history and physical examination, lead to the diagnosis of treatable disease in most women with abnormal uterine bleeding.

If the case is complex or resistant to initial treatment, transvaginal sonography and hysteroscopy can be helpful in contributing to the management of abnormal uterine bleeding. In a recent study (Langer et al, 1997) of the value of transvaginal sonography in identifying endometrial abnormalities in menopausal women, it was determined to be a sensitive, though not a specific, test for identifying serious endometrial lesions. Transvaginal sonography has revealed that endometrial thickness less than 5 mm in diameter is almost never associated with endometrial disease. Although endometrial thickness in most patients with endometrial disease is greater than 5 mm, many women on estrogen therapy who are disease free also have endometriums that are greater than 5 mm thick.

An important advantage of transvaginal sonography is that it can identify lesions of the uterus (leiomyomata, endometrial polyps, adenomyosis) and the ovary (ovarian tumors) that cannot be identified by endometrial biopsy (Dubinsky et al, 1997). An advanced technique, saline infusion uterine sonography, may increase the sensitivity and specificity of transvaginal sonography and is best performed during the proliferative (follicular) phase of the menstrual cycle. The appearance of the proliferative phase ensures that pregnancy has not occurred and minimizes the sonography signature of the normal endometrium. The uterus is cannulated, and sterile saline or a solution of 1.5% glycine is infused at a rate of 5 to 30 mL/min. Polyps and other intracavitary lesions are well outlined by the anechoic saline.

Office hysteroscopy is an alternative method of directly visualizing the endometrial cavity. In one direct comparison of office hysteroscopy versus transvaginal sonography for the evaluation of abnormal uterine bleeding, it is reported (Towbin et al, 1996) that transvaginal sonography is specific (90%) but not sensitive (54%), whereas office hysteroscopy is sensitive (79%) and specific (93%). In another study (Widrich et al, 1996) of the usefulness of office hysteroscopy versus saline infusion sonography, it is reported that both methods are specific and sensitive in diagnosing lesions that cause abnormal uterine bleeding. These studies suggest that office hysteroscopy and saline infusion sonography are the two best methods for evaluating abnormal uterine bleeding.

Hormonal Abnormalities that Cause Abnormal Uterine Bleeding

Normal cyclic uterine bleeding requires the sequential appearance of estrogen alone, which promotes endometrial growth, followed by progesterone, which causes differentiation of the endometrium. As noted earlier, the cessation of estrogen and progesterone secretion (demise of the corpus luteum) initiates menstrual sloughing of the endometrium. The key factors that ensure normal menstrual cyclicity are the sequence of estrogen stimulation of the endometrium followed by progesterone-induced differentiation. Processes that interfere with this normal sequence often result in abnormal uterine bleeding. The most common process that interferes with this normal sequence is constant estrogen stimulation in the absence of cyclic progesterone exposure. This can occur because of endogenous hormonal abnormalities (anovulation) or exogenous administration of estrogen.

Dysfunctional uterine bleeding is the term used to describe abnormal bleeding caused by hormonal abnormalities in the absence of pregnancy, tumor, infection, or coagulopathy. Dysfunctional uterine bleeding is often associated with anovulation and continuous ovarian estrogen production. In elite women athletes, anovulation and amenorrhea often develop, and low levels of GnRH result in little ovarian estrogen production. Although many of these women are anovulatory, abnormal uterine bleeding does not develop because their estrogen levels are too low to stimulate endometrial growth. In contrast, some women with polycystic ovary syndrome produce significant amounts of continuous ovarian estrogen, but they are anovulatory and do not produce progesterone. These women have a high risk for dysfunctional uterine bleeding. In summary, dysfunctional uterine bleeding occurs most often in anovulatory women in whom significant amounts of ovarian estrogen are produced. Dysfunctional uterine bleeding usually does not develop in anovulatory women in whom ovarian estrogen is not produced.

Continuous ovarian estrogen production associated with anovulation occurs and is diagnosed most commonly in adolescent and perimenopausal women. In adolescents, the hypothalamus begins to secrete GnRH once a critical body mass (weight) is achieved. The GnRH secretion stimulates LH and FSH secretion, which causes an increase in ovarian estrogen production, but ovulation may not occur. Continuous estrogen exposure results in endometrial growth. The absence of ovulation and progesterone exposure prevents the proper maturation of the endometrium and may result in abnormal uterine bleeding. In adolescents who are not pregnant, abnormal uterine bleeding is almost always the result of a hormonal abnormality (anovulation) or coagulopathy.

As it does in adolescents, dysfunctional uterine bleeding develops in perimenopausal women because of the continuous exposure to estrogen without similar exposure to progesterone. In perimenopausal women, the ovary becomes depleted of healthy follicles and oocytes. Because of the low number of follicles in the ovary, FSH levels become abnormally elevated. This stimulates estrogen production from the few remaining ovarian follicles. These "aged" follicles are often unable to grow to a size that initiates ovulation. The hormonal milieu is characterized by continuous estrogen unopposed by progesterone. Frequently, endometrial cancer or endometrial hyperplasia is the cause of uterine bleeding in perimenopausal women. Therefore, all perimenopausal women with abnormal uterine bleeding must have an endometrial biopsy specimen taken. They should not be treated with hormones until endometrial biopsy results are available.

Long-term exposure to estrogen unopposed by progesterone is associated with a high risk for dysfunctional uterine bleeding. In most women, the ovary is the major source of estrogen production. However, estrogen can also be produced in fat tissue by the extraovarian aromatization of androstenedione to estrone. In markedly obese women, the excess adipose tissue results in abnormally increased extraovarian estrogen production. Because obesity is also associated with anovulation, obese women are at high risk for abnormal uterine bleeding.

Before making a diagnosis of dysfunctional uterine bleeding in the three groups of women at greatest risk for it (adolescents, perimenopausal women, obese women), the clinician must be sure that pregnancy, tumor, and infection are not the cause of bleeding. If long-term estrogen exposure unopposed by progesterone is the cause of bleeding, therapy is directed to the replacement of adequate amounts of progesterone. The method of progesterone replacement used to treat dysfunctional uterine bleeding depends on the patient's clinical condition. For the adolescent, oral contraceptives provide an excellent means of replacing progesterone deficiency. For the perimenopausal woman, the administration of an oral progestogen for 10 to 14 days each month helps regulate endometrial cyclicity. Many different oral progestins can be used for this purpose. One of the most common is medroxyprogesterone acetate (10 mg/day for 10 to 14 days each month).

For the woman with anovulation and dysfunctional uterine bleeding who desires fertility, ovulation induction with clomiphene citrate or gonadotropins will cause ovulation, endogenous progesterone production, and possibly pregnancy. Many forms of progesterone replacement are available. The oral administration of "natural" progesterone results in low levels of progesterone in the blood because of intestinal and hepatic metabolism. However, natural progesterone can be given intramuscularly (100 mg each month) or intravaginally (25 mg 3 times daily for 10 days each month). The expense of progesterone vaginal suppositories limits the practicality of this dosage form.

Many synthetic progestins that are well absorbed through the oral route have been produced. Medroxyprogesterone acetate and megestrol acetate are two synthetic progestins that are structurally similar to progesterone (Fig. 3-23, A and B). Typically, medroxyprogesterone is administered at a dose of 10 or 20 mg daily for 10 to 14 days. This duration of therapy is recommended because courses of progestin therapy shorter than 10 days can fail to prevent the appearance of endometrial hyperplasia. Courses of progestin therapy are repeated every month or every other month until the patient begins to ovulate spontaneously.

Norethindrone, norethindrone acetate, and norgestrel are three synthetic progestins that are structurally similar to progesterone and testosterone (Fig. 3-23, C and D). Because of the structural similarities among norethindrone, norethindrone acetate, norgestrel, and testosterone, the three synthetic progestins have androgenic actions. All three lower

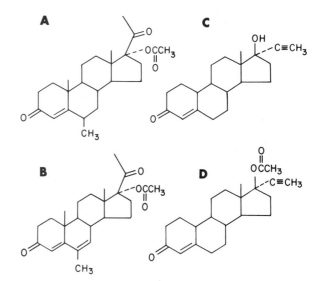

Fig. 3-23. Chemical structures. **A,** Medroxyprogesterone acetate. **B,** Megestrol acetate. **C,** Norethindrone. **D,** Norethindrone acetate.

HDL levels at dosages commonly used. Decreased HDL levels may be associated with an increased risk for atherosclerosis. In general, medroxyprogesterone acetate and megestrol acetate are the preferred agents for the treatment of abnormal uterine bleeding. If norethindrone acetate is used in the treatment of dysfunctional uterine bleeding, it is usually prescribed at a dosage of 5 mg/day for 10 to 14 days.

Occasionally, abnormal uterine bleeding is caused by the administration of hormones. The long-term administration of exogenous estrogen often results in abnormal uterine bleeding (long-term estrogen unopposed by progesterone). This clinical occurrence is so widely known that it is unusual to find a woman with an intact uterus treated with unopposed estrogen. Approximately 20% of women receiving danazol, an attenuated androgen, have irregular uterine bleeding. In these women, endometrial biopsy specimens usually demonstrate atrophic endometrium.

An unusual endocrine cause of dysfunctional uterine bleeding is hyperthyroidism or hypothyroidism. Women with dysfunctional uterine bleeding who do not respond to the standard therapy should be screened for thyroid disease through detailed history, physical examination, and thyroid function tests.

Abnormal Uterine Bleeding Caused by Infection

Infections of the endometrium are characterized grossly by hyperemia and microscopically by edema and white blood cell infiltration. Disruption of vascular integrity by the infection can result in abnormal uterine bleeding. Bleeding caused by endometritis is usually characterized by intermittent spotting, not severe hemorrhage.

When compared with the fallopian tube, the endometrium is relatively resistant to infection. Incomplete spontaneous or therapeutic abortion can cause endometrial infection from *Escherichia coli*, *Pseudomonas aeruginosa*,

Enterococcus spp., and *Bacteroides* spp. These infections are best treated by broad-spectrum antibiotic therapy and by dilatation and curettage. Endometritis not associated with a recent pregnancy may be caused by *Chlamydia* spp. or *Mycoplasma* spp. Patients with infection can be treated with tetracycline (250 mg orally 4 times daily for 3 weeks) or doxycycline (100 mg orally 2 times daily for 2 to 3 weeks).

Abnormal Uterine Bleeding Caused by Coagulopathies

The initial step in clot formation is the formation of a platelet plug. Diseases that inhibit platelet aggregation or decrease platelet number may be associated with abnormal uterine bleeding. Thrombocytopenia can be caused by a variety of diseases, including acute and chronic leukemia, lymphoma, and idiopathic thrombocytopenic purpura. The most common cause of thrombocytopenia is treatment with high-dose chemotherapeutic agents such as cyclophosphamide. Von Willebrand disease is a disorder of platelet aggregation and clot formation caused by an abnormal factor VIII. Abnormal uterine bleeding caused by coagulopathies is best treated by correcting the underlying abnormality. Too often, however, this is not possible.

An alternative approach to treat thrombocytopenia is to produce a quiescent endometrium that does not undergo menstrual cycles and will not undergo withdrawal bleeding. This can be accomplished by long-term GnRH agonist therapy or with combined estrogen-progestogen oral contraceptives. The GnRH agonists produce paradoxic inhibition (downregulation) of pituitary gonadotropin production and cause the cessation of ovarian estrogen production. In a hypoestrogenic environment, the endometrium becomes inactive. Another approach is to use combined estrogen-progestin oral contraceptives to prevent menstrual bleeding during an episode of thrombocytopenia. This approach is of special benefit to women administered cyclic courses of chemotherapeutic agents, such as cyclophosphamide, because the oral contraceptives prevent menstrual bleeding during the thrombocytopenic episodes that follow chemotherapy. After the thrombocytopenic episode, the oral contraceptives are stopped and a "normal" withdrawal bleed is initiated.

Treatment of Life-Threatening Uterine Bleeding

Occasionally, women come to the emergency room of a hospital with life-threatening vaginal bleeding. Rapid evaluation and therapy are required to minimize morbidity and mortality. Initial evaluation should include CBC; coagulation studies (prothrombin time, partial thromboplastin time); rapid, sensitive pregnancy testing; and, if indicated, endometrial curettage. Coagulopathies require correction with the appropriate replacement products (platelets or fresh frozen plasma). If the physical examination or ultrasonography shows the uterus to be structurally normal, if the pregnancy test result is negative, and if the dilatation and curettage does not slow bleeding, aggressive hormonal therapy may be required. Conjugated estrogens (25 mg intravenously every 4 hours for 3 doses) have been successful in the treatment of life-threatening uterine hemorrhage that is not caused by pregnancy or tumor. Alternatively, large dosages of a combined estrogen-progestin medication may be used. For example, 0.05 mg ethinyl estradiol plus 0.5 mg of norgestrel (Ovral) given 4 times daily for up to 7 days may slow the bleeding. In severe cases of uterine bleeding in which conventional therapy has failed, angiographic embolization of the uterine arteries may help control the bleeding. In some patients, hysterectomy may be required to treat an episode of life-threatening uterine bleeding.

DYSMENORRHEA

Dysmenorrhea, or painful menstruation, is one of the most common gynecologic problems. Approximately 50% of all women experience dysmenorrhea, and approximately 1% of women of reproductive age are incapacitated for 1 to 3 days each month because of severe dysmenorrhea. For clinical purposes, dysmenorrhea is often divided into two broad categories: primary and secondary. Primary dysmenorrhea is the presence of painful menstruation in the absence of demonstrable pelvic disease. Secondary dysmenorrhea is the occurrence of painful menstruation caused by pelvic disease, such as endometriosis, chronic pelvic inflammatory disease, or uterine leiomyomata. It is often difficult to differentiate between primary and secondary dysmenorrhea from the history and physical examination. Trials of empirical drug therapy and diagnostic laparoscopy are often necessary to discover the cause.

In primary dysmenorrhea, the pain characteristically begins with the onset of menstruation and lasts for 12 to 72 hours. Usually confined to the lower abdomen, the pain, described as cramps that are intermittently intense, is most intense in the midline. In some women, back pain and thigh pain may be severe. Oftentimes nausea, diarrhea, fatigue, headache, and a general sense of malaise accompany the abdominal pain. Pain is usually most severe on the first day of menstruation and gradually diminishes.

Evidence suggests that prostaglandin F_{2a} (PGF_{2a}) and prostaglandin E_2 (PGE_2), released from the endometrium at the time of menstruation, cause primary dysmenorrhea (Ylikorkala and Dawood, 1978). Prostaglandin F_{2a} and PGE_2 are derivatives of the fatty acid arachidonic acid. The sequential stimulation of the endometrium by estrogen and then by progesterone results in a dramatic increase in prostaglandin production by the endometrium. During menstruation the endometrial cells undergo lysis and release PGF_{2a} and PGE_2. Prostaglandins induce smooth muscle contraction (or relaxation) in many diverse tissues. Uterine smooth muscle contractions induced by the prostaglandins produce the colicky, spasmodic, laborlike lower abdominal and back pain characteristic of dysmenorrhea. Prostaglandin-induced uterine contractions can last many minutes and may produce intrauterine pressures greater than 60 mm Hg. When uterine pressure exceeds mean arterial pressure for a prolonged period of time, uterine ischemia ensues. Uterine ischemia results in the accu-

Table 3-3   Inhibitors of Prostaglandin Synthesis Commonly Used in the Treatment of Dysmenorrhea

Drug Class	Drug	Standard Dosage
Fenamates	Mefenamic acid	500-mg loading dose; 250 mg 4 times daily
	Flufenamic acid	100 to 200 mg 3 times daily
	Tolfenamic acid	133 mg 3 times daily
Phenylpropionic acid	Ibuprofen	400 mg 4 times daily
	Naproxen sodium	550-mg loading dose; 275 mg 4 times daily
	Ketoprofen	50 mg 3 times daily

mulation of anaerobic metabolites that can stimulate the small type-C pain neurons. In many ways, primary dysmenorrhea is like "angina" of the uterus.

The hypothesis that prostaglandins released from the endometrium cause primary dysmenorrhea is supported by the observation that endometrial concentrations of PGE_2 and PGF_{2a} correlate with the severity of dysmenorrhea. In general, women with the highest endometrial concentrations of PGF_{2a} and PGE_2 have the most severe dysmenorrhea (Chan et al, 1979).

Many factors can modulate prostaglandin-induced uterine contractions. For example, strenuous exercise can increase uterine tone (possibly because of decreased uterine blood flow). Many women athletes note that strenuous exercise at the time of menstruation increases the severity of their dysmenorrhea. Other women report that caffeine ingestion can decrease the severity of dysmenorrhea. Caffeine may increase uterine cyclic adenosine monophosphate levels that result in decreased uterine tone. In addition to stimulating uterine contractions, PGF_{2a} and PGE_2 can cause contraction of bronchial, bowel, and vascular smooth muscle that produces bronchoconstriction (asthma), diarrhea, and hypertension. As noted earlier, diarrhea is commonly associated with primary dysmenorrhea.

High rates of endometrial prostaglandin production require the sequential stimulation of the endometrium by estrogen and then by progesterone. Usually women who menstruate without ovulating (hence, there is no progesterone) do not have primary dysmenorrhea. In most girls the menses that immediately follow menarche (approximate age, 12 years) are often anovulatory because of the immaturity of the hypothalamic-pituitary axis. Because regular ovulatory cycles may not begin until 2 to 5 years after menarche, in many adolescents primary dysmenorrhea begins a few years after menarche.

Secondary dysmenorrhea is the occurrence of painful menstruation caused by pelvic abnormalities, such as endometriosis or chronic pelvic inflammatory disease. The major goal of the clinical evaluation of dysmenorrhea is to identify whether the process is primary or secondary. Although it is difficult to differentiate between primary and secondary dysmenorrhea based on history and physical examination, many women with secondary dysmenorrhea re-

port that the dysmenorrhea began after age 20, often lasts for 5 to 7 days each month, and has increased in severity over time. In addition, women with secondary dysmenorrhea usually report pelvic pain at times other than menses. By definition, women with primary dysmenorrhea have normal pelvic examination results. Women with secondary dysmenorrhea may also have normal pelvic examination results if the pelvic abnormality cannot be palpated (stage I endometriosis, adenomyosis, pelvic adhesions). Some women with secondary dysmenorrhea have markedly abnormal pelvic examination results. In those patients, appropriate clinical action (ultrasonography, diagnostic laparoscopy, exploratory laparotomy) should be immediately undertaken. For example, a woman with dysmenorrhea and a pelvic examination suggestive of severe endometriosis (cul-de-sac induration, uterosacral ligament modularity, adnexal masses) should be scheduled for laparoscopy to confirm the diagnosis. In the evaluation of a woman with dysmenorrhea, pelvic ultrasonography may help to identify uterine (fibroid) or adnexal masses (hydrosalpinx) that cannot be palpated on pelvic examination. In women with secondary dysmenorrhea, a CBC and an erythrocyte sedimentation rate (ESR) may raise the suspicion of chronic pelvic inflammatory disease (high white blood cell count and high ESR).

Dysmenorrhea in a woman who has a history of primary dysmenorrhea and normal pelvic examination results is treated as primary dysmenorrhea. If aggressive therapy for primary dysmenorrhea fails to relieve the pain, additional studies (ultrasonography, laparoscopy) should be considered to determine whether a cause of secondary dysmenorrhea is present. As previously noted, the cause of primary dysmenorrhea is elevated endometrial prostaglandin production. Therefore, therapy for primary dysmenorrhea should be directed at reducing endometrial prostaglandin production. Anti-inflammatory agents that directly inhibit prostaglandin production or action (ibuprofen) and agents that suppress ovulation (oral contraceptives) are effective in reducing endometrial prostaglandin production. Table 3-3 lists inhibitors of prostaglandin production that have been successful in the treatment of dysmenorrhea. All these agents inhibit the cyclooxygenase enzyme. Mefenamic acid also directly blocks activation of the prostaglandin receptor. Table 3-3 lists the agents associated with a low incidence of serious adverse effects, and most are available without a prescription. Side effects of the prostaglandin synthesis inhibitors include gastrointestinal irritation and ulceration, nausea, prolonged bleeding time, renal papillary necrosis, and decreased renal blood flow.

Usually, therapy for dysmenorrhea is initiated with ibuprofen, 400 mg orally 4 times a day. Therapy is initiated either just before menses (for women who can accurately predict when it begins) or at the beginning of menses. Therapy usually lasts 3 to 4 days. If ibuprofen (an arylpropionic acid derivative) fails to be effective, a drug in the fenamate class (mefenamic acid) can be tried. If naproxen is to be used in the treatment of primary dysmenorrhea, the sodium salt is preferred because it is absorbed more rapidly and reaches a higher peak plasma level than the acid form.

Oral contraceptives contain a combination of estrogen (ethinyl estradiol) and progestogen (19-norprogestin). Oral contraceptives suppress endometrial prostaglandin production by inhibiting ovulation (no endogenous progesterone production) and by preventing normal synchronous endometrial growth and differentiation (constant estrogen and progestogen production prevents normal endometrial growth). If therapy for 3 to 6 months fails to produce a significant decrease in dysmenorrhea, the clinician should carefully review the history and physical examination results to be sure a cause of secondary dysmenorrhea has not been overlooked. Pelvic ultrasonography and diagnostic laparoscopy should be considered if the patient does not respond to treatment with prostaglandin synthesis inhibitors. Two studies of chronic pelvic pain, one in a population of adolescent girls and one in a population of adult women, demonstrate the importance of performing diagnostic laparoscopy in women with chronic pelvic pain that does not respond to supportive therapy (Goldstein et al, 1980; Kresch et al, 1984). Both studies show that significant numbers (more than 30%) of women with chronic pelvic pain have documented pelvic abnormalities (adhesions, endometriosis, pelvic inflammatory disease) that account for the pain.

An evolving concept is that empirical treatment of presumptive endometriosis, a cause of secondary dysmenorrhea, can be instituted with a GnRH agonist analogue before laparoscopy. Proponents of this approach believe that laparoscopy often fails to identify subperitoneal implants of endometriosis (failure of diagnosis) and that laparoscopy often is ineffective in treating all endometriosis implants (failure of treatment). If failure of diagnosis and treatment occur with laparoscopy, it may be reasonable to use a 3-month trial of GnRH agonists as empiric therapy for presumed endometriosis (Barbieri, 1997).

PREMENSTRUAL SYNDROME

Premenstrual syndrome (PMS) can be defined as the cyclic recurrence during the luteal phase of the menstrual cycle of a combination of distressing physical, psychologic, or behavioral changes that interfere with family, social, or work-related activities. In approximately 1% of women of reproductive age, PMS is so severe that it threatens their work and interpersonal relationships. Premenstrual syndrome is most common in women 20 to 45 years of age. Symptoms of PMS are diverse. They include pain (headache, cramps, fatigue); water retention (weight gain, swelling, painful breasts); negative affect (depression, crying, loneliness, irritability); autonomic reactions (cold sweats, dizziness, fainting); behavioral changes (decreased efficiency, difficulty concentrating, lowered motor coordination); and somatization (feelings of suffocation, chest pain, ringing in the ears, blind spots, blurry vision, numbness, tingling). To order these diverse symptoms and signs, Abraham (1983) devised a classification schema consisting of four categories (Box 3-2). These categories are not all inclusive, but they do help the clinician organize history taking for patients with PMS.

The first step in the diagnosis of PMS is to have the patient keep a prospective diary of daily symptoms for 2 months. If examination of the diary reveals no symptom-free week in the early follicular phase (just after menses), a chronic psychiatric disorder such as major depression or anxiety should be strongly suspected. To arrive at a diagnosis of PMS, the diary should demonstrate that the symptoms are temporally clustered before menses (luteal phase) and that they markedly diminish 2 or 3 days after the initiation of menses. In addition to luteal-phase symptoms, some women with PMS have periovulatory exacerbation of symptoms.

BOX 3-2
ABRAHAM'S (1983) CLASSIFICATION OF PREMENSTRUAL SYNDROME

A Anxiety
    Nervous tension
    Mood swings
    Irritability
    Anxiety
C Cravings
    Headache
    Craving for sweets
    Increased appetite
    Heart pounding
    Fatigue
    Dizziness or faintness
D Depression
    Depression
    Forgetfulness
    Crying
    Confusion
    Insomnia
H Water-related symptoms
    Weight gain
    Swelling of extremities
    Breast tenderness
    Abnormal bloating

Approximately 30% of women who seek treatment for PMS have a separate psychiatric disorder, such as major depression. As just noted, these women can often be identified by the absence of a symptom-free week in the follicular phase of the menstrual cycle. Some experienced practitioners suggest that all women with symptoms consistent with PMS complete a screening questionnaire for depression, such as Beck's Depression Inventory. For a diagnosis of major depression, five or more symptoms of depression must be present for at least 2 weeks. The diagnosis of premenstrual dysphoric disorder requires the presence of three or four symptoms of depression associated with the luteal phase of the menstrual cycle. In summary, the diagnosis of PMS is a two-step process. The first step involves obtaining a prospective diary of daily symptoms, and the second involves screening for chronic psychiatric problems, such as major depression.

The cause of PMS is not understood. Numerous theories have been proposed—estrogen excess, progesterone deficiency, fluid retention, vitamin B_6 deficiency, hyperprolactinemia, hormone allergies, and prostaglandin abnormalities—but none have been proven. A popular theory is that progesterone or metabolites of progesterone interact with neurotransmitters and ion channels in the brain. Recent experiments suggest that metabolites of progesterone may modulate neural γ-aminobutyric acid receptors (a common neural ion channel). Another hypothesis is that abnormalities of endogenous neural opioid peptides develop in some women and result in symptoms of endogenous opioid withdrawal in the late luteal phase of the menstrual cycle. Investigators (Reid and Yen, 1981) have, in fact, demonstrated abnormally low levels of circulating opioid peptides in women with PMS in the late luteal phase of the menstrual cycle. The symptoms are probably caused by the complex interaction of ovarian hormones, central neurotransmitters, and the autonomic nervous system.

Schmidt et al (1998) recently reported that either estrogen or progesterone appears to trigger PMS symptoms. They treated women with and without PMS with a GnRH agonist analogue. After the suppression of ovarian steroidogenesis by a GnRH agonist analogue, 10 of 18 women with PMS had significant relief of their menstrual cycle–associated symptoms. The investigators continued treatment with the GnRH agonist and replaced estrogen or progesterone. Women with PMS noted the return of their symptoms, such as sadness, with the replacement of either estrogen or progesterone. Women without PMS reported no adverse symptoms when estradiol or progesterone was replaced. This study suggests that in susceptible women, normal plasma concentrations of estrogen or progesterone can trigger deterioration in mood. The mechanisms that subserve this observation remain to be identified.

Therapy for PMS should include a comprehensive program of education, psychologic counseling and support, exercise, dietary assessment, and, if necessary, pharmacologic intervention. Effective dietary considerations include minimizing the daily intake of alcohol, nicotine, simple sugars, caffeine, and salt. Exercise programs and psychological counseling can help the woman with PMS regain control of her life. Many pharmacologic agents have been used in the treatment of PMS. Because placebo therapy can cause significant improvements in PMS, controlled clinical trials are absolutely necessary before a drug can be accepted as effective (Maddocks et al, 1986). Progesterone therapy is reported to be effective in the treatment of PMS in noncontrolled trials (Dalton, 1977). However, results of randomized clinical trials demonstrate that progesterone is no better than placebo in the treatment of PMS (Maddocks et al, 1986). Seven agents are effective in the treatment of PMS: mefenamic acid, γ-linoleic acid, GnRH agonists, danazol, alprazolam, fluoxetine, and diuretics (spironolactone). The use of each agent in the treatment of PMS is described here.

Mefenamic acid is a nonsteroidal, antiinflamatory agent that inhibits prostaglandin synthesis and competes for binding at the prostaglandin receptor site. In addition to its use in PMS, mefenamic acid is of value in the treatment of pelvic pain. For the treatment of PMS, mefenamic acid is usually administered as a 500-mg loading dose followed by 250 mg 4 times daily for up to 7 days. Prolonged administration of mefenamic acid is not recommended because it can result in decreased renal blood flow and renal papillary necrosis. Common side effects of mefenamic acid therapy include diarrhea, nausea, vomiting, and drowsiness. Mefenamic acid is especially effective in relieving the pain associated with PMS.

γ-Linoleic acid (evening primrose oil) is a dietary supplement especially useful in the treatment of breast tenderness, bloating, weight gain, and edema associated with PMS. It is a precursor of prostaglandin E_1 (PGE_1) and may be effective in the treatment of PMS because it alters prostaglandin production and metabolism. A standard dose is 3 g/day in the late luteal phase of the cycle. Evening primrose oil is available without a prescription in stores that specialize in dietary supplements.

GnRH agonists such as nafarelin and leuprolide are useful for the treatment of severe PMS (Muse et al, 1984). Synthetic changes in amino acids 6 and 10 of the hypothalamic decapeptide GnRH produce agents with long half-life and high affinity for the pituitary GnRH receptor. Long-term administration of these compounds produces a transient stimulation of pituitary LH and FSH secretion and paradoxically results in the complete suppression of LH and FSH secretion. Therefore, long-term administration of a GnRH agonist produces an anovulatory, amenorrheic state that results in the relief of PMS symptoms in approximately 50% of patients (Hammarback and Backstrom, 1988; Brown et al, 1994). The major side effects of the GnRH agonists are attributable to hypoestrogenism (accelerated bone loss, hot flushes, dry vagina). Effective dosages of the GnRH agonists are 3.75 mg leuprolide depot administered every 4 weeks, 0.5 mg leuprolide administered subcutaneously each day, or 200 μg nafarelin administered intranasally twice a day.

Danazol, an attenuated androgen, has been demonstrated to be effective in the treatment of PMS in randomized, controlled trials (Sarto et al, 1987; Hahn et al, 1995).

Alprazolam is a member of the benzodiazepine class of psychoactive agents. The molecular action of alprazolam is unknown, but all benzodiazepines cause a dose-related depressant effect on the central nervous system. Alprazolam is especially effective in the treatment of anxiety caused by PMS. The recommended dosage is 0.25 mg 3 times a day during the late luteal phase of the cycle. The dose can be titrated to the needs of the patient. A major side effect of alprazolam is drowsiness. In some patients discontinuance of benzodiazepines can produce withdrawal symptoms that include insomnia, dysphoria, abdominal cramps, sweating, tremors, and convulsions. After prescribing alprazolam for the treatment of PMS, the clinician must carefully screen for the occurrence of withdrawal symptoms. If withdrawal symptoms occur, the drug should be permanently discontinued.

Fluoxetine is a serotonin reuptake inhibitor approved for the treatment of major depression. In a double-blind, placebo-controlled, cross-over study, Wood et al (1991) demonstrate that daily fluoxetine (20 mg) is superior to placebo in reducing symptoms of depression, anger, and anxiety. A preliminary follow-up study suggests that limiting fluoxetine therapy to the luteal phase of the cycle may be as effective in the treatment of PMS as therapy throughout the follicular and luteal phases of the cycle. The most common side effects caused by fluoxetine include nervousness, insomnia, drowsiness, nausea, and anorexia.

In women with significant premenstrual weight gain (more than 1.5 kg), short-term diuretic therapy may help relieve the symptoms of bloating, edema, and breast fullness. Metolazone (2.5 mg/day) and spironolactone (25 mg 4 times a day) administered during the late luteal phase of the menstrual cycle have been shown to be effective in the treatment of PMS. All diuretics can produce electrolyte imbalance, and women given diuretics for PMS should be evaluated for electrolyte abnormalities.

Three agents reported to be successful in the treatment of PMS in uncontrolled trials are progesterone, oral contraceptives, and lithium. However, controlled clinical trials have failed to demonstrate consistently a beneficial effect of these agents. For example, in a controlled, randomized trial, progesterone supplementation was shown to have no beneficial effects when compared to a placebo (Freeman et al, 1990). Until further research is completed, these agents are not recommended for the treatment of PMS.

Vitamin B_6 in dosages of 500 mg/day is effective in the treatment of PMS. However, at this dosage level, vitamin B_6 therapy may be associated with the onset of sensorineural deficits. Given the potentially serious side effects of high-dose vitamin B_6 therapy, its use is not recommended.

Bromocriptine is a dopamine agonist that is extremely effective in the treatment of hyperprolactinemia. The majority of controlled clinical trials, however, do not suggest that it is of significant value in the treatment of PMS. If used in the treatment of PMS, it should probably be reserved for women with symptoms isolated to the breast. Pharmacologic therapy should not be an isolated intervention in the treatment of PMS but should be part of a comprehensive program of diet, exercise, and counseling.

The cause of PMS is unknown. It is likely that important discoveries are to come that will explicate the biologic mechanisms that cause PMS. These discoveries will be beacons, guiding translational scientists to develop new, specific, and effective treatments for PMS.

REFERENCES

Abraham GE: Nutritional factors in the etiology of the premenstrual tension syndromes. *J Reprod Med* 1983; 28:446.

Allen SE, Potter HD, Azziz R: Prevalence of hyperandrogenemia among nonhirsute oligo-ovulatory women. *Fertil Steril* 1997; 67:569-572

Bakiri F, Benmiloud M: Antidiuretic function in Sheehan's syndrome. *Br Med J* 1984; 289:579-580.

Bakiri F, Benmiloud M, Vallotton MB: Arginine vasopressin in postpartum panhypopituitarism: Urinary excretion and kidney response to osmolar load. *J Clin Endocrinol Metab* 1984; 58:511-515.

Barbieri RL: Primary gonadotropin-releasing hormone agonist therapy for suspected endometriosis. *Am J Managed Care* 1997; 3:285-290.

Barbieri RL: The maternal adenohypophysis. In Tulchinsky D, Little BA, editors: *Maternal fetal endocrinology*, Philadelphia, 1994, WB Saunders.

Barbieri RL: Endocrinology of pregnancy. In Yen SSC, Jaffe RB, Barbieri RL, editors: *Reproductive endocrinology*, Philadelphia, 1999, WB Saunders.

Barbieri RL, Cooper DS, Daniels GH, et al: Prolactin responses to thyrotropin releasing hormone in patients with hypothalamic pituitary disease. *Fertil Steril* 1985; 43:66-73.

Barbieri RL, Gao X: Presence of 17 beta-hydroxysteroid dehydrogenase type 3 messenger ribonucleic acid transcript in an ovarian Sertoli-Leydig cell tumor. *Fertil Steril* 1997; 68:534-537.

Barbieri RL, Ryan KJ: Bromocriptine, endocrine pharmacology, and therapeutic applications. *Fertil Steril* 1983; 39:727.

Belsey EM, Pinol AP: Menstrual bleeding patterns in untreated women. *Contraception* 1997; 55:57-65.

Bergh T, Nillius SJ, Wide L: Clinical course and outcome of pregnancies in amenorrheic women with hyperprolactinemia and pituitary tumors. *Br Med J* 1978; 1:875.

Bohlke K, Cramer DW, Barbieri RL: The relation of luteinizing hormone levels to body mass index in premenopausal women. *Fertil Steril* 1998; 69:503-504.

Brown CS, Ling FW, Anderson RN, et al: Efficacy of depot leuprolide in premenstrual syndrome: Effect of symptom severity and type in a controlled clinical trial. *Obstet Gynecol* 1994; 84:779-786.

Chan WY, Dawood MY, Fuchs F: Relief of dysmenorrhea with the prostaglandin synthetase inhibitor ibuprofen: effect of prostaglandin levels in menstrual fluid. *Am J Obstet Gynecol* 1979; 135:102.

Chandler MH, Schuldheisz S, Phillips BA, et al: Premenstrual asthma: The effect of estradiol on symptoms, pulmonary function and beta-2 receptors. *Pharmacotherapy* 1997; 17:224-234.

Cooper GS, Sandler DP: Long term effects of reproductive age, menstrual cycle patterns on peri- and postmenopausal fracture risk. *Am J Epidemiol* 1997; 145: 804-809.

Corenblum B, Donovan L: The safety of physiological estrogen plus progestin replacement therapy with oral contraceptive therapy in women with pathological hyperprolactinemia. *Fertil Steril* 1993; 59:671.

Dalton K: *The premenstrual syndrome and progesterone therapy.* London: William Heinemann, 1977.

DiZerga GS, Hodgen GD: Folliculogenesis in the primate ovarian cycle. *Endocr Rev* 1981; 2:27.

Dorrington JH, Armstrong DT: Effects of FSH on gonadal functions. *Recent Prog Res* 1979; 35:301.

Dubinsky TJ, Parvey HR, Maklad N: The role of transvaginal sonography and endometrial biopsy in the evaluation of peri- and postmenopausal bleeding. *Am J Roentgenol* 1997; 169:145-149.

Erickson GF, Nakatani A, Ling N, et al: Localization of insulin-like binding protein-5 in rat ovaries during the estrous cycle. *Endocrinology* 1992; 130:1867-1878.

Erickson GF, Nakatani A, Ling N, et al: Cyclic changes in insulin-like growth factor 4 messenger RNA in the rat ovary. *Endocrinology* 1992; 130:625-636.

Freeman E, Rickels K, Sondheimer SJ, et al: Ineffectiveness of progesterone suppository treatment for premenstrual syndrome. *JAMA* 1990; 264:349-353.

Giudice LC: Insulin-like growth factors and ovarian follicular development. *Endocr Rev* 1991; 13:641.

Goldstein DP, deCholnsky C, Emans SJ, et al: Laparoscopy in the diagnosis and management of pelvic pain in adolescents. *J Reprod Med* 1980; 24:251.

Hahn PM, Van Vugt DA, Reid RL: A randomized placebo controlled crossover trial of danazol for the treatment of premenstrual syndrome. *Psychoneuroendocrinology* 1995; 20:193-209.

Hammarback S, Backstrom T: Induced anovulation as a treatment of premenstrual syndrome: A double blind cross-over study with GnRH agonist versus placebo. *Acta Obstet Gynecol Scand* 1988; 67:159-166.

Hoffman M, Runnebaum B, Gerhard I: Effects of weight loss on hormone profile in obese infertile women. *Human Reprod* 1996; 11:1884-1191.

Holmgren U, Bergstrand G, Hagenfeldt K, et al: Women with prolactinoma: Effect of pregnancy and lactation on serum prolactin and on tumor growth. *Acta Endocrinol* 1986; 111:452.

Jialal I, Naidoo C, Norman RJ, et al: Pituitary function in Sheehan's syndrome. *Obstet Gynecol* 1984; 63:15.

Kelsey JL, Gammon MD, John EM: Reproductive factors and breast cancer. *Epidemiol Rev* 1993; 15:36-47.

Khoury SA, Reame NE, Lelch RP, et al: Diurnal patterns of pulsatile luteinizing hormone secretion in hypothalamic amenorrhea. *J Clin Endocrinol Metab* 1987; 64:755.

Knobil E: The neuroendocrine control of the menstrual cycle. *Recent Prog Horm Res* 1980; 36:53.

Konopka P, Raymond JP, Merceron RE, et al: Continuous administration of bromocriptine in the prevention of neurological complications in pregnant women with prolactinomas. *Am J Obstet Gynecol* 1983; 146:935.

Koyama H: Cyclophosphamide-induced ovarian failure. *Cancer* 1977; 39:1403.

Kresch AJ, Seiter DB, Scas LB, et al: Laparoscopy in 100 women with chronic pelvic pain. *Obstet Gynecol* 1984; 64:672.

Landis CA, Harsh G: Clinical characteristics of acromegalic patients whose pituitary tumors contain mutant Gs protein. *J Clin Endocrinol Metab* 1990; 71:1416.

Langer RD, Pierce JJ, O'Hanlan KA, et al: Transvaginal ultrasonography compared with endometrial biopsy for the detection of endometrial disease. *N Engl J Med* 1997; 337:792-798.

Maddocks S, Hahn P, Moller F, et al: A double-blind placebo-controlled trial of progesterone vaginal suppositories in the treatment of premenstrual syndrome. *Am J Obstet Gynecol* 1986; 154:573.

McGregor AM, Scanlon MF, Hall R, et al: Effects of bromocriptine on pituitary tumor size. *Br Med J* 1979; 2:700.

McNatty KP, Smith DM, Makrus A, et al: The microenvironment of the human antral follicle. *J Clin Endocrinol Metab* 1979; 49:851-860.

Molitch M: Pregnancy and the hyperprolactinemic woman. *N Engl J Med* 1985; 312:1364.

Molitch ME, Elton RL, Blackwell RE, et al: Bromocriptine as a primary therapy for prolactin secreting macroadenomas: Results of a prospective multicenter study. *J Clin Endocrinol Metab* 1985; 60:698.

Morales AJ, Laughlin GA, Butzow T, et al: Insulin, somatotropic and luteinizing hormone axes in non-obese and obese women with PCOS: common and distinct features. *J Clin Endocrinol Metab* 1996; 81:2854-2864.

Muse KN, Cetel NS, Futterman LA, et al: The premenstrual syndrome: The effects of medical oophorectomy. *N Engl J Med* 1984; 311:1345.

Nakamura T, Takio K, Eto Y, et al: Activin-binding protein from rat ovary is follistatin. *Science* 1990; 247:836-838.

Noyes RW, Hertig AT, Rock J: Dating the endometrial biopsy. *Fertil Steril* 1950; 1:3.

Parsons TF, Pierce JG: Glycoprotein hormones: Structure and function. *Annu Rev Biochem* 1981; 50:465.

Pelletier G, Robert F, Hardy J: Identification of human anterior pituitary cells by immunoelectron microscopy. *J Clin Endocrinol Metab* 1978; 46:534.

Raymond JP, Goldstein E, Knopoka P, et al: Follow up of children born of bromocriptine treated mothers. *Horm Res* 1985; 22:239.

Rebar RW, Connolly HV: Clinical features of young women with hypergonadotropic amenorrhea. *Fertil Steril* 1990; 53:804-810.

Reid RL, Yen SSC: Premenstrual syndrome. *Am J Obstet Gynecol* 1981; 139:85.

Ruchhoft EA, Elkind-Hirsch KE, Malinak R: Pituitary function is altered during the same cycle in women with PCOS treated with continuous or cyclic oral contraceptives or a gonadotropin releasing hormone agonist. *Fertil Steril* 1996; 66:54-60.

Ryan KJ, Petro Z: Steroid biosynthesis by human ovarian granulosa and thecal cells. *J Clin Endocrinol Metab* 1966; 26:46.

Ryan KJ, Petro Z, Kaiser J: Steroid formation by isolated and recombined ovarian granulosa and thecal cells. *J Clin Endocrinol Metab* 1968; 28:355.

Ryan KJ, Smith OW: Biogenesis of steroid hormones in the human ovary. *Recent Prog Horm Res* 1965; 21:367.

Sarto AP, Miller EJ, Lundblad EG: Premenstrual syndrome: Beneficial effects of periodic, low dose danazol. *Obstet Gynecol* 1987; 70:33-36.

Savard K, Marsh JM, Rice BF: Gonadotropins and ovarian steroidogenesis. *Recent Prog Horm Res* 1965; 21:285.

Schmidt PJ, Nieman LK, Danaceau MA, et al: Differential behavioral effects of gonadal steroids in women with and in those without premenstrual syndrome. *N Engl J Med* 1998; 338:209-216.

Sheehan HL, Whitehead R: The neurohypophysis in postpartum hypopituitarism. *J Pathol* 1965; 85:145.

Thorner MO: Medical treatment of prolactinomas. *J Clin Endocrinol Metab* 1997; 82:997-999.

Towbin NA, Gviazda IM, March CM: Office hysteroscopy versus transvaginal ultrasonography in the evaluation of patients with excessive uterine bleeding. *Am J Obstet Gynecol* 1996; 174:1678-1682.

Treloar AE, Boynton RE, Borghild BG, et al: Variations of the human menstrual cycle through reproductive life. *Int J Fertil* 1967; 12:77.

Tsonis CG, Sharpe R: Dual control of follicle-stimulating hormone. *Nature* 1986; 321:724-725.

Tureck RW, Strauss JF III: Progesterone synthesis by luteinized human granuloma cells in culture: The role of de novo sterol synthesis and lipoprotein-carried sterol. *J Clin Endocrinol Metab* 1982; 54:367.

Waldstreicher J, Santoro NF, Hall JE, et al: Hyperfunction of the hypothalamic-pituitary axis in women with polycystic ovarian disease. *J Clin Endocrinol Metab* 1988; 66:165.

Webster J, Piscitelli G, Polli A, et al: A comparison of cabergoline and bromocriptine in the treatment of hyperprolactinemic amenorrhea. *N Engl J Med* 1994; 331:904-909.

Whitehead R: The hypothalamus in post-partum hypopituitarism. *J Pathol* 1965; 86:55.

Widrich T, Bradley LD, Mitchinson AR, et al: Comparison of saline infusion sonography with office hysteroscopy for the evaluation of the endometrium. *Am J Obstet Gynecol* 1996; 174:1327-1334.

Wilcox AJ, Weinberg CR, Baird DD: Timing of sexual intercourse in relation to ovulation. *N Engl J Med* 1995; 333:1517-1521.

Wilson C: The case for initial surgical removal of certain prolactinomas. *J Clin Endocrinol Metab* 1997; 82:999-1000.

Wood SH: Treatment of premenstrual syndrome with fluoxetine: A double blind, placebo controlled, crossover study. *Obstet Gynecol* 1991; 80:339.

Ylikorkala O, Dawood MY: New concepts in dysmenorrhea. *Am J Obstet Gynecol* 1978; 130:833.

Zhou J, Bondy C: Anatomy of the human ovarian insulin-like growth factor system. *Biol Reprod* 1993; 48:467.

CHAPTER

4

The Vulva

MICHAEL G. MUTO

KEY ISSUES

1. Systemic and local diseases may affect the integrity of vulvar skin.
2. There is little correlation between appearance and histopathology of a vulvar lesion.
3. Biopsy specimens should be taken of all vulvar lesions before therapy is initiated.
4. Vulvar cancer is a preventable disease.

GENERAL CONSIDERATIONS

The vulva and external genitalia include the mons, labia majora and minora, clitoris, vestibule, and urethral meatus. Vulvar skin is predisposed to numerous abnormalities that reflect local and systemic disease. Skin in this region is intrinsically more sensitive and more easily injured than skin in other locations of the body (Pincus and McKay, 1993). This is in part because the vulvar skin is in a dependent position and is, therefore, more susceptible to edema. In addition, normal secretions of the vagina and vulvar glands create a moist environment that can lead to maceration and loss of skin integrity. Many systemic toxins, such as the chemical carcinogens in cigarette smoke, may be concentrated numerous times more than blood levels in vulvar secretions. Finally, the vulvar skin is prone to infection through sexually transmitted diseases, many of which may contribute to the development of preinvasive and invasive neoplasia.

Vulvar hygiene is an important part of the care and cure of many diseases and syndromes. Basic hygiene includes daily washing with a mild, nondrying soap and the avoidance of tight, impermeable underclothes and of most so-called feminine hygiene products.

Diagnoses of vulvar disease are often delayed because of patient procrastination and embarrassment in seeking treat-

ment, professional omission or neglect, and ineffective treatment. Delays in diagnosis, however, can influence infectious morbidity and malignant mortality rates. Accurate diagnosis begins with a thorough history to determine the nature, site, and duration of specific symptoms and of general symptoms and problems. Inquiries should be made about discharge, diarrhea, topical contacts of any kind, medications, contraceptives, sexual practices, clothing, and stress or anxiety. Physical examination should include examination of the oral mucosa, scalp, skin, nails, and pubic hair. It is insufficient to allay symptoms temporarily. The cause of the disorder should be found and specific therapy instituted.

Magnification is helpful in evaluating contours (ulcers or exophytic growths) and blood vessels. Vessels are not as easily visualized through keratinized epithelium, but Iverson (1981) found abnormal vessels in 58% of patients with vulvar carcinoma in situ. In addition to enhancing the choices for biopsy, magnification can help detect parasites or nits. Dermatologists favor twofold to fourfold magnification with a large illuminated lens. Gynecologists magnify 7.5-fold to fourteenfold with a colposcope ("vulvoscope").

ANATOMY AND HISTOLOGY
Mons and Labia

The mons consists of an accumulation of subcutaneous fat in a rounded pad overlying the symphysis pubis. The typical female escutcheon of hair over the mons is triangular and usually does not extend upward along the abdomen, although there is much variation depending on racial and familial traits.

The labia majora (and mons) form the outer extent of the external genitalia. Vulvar folds continue cephalad toward the lower abdomen and fuse in the midline as the mons pubis or anterior commissure. The union of the labia majora caudally is the posterior commissure and the posterior extent of the vulva (Fig. 4-1).

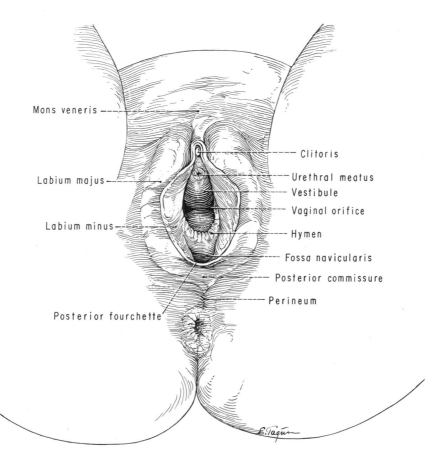

Fig. 4-1. External genitalia of the female.

The outer skin contains many sebaceous, apocrine, and sweat (eccrine) glands, and it is covered with hair lateral to the pilosebaceous line along the crest. Pronounced glandular and adnexal development accounts for the frequency of sebaceous cysts and hair follicle infections.

The blood supply of the labia majora is derived from the internal pudendal artery through the posterior labial branch and from a small branch of the obturator artery. Veins have approximately the same source, but they also communicate with the vesicovaginal plexus and the inferior hemorrhoidal veins.

The pudendal nerve, derived from the second to fourth sacral nerves, yields the perineal branch, from which the posterior labial nerve arises. The latter innervates the labia majora and the lateral portion of the urethral triangle (Fig. 4-2).

The labia minora consist of two medial folds proximal to each other and sharing a convex-free border. They extend from the prepuce and frenulum of the clitoris to join the labia majora posteriorly as they terminate in the posterior fourchette. Between this fourchette and the hymenal ring is a curved depression, the fossa navicularis (Fig. 4-1). Labia minora are duplications of skin, not of mucosa.

Skin of the labia minora contains abundant pigment and blood vessels. The blood supply is derived from the labial vessels and from the dorsal artery to the clitoris, which is a terminal branch of the internal pudendal artery. The nerve supply is the same as that of the labia majora. Immediately preceding and during coitus, the labia become moist and lubricated with secretions from vestibular and sebaceous glands.

Labia minora have a specific role in the process of urination. After vulvectomy, uncontrolled "spraying" is common.

Clitoris

The clitoris is composed of two roots that traverse the pubic rami to unite posteriorly to the symphysis in the clitoral body, which terminates in the upper portion of the vestibule as the glans. Although clitoral roots and body are covered by overlying muscle, the glans is exposed. Figure 4-2 illustrates the relationship of the root of the clitoris to the overlying ischiocavernosus muscle. The roots, or crura, are 3 to 4 cm long in the flaccid state, but in erection they are 4.5 to 5 cm long. The body is 2.5 to 3 cm long and is surrounded by a connective tissue capsule of fibroelastic tissue, the clitoridean fascia. Unlike the penis, the clitoris contains no corpus spongiosum, and it has less erectile tissue.

The function of the clitoris is that of a sexual "nerve center." Before contact, sexual stimulation causes vascular engorgement and enlargement, so that when the penis is inserted the clitoris becomes particularly sensitive to the motion of the shaft. Orgasm in the female may be brought about by this stimulation, even in the absence of the vagina;

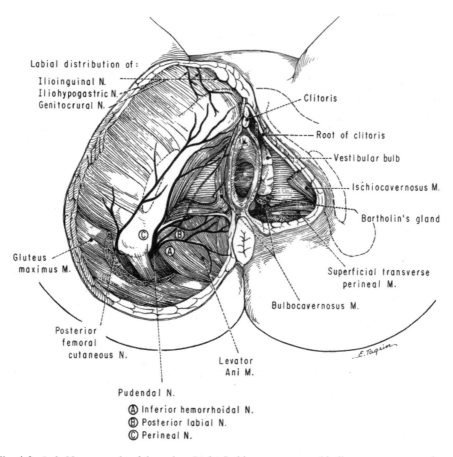

Labial distribution of:
Ilioinguinal N.
Iliohypogastric N.
Genitocrural N.

Clitoris

Root of clitoris

Vestibular bulb

Ischiocavernosus M.

Bartholin's gland

Superficial transverse perineal M.

Bulbocavernosus M.

Levator Ani M.

Gluteus maximus M.

Posterior femoral cutaneous N.

Pudendal N.
Ⓐ Inferior hemorrhoidal N.
Ⓑ Posterior labial N.
Ⓒ Perineal N.

Fig. 4-2. *Left:* Nerve supply of the vulva. *Right:* Ischiocavernosus and bulbocavernosus muscles have been reflected to show the anatomy of the clitoris and the vestibular bulbs.

it consists of an interrelated reflex resulting in forceful contractions of voluntary and involuntary musculature of the pelvis and pelvic viscera. After orgasm has been experienced and a conditioned reflex established, the presence of the clitoris is not absolutely necessary. Women who have had vulvectomy with excision of the clitoris are capable of experiencing orgasm. However, major sexual problems are common, as they are with women who have undergone "female circumcision."

Arteries of the clitoris arise from the internal pudendal. Veins correspond to arteries except for the large dorsal vein of the clitoris, which runs beneath the arcuate ligament of the symphysis through a small notch and which communicates with the pelvic veins. Lymphatics coursing along this plexus may play a role in the dissemination of vulvar cancer to the pelvic lymph nodes.

Vestibule and Vulvar Glands

Situated just inside the labia minora, the vestibule (introitus) is an elliptical space into which multiple glands open (Woodruff and Friedrich, 1985). Bartholin's glands are the homologue of bulbourethral glands in the male. They secrete mucus, particularly during sexual stimulation. Situated at each side of the vaginal orifice, distal to the hymen, the glands are normally small and can be palpated only in thin

women or if they become enlarged by inflammation or tumor. Duct openings are in the posterolateral introitus at the 5- and 7-o'clock positions. Rapid growth occurs at puberty, and shrinkage occurs after menopause.

Periurethral ducts are the external orifices of the Skene's glands situated beneath the urethral floor. Duct orifices are small, usually grossly visible crypts just lateral and posterior to the urethral meatus. They are the rudimentary homologue of the prostate gland and are commonly invaded by lower genital organisms, such as the gonococcus. When the glands are infected, pus may be expressed from the openings.

Vestibular Bulbs

Vestibular bulbs correspond to the corpus spongiosum of the male and consist of truncated masses of erectile tissue on either side of the vaginal orifice. They are situated above the interior fascia of the pelvic diaphragm and below the bulbocavernosus muscles (Fig. 4-2).

Hymen

The hymen is an irregular membranous fold of varying thickness that partially occludes the vaginal orifice. It extends from the floor of the urethra to the fossa navicularis and may be complete (imperforate), absent, incomplete, or cribriform. The hymen may be avulsed from examination,

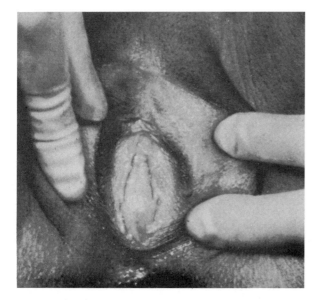

Fig. 4-3. Imperforate hymen.

trauma, surgery, or coitus. Usually irregular remnants persist, which form a fleshy fringe about the vaginal opening (the carunculae multiforma) (see Fig. 4-1).

Developmental defects, often unnoticed until menarche or later, can affect the hymen. An imperforate hymen (Fig. 4-3) is usually noticed at menarche, when menstrual blood accumulates behind the membrane with the resultant hematocolpos and hematometra. A rigid hymen can cause dyspareunia. It may be the result of an excess amount of tough, fibrous tissue or of the presence of multiple small orifices, none of which is large enough to admit the penis. If not modified by gradual dilatation, surgical correction is required.

Urethra

Just inferior to the clitoris, the urethral meatus may be visualized by separating the labia minora. It has a cleftlike appearance with slightly raised lateral margins, and it is the uppermost structure of the vestibule (see Fig. 4-1).

Malformations of the urethra include stenosis, diverticula, and hypospadias. Mild degrees of stenosis are fairly common and usually cause no symptoms. Some patients may have tenesmus and recurrent cystitis from urinary retention. Urethral dilation and treatment of the cystitis bring marked relief to the patient. Diverticula result from incomplete development of the urethrovaginal septum. There may be single or multiple outpouchings of the urethra along its inferior surface that lack connection with the vagina. Diagnosis is made by applying firm pressure on the diverticulum to express urine or pus. Treatment is surgical excision.

INJURIES
Accidents

Accidental injuries to the vulva may result from blunt or penetrating trauma. They usually occur in young girls and often result from straddle injuries. Such blows may rupture the venous plexi, vestibular bulb, or vulvar varicosities. Bleeding may result in small contusions or massive, life-threatening vulvar and retroperitoneal hematomas.

As in the evaluation of any traumatic injury, the clinician should make every attempt to reconstruct the accident accurately to anticipate the possible extent of injury. For example, a vulvar hematoma from riding a mechanical bull is caused by shearing forces of the labial fat against the underlying pubic bone. Tears in the periclitoral veins and the superficial venous plexi can be anticipated in such an injury. On the other hand, a fall onto a tree limb or a picket fence may result in superficial and penetrating injury with arterial bleeding. High-speed impact, reported in water skiing accidents, may result in pelvic fractures. When the patient is unable to report the nature of the accident, witnesses should be sought.

After determining the mechanism of injury, the physician must assess the extent. If the patient has a hematoma, the volume of blood contained within it should be estimated and serial examinations performed to determine whether it is expanding. Small contusions are best treated with the application of cold compresses. Large hematomas, particularly those that are expanding or are associated with hypotension, should be evacuated and packed to control bleeding, reduce the risk for infection, and limit pressure necrosis of the overlying skin. Broad-spectrum antibiotics are indicated. A Foley catheter or a suprapubic tube may be required if the urethra is injured or obstructed. Careful inspection of the urethra, clitoris, vagina, perineum, and anus should be performed to rule out perforating injuries. An inadequate examination of the patient while she is awake requires another examination under anesthesia.

Continued blood loss that is not apparent may herald the formation of an expanding retroperitoneal hematoma. Abdominal-pelvic computed tomography can may help detect and manage such hematomas. Injuries to the urinary tract may require gravity cystography, intravenous pyelography, or cystoscopy. Finally, if injuries result from high-speed accidents or violence, pelvic bone fractures must be ruled out.

Coital Injuries

Hymeneal lacerations at the coitarche are usually minor, but occasionally they result in massive bleeding. Lacerations caused by forced entry, such as too vigorous sexual activity, rape, or sexual molestation, may be far more extensive. A thorough discussion of coital injuries in the young is presented in Chapter 12. As with accidental injuries, meticulous examination to assess the extent of the injury is essential. When dealing with the consequences of traumatic sexual acts, the physician must demonstrate extraordinary sensitivity and tact. If sex was consensual, the patient and her partner may be deeply embarrassed by the injury and withhold information vital to rendering appropriate care. If sexual molestation or rape is suspected, the physician must pay strict attention to the collection of evidence as outlined in the institution's rape protocol. When dealing with self-inflicted injuries, psychiatric counseling should be obtained to establish whether the patient is a threat to herself or to others.

INFECTIONS AND SEXUAL DISEASES

Syphilis, gonorrhea, herpes, and acquired immunodeficiency syndrome (AIDS) are covered in detail in Chapter 18. Human papillomavirus (HPV) is covered in detail in Chapter 6. Infections that are primarily vaginal are covered in Chapter 5. This section focuses on infections that have manifestations unique to the vulva.

General principles are as follows:
1. Any persistent lesion should be evaluated for its infectious or neoplastic cause.
2. One sexually transmitted disease places the patient at higher risk for others; therefore, cultures should be taken for chlamydia and gonorrhea. Serologic tests should be performed for hepatitis B, herpes, human immunodeficiency virus (HIV), and syphilis. Biopsy specimens should be taken of any endophytic or ulcerative lesion and of any exophytic lesion that is not a "typical" condyloma in appearance or behavior.
3. The public health is best served when disease is diagnosed and treated in sexual partners.

Condyloma Acuminata

Anogenital HPV and oncogenesis are discussed in Chapter 6. This chapter focuses on the diagnosis and treatment of vulvar condyloma acuminata. Human papillomavirus is the most prevalent and one of the most contagious genital infections. In the United States, approximately 40 million men and women are infected, and at least 1 million more become infected each year (Reichman and Bonner, 1990). These figures may be a conservative estimate because most infected persons are asymptomatic and do not have condylomas.

Vulvar condyloma (Fig. 4-4) is part of a regional anogenital infection that requires diagnosis and treatment.

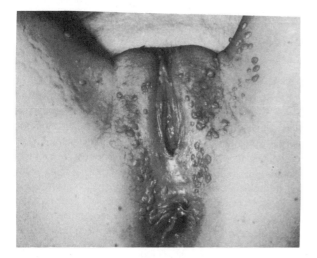

Fig. 4-4. Condylomata acuminata.

This means that patients with vulvar condylomas need the following:
1. A definitive diagnosis must be made. "Typical" vulvar condylomas do not require histologic diagnosis initially, but biopsy specimens should be taken liberally if there is any variation from the typical acuminate condyloma or if it persists for more than 2 months despite treatment (Fig. 4-5).
2. The entire lower genital-anal tract should undergo colposcopy for occult squamous intraepithelial neoplasia.
3. Screening should be performed for associated sexually transmitted disease.

Treatment

There is no effective systemic, antiviral agent for the treatment of anogenital HPV infections. Therefore, therapy must be directed at the removal of macroscopic condylomas. The appropriate treatment of vulvar condylomas is determined by their size and location and by whether they are primary, persistent, or recurrent.

Medical therapy is most effective in small-volume primary condyloma infections. Agents such as bichloroacetic acid and trichloroacetic acid work well on flat condyloma without significant keratinization. Podophyllotoxin 0.5% may be self-administered and is safe and efficacious for small, solitary warts (Bonner et al, 1994; Reichman and Binnez, 1990). Topical 5-fluorouracil (5-FU) has been used for treatment and prevention, but it causes severe vulvar burns and is not a first-line agent. Interferon may induce dramatic local responses, but its duration of response is short and it requires frequent intralesional injection by health professionals (Reid and Greenberg, 1991). Recently, 5% imiquimod cream, a topical immunostimulant, has been demonstrated to be effective and safe in a prospective, double-blind placebo-controlled trial of 311 patients with external anogenital warts (Edwards et al, 1998). Trials comparing this novel topical agent to standard treatments are not yet reported.

Surgical therapy may be either ablative or excisional. Ablative therapeutic options include cryosurgery and laser vaporization. Vulvar cryosurgery lacks precision, and effects are lost rapidly with large warts. In experienced hands and controlled by colposcopy, laser vaporization affords the surgeon the greatest number of options in the treatment of warts, and it is the preferred method of treatment for large discrete warts (Reid, 1985; Dorsey, 1984). Sometimes enormous warts must be surgically excised.

Treating persistent or recurrent condylomas is challenging, and the need for an effective systemic, antivirotic agent is clear. Until one is discovered, the best regional therapy is topical 5-FU. Topical 5-FU is well tolerated when administered carefully, but overdosing can result in painful chemoinflammation. Mild chemoinflammation cannot always be avoided, and this risk must be acceptable to patient and physician or 5-FU should not be used. Preoperative and postoperative administration of 5-FU is a useful surgical adjunct for persistent or recurrent condylomas (Krebs, 1986). During pregnancy, trichloroacetic acid and laser treatment can be

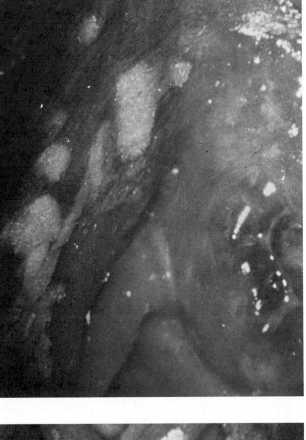

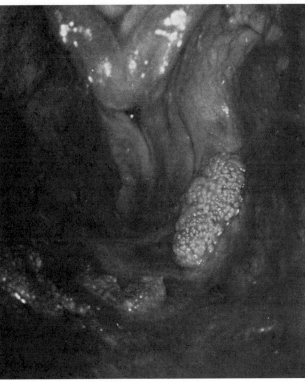

Fig. 4-5. A, Human papillomavirus only at 11 o'clock. **B,** Moderate wartlike dysplasia at 5 o'clock. (From Sillman FH: 5-fluorouracil/chemosurgery for intraepithelial neoplasia of the lower genital tract. *Obstet Gynecol* 1981; 58:356, and Sillman FH: Anogenital papillomavirus infection and neoplasia in immunodeficient women. *Obstet Gynecol Clin North Am* 1987; 14:537.)

used safely for debulking condylomas. If condylomas are persistent or recurrent, HIV testing is especially encouraged.

Fungal Infections

The vulvovaginal area harbors numerous fungi. Normal floral balance and cellular immunity maintain a healthy homeostasis. Lowered resistance, increased heat, friction, or excessive perspiration can upset the normal balance, and fungi may become pathogens. Predisposing causes are pregnancy, oral contraceptives, broad-spectrum antibiotics, diabetes and other chronic diseases, and immunosuppression. These should be investigated when a fungal infection is diagnosed. The initial nidus is often the vagina, especially during the reproductive years. Occasionally, adjacent intertrigo or the vulva itself can be the initial site. Common forms are candida and tinea.

Candida

Nine fungi have been found to cause mycotic vulvitis. The most common normal and pathogenic type is *Candida albicans* (monilia), which causes 66% to 75% of vulvovaginal fungal infections. Infection can begin as an erythema or a reddish papule that later becomes vesicular or pustular. After rupture, a moist, red membrane remains. Secondary infection is common, and the vagina and vulva can become markedly edematous and tender. The vulva may be covered with a tenacious gray-white frosting (Fig. 4-6), or there may be marked inflammation caused in part by repetitive scratching. The most common symptom is intense pruritus. A white, curdlike vaginal discharge may develop as the infection becomes more severe. If chafing occurs, secondary dermatitis of the thighs may result. Intercourse may be painful or impossible because of swelling, abrasion, and inflammation, and walking may be uncomfortable because of chafing.

In some patients these characteristics of *Candida* infection are so obvious that they may be identified by inspection alone. Diagnosis is more difficult in the older patient with an

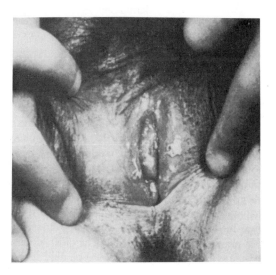

Fig. 4-6. Candidiasis of the vulva.

infection in the early stages or when there is a secondary bacterial infection.

Diagnosis. Diagnosis is made when "budding" can be seen on the hyphea on wet smear, Gram stain, or culture. A dark brown or black growth occurs on Nickerson's medium in approximately 48 hours if *Candida* organisms are present.

Treatment. Imidazole in cream and suppository forms is effective and should be used in the vagina and on the vulva. Cool sitz baths help relieve pruritus and irritation. Hydroxyzine taken at bedtime is helpful for pruritus-induced insomnia. Among patients with persistent or recurrent infections, systemic diseases should be ruled out and substitutions made for oral contraceptives. Cultures should be taken from the patient and her partner to test for specific fungi, and appropriate treatment should be instituted. A broad-spectrum triazole (Terconazole) may be appropriate (Lancutsen, 1991). Short courses of a prophylactic, postmenstrual antifungal agent may help. The gastrointestinal tract is a ready source; therefore, oral nystatin (or ketoconazole) may also be added. A culture test should again be taken 2 weeks after therapy for *C. albicans* infection.

Tinea

Dermatophytes grow on dead, superficial, keratinized layers of the skin (Fitzpatrick, 1992). Tinea is well known to many parts of the body. Tinea capitis, tinea corporis (ringworm), tinea pedis (athlete's foot), and tinea cruris (jock itch) occur more commonly in males (Kaufman, 1989).

Tinea cruris usually is caused by *Epidermophyton floccosum* (or by *Trichophyton rubrum*). It is characterized by superficial pale-pink to bright-red lesions with well-defined scaly borders. Central clearing led to the term *ringworm*. Through coalescence, the vulvar skin, thighs, and pubis may become involved. After periods of scratching or maceration, the process may resemble a "weeping" type of eczema.

Diagnosis. Diagnosis is made with potassium hydroxide, microscopic examination of scrapings showing nonbudding hyphae (spores are not seen), Gram stain, or culture on Sabouraud's maltose agar (Kaufman, 1989). In office practice, scrapings plated on a dermatophyte test medium result in colonies that change from yellow to red. This is in contrast to *C. albicans*, in which color change is rare.

Treatment. Treatment consists of topical imidazole and aeration to reduce warmth and humidity. After reevaluating for predisposing causes, systemic griseofulvin or ketoconazole may be a needed adjunct in the treatment of chronic, intractable tinea.

Intertrigo

The diagnosis of intertrigo is arrived at after excluding primary fungal infection, contact dermatitis, eczema, psoriasis, and seborrheic dermatitis. It can result from maceration in folds, where drying and corticoids can help, or it can have a superimposed fungal (or other) infection. Its clearance requires keeping the area clean and dry and diagnosing and treating any fungal infection.

Parasites
Scabies

Millions of people are infected each year with the female itch mite, *Sarcoptes scabiei*. Transmission is by close contact that is not necessarily sexual. Pruritus begins approximately 1 month after the initial infection. Examination reveals papular lesions on the hands, wrists, other joints, axillae, nipples, umbilicus, and pubis. Pruritus may be intense and is usually nocturnal. The neck and head are seldom involved.

Diagnosis. Diagnosis is confirmed by light-gray, threadlike burrows (magnification is helpful) and by obtaining eggs or a mite (dark spot at the end of burrow) with a needle for microscopic examination in an oil preparation.

Treatment. Treatment begins with rubbing the scabicide permethrin (or lindane) into the skin and under the fingernails. The patient must then bathe after 12 hours and change and decontaminate bedding, towels, and clothing daily until remission. Medication must be repeated in 1 week. Severe dermatitis should be treated with soothing baths and lotions. If this is a secondary infection, it should also be treated with topical antibiotics, oral erythromycin, or dicloxacillin. Sexual partners and close contacts (including pets) should be examined and treated.

Pediculosis pubis

The pubic louse *(Phthirius pubis)* infects more than 1 million people each year in the United States. It pierces the skin, and its "saliva" can produce severe, allergic pruritus and erythema (Billstein, 1988). The disease is most easily spread through coitus, but it can be spread by any kind of contact, including contact with towels or bedding.

Diagnosis. Diagnosis is made by removing a hair that carries an egg-filled nit or by capturing a crab-shaped ectoparasite and examining it microscopically.

Treatment. Treatment is permethrin (or lindane) and should be administered to patient and sexual partner.

Other Infections
Chancroid

Chancroid is caused by *Hemophilus ducreyi*. Approximately 4000 patients are infected each year in the United States. More men than women are infected (7-to-1 ratio) because transmission is mainly through prostitutes. The incubation period is 4 to 10 days. Infection begins as a papule that soon becomes a painful, nonindurated (soft) ulcer with irregular, undermined red edges and a necrotic base, best seen with a vulvoscope. The ulcers are deeper and wider than those of syphilis and herpes. One third to one half of patients have multiple ulcers (Faro, 1989).

Diagnosis. Diagnosis is usually made clinically. Gram stain can be helpful, but the characteristic "school of fish" arrangement of the gram-negative bacilli is not specific. Organisms may be cultured from ulcers or aspirate from infected nodes, but growth is difficult, and at this time there is no serologic test. Exclusion of herpes and syphilis supports the diagnosis, but 20% of patients with chancroid have syphilis, herpes, or HIV infection.

Treatment. Treatment is oral azithromycin 1 g or erythromycin 500 mg for a week, or 250 mg ceftriaxone intramuscularly. Sexual partners should be treated.

Lymphogranuloma Venereum

Lymphogranuloma venereum (LGV) is caused by *Chlamydia trachomatis*. It is found primarily in the tropics; approximately 500 cases are diagnosed in the United States each year. Inoculation occurs only through a disrupted epithelium (Faro, 1989). After an incubation period of as much as 4 weeks, a genital papule appears. After that a small ulcer appears, perhaps for a few days, that may be asymptomatic and heal spontaneously. Approximately 2 weeks later, after prodromal systemic symptoms of fever and malaise, the infection takes hold in the principal site—the lymph nodes. Painful, suppurative, inguinal adenitis develops with subsequent necrosis, abscess formation (buboes), and, later, ulcerations and draining sinuses. Fibrous bands, including Poupart's ligament, indent the buboes and form the characteristic genital-inguinal grooves. Fibrosis and scarring are late manifestations, and lymphatic obstruction can result in marked edema of the vulva. Lymphatic extension to adjacent organs may produce abscesses around the strictures of the urethra, anus, and rectum. The late disfigurement and destruction of infected structures may suggest suppurative hidradenitis or Crohn disease. Both spare the labia minora.

Diagnosis. Diagnosis is usually made clinically with a complement fixation test. Culture from aspirated buboes and an immunofluorescent test with monoclonal antibodies are available in certain laboratories. If there are hard, enlarged lymph nodes, it is important to rule out carcinoma and lymphoma.

Treatment. Treatment includes local cleansing. Buboes should be aspirated; incising promotes chronic fistula formation. Tetracycline should be given for at least 3 weeks and continue until remission. In chronic LGV, antibiotics are less effective. For severe deformities, vulvectomy or colostomy may be necessary.

Granuloma Inguinale

Granuloma inguinale is a chronic granulomatous, mainly tropical disease rarely found in the United States (fewer than 50 cases per year). The etiologic agent is *Calymmatobacterium* (Donovania) *granulomatis*. The incubation period is 2 to 12 weeks. Transmission can occur without sexual contact. The disease begins as a small, painless papule that gradually becomes a serpiginous, red, raised, irregular, velvety, friable ulcer. If not treated, subcutaneous granulomas and other ulcers develop that become secondarily infected. Infections and granulomas can ultimately lead to scarring, edema, and tissue destruction (Fig. 4-7). The carcinogenic significance of granuloma inguinale is still in doubt.

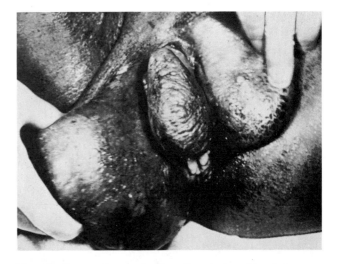

Fig. 4-7. Severe edema and vulvar distortion resulting from granuloma inguinale.

Diagnosis. Diagnosis is established by finding Donovan bodies—groups of bacilli—in Wright stains of scrapings or biopsy.

Treatment. Treatment is 1 g tetracycline daily for at least 2 weeks until healing occurs. Occasionally, late, marked edema and damage necessitate vulvectomy.

Molluscum

Molluscum contagiosum is a pox virus that has an incubation period of approximately 1 month. Infection can occur without sexual contact. This rare, usually asymptomatic, sometimes pruritic infection is seen with increasing frequency because of AIDS and the increasing use of immunosuppressive drugs for certain diseases and types of transplant surgery. Because the lesions are asymptomatic and amorbid, national statistics are not kept. Typical lesions are small (2 to 5 mm), dome-shaped, waxy, flesh-colored papules with a smooth surface. Mature lesions often have a central dimple.

Diagnosis. Diagnosis is confirmed cytologically and histologically by unroofing and expressing or by curetting the waxy contents onto a slide and finding molluscum bodies—dark, intracytoplasmic inclusions within epithelial cells (Fig. 4-8).

Treatment. Treatment of choice is incision with a large needle and curettage to remove the infected cells and debris. Other therapies include liquid nitrogen, chloracetic acid, and cantharidin. Gentle electrodesiccation or laser therapy should be used with care because more than the minimal necessary surgery can cause scarring.

Folliculitis

Folliculitis may appear on the vulva, as on any hair-bearing skin surface. The initial lesion is papular and results from obstruction and infection of the hair follicle and the adjacent pilosebaceous unit. This may progress to a pustule. When fluctuant, these abscesses should be drained and a wick

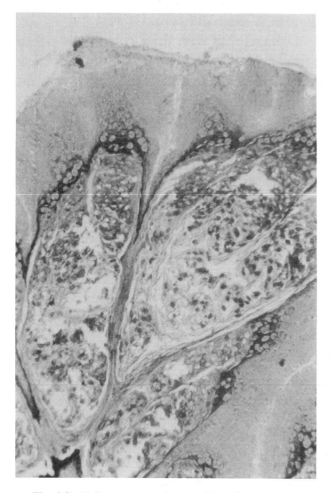

Fig. 4-8. Molluscum contagiosum with molluscum body.

placed to allow continued drainage. Surrounding erythema is common, but cellulitis is rare. Infection may be more aggressive among patients who are elderly, diabetic, irradiated, or otherwise immunosuppressed. If symptoms persist, antibodies should be instituted and inpatient management considered (Friedrich, 1983).

Necrotizing Fasciitis

Necrotizing fasciitis and the associated progressive bacterial synergistic gangrene represent the most dangerous of all vulvar infections. Necrotizing fasciitis is a rapidly progressive, often fatal infection that may develop at a site of minimal trauma or previous localized infection. Risk factors for the development of necrotizing fasciitis include diabetes mellitus, arteriosclerosis, previous vulvar surgery, irradiation, or immunosuppression (Roberts, 1987). It may also develop spontaneously in patients with neutropenia or with vulvar carcinoma (Adelson et al, 1991; Hoffman and Turnquist, 1989). The infection is polymicrobial and often is associated with anaerobic streptococcus and enterococci.

Diagnosis. In a recent study of 29 nonpregnant women with necrotizing fasciitis of the vulva, a delay in diagnosis of more than 48 hours was associated with a 78% mortality

rate. Nearly all the deaths occurred in women with diabetes or when the infections were misdiagnosed as mild labial cellulitis (Stephenson et al, 1992).

Clinical symptoms suggestive of necrotizing fasciitis include pain out of proportion to the clinical findings. Signs include pallor and edema of the overlying skin, paresthesia, anesthesia, and crepitance. A grey "fish water" discharge may also be noted. Finally, signs of sepsis, including hypotension, become apparent.

Treatment. Treatment must be aggressive and must include fluid resuscitation, arterial and pulmonary artery monitoring, rapid institution of broad-spectrum antibiotics, and immediate surgical debridement. It is not unusual to remove enormous areas of damaged soft tissue from the vulva, medial thigh, and anterior abdominal wall. Pink, bleeding tissue indicates an adequate surgical margin. Frozen-section analysis of margins may help to guide the limits of resection. Debrided areas should be packed, not closed, to allow for the inevitable secondary debridement procedures. If the process extends to the endopelvic fascia, the prognosis is grim.

Hidradenitis Suppurativa

Hidradenitis suppurativa is an infection resulting from mixtures of *Staphylococcus, Streptococcus,* and occasionally coliform organisms. The disease results from plugging of the sweat glands by keratin, subsequent rupture, and secondary infection with abscess formation, ultimately leading to the development of fistulous tracts. It is not seen before puberty. The disease primarily affects the labia majora and intercrural folds, occasionally the mons, and rarely the clitoris or labia minora. Because of the cyclic nature of the disease in the early stages, it may respond favorably to the use of intermittent oral estrogens or cyclic oral contraceptives. Once the disease progresses to the suppurative phase, multiple abscesses form. These abscesses can drain spontaneously or be drained surgically. Chronic drainage leads to deep scarring. The treatment of choice is wide surgical excision that spares the labia minora, the clitoris, and the prepuce, and the next is skin grafting (Bhaha, 1984).

Fox-Fordyce Disease

Fox-Fordyce disease is also papular, limited to the sweat glands, and develops secondary to plugging. It is thought that subsequent extravasation of sweat into the epidermal tissue results in the intense pruritus that accompanies the lesion. The axilla may be simultaneously involved with the same process, and there appears to be some relationship between pruritus and a particular time in the menstrual cycle. Treatment with cyclic oral contraceptives may be successful. Occasional relief using topical antibiotics has been reported (Feldmann, 1992).

SYSTEMIC DISEASES

Vulvar skin shares much in common with other skin and thus could merit a vulvar dermatology textbook; its unique location and sensitive nature can make it a sentinel skin site, or even a first body site, to signal a systemic or skin disease. The following common, systemic diseases affect the vulva.

Acquired Immunodeficiency Syndrome

Patients with AIDS may have a host of skin diseases that appear on the vulva. Kaposi sarcoma may be the most specific, and AIDS ulcers are likely to be genitally located (Covino and McCormack, 1990). Many infections can become florid vulvar problems: monilia, herpes, HPV, molluscum, and more. Systemic diseases that rarely appear on the vulva (such as tuberculosis) are more likely in immunosuppressed patients.

Blood Dyscrasias

Leukemia, aplastic anemia, and agranulocytosis may cause vulvar ulceration. These ulcers are deep, well-demarcated oval lesions usually covered with thin, gray membranes. They have also been found after the administration of bone marrow–depressing drugs (for example, methotrexate). Ulcers heal spontaneously after cessation of the drug. In pernicious anemia, vulvar ulceration and hyperpigmentation may be part of the general tissue hypovitaminosis and devitalization. Other blood diseases (anemias, polycythemia, dyscrasias) can be associated with nonspecific vulvar changes.

Circulatory Disturbances

The most common disturbances are edema and varicose veins. With no muscular "pump," marked edema may be found in the presence of generalized anasarcas, lymphatic obstruction, inflammation, or pelvic tumors.

Problematic varicose veins are rare outside pregnancy. Hemorrhoids and leg varicosities are especially prominent during the last trimester. Symptoms may include burning, itching, and heaviness of the vulva. Relief can come with pressure against the vulva from a sanitary napkin or foam rubber. Rest, with legs and hips elevated at or above the heart, is necessary. On rare occasion, varices may require excision. After delivery, the veins become smaller and usually asymptomatic. An angioma may occasionally produce unilateral vulvar swelling.

Diabetes

Diabetic vulvitis (usually fungal) may be the first sign of diabetes, or it may arise when known diabetes is inadequately controlled. Symptoms include acute erythema and pruritus, edema (sometimes), burning as urine strikes the inflamed vulva, and associated monilial vaginitis (frequently). Hyperkeratosis ensues with time. Red, inflamed areas appear interspersed with white opaque patches.

Control of diabetes, together with antifungal agents applied to the vagina and the vulva, provide improvement within a week. Low-potency, topical, short-term corticoids can be used, if necessary, to control severe pruritus, inflammation, and squamous hyperplasia. Meticulous care of the skin is essential.

Uremia

Late-stage renal disease may result in uremic frost of the vulva and the mouth. Labial surfaces are covered with a gray-white-brown membrane containing urea and uric acid deposits. Treatment consists of local cleansing and correction of renal failure.

Vitamin Deficiencies

In the United States, vitamin deficiencies usually result from anorexia and malabsorptive states, debility, or chronic diseases. Deficiencies of vitamins A, B (especially niacin or riboflavin), and C can cause chronic vulvitis. The skin can be dry and scaly or fissured and ulcerated. Excess vitamin A can cause erythematous, exudative dermatitis.

Autoimmune Diseases
Crohn Disease (Regional Enteritis)

Crohn disease is found primarily in the ileum. Early symptoms are low-grade fever, abdominal pain, and diarrhea. On occasion patients may seek treatment for draining sinuses or abscesses in the anogenital region. Approximately one fifth of patients have anogenital involvement, primarily of the anoperineum and rarely of the labia majora (Kim et al, 1992; Patton et al, 1990). Anogenital Crohn disease can be the terminus of a bowel fistula or it can be metastatic and have no bowel connection (Levine et al, 1982). Constitutional symptoms often include low fever, diarrhea, fatigue, and weight loss.

Diagnosis. Diagnosis is confirmed by radiologic evidence of bowel disease and communicating sinuses. Differential diagnoses include hidradenitis suppurativa, lymphogranuloma venereum, granuloma inguinale, tuberculosis, and Behçet syndrome.

Treatment. Treatment. Surgical treatment alone is usually futile; the disease may become progressively more destructive with the creation of a cloaca. Treatment of the primary disease is essential and usually requires steroids plus antibiotics and the removal of involved parts of the bowel, if necessary. Biopsy findings of the anogenital lesions reveal nonspecific, noncaseating, granulomatous change. Ulcers and sinus tracts should be debrided and cleansed frequently with a povidone-iodine solution and hydrogen peroxide. As healing progresses, wide excision of the sinus tracts may be necessary and usually provides good results.

Behçet Syndrome

This syndrome is a triad of ulcerations of buccal and vulvar epithelium and anterior uveitis. There can be multiple other manifestations, particularly arthritis and vasculitis. Ulcers are often small but deep, and they tend to come and go spontaneously.

Diagnosis. Diagnosis is made clinically by characteristic, recurrent oral and vulvar ulcers and uveitis. Differential diagnoses include herpes, syphilis, lichen planus, lupus, pemphigus, and Stevens-Johnson syndrome. Biopsy of vulvar ulcers reveals nonspecific inflammation and vasculitis.

Treatment. Treatment is careful cleansing; corticosteroids may be helpful. There have been reports (Hewett, 1971) that high estrogen oral contraceptives might help. Surgery is contraindicated unless the vulvar lesions are incapacitating.

NONNEOPLASTIC EPITHELIAL DISORDERS

In 1987 the International Society for the Study of Vulvar Disease adopted three classifications (McKay, 1991) for benign epithelial disorders: lichen sclerosus, squamous hyperplasia, and other dermatoses. Although the first two are mainly vulvar, the latter are *general skin dermatoses* and are described in the following sections.

Psoriasis

Psoriasis is an incurable, inflammatory dermatosis characterized by light red plaques covered by a silvery scale. Approximately 5 million people in the United States have it; genetic predisposition appears to be activated by trauma, infection, or stress.

Psoriasis may involve the vulva, although the more common sites are the scalp, nails, extensor surfaces of the elbows and knees, and sacrum; the face is spared. Scratching can produce characteristic signs, including the appearance of small papules in a row of microtrauma and punctate as capillaries are disrupted.

As with all scaly dermatoses, the vulvar environment makes lesions less scaly, less white, and more noticeably red. Psoriasis has periods of exacerbation and remission.

Diagnosis

Diagnosis can be made by inspection; biopsy confirms it. Microscopic evaluation reveals parakeratosis, rete peg elongation with clubbing, and microabscesses in the stratum corneum. Differential diagnoses include seborrheic or reactive dermatitis, fungi, lymphoma, vulvar intraepithelial neoplasia, and Paget disease.

Treatment

Treatment is with ultraviolet light (natural or artificial), tars, or salicylic acid (2% to 10%) ointments. Short-term, topical, fluorinated corticosteroid ointments are helpful. Long-term use of topical corticosteroids is best avoided to minimize fibrosis and atrophy. In severe cases, methotrexate can help slow the rapid cell turnover; stress relief may also help.

Seborrheic Dermatitis

Seborrheic dermatitis is a red, scaly rash appearing in areas of skin where there is a high concentration of sebaceous glands. However, it is not a disease of the sebaceous glands. The skin appears oily and has a white-yellow-red tinge, and greasy-looking plaques may occur. Common sites include the scalp (dandruff is often the initial sign), central face and trunk, and various folds (including behind the ears and the

groin). The labia majora, mons, and perianus are rarer sites and are sometimes pruritic.

Diagnosis

Diagnosis is by appearance, distribution, and elimination (for example, negative findings on a potassium hydroxide slide). Histology is nonspecific, and biopsy is not usually necessary. Differential diagnoses include psoriasis, fungi, reactive dermatitis, squamous hyperplasia, and Paget disease. Asymmetry of this lesion is the exception, and, if that appears, an alternative diagnosis should be considered.

Treatment

The disease is incurable, but it may be ameliorated with good hygiene, Burow's solution, and topical steroids. Topicals are best applied after a bath or a shower, when the keratin has softened. Ketoconazole can improve the condition because of the association with *Pityrosporum* species.

Lichen Planus

Lichen planus is inflammatory dermatosis of unknown origin. It is characterized by multiple, small, purple, polygonal papules that are shiny, not scaly. There are usually associated lesions elsewhere on the body, especially flexor surfaces (wrists, ankles, and thighs). Lesions on internal sites (mouth, medial vulva, vagina), which are usually involved, are white and lacy. Lichen planus can produce inflamed, erosive vaginitis.

Diagnosis

Diagnosis is based on the biopsy specimen, which shows hyperkeratosis, absence of parakeratosis, saw-toothed rete pegs, and a characteristic band of chronic inflammatory cells in the upper dermis (Fig. 4-9). There seems to be some relation to an autoimmune cell–mediated response because the

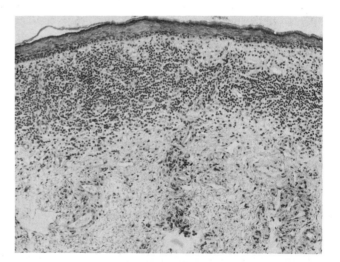

Fig. 4-9. Lichen planus.

disease is common among patients who have had bone marrow transplants with graft-versus-host reaction.

Differential diagnoses are psoriasis, vulvar intraepithelial neoplasia, and Kaposi sarcoma.

Treatment

Treatment with topical steroids and retin-A relieves pruritus and cutaneous lesions. Vulvovaginal lesions are often refractory; vaginal stenosis and atrophy can ensue.

Reactive Dermatitis

Dermatitis may be caused by direct contact with any laundry material, deodorant, toilet paper additives, feminine hygiene product, local contraceptives, or skin allergens such as poison ivy and nail polish. A careful history that includes exposure to these and the appropriate chronology is crucial. Contact dermatitis is confluent at the contact site.

The vulva can also be vulnerable to ingested allergens. Although they may respond, other skin sites may be less sensitive. Most times the initial reaction is pruritus. After that the reactions are erythema and edema, which can become vesicular, and then ulcerations and weeping when the reaction is severe. Later hyperkeratotic, scaly whitening can ensue.

Diagnosis

Diagnosis can be difficult when an irritant, allergen, or other disease (psoriasis, seborrheic dermatitis, fungi, squamous hyperplasia) is not obvious. The reaction may not be to the main substance but to its vehicle, preservative, or other ingredient. Marren et al (1992) conducted patch testing with 78 possible allergens but seldom found it to be of significant help.

Treatment

Treatment includes elimination of the offending agent. During the acute phase, the application of cool Burow's compresses, ice, corticosteroid cream, antihistamine, and short-term antipruritics (hydroxyzine) are helpful.

Vulvar Dermatoses
Lichen Sclerosus

Lichen sclerosus is an atrophic change that usually occurs in postmenopausal women. The main symptom, if any, is pruritus. It can appear in children but remits after the menarche. The skin thins to a dry, shiny, fragile, finely wrinkled, parchmentlike appearance, and the external genitalia contract and lose their shape and definition. White patches fuse into a symmetric keyhole pattern, often encompassing the perianus (Fig. 4-10). Telangiectasia and midline skin splits are common. Histologically, the epidermis is thin with flattened rete pegs (Fig. 4-11). The dermis is edematous and hyalinized and has lost elastic fibers. There is a chronic inflammatory infiltrate in the lower dermis (Pincus and McKay, 1993).

Autoimmunity may play a role in the development of lichen sclerosus. Patients with lichen sclerosus have an in-

creased incidence of autoimmune antibodies and diseases; the main mechanism, however, may be testosterone deficiency or dysfunction. The principal trophic hormone for the ectoderm-derived skin is testosterone (for the Müllerian-derived epithelium, it is estrogen). Friedrich and Kalra (1984) suggest that reduced 5α-reductase activity, the enzyme that converts free testosterone to the more potent dihydrotestosterone, may contribute to the development of lichen sclerosus.

In older women there is an association between lichen sclerosus and invasive cancer (Crum, 1992; Leibowitch et al, 1990). Lynch (1987) estimates that invasive cancer develops in 4% of patients with lichen sclerosus, a tenfold increased risk. Whether lichen sclerosus plays an etiologic role in carcinogenesis is unknown.

Diagnosis. Diagnosis can be made by inspection, but biopsy is confirmatory and will determine whether there

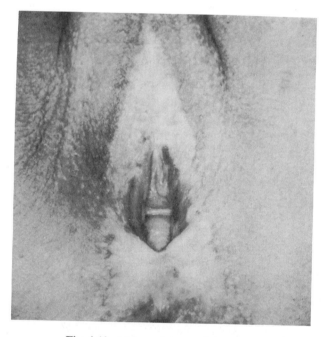

Fig. 4-10. Lichen sclerosus of the vulva.

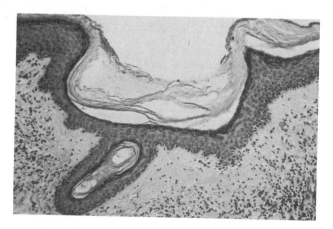

Fig. 4-11. Histologic appearance of lichen sclerosus.

is a hyperplastic or a neoplastic component that influences treatment.

Treatment. Treatment is replacement of the deficient hormone. Testosterone propionate (2%) in petrolatum should be applied twice daily until the condition is in remission, which may not occur until after several months of use. Maintenance therapy (twice weekly) is needed indefinitely. Androgenic side effects, such as clitoral hypertrophy, increased libido, and hirsutism, merit surveillance and adjustment of dosage. Estrogen is not helpful. If pruritus is severe, it is best controlled with corticoid cream. This should be used only briefly because it compounds the atrophy.

Squamous Hyperplasia

Squamous hyperplasia is a chronic reactive disorder to problems such as chronic fungal vulvitis (with or without diabetes), allergies, or unknown stimuli. Pruritus and the chronic trauma of scratching play an important role in the development.

Diagnosis. Diagnosis begins by searching for any initiating factor(s). Inflammation (Fig. 4-12), often whitening, excoriation, increased skin markings, and lichenification are present (Lynch, 1987). There are nonspecific histologic changes of hyperkeratosis, lengthening of rete pegs, and chronic inflammation (Fig. 4-13).

Differential diagnoses are lichen sclerosus, psoriasis, seborrheic dermatitis, vitiligo, tinea, and vulvar intraepithelial neoplasia. Biopsy is essential to rule out the latter.

Treatment. Treatment is most effective if an inciting cause can be found and corrected. Additional nonspecific therapy begins with potent, fluorinated corticoids (for 6 weeks or less) to relieve pruritus and to reduce the hyperplasia. After symptoms are relieved, nonfluorinated corticoids of lower potency should be substituted while the dosage is tapered as indicated. General hygiene and antipruritic medicines to break the itch-scratch cycle are needed. Red lesions brought on by psoriasis, seborrheic dermatitis, and fungi become thicker, more scaly, and whiter on the lateral vulva.

Purple lesions are indicative of lichen planus, Kaposi sarcoma, and hemangiomas. *Dark* lesions are rare in black women; in white women, 10% to 12% of gynecology patients have "dark" lesions (Rock, 1992). Forty percent of these lesions are lentigines, 20% are nevi, and 10% are vulvar intraepithelial neoplasia.

ULCERS

Ulcers may form from neoplastic processes, chronic infections, or trauma, including scratching. One third of carcinomas ulcerate (Friedrich, 1983). Cytology, colposcopy, and biopsy, especially of persistent lesions, are helpful in the diagnosis. Because ulcers do not have keratinized surfaces, smears can be particularly useful with chancroid, herpes, syphilis (dark field), granuloma inguinale, and neoplasia. Biopsy may lead to the diagnosis of rare tumors, such as basal cell carcinoma, granular cell myoblastoma, or hidradenoma (Friedrich, 1983).

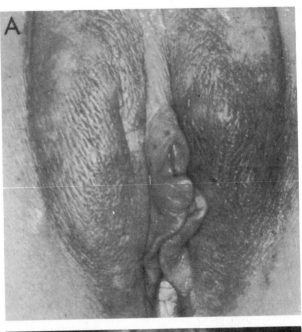

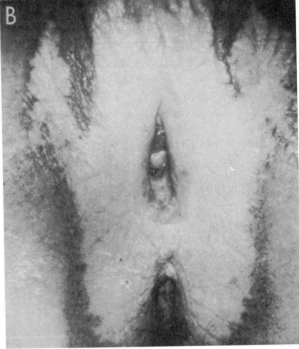

Fig. 4-12. Squamous hyperplasia. **A,** Edema and lichenification of early stage. **B,** Area under the secretory cylindrical cells.

Kraus (1990) emphasizes that infectious ulcers are secondary lesions. They follow *vesicles* (herpes), *papules* (syphilis, chancroid, granuloma inguinale, LGV), or *pustules* (folliculitis). Therefore, the patient's history just before ulceration, report of self-examination (preferably with a photograph), or early professional inspection are all diagnostically helpful. Ulcers from AIDS have been described, as has the increased susceptibility to other ulcerative infections. Rarely is a syndrome such as Behcet's the cause. Soli-

1. Conduct a brief history taking and physical examination. If a vulvar lesion is present, vulvoscopy should be performed and a biopsy should be obtained. If no lesion is present, rule out local infections (vulvovaginitis).
2. If no infectious agent is identified, a comprehensive history and physical examination are mandated. Pruritus may result from diabetes mellitus, renal or hepatobiliary disease, gout, nutritional deficiency, or allergies.
3. If no systemic or localized disease processes are identified, consider psychosexual or psychiatric disorders. In particular, consider the possibility of past or ongoing sexual abuse.

Treatment

The first step in the treatment of vulvar pruritus is to break the itch-scratch cycle (Fischer, 1995). Chronic trauma associated with scratching produces a hyperplastic dermatopathologic lesion that is pruritic. Topical corticoids or a systemic antipruritic such as hydroxyzine or amitriptyline, particularly at bedtime, can be effective. General vulvar hygiene and cool compresses may also help. Topical lidocaine offers only transient relief and may cause a local burning sensation before anesthesia is induced. Denervating procedures, such as local ethanol injections, are not recommended.

Vulvar Vestibulitis

Vulvar vestibulitis is characterized by tenderness and erythema of the vestibule. The only consistent histologic finding is that of chronic inflammation (Pyka, 1988). Despite the use of special stains and cultures, no specific organisms have been identified. In addition, there is no histologic evidence of allergic reaction.

Treatment is ill defined. Antibiotics, corticoids, retinoids, chloracetic acid, 5-FU, and laser therapy have all proven ineffective. Spontaneous remissions may occur in as many as 50% of patients. Vestibulectomy, particular complete resection of the vulvar skin, improves symptoms in some patients, but there are substantial risks of scarring, introital narrowing, and dyspareunia (Mann, 1992).

TUMORS AND BENIGN GROWTHS
Vulvar Tumors

Benign vulvar tumors may be cystic or solid. Cystic tumors include Bartholin's duct cyst or abscess, hydrocele, or hernia. Conditions such as endometriosis may also give rise to vulvar masses. The most common solid tumors of the vulva include lipomas, fibromas, and hidradenomas. Less common tumors include lymphangiomas, hemangiomas, and myxomas. Although these tumors are benign, they may achieve significant size and cause disability.

Bartholin's Cyst and Abscess

The Bartholin's gland undergoes cystic dilation when it becomes obstructed as a result of chronic inflammation. It is uncommon for a Bartholin's cyst to cause significant

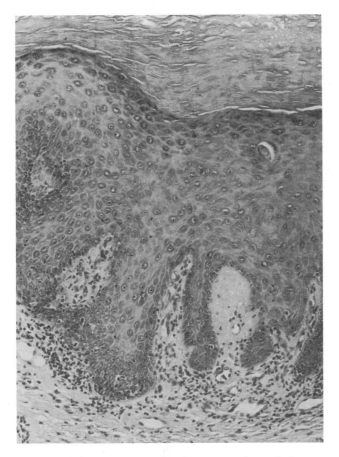

Fig. 4-13. Histologic changes in squamous hyperplasia.

tary ulcers suggest neoplasia, syphilis, and LGV. Multiple ulcers suggest herpes, chancroid, and granuloma inguinale (trauma or allergy). Pain and tenderness suggest herpes and chancroid. Nontender ulcers suggest neoplasia, syphilis, granuloma inguinale, and LGV.

VULVAR PRURITUS, VULVODYNIA, AND VESTIBULITIS

Vulvar pain and itching are among the most common gynecologic complaints. Vulvodynia is estimated to affect approximately 200,000 women in the United States (Brody, 1993; Paavonen, 1995). Unfortunately, little is known about these chronic disabling syndromes. As in most multifactorial syndromes, a diagnosis is established only through the exclusion of infections and neoplastic and traumatic causes. Chronic vulvar discomfort may be a somatic manifestation of psychosexual or psychiatric disorders (Pincus, 1992; McKay, 1992). A methodical approach to diagnosis and treatment is most likely to result in clinical improvement.

Pruritus Syndrome

Itching may be associated with nearly all the conditions listed in this chapter. An orderly diagnostic approach should include these steps:

symptoms. It becomes painful when an abscess develops, but it requires drainage only if it impairs walking or intercourse. Infection tends to be polymicrobial, and there is gonococcal involvement 20% to 30% of the time (Woodruff, 1987). Rapid amelioration of symptoms results from any abscess incision and drainage procedure (usually under local anesthesia). Every attempt should be made to incise the abscess at or behind the hymenal ring. This prevents vulvar scarring and allows packing or catheter placement within the vagina, where it is far more controllable. Placement of a WORD catheter through a 6-mm, Keyes-punched hole allows for thorough drainage and for the formation of an epithelialized tract for additional cyst or duct drainage. This tiny, balloon-tipped device can be placed in the abscess cavity; the tip is then inflated with saline. The catheter is left in for 3 weeks and is removed in an outpatient setting. Such a device is particularly suited for recurrent Bartholin's abscesses.

For recalcitrant abscesses not responsive to catheter drainage, marsupialization may be performed by surgically creating a large fenestration in the gland behind the hymenal ring. The edges of this opening are sutured to the skin to maintain patency. With the widespread use of the WORD catheter, marsupialization rarely is required.

Vaginal dryness or dyspareunia are uncommon results of chronic Bartholin's abscesses and loss of lubrication. If a scar or a mass exists after the acute infection has subsided, it may be necessary to excise the entire gland. This procedure involves dissection deep within the vulva close to the pudendal vessels and venous plexi of the vestibular bulb. Significant blood loss is possible. Finally, abscess formation in the postmenopausal patient may be secondary to malignancy. A biopsy of the cyst wall or cyst excision is recommended in these patients.

Hernia of the Canal of Nuck

The round ligament, the anlage of the gubernaculum in the male, leaves the pelvis through the canal of Nuck and terminates in the apex of the labia majora. The ligament carries its peritoneal investments through the external inguinal ring. Hydroceles, cysts, and hernias may form along this tract and resemble cystic vulvar tumors. Although sometimes confused with Bartholin's cysts, these cystic tumors are more anterior within the labia majora and are often bilateral. Bartholin's cysts tend to split the labia minora and are unilateral. This difference in anatomic location has practical implications—attempting to incise and drain a hernia sac may lead to bowel injury. Drainage of a hydrocele or cyst inevitably is ineffective. Hernia repair in the canal of Nuck includes dissection of the hernia sac, high ligation, and reinforcement of the external inguinal ring.

Endometriosis

Implants of endometriosis may occur along the canal of Nuck, in the labia, or at the site of previous episiotomy scars or other surgery. These lesions may be cystic or partially

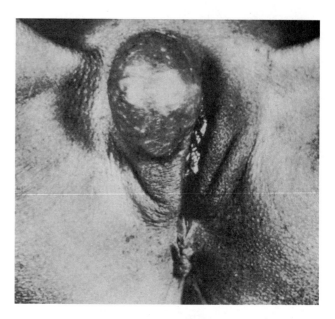

Fig. 4-14. Vulvar hidradenoma.

solid. Inflammatory changes may be cyclic. Treatment is surgical excision and either medical or surgical management of the underlying disorder.

Lipoma

A lipoma is a benign tumor that arises from the fatty tissue of the labia majora or the mons veneris, and it usually grows slowly. It causes no symptoms unless its size is excessive. When this occurs, the mass acquires a pedicle and hangs from the groin or vulva as a pendulum. If the pedicle is wide, it may resemble a hernia. Some lipomas become gigantic, but usually they are no larger than 10 to 12 cm. Liposarcomas are rare. Nevertheless, the lesion should be excised because difficulty in walking or coitus will eventually occur.

Fibroma

A fibroma is a lesion that usually develops as a firm nodule on the labia majora, which then enlarges and develops a pedicle that may hang down for several inches (or feet). Ulceration and necrosis of the distal portion may occur. The circumscription of the lesion and the absence of mitotic figures and giant cells are usually sufficient to indicate benignity. These lesions should be removed mainly for cosmetic effect.

Hidradenoma

A hidradenoma is a benign, slow-growing, sweat gland tumor, whose histology simulates that of an adenocarcinoma. It usually measures 1 to 2 cm in diameter, and it has a slightly raised, brown surface that may be umbilicated (Fig. 4-14). The lesion may become large, and cystic changes may occur. Histologically, this is an adenoma of the vulvar apocrine glands. It is not connected with the epider-

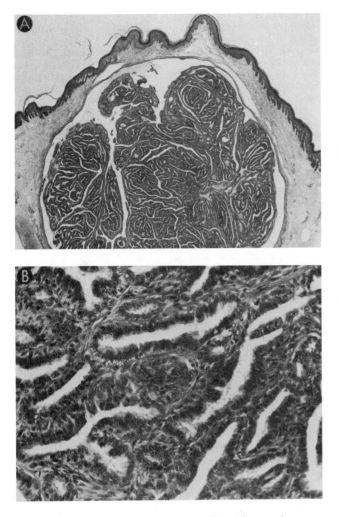

Fig. 4-15. Hidradenoma. **A,** Low-power photomicrograph. **B,** High-power photomicrograph showing myoepithelial cells under the secretory cylindrical cells.

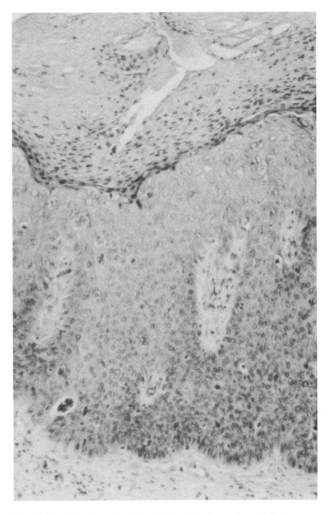

Fig. 4-16. Carcinoma in situ of the vulva beneath a thick, hyperkeratotic patch.

mis and is usually well encapsulated. This lesion is almost always benign, but because a few hidradenocarcinomas have been reported, all should be excised and submitted for biopsy (Fig. 4-15).

VULVAR INTRAEPITHELIAL NEOPLASIA

Vulvar intraepithelial neoplasia is diagnosed more often now than it was in the past, and it is appearing in younger women. Although the mean age of invasive vulvar carcinoma has remained stable (early 60s), the mean age of patients with vulvar carcinoma in situ has dropped from 53 to 42 years in the past 30 years (Woodruff, 1991).

The natural history of vulvar neoplasia is not as well known as is that of the cervix. The mean age of patients with vulvar carcinoma in situ is 20 years younger than it is for those with invasion. Progression to invasion may occur at any time; hence, prompt diagnosis and treatment are mandated.

Etiology

Vulvar intraepithelial neoplasia (VIN) is a dichotomous disease (Crum, 1992). In young women, it is invariably associated with HPV 16, and to a lesser extent HPV 18 and 31. This disease often occurs in multifocal sites on the vulva, and it may occur in conjunction with vaginal and cervical squamous neoplasias. In older women, VIN often is unifocal and less commonly associated with HPV. Immunosuppression and cigarette smoking are risks for progression to invasive disease (Daling, 1992).

Diagnosis

The diagnosis of VIN is made by directed biopsy (Figs. 4-16, 4-17). Any symptomatic vulvar lesion should undergo immediate biopsy; however, nearly 20% of patients with VIN have no symptoms at all (Bernstein, 1983). Careful inspection of the vulva during the pelvic examination is required to detect the sometimes subtle color changes associated with this disease. Vulvar colposcopy after a 5-minute soak with

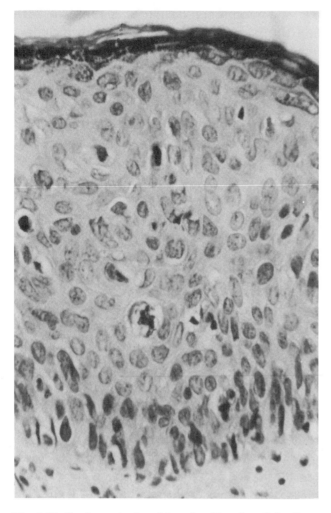

Fig. 4-17. Carcinoma in situ of the vulva. Note the cellular disarray, abnormal mitoses, and dyskeratosis.

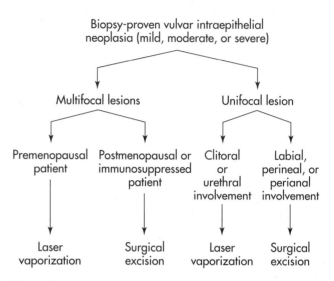

Fig. 4-18. Algorithm for the treatment of vulvar intraepithelial neoplasia.

5% acetic acid can be helpful (Iverson, 1981). A 4-mm Keyes punch biopsy device is ideal for directed vulvar biopsies.

Treatment

The mainstay of therapy for VIN is surgery, whether it be excisional or ablative. The choice of treatment is based on the topography of the lesion, the focality of the lesion, and the underlying risk for coexisting invasive cancer (Fig. 4-18). Young women often have multifocal disease in association with multiple lower genital tract sites. Preservation of normal vulvar anatomy is of paramount importance. In addition, unless the patient is immunosuppressed, the likelihood of coexisting invasive cancer is low. Laser vaporization is an ideal treatment because it allows for highly tailored treatment with minimal scar formation. There is substantial pain after surgery, however, and care of the surgical sites is critical to prevent secondary infections.

Unifocal lesions with a higher risk for coexisting invasive cancer are more likely to develop in older women. They should be excised whenever possible to ensure adequate sampling. When they are confined to the labia, the procedures are quick and healing is rapid. There is substantially less pain and disability than with laser treatments. However, because full-thickness skin is removed, the vulvar anatomy is disturbed.

Treatment of the periclitoral, urethral, and perineal areas is particularly difficult, and some patients have protracted severe pain, dyspareunia, and loss of sensation. Only in extreme, refractory VIN is skinning vulvectomy with reconstruction required. Prophylactic 5-FU therapy may help prevent recurrent VIN in recalcitrant cases (Krebs, 1986; Reid, 1990).

MALIGNANT NEOPLASMS

Malignant neoplasms of the vulva are uncommon and represent 5% of all malignancies of the female genital tract. Ninety percent of cancers are squamous, arising on the labia majora, minora, or vestibule. Less often, adenocarcinomas may arise in adnexal structures, Bartholin's glands, and even ectopic breast tissue. The vulva may develop skin malignancies, including melanoma, basal cell carcinoma, and Paget disease.

Squamous Cell Carcinoma
Epidemiology

Squamous cell carcinoma is a disease of postmenopausal women (mean age, 61.1 years). Unlike the incidence of vulvar intraepithelial neoplasia, which has doubled, the incidence of invasive carcinoma has remained constant. It may be that women with VIN are not yet old enough for invasive lesions to develop, and the incidence may rise over the next decade. Alternatively, aggressive therapy currently used for vulvar intraepithelial neoplasia lesions may prevent invasion; however, vulvar intraepithelial neoplasia may not represent a continuum to invasion (Brinton et al, 1990).

Risk factors for the development of invasive squamous cancer include chronic inflammatory diseases of the vulva, such as some vulvar dystrophies, poor hygiene, and age greater than 70 years. Risk factors commonly associated with cervical cancer— including number of sexual partners, abnormal results on Papanicolaou smear, anogenital HPV or neoplasm, smoking, and immunosuppression—increase the risk for invasive vulvar cancer (Daling, 1992).

Mode of Spread

The mode of cancer spread is important to consider in designing diagnostic and therapeutic approaches. Cancers may spread by direct extension, implantation, and lymphatic or vascular dissemination. Squamous cancers of the vulva spread predominantly by direct extension and lymphatic dissemination. Therefore, knowing the lymphatic drainage of the vulva is crucial to understanding the biologic behavior of the tumor and the rationale for therapy.

Lymphatics from the external genitalia, including the labia, vestibule, and lower vagina, drain to the superficial inguinal lymph nodes. These nodes are located in the femoral triangle defined superiorly by the inguinal ligament, medially by the adductor longus, and laterally by the sartorius muscle. Clustered around the superficial saphenous vein, the nodes then drain to the deep or femoral nodes. The most superior deep femoral node, lying just beneath the inguinal ligament, is Cloquet's node. At one time Cloquet's node was thought to be a sentinel node, which, when positive, necessitated the removal of the pelvic lymph nodes. With the introduction of pelvic radiotherapy, pelvic lymph node dissection for carcinoma of the vulva became less necessary, and the clinical importance of Cloquet's node has been diminished.

The deep femoral nodes ultimately drain to the external iliac, common iliac, and aortic nodal groups. Although some lymphatic channels from the clitoris have been shown to drain directly to the deep femoral nodes, the clinical significance of these anatomic findings is unclear.

Classification and Staging

The current system for staging squamous cell carcinoma of the vulva is based on a surgical staging system. Staging reflects the known biologic behavior of the disease, its pattern of growth, and new prognostic variables, including the number and location of involved lymph nodes (Table 4-1). Determination of an accurate surgical stage is of great value in prognosis, therapy, and uniform reporting of data.

Histologic Grade

Squamous carcinoma tumors of the vulva are generally well differentiated to moderately differentiated (Fig. 4-19). The degree of differentiation is important in predicting biologic behavior of the tumors. Well-differentiated tumors are characterized by minimal cytologic atypia and a tendency

Table 4-1   FIGO Staging for Carcinoma of the Vulva

Stage 0	Tis	Carcinoma in situ, intraepithelial carcinoma
Stage I	T1 N0 M0	Tumor confined to the vulva or perineum; less than or equal to 2 cm in greatest dimension; nodes are not palpable
Stage II	T2 N0 M0	Tumor confined to the vulva or perineum; more than 2 cm in greatest dimension; nodes are not palpable
Stage III	T3 N0 M0 T3 N0 M0 T1 N1 M0 T2 N1 M0	Tumor of any size with: adjacent spread to the lower urethra, vagina, anus and/or unilateral regional lymph node metastasis
Stage IVA	T1 N2 M0 T1 N2 M0 T3 N2 M0 T4 any N M0	Tumor invades upper urethra, bladder mucosa, rectal mucosa, or pelvic bone with or without bilateral regional node metastasis
Stage IVB	Any T Any N, M1	Any distant metastasis, including pelvic lymph nodes

From American Joint Committee on Cancer: *Manual for staging cancer,* ed 4, Chicago, 1992, The Committee.

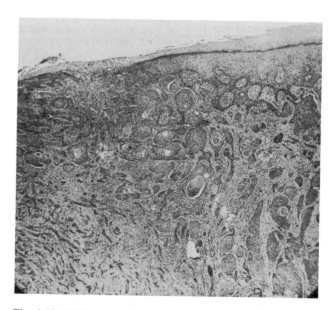

Fig. 4-19. High-power photomicrograph of carcinoma of the vulva. (Courtesy Armed Forces Institute of Pathology, no. 70121.)

toward keratinization. Often, these tumors form epithelial "pearls" that are composed of concentric layers of squamous cells. In contrast, undifferentiated cells are characterized by scant cytoplasm and marked nuclear pleomorphism. Such anaplastic cells are often seen deeply invading the underlying stroma in smears or clusters. There are multiple bizarre mitotic figures and a lack of keratin.

The grade of squamous cancers is defined by the ratio of differentiated and undifferentiated regions within the tumor. Grade 1, or well-differentiated tumors, show no regions of undifferentiation, whereas grade 3 tumors are composed of greater than 50% undifferentiated cells. Squamous cancer grade is a strong predictor of biologic behavior. Increasing dedifferentiation comes with an increasing tendency for deep invasion, lymphatic or vascular space involvement, and regional nodal spread.

Treatment

Squamous carcinoma of the vulva is generally a local malignancy with a predilection for sequential nodal involvement. Distant metastases are uncommon in the absence of advanced local disease. Since the introduction of radical vulvectomy and inguinal lymphadenectomy by Taussig in 1940, the radical surgical approach has often been successful (Heaps et al, 1990; Taussig, 1940; Way, 1960).

As more knowledge of the factors affecting outcome has been obtained, there has been an evolution toward surgery that is more tailored. For appropriately selected patients, this offers a less mutilating, less morbid, but equally effective result. When first described by Taussig, the vulva was removed in continuity with inguinal and femoral nodal tissue. To eliminate the possibility of leaving lymphatic metastases between vulva and groin, the intervening skin bridges were removed, resulting in a butterfly-shaped skin defect. Understanding that the mode of metastatic spread was embolic rather than by contiguous growth allowed for the development of the three-incision technique, which dramatically reduced overall morbidity and had no impact on recurrence or survival (Hacker et al, 1981).

Recently, the radical vulvectomy has been modified further for patients with small, lateral lesions. Radical, wide local excision combined with ipsilateral, superficial inguinal lymphadenectomy now appears appropriate in selected patients.

Treatment Based on Stage

Early-stage disease: For patients with small (less than 2 cm) lateral lesions, a radical wide local excision with ipsilateral groin node dissection is an appropriate initial procedure. If a positive node is detected at the time of frozen section of the ipsilateral nodes, the contralateral inguinal nodes must be explored (Burke et al, 1990). If surgical margins on the vulva are within 1 cm, or two or more inguinal nodes are positive for metastasis, adjuvant radiotherapy to the vulva, pelvic nodes, or inguinal nodes may be required (Thomas et al, 1987).

For patients with early but centrally located lesions, three-incision radical vulvectomy is preferred. Once again, adjuvant radiotherapy may be required for close vulvar margins or multiple positive inguinal nodes.

Management of Advanced Vulvar Cancer

For patients with advanced vulvar lesions involving the urethra, anal sphincter, or vagina, a primary surgical approach would involve an extensive resection or possible exenteration. An alternative is to use local radiotherapy or a combination of chemotherapy and radiation. Such neoadjuvant chemoradiation therapy has been shown to reduce tumor bulk dramatically and to allow for more limited surgical resection (Perez et al, 1987). A similar strategy may be used for patients with fixed inguinal lymph nodes.

Treatment of Microinvasive Carcinoma of the Vulva

There is a subset of vulvar carcinomas with virtually no risk for nodal spread. Such microinvasive lesions can be managed in a nonradical way. Microinvasive lesions were initially defined as those demonstrating less than 5 mm of invasion. Given that 50% of all vulvar cancers are less than 5 mm thick and that 20% of these metastasize, such a definition is inappropriate.

A Gynecologic Oncology Group study (Sedlis et al, 1987) better defined the term *microinvasive vulvar cancer*. That definition bases it not only on the thickness of the primary lesion but also on its size, degree of differentiation, location, presence of vascular space involvement, and clinical status of regional lymph nodes.

It is now clear that well-differentiated squamous cell tumors less than 1 mm in thickness and distant from the clitoris or perineum have virtually no risk for metastasis to the ipsilateral groin nodes. This is particularly true in the absence of lymphatic or vascular space involvement or of clinically palpable lymph nodes. It is, therefore, appropriate to offer wide local excision without lymphadenectomy to this subset of patients with vulvar cancer (Sedlis et al, 1987).

PAGET DISEASE

Since it was first described in 1895, the origin, biologic behavior, and optimal management of Paget disease of the vulva have remained controversial (Dubrieuilh, 1901). Unlike Paget disease of the breast, a cutaneous manifestation of underlying ductal carcinoma, vulvar Paget is associated with underlying carcinoma only 25% of the time. This suggests a different natural history and malignant potential for vulvar Paget when it is compared with breast or other extramammary sites in which the association with underlying carcinoma is high (Sitakalin et al, 1985).

Paget cells may develop from an intraepithelial site, such as apocrine cells (Mazoujin, 1984). Results of recent immunocytochemistry studies using a panel of monoclonal antibodies specific for cytokeratins have added support to this hypothesis (Bacchi et al, 1997). An apocrine cell of origin is consistent with the observation that Paget disease is often multicentric and multifocal (Taylor, 1975).

Invasive adenocarcinomas associated with Paget disease may occur within, beneath, or distant from the epithelial lesion. There may be a coexisting underlying adenocarcinoma of the vulva, and there are usually contiguous adnexal carcinomas that may be palpable beneath the epithelial changes. Carcinoma may develop distant from the site of the intraepithelial lesion, such as carcinoma of the breast, cervix, colon, or skin (Fauer, 1990). Paget cells rarely invade directly from the intraepithelial site, but metastatic Paget disease may develop up to 10.8 years after local resection (Hart and Millman, 1977).

Paget disease accounts for less than 1% of vulvar malignancies. It is most often a disease of the seventh decade of life, characterized by red raised lesions that are often dotted with pale white "islands" of epithelium. Lesions may occur at any site on the vulva or perineum. Extension to the mons or thigh has been reported. Paget is a difficult disease to eradicate because of its propensity to recur despite free excisional margins.

As with any other vulvar lesion, directed biopsy, either excisional or with Keyes punch, is mandatory to establish the diagnosis (Fig. 4-20). Once the diagnosis is confirmed, management of the disease must take into account the risk for malignancy within, beneath, or distant from the Paget lesion. Papanicolaou smear, breast examination, and mammography are all critical elements of the preoperative evaluation. A wide local excision of the lesion, including 0.5 to 1 cm of underlying fat, should be performed if no vulvar mass is present. Any mass beneath the lesion should be fully excised and submitted for histopathologic evaluation to rule out an underlying malignancy.

Frozen sections of the surgical resection margins should be obtained. Although the margins of the Paget lesion may appear clear, Pagetoid cells often extend beyond the margin of the resection. Negative resection margins (wide and deep)

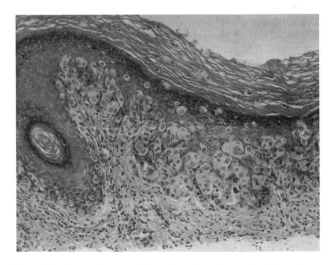

Fig. 4-20. Paget disease of the vulva, showing marked hyperkeratosis and parakeratosis. Large, irregular cells are seen in the basal layer of the epidermis and infiltrating the upper layers. Paget cells contain clear, vacuolated cytoplasm and vesicular nuclei that vary in size, shape, and staining quality.

significantly reduce the risk for local recurrence. Extensive resection may necessitate skin grafting.

The role of laser ablation in Paget disease is controversial. Laser surgery is best suited for the treatment of recurrent disease in which underlying adenocarcinoma has already been ruled out by wide local excision. It may also be useful for patients in whom grossly negative but histologically positive margins extend to the paraclitoral, urethral, anal, or other sensitive areas, where delicate and precise surgical procedures are preferred (Ewing, 1991). Regardless of the treatment selected, frequent follow-up is required because of the high recurrence rate.

MELANOMA

Malignant melanoma accounts for 2% of all vulvar malignancies. The average age at diagnosis is 57 years, but melanoma may affect women as young as 20 years of age. In a recent survey in Sweden of 219 consecutive patients with malignant vulvar melanoma, 75% of the patients were older than 60. Most lesions involve the clitoris and the labia minora and are usually noticed by the patient because of enlargement of a preexisting mole or because of bleeding or pruritus.

Vulvar melanomas may display two patterns of growth, either superficial spreading or modular. Superficial spreading melanoma has a protracted intraepithelial growth phase that is followed by stromal invasion, whereas nodular melanomas involve vertical growth that results in rapid and deep invasion. Because management and prognosis are based largely on the depth of invasion, the diagnosis should be made by excisional biopsy. Microstaging of vulvar melanomas is based on the depth of skin involvement. Because of variations in vulvar skin, staging that takes into account lesion thickness correlates best with prognosis (Table 4-2).

Therapy for vulvar melanoma remains controversial largely because of the rarity of lesions and the lack of a consistent strategy. In the past, radical vulvectomy with inguinal lymphadenectomy has been used. Unfortunately, radical resection does not eliminate the risk for local recurrence, which happens 30% to 42% of the time (Ragnansson-Olding, 1993; Podratz et al, 1983). Davidson et al (1987) reviewed the outcomes of 32 patients with vulvar melanoma.

Table 4-2	Vulvar Melanoma Staging	
Level	Description	Corrected 5-Year Survival Rate (%)
I	Intraepithelial	100
II	1 mm from granular layer	100
III	1-2 mm from granular layer	40
IV	2 mm from granular layer	40
V	Into subcutaneous fat	20

They found that the 5-year survival rate, local control rate, and disease-free interval were not affected by type of surgical procedure, whether it was local resection, simple vulvectomy, or radical vulvectomy with inguinal lymphadenectomy. Confusing the issue is the fact that 5-year survival rates for melanoma do *not* equate with cure. In one series with a 10-year follow-up, 50% of patients alive at 5 years died by the tenth anniversary of their diagnoses. Based on these observations, regional lymph node sampling may yield important prognostic information but is unlikely to have an impact on survival.

A prudent recommendation is to tailor the surgical resection based on thickness of the melanoma. A radical local excision with 2-cm margins should be performed for melanomas less than or equal to 1 mm from the granular layer (Chung level 2), (Chung, 1975) and a radical local excision with 3-cm margins should be used for more deeply invasive lesions (levels 3 and 4). Superficial (level 1) lesions may be treated with simple excision. Although controversial, dissection of the regional nodes is recommended.

Carcinoma of Bartholin's Gland

Adenocarcinomas arising in Bartholin's gland are rare. A cystic mass in the lateral walls of the vestibule is far more likely to represent a benign condition than a malignancy. Bartholin's gland rarely exceeds 1 cm, and it undergoes gradual involution in women older than 30 years of age. Therefore, the occurrence of an enlarged vulvar mass in an older woman, particularly if she is postmenopausal, is worrisome. It is recommended that incision and drainage of a presumed Bartholin's cyst or cyst abscess in a postmenopausal woman be accompanied by a biopsy taken from the cyst wall.

Carcinoma of Bartholin's gland may derive from the transitional cells that line the duct or from the mucin-secreting cells of the gland itself. Mucus-secreting tumors tend to be less aggressive than transitional-cell carcinomas.

Unfortunately, Bartholin's gland carcinomas arise deep within vulvar tissue rich with lymphatic and vascular supplies, and metastasis to inguinal and pelvic lymph nodes is common. Radical hemivulvectomy, ipsilateral inguinal lymphadenectomy, and adjuvant radiotherapy to pelvic node groups are recommended.

Basal Cell Carcinoma

Despite its status as the most common tumor of the skin, vulvar basal cell carcinoma is rare. Lesions have a characteristic pearly-grey appearance with marked telangiectasis. Brown or black pigmentation may be observed, and central ulceration is not uncommon. Bilateral tumors have been reported (Stiller et al, 1993).

Basal cell carcinoma is a locally aggressive epidermal tumor that rarely metastasizes. However, it is important to examine the inguinal nodes and to resect any suspicious node. When local nodes are not suspicious, a wide local excision is adequate therapy for the primary lesion. Care in obtaining histologically negative margins will dramatically reduce the risk for local recurrence. The prognosis after complete local resection is excellent.

Sarcomas

Sarcomas may arise from any connective tissue component of the vulva. Epithelioid sarcomas, which occur in young women and may mimic Bartholin's cyst, are more aggressive when they develop on the vulva. Rapid progression and death ensue. Kaposi sarcoma tumors, associated with AIDS, are small vulvar papilloma. Regardless of the histologic type of sarcoma, radical surgery is ineffective and the prognosis is poor.

Verrucous Carcinoma

Verrucous carcinoma of the vulva affects postmenopausal women. It is a locally invasive, slow-growing tumor characterized by a cauliflower-like, or verrucoid, growth pattern. The lesion may be very large and cause severe genital itching. Histologic features include papillary bands of highly differentiated, hyperkeratotic epithelia with abrupt transitions to normal skin. Superficial biopsy specimens of these large lesions may be misleading. In this type of tumor, the fibrovascular cores that are so prominent in benign condyloma are limited to the superficial layers of the verrucous carcinoma.

Wide local excision with negative margins is appropriate if there are no clinically suspicious nodes. For patients who have recurrent disease, regional lymph node dissection is advocated. Local radiation therapy may cause anaplastic transformation of this tumor and is contraindicated. Once local control of the tumor is achieved, the prognosis is excellent.

ACKNOWLEDGMENTS

We acknowledge the legacy of this chapter from Dr. Thomas Leavitt, Jr. We are grateful to him for his advice on the current edition and for the many kind and generous hours he devoted to our training as residents and fellows, and we thank Dr. Frederick Sillman for his contributions to the previous edition. We also thank Drs. Christopher P. Crum and Harley Haynes for their expertise and help concerning the pathology and dermatology, respectively, of these diseases.

REFERENCES

Adelson MD, Miranda FR, Strumpf KB: Necrotizing fasciitis: a complication of squamous cell carcinoma of the vulva. *Gynecol Oncol* 1991; 42:98.

Andersen WA, Franquemont DW, Williams J, et al: Vulvar squamous cell carcinoma and papilloma viruses: Two separate entities? *Am J Obstet Gynecol* 1991; 165:329-335.

Arndt KA: Lichen planus. In Fitzpatrick TB, et al: *Dermatology in general medicine,* ed 4, New York, 1993, McGraw-Hill.

Bacchi CE, Goldfogel GA, Greer BE, et al: Paget's disease and melanoma of the vulva: Use of a panel of monoclonal antibodies to identify cell type and to microscopically define adequacy of surgical margins. *Gynecol Oncol* 1992; 46:216-221.

Bernstein SG, Kovacs BR, Townsend DE, et al: Vulvar carcinoma in situ. *Obstet Gynecol* 1983; 61(3):304-307.

Bhaha NN, Bergman A, Broen EM: Advanced hidradenitis suppurative of the vulva: A report of 3 cases. *J Reprod Med* 1984; 29:436.

Billstein SA: Human lice. In Holmes KK, et al: *Sexually transmitted diseases,* ed 2, New York, 1990, McGraw-Hill.

Bonnez W, Elswick RK Jr., Bailey-Fairchione A, et al: Efficacy and safety of 0.5% podofilox solution in the treatment and suppression of anogenital warts. *Am J Med* 1994; 96:420-425.

Bornstein S, Kaufman RH: Combination of surgical excision and carbon dioxide laser vaporization for multifocal vulvar intraepithelial neoplasia. *Am J Obstet Gynecol* 1988; 158:459-464.

Bornstein J, Pascal B, Abramovici HZ: The common problem of vulvar pruritus. *Obstet Gynecol Surv* 1993; 48:111-118.

Brinton LA, Nasca PC, Malin K, et al: Case-control study of cancer of the vulva. *Obstet Gynecol* 1990; 75:859-866.

Burke TW, Stringer CA, Gershensen DM, et al: Radical wide excision and selective inguinal node dissection for squamous cell carcinoma of the vulva. *Gynecol Oncol* 1990; 38:328-332.

Chung AF, Woodruff JD, Lewis JL: Malignant melanoma of the vulva; A reprint of 44 cases. *Obstet Gynecol* 1975; 45:638.

Covino JM, McCormack WM: Vulvar ulcer of unknown etiology in a human immunodeficiency virus-infected woman: Response to treatment with zidovudine. *Am J Obstet Gynecol* 1990; 163:116-118.

Cruikshank SH, McLauchlan L: A de novo case of vulvar synergistic necrotizing fasciitis. *Obstet Gynecol* 1987; 69:516.

Crum CP: Carcinoma of the vulva: Epidemiology and pathogenesis. *Obstet Gynecol* 1992; 79:448-454.

Daling JR, Sherman KJ, Hislop TG, et al: Cigarette smoking and the risk of anogenital cancer. *Am J Epidemiol* 1992; 135:180-189.

Davidson T, Kissin M, Westung G: Vulvovaginal melanoma—should radical surgery be abandoned? *Br J Obstet Gynecol* 1987; 94:473-476.

DiSaia PJ, Rutledge F, Smith JP: Sarcoma of the vulva: Report of 12 patients. *Obstet Gynecol* 1971; 38:180-184.

Dubreuilh W: Paget's disease of the vulva. *Br J Dermatol* 1901; 13:407-413.

Edwards L, Ferenczy A, Eron L: Self-administered topical 5% imiguimod cream for anogenital warts. HPV Study Group: Human papilloma virus. *Arch Dermatol* 1998; 134:25-30.

Ewing TL: Paget's disease of the vulva treated by combined surgery and laser. *Gynecol Oncol* 1991; 43:137-140.

Faro S: Lymphogranuloma venereum, chancroid, and granuloma inguinale. *Obstet Gynecol Clin North Am* 1989; 16:517-530.

Feldmann R, Masouye I, Chavas P: Fox-Fordyce disease: Successful treatment with topical clindamycin in alcoholic propylene glycol solution. *Dermatology,* 1992; 184:310.

Ferenczy A: Comparison of CO, laser ablation and loop electrosurgical excision procedure for the treatment of vulvar intraepithelial neoplasia [SGO abstract]. *Gynecol Oncol* 1992; 45:76.

Feuer GA, Shotchuk M, Calanog A: Vulvar Paget's disease—the need to exclude an invasive lesion. *Gynecol Oncol* 1990; 38:81-89.

Fischer G, Spurrett B, Fischer A: The chemically syndromatic vulva: aetiology and management. *Br J Obstet Gynaecol* 1985; 102:773-779.

Fitzpatrick TB, et al, editors: *Color atlas and synopsis of clinical dermatology,* ed 2, New York, 1992, McGraw-Hill.

Fitzpatrick TB, et al, editors: *Dermatology in general medicine,* ed 4, New York, 1993, McGraw-Hill.

Friedrich EG Jr: *Vulvar disease,* ed 2, Philadelphia, 1983, WB Saunders.

Friedrich EG Jr: Vulvar disease. In *Major problems in obstetrics and gynecology,* vol 9, ed 2, Philadelphia, 1983, WB Saunders.

Friedrich EG Jr, Kalra PS: Serum levels of sex hormones in vulvar lichen sclerosus and the effect of topical testosterone. *N Engl J Med* 1984; 310:488-491.

Gianini GD, Method MW, Christman JE: Traumatic vulvar hematomas: Assessing and treating non-obstetric patients. *Postgrad Med* 1991; 89:115.

Goetsch MF: Vulvar vestibulitis: Prevalence and historic features in a general gynecologic practice population. *Am J Obstet Gynecol* 1991; 164:1609-1614.

Hacker NF, Leuchter RS, Benek JS, et al: Radical vulvectomy and bilateral inguinal lymphadenectomy through separate groin incisions. *Obstet Gynecol* 1981; 58:574-579.

Hart W, Millman J: Progression of intraepithelial Paget's disease of the vulvar to invasive carcinoma. *Cancer* 1977; 40:2333-2337.

Heaps JM, Fu YS, Montz FJ, et al: Surgical-pathologic variables predictive of local recurrence in squamous carcinoma of the vulva. *Gynecol Oncol* 1990; 38:309-314.

Hewett AB: Behcet's disease. Alleviation of buccal and genital ulceration by an oral contraceptive agent. *Br J Vener Dis* 1971; 47(1):52-53.

Hoffman MS, Turnquist D: Necrotizing fasciitis of the vulva during chemotherapy. *Obstet Gynecol* 1989; 74:483.

Holmes KK, Sparling PF, et al: *Sexually transmitted diseases,* ed 2, New York, 1990, McGraw-Hill.

Horowitz BJ: Interferon therapy for condylomatous vulvitis. *Obstet Gynecol* 1989; 73:446-448.

Horowitz BJ: Mycotic vulvovaginitis. *Am J Obstet Gynecol* 1991; 165:1188-1192.

Iverson T, Abeler V, Kolstad P: Squamous carcinoma in situ of the vulva: A clinical and histopathologic study. *Gynecol Oncol* 1981; 11:224.

Kim NI, Eom JY, Sim WY, et al: Crohn's disease of the vulva. *J Am Acad Dermatol* 1992; 27:764-765.

Kraus SJ: Diagnosis and management of acute genital ulcers in sexually active patients. *Semin Dermatol* 1990; 9:160-166.

Krebs HB: Prophylactic topical 5-fluorouracil following treatment of human papilloma-associated lesions of the vulva and vagina. *Obstet Gynecol* 1986; 68:837-841.

Leibowitch M, Neill S, Pelisse M, et al: The epithelial changes associated with squamous cell carcinoma of the vulva: A review of the clinical, histologic, and viral findings in 78 women. *Br J Obstet Gynaecol* 1990; 97:1135-1139.

Levine EM, Barton JJ, Grier EA: Metastatic Crohn's disease of the vulva. *Obstet Gynecol* 1982; 60:395-397.

Lynch PJ: Vulvar dystrophies and intraepithelial neoplasias. *Dermatol Clin* 1987; 5:789-799.

Mandell GE, Douglas RG Jr, Bennett JE, editors: *Principles and practice of infectious diseases,* ed 3, New York, 1990, Churchill Livingstone.

Mann MS, Kaufman RH, Brown D Jr., et al: Vulvar vestibulitis: Significant clinical variables and treatment outcome. *Obstet Gynecol* 1992; 79:122-125.

Marren P, Wojnarowska F, Powell S: Allergic contact dermatitis and vulvar dermatoses. *Br J Dermatol* 1992; 126:52-56.

Mazoujian G, Pinkus GS, Mangensen DE: Extramammary Paget's disease: evidence of an apocrine origin. *Am J Surg Pathol* 1984; 8:43-50.

McKay M: Vulvitis and vulvovaginitis: Cutaneous considerations. *Am J Obstet Gynecol* 1991; 165:1176-1182.

McKay M: Vulvodynia: Diagnostic patterns. *Dermatol Clin* 1992; 10:423-433.

Morrow CP, Pisaia PJ: Malignant melanoma of the female genitalia: A clinical analysis. *Obstet Gynecol Surv* 1976; 31:233-271.

Paavonen J: Vulvodynia—a complex syndrome of vulvar pain. *Acta Obstet Gynecol Scand* 1985; 74:243-247.

Pack GT, Oropeza R: A comparative study of melanomas and epidermoid carcinomas of the vulva. *Rev Surg* 1967; 24:305-324.

Patton LW, Elgart ML, Williams CM: Extraintestinal Crohn's disease of the vulva. *Arch Dermatol* 1990; 126:1351-1354.

Perez CA, Grigsby PW, Galakatos A, et al: Radiation therapy in the management of carcinoma of the vulva with emphasis on conservative therapy. *Cancer* 1993; 71:3707-3716.

Pincus SH: Vulvar dermatoses and pruritus vulvae. *Dermatol Clin* 1992; 10:297-308.

Pincus SH, McKay M: Disorders of the female genitalia. In Fitzpatrick TB, et al, editors: *Dermatology in general medicine,* ed 4, New York, 1993, McGraw-Hill.

Plentl AA, Friedman EA: *Lymphatic system of the female genitalia,* Philadelphia, 1971, WB Saunders.

Podratz KC, Gaffey TA, Symmonds RE, et al: Melanoma of the vulva: An update. *Gynecol Oncol* 1983; 16:153-168.

Pyka RE, Wilkinson EJ, Fridrich EG Jr., et al: The histopathology of vulvar vestibulitis syndrome. *Int J Gynecol Pathol* 1988; 7:249-257.

Rader JS, Leake JF, Dillon MB: Ultrasonic surgical aspiration in the treatment of vulvar disease. *Obstet Gynecol* 1991; 77:573-576.

Ragnarsson-Olding B, Johansson H, Rutqvist LE, et al: Malignant melanoma of the vulva and vagina: Trends in incidence, age distribution, and long term survival among 245 consecutive cases in Sweden 1960-1984. *Cancer* 1993; 71:1893-1897.

Reichman RC, Bonnez W: Papillomaviruses. In Mandell GE, et al, editors: *Principles and practice of infectious diseases,* ed 3, New York, 1990, Churchill Livingstone.

Reid R: Superficial laser vulvectomy, I: The efficacy of extended superficial ablation for refractory and very extensive condylomas. *Am J Obstet Gynecol* 1985; 151:1047-1052.

Reid R: Laser surgery of the vulva. *Obstet Gynecol Clin North Am* 1991; 18:491-510.

Reid R, Greenberg MD, Lorincz AT: Superficial laser vulvectomy, IV: Extended laser vaporization and adjunctive 5-fluorouracil therapy of human papillomavirus-associated vular disease. *Obstet Gynecol* 1990; 76:439-448.

Reid R, Greenberg MD: Human papillomavirus-related diseases of the vulva. *Clin Obstet Gynecol* 1991; 34:630-650.

Roberts DB: Necrotizing fasciitis of the vulva. *Am J Obstet Gynecol* 1987; 157:568.

Rock B: Pigmented lesions of the vulva. *Dermatol Clin* 1992; 10:361-370.

Secor RM, Fertitta L: Vulvar vestibulitis syndrome. *Nurse Pract Forum* 1992; 3:161-168.

Sedlis A, Homesley H, Bundy BN, et al: Positive groin lymph nodes in superficial squamous cell vulvar cancer: A Gynecologic Oncology Group Study. *Am J Obstet Gynecol* 1987; 156:1159-1164.

Sillman FH, Sedlis A: Anogenital HPV/neoplasia in immunosuppressed women: An update. *Dermatol Clin North Am* 1991; 9:353-369.

Simonsen E, Johnsson JE, Trope C, et al: Basal cell carcinoma of the vulva. *Acta Obstet Scand* 1985; 64:231-234.

Sitakalin C, Ackerman AB: Mammary and extramammary Paget's disease. *Am J Dermatopathol* 1985; 7:340.

Soper DE, Patterson JW, Hurt WG et al: Lichen planus of the vulva. *Obstet Gynecol* 1988; 72:74-76.

Stephenson H, Dotters DJ, Katz V, et al: Necrotizing fasciitis of the vulva. *Am J Obstet Gynecol* 1992; 166:1324.

Stiller M, Klein W, Dorman R, et al: Bilateral vulvar basal cell carcinomata. *J Am Acad Dermatol* 1993; 28: 836-838.

Taussig FJ: Cancer of the vulva. *Am J Obstet Gynecol* 1940; 40:764-767.

Tayor PT, Stenwig JT, Klausen H: Paget's disease of the vulva. *Gynecol Oncol* 1975; 3:46-60.

Thomas G, Dembo A, DePetrillo A, et al: Concurrent radiation and chemotherapy in vulvar carcinoma. *Gynecol Oncol* 1987; 34:263-267.

Thomas GM, Dembo AJ, Bryson SC, et al: Changing concepts in the management of vulvar cancer. *Gynecol Oncol* 1991; 42:9-21.

Turner MLC, Marinoff SC: Pudendal neuralgia. *Am J Obstet Gynecol* 1991; 165:1233-1235.

Ulbright TM, Brokaw SA, Stehman FB, et al: Epithelioid sarcoma of the vulva. *Cancer* 1983; 52:1462-1469.

Van Cutsem J: The in vitro activity of terconazole against yeasts: its topical long-acting therapeutic efficacy in experimental vaginal candidiasis in rats. *Am J Obstet Gynecol* 1991; 165:1200-1206.

Vermesh M, Deppe G, Zbella E: Non-puerperal traumatic vulvar hematoma. *Int J Gynaecol Obstet* 1984; 22:217-219.

Way S: Carcinoma of the vulva. *Am J Obstet Gynecol* 1960; 79:692-697.

Wilkinson EJ, editor: *Pathology of the vulva and vagina,* New York, 1987, Churchill Livingstone.

Wilkinson EJ, Friedrich EG Jr: Diseases of the vulva. In Kurman RJ, editor: *Blaustein's pathology of the female genital tract,* ed 3, New York, 1987, Springer-Verlag.

Winkelmann SE, Llorens AS: Metastatic basal cell carcinoma of the vulva. *Gynecol Oncol* 1990; 38:138-140.

Woodruff JD: The vulva. In Rosenwaks Z, Benjamin F, Stone ML, editors: *Gynecology principles and practice,* New York, 1987, Macmillan.

Woodruff JD: Carcinoma in situ of the vulva. *Clin Obstet Gynecol* 1991; 34:669-676.

Woodruff JD, Friedrich EG Jr: The vestibule. *Clin Obstet Gynecol* 1991; 29:134-141.

CHAPTER

The Vagina

JOAN M. BENGTSON

KEY ISSUES

1. Dyspareunia may have either organic or functional causes, including vaginismus.
2. Vaginal malformations are often associated with upper genital tract and renal abnormalities.
3. Diethylstilbestrol-associated vaginal abnormalities include adenosis, clear cell adenocarcinoma, and structural abnormalities.
4. The vagina is a rare site of genital tract malignancy, and most lesions are metastatic.

The vagina is a fibromuscular tube that extends from the vulva to the uterine cervix. The walls of the tube are normally apposed, but they create potential space in the midpelvis to allow for coitus. The vagina is the interface between the environment and the upper generative tract.

The functions of the vagina are to provide an outflow duct for menstrual discharge, to receive the penis during intercourse, and to form the lowermost part of the birth canal. Clinically, it provides access to upper genital tract structures. Diagnostic procedures that use the vaginal space include bimanual examination of the uterus and adnexae, culdocentesis, and vaginal probe ultrasonography. Therapeutically, surgical drainage and excision of pelvic abnormalities may be performed through the vagina (Hovsepian, 1997).

Localized vaginal infections and defects of vaginal support are fairly common. However, the vagina is otherwise resistant to disease and, therefore, is easily overlooked during routine examination. Symptoms are often manifested late, even when patients have significant disease, because they may neglect routine screening, especially after menopause. Thus it is important for clinicians to remain vigilant and to incorporate careful evaluation of the vagina in the routine examination and to pursue prompt evaluation of any abnormal findings.

Clinical evaluation of the vagina is conducted through careful inspection and palpation. The patient usually assumes the dorsal lithotomy position with her feet resting in stirrups. The introitus is observed by gently separating the labia. Look for discrete mucosal lesions, evidence of bleeding, swelling, or prolapse of vaginal mucosa through the opening. A vaginal speculum is used to inspect the vault. It should be moistened with warm water and positioned by inserting the blades into the vaginal space in the anteroposterior diameter. The tip of the speculum is directed toward the sacrum. Any pressure is directed down and away from the sensitive urethral tissues. As the speculum is inserted, the handle is rotated from the lateral to the posterior position so the blade tips come to rest in the anterior and posterior fornices. The anterior and posterior walls are now retracted, allowing for inspection of the lateral walls and cervix. The anterior and posterior walls are observed by rotating the blades laterally as the speculum is withdrawn. Thus the entire surface of the vaginal cylinder is visualized.

Submucosal lesions may not be detected by visual inspection alone. The vagina should also be systematically palpated to exclude cysts, induration, urethral diverticuli, and other focal irregularities. Pelvic floor muscle tone may be assessed by having the patient contract the vaginal constrictor muscles while the examining fingers are in place. Support defects are localized after the patient bears down with a Valsalva maneuver. Finally, palpation of the rectovaginal septum and cul-de-sac of Douglas are accomplished through rectovaginal examination.

ANATOMY AND PHYSIOLOGY

Knowledge of anatomy and physiology assists in understanding the symptoms that result from diseases in the vagina and adjacent structures. Vaginal length is variable, but it usually ranges from 8 to 10 cm. In a standing position its orientation is not vertical. Rather it is directed cephalad

81

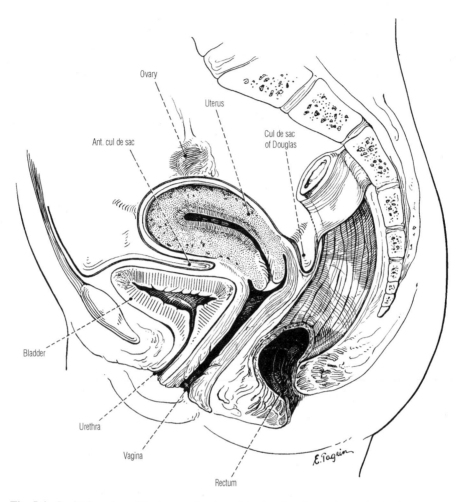

Fig. 5-1. Sagittal section of the human female pelvis showing the vagina and related structures.

and posterior toward the sacrum at approximately a 45° angle, and it rests on the perineal body (Fig. 5-1). Anteriorly the vagina is closely related to the bladder and urethra. Posteriorly it is apposed to the peritoneal cul-de-sac of Douglas at its upper third, the ampulla of the rectum at its middle third, and the perineal body at its lower third. The cul-de-sac of Douglas is clinically important in its relationship with the vagina because it provides a route of access to the peritoneal cavity. The perineal body, too, is important because it provides a central point of insertion for the supporting musculature of the urogenital diaphragm and the pelvic floor.

The vaginal mucosa is uniformly pink. If there is adequate estrogen stimulation, the inner aspect of the vaginal tube appears as multiple circumferential folds called rugae. Rugae allow for the remarkable ability of the vaginal vault to stretch. At the junction of the vagina and the vulva is the hymen. Its appearance is variable; it may form a complete membrane occluding the vagina or an incomplete membrane, or it may be cribriform. If it is ruptured, irregular fragments may persist as the carunculae hymenales.

Histologically, three layers can be distinguished in the vagina: mucous membrane, muscularis, and adventitia

(Sedlis and Robboy, 1987). The mucous membrane is a nonkeratinized, stratified, squamous epithelium (Fig. 5-2). The epithelium is several cell layers thick and is surrounded by a dense layer of fibroelastic tissue generously supplied with blood vessels and lymphatics. It functions as erectile tissue during sexual arousal. The mucosa has no glandular elements or hair follicles. In marked contrast to the nearby vulvar skin, the vagina has few sensory nerve endings and therefore is relatively asensory. Deep to the mucous membrane is the muscularis, which consists of an inner circular and an outer longitudinal layer of smooth muscle. The adventitial layer consists of dense connective tissue, nerves, and blood vessels. It is continuous with the endopelvic fascia, and the supporting connective tissue layer invests all the pelvic viscera and muscles.

Vaginal physiology depends on an appropriate hormonal and bacteriologic milieu. The vagina is a target organ for ovarian estrogen. Estrogen induces proliferation and maturation of the stratified squamous epithelium. Three cell types are seen that demonstrate progressive maturation as they are displaced upward by proliferation of the basal stratum germinativum (Blaustein, 1987). They are parabasal cells, in-

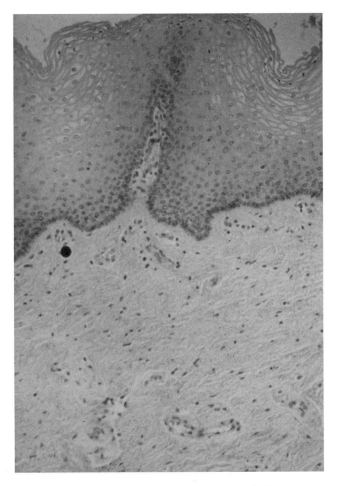

Fig. 5-2. Photomicrograph showing normal vaginal mucosa.

termediate cells, and superficial cells. A sample of vaginal epithelial cells may be studied to determine the presence of an estrogen effect. By gently scraping the lateral wall of the upper third of the vagina with a spatula, the sample can be collected, smeared thinly on a slide, fixed, and submitted for cytologic analysis. The estrogen effect is expressed as the *maturation index,* reported as the ratio of the three cell types. Estrogen stimulation results in a predominance of mature superficial cells.

A wide variety of bacteria can be cultured from the normal vagina (Larsen, 1993). Number and type depend in part on the culture medium used. *Lactobacillus* species, *Staphylococcus epidermidis*, diphtheroids, and aerobic and anaerobic streptococci are most frequently isolated. Competition for nutrients is an important mechanism that allows abnormal organisms to remain in numbers insufficient to cause clinical infection.

Estrogen also stimulates glycogen storage in the epithelium. Glycogen stored in the intermediate and the superficial cells serves as a substrate for carbohydrate metabolism by the bacterium *Lactobacillus vaginalis*. The product of fermentation is lactic acid, which maintains the low vaginal pH (normal, 3.5 to 4.5). Acidity, in turn, favors continued growth of the nonpathogenic *Lactobacillus* species and in-

hibits colonization by more virulent organisms. Disruption of the normal environment may result in infectious vaginitis. This topic is covered in detail in Chapter 18.

Atrophic Vaginitis

Atrophic vaginitis results from hypoestrogenemia. Although atrophic vaginitis typically occurs after menopause because of the absolute lack of estrogen, it may also occur during pregnancy, lactation, and other progesterone-dominant states. In the absence of estrogen stimulation, the mucous membrane is thin and subject to traumatic injury. Decreased estrogen also diminishes the collagen content of the pelvic support tissues, which may lead to support disorders (Brincat et al, 1987). Transudation across the epithelium is the primary way physiologic vaginal fluids are produced, though small amounts are also produced by cervical and vestibular gland secretions. Hormonal status and erotic stimuli influence fluid amounts and composition. Estrogen deprivation causes a decrease in blood flow to the paravaginal tissues that reduces tissue turgor and depresses production of vaginal fluids in basal and aroused states (Forsberg, 1995).

Symptoms of atrophic vaginitis include painful intercourse (dyspareunia), dryness, pruritus, and abnormal bleeding. If the urothelium is affected (urogenital atrophy), patients may also report urinary urgency. The mucosa is pale, and rugae cannot be observed. The vagina is dry and nonpliant. Placement of a speculum may be painful.

Treatment with local or systemic estrogens reverses the patient's tissue changes and relieves symptoms. When estrogen is administered locally as a vaginal cream, an irregular absorption pattern and poorly predictable systemic effects may result (Forsberg, 1995). Long-term use is discouraged in favor of systemic administration. If topical estrogen is used, a low dosage (1 g conjugated equine estrogen cream intravaginally every other day) is recommended. Recently, an estrogen-impregnated polymer ring (Estring; Pharmacia and Upjohn, Kalamazoo, MI) was developed for local estrogen delivery. The ring is inserted into the vault and remains in place for 3 months. It provides continuous release of estradiol in dosages reported to cause minimal systemic absorption (Johnston, 1996).

Women who cannot or will not use estrogen can obtain symptomatic treatment of atrophy with vaginal lubricants (Hendrix, 1997). Replens (Parke-Davis, Morris Plains, NJ), K-Y jelly (Ortho Pharmaceutical, Raritan, NJ), and Astroglide (Biofilm, Vista, CA) are examples of water-based emollients that can be applied as needed. It is best to avoid preparations that contain fragrances and other irritants. Oil-based preparations may clog vulvar glands and lead to folliculitis so their use is similarly discouraged.

Dyspareunia

Dyspareunia has various causes. Some of them and an approach to evaluating the patient with dyspareunia are shown in Figure 5-3.

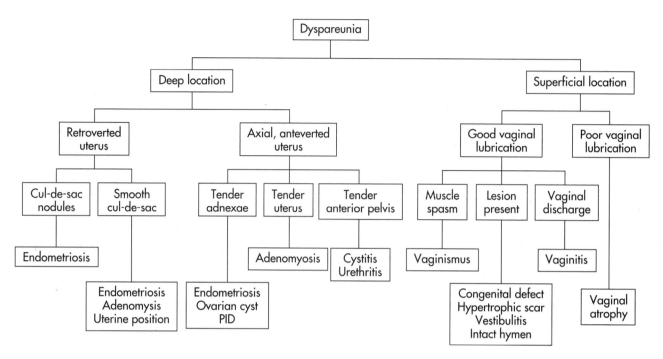

Fig. 5-3. Algorithm for evaluation of the patient with dyspareunia.

Evaluation begins with careful history taking. Most patients do not spontaneously report dyspareunia, and it must be gently elicited by the clinician. Important characteristics of the pain are its location (superficial, deep), chronicity, and associated symptoms. The physical examination must be conducted with great care and be directed toward identifying structural causes.

Palpation of tender, contracted constrictor muscles helps to determine vaginismus as a cause. Vaginismus is the involuntary spasm of the vaginal constrictor or levator ani muscles during attempted penetration of the vaginal vault. The condition is thought to be psychologically mediated through the mechanisms of fear of injury, guilt about sexuality, or dissatisfaction with the relationship (Scholl, 1988).

Treatment of dyspareunia depends on its cause. Pain secondary to an organic condition is best managed by treating the underlying disease. Vaginismus is managed by desensitization techniques performed in a supportive setting. Gradual self-dilation of the vault that reinforces the patient's control is effective treatment in most cases. Sets of soft rubber vaginal dilators of increasing size are available to assist the process. Often it is appropriate to combine their use with psychotherapy.

MALFORMATIONS

Embryologically, the vagina forms when the distal, fused, müllerian (paramesonephric) ducts attach to the urogenital sinus and stimulate a bilateral proliferation of cells in the dorsal wall called the sinovaginal bulbs (Koff, 1933). Additional proliferation results in the formation of a solid midline cord of cells called the vaginal plate (Fig. 5-4).

Canalization of the vaginal plate occurs as the central cells degenerate. This begins at the urogenital sinus and proceeds cranially to form the vault. The process is completed by approximately the fifth month. The lumen of the vagina remains separated from the lumen of the urogenital sinus by the formation of the hymen. Vaginal malformations occur when normal embryologic processes are disrupted. They may be classified as agenesis, failure of lateral fusion, or failure of canalization.

Vaginal Agenesis

Vaginal agenesis (the Rokitansky-Küster-Hauser syndrome), which results from müllerian duct agenesis, occurs in 1 in 4000 to 5000 female births (Griffin et al, 1976). It affects the development of a variable portion of the müllerian duct. Although the cause is unknown, it does not appear to be a single gene defect or a known teratogenic effect (Lindenman et al, 1997). Vaginal agenesis is usually associated with uterine agenesis, but 8% of patients have a rudimentary bipartite uterus with a functional endometrium (Wiser and Bates, 1984).

Clinical presentation depends on the absence or presence of a functioning uterus. The typical patient is in her teens and has primary amenorrhea (Reindollar et al, 1981). Alternatively, if endometrial tissue is involved, she may have cyclic pain. Ovarian function is normal and may induce cyclic shedding of the endometrium. However, because there is no outflow tract, the menstrual products are retained and cause symptoms. If retrograde flow of the menstrual endometrium occurs, endometriosis may result.

Patients display normal growth and development of secondary sexual characteristics, including the external geni-

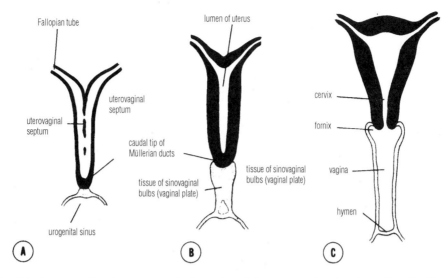

Fig. 5-4. Schematic drawing showing the formation of the uterus and vagina. **A,** At 9 weeks. Note the disappearance of the uterovaginal septum. **B,** At the end of the third month. Note the tissue of the sinovaginal bulbs, extending between the uterus and the urogenital sinus. **C,** Newborn. The vagina and the fornices are formed by vacuolization of the tissue of the sinovaginal bulbs. (From Sadler TW: *Langman's medical embryology,* ed 5, Baltimore, 1985, Williams & Wilkins.)

talia. Examination of the vaginal area reveals a mucosal wall beyond the introitus. A vaginal dimple may be present. Rectal examination usually demonstrates the absence of a uterus, although ultrasonography should be performed to confirm the diagnosis. Renal and skeletal anomalies are often associated and should be diagnosed by appropriate imaging techniques (Forstner and Hricak, 1994).

The differential diagnosis includes imperforate hymen and testicular feminization (androgen insensitivity) syndrome. In the former, a uterus is present and can usually be detected by physical examination or imaging studies. Patients with congenital absence of the vagina are distinguished from patients with testicular feminization by their normal female karyotype and normal serum testosterone levels.

The goal of treatment for patients with vaginal agenesis is to create a vaginal vault adequate for sexual function; menstrual and reproductive function usually will not be possible. Surgical and nonsurgical approaches are reported. The Frank nonsurgical method for the formation of a vagina involves the application of vaginal dilators to the introital region. Intermittent pressure is applied with progressively longer and wider dilators. This technique requires considerable cooperation and diligence from the patient, but it achieves good results without complications (Lindenman et al, 1997). McIndoe vaginoplasty involves surgical dissection of the areolar tissues in the potential vaginal space followed by placement of a split-thickness skin graft to achieve epithelialization (Meyers, 1997). If a rudimentary uterine anlage brings the onset of symptoms, the anlage should be surgically removed. Only the rare patient with an intact uterus has a chance of becoming pregnant. Surgery that incorpo-

rates uterine conservation is preferred in this group (Bates and Wiser, 1985).

Failure of Lateral Fusion

Failure of lateral fusion of the paramesonephric ducts results in longitudinal septae. As with agenesis, the extent of the developmental abnormality can be variable. There may be only a partial, distal fibromuscular band in the sagittal plane of the vagina. In the extreme situation, there may be duplication of all the müllerian derivatives, and the patient will have two uterine horns, two cervices, and two vaginas (Buttram, 1983). Abnormalities are classified as obstructive or nonobstructive. If the hemivagina created by the septum does not communicate with the introitus, there is obstruction of the ipsilateral uterine horn. If the uterus has a functioning endometrium, painful hematocolpos and hematometra may occur with menstruation. Because the contralateral horn continues to discharge its menstrual effluent normally, this diagnosis may not be considered unless careful physical examination reveals a tender mass.

Treatment is individualized according to the lesion and the symptoms. Obstructive lesions require surgical resection of the septum to resolve the hematocolpos and to prevent endometriosis. Surgery is also required for dyspareunia. Asymptomatic septae do not require treatment.

Failure of Canalization

Failure of canalization of the vaginal plate results in transverse septae. The incidence is reported as 1 in 30,000 to 80,000 females (Rock and Azziz, 1987). Septae may develop at any level of the vagina; occasionally, there may be more than one. A fibromuscular membrane covered with squamous epithelium, the septum may be partial, forming a constricting band, or complete, resulting in obstruction.

Diagnosis usually is made at menarche, when cyclic abdominal pain from retained menstrual blood prompts an evaluation. Imaging studies should include a pelvic ultrasonogram to delineate the septal thickness and to confirm a normal uterus and normal ovaries and an intravenous pyelogram to exclude renal anomalies and ureteral obstruction. Treatment requires surgical resection of the septum and reanastomosis of the upper and lower vaginal vaults.

The hymen probably forms at the junction of the vaginal plate and the urogenital sinus. If a normal lumen fails to develop and the hymen remains imperforate, retained menstrual blood and/or dyspareunia can result. Surgical treatment consists of a cruciate incision in the membrane and resection of the resultant triangular membranous flaps.

DISORDERS OF PELVIC SUPPORT

The vagina is a potential space in the pelvic floor through which the pelvic organs may descend under the influence of gravity if they are not properly suspended from the bony pelvis. In the erect posture, the axis of the vagina normally assumes a 45° angle from the vertical plane. Therefore, gravitational forces are not applied directly parallel to the vaginal tube, toward the introitus, but are absorbed along its length by various muscular, fascial, and ligamentous supports. Damage to these structures from acute or chronic injury results in the clinical condition called prolapse. A thorough discussion of disorders of pelvic support is included in Chapter 22.

BENIGN CONDITIONS OF THE VAGINA

Benign tumors of the vagina are uncommon. They are often asymptomatic and are detected only on pelvic examination. They may be solid masses or cysts. Small asymptomatic cysts do not require treatment. Larger cysts may occlude the vault and cause dyspareunia or pelvic pressure, and surgical excision is necessary. Solid tumors should always be excised, and a biopsy specimen should be studied to establish a diagnosis based on its histology and to exclude malignancy.

Vaginal cysts form from remnants of the mesonephric duct or arise as epithelial inclusion cysts. In normal female development, the mesonephric ducts undergo degeneration because of a lack of androgenic support. When remnants persist, they may form Gartner's duct cysts, which are typically located along the lateral walls of the vagina in the submucosal tissues. Histologically, the cysts are lined with a single layer of cuboidal or columnar cells that secrete mucinous material. The differential diagnosis includes epithelial inclusion cysts and suburethral diverticulum. Diverticuli are usually located directly along the course of the urethra in the 12 o'clock position. Treatment by surgical excision is preferred in most cases. Occasionally, a Gartner's duct cyst may dissect deeply into the paravaginal tissues, making excision difficult and bloody. In such cases, incision, drainage, and marsupialization of the cyst wall are preferred to excision if treatment is required.

Epithelial inclusion cysts arise from vaginal epithelia buried under the mucosa during healing from a traumatic injury. Obstetric laceration and episiotomy are common antecedents. The vaginal mucosa is not secretory. However, if the tissue remains viable, cell turnover and desquamation will occur. Subsequent degeneration of the cellular material results in the accumulation of a thick, cheesy substance. These cysts are distinguished from Gartner's duct cysts because of their contents, histology (stratified squamous epithelium), and location (Sedlis and Robboy, 1987). They usually develop in the lower third of the vagina on the posterior or posterolateral wall.

Solid tumors are more rare and arise from the connective tissue elements of the vagina. Clinically, they appear as polypoid growths or as firm, nontender masses, often within the rectovaginal septum (Robboy and Welch, 1991). Histologic examination usually reveals smooth muscle elements (leiomyoma), fibrous tissue (fibromyoma), or mixed patterns. Skeletal muscle elements (rhabdomyoma) occasionally are identified. Surgical excision to exclude malignancy is the appropriate management (Tavossoli and Norris, 1979).

The vagina is a relatively common site for extraperitoneal endometriosis, though overall incidence in the vagina is low (Azzena et al, 1996). Patients may have cyclic pain and dyspareunia. Implants often form small, dark blue cysts that may be tender to palpation. Diagnosis is established by examination of the biopsy specimen, and treatment is surgical excision or hormonal therapy.

The squamous epithelium of the vagina may become infected with certain types of the human papillomavirus that result in condylomas. These soft, verrucous tumors may occur singly, in small clusters, or as confluent growths. Lesions may appear on the cervix, vulva, and perianal skin, and treatment may be difficult. Podophyllin, a cytotoxic agent widely used to treat vulvar condyloma, is not recommended for vaginal therapy. Excessive absorption may result in neurotoxicity. Chemical cauterization with trichloroacetic acid may be used, but other treatments include laser ablation, cryocautery, and interferon therapy (Smotkin, 1993).

DIETHYLSTILBESTROL-ASSOCIATED VAGINAL ABNORMALITIES

In 1971 Herbst et al described an increased risk for clear cell adenocarcinoma of the vagina in young women with in utero exposure to diethylstilbestrol (DES). A synthetic estrogen, DES was administered in the mid-1940s to prevent miscarriage in some women with high-risk pregnancies. Before 1970 only rare cases of clear cell adenocarcinoma had been reported. After recognition of its relationship with DES, a registry was established that now contains the names of more than 500 patients with clear cell adenocarcinoma of the vagina and cervix (Melnick et al, 1987). Exposure to DES during gestation has been confirmed in as many as 88% of patients, although maternal recall of the exposure is not reliable (Sharp et al, 1990).

The risk for clear cell adenocarcinoma among exposed females is approximately 1 in 1000 (Giusti et al, 1995). Although risk increases inversely with gestational age at exposure, it is not clearly associated with total dosage. Occurrence of the cancer appears to be age related. The median age at diagnosis is 19 years, and more than 90% of the diagnoses have been made among patients between 15 and 27 years. Prognosis for survival is related to the extent of disease at the time of diagnosis. For instance, the 5-year survival rate for patients with tumors confined to the vaginal wall (stage I) is approximately 90% (Robboy and Welch, 1991). Therapeutic modalities include surgery, radiation, chemotherapy, and combined approaches.

Clear cell adenocarcinoma of the vagina is not the only DES-related abnormality of the genital tract. Vaginal adenosis and structural anomalies occur more often in this group of patients than in nonexposed controls (Giusti et al, 1995; Senekjian et al, 1988). Vaginal adenosis is the presence of glandular-columnar epithelia and their mucinous secretory products in the vagina. Prevalence in DES-exposed women is more than 90%. The strong association between adenosis and prenatal exposure to DES suggests that the drug interferes with normal vaginal development. The precise mechanism is unknown, but the replacement of müllerian columnar epithelium by upward-growing squamous epithelium from the urogenital sinus may be impeded (Ufelder and Robboy, 1976).

Adenosis is most often encountered on the upper, anterior vaginal wall and may continue to the cervical portio to form a cervical ectropion. It is granular and red, in contrast to the smooth, pink squamous mucosa. Sometimes it is submucosal and can be detected only by careful palpation of the vaginal walls. Vaginal adenosis is usually asymptomatic, but it may cause excessive vaginal secretions. Over time it may regress as the columnar epithelium is converted to squamous epithelium by metaplasia. It is usually found with clear cell adenocarcinomas, but the progression of adenosis to cancer has not been documented (Ghosh and Cera, 1983). Adenosis should be observed carefully by cytologic and clinical examinations, but treatment is required only for symptoms.

Structural anomalies related to DES exposure have been described for the vagina, cervix, uterus, and fallopian tubes. A transverse ridge of tissue, called a hood or a collar, may develop. In addition, a cockscomb cervix or pseudopolyp may develop on the exocervix. The polypoid appearance results from a thick, constricting stromal groove encircling the exocervix and causing protrusion of the endocervical tissue. The cervix may be hypoplastic, and the vaginal fornices may be absent or poorly developed. Changes in the endometrial cavity include reduction in size, reformation to a T-shape, and development of constrictions. Fallopian tube abnormalities include a withered, foreshortened, and convoluted appearance. The clinical implication of these structural changes is an adverse effect on reproductive potential. Fertility rates may be decreased in this group of women; after conception, they are also at increased risk for spontaneous abortion, ectopic pregnancy, and preterm delivery (Senekjian et al, 1988).

Women with in utero DES exposure may have increased risk for cervical and vaginal intraepithelial neoplasia (Robboy et al, 1984). Because the cervix is an area of active metaplastic growth, the more extensive transformations that occur on the cervices of women exposed to DES may predispose them to these abnormalities. Thus far no increase in squamous cell carcinoma has been documented (Faber et al, 1990). However, as these patients grow older and approach the age of peak incidence of invasive cancer, close follow-up is required.

VAGINAL INTRAEPITHELIAL NEOPLASIA

Vaginal intraepithelial neoplasia (VAIN) is uncommon. However, in recent decades this diagnosis has been made with increased frequency, probably because of the more extensive cytologic screening that takes place even in women who have undergone hysterectomy. The incidence of VAIN is approximately 0.2 to 0.3 per 100,000 women (Wharton et al, 1996), which is approximately one third the rate for invasive lesions. Patient age ranges from 25 to 80 years, and the mean age is 50 to 55 years. Carcinogenic agents responsible for squamous cell neoplasms of the lower genital tract are unknown. Factors that have been implicated, however, include infection with human papillomavirus and exposure to radiation (Audet-Lapointe et al, 1990).

A striking association in reported series of patients with VAIN is neoplasia at another genital tract site. Evidence of another genital tract neoplasm occurs in 50% to 75% of patients (Lenehan et al, 1986; Benedet and Sanders, 1984). Most of the earlier or concomitant neoplastic lesions are squamous and involve the cervix or vulva. This is cited as support for the hypothesized "field response" of the squamous epithelium of the lower genital tract (Marcus, 1960). According to this theory, tissues with a common embryologic origin share susceptibility to common carcinogens. The urogenital sinus is the ultimate source of the epithelium of the vulva, vagina, and cervix. Under certain conditions, neoplasms that arise in these tissues develop as multicentric lesions, not as the result of neoplastic transformation of a single cell. Alternatively, the association may be the result of the incomplete treatment of occult contiguous spread from the primarily affected organ. Thus failure to make an initial diagnosis that indicates the true extent of a single neoplasm may result in misdiagnosis of a field response. Regardless of cause, the important clinical implication is the need for careful evaluation and follow-up of the entire lower genital tract whenever a patient has a neoplasm of the vulva, vagina, or cervix.

Except in occasional patients with postcoital staining or vaginal discharge, VAIN is asymptomatic. Sometimes the astute clinician will detect a mucosal lesion on physical examination; in most patients, however, Papanicolaou smears are abnormal, and this is what prompts diagnostic evaluation. Diagnosis is established by colposcopically directed biopsies. Because colposcopic examination of the vagina is difficult, a vaginal speculum must be repositioned enough times to visualize the entire mucosal surface (Davis, 1993). The lesions found in patients with VAIN tend to be multifocal, and they usually occur in the upper third of the vagina. Colposcopic findings are similar to those seen in cervical intraepithelial neoplasia and include white epithelium, punctation, and mosaicism. White lesions may become more obvious after the application of 3% acetic acid solution to the mucosa. An iodine stain, such as Schiller's solution, may also be used to demonstrate abnormal areas. Normal vaginal epithelial cells stain brown because of the high glycogen content. Dysplastic cells often contain less glycogen and, therefore, do not take up the dye.

Findings on histologic examination are confined to the surface epithelial cells. Neoplastic changes include the presence of abnormal mitotic figures, nuclear pleomorphism, and loss of polarity. The degree of severity is determined by the depth of epithelial involvement. If only the lower third of the cell layers of the squamous epithelium is affected, it is graded VAIN I, or mild; involvement of the middle third is graded VAIN II, or moderate; and involvement of the upper third is graded VAIN III, or severe. Involvement of the full thickness of the epithelium is called vaginal carcinoma in situ.

Vaginal intraepithelial neoplasia is considered a premalignant lesion analogous to cervical in situ lesions. However, because of its lower incidence, there is less information regarding the magnitude of premalignant potential, transition times, and factors influencing the transition. Once diagnosed, treatment is necessary to prevent progression (Fig. 5-5). Several treatment options exist. The rationale for all modalities is to excise or destroy the dysplastic cells and to cause minimal damage to the normal epithelium and submucosa. The age of the patient, the desire for future sexual function, and the extent of disease will determine the choice of treatment.

Surgical excision has been the mainstay of therapy. This may involve wide local excision with primary repair for an isolated lesion, or it may involve total vaginectomy if the disease is widespread (Hoffman et al, 1992; Patsner, 1993). If a woman is no longer sexually active, repair after vaginectomy may be made by colpocleisis. Otherwise repair necessitates the formation of a neovagina using a split-thickness skin graft. Surgical treatment is successful in more than 80% of patients, but recurrences have been reported that involve even the skin grafts (Gallup et al, 1987a).

Chemotherapy with topical 5-fluorouracil (5-FU) is effective for treating most in situ VAIN lesions. Its advantage is that it involves the entire epithelial surface at risk from this potentially multifocal disease. A pyrimidine analogue that blocks DNA synthesis, especially in rapidly proliferating tissues, its effect occurs locally by ulceration and erosion and then by reepithelialization. Side effects include pain, vulvar irritation, and dysuria. One disadvantage to using chemotherapy rather than surgery is the unavailability of a histologic specimen to exclude concomitant invasive disease. However, the reported results with 5-FU suggest remission rates of 80%, a value that compares favorably with those obtained surgically (Krebs, 1989).

Another way to treat VAIN is with the carbon dioxide laser, which was initially used to ablate isolated lesions. Carbon dioxide laser treatment averts vulvitis, which has been associated with 5-FU, and excellent functional results are reported. Again, however, no specimen is available for histologic analysis. Therefore, laser therapy requires exhaustive colposcopic examination before treatment to exclude invasive cancer.

MALIGNANT NEOPLASMS

Only 1% to 2% of genital tract cancer originates in the vaginal tissues; the highest percentage is squamous cell carcinoma. Other types of primary cancer include melanoma, sarcoma, adenocarcinoma, and endodermal sinus tumors. Most malignant vaginal lesions are secondary. They occur as extensions of cervical or vulvar carcinoma, or as metastatic cancers that usually arise in the bladder, rectum, uterus, or ovary.

Squamous Cell Carcinoma

Squamous cell carcinoma accounts for approximately 90% of primary vaginal cancers. Patient age ranges from 30 to 90 years, and the average age at diagnosis is approximately 60 years. The causes of this tumor are unknown. One theory suggests that prolonged exposure of the mucosa to irritants has a causative role (Schraub et al, 1992). No data are available to substantiate such a relationship, nor has a relationship been proven between vaginal cancer and pessary use, prolapse, or similar potentially chronic irritants. Other factors implicated are pelvic radiation and viral infection (Merino, 1991).

Symptoms most often attributed to vaginal cancer are abnormal bleeding or blood-tinged discharge. Bleeding may occur only with intercourse or douching. Anterior wall lesions may cause urinary symptoms, such as frequency, dysuria, and hematuria. Rectal involvement from a posterior wall tumor may manifest as tenesmus, melena, or pain. Many patients report no symptoms, and the diagnosis is then established by pelvic examination. Occasionally, small lesions are detected colposcopically in response to abnormal cytologic smear findings. The vaginal

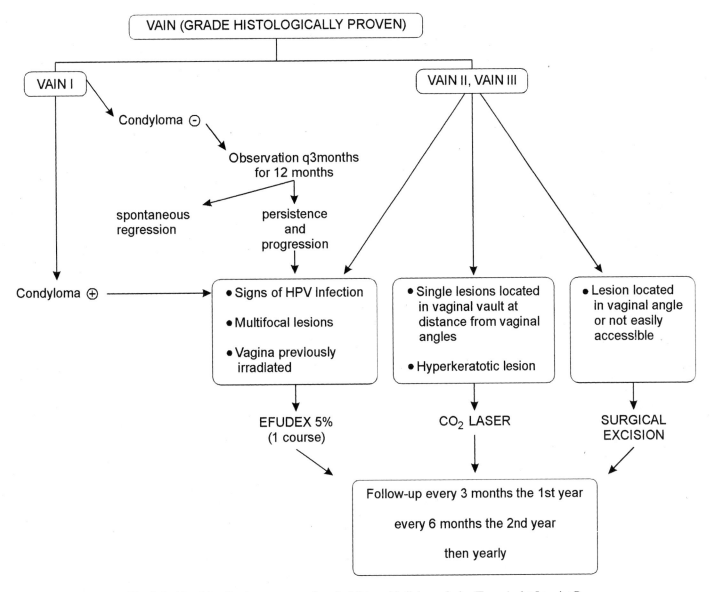

Fig. 5-5. Algorithm for the treatment of vaginal intraepithelial neoplasia. (From Audet-Lapoint P, Body G, Vauclair R, et al: Vaginal intraepithelial neoplasia. *Gynecol Oncol* 1990; 6:232-239.)

vault is highly distensible and can accommodate a relatively large lesion before symptoms ensue. For this reason, and because many older patients avoid seeking medical care despite symptoms, diagnosis is often delayed (Benedet, 1991). This is unfortunate because vaginal cancer occurs in a clinically accessible site, and there is an opportunity for early diagnosis and treatment.

Lesions vary and may appear as exophytic growths, superficial plaques, or ulcers. A diagnosis of vaginal cancer is confirmed by a biopsy that shows neoplastic epidermoid cells invading the submucosal tissues and the vascular and lymphatic spaces. Usually there is an associated inflammatory infiltrate. Histologic grade may be based on the degree of differentiation, but this does not give reliable prognostic information (Dixit et al, 1993).

Vaginal squamous cell carcinoma spreads by contiguous growth through the lymphatic vasculature. Local growth occurs initially in the submucosal layers, and there is gradual extension to the paracolpos, bladder, and rectum. Metastatic spread through the lymphatics follows a pattern that depends on the location of the primary lesion (Fig. 5-6). Tumors located in the upper vagina tend to spread into the pelvic lymph nodes (iliac, hypogastric, and obturator groups), as they do in cervical cancer. Tumors arising in the lower vagina often metastasize first to the femoral and inguinal lymph nodes, as they do in vulvar cancer. Lymphatic involvement is observed in approximately one fourth of patients at the time of diagnosis (Sedlis and Robboy, 1987).

Staging is based on a careful patient history and clinical examination. In addition, chest x-ray, intravenous pyelogram,

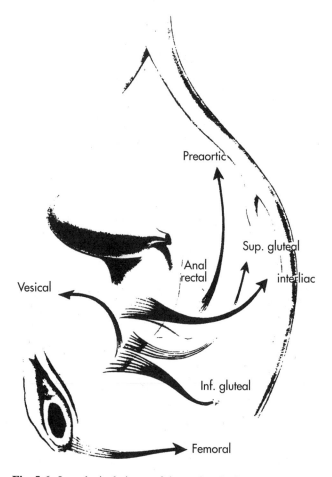

Fig. 5-6. Lymphatic drainage of the vagina. In the upper part of the vagina, it follows the cervical drainage pattern to the pelvic lymph nodes. In the lower part of the vagina, it follows the vulvar drainage pattern to the femoral nodes. (From Plentl AA, Freidman EA: *Lymphatic system of the female genitalia: The morphologic basis of oncologic diagnosis and therapy,* Philadelphia, 1971, WB Saunders.)

Table 5-1 International Federation of Gynecology and Obstetrics Classification of Vaginal Cancer

Stage	Location of Carcinoma
0	In situ
I	Limited to the vaginal wall
II	Involving the subvaginal tissues but not extending to the pelvic wall
III	Extending to the pelvic wall
IV	Extending beyond the true pelvis or involving the mucosa of the bladder or rectum. (Bullous edema alone does not permit allotment of a case to stage IV.)
IVA	Involving adjacent organs (bladder, rectum)
IVB	Involving distant organs

barium enema, cystoscopy, and proctosigmoidoscopy are performed to determine local or distant spread. The staging system is based on the recommendations of the International Federation of Gynecology and Obstetrics (Table 5-1). The distribution of patients among the stages varies with the different series reported. Typically, 30% to 40% of patients have stage III or IV disease (Kirkbride et al, 1995; Gallup et al, 1987b; Eddy et al, 1991).

Radiation treatment is the primary therapy for vaginal squamous cell carcinoma, though in some patients surgery is an option. Each therapeutic plan should be individualized according to the following factors: extent of disease, patient's general health, desire for vaginal function, and childbearing status. In addition, the proximity of the vagina to the bladder and rectum must be known to minimize complications.

Radiation therapy uses a combined approach of external radiation therapy and local implants (Podczaski and Herbst, 1993). The normal vaginal mucosa is relatively radioresis-

tant, but the proximity of the radiosensitive bladder and the rectal tissues results in radiation complications in approximately 15% to 25% of patients (Kirkbride et al, 1995; Pezez and Camel, 1982; Gallup et al, 1987b). Complications include proctitis, rectovaginal and vesicovaginal fistulae, and strictures. They occur more often in patients who have advanced disease and are administered higher doses of irradiation.

Surgical excision as primary therapy applies only to small, localized tumors located in the upper third of the vagina. Tumors arising on the posterior vaginal wall are more easily resected than those that arise anteriorly, near the more intimate attachment of the bladder. Reported treatments consist of radical hysterectomy with vaginectomy and excision of the pelvic lymph nodes, radical vaginectomy, and wide local excision. Surgery may be used adjunctively to treat advanced disease or recurrences after radiation therapy.

The prognosis for patients with vaginal squamous cell carcinoma depends primarily on the extent of disease at the time of diagnosis (Benedet, 1991). Stage I disease treated with radiation therapy results in 5-year survival rates of 80% to 90%. Five-year survival rates are 45% to 58% for stage II disease, 25% to 40% for stage III disease, and up to 10% for stage IV disease. The overall 5-year survival rate is approximately 45%.

Other Malignancies

Malignant melanoma may arise from vaginal melanocytes. This is a rare form of tumor, and it comprises less than 1% of all melanomas in women (Ragnarsson-Olding et al, 1993). Patients may be asymptomatic or they may have a mass, discharge, or vaginal bleeding. Tumor appearance is variable, ranging from a flat, spreading lesion to a heaped-up polypoid mass. Most lesions are pigmented. Diagnosis must be confirmed by histologic evaluation of a biopsy specimen.

The prognosis for patients with vaginal melanoma is poor. The disease is often well advanced by the time the diagnosis is made. Tumors are not responsive to radiation therapy, and effective chemotherapeutic agents have not been identified. Radical surgical therapy, including lymph node dissection if the primary tumor is more than superficially invasive, is the treatment most often recommended (Trimble, 1996).

Adenocarcinoma of the vagina associated with in utero DES-exposure was discussed earlier in this chapter. A much rarer type of vaginal adenocarcinoma is the endodermal sinus tumor (Young and Scully, 1984), which occurs exclusively in infants, usually in those younger than 2 years. The tumor probably arises from extragonadal germ cells. Endodermal sinus tumors occurring in the vagina may secrete alpha-fetoprotein, as do their ovarian counterparts. This is a useful marker to monitor disease activity among patients undergoing treatment. Combination therapy consisting of surgery with chemotherapy has resulted in long-term survival in several patients. The most commonly used chemotherapeutic agents are vincristine, actinomycin D, and cyclophosphamide.

Sarcomas are rare and account for less than 2% of vaginal malignancies. There are two types, based on age predilection (Sulak et al, 1988). Sarcoma botryoides (embryonal rhabdomyosarcoma) is usually found in children younger than 2 years. Tumors form friable clusters of polypoid masses that protrude from the vagina. They are often multicentric and appear to arise from the vaginal subepithelium. Histologically, there is diffuse proliferation of spindled neoplastic cells mixed with embryonic, striated muscle cells. Clinically, they are aggressive tumors, and the prognosis is poor. The traditional therapy has been radical surgery. However, a multimodal approach combining less radical surgery with chemotherapy or radiation therapy may offer equal efficacy with less morbidity (Hicks and Piver, 1992).

The second form of vaginal sarcoma develops in adults as a varied group of histologic types. The most common is the smooth-muscle tumor, leiomyosarcoma. Others are classified as fibrosarcomas, reticulum cell sarcomas, malignant schwannomas, müllerian stromal sarcomas, and mixed-cell types; all have a poor prognosis. One series reported a 5-year survival rate of 23% (Davos and Abell, 1976). The rarity of these tumors makes an evaluation of treatment regimens difficult. Treatment is usually radical surgical excision supplemented by radiation therapy to control local disease.

Metastatic cancer occurs more often in the vagina than does primary disease. Contiguous spread from the uterine cervix accounts for metastases. Other sites of primary malignancy that may involve the vagina include vulvar, endometrial, ovary, bladder, urethral, rectal, and malignant trophoblastic disease.

REFERENCES

Audet-Lapoint P, Body G, Vauclair R, et al: Vaginal intraepithelial neoplasia. *Gynecol Oncol* 1990; 6:232-239.

Azzena A, Ferrara A, Castellen L, et al: Vaginal endometriosis: Two case reports and a review of the literature on rare urogenital sites. *Clin Exp Obstet Gynecol* 1996; 23:94-98.

Bates GW, Wiser WL: A technique for uterine conservation in adolescents with vaginal agenesis and a functional uterus. *Obstet Gynecol* 1985; 66:290-294.

Benedet JL: Vaginal malignancy. *Curr Opinion Obstet Gynecol* 1991; 3:73-77.

Benedet JL, Sanders BH: Carcinoma in situ of the vagina. *Am J Obstet Gynecol* 1984; 148:695-700.

Blaustein RL: Cytology of the female genital tract. In Kurman RJ, editor: *Blaustein's pathology of the female genital tract,* New York, 1987, Springer-Verlag.

Brincat M, Versi E, Moniz CF, et al: Skin collagen changes in postmenopausal women receiving different regimens of estrogen therapy. *Obstet Gynecol* 1987; 70:123-127.

Buttram VC: Müllerian anomalies and their management. *Fertil Steril* 1983; 40:159-163.

Davis GD: Colposcopic examination of the vagina. *Obstet Gynecol Clin North Am* 1993; 20:217-229.

Davos I, Abell MR: Sarcomas of the vagina. *Obstet Gynecol* 1975; 47:342-350.

Dixit S, Singhal S, Baboo HA: Squamous cell carcinoma of the vagina: A review of 70 cases. *Gynecol Oncol* 1993; 48:80-87.

Eddy GL, Marks RD, Miller MC, et al: Primary invasive vaginal carcinoma. *Am J Obstet Gynecol* 1991; 165:292-298.

Faber K, Jones M, Tarraza HM: Invasive squamous cell carcinoma of the vagina in a diethylstilbestrol-exposed woman. *Gynecol Oncol* 1990; 37:125-128.

Forsberg J-G: A morphologist's approach to the vagina-age-related changes and estrogen sensitivity. *Maturitas* 1995; 22:S7-S15.

Forstner R, Hricak H: Congenital malformations of uterus and vagina. *Radiologe* 1994; 34:397-404.

Gallup DG, Castle CA, Stock RJ: Recurrent carcinoma in situ of the vagina following split-thickness skin graft vaginoplasty. *Gynecol Oncol* 1987a; 26:98-102.

Gallup DG, Talledo E, Shah KJ, et al: Invasive squamous cell carcinoma of the vagina: A fourteen year study. *Obstet Gynecol* 1987b; 69:782-785.

Ghosh TK, Cera PJ: Transition of benign vaginal adenosis to clear cell carcinoma. *Obstet Gynecol* 1983; 61:126-130.

Giusti RM, Iwamoto K, Hatch EE: Diethylstilbestrol revisited: A review of the long-term health effects. *Ann Intern Med* 1995; 122:778-788.

Given FT: Posterior culdoplasty: Revisited. *Am J Obstet Gynecol* 1985; 153:135-139.

Griffin JE, Creighton E, Madden JD, et al: Congenital absence of the vagina: The Mayer-Rokitansky-Kuster-Hauser syndrome. *Ann Int Med* 1976; 85: 224-236.

Hendrix SL: Nonestrogen management of menopausal symptoms. *Endocrinol Metab Clin North Am* 1997; 26:379-390.

Herbst AL, Ulfelder H, Poskanzer DC: Adenocarcinoma of the vagina: Association of material stilbestrol therapy with tumor appearance in young women. *N Engl J Med* 1971; 284:878-881.

Hicks ML, Piver MS: Conservative surgery plus adjuvant therapy for vulvovaginal rhabdomyosarcoma, diethylstilbestrol clear cell adenocarcinoma of the vagina, and unilateral germ cell tumors of the ovary. *Pediatr Adolesc Gynecol* 1992; 19:219-233.

Hoffman MS, DeCesare SL, Roberts WS, et al: Upper vaginectomy for in situ and occult, superficially invasive carcinoma of the vagina. *Am J Obstet Gynecol* 1992; 166:30-33.

Hovsepian DM: Transrectal and transvaginal abscess drainage. *J Vasc Interv Radiol* 1997; 8:501-515.

Johnston A: Estrogens—pharmacokinetics and pharmacodynamics with special reference to vaginal administration and the new estradiol formulation Estring. *Acta Obstet Gynecol Scand Suppl* 1996; 163:16-25.

Kirkbride P, Fyles A, Rawlings GA, et al: Carcinoma of the vagina—experience at the Princess Margaret Hospital (1974-1989). *Gynecol Oncol* 1995; 56:435-443.

Koff AK: Development of the vagina in the human fetus. *Contrib Embryol* 1933; 24:61-90.

Krebs HB: Treatment of vaginal intraepithelial neoplasia with laser and topical 5-fluorouracil. *Obstet Gynecol* 1989; 73:657-660.

Larsen B: Vaginal flora in health and disease. *Clin Obstet Gynecol* 1993; 36:107-121.

Lenehan PM, Meffe F, Lickrish GM: Vaginal intraepithelial neoplasia: Biologic aspects and management. *Obstet Gynecol* 1986; 68:333-337.

Lindenman E, Shepard MK, Pescovitz OH: Müllerian agenesis: An update. *Obstet Gynecol* 1997; 90:307-312.

Marcus SL: Multiple squamous cell carcinomas involving the cervix, vagina and vulva: The theory of multicentric origin. *Am J Obstet Gynecol* 1960; 80:802-812.

Melnick S, Cole P, Anderson D, et al: Rates and risks of diethylstilbestrol-related clear-cell adenocarcinoma of the vagina and cervix. *N Engl J Med* 1987; 316:514-516.

Merino MJ: Vaginal cancer: The role of infectious and environmental factors. *Am J Obstet Gynecol* 1991; 165:1255-1262.

Meyers RL: Congenital anomalies of the vagina and their reconstruction. *Clin Obstet Gynecol.* 1997; 40:168-180.

Patsner B: Treatment of vaginal dysplasia with loop excision: Report of five cases. *Am J Obstet Gynecol* 1993; 169:179-180.

Perez CA, Camel HM: Long term follow up in radiation therapy of carcinoma of the vagina. *Cancer* 1982; 49:1308-1315.

Podczaski E, Herbst AL: Cancer of the vagina and fallopian tube. In Knapp RC, Berkowitz RS, editors: *Gynecologic oncology,* ed 2, New York, 1993, McGraw-Hill.

Ragnarsson-Olding B, Johansson H, Rutqvist L, et al: Malignant melanoma of the vulva and vagina. *Cancer* 1993; 71:1893-1897.

Reindollar RH, Byrd JR, McDonough PG: Delayed sexual development: A study of 252 patients. *Am J Obstet Gynecol* 1981; 140:371-380.

Robboy SJ, Noller KL, O'Brien P, et al: Increased incidence of cervical and vaginal dysplasia in 3980 diethylstilbestrol-exposed young women. *JAMA* 1984; 252:2979-2983.

Robboy SJ, Welch WR: Selected topics in the pathology of the vagina. *Human Pathol* 1991; 22:868-876.

Rock JA, Azziz R: Genital anomalies in childhood. *Clin Obstet Gynecol* 1987; 30:682-696.

Scholl GM: Prognostic variables in treating vaginismus. *Obstet Gynecol* 1988; 72:231-235.

Schraub S, Sun XS, Maingon PH, et al: Cervical and vaginal cancer associated with pessary use. *Cancer* 1992; 69:2505-2509.

Sedlis A, Robby SJ: Diseases of the vagina. In Kurman RJ, editor: *Blaustein's pathology of the female genital tract,* New York, 1987, Springer-Verlag.

Senekjian EK, Potkul RK, Frey K, et al: Infertility among daughters either exposed or not exposed to diethylstilbestrol. *Am J Obstet Gynecol* 1988; 158:493-498.

Sharp GB, Cole P, Anderson D, et al: Clear cell adenocarcinoma of the lower gential tract: Correlation of mother's recall of diethylstilbestrol history with obstetrical records. *Cancer* 1990; 6:2215-2220.

Smotkin D: Human papillomavirus infection of the vagina. *Clin Obstet Gynecol* 1993; 36:188-194.

Sulak P, Barnhill D, Heller P, et al: Nonsquamous cancer of the vagina. *Gynecol Oncol* 1988; 29:309-320.

Tavossoli FA, Norris HJ: Smooth muscle tumors of the vagina. *Obstet Gynecol* 1979; 53:689-693.

Trimble EL: Melanomas of the vulva and vagina. *Oncology* 1996; 10:1017-1023.

Ulfelder H, Robboy SJ: The embryologic development of the human vagina. *Am J Obstet Gynecol* 1976; 126:769-776.

Wharton JT, Tortolero-Luna G, Linares AC, et al: Vaginal intraepithelial neoplasia and vaginal cancer. *Obstet Gynecol Clin North Am* 1996; 23:325-345.

Wiser WL, Bates GW: Management of agenesis of the vagina. *Surg Obstet Gynecol* 1984; 159:108-112.

Young RH, Scully RE: Endodermal sinus tumor of the vagina: A report of nine cases and review of the literature. *Gynecol Oncol* 1984; 18:380-392.

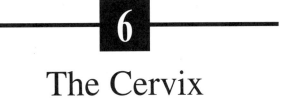

The Cervix

ELLEN E. SHEETS

KEY ISSUES

1. The ectocervix is covered by squamous epithelium that abuts the glandular epithelium of the endocervix at the transformation zone.
2. Cervical neoplasia forms at the transformation zone.
3. Human papillomavirus is now recognized as the causative agent of cervical preinvasive and invasive cancer.
4. Abnormal findings on Papanicolaou smears usually signify preinvasive cervical disease and mandate colposcopic evaluation.
5. The classic clinical symptoms of invasive cervical cancer are abnormal uterine bleeding, specifically postcoital bleeding, and discharge.

EMBRYOLOGY

The cervix begins to develop at approximately 12 weeks' gestation. Before that, at 3 weeks' gestation, the müllerian (paramesonephric) duct system begins to develop as an invagination of the coelomic epithelium lateral to the wolffian (mesonephric) duct. Initially these paired ducts run caudally, but at 6 weeks' gestation they turn medially to meet in the midline, after which they again run caudally to reach the urogenital sinus at approximately 8 weeks' gestation (Fig. 6-1). The point of contact between the now-fused müllerian ducts and the urogenital sinus enlarges to form the müllerian tubercle, and the wolffian ducts enter the sinus immediately lateral to the tubercle.

Evagination of the sinus between the wolffian ducts and the müllerian tubercle produces the sinovaginal bulbs, which proliferate to form the vaginal plate or vaginal cord. This solid plate advances in a caudal-cranial direction and obliterates the fused müllerian ducts (vaginal canal) as the müllerian epithelium degenerates. At 11 weeks' gestation,

cavitation begins in a caudal-cranial direction, and the vaginal lumen is created. Simultaneously, a constriction appears between the developing corpus and cervix, and the cervix is identified by thickened fusiform of the surrounding mesenchyme (Fig. 6-2). Cranial proliferation of the vaginal plate around the developing cervix forms the vaginal fornices, which are well delineated by 21 weeks' gestation (Ferenczy, 1982; Langman, 1981).

Abnormalities in the development or fusion of one or both müllerian ducts may result in malformations of the cervix. These include a double cervix with a septate or bicornuate uterus in conjunction with a normal or a double vagina; a double cervix with uterus didelphys; or, rarely, complete atresia of the cervix (Fig. 6-3).

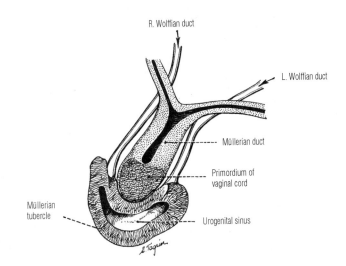

Fig. 6-1. Formation of the lower portion of the vagina. The müllerian tubercle is formed as the terminal ends of the müllerian ducts impinge on the urogenital sinus. Thus the vagina has two origins, one from the müllerian tubercle and one from outgrowths of the urogenital sinus.

The development of epithelium in the vagina and cervix is most likely müllerian in origin (Gondos, 1985). In the fetus exposed to in utero diethylstilbestrol (DES), the estrogen effect causes heterotopic columnar epithelium to form in the adult vagina (Stillman, 1982).

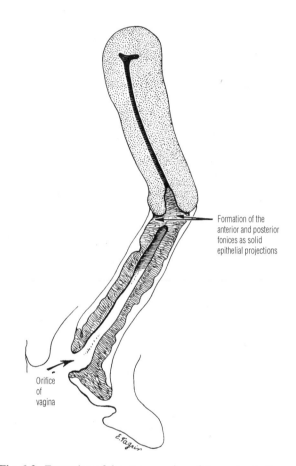

Formation of the anterior and posterior fonices as solid epithelial projections

Orifice of vagina

Fig. 6-2. Formation of the upper portion of the vagina in the 151-mm embryo. At this stage the cranial end of the vagina contains two solid epithelial projections that become the anterior and the posterior fornices.

ANATOMY

The cervix (which means *neck* in Latin) is the narrowed, most caudad portion of the uterus (Fig. 6-4). It measures approximately 2.5 to 3 cm in length in the adult nulligravida and is contiguous with the inferior aspect of the uterine corpus; the point of juncture is known as the isthmus. The vagina is attached obliquely around the center of the cervical periphery and divides the cervix into two segments—an upper supravaginal portion and a lower vaginal portion. The cervix enters the vagina at an angle through the anterior vaginal wall. The supravaginal segment of the cervix is separated anteriorly from the bladder by the pubovesicocervical fascia. Laterally, at the same level, the cervix is in continuity with the paracervical ligaments or cardinal ligaments of Mackenrodt, which contain the uterine artery and vein. The cervical lymphatic vessels primarily drain lateral to the hypogastric, obturator, and external iliac nodes, but they also drain anterior to the posterior bladder wall nodes and posterior to the presacral nodes. Innervation of the cervix arises from the superior, middle, and inferior hypogastric plexuses and is primarily limited to the endocervix and the deeper areas of the exocervix. This accounts for the relative insensitivity to pain of the exocervix (Ferenczy, 1982).

The vaginal portion (portio vaginalis, exocervix, ectocervix, or anatomic portio) projects into the apex of the vagina, between the anterior and posterior fornices, as a convex prominence of elliptical shape. A small aperture, usually round or slitlike in the nullipara, is in the center of the projection and constitutes the external os. This orifice joins the uterine cavity with the vagina and is surrounded by the anterior and posterior lips. The cervical canal extends from the external os to the anatomic internal os, where it connects with the uterine cavity. It is fusiform, or spindle shaped, and measures approximately 8 mm at its greatest width.

The isthmus is defined as that area of the uterus that lies between the anatomic internal os above and the histologic internal os below. The latter is defined as the area of transition from the endometrial to the endocervical glands. The

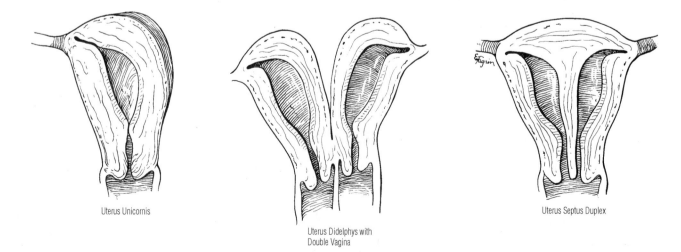

Uterus Unicornis

Uterus Didelphys with Double Vagina

Uterus Septus Duplex

Fig. 6-3. Major congenital anomalies of the uterus.

isthmic musculature is thinner than that of the corpus and facilitates effacement and dilation during labor. This area is often called the lower uterine segment during pregnancy and labor.

PHYSIOLOGY

The cervix functions passively as a segment of the birth canal and as a channel for menstrual discharge. Its primary physiologic function is the secretion of mucus, which facilitates the transport of spermatozoa and subsequently acts as a plug to seal the gravid uterine cavity from the external environment.

This cervical mucus is subject to profound cyclic changes in relation to the levels of circulating ovarian hormones. In the immediate postmenstrual phase, when the circulatory level of estrogen is low, and in the postovulatory period under the influence of progesterone, the cervical mucus is sparse, thick, and viscid. If it is allowed to dry on a slide, abundant vaginal and cervical cells, leukocytes, and mucous particles can be seen. From the eighth day of the cycle until ovulation, under the stimulation of rising levels of estrogen, the amount of mucus increases, its viscosity decreases, and it becomes highly permeable to spermatozoa. Just before ovulation the mucus is glassy, transparent, and highly elastic.

PHYSIOLOGIC ALTERATIONS
Changes in Endocervical Mucosa

During the latter part of intrauterine development, when growth of the cervix is accelerated as a result of high levels of circulating estrogens, such growth is not shared by the corpus. At birth the cervix:corpus ratio may approach 3:1. After birth there is a rapid regression in cervical length; this returns to the more normal cervix:corpus ratio seen in the adult. During the third trimester, endocervical cell shape changes from cuboidal to tall columnar (with evidence of

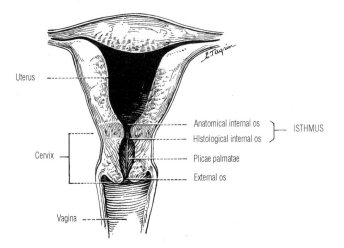

Fig. 6-4. Frontal section of the uterine cervix and corpus.

mucin secretion), and the mucosa deeply infolds into the stroma to form clefts or glands. This excessive proliferation of endocervical mucosa after 28 weeks' gestation produces the congenital eversion, or overgrowth, of endocervical glands, seen in 50% of newborn girls. In contrast, the endometrium is incompletely developed, usually inactive, and has only a few tubular glands. In the newborn, squamous cells of the exocervix, which are well stratified and contain abundant glycogen, are similarly affected by maternal estrogens. At puberty, with the stimulation of estrogen from the developing ovarian follicles, these changes presumably occur again, although adequate morphologic studies in this age group are lacking (Langman, 1981).

During the childbearing years, endocervical glands are found just below the internal os and extend just beyond the external os, onto the anatomic portio, which creates the so-called cervical erosion. In women older than 40 years of age, as a result of waning ovarian activity, the endocervical mucosa ascends the canal. During the menopausal years, the lowest glands—the original squamocolumnar junction and the transformation zone—are at or above the anatomic external os. Coppleson and Reid (1967) and Song (1964) attribute the downward shift and eversion of the endocervix to an increase in mucosal volume during the years when estrogen stimulation is maximal. This explains the increase in eversions noted after the first pregnancy (Fig. 6-5).

HISTOLOGY

Careful consideration of cervical histology will allow us to understand how and where benign, precancerous, and cancerous lesions of the cervix occur. The cervix is essentially composed of two different types of epithelium: squamous and columnar. The area of transition between these two epithelial types gives rise to the three histologic zones: the histologic portio, the transitional or transformation zone, and the histologic endocervix. In addition, it is in the transition from columnar to squamous epithelium that precancerous and cancerous lesions can arise.

Histologic Portio

The histologic portio is defined as a cervical stroma devoid of glands and covered by stratified squamous epithelium (Fig. 6-6). This epithelium is 15 to 20 cells thick, and there is a progressive and orderly maturation from the lowest basal layer through the prickle cell layer to the superficial zone, where cornification occurs under estrogenic stimulation.

The basal layer (stratum germinativum), responsible for epithelial regeneration, consists of a single row of small, cylindrical cells with large nuclei and scanty cytoplasm. Mitotic figures may occasionally be seen. Above the basal cells is a layer of larger polyhedral cells, 4 to 10 cells thick, arranged in an irregular mosaic pattern and interconnected by numerous tonofilament-desmosomal complexes. These characteristic intercellular bridges have led to the

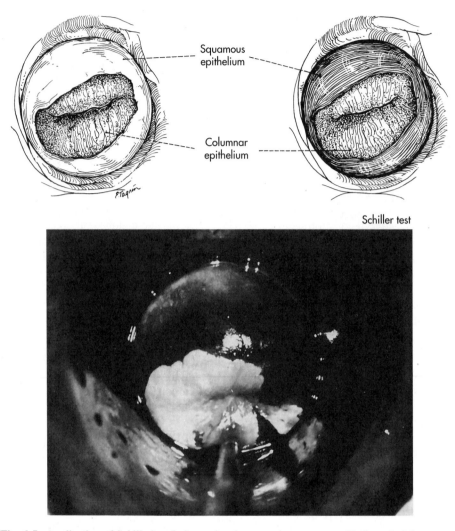

Squamous
epithelium

Columnar
epithelium

Schiller test

Fig. 6-5. Application of Schiller's solution stains the normal squamous epithelium dark brown. Endocervical epithelium does not stain.

designation *prickle cells,* and their location has led to the designation *parabasal cells.*

Above the parabasal cells is a layer of larger oval or navicular cells with relatively small nuclei. These cells are involved in ascending maturation, during which nuclear size remains constant while cytoplasmic volume gradually increases. This layer is called the intermediate, clear cell, or navicular zone. The most superficial layer, the stratum corneum, consists of flattened, elongated cells with small pyknotic nuclei. These are the cornified cells, or squames, seen in cytologic smears. The superficial and intermediate cells are rich in glycogen but appear clear in histologic sections because the glycogen is washed out during fixation.

The basal layer is usually regular and does not show the rete peg formation seen in the vulva and the vagina. The cervical squamous epithelium rests on a basement membrane. This membrane is inconsistently seen under the light microscope and appears to consist of condensed stromal collagen. The underlying fibrous connective tissue stroma contains a lush capillary network at the epithelial junction that includes

scattered papillae extending upward into the epithelium (Forsberg, 1965).

Transformation Zone

The transformation zone lies between the histologic portio and the endocervical mucosa, and it consists of endocervical stroma and glands covered by squamous epithelium. The squamous epithelium comes to lie on the endocervical stroma as a result of several physiologic or pathologic processes. Although these processes cause upward displacement of the squamocolumnar junction, the junction between the histologic portio and the transformation zone is dependent on age, estrogen influence, and previous trauma or surgery to the cervix. With Figure 6-4 as a guide, the transformation zone may be located on the vaginal portion of the cervix, at the external os, or above the external os within the cervical canal. Therefore, one should not equate the location of the histologic transformation zone with the location of the anatomic external os. The importance of the location of this zone will become apparent in the section on colposcopy.

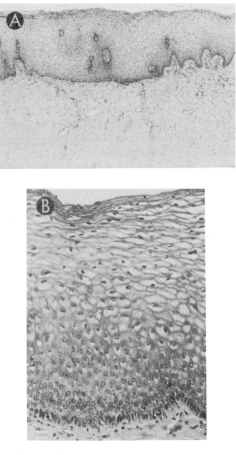

Fig. 6-6. **A,** Normal exocervix at low-power magnification (×50). **B,** High-power magnification (×150) shows process of stratification and cornification.

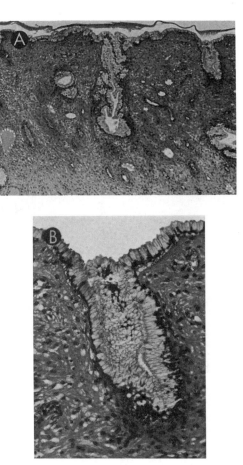

Fig 6-7. **A,** Normal endocervix at low-power magnification (×50). **B,** High-power magnification (×150) shows typical high columnar epithelium.

Histology of the Endocervix

Histologically, the endocervix is lined by a single layer of tall, columnar epithelial cells characterized by dense, basal nuclei and cytoplasm that stains pale pink in standard hematoxylin-eosin preparations (Fig. 6-7). Two cell types are present in this epithelium: prevalent mucus-secreting cells and scattered ciliated cells located in patches within the cervical canal and in gland orifices. These endocervical glands are actually formed by complex, cleftlike infoldings of the epithelium, which appear as simple glandular units in histologic section (Ferenczy, 1982; Fluhmann, 1960). Although this concept renders the term *gland* a misnomer, reference to endocervical glands persists. The cleft arrangement increases the surface area of the endocervical mucosa and permits the increased production of mucus that is dependent on estrogen. Maximal production and secretion of mucus occurs before ovulation. Most early neoplastic cervical lesions in women of childbearing age occur on the anatomic portio, where they are readily available for biopsy. Histopathologic evaluation of the biopsy specimen reveals that the majority of these lesions actually involve the transformation zone as endocervical glands will be seen in the transformation zone.

Histologically, the cervix differs from the body of the uterus because a small intraabdominal portion is covered by peritoneum. Approximately 85% of the cervix is made up of fibrous connective tissue. The cervix has no venous sinuses. Cervical mucosa does not undergo the marked menstrual changes the endometrium undergoes; however, it does undergo some cyclic changes that are dependent on estrogen and progesterone. The vaginal cervix is covered by stratified squamous epithelium.

Squamous Metaplasia and Epithelialization

After menarche and through the reproductive period, the previously described cervical ectropion essentially disappears, and the squamocolumnar junction moves out of view within the cervical canal. Two mechanisms for replacement of the endocervical eversion by squamous epithelium have been proposed as the histogenesis of the transformation zone. Because virtually every cervical squamous neoplasm originates in the transformation zone, histogenesis provides insight into the oncogenesis of cervical neoplasia.

The first mechanism, termed squamous metaplasia, is the result of a process known as subcolumnar reserve cell metaplasia. These reserve cells are undifferentiated, spherical, or

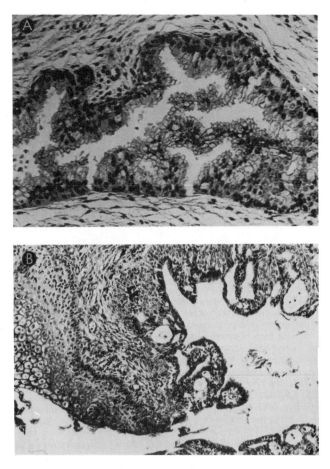

Fig. 6-8. A, Hyperplasia of reserve cells in the endocervix.
B, Squamous metaplasia from reserve cells of the endocervix
at the histologic external os. Normal stratified squamous epithelium is seen at the left. (Courtesy Drs. Louis M. Hellman and
Alexander Rosenthal.)

polygonal cells with plump, centrally placed, dark-staining
nuclei and scant cytoplasm. They come to lie beneath the
columnar epithelium, and their origin is controversial. It has
been proposed that reserve cells derive from either embryonal rests of urogenital sinus epithelium, direct or indirect
metaplasia of columnar cells, basal cells of the portio, or
stromal cells. Coppleson and Reid (1967) suggest that the
metaplastic process is initiated by the exposure of the endocervical mucosa to the lower pH of the vagina and that
estrogen plays a crucial role by promoting endocervical hyperplasia and prolapse and by acidifying the vaginal environment. In support of this mechanism, Hellman et al (1954)
found a striking increase in reserve cell hyperplasia and
metaplasia after the administration of large doses of estrogen to postmenopausal women.

Once reserve cell hyperplasia and metaplasia occur
(Fig. 6-8), the overlying columnar epithelium sloughs off.
The epithelium initially differentiates into a multilayered,
immature, squamous epithelium and then differentiates into
mature, stratified, squamous epithelium.

The second mechanism by which squamous epithelium
comes to overlie endocervical stroma is termed squamous
epithelialization (Johnson et al, 1964). The initiating event
may be true pathologic erosion of the distal endocervix
followed by an ingrowth or overglide of portio squamous
cells. In the early stages of this process, the squamous epithelium may be seen as a tenuous strand of immature
squamous cells, gradually decreasing in height as they are
stretched over an otherwise denuded and inflamed stroma.
Others (Ferenczy, 1982; Johnson et al, 1964) have shown
that the squamous epithelium of the portio may grow beneath the adjacent, intact endocervical epithelium and that
there may be loss of the overlying columnar cells on maturation and stratification of the squamous elements. As
with many reparative and regenerative processes, mitotic
activity with associated basal cell hyperplasia may be
considerable, although the atypia of malignancy is absent.
The extension of the new epithelium over the mouth of
the endocervical gland may result in occlusion and the
formation of mucinous retention (nabothian) cysts. These
are grossly visible on the portio as spherical elevations or
small cysts 2 to 10 mm in diameter (Fig. 6-9). Microscopic observation reveals that the cystic space is lined
with low cuboidal or flattened endocervical cells.

BENIGN CERVICAL LESIONS
Cervical Polyps

Cervical polyps usually develop in the endocervix as a result
of chronic papillary endocervicitis. They are soft, spherical,
glistening red masses that measure several millimeters to
several centimeters (Fig. 6-9). Often they are friable, and
they may be associated with profuse leukorrhea secondary
to the underlying endocervicitis. Histologically, they are
composed of endocervical epithelia with a fibrovascular
stalk. Differential diagnoses include polypoid fragments
of endocervical carcinoma or carcinosarcoma protruding
through the os, retained products of conception, grapelike
swellings of sarcoma botryoides that occasionally originate
in the cervix, and prolapsing submucous fibroids or endometrial polyps. Most cervical polyps can be grasped with
a clamp and twisted free, and the base can be cauterized for
hemostasis. All cervical polyps should be submitted for
evaluation, though malignancy is rare.

Leiomyomas

Leiomyomas, or fibroids, are the most common uterine tumors. Cervical involvement occurs in as many as 8% of
patients. Cervical leiomyomas are grossly and histologically identical to those found in the corpus. Although they
are often incidental findings on physical examination, if
allowed to grow excessively they may cause bowel or
bladder symptoms, dyspareunia, or dystocia in labor. The
treatment for symptomatic fibroids is either myomectomy
or hysterectomy.

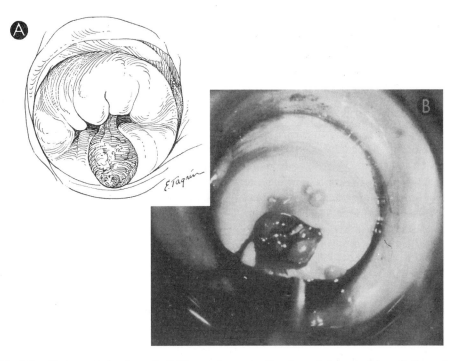

Fig. 6-9. Endocervical polyps. **A,** Solitary polyp protruding through the external os. **B,** Several endocervical polyps occluding the exocervix. Several nabothian (mucous) cysts are seen on the portio epithelium.

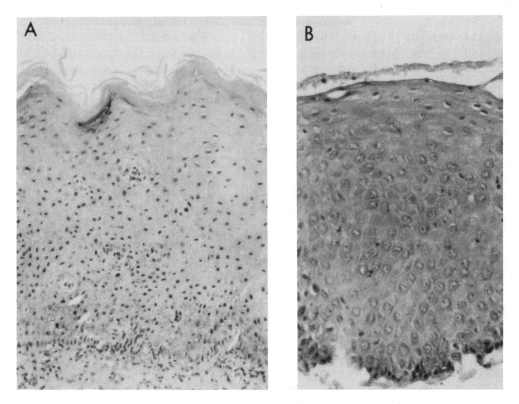

Fig. 6-10. A, Hyperkeratosis (×120). Normal ascending cellular maturation with a thickened keratin layer can be seen. **B,** Parakeratosis (×200). Pyknotic nuclei are evident within the keratin layer (×260). (Courtesy Dr. Robert Ehrmann and the Division of Women's and Perinatal Pathology, Brigham and Women's Hospital, Boston.)

Keratinization

Because keratinization is not a physiologic property of cervical squamous epithelium, any sign of it must be considered abnormal, though some degree of focal keratinization may occasionally be observed in the absence of other abnormalities. Hyperkeratosis and parakeratosis usually appear grossly visible as white, raised plaques (leukoplakia) on the portio. Microscopically, hyperkeratosis exhibits a thickened layer of keratin, scant intraepithelial glycogen, and no cytologic atypia. It may only be seen among patients with procidentia. Parakeratosis, evidenced by white cervical lesions that are the most common abnormality of keratinization, exhibits features that are similar to those of hyperkeratosis but retains pyknotic nuclei in the keratin layer (Fig. 6-10). There is no evidence to indicate that either hyperkeratosis or parakeratosis is premalignant or predisposes to cervical malignancy. However, white lesions of the cervix cannot be diagnosed solely by gross observation. Occasionally, keratinization of squamous cell cervical cancer appears as a white lesion. Therefore, all white lesions of the cervix must undergo biopsy for tissue diagnosis.

Herpes Simplex Virus

Herpesvirus hominis types 1 and 2, the etiologic agents of genital herpes, belong to the group of herpes viruses found in almost every animal species studied. These are large DNA viruses, five of which are associated with disease in humans: herpes simplex virus (HSV) types 1 and 2, varicella-zoster virus, cytomegalovirus, and Epstein-Barr virus. Infection requires direct contact followed by an incubation period of 1 to 45 days (average, 6 days). Clinically, herpes genitalis may be conveniently divided into either primary or recurrent infection, the former indicating infection resulting from the first exposure to either HSV type 1 or 2 and the latter indicating any subsequent infection.

Multiple painful vesicles, usually measuring 1 to 2 mm, appear on an erythematous background; these rapidly erode and coalesce to form large ulcers. The cervix is involved in 80% of primary infections, and manifestations include nonspecific inflammation, vesicles, ulcers, or occasionally fungating masses that are indistinguishable from invasive cervical carcinoma. Vaginal discharge is a common symptom. Complete healing requires several weeks as the symptoms and lesions slowly resolve. Recurrent pelvic infections involve the cervix less commonly than do primary infections. Culture of an area of involvement confirms the diagnosis.

CERVICAL NEOPLASIA

Cervical neoplasia is a neoplastic alteration of a normal physiologic change that occurs in the cervical epithelium (such as metaplasia). This alteration ranges from minor changes in the epithelium (low-grade cervical intraepithelial neoplasia), to full-thickness involvement of the epithelium (cervical carcinoma in situ), to invasive cervical cancer.

Many investigators feel that cervical neoplasia represents a continuum of disease and that lesions that are preinvasive (confined to the epithelium) can spontaneously regress to normal epithelium or progress to invasive cancer.

Epidemiology

The earliest epidemiologic studies of cervical neoplasia were conducted in 1842 by Rigoni-Stern. He showed that the incidence of cervical carcinoma was higher in married and widowed women and lower in women who never married and among nuns in certain religious orders (Rigoni-Stern, 1976). Since then numerous epidemiologic studies have been conducted on the association between cancer of the cervix and coitus. Handley (1936) looked at the role of circumcision in relation to cervical cancer. He found a lower incidence of cervical cancer among subsets of ethnic groups that practiced circumcision than among those who did not. Kessler (1976, 1981) further advanced the concept of a "high-risk male." In a comparison study with a control population, he found a severalfold increase in risk for cervical carcinoma among women whose husbands were previously married to women with cervical carcinoma.

Since the 1980s, it has become generally accepted that the passage of human papillomavirus (HPV) sexually causes precancerous and cancerous changes in cervical epithelium. Overwhelming epidemiologic data support a causative role for HPV, although the exact mechanism leading to neoplastic change remains unknown. Even when all other risk factors are considered, the presence of HPV infection is the leading risk factor for the development of cervical cancer and its precursors (Schiffman et al, 1993).

When evaluating nonsexual factors that could increase the incidence of cervical neoplasia, sexual factors have to be controlled. The most commonly considered nonsexual risk factors are cigarette smoking, diet, and use of oral contraceptives. Currently, the most significant dietary factor appears to be blood folate levels.

For cigarette smoking, the mechanism underlying the increased risk appears to be related to specific smoking-related mutagens in the cervix and in cervical mucus (Yang, 1997; Prokopczyk, 1997). The greatest problem in evaluating the clinical risk for cigarette smoking and the development of cervical neoplasia is controlling for confounding factors. Although most case-controlled studies indicate a relative increased risk of 1.5 to 14 for preinvasive or invasive disease (La Vecchia, 1986; Nischan, 1988), Phillips et al (1994) used a simulation approach to control further for confounding variables. They found that with this added measure of control, they could not support the concept that cigarette smoking alone enhances the risk for cervical preinvasive or invasive disease. From these analyses, one can only conclude that prospective data are needed to define completely the role of cigarettes.

Butterworth et al (1992) published one of the first case-controlled studies looking at a range of dietary issues and the development of cervical precancer. They found that low red blood cell folate levels place patients at greater risk for precancerous changes once they are infected with HPV. However, in a case-controlled study looking at dietary risk in women with invasive cervical cancer, Potischman et al (1991) found no differences in serum folate levels between patients and controls. Others have found retrospectively that red blood cell folate levels are a relative risk factor for precancerous changes (Kwasniewska, 1997; Harper, 1994). Prospective trials, especially among women who also take oral contraceptives, would be of help in determining the true significance of the folate data thus far (Butterworth, 1982).

The role that oral contraceptives may play in the development of cervical neoplasia is difficult to evaluate. Not only do the traditional sexual risk factors require control, but also what type of birth control is used. Women who use barrier contraceptives may have some degree of protection over those who do not. Studies that control for all these factors indicate that the longer a woman uses oral contraceptives, the greater is her risk for cervical cancer. In data published in 1993 from a multinational hospital-based, case-controlled study, the World Health Organization reports a 1.5 relative adjusted risk when oral contraceptives are used for 5 or more years (World Health Organization, 1993). These data are reinforced by Ye et al (1995), who find similar results in women who use oral contraceptives for more than 5 years. The mechanism by which oral contraceptives can increase risk may be the prolongation of HPV infection, allowing for other cellular events to occur and giving rise to a precancerous state (von Knebel Doeberitz, 1997).

Human Papillomavirus

Since its first suggestion in the 1970s, the association between HPV and cervical neoplasia has been essentially irrefutable because of the overwhelming epidemiologic evidence that now exists (Bosch et al, 1995; Lowy et al, 1994). The Papovaviridae family is composed of two branches. Simian virus 40 and polyomavirus make up one side, and the papillomaviruses make up the other. Human papillomaviruses are 8000-kilobase DNA viruses composed of many different subtypes. Each subtype represents a virus that has less than 50% DNA base sequence homology with other types.

More than 80 distinct types of HPV have been identified (Volter et al, 1996). Each appears to have a preference for a certain epithelial surface. For example, HPV type 1 is involved in plantar warts, whereas HPV types 5 and 14 are involved in a rare external skin disease, epidermodysplasia verruciformis. HPV types 6, 11, 16, 18, 31, 35, and some types in the 50s are found in genital epithelial surfaces.

In the genital tract, HPV types can be broken down into two groups: those with low oncogenic potential (HPV types 6, 11, 35) and those with high oncogenic potential (HPV types 16, 18, 31, some 50s). Low-risk HPVs are associated with condylomata and low-grade precancers. High-risk HPVs are associated with high-grade precancers and invasive cancer. Although most of these lesions fall into one HPV category and follow the general trends, this is not an absolute. Hence, precancerous or cancerous lesions can be of more than one HPV type or can be associated with HPV type 6 or 11 and vice versa (Bergeron et al, 1987). This ability of HPV categories to be common to all types of clinical lesions leads to difficulty in predicting which patient will be at risk for a serious clinical problem if the clinician relies solely on HPV type. Adding to this dilemma is the well-known fact that HPV can remain dormant in normal-appearing skin (Ferenczy et al, 1985), which further decreases the predictive value of screening women for HPV types (Grunebaum et al, 1983). Readers interested in additional detail are referred to appropriate reviews (Howley, 1991; Alani and Munger, 1998).

Our understanding of HPV infections is greatly hampered by the lack of a culture system for the virus. For reasons yet unknown, the mature viral particle for HPV requires the permissive environment of a mature keratinocyte to form and replicate.

Preinvasive Cervical Lesions

Human papillomavirus changes of the cervical epithelium were first noted as condylomata, or exophytic veneral warts. Microscopic examination reveals that condylomata are characterized by papillomatosis, acanthosis, lengthening and thickening of the rete pegs, submucosal capillary proliferation, and koilocytes. First described by Koss and Durfee (1956), koilocytes exhibit hyperchromasia, multinucleation, and perinuclear cytoplasmic vacuolization (Fig. 6-11). Initially, koilocytes were thought to be pathognomonic of HPV infections, but as the understanding of HPV expanded because of DNA hybridization, this constant association was called into doubt. Meisels et al (1977) are the first investigators to find cervical lesions that have koilocytotic atypia and other features suggestive of condylomata, but not the typical gross papillary features. In this study of 152 cervical cytologic smears diagnosed with mild precancerous changes, they also found that 70% of the smears exhibit changes suggestive of HPV infection. This finding led the authors to consider koilocytotic atypia as an early phase in the natural history of cervical neoplasia.

The initial histologic descriptions of the preinvasive cervical lesions use the categories of mild, moderate, and severe dysplasia, or abnormal growth (Reagan et al, 1969). The concept that these epithelial lesions represent a continuum of change, starting with mild dysplasia and advancing through severe, led Richart (1966) to introduce the concept of cervical intraepithelial neoplasia (CIN). Evidence in support of Richart's classification comes from the finding of aneuploid changes in the nuclei of dysplastic cells—the same chromosomal changes usually associated with malignant tumors but not with benign tumors. Autoradiographic studies demonstrate a steady increase in the mitotic activity

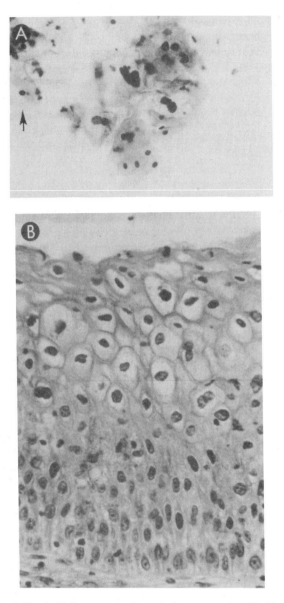

Fig. 6-11. A, Koilocytes on a Papanicolaou smear (×320). The nuclei are hyperchromatic and show characteristic, perinuclear, cytoplasmic vacuolization. Multinucleated forms are evident. A normal, superficial cell is shown for comparison (*arrow*). **B,** Flat condyloma. (×530). Koilocytotic changes can be seen in the superficial layers. (Courtesy Dr. Robert Ehrmann and the Division of Women's and Perinatal Pathology, Brigham and Women's Hospital, Boston.)

of these lesions that corresponds exactly with the degree of histologic dedifferentiation and maturation present (Richart, 1963). This is consistent with the postulate that CIN represents stages in a continuum of disease.

Histologically, these preinvasive lesions span a range of severity from a mild loss of polarity with a high degree of cellular differentiation and few mitoses (mild dysplasia or CIN I) to a lesion involving the full thickness of the epithelium, termed severe dysplasia, CIN III, or

carcinoma in situ (CIS). The latter shows marked cytologic and nuclear atypia and increased mitotic activity but retains some degree of epithelial maturation (Fig. 6-12). The differentiation between CIN III and CIS is considered technical only in that the diagnoses are biologically identical. The diagnosis of CIS traditionally requires that the histology reveal identification of minimal cellular flattening in the most superficial cell layers of the epithelium (Fig. 6-13).

In multiple series of untreated patients with CIS (diagnosed on biopsy) who were followed up conservatively, the progression to invasive carcinoma occurred in as many as 70% of patients (Kolstad and Klem, 1976; Spriggs and Boddington, 1980). Observed progression of lesser forms of preinvasive lesions to CIS is reported in 5% to 60% of patients, and this variation in percentages appears to result from differences in the criteria used to define each lesion and varying periods of follow-up (Christopherson and Gray, 1982; Richart, 1966).

These reports also suggest that preinvasive lesions regress in as many as 50% of patients. It has been shown that taking a biopsy specimen may remove the lesion entirely or that the inflammatory process that accompanies repair at the biopsy site may destroy remaining areas of atypicality, thereby giving the clinical impression of regression. More recent studies, in which patients were diagnosed cytologically and then followed up cytologically and colposcopically (thereby eliminating the "biopsy effect"), confirm the progression of preinvasive lesions to CIS in 40% to 60% of patients and spontaneous regression rates as high as 30% for low-grade CIN. The more severe the precancerous change, the higher the rate and speed of progression toward CIS and the lower the rate of regression. The average age of patients with low-grade CIN is consistently 5 to 10 years younger than that of patients with CIS, who are in turn of an average age 10 to 15 years younger than patients with invasive squamous cell carcinoma (Meanwell, 1988).

Histologic and colposcopic observations have established that the transformation zone is where virtually every preinvasive disease originates. Lesions are thought to arise from the basal cells of the transformation zone. If progression occurs, this can result in large-cell nonkeratinizing squamous cell carcinoma. Small-cell carcinoma is thought to arise from the subcolumnar reserve cells of the endocervical canal, whereas large-cell keratinizing carcinoma is thought to arise from the basal cells of the native squamous epithelium. Large-cell nonkeratinizing squamous carcinoma is the most common histologic type seen, which supports the observation that the majority of CIN originates in the transformation zone.

Although some preinvasive lesions regress spontaneously or regress after biopsy, a percentage progresses to invasion. Until we can accurately predict when preinvasive disease will progress, regress, or remain stable, these lesions must be considered premalignant, and the patient must be evaluated, treated, and followed up appropriately. The patient's

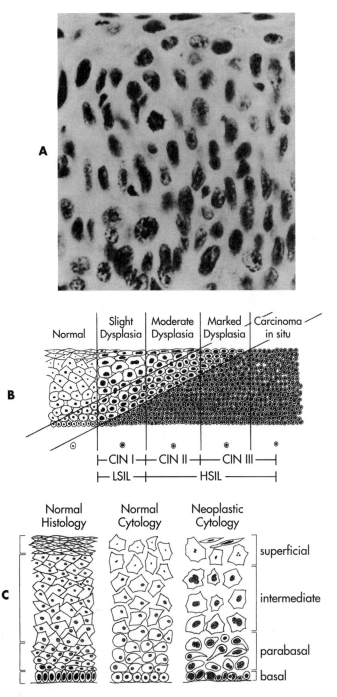

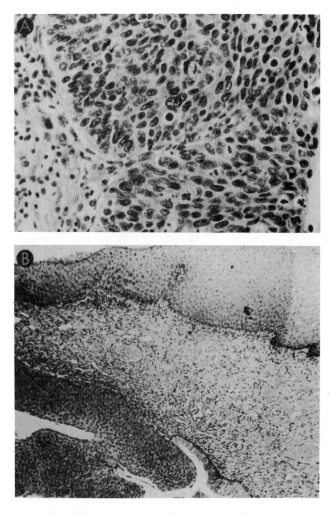

Fig. 6-13. A, Carcinoma in situ (CIS) of cervix. **B,** CIS of cervix with gland involvement. An area of parakeratosis is seen at the upper right. (**A** from Hertig AT, Gore HM: Tumors of the female sex organs, fasc 33, *Atlas of tumor pathology,* Washington, DC, 1960, Armed Forces Institute of Pathology.)

Fig. 6-12. A, High-power (×150) magnification of carcinoma in situ (CIS) of cervix. **B,** Diagrammatic representation of changes in cellular morphology from slight dysplasia to CIS. Nuclear-cytoplasmic ratios are shown at the bottom. **C,** Diagrammatic representation of exfoliated cells from the normal cervix compared with variations of exfoliated cells from the neoplastic cervix. (**B** and **C** courtesy Dr. Paul A. Younge.)

age and desire for fertility, and presence or absence of other pelvic disease must be taken into account.

Recently, preinvasive lesions have undergone a further descriptive transition. With the advent of the Bethesda System for reporting cervical cytology specimens (Kurman et al, 1991) came a transition for preinvasive histology as well.

Essentially, the diagnoses of HPV infection and CIN I were categorized as low-grade squamous intraepithelial lesions (LSIL). CIN II/III and CIS were categorized as high-grade squamous intraepithelial lesions (HSIL). Since the identification of these categories, there have been numerous reports correlating histologic diagnoses with HPV DNA type. When LSIL/HSIL categories are used, a strong correlation is seen between low oncogenic risk viruses 6 and 11 and the diagnosis of LSIL, whereas HSIL has a strong correlation with HPV 16 (Genest et al, 1993; Tabbara et al, 1992).

Adenocarcinoma In Situ

Although the transition of normal squamous epithelium through invasive squamous cell cervical cancer has been well defined histologically, this is not true for its glandular counterpart. First described in 1953 (Friedell and McKay, 1953), adenocarcinoma in situ (ACIS) still does not have a well-defined precursor lesion. Histologically,

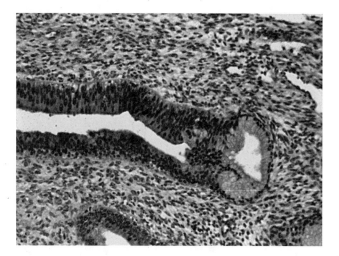

Fig. 6-14. Adenocarcinoma in situ extending into an endocervical crypt. A remnant of the normal columnar epithelium is at the base. Extending upward within the confines of the crypt is a stratified epithelium with nuclear atypia and mitotic activity, characteristic of neoplastic glandular epithelium. (Courtesy Dr. Christopher Crum.)

it is a full-thickness abnormality of the glandular epithelium that generally arises at the transformation zone (Fig. 6-14). In a discussion of the anatomic distribution of cervical ACIS, Bertrand et al (1987) stress that the depth of excision for the treatment of ACIS must be at least 2.5 cm into the endocervical canal. In their series, they advocate conservative management for women who have undergone treatment and are found to have adequate negative margins. More recent reports question the validity of negative margins at the time of conization of the cervix for ACIS, implying that hysterectomy is needed (Poyner et al, 1995). Unfortunately, few, if any, of the recent reports examine depth of excision and publish those findings. Although criteria exist for the cytologic diagnosis of ACIS on Papanicolaou smear (Lee et al, 1997b), most are found at the time of evaluation for squamous intraepithelial lesions (Bertrand et al, 1987).

Diagnosis of Cervical Neoplasia

The contribution of the late George Papanicolaou to the field of cancer detection was outstanding. In studying cells exfoliated from the female genital tract in the late 1920s, Papanicolaou noted characteristic cellular changes associated with cervical carcinoma. These cellular abnormalities included anomalies of staining reaction, pleomorphism, nuclear irregularity, hyperchromasia, the presence of multiple nucleoli, and an increased nuclear-cytoplasmic ratio (Fig. 6-15). As with so many important discoveries, fully 20 years elapsed before Papanicolaou's cytologic technique (the Papanicolaou smear) was accepted as a cancer-screening technique.

The technique used in obtaining a Papanicolaou smear is important because it can significantly decrease false-

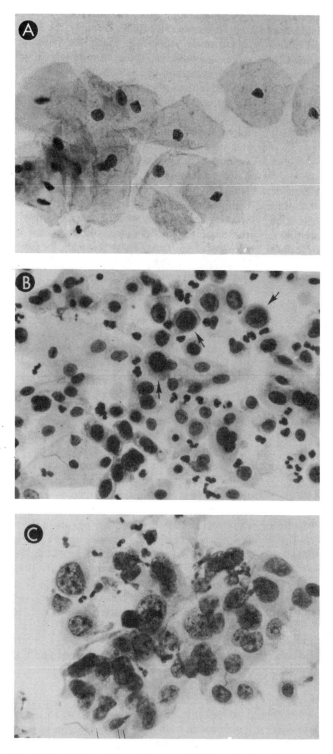

Fig. 6-15. A, Class I (no malignant cells) Papanicolaou smear, benign (×320). Normal polygonal superficial cell, with small pyknotic nuclei. **B,** Class IV (suspicious for cancer) Papanicolaou smear, carcinoma in situ (×320). Neoplastic cells are uniformly large, with hyperplastic nuclei and an increased nuclear-cytoplasmic ratio *(arrows)*. **C,** Class V Papanicolaou smear, invasive cancer (×320). Nuclei exhibit coarse, clumped chromatin and may contain multiple nucleoli. Marked pleomorphism and atypical mitotic figures may be seen. (Courtesy Dr. Robert Ehrmann and the Division of Women's and Perinatal Pathology, Brigham and Women's Hospital, Boston.)

negative and inadequate sampling rates. Papanicolaou smears should be obtained before digital examination with the patient in the lithotomy position. Lubricants, which spoil the staining characteristics of the cells, cannot be used during insertion of the speculum. Douches dilute and wet the cells and should be avoided for 24 hours before a Papanicolaou smear is to be taken. Recent data indicate that the ectocervical area should be sampled first by using a spatula and the endocervical area sampled last using an endocervical brush. This sequence decreases the incidence of obscuring blood on the Papanicolaou smear because the endocervical brush tends to irritate the epithelium (Eisenberger et al, 1997). Both should be smeared onto a glass slide as soon as possible. The most effective technique for transferring cells from the endocervical brush is to roll the brush as the sample is smeared onto the slide. Air-drying artifact is the most common error in the Papanicolaou smear technique. This can be decreased by quick and thorough fixation of the slide after the sample is plated. Hold the can of fixative spray approximately 12 inches from the surface of the slide. Spraying too close can destroy the cells and lead to additional artifacts.

False-negative Papanicolaou smear findings occur when the diagnosis of the cytology specimen is normal but the cervical epithelium is actually abnormal. The most common cause of false-negative findings is sampling error. Some intraepithelial lesions do not shed cells well, or they are small enough to be missed on sampling. Less common sources of false-negative findings are errors in screening or interpretation (Gay et al, 1985; Wilkinson, 1990).

Initially, the Papanicolaou smear was used to detect invasive asymptomatic cervical cancer. As the concept of preinvasive disease was recognized, the Papanicolaou smear classification system was revised to reflect the preinvasive disease diagnoses. Once an abnormality is found, the patient undergoes further evaluation by colposcopy and biopsy of the cervix.

The effects of Papanicolaou smear screening have been well documented. It is estimated that screening every 3 years for women who are between the ages of 20 and 65 years decreases the incidence and mortality rate of invasive cervical cancer by approximately 90% (Eddy, 1990). Factors that affect mortality from cervical cancer include a population's natural incidence of the disease, preclinical stage duration, sensitivity and specificity of the screening process, and quality of treatment available for women with diagnoses of preinvasive and invasive cancer (Klassen et al, 1989). Studies have been conducted to evaluate the age at which women should undergo screening, how frequently they should be screened, at what age screening should cease, and who should perform the screening examination.

There is little debate about when a woman should start to undergo periodic screening. Most clinicians agree that once regular intercourse begins, the risk for preinvasive disease is present. How often a Papanicolaou smear should be taken after the initiation of periodic screening is unclear. In 1988 the American College of Obstetrics and Gynecology, in conjunction with the American Cancer Society and several other cancer organizations, agreed on recommendations for Papanicolaou smear screening intervals (ACOG, 1988; ACOG 1989). They conclude that every woman should have a Papanicolaou smear annually after age 18 years or after the onset of sexual activity. If three consecutive Papanicolaou smears and pelvic examinations 1 year apart are entirely normal, the screening interval can be lengthened at the discretion of the physician. They do not recommend lengthening the interval if the patient or her sexual partner has had more than one other sexual partner. These recommendations do not apply to women followed up for abnormal Papanicolaou smear findings or after treatment of such. Clinicians must stress to their patients the importance of screening and of pelvic examinations because other reproductive tract cancers may be found.

New Papanicolaou Smear Technologies

To decrease the number of false-negative Papanicolaou smears, new technologies for screening or preparing the Papanicolaou smear were approved by the Food and Drug Administration (FDA) in 1995 and 1996. Both the PAPNET system (Neuromedical Systems) and the AutoPap 300 (Neopath) rescreen Papanicolaou smears read as normal, and they try to identify the false-negative interpretation errors. In contrast, the ThinPrep PapTest (Cytic), which was approved by the FDA in 1996, is a new Papanicolaou smear preparation technique. All these new systems are claimed to decrease the false-negative Papanicolaou smear rate (Koss et al, 1994; Colgan et al, 1995; Lee et al, 1997a).

The PAPNET system rescreens conventionally prepared Papanicolaou smears read conventionally as within normal limits. Using a two-step process that involves a primary algorithmic classifier that locates cells and extracts morphologic features, it screens these areas using a neural network-based computer system. From the images reviewed, the system identifies 128 images that require repeat human review. The review is conducted initially by screening the video images, but the slide itself can be rescreened. The person performing the evaluation decides whether any of the areas identified are abnormal and require a change of diagnosis based on the Papanicolaou smear (Koss et al, 1994).

In the AutoPap 300 system, conventional Papanicolaou smears read as normal are rescreened using an algorithmic classifier that also tries to determine the degree of abnormality in a given area of the Papanicolaou smear slide. The device records the coordinates of the area and leads the cytotechnologist or the cytopathologist back to the area of abnormality. Again, the screener determines whether there is an abnormality that necessitates a change in diagnosis (Colgan et al, 1995).

When using the ThinPrep Pap Test, a conventional Papanicolaou smear is not performed. The technique for obtaining a Papanicolaou smear improves with the ThinPrep test. Using a spatula and a brush or a cervical broom, the cervical area is sampled and the devices are rinsed in a fixative solution. The slide is then automatically made in the laboratory, which decreases the possibility of air-drying artifacts. It is then stained and read by a technician or a cytopathologist (Lee et al, 1997a).

Although each system claims to reduce significantly the rate of false-negative Papanicolaou smears, their acceptance in the health care market is slow because they cost more than conventional Papanicolaou smears. It will take additional studies to define their roles in cervical cancer screening, but they may be used widely in the next few years.

Evaluation of the Abnormal Papanicolaou Smear

One must remember that a Papanicolaou smear is a screening tool. It does not render a formal diagnosis of a cervical epithelial abnormality. Histologic diagnosis is required when an abnormal finding is obtained. In the United States, the next step in evaluating an abnormal finding is to perform colposcopy and directed biopsy of the cervix.

Colposcopy and Cervical Biopsy

Colposcopy was developed by Hinselman in 1925 to localize small ulcerations that he theorized represented small cervical neoplasms. He found, however, that the low-power (×6 to ×40) binocular magnification of the colposcope revealed not neoplastic cervical epithelium but alterations of the underlying stromal vasculature. These alterations from the neoplastic process could then be visualized through the thin epithelial layer. The degree of alteration in vascular pattern, in intercapillary distance, and in surface color and texture was found to correlate well with the severity of the neoplastic process. These patterns are enhanced by applications of 3% acetic acid to the cervical epithelium. Use of 3% acetic acid not only cleanses the epithelium, but also causes the precipitation of nucleic proteins in the superficial layers. This leads to the classic aceto-white epithelium that is one of the features of abnormal epithelium.

Adequate colposcopic evaluation requires complete visualization of the transformation zone and of the lesion in question and correlation between the cytologic and histologic diagnoses and the clinical impression of the colposcopist. The cervix is visualized with a speculum and adequately illuminated. Repeating the Papanicolaou smear immediately before a colposcopy is not cost-effective and is not recommended (Spitzer et al, 1997). After visualization and illumination, the cervix is carefully cleaned and soaked with 3% acetic acid. It is generally thought that the most common error in colposcopy is not keeping the cervix adequately soaked with acetic acid, leading to the overlooking of abnormal areas. Endocervical curettage is obtained before biopsies are taken on the cervical portio to reduce the number of curettages contaminated by detached fragments of cervical epithelium. A rectangular biopsy specimen is obtained using a Kevorkian or Younge biopsy punch and is then immediately fixed. Bleeding after biopsy may be controlled by pressure, cauterization with silver nitrate or ferrous subsulfate

(Monsel's solution), packing with oxidized regenerated cellulose, or suturing if required. The patient is instructed to avoid douching, tampons, and intercourse for 5 days after biopsy. Almost 90% of women with abnormal cytologic findings may be adequately evaluated with colposcopy.

Cervical biopsy is perhaps the most common minor surgical procedure performed by the gynecologist. Simple and relatively painless, it may be performed as part of the routine office examination. Contraindications to cervical biopsy are limited to acute pelvic inflammatory disease and acute cervicitis. Pregnancy is not a contraindication to biopsy. Perhaps 85% to 90% of all patients with preinvasive cervical disease may have lesions limited to the portio and yet meet the criteria obviating conization.

When to Evaluate the Abnormal Papanicolaou Smear

The classification of smear abnormalities has evolved over the decades since Papanicolaou first described his classes of smear diagnoses (Table 6-1). When the concept of preinvasive disease was introduced in the late 1950s, the Papanicolaou smear diagnoses were changed to reflect cervical intraepithelial designations. In 1988, a workshop was convened by the National Cancer Institute to address

Table 6-1   Comparison of the Cervical Intraepithelial Neoplasia Papanicolaou Smear Classification and the Bethesda System

Modern Classification	Bethesda System
Squamous Lesions	
No evidence of malignant cells	No evidence of malignant cells
Atypical cells, possibly inflammatory	Atypical squamous cells of undetermined significance (ASCUS) (this term should not include inflammatory cells)
HPV effect, CIN grade I	Squamous intraepithelial lesion, low grade (LSL)
CIN grade II/III, CIS	Squamous intraepithelial lesion, high grade (HSIL)
Squamous cell cancer	Squamous cell cancer
Glandular Lesions	
Atypical glandular cells	Atypical glandular cells of undetermined significance (AGCUS) (should be divided into endocervical or endometrial; origin may include adenocarcinoma in situ [ACIS])
Adenocarcinoma	Adenocarcinoma

HPV, human papillomavirus; *CIN,* cervical intraepithelial neoplasia; *CIS,* carcinoma in situ.

standardization of cervical and vaginal cytopathology reports. This new system of classification came to be known as the Bethesda System (TBS). Its relationship to the previous categories of cervical intraepithelial neoplasia is illustrated in Table 6-1. The term *squamous intraepithelial lesion* now replaces the old category of cervical intraepithelial neoplasia. Modifications of the system have occurred over the years, and now TBS is widely accepted and used in the United States and Western Europe (National Cancer Institute Workshop, 1989).

The categories of LSIL and HSIL have been refined enough to be reproducible and reflective of HPV type (Genest et al, 1993). This has allowed for the development of guidelines indicating how and when to evaluate each abnormal diagnosis with TBS. The algorithms show schematically the approach to each diagnosis (Fig. 6-16). However, the absolute threshold for initial evaluation by colposcopy is not well defined and will vary from one clinician to another. In general, evaluation by colposcopy should occur when a patient has had a second Papanicolaou smear within a 2-year period that shows atypical squamous cells of undetermined significance, or when the smear shows squamous epithelial lesions of low or greater grade. All atypical glandular cells of undetermined significance, or any greater glandular lesion, should undergo colposcopy at once (Kurman et al, 1994).

Therapy for Preinvasive Cervical Disease

Deciding when to treat preinvasive disease of the cervix is controversial. Since the advent of TBS, histology now is read as squamous intraepithelial lesions with the same morphological criteria as in cytology (Tabbara et al, 1992). In general, most clinicians treat HSIL in the patient who is not pregnant, but they reserve treatment for pregnant patients

until after delivery. Whether LSIL should be treated represents the boundary of controversy. Most clinicians allow a patient with a small (two or fewer quadrants of the cervix involved) LSIL to be monitored for 1 to 2 years after histologic diagnosis. This approach is based on the presumption of regression for LSIL, particularly in young women in their 20s and 30s (Koutsky, 1997).

The approach to treatment of preinvasive cervical neoplasia has undergone dramatic changes over the past several decades as the pathogenesis of cervical neoplasia has become better understood. Treatment in general has become less aggressive, and preinvasive disease is rarely treated with removal of the uterus. Most clinicians favor office procedures such as laser therapy, cryosurgery, or simple loop excision of the transformation zone. Cold-knife cervical conization is reserved for ruling out invasive disease in three groups of patients: those in whom colposcopy results are unsatisfactory, those in whom adenocarcinoma in situ is found, or those in whom Papanicolaou smears indicate possible invasion. Hysterectomy still plays a role in treatment, but it is reserved for patients who have completed childbearing and who have severe precancerous lesions that have been resistant to repetitive treatment and for patients who have deep margins of conization with HSIL or ACIS.

Cryocauterization

This technique appears to be the simplest and safest outpatient modality developed. It uses a cryoprobe cooled by carbon dioxide to inflict necrosis on the surface epithelium. Probes of various shapes are available for different cervices. After treatment a watery discharge is common, but it resolves in several weeks. Reepithelialization begins immediately and is virtually complete in 6 weeks (Creasman et al, 1981). The most common technique for cryosurgery is to

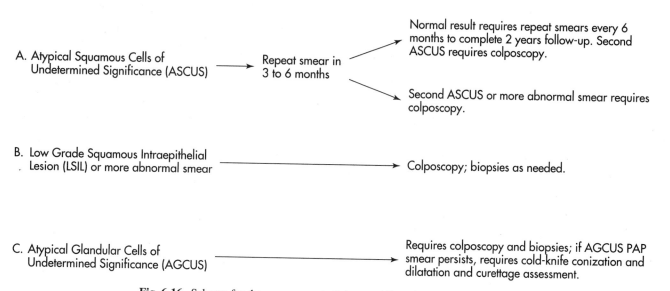

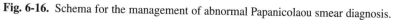

Fig. 6-16. Schema for the management of abnormal Papanicolaou smear diagnosis.

freeze the cervix for 3 minutes, allow it to thaw for 5 minutes, and perform a second freeze for 3 minutes. When properly performed, cryocautery produces necrosis to a depth of 5 to 6 mm, which should theoretically destroy more than 99% of the involved glands (Anderson and Hartley, 1980).

Criticism of cryocauterization has resulted from reports that invasive carcinoma sometimes develops after the procedure. This implies that residual neoplasms were buried during the reparative process and progressed to invasion undetected by cytologic or colposcopic techniques. In a review of eight such incidences, Sevin et al (1979) found that seven of these patients did not undergo pretreatment endocervical curettage, five did not undergo biopsy, and one biopsy was misinterpreted and the true results pointed to invasive carcinoma. Only three patients in this study underwent colposcopic examination. The implication is that these "failures" resulted from inadequate initial evaluations rather than the consequences of cryocauterization.

Laser Therapy

Laser light is generated by electricity running through gas; generally, carbon dioxide is used to treat lower genital tract lesions. Laser therapy produces a coherent or in-phase parallel beam of light of very high energy that is capable of instantly boiling water and thus vaporizing cells. Originally, the laser was focused to eradicate the lesion itself, which spared the remaining cervix. However, failure rates averaged 10% to 30%, and it became clear that the entire transformation zone could be vaporized safely to a depth of 5 to 7 mm to yield cure rates exceeding 90% (Townsend and Richart, 1983). The major drawbacks of this technique are the cost of the laser apparatus and the greater skill required when compared with cryocauterization. Proponents cite less cervical scarring with laser therapy than with cryocauterization. The major benefit from less scarring is the ability to achieve adequate colposcopic evaluation after laser therapy. In younger women of childbearing age, the need for conization is reduced by the need to repeat colposcopy should abnormal cytologic smear results be obtained in the future.

Large-Loop Excision of the Transformation Zone

Prendiville et al (1986, 1989) and others (Murdoch et al, 1992) describe the results of excising the cervical transformation zone using a thin-wire loop and a blended form of electrocautery. The advantages of this technique are that an additional histologic specimen can be obtained and that the procedure can be performed in the office with the patient under local anesthesia. Wright et al (1992) were responsible for popularizing this technique in the United States in the early 1990s.

Technique. Large-loop excision of the transformation zone is often performed in Western Europe as a "see-and-treat" procedure. Patients undergo colposcopy for abnormal Papanicolaou smear results, cervical lesions are identified, and loop excision of the transformation zone is immediately performed. However, this approach has not been as popular in the United States (Murdoch et al, 1992). Most clinicians think it is important that each patient meet the same criteria for outpatient ablative therapy. When this happens, the success rate of large-loop excision is greater than 90%.

During the procedure the patient is placed in the dorsal lithotomy position and is grounded for electrocautery. A speculum insulated for electrical current is used to visualize the cervix. Excision margins are usually defined by iodine staining, though colposcopy can be used. Local anesthetic with 1:100,000 epinephrine is administered in the cervical stroma. A wire loop large enough to remove at least the diseased area on a single lip of the cervix is used. It is preferable to use a single-pass technique. The specimen is sent to pathology department for further evaluation.

It can be difficult to interpret the margins of resection either because of lack of orientation or because of thermal damage. Unless invasive cancer is identified, most clinicians follow up even for margins thought to be involved with preinvasive disease. The patient is evaluated 4 months after the procedure by Papanicolaou smear, colposcopy, endocervical curettage, and cervical biopsy when appropriate. If results are normal, careful follow-up with Papanicolaou smears is continued every 4 months for a year. If results remain normal, 6-month follow-ups and eventually annual follow-ups are recommended (Murdoch et al, 1992; Wright et al, 1992).

Cervical Conization

Cervical conization is the standard against which all outpatient evaluation techniques must be weighed. Properly performed conization removes the entire transformation zone and nearly the entire endocervical canal, and it provides the pathologist with the maximum amount of tissue to rule out invasive carcinoma. Drawbacks of this procedure include the need for anesthesia, a complication rate approaching 10% (primarily postoperative hemorrhage), and possible adverse effects on fertility.

Technique. After the administration of adequate general or regional anesthesia, the patient is placed in the dorsal lithotomy position. The vagina and perineum are prepared with povidone-iodine (Betadine, Purdue Frederick Co.), and the cervix is visualized. Colposcopy or Schiller's test is performed to delineate the extent of disease on the portio. Lateral-angle sutures are placed into the stroma of the cervix at the 3 and 9 o'clock positions to ligate the descending branches of the uterine artery. Some clinicians infiltrate the cervix with dilute solutions of 20 U vasopressin in 20 mL normal saline or bupivacaine (Marcaine, Sanofi Winthrop Pharm.) hydrochloride with epinephrine 1:200,000 to aid hemostasis.

The mucosa is incised circumferentially while a margin of 2 to 3 mm is maintained beyond the lesions (as delineated by colposcopy or Schiller's staining). A cone-shaped specimen 1.5 to 1.8 cm in length and encircling the endocervical canal is excised. A uterine probe may be placed within the canal to aid in the dissection. Once the specimen is removed, a suture is placed at the 12 o'clock position in the stroma of the specimen to aid in orientation of the abnormality. The uterus is then sounded and dilated, and an endometrial sample is taken as desired.

Bleeding is usually minimal with this technique. Bleeding points may be electrocauterized or ligated with size-0 chromic sutures in a figure-eight pattern. The canal is then packed with Surgicel (Johnson & Johnson Medical, Inc.) which is gently tied in place with the long ends of the lateral sutures. Generally, conization is conducted on an outpatient basis; the patient is observed until the anesthetic wears off. The patient is then discharged with instructions to avoid douching, use of tampons, and intercourse for 3 weeks.

Conization for any degree of SIL has a cure rate of 98% when surgical margins are normal; thus, it requires no additional therapy. Close follow-up is suggested, and it includes Papanicolaou smears every 3 months for 1 year and every 6 months thereafter. Given the 70% to 80% cure rate reported after conization with abnormal margins, conservative management with serial endocervical sampling, colposcopy, and cytology is acceptable if patient compliance can be expected. Otherwise re-conization or hysterectomy is indicated. Before surgery, if colposcopy or Schiller's staining shows the upper vagina to be normal, there is no need for a wide vaginal cuff.

Invasive Cancer

Fifty years ago carcinoma of the cervix was the leading cause of death from malignant disease in American women. Since 1940, however, the mortality rate from cervical carcinoma has declined by more than 50%. Yet it still ranks sixth in cancer mortality, and it results in an estimated 4500 deaths each year in the United States. In addition, each year in the United States 12,500 new cases of invasive cervical carcinoma are diagnosed, with the peak incidence in women between ages 45 to 55 years of age, and more than 44,000 new cases of in situ cervical carcinoma are diagnosed. Despite the recognition of a significant preinvasive phase and the availability of screening methods, cervical neoplasia remains a major health problem.

The incidence of cervical cancer varies according to geographic area and race. Cervical cancer is the leading cause of cancer death among women in underdeveloped countries. In the United States the incidence rate for black, Hispanic, and American Indian women is approximately two times higher than it is for white women. The risk for women of Asian-Pacific origin is similar to that for white women (Eddy, 1990). Results from the 1987 U.S. National Health Interview Survey indicate that black women are screened at rates comparable to or higher than those for white women through age 69. Screening rates for Hispanic women are lower than they are for white women. Why black women have a higher incidence rate for cervical cancer is unknown (Harlan et al, 1991).

Symptoms and Diagnosis

There are no specific symptoms that characterize cervical cancer, especially in its early stages. Irregular vaginal bleeding, postcoital bleeding, or both may be noted, or there may be only a pink discharge that is occasionally odorous. Abnormal vaginal bleeding may first be noted as a prolonged menstrual period or as profuse flow at the time of a normal period. As the disease progresses, an initially scant serosanguineous discharge may become grossly hemorrhagic. A common symptom is the daily appearance of a little blood, usually noted after voiding. In the advanced stages of cancer, a characteristic bloody, malodorous discharge, together with pain from fistula formation or nerve irritation, may develop. Pain is a late symptom and is typical of a sciatic distribution that radiates down the back of the buttock, thigh, and knee. Endophytic tumors may cause little or no bleeding or discharge; however, the cancer may spread rapidly to the sacral plexus and produce severe pain. These symptoms, if they result from cervical cancer, become manifest when lesions are of moderate size.

The gross clinical appearance of invasive cervical lesions is generally of two types: exophytic (proliferative) and endophytic (ulcerating). The exophytic lesion may involve the entire cervix and have a cauliflowerlike appearance, whereas the endophytic lesion has a predilection to invade upward into the endocervical canal, often expanding the lower uterine segment and giving rise to the so-called barrel-shaped cervix. Although an endophytic lesion may infiltrate the tissue adjacent to the cervix earlier than an exophytic tumor, either type may extend into the parametrium and involve the uterosacral ligaments or may spread into the vaginal mucosa and down the vaginal canal. This spread causes the tissues to feel firm and nodular. Similarly, the rectum and the bladder may be infiltrated by tumor. Metastatic spread toward the bladder usually involves the vesicovaginal septum and the formation of bullous edema of the bladder before actual involvement of the bladder mucosa. Posterior spread involves the rectovaginal septum, and only late in the disease is the rectal mucosa involved.

Differential Diagnosis

Lesions most commonly confused with cervical cancer are eversions, polyps, papillary endocervicitis, and papillomas. Tuberculosis, syphilitic chancres, and granuloma inguinale rarely involve the cervix, though it may be impossible to differentiate these benign lesions from early invasive cancer by any method other than biopsy. In many patients, repeat or multiple biopsies are necessary before a final diagnosis can be made. This has been particularly true in papillomas of the cervix, which are often difficult to distinguish from low-grade papillary carcinomas.

Secondary carcinoma of the cervix may occur by direct extension from the corpus or the vagina. Metastatic ovarian, bladder, and breast carcinomas have also been reported, though breast cancer may first spread to the ovary and then to the cervix. Lymphoma, particularly histiocytic lymphoma, may appear to be a cervical tumor.

Pathology

Squamous cell carcinoma accounts for 80% the incidences of invasive cervical cancer. Adenocarcinoma accounts for approximately 10% to 15%, and the remainders are sarcomas and primary or secondary lymphomas. The incidence of adenocarcinoma is reported to be 25% in women younger than 35 years (Berkowitz et al, 1979).

Wentz and Reagan (1959) divided squamous cell carcinoma into three types: keratinizing, nonkeratinizing, and small-cell carcinoma. Keratinizing cells show foci of keratinization with cornified "pearls." Nonkeratinizing cells have well-demarcated tumor-stromal borders but no evidence of keratinization or cornified pearls. The small-cell type consists of small, round, or spindle-shaped cells with poorly defined tumor-stromal borders. Although they account for only 1% to 2% of all cervical cancers, small-cell cervical cancers should be recognized as a group that covers a wide variety of subtle, histologically different cancers that have markedly different clinical outcomes.

The significant features differentiating invasive cancer from high-grade intraepithelial lesions are the breakdown of the basement membrane and the involvement of the stroma. Nests and clusters of epithelial cells can be seen scattered in an irregular pattern within a stroma infiltrated by inflammatory cells (Fig. 6-17, *A*). Individual cells of invasive squamous cell carcinoma show the same characteristics described for in situ cancer, namely, loss of stratification and polarity with numerous atypical mitotic figures, pleomorphism, nuclear hyperchromatism (Fig. 6-17, *B*), and dyskaryosis. Giant tumor cells may be found with areas of necrosis and cellular degeneration.

The typical appearance of cervical adenocarcinoma is shown in Fig. 6-17. Adenocarcinoma arises from the columnar cells lining the endocervical canal and glands. Glandular elements are greatly increased, and they show marked variation in size and shape. Cellular pleomorphism, nuclear enlargement and hyperchromatism, and increased mitotic activity with areas of necrosis and degeneration are seen. Adenosquamous carcinoma consists of intermingled malignant squamous epithelial cells and malignant glandular structures. If the squamous component appears benign, the tumor is referred to as an adenoacanthoma.

Mode of Spread of Cervical Cancer

Carcinoma of the cervix spreads principally by direct local invasion and through the lymphatic system. Tumor growth commonly occurs by contiguous spread to the vagina and uterine cavity and laterally through the cardinal and uterosacral ligaments. Lateral spread may occur within the substance of the ligaments or in the areolar tissue adjacent to them. Laterally extending carcinoma may encompass and obstruct the ureters as they traverse the paracervical region and ultimately cause hydroureter, hydronephrosis, and even-

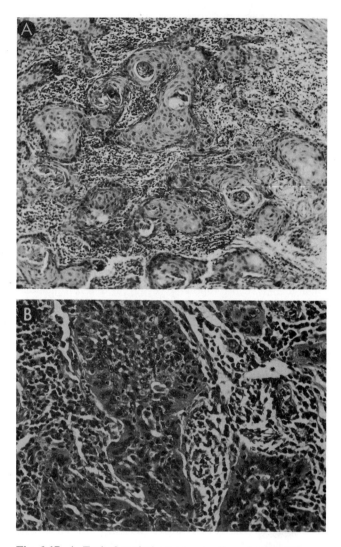

Fig. 6-17. **A,** Typical grade 1 squamous cell carcinoma of the cervix. There is extensive keratinization with "pearl" formation and lymphocytic infiltration of the stroma. **B,** Grade 2 squamous cell carcinoma of the cervix. Several nests of malignant cells show pleomorphism, nuclear hyperchromatism, and atypical mitotic figures. (**A** from Hertig AT, Gore HM: Tumors of the female sex organs, fasc 33, *Atlas of tumor pathology,* Washington, DC, 1960, Armed Forces Institute of Pathology.)

tual loss of kidney function. This may lead to uremia and eventually to death. The cancer may traverse the paravaginal fascia with extension into the bladder or bowel and can result in vesicovaginal or rectovaginal fistulas.

Plentl and Friedman (1971) evaluated pelvic node metastases in cervical cancer by stage and found 15.4% of the nodes to be positive in stage I, 28.6% to be positive in stage II, and 47% to be positive in stage III. They also note that the preferential course of metastatic spread is to the external iliac, hypogastric, and obturator lymph nodes. The next most commonly involved groups are the common iliac, parametrial, and paracervical lymph nodes. The posterior channels that drain to the sacral and the periaortic nodes are less commonly used pathways for tumor dissemination. It appears that the parametrial and paracervical nodes are often skipped in the transit of tumor emboli to the more preferred distal sites.

Pretreatment laparotomy has defined the spread of cervical carcinoma beyond the pelvis. The incidence of periaortic node metastases is approximately 6% in stage IB, 14% in stage IIA, 22% in stage IIB, and 33% in stage IIIB disease (Lagasse, 1980). Buchsbaum reports 23 patients with abnormal aortic nodes who underwent left scalene node biopsy, of which 8 (34.8%) were abnormal (Buchsbaum, 1979). The sites of distant organ metastases in order of frequency are lung, liver, and bone.

Clinical Staging of Cervical Cancer

Clinical staging remains the most important prognostic criterion in determining the patient's response to therapy. The staging process includes pelvic and rectal examination under anesthesia, chest x-ray, routine liver function tests, and evaluation of the urinary tract by either intravenous pyelogram or computed tomography (CT) with intravenous dye. Proctoscopy and cystoscopy are reserved for patients with advanced disease or for whom radiation therapy is planned. Contiguous spread of cervical cancer into the vagina, adjacent parametrium, and pelvic organs is characteristic in the natural history of this disease and forms the basis for clinical staging. All these studies are generally available worldwide and report the standard approach to staging.

Once all the data are obtained, they are used to assign a clinical stage of disease as outlined by the International Federation of Gynecologists and Obstetricians (FIGO; Box 6-1). In the United States, often a computed tomogram with intravenous contrast is used in lieu of an intravenous pyelogram. Information obtained on intraabdominal lymph node sampling cannot be used in clinical staging. However, these data may alter clinical management; therefore, any abnormalities or lymph node enlargements should be sampled by external CT-guided biopsies. *Final staging cannot be changed once therapy has begun.*

Certain difficulties and misinterpretations are unavoidable in clinical staging. On occasion the examiner may interpret pelvic inflammatory processes or scarring from endometriosis as a tumor, thereby "overstaging" the disease. Conversely, the lateral pelvis may be soft when palpated, but abnormal lymph nodes may be found during surgery. Thus, staging will vary with the experience of the examiner. Discrepancies between the clinical staging and the surgical findings have been reported in as many as 25% to 40% of patients (Piver and Barlow, 1974).

It is for this reason that some investigators elect to perform laparotomy before they institute therapy and to determine the presence of metastases to the aortic nodes or other sites beyond the pelvis. Extending the field of treatment to include involved nodal groups is then performed in the hope of improving survival. Although the complication rates have been minimized by extraperitoneal approaches, pretreat-

---

BOX 6-1
INTERNATIONAL FEDERATION OF GYNECOLOGISTS AND OBSTETRICIANS: CLINICAL STAGING OF INVASIVE CERVICAL CANCER

Stage 0
   Carcinoma in situ

Stage I
   Carcinoma confined to the cervix

Stage IA
   Preclinical carcinoma; diagnosis only by microscopy

Stage IA-1
   Microscopically measured invasion of stroma less than or equal to 3-mm depth; 7-mm horizontal spread maximum; lymphovascular space involvement does not alter stage

Stage IA-2
   Microscopically measured invasion of stroma greater than 3 mm to less than or equal to 5 mm; 7-mm horizontal spread maximum; lymphovascular space involvement does not alter stage

Stage IB
   Clinically confined to the cervix; all preclinical greater than stage IA2

Stage IB-1
   Clinical lesion not greater than 4 cm diameter

Stage IB-2
   Clinically confined to cervix; greater than 4 cm diameter

Stage II
   Carcinoma extends beyond the cervix but has not extended to the pelvic wall; it involves the vagina but not the lower third

Stage IIA
   No obvious parametrial involvement

Stage IIB
   Obvious parametrial involvement

Stage III
   Carcinoma has extended to the pelvic wall; on rectal examination there is no cancer-free space between the tumor and the pelvic wall; tumor involves the lower third of the vagina; all patients have hydronephrosis or nonfunctioning kidney

Stage IIIA
   Does not involve pelvic wall

Stage IIIB
   Involves pelvic wall

Stage IV
   Carcinoma has extended beyond the true pelvis or has clinically involved the mucosa of the bladder or rectum; bullous edema is not classified as stage IV

Stage IVA
   Spread of the growth to adjacent organs

Stage IVB
   Spread to distant organs

ment laparotomy has not been shown to increase the survival rates of these patients. More recently, with advances in operative laparoscopy, these same nodal dissections may be performed as outpatient surgical procedures. It remains to be seen whether these staging lymphadenectomies will have an impact on overall survival rates.

Treatment

Conventionally, cervical cancer has been treated with either radical surgery (i.e., radical hysterectomy with pelvic lymph node dissection) or radiation therapy. In certain instances, hysterectomy is performed after radiation therapy. This approach is used when the patient has bulky central pelvic disease because radiation therapy is compromised during the sterilization of such disease. This includes cervical adenocarcinomas that have a propensity to endophytic growth and enlargement of the lower uterine segment and the so-called barrel-shaped cervix that similarly exhibits infiltration and expansion of the lower uterine segment.

Because of the success in managing head and neck squamous cell cancer, a neoadjuvant approach to the management of bulky squamous cervical tumors has been advocated. Tumor cytoreduction through cytotoxic chemotherapy is performed before definitive treatment with radiation therapy or radical surgery. Chemotherapeutic agents also may be used as radiation sensitizers to enhance responses in patients with advanced disease.

Radical Surgery

In the late 1800s, Wertheim of Vienna was the first to perform surgery as a treatment for invasive cervical cancer. Wertheim (1907) reported an 18.9% mortality rate after surgery in his first 500 patients. Because of the high morbidity and mortality rates associated with surgery in that era and because of the discovery of radium by the Curies and of its tissue effects by Becquerel, radiation therapy became the standard treatment modality for invasive cervical cancer. The radical surgical approach, however, was kept alive and was refined by centers in Japan, Germany, Austria, and England. Radical vaginal hysterectomy was introduced in 1901 by Schauta to minimize the morbidity and mortality rates associated with abdominal radical or Wertheim hysterectomy (Schauta, 1902). This procedure permitted wide excision of the parametrial tissues but was limited by the obvious inability to perform a lymph node dissection. Joseph Meigs reintroduced and popularized radical hysterectomy in the United States (Meigs, 1944). A decade later, Liu and Meigs (1955) reported a mortality rate of 1.7% in their first 500 patients.

Radical Hysterectomy. Radical hysterectomy requires removal of the uterus, cervix, parametrial tissues, and upper vagina in conjunction with a pelvic lymphadenectomy from the bifurcation of the iliac vessels to approximately the level of the inguinal ligament. The higher chains and the common iliac and paraaortic areas may be investigated at the discretion of the operating surgeon. Because cervical cancer rarely

metastasizes to the ovaries, they may be preserved in younger patients to avoid the need for replacement therapy. The difficulty in this operation revolves around the need to preserve the integrity and function of the adjacent structures—sidewall vessels, bladder, rectum, and ureters—and at the same time remove enough tissue to ensure clearance of the cancer.

Prophylactic antibiotics and pneumatic calf-compression boots are used routinely. Surgery may be performed through either a low midline or a low transverse muscle-splitting incision. The latter incision provides excellent exposure to the pelvic sidewalls and permits the common iliac nodes and the low paraaortic chain to be dissected. The abdomen and pelvis are carefully explored to exclude the presence of metastatic disease. Biopsy specimens are taken of suspicious lymph nodes in the common iliac or aortic chains and are sent for frozen-section evaluation. Metastatic disease in these areas should be marked with clips for assistance in planning radiation therapy, and surgery should not be performed. Similarly, parametrial (cardinal and uterosacral ligaments), vesicouterine, and rectouterine tissues should be carefully evaluated. Extension to these areas suggests the need for primary radiation therapy.

The mortality rate from radical hysterectomy is 1% or less in appropriately skilled hands; otherwise, the morbidity rate may approach 30%. Complications from radical hysterectomy result in large part from the extent of dissection required. Bladder dysfunction may be seen in 10% to 20% of patients because of denervation injury. Although usually transient, urinary stasis may result in chronic cystitis, ureteritis, and pyelonephritis. Occasionally, a patient may incur permanent bladder paralysis but can learn to control micturition with a semiautomatic bladder that empties itself with voluntary abdominal pressure. Urinary tract fistulas, either ureteral or vesicular, are a result of vascular compromise and may occur in 1% to 2% of patients. Thromboembolic sequelae are in great part averted by pneumatic compression boots. Subcutaneous low-dose heparin is not as effective as compression boots and may increase the risk for the developoment of lymphocysts after pelvic lymph node dissection.

Radiation Therapy

Radiation therapy is administered in most clinics in two forms: external beam whole pelvic radiation and transvaginal intracavitary cesium. The ability to cure cervical cancer with an acceptable level of complication is contingent on intracavitary or interstitial techniques that permit high-dose delivery to the cervix and vagina while minimizing the dosage to the bladder or the rectum.

External beam whole pelvic radiation is generally delivered to the patient in divided doses for 4 to 5 weeks on an outpatient basis. Current dosage conventions for external radiation are defined by the international system of weights and measures (SI). In the past, radiation dosages were defined by the rad, the radiation-absorbed dose. Recently, the SI designated the term *gray* (Gy) to represent the absorbed dose, and this is equivalent to 100 rads. Therefore, 1 rad equals 1 cGy. Most centers administer radiation in single doses of 180 to 200 cGy each weekday, until an accumulative dose of 4500 to 5000 cGy to the pelvis is achieved.

Transvaginal applicators allow significantly larger doses of radiation to the surface of the cervix. Most applicators are placed in the vagina at the time of examination under anesthesia. The cervix is dilated, and a hollow tube (tandem) is placed in the endocervical canal to the fundus. Two small, hollow, round applicators (ovoids) are placed externally to the cervix in the side vaginal fornices. The bladder and rectum are packed away from the applicators using gauze.

Although external beam therapy is limited to 4500 to 5000 cGy because of the tolerance of other pelvic organs, the surfaces of the cervix and the vagina can tolerate up to 15,000 to 20,000 cGy. Typically, 4000 to 8000 additional cGy can be given to the cervix by transvaginal application. This represents a total cervical tumor dose that is between 10,000 and 15,000 cGy. It is estimated that 10,000 cGy or more is necessary to sterilize a squamous cell tumor.

Radiation therapy entails a moderate incidence of complications because of either inherent sensitivity or improper application. The most common difficulties after radiation treatment are cystitis and proctitis. Cystitis is usually delayed 1 year or more after treatment and is characterized by marked frequency, urgency with occasional incontinence, nocturia, dysuria, and hematuria. Results of urine specimens and cultures are usually normal, but the cystoscopic examination is diagnostic. Bladder mucosa is pale and smooth, blood vessels appear constricted, and there is a loss of normal elasticity resulting in diminished bladder capacity. Cystitis is caused by the late effects of radiation therapy, namely, gradual obliteration of capillaries and scarring of supportive tissues. Treatment is often unsatisfactory and protracted, but some relief may be obtained with antispasmodics and with bladder irrigation using dilute silver nitrate or analgesic oily solutions.

Proctitis usually occurs shortly after cesium administration, but it is usually transient. Symptoms include diarrhea, tenesmus, and painful defecation. Relief is obtained with a preparation of diphenoxylate hydrochloride and atropine sulfate (Lomotil, G.D. Searzle & Co.) or with paregoric. Analgesic rectal suppositories are useful if tenesmus persists, and some patients benefit from steroid enemas. In a few patients the radiation reaction may be delayed a year or more, and they may have constipation, diarrhea, and rectal bleeding. Extensive fibrosis may seriously diminish the caliber of the rectosigmoid region so that colostomy is occasionally necessary.

Vesicovaginal and rectovaginal fistulas only rarely result from radiation therapy. Usually they form out of tumors or the destruction of tumor areas by irradiation. However, poor positioning of the intracavitary applicator or an overdose may result in a fistula in the absence of cancer. This is not the fault of the methods but of the technique (Stryker et al, 1988).

Pelvic inflammatory disease prohibits the use of either intracavitary cesium or external radiation; the disease may be markedly activated or aggravated and may lead to tubo-ovarian abscesses, septicemia, and occasionally death. If pyometra is found at the time of uterine curettage, it should be drained and antibiotics should be given until there is no more evidence of infection. If inflammatory tubo-ovarian masses are present, a salpingo-oophorectomy should be carried out before radiation therapy.

Vaginal stenosis may develop after radiation treatment. This may be prevented in younger women by frequent examinations and by breaking up the thin synechiae as they develop. Coitus will aid in keeping the vagina of normal size. In older women, the vagina usually closes off so that the cervix is no longer available for inspection or cytologic examination. This may restrict vaginal sexual activity, and it prevents adequate follow-up by means of vaginal smears. Many of these problems may be minimized or prevented if patients undergoing radiation therapy routinely use vaginal dilators.

Other effects of radiation therapy include late small-bowel obstruction and perforation and loss of ovarian function before menopause. Loss of hormonal function typically occurs at 1000 cGy or higher and can result in decreased libido and menopausal symptoms. Estrogen replacement therapy is recommended for most patients undergoing radiation therapy for cervical cancer. This is not considered a hormonally responsive tumor, and there is no evidence that such therapy brings about a recurrence of cervical cancer.

Bowel obstruction or perforation may occur as late as 10 years after therapy. Often the patient may note vague lower abdominal cramps, irregular bowel habits, and blood in the stool. Roentgenogram findings may be entirely normal, but exploration will reveal multiple loops of small bowel adherent to each other and to adjacent structures. In the more severe forms, arteriolar occlusion may result in localized areas of necrosis with perforation. It is well to remember this possible complication of radiation therapy in the differential diagnosis of an acute abdomen.

Neoadjuvant Chemotherapy

In response to the limited success in treating locally advanced squamous cervical carcinoma, protocols using chemotherapy as an initial treatment step have been devised and at least preliminarily tested. The concept behind neoadjuvant chemotherapy is to decrease the central tumor bulk in stage IB2 and beyond, potentially making those patients amenable to radical surgery or more responsive to radiation therapy. Results of several outcome studies have been published (Sardi et al, 1997; Colombo et al, 1998), and the consensus is that tumors that are 4 cm or smaller do not experience a survival benefit after neoadjuvant therapy and surgery compared to surgery alone. Patients whose tumors are larger than 4 cm have potential survival benefit if the therapy results in a surgical procedure that has negative margins. The ultimate answer regarding this treatment modality awaits a prospective clinical trial.

Appropriate Therapy Based on Clinical Staging

To a degree, the management of invasive cervical cancer is stage dependent. Stage I/IIA disease allows for the option of surgical management or radiation therapy. Traditionally, however, disease at stage IIB and beyond requires treatment with radiation. Within stage I disease, it is important to realize that both surgery and radiation provide the same chance for cure. How to decide which to use depends on patient age (those younger than 65 years have surgery; those older than 65 years have radiation only), body habitus (obesity can preclude surgery), hormonal function (surgery can preserve function), and underlying medical problems (Landoni, 1997).

Stage IA. The concept of minimally invasive or microinvasive cervical carcinoma was first suggested by Mestwerdt in 1947. He suggested that patients with minimal degrees of invasion (3 to 5 mm below the basement membrane) are at virtually no risk for either parametrial spread or lymph node involvement and can be treated with simple hysterectomy (Fig. 6-18). The critical issue is to identify which group of patients would benefit from more conservative therapy. The Society of Gynecologic Oncologists (SGO) has proposed the following definition: A microinvasive lesion is one in which neoplastic epithelium invades the stroma in one or more places to a depth of 3 mm or less below the base of the epithelium and in which lymphatic or vascular involvement is not demonstrated. When this definition of microinvasive cervical cancer is used, the risk for lymph node involvement is less than 1% (Seski et al, 1977). In most centers a total extrafascial hysterectomy performed either abdominally or vaginally without lymph node dissection may be considered adequate treatment.

In 1995 the Staging Committee of FIGO developed specific criteria for defining minimally invasive or microinvasive cervical carcinoma (see Box 6-1). Stage IA-1 was defined as preclinical cancer with a maximum depth of invasion from the basement membrane of 3 mm and maximum lateral spread of 7 mm. This depth of invasion is now more aligned with the SGO definition. Although stage assignment must be made according to the FIGO system, patient management in this country is still based on the SGO definition.

Preliminary data indicate that cone biopsy alone may be adequate therapy for patients whose lesions match the SGO definition. This should only be considered in patients who desire to retain fertility, whose cone margins are free of disease, in whom compliance for Papanicolaou smear follow-up is expected, and who have been provided appropriate counseling and have given informed consent (Copeland and Silva, 1992). Microinvasive carcinoma may also be treated with intracavitary radioactive sources alone (7000 to 9000 cGy in one or two insertions). However, many of these patients are young, and surgical treatment is preferred because it preserves normal ovarian function.

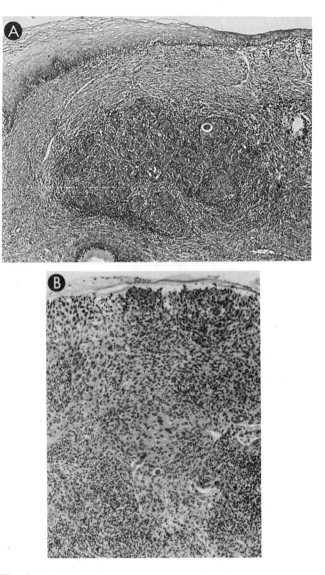

Fig. 6-18. A, Microinvasive carcinoma underlying normal portio epithelium. No other areas of invasion can be found in this cervix. Carcinoma in situ (CIS) from which this miniature cancer must have arisen was found in the endocervix. **B,** Late stromal invasion characterized by a confluence of invasive buds into an inflamed stroma. The surface epithelium is absent on the right, but overlying CIS is visible on the left.

Stages IB and IIA. Patients with stage IB or IIA carcinoma (confined to the upper vagina) may be treated with radical surgery or radiation therapy. Overall the survival for stage IB cervical cancer treated with radiation therapy or radical surgery is approximately 85% at 5 years. For stage IIA lesions, survival with either modality approaches 75%. Patients with extensive stage IIA disease are routinely treated with radiation therapy. If radical hysterectomy and node dissection reveal involvement of the pelvic nodes, patients are often treated with postoperative pelvic radiation therapy, though there is little evidence that this approach improves survival rates. It does appear to increase the likelihood of pelvic control (SGO Panel Report, 1980).

Within the stage IB grouping, lesion size must be taken into consideration when deciding on treatment. In one large series of women treated by radical hysterectomy, Piver and Chung (1975) report a 5-year survival rate of 85% for those with stage IB lesions up to 3 cm in diameter but only a 66% survival rate for those with tumors 4 to 5 cm in diameter. In a later study Van Nagell et al (1979) found that for stage I lesions larger than 2 to 5 cm in diameter, the failure rate was 24% for surgery and only 11% for radiation. These studies suggest that stage I lesions larger than 3 cm are best treated with radiation therapy, though it has been shown that increasing tumor size may be associated with reduced survival rates even in patients treated with radiation therapy (Patanaphan and Poussin-Rusillo, 1986; Stehman and Bundy, 1991). Based on these data and because of the technical difficulties in radically excising large lesions, patients with tumors larger than 3 cm are usually treated with radiation therapy.

Bloss et al (1992) at the University of California, Irvine Medical Center report on bulky cervical carcinoma greater than 4 cm in patients treated with radical hysterectomy and node dissection. Adjuvant radiotherapy was tailored to the clinical status and was based on such variables as nodal involvement, deep invasion, and close margins. Morbidity outcomes were similar to their experiences with radical hysterectomy for smaller lesions: 50% of the patients underwent radiotherapy, and 70% of those survived 5 years.

Patients with stage IB or IIA disease not amenable to radical surgery are usually treated with radiation therapy. If the initial bulk of disease is minimal, the tandem and ovoid can be used first, which decreases the amount of external beam therapy. If the initial bulk of disease is large, then external beam therapy is delivered to achieve maximum tumor shrinkage in preparation for brachytherapy. Neoadjuvant chemotherapy may also be considered for these patients. Depending on tumor size, many patients are able to undergo surgery chemo-cytoreduction.

Barrel-shaped cervix. Among patients treated with a single therapy, the probability of pelvic failure increases with increasing tumor size. If the therapy has been surgery, the risk for nodal involvement increases with increasing bulk. With radiation therapy, failure can result because of the inability of radiation to sterilize bulky tumor masses that probably contain hypoxic (radiation-resistant) areas. Reports suggest that conservative hysterectomy after radiation therapy to remove the bulky, central stage I disease may improve local control and increase survival (Gallion, 1985). This technique is often used in the management of endocervical adenocarcinoma that has a propensity for endophytic growth with upward involvement and expansion of the lower uterine segment.

Stages IIB, III, and IVA. Patients with stage IIB, III, or IVA cervical carcinoma are best treated with radiation therapy techniques because adequate dissection beyond the boundaries of the tumor is not technically feasible. External beam therapy is expanded to encompass the common iliac nodes, the upper half of the vagina, and the central pelvis. Stage IIB may be treated with 4000 cGy to the pelvis and an additional parametrial boost to 1000 cGy delivered before or after intracavitary treatment. This results in a slightly higher dosage to the medial parametria-lateral cervix. The 5-year survival rate for stage IIB disease treated in this fashion is 60% to 65%.

Treatment of stage III disease requires a higher dosage provided by external therapy. For example, 5000 cGy to the whole pelvis with an additional parametrial boost of 1000 to 1500 cGy to the involved sides may be prescribed. This is followed by one intracavitary treatment to the nodal areas providing a total dosage of 6500 to 7000 cGy and to the medial parametrial-lateral cervix of 8500 to 9500 cGy. In all circumstances the higher the dosage that can be provided by intracavitary therapy, the lower the dosage delivered to the bladder and rectum. The 5-year survival rate for patients with stage III disease ranges from 25% to 40%. Patients with stage IVA cancer (bladder or rectum) can be treated with either high-dose radiation therapy or exenterative surgery. A neoadjuvant approach may be considered for patients with advanced stage disease.

Stage IVB. Patients diagnosed with distant metastases at the initial visit are rarely cured, given the limitations of conventional treatment modalities. The exception is the patient with disease that has spread to an area that can be aggressively irradiated. For example, patients with extrapelvic disease limited to the para-aortic chain may undergo extended field radiotherapy; the cure rates are in the 20% to 30% range at 5 years (Potish et al, 1984). Morbidity and mortality rates of extended field radiation therapy after para-aortic dissection is high, usually because of gastrointestinal dysfunction. The typical patient with stage IVB disease undergoes systemic cytotoxic chemotherapy. Although the anecdotal patient may do well, the prognosis for this stage is dismal.

Recurrent Cervical Carcinoma

When cancer of the cervix recurs, it is usually within 2 to 3 years of primary treatment. Symptoms may include vaginal bleeding, bloody discharge, hematuria, dysuria, constipation, melena, pelvic and leg pain, edema of the leg, and fistulas. If sacral backache or pain of sciatic distribution occurs, it is invariably caused by tumors of the sacral plexus. Costovertebral angle and flank pain may herald the development of ureteral obstruction and pyelonephritis. There is usually associated lassitude, anorexia, weight loss, and anemia. Diagnosis may be simplified by routine cytologic studies on follow-up examination because tumor cells may be detected before symptoms develop. This is applicable to recurrence in the vagina and cervix only because a tumor in the pelvic nodes or broad ligament does not exfoliate tumor cells into the vaginal vault. In most patients the diagnosis depends on an evaluation of symptoms and a careful pelvic examination. Progressively firm nodularity in the paracervical and uterosacral area, felt best on rectal examination, is usually pathognomonic of a viable tumor.

Cervical or vaginal vault (central) recurrences should always be confirmed by biopsy. Computed axial tomography is useful for defining a tumor in enlarged lymph nodes and distant metastases. Abnormalities on the excretory urogram, such as the development of hydroureter and hydronephrosis, suggest periureteral compression by tumor—though radiation fibrosis may produce the same condition and may be amenable to surgical correction by ureteral implantation or urinary diversion.

Anatomic sites of treatment failure correlate closely with tumor stage and volume. With adequate local resection or satisfactory dosimetry, any recurrences are rare in small-volume stage I or IIA disease. Patients with more extensive pelvic disease generally experience treatment failure and recurrence because of the difficulty of controlling a bulky tumor with radiation therapy alone. Improved radiotherapy techniques have improved our ability to attain local control. However, because of the high incidence of failure among patients with advanced-stage disease, effective systemic therapy is needed for an impact on long-term survival.

Patients with recurrent cervical cancer may be treated for cure only if the disease is confined to the pelvis. In general, patients who have central recurrence after radical hysterectomy are treated with radiation therapy. This combines external beam therapy with an intracavitary or an interstitial approach. Salvage rates approaching 50% have been reported, though it may be difficult to salvage patients with massive central recurrence by using radiotherapy alone (Deutsch and Parsons, 1974).

Patients who have previously been treated with radiotherapy may be treated now only by radical pelvic surgery. Patients with minimal disease may be considered for radical hysterectomy, though the complication rate related to fistula formation may be as high as 50% and permanent diversion is required for correction. Most patients, however, require ultraradical, multivisceral pelvic resection, or pelvic exenteration. This procedure entails resection of the bladder, distal ureters, rectum, vagina, internal genitalia, and parametrial tissues, and diversion of the urinary stream to a permanent conduit and the fecal stream to a colostomy. Vaginal reconstruction may be performed at the time of exenteration. Similarly, low rectal anastomosis or construction of a continent urinary conduit may make this procedure more acceptable to the patient. Because of the extensive nature of this surgery and the permanent changes in organ function and body image, exenteration should be performed for cure. If the disease is extrapelvic or there is extension to the pelvic sidewalls or lymph nodes, the disease is inoperable and the prognosis dismal. Morley (1984) reported on the use of pelvic exenteration for treating recurrent cervical cancer. Of more than 90 patients, 75% were treated with total pelvic exenteration; based on the location of the tumor, the remainder were treated with either resection of the bladder anteriorly or excision of the bowel posteriorly. The 5-year

survival rate for recurrent carcinoma of the cervix in his series was 63%.

Ureteral compression in the pelvis or near the kidney, with uremia, pyelonephritis, or both, is a major cause of death and is found in approximately 50% of patients. Other causes of death are infection (peritonitis, pelvic abscess, septicemia), uncontrolled hemorrhage, and extrapelvic metastases. Patients treated for cardiac failure sometimes have severe pulmonary edema together with edema of the arms and neck. Usually there is redness in the face and neck caused by superior vena caval obstruction from metastatic cervical cancer.

In 13% of deaths from cancer of the cervix, the cause is gastrointestinal tract involvement that usually manifests itself as large-bowel obstruction at the rectosigmoid level. Occasionally, perforation of the large or small bowel results in fatal peritonitis. Jaundice caused by extensive terminal hepatic metastases may be noted.

Chemotherapy. Various single agents have been used in the treatment of women with recurrent squamous cell carcinoma of the cervix, with cisplatin uniformly yielding response rates of 25% to 30%. Other active agents include 5-fluorouracil, mitomycin, ifosfamide, doxorubicin hydrochloride, vincristine, and bleomycin. In general the response rates with combination therapy are higher, but the cost is increased toxicity (Jobson et al, 1981). Most combinations include platinum, and response rates often range from 50% to 70% (Alberts and Mason-Liddil, 1989; Kumar and Bhargava, 1991; Rotmensch and Senekjian, 1988). Although these appear to be acceptable results, the durations of response—4 to 6 months—are dismally short. Only the occasional patient reaches complete response. Several factors contribute to these poor results:

- Pelvic radiation therapy compromises bone marrow reserve.
- Renal insufficiency secondary to tumor recurrence or radiation fibrosis limits adequate drug dosing.
- Radiation fibrosis or vascular distortion associated with radical surgery may impair drug delivery.

To bypass these issues, up-front chemotherapy used neoadjuvantly or as a radiation sensitizer is gaining widespread acceptance. Additionally, chemotherapy with or without radiation therapy is sometimes used for patients who are node positive after radical hysterectomy and node dissection (Tattersall and Ramirez, 1992).

Carcinoma of the Cervix During Pregnancy

Cervical cancer occurs in aproximately 0.01% of pregnant patients. Therapeutic decisions are based on cancer stage, pregnancy trimester, and patient preference. Although pregnancy does not have a detrimental effect on the course of the disease, nor does vaginal delivery affect prognosis, it is essential that the diagnosis be made promptly because delay in treatment can alter prognosis.

Before the third trimester, treatment is based on disease stage. For stage I and IIA lesions, the acceptable therapy is radical hysterectomy with pelvic lymph node dissection. If radiation therapy is planned, one of two courses is followed: the uterus may be evacuated at the time of the first radium application or whole-pelvis irradiation may be started. If abortion has not been performed or has not occurred spontaneously, the uterus is evacuated surgically after the completion of external irradiation during radium application.

Late in the second trimester, therapy may be delayed until fetal viability is assured. For stage I and IIA lesions, classic cesarean section is performed and is followed immediately by radical hysterectomy and pelvic lymph node dissection. In more advanced stages, external radiation is delivered after cesarean section. This usually requires a delay of 7 to 10 days while the abdominal incision heals. After the completion of external radiation therapy, intracavitary radiation is used, as outlined earlier, for the appropriate stage.

Clear Cell Adenocarcinoma of the Cervix

The incidence of clear cell adenocarcinoma in women exposed in utero to DES is 1:1000. This low-risk level indicates that DES is not a complete carcinogen but that it requires some other factor to induce cancer. Cancer has developed in women as young as 16 to 27 years (median age, 19 years). Follow-up of the DES-exposed women consists of annual Papanicolaou smears from the cervix and the vaginal walls and careful palpation of the vaginal walls for evidence of adenosis or masses (Committee on Gynecologic Practice, 1993).

Controversy remains over whether intraepithelial neoplasia of the vagina or the cervix is more likely to develop in DES-exposed women or in nonexposed women. Because the evidence is inconclusive either way, yearly Papanicolaou smears are recommended for all women, with referral for colposcopy if an abnormality appears (Committee on Gynecologic Practice, 1993). In women who took DES during pregnancy, there is a 1.35% increased relative risk of breast cancer. This risk does not increase with age (Colton et al, 1993).

Treatment of cervical clear cell adenocarcinoma is similar to that outlined for squamous cell carcinoma of the cervix. However, because most of these patients are young, the preferred therapy is radical hysterectomy and pelvic lymph node dissection if they have stage I or IIA disease. Ovarian conservation is maintained; if the vagina is involved, vaginectomy followed by reconstruction provides excellent functional results. The overall survival rate for women with DES-associated clear cell carcinoma is 80%. In those with stage I disease, the 5-year survival rate exceeds 90%.

Although most DES-related clear cell carcinomas recur within 3 years of initial treatment, late recurrences have been reported. Burks et al (1990) report that the longest interval to recurrence is 17 years after initial therapy; they recommend long-term yearly follow-up with periodic chest x-rays. Pulmonary and supraclavicular nodal metastases are more common than squamous cell carcinoma of either the cervix or the vagina. If there is local recurrence without

sidewall involvement, pelvic exenteration may be considered. If aortic or pelvic nodes are involved, exenteration is contraindicated (Knapp, 1984).

Carcinoma of the Cervical Stump

In past decades subtotal hysterectomy has been performed less often, and removal of the stump accounts for a decreased incidence of cervical stump cancer. With increased interest in minimally invasive surgery and attempts to preserve sexual function, resulting in retention of the cervix, the possiblility of an increase in stump cancer is present.

Carcinoma of the cervical stump poses special challenges to the treating physician, both from a surgical and a from radiotherapeutic standpoint. Radical cervicectomy and pelvic lymph node dissection may be performed. However, earlier surgery may have introduced fibrosis and scarring to the retroperitoneum, significantly increasing the difficulty of ureteral dissection. Morbidity rates and outcome, however, are similar to those reported for treatment by radical hysterectomy (Creadick, 1958).

Radiotherapy may be compromised by the inability to use a uterine tandem, which is critical in dosing the central tumor and the medial parametrium. Transvaginal or interstitial therapy is common when a tandem cannot be used, and, in most circumstances, the dose administered by external beam to the pelvis must be increased. These changes in dose, and the likelihood of adhesions to the bowel at the vaginal apex, suggest that survival may be compromised by increased complications. Survival rates in most series, however, are similar to those seen among patients with intact uteri, though the complication rate may be modestly increased (Oats, 1976; Wimbush and Fletcher, 1969).

Incidental Invasive Cervical Carcinoma Found at Conservative Hysterectomy

Invasive carcinoma may be found after hysterectomy has been performed for benign indications. This occurs if emergency surgery has precluded complete cervical evaluation, if evaluation was inadequate before elective surgery, or if hysterectomy is performed in response to false-negative Papanicolaou test results. Prognosis is related to the extent of tumor. Patients with apparently minimal disease confined to the cervix do well. In contrast, patients with more extensive disease do poorly (Andras and Fletcher, 1973). Patients treated with radiation therapy may have problems similar to those encountered when treating stump cancer. With exploration, it may be found that radical parametrectomy and node dissection obviate the increased complications associated with radical radiotherapy (Orr, 1986).

Cervical Adenocarcinoma

In the past, cervical adenocarcinomas accounted for perhaps 5% of the total number of invasive cervical cancers treated in the United States (Fig. 6-19). This relative proportion has increased, with glandular tumors accounting for 10% to 20% of the total. In part this arises from an absolute

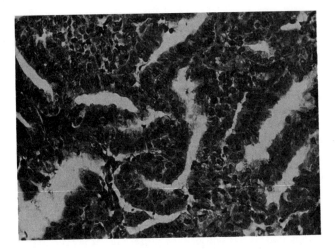

Fig. 6-19. Adenocarcinoma of the cervix. Malignant cells are arranged in a glandular pattern. The typical columnar appearance of the cell has been lost, and numerous cells show atypical mitoses.

decrease in the number of squamous cell carcinomas and a probable absolute increase in the number of adenocarcinomas. From a diagnostic standpoint, early diagnosis is difficult. The false-negative rate of Papanicolaou testing may be as high as 80% despite occult cervical adenocarcinoma. Many patients are diagnosed once symptoms of bleeding or discharge are noted (Hurt, 1977).

These lesions arise from the endocervical epithelium and have a propensity for endophytic growth and upward spread to the lower uterine segment. Often this gives rise to bulky tumors in a barrel-shaped distribution. The pattern of spread is otherwise similar to that seen with squamous tumors. A higher local failure rate for these tumors after treatment with radiation therapy suggests that they are relatively radiation resistant compared with the squamous lesions. However, the higher local failure rate probably results from higher tumor volume secondary to its distinctive pattern of spread. As a result, many investigators recommend a combined-modality approach with radiotherapy followed by simple hysterectomy, similar to what is recommended for patients with barrel-shaped squamous cell carcinoma of the cervix (Berek and Castaldo, 1981). Combined radical hysterectomy and node dissection remains an excellent treatment option, and it minimizes the problems surrounding extensive central uterine disease. Patients with recurrent disease undergo treatment similar to that used for patients with squamous tumors. The role of chemotherapy, however, is yet to be defined because the agents now available have little effect on these lesions.

Small-Cell and Neuroendocrine Small-Cell Carcinoma

Small-cell carcinoma of the cervix accounts for 1% to 6% of all cervical cancer. Additional classification by the pathologist is small-cell squamous cell carcinoma, which is managed similarly to other cervical squamous cancers, and neuroendocrine small-cell carcinoma, which requires more aggressive therapy and carries a dismal prognosis. These latter tumors may arise from either the argyrophil cells of the cervix (part of the amine precursor uptake and decarboxylation system) or from subcolumnar reserve cells, and they are histologically identical to oat cell carcinoma of the lung. They have a high propensity for early lymphatic and systemic spread and are treated aggressively with a combined-modality approach that includes surgery, radiation, and chemotherapy (Sheets et al, 1988).

Cancer Metastatic to the Uterine Cervix

A variety of tumors may metastasize to the cervix, and cervical cytology may be the first indication of a malignancy. Endometrial, bladder, and rectal cancer may spread directly to the cervix. Intraabdominal cancer may involve the cervix as a sequelae of extensive pelvic involvement and extension through the vagina, uterus, or uterosacral ligaments. On occasion, hematogenous spread may extend to the uterus or cervix from such sites as the breast or lung. Therapy is aimed at the primary site of origin.

REFERENCES

Alani R, Munger K: Human papillomaviruses and associated malignancies. *J Clin Oncol* 1998; 16:330-337.

Alberts DS, Mason-Liddil N: The role of cisplatin in the management of advanced squamous cell cancer of the cervix. *Semin Oncol* 1989; 16:66-78.

American College of Obstetrics and Gynecology: ACOG and other organizations draw closer on frequency of pap smears. *ACOG Newsletter* 1988; 32:1-5.

American College of Obstetrics and Gynecology: *Recommendation on frequency of Pap test screening*, ACOG Committee Opinion 152, Washington DC, 1995, Author.

Anderson MC, Hartley RB: Cervical crypt involvement by intraepithelial neoplasia. *Obstet Gynecol* 1980; 55:546-550.

Andras EJ, Fletcher GH: Radiotherapy of carcinoma of the cervix following simple hysterectomy. *Am J Obstet Gynecol* 1973; 115:647-651.

Anonymous: 1988 Bethesda System for reporting cervical/vaginal cytologic diagnoses. *JAMA* 1989; 262:931-934.

Berek JS, CastaldoTW: of the uterine cervix. *Cancer* 1981; 48:2734-2741.

Bergeron C, Ferenczy A, Shah KV, Naghashtar Z: Multicentric human papillomavirus infections of the female genital tract: Correlation of viral types with abnormal mitotic figures, colposcopic presentation and location. *Obstet Gyencol* 1987; 69:736-742.

Berkowitz RS, Ehrmann RL, Lavizzo-Mourey R, Knapp RC: Invasive cervical cancer in young women. *Gynecol Oncol* 1979; 8:311-316.

Bertrand M, Lickrish GM, Colgan TJ: The anatomic distribution of adenocarcinoma in situ: Implications for treatment. *Am J Obstet Gynecol* 1987; 71:842-846.

Bloss JD, Berman ML, Mukhererjee J et al: Bulky stage IB cervical carcinoma managed by primary radical hysterectomy followed by tailored radiotherapy. *Gynecol Oncol* 1992; 47:21-27.

Bosch FX, Manos MM, Munoz N, et al: Prevalence of human papillomavirus in cervical cancer: A worldwide perspective. *J Natl Cancer Inst* 1995; 87:796-802.

Buchsbaum HJ: Extrapelvic lymph node metastases in cervical carcinoma. *Am J Obstet Gynecol* 1979; 133:814-824.

Burks RT, Schwartz AM, Wheeler JE, Antonioli D: Late recurrence of clear-cell adenocarcinoma of the cervix, II: Case report. *Obstet Gynecol* 1990; 76:525-527.

Butterworth CE Jr, Hatch KD, Gore H, et al: Improvement in cervical dysplasia associated with folic acid therapy in users of oral contraceptives. *Am J Clin Nutr* 1982; 35:73-82.

Butterworth CE Jr, Hatch KD, Macaluso M, et al: Folate deficiency and cervical dysplasia. *JAMA* 1992; 267:528-533.

Christopherson WM, Gray LA: Dysplasia and preclinical carcinoma of the uterine cervix: Diagnosis and management. *Semin Oncol* 1982; 9:265-279.

Colgan TJ, Patten SF, Lee JSJ: A clinical trial of the AutoPap 300 QC system for quality control of cervicovaginal cytology in the clinical laboratory. *Acta Cytol* 1995; 39:1191-1198.

Colombo A, Landoin F, Maneo A, et al: Neoadjuvant chemotherapy to radiation and concurrent chemoradiation for locally advanced squamous cell carcinoma of the cervix: A review of the recent literature. *Tumori* 1998; 84:229-237.

Colton T, Greenberg ER, Noller K, et al: Breast cancer in mothers prescribed diethylstilbestrol in pregnancy: Further follow-up. *JAMA* 1993; 269:2096-2100.

Committee on Gynecologic Practice: Diethylstilbestrol. *ACOG Committee Opinion* 1993; 131:1.

Copeland LJ, Silva EG: Superficially invasive squamous cell carcinoma of the cervix. *Gynecol Oncol* 1992; 45:307-312.

Coppleson M, Reid BL: *Preclinical carcinoma of the cervix uteri,* New York, 1967, Pergamon Press.

Creadick RN: Carcinoma of the cervical stump. *Am J Obstet Gynecol* 1958; 75:564-567.

Creasman WT, Clarke-Pearson DL, Weed JC et al: Results of outpatient therapy of cervical intraepithelial neoplasia. *Gynecol Oncol* 1981; 12:5306-5316.

Deutsch M, Parsons JA: Radiotherapy for carcinoma of the cervix recurrent after surgery. *Cancer* 1974; 34:2051-2055.

Eddy DM: Screening for cervical cancer. *Ann Intern Med* 1990; 113:214-226.

Eisenberger D, Hernandez E, Tener T, Atkinson BF: Order of endocervical and ectocervical cytologic sampling and the quality of the papanicolaou smear. *Obstet Gynecol* 1997;90:755-758.

Ferenczy A: Anatomy and histology of the cervix. In Blaustein A, editor: *Pathology of the female genital tract,* ed 2, New York, 1982, Springer-Verlag.

Ferenczy A: Comparison of cryo- and carbon dioxide laser therapy for cervical intraepithelial neoplasia. *Obstet Gynecol* 1995; 66:793-797.

Ferenczy A, Mitao M, Nagai N,et al: Latent papillomavirus and recurring genital warts. *N Engl J Med* 1985; 313:784-788.

Fluhmann CF: Developmental anatomy of the cervix uteri. *Obstet Gynecol* 1960; 15:62-69.

Forsberg JG: Cervicovaginal epithelium: Its origin and development. *Am J Obstet Gynecol* 1973; 115:1025-1043.

Friedell GH, McKay DG. Adenocarcinoma in situ of the endocervix. *Cancer* 1953; 6:887-897.

Gallion HH, Van Nagell Jr., JR, Donaldson ES, et al: Combined radiation therapy and extrafascial hysterectomy in the treatment of stage IB barrel-shaped cervical cancer. *Cancer* 1985; 56:262-265.

Gay JD, Donaldson LD, Goellner JR: False-negative results in cervical cytologic studies. *Acta Cytol* 1985; 24:1043-1046.

Genest DR, Stein L, Cibas E, et al: A binary (Bethesda) system for classifying cervical cancer precursors: Criteria, reproducibility, and viral correlates. *Hum Pathol* 1993; 24:730-736.

Gondos B: Development of the reproductive organs. *Ann Clin Lab Sci* 1985; 15:363-373.

Grunebaum AN, Sedlis A, Sillman F, et al: Association of human papillomavirus infection with cervical intraepithelial neoplasia. *Obstet Gynecol* 1983; 62:448-455.

Handley WS: The prevention of cancer. *Lancet* 1936; 1:987.

Harlan LC, Bernstein AM, Kessler LG: Cervical cancer screening: Who is not screened and why? *Am J Public Health* 1991; 81:885-890.

Harper JM, Levine AJ, Rosenthal DL, et al: Erythrocyte folate levels, oral contraceptive use and abnormal cervical cytology. *Acta Cytol* 1994; 38:324-30.

Hellman LM, Rosenthal AH, Kistner RW, Gordon R: Some factors influencing the proliferation of the reserve cells in the human cervix. *Am J Obstet Gynecol* 1954; 67:899-915.

Howley PM: Role of the human papillomaviruses in human cancer. *Cancer Res* 1991; 51:5019S-5022S.

Hurt GW, Silverberg SG, Frable WJ, et al: Adenocarcinoma of the cervix: Histologic and clinical features. *Am J Obstet Gynecol* 1977; 129:304-315.

Jobson VW, Muss HB, Thigpen JT, et al: Chemotherapy of advanced squamous carcinoma of the cervix: A phase I-II study of high-dose cisplatin and cyclophosphamide. *Am J Clin Oncol* 1981; 7:341-345.

Johnson LD, Nickerson RJ, Easterday CL, et al.: Epidemiologic evidence for the spectrum of change from dysplasia through carcinoma in situ to invasive cancer *Cancer* 1964; 22:901-914.

Kassirer E: Impace of the Walton report on cervical cancer screening programs in Canada. *Can Med Assoc J* 1980; 122:417-423.

Klassen AC, Celentano DD, Brookmeyer R: Variation in the duration of protection given by screening using the Pap test for cervical cancer. *J Clin Epidemiol* 1989; 42:1003-1011.

Kessler II: Human cervical cancer as a venereal disease. *Cancer Res* 1976; 36:783-791.

Kessler II: Etiological concepts in cervical carcinogenesis. *Gynecol Oncol* 1981; 12:S7-S24.

Knapp RC: Clear cell carcinoma of the vagina. In Heintz APM, Griffiths CT, Trimbos JB, editors: *Surgery in gynecological oncology,* The Hague, 1984, Martinus Nijhoff.

Kolstad P, Klem V: Long term follow-up of 1121 cases of carcinoma in situ. *Obstet Gynecol* 1976; 48:125-129.

Koss LG, Durfee GR: Unusual patterns of squamous epithelium of uterine cervix: Cytologic and pathologic study of koilocytotic atypia. *Ann NY Acad Sci* 1956; 63:1235-1238.

Koss LG, Lin E, Schreiber K, et al: Evaluation of the PAPNET cytologic screening system for quality control of cervical smears. *Am J Clin Pathol* 1994; 101:220-229.

Koutsky L: Epidemiology of genital human papillomavirus infection. *Am J Med* 1997; 102:3-8.

Kumar L, Bhargava VL: Chemotherapy in recurrent and advanced cervical cancer. *Gynecol Oncol* 1991; 40:107-111.

Kurman RJ, Henson DE, Herbst AL, et al: Interim guidelines for management of abnormal cervical cytology. *JAMA* 1994; 271:1866-1869.

Kurman RJ, Malkasian GD Jr, Seidlis A, Solomon D: From Papanicolaou to Bethesda: The rationale for a new cervical cytologic classification. *Obstet Gynecol* 1991;77:779-782.

Kwasniewska A, Tukendorf A, Semczuk M: Folate deficiency and cervical intraepithelial neoplasia. *Eur J Gynaecol Oncol* 1997; 18:526-530.

Lagasse LD, Creasman WT, Shingleton HM, et al: Results and complications of operative staging in cervical cancer: Experience of the Gynecologic Oncology Group. *Gynecol Oncol* 1980; 9:90-98.

Landoni F, Manco A, Colombo A, et al: Randomized study of radical surgery versus radiotherapy for stage Ib-Iia cervical cancer. *Lancet* 1997; 350:535-540.

Langman J: *Medical embryology,* Baltimore, 1981, Williams & Wilkins.

La Vecchia C, Franceschi S, Decarli A, et al: Cigarette smoking and the risk of cervical neoplasia. *Am J Epidemiol* 1986; 123:22-29.

Lee KR, Ashfaq R, Birdsong GG, et al: Comparison of conventional Papanicolaou smears and a fluid-based, thin-layer system for cervical cancer screening. *Obstet Gynecol* 1997a; 90:278-284.

Lee KR, Minter LJ, Granter SR: Papanicolaou smear sensitivity for adenocarcinoma in situ of the cervix: A study of 34 cases. *Am J Clin Pathol* 1997b; 108:114-118.

Lowy DR, Kirnbauer R, Schiller JT: Genital human papillomavirus infection. *Proc Natl Acad Sci USA* 1994; 91:2436-2440.

Lui W, Meigs JV: Radical hysterectomy and pelvic lymphadenectomy. *Am J Obstet Gynecol* 1955; 69:1-32.

Meanwell CA: The epidemiology of human papillomavirus infection in relation to cervical cancer. *Cancer Surv* 1988; 7:481-497.

Meigs JV: Carcinoma of the cervix: The Wertheim operation. *Surg Gynecol Obstet* 1944; 78:1-24.

Meisels A, Fortin R, Roy M: Condylomatous lesions of the cervix, II: Cytologic, colposcopic, and histopathologic study. *Acta Cytol* 1977; 21:379-390.

Morley CW: Pelvic exenteration in the treatment of recurrent cervical cancer. In Heintz APM, Griffiths CT, Trimbos JB, editors: *Surgery in gynecologic oncology,* The Hague, 1984, Martinus Nijhoff.

Murdoch JB, Morgan PR, Lopes A, Monaghan JM: Histological incomplete excision of CIN after large-loop excision of the transformation zone (LLETZ) merits careful follow up, not retreatment. *Br J Obstet Gynaecol* 1992; 99:990-993.

National Cancer Institute Workshop. The 1988 Bethesda System for reporting cervical/vaginal cytologic diagnoses—report of the 1991 Bethesda Workshop. *JAMA* 1989; 262:931-934.

Nischan P, Ebeling K, Schindler C: Smoking and invasive cervical cancer risk: Results from a case-control study. *Am J Epidemiol* 1988; 128:74-77.

Oats JJ: Carcinoma of the cervical stump. *Br J Obstet Gynaecol* 1976; 83:896-900.

Orr JW: Surgical treatment of women found to have invasive cervical cancer at the time of total hysterectomy. *Obstet Gynecol* 1986; 68:353-355.

Patanaphan V, Poussin-Rusillo H: Cancer of uterine cervix stage IB treatment results and prognostic factors. *Cancer* 1986; 57:866-870.

Phillips AN, Smith GD: Cigarette smoking as a potential cause of cervical cancer: Has confounding been controlled? *Int J Epidemiol* 1994; 23:42-49.

Piver MS, Barlow JJ: Paraaortic lymphadenectomy in staging patients with advanced local cervical cancer. *Obstet Gynecol* 1974; 43:544-548.

Piver MS, Chung WS: Prognostic significance of cervical lesion size and pelvic node metastases in cervical carcinoma. *Obstet Gynecol* 1975; 46:507-510.

Plentl AA, Friedman EA: Lymphatic system of the female genetalia: The morphologic basis of oncologic diagnosis and therapy. *Major Pnbl Obstet Gynecol* 1971; 2:1-223.

Potischman N, Brinton LA, Laiming VA, et al: A case-control study of serum folate levels and invasive cervical cancer. *Cancer Res* 1991; 18:4785-4789.

Potish RA, Twiggs LB, Adcock LL, Prem KA: The utility and limitations of decision theory in the utilization of surgical staging and extended field radiotherapy in cervical cancer. *Obstet Gynecol Surv* 1984; 39:555-562.

Poyner EA, Barakat RR, Hoskins WJ: Management and follow-up of patients with adenocarcinoma in situ of the uterine cervix. *Gynecol Oncol* 1995; 57:158-162.

Prendiville W, Cullimore J, Norman S: Large loop excision of the transformation zone (LLETZ): A new method of management for women with cervical intraepithelial neoplasia. *Br J Obstet Gynecol* 1989; 96:1054-1060.

Prendiville W, Davies R, Berry PJ: A low voltage diathermy loop for taking cervical biopsies: A qualitative comparison with punch biopsy forceps. *Br J Obstet Gynaecol* 1986; 93:773-776.

Prokopczyk B, Cox JE, Hoffmann D, et al: Identification of tobacco-specific carcinogen in the cervical mucus of smokers and nonsmokers. *J Natl Cancer Inst* 1997; 89:868-873.

Reagan JW, Ng AB, Wentz WB: Concepts of genesis and development in early cervical neoplasia. *Obstet Gynecol Surv* 1969; 24:860-874.

Richart RM: A radioautographic analysis of cellular proliferation in dysplasia and carcinoma in situ of the uterine cervix. *Am J Obstet Gynecol* 1963; 86:925-930.

Richart RM: Influence of diagnostic and therapeutic procedures in the distribution of cervical intraepithelial neoplasia. *Cancer* 1966; 19:1635-1638.

Rotmensch J: Cervical sarcoma: A review. *Obstet Gynecol Surv* 1983; 38:456-465.

Rotmensch J, Senekjian EK: Evaluation of bolus cis-platinum and continuous 5-fluorouracil infusion for metastatic and recurrent squamous cell carcinoma of the cervix. *Gynecol Oncol* 1988; 29:76-81.

Sardi JE, Giaroli A, Sananes C, et al: Long-term follow-up of the first randomized trial using neoadjuvant chemotherapy in stage Ib squamous carcinoma of the cervix: The final results. *Gynecol Oncol* 1997; 67:61-69

Schiffman MH, Bauer HM, Hoover RN, et al: Epidemiologic evidence showing that human papillomavirus infection causes most cervical intraepithelial neoplasia. *J Natl Cancer Inst* 1993; 12:958-963.

Seski JC, Abell MR, Morley GW: Microinvasive squamous carcinoma of the cervix. *Obstet Gynecol* 1977; 50:410-414.

Sevin BU, Ford JH, Girtanner RD, et al: Invasive cancer of the cervix after cryosurgery: Pit-falls of conservative management. *Obstet Gynecol* 1979; 53:465-471.

SGO Panel Report: Is pelvic radiation beneficial in the postoperative management of stage IB squamous cell carcinoma of the cervix with pelvic node metastasis treated by radical hysterectomy and pelvic lymphadenectomy? *Gynecol Oncol* 1980; 10:105.

Sheets EE, Berman ML, Hrountas CK, et al: Surgically treated early-stage neuroendocrine small-cell cervical carcinoma. *Obstet Gynecol* 1988; 71:1-10.

Song J: *The human uterus: Morphogeneis and embryological basis for cancer,* Springfield, Ill., 1964, Charles C Thomas.

Spitzer M, Ryskin M, Chernys AE, Shifrin A: The value of repeat pap smear at the time of initial colposcopy. *Gynecol Oncol* 1997; 67:3-7.

Spriggs AI, Boddington MM: Progression and regression of cervical lesions: Review of smears from women followed without initial biopsy or treatment. *J Clin Pathol* 1980; 33:517-522.

Stehman FB, Bundy BN: Carcinoma of the cervix treated with radiation therapy, I: *Cancer* 1991; 67:2776-2785.

Stillman RJ: In utero exposure to diethylstilbestrol: Adverse effects on the reproductive tract and reproductive performance and male and female offspring. *Am J Obstet Gynecol* 1982; 142:905-921.

Stryker JA, Bartholomew M, Velkey DE, et al: Bladder and rectal complications following radiotherapy for cervical cancer. *Gynecol Oncol* 1988; 29:1-11.

Tabbara S, Saleh AD, Anderson WA, et al: The Bethesda classification for squamous intraepithelial lesions: Histologic, cytologic, and viral correlates. *Obstet Gynecol* 1992; 79:338-346.

Tattersall MHN, Ramirez C: A randomized trial of adjuvant chemotherapy after radical hysterectomy in stage IB-IIA cervical cancer patients with pelvic lymph node metastases. *Gynecol Oncol* 1992; 46:176-181.

Townsend DE, Richart RM: Cryotherapy and carbon dioxide laser management of cervical intraepithelial neoplasia: A controlled comparison. *Obstet Gynecol* 1983; 61:75-78.

Van Nagell Jr., JR, Rayburn W, Donaldson ES, et al: Therapeutic implications for patterns of recurrence in cancer of the uterine cervix. *Cancer* 1979; 44:2354-2361.

Volter C, He Y, Delius H, et al: Novel HPV types present in oral papillomatous lesions from patients with HIV infection. *Int J Cancer* 1996; 66:453-456.

von Knebel Doeberitz M, Spitkovsky D, Ridder R: Interactions between steroid hormones and viral oncogenes in the pathogenesis of cervical cancer. *Verh Dtsch Ges Pathol* 1997; 81:233-239.

Wertheim E: The radical abdominal operation in carcinoma of the cervix uteri. *Surg Gynecol Obstet* 1907; 4:1.

Wilkinson EJ. Pap smears and screening for cervical neopasia. *Clin Obstet Gynecol* 1990;33:817-825.

Wimbush PR, Fletcher GH: Radiation therapy of carcinoma of the cervical stump. *Radiology* 1969; 93:655-659.

World Health Organization: Invasive squamous-cell cervical carcinoma and combined oral contraceptives: Results from a multinational study: WHO collaborative study of neoplasia and steroid contraceptives. *Int J Cancer* 1993; 55:228-236.

Wright TC Jr, Gagnon S, Richart RM, Ferenczy A: Treatment of cervical intraepithelial neoplasia using the loop electrosurgical excision procedure. *Obstet Gynecol* 1992; 79:173-178.

Yang X, Nakao Y, Pater MM, et al: Expression of cellular genes in HPV16-immortalized and cigarette smoke condensate-transformed human endocervical cells. *J Cell Biochem* 1997; 66:309-321.

Ye Z, Thomas DB, Ray RM: Combined oral contraceptives and risk of cervical carcinoma in situ: WHO collaborative study of neoplasia and steroid contraceptives. *Int J Epidemiol* 1995; 24:19-26.

zur Hausen H: Papillomaviruses in human cancers. *Mol Carcinog* 1988; 1:147-150.

CHAPTER

The Uterine Corpus

SARAH FELDMAN
ELIZABETH A. STEWART

KEY ISSUES

1. Abnormal uterine bleeding is an important indicator of uterine disease, and it requires thorough evaluation that is dependent on a patient's menopausal status.
2. Uterine leiomyomas or fibroids are benign uterine neoplasms that are a major cause of abnormal uterine bleeding in premenopausal women.
3. Endometrial hyperplasia with atypia is a premalignant disease of the uterus; its incidence is associated with conditions of excessive estrogen, including obesity, chronic anovulation and exogenous estrogen.
4. Eighty percent of patients with endometrial cancer seek medical help because of abnormal vaginal bleeding.
5. Hysterectomy is often the treatment of choice for a number of uterine conditions and outcomes; research suggests most women are happy with their decision to proceed with this option.
6. Medical and gynecologic history, size and mobility of the uterus, surgeon skill, and patient preference all factor into the decision to pursue hysterectomy or the many alternatives to hysterectomy available today.

The uterine corpus, the focus of this chapter, consists of the thick, muscular myometrium and the thin, hormonally responsive lining epithelium, the endometrium. The lower portion of the uterus, the cervix, though anatomically continuous, is considered functionally different and is described in detail in Chapter 6. The uterine corpus allows for the cyclic physiologic changes that characterize menstruation, and, after successful fertilization, it serves to sustain, protect, and ultimately deliver the fetus.

Pathophysiologic processes are also important to the study of the uterus. The myometrium gives rise to the most common solid tumor in women, the leiomyoma, which is a major source of abnormal uterine bleeding and a major in-

dication for hysterectomy. The endometrial cavity is often the site of hyperplasia and neoplasia. Because the uterine cavity is readily available for thorough investigation and many of these problems are evident when there is abnormal uterine bleeding, such conditions lend themselves to early diagnosis. Understanding of the anatomy of the uterine corpus, of benign, premalignant, and malignant conditions, and of operative and nonoperative techniques to evaluate the uterus is essential for the clinician involved in the care of women.

CLINICALLY RELEVANT ANATOMY

A muscular, hollow organ, the uterus (Fig. 7-1) lies in the true pelvis between the bladder and the rectum. The cephalic portion of the corpus is known as the fundus. Fallopian tubes enter the fundus laterally in a region termed the cornua. Thus, a portion of the fallopian tube traverses the myometrium and can be clinically important in cornual ectopic pregnancies (Chapter 8). The cavity of the corpus is continuous with that of the endocervix; in women of reproductive age, its average depth is approximately 6 cm, and its capacity is 3 to 8 mL. It is smaller before menarche and after menopause.

The urinary bladder rests anteriorly on the lower uterine segment. Posterior to the uterus is a space between the posterior uterus and vagina and the colon, often termed the *pouch of Douglas,* or the *cul-de-sac.* Ovaries and tubes often occupy this space. The peritoneum covering the anterior and the posterior surfaces of the uterus comes together to form the broad ligament. This broad ligament is, therefore, a double layer of peritoneum that extends from the lateral surface of the uterus outward to the pelvic wall, and it contains blood vessels, lymphatics, and the ureter. The most inferior portion is thickened and contains a condensation of connective tissue and muscle fibers called the cardinal ligament or the parametrium. Uterine vessels approach the lateral aspect of the cervix in the cardinal ligament, an anatomic point of importance in total hysterectomy. Between the ovary and the fallopian tube is the mesosalpinx, the portion of the broad ligament that contains many small blood vessels.

Round ligaments, embryologic anlages of the gubernaculum in the male, consist principally of bands of muscle tissue that extend laterally from the anterolateral aspect of the fundus. They provide little pelvic support and primarily serve as anatomic markers of the uterine fundus when the uterine anatomy is distorted. Uterosacral ligaments arise from the posterior wall of the uterus at the level of the internal cervical os, pass dorsally around the rectosigmoid, insert onto the sacrum, and provide support for the uterus. The uterus is composed of three separate and distinct layers: the serosa, an outer peritoneal covering; the myometrium, an inner layer of smooth muscle; and the endometrium, the mucous membrane lining the cavity (Fig. 7-2). The uterine serosa is continuous with the peritoneum.

Because it receives branches from uterine and ovarian arteries, the uterus has a dual blood supply (Fig 7-3). The uterine artery is derived from the hypogastric anterior trunk. It crosses over the ureter at the level of the internal os of the cervix and divides into ascending and descending limbs. The ascending limb runs tortuously upward, between the leaves of the broad ligament, and supplies horizontal anterior and posterior branches to the cervix and the corpus. The descending branch of the uterine artery turns inferiorly and supplies the vagina from the lateral aspect. It anastomoses freely with the vaginal artery along its course. The ovarian arterial supply also has branches that anastomose with the ascending limb of the uterine artery.

Endometrium

Processes of menstruation and pregnancy give singular importance to an understanding of the anatomic vascular pattern of the endometrium. A series of radial arteries branches off at right angles from the uterine artery as it courses along the corpus (Fig. 7-3). These radial arteries branch in the inner third of the myometrium into straight and spiral (coiled) vessels. Straight arteries pass only as far as the basal layer of the endometrium and terminate in capillaries. Spiral arteries, however, follow a coiled course throughout the thickness of the endometrium, develop into a few branches in the endometrium, then fork and give rise to superficial capillaries just below the surface epithelium. These capillaries form plexuses in the stroma and a meshwork around the glands. In the superficial layer of the endometrium, the capillaries form sinuslike dilations known as lakes. Blood is returned through small veins that drain these vascular lakes and capillary plexuses. It should be remembered that the vascular pattern is a dynamic one and includes constant proliferation and regression. Specific morphologic details are considered in the section on menstruation.

Although the prime function of the straight arteries is to supply the basal endometrium, they may also support regeneration of the lower portion of the functional layer. Coiled arteries alone supply blood to the superficial third of

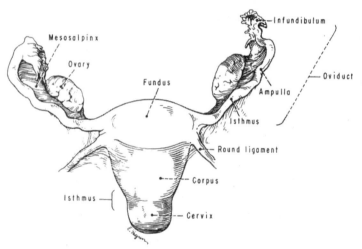

Fig. 7-1. Anterior view of uterus.

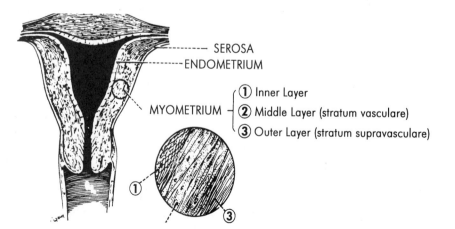

Fig. 7-2. Structure of uterus.

the endometrium and most of the blood to the middle third. Some straight arteries may be converted to coiled ones and later to straight ones. Thus it is possible that the blood supply of the endometrium could regenerate and develop specificity of function even after complete curettage.

Lymphatics of the uterine corpus proceed in four or five channels through the broad ligament just below the oviducts, then upward along the ovarian vessels, and they terminate in the aortic nodes. Lymphatics from the lower uterine segment anastomose with adjacent lymph channels from the cervix and drain to the obturator, iliac, hypogastric, and sacral nodes. A third route of lymphatic drainage, especially from the fundal area, is through the round ligament to the superficial inguinal nodes.

Abnormal Uterine Bleeding

Many pathologic conditions of the uterus become manifest with abnormal uterine bleeding. Thus, the evaluation of bleeding abnormalities is essential for the clinical care of women (Figs. 7-4 and 7-5). For women of reproductive age, deviation from the normal menstrual cycle is often the clue to pathologic conditions (see Chapter 3) (Fig. 7-4). Most in-

cidences of abnormal menstrual bleeding in women of reproductive age result from hormonal abnormalities caused by oligoovulation or pregnancy. However, abnormalities arising from either the endometrial layer (endometrial polyps, hyperplasia, or cancer) or the myometrial layer (uterine leiomyomas, adenomyosis, or sarcomas) can cause abnormal uterine bleeding. In addition, because cervical bleeding cannot easily be differentiated from uterine bleeding, a Papanicolaou smear should be part of any evaluation. Older women and women of increased body mass have a greater risk for endometrial hyperplasia and endometrial cancer, so a more diligent effort to exclude these diseases in this group of patients is warranted. For adolescents with menorrhagia, evaluation for bleeding disorders should be considered because the incidence of bleeding disorders in this group is relatively high (Claessens and Cowell, 1981). Evaluation of abnormal uterine bleeding in premenarchal girls is discussed in Chapter 12.

Any vaginal bleeding in postmenopausal women should be thoroughly investigated to exclude the possibility of neoplasia (Fig. 7-5). Endometrial biopsy is the most cost-effective initial strategy for the evaluation of postmeno-

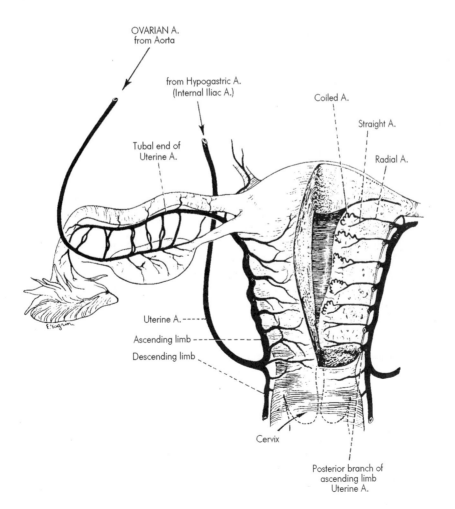

Fig. 7-3. Blood supply to the uterus.

Abnormal uterine bleeding in premenopausal women

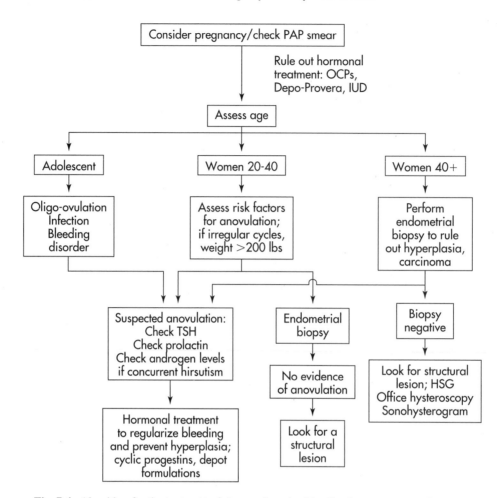

Fig. 7-4. Algorithm for the treatment of abnormal uterine bleeding in premenopausal women.

pausal bleeding (Akkad et al, 1995, Feldman et al, 1993). In fact, endometrial biopsy is cost effective regardless of the amount or the duration of bleeding (Feldman et al, 1993; Feldman et al, 1995).

For a postmenopausal patient in whom the initial office biopsy shows insufficient tissue, further evaluation of her underlying risk for endometrial cancer or complex atypical hyperplasia is warranted. There are two ways to assess risk. A vaginal probe ultrasound can provide information on endometrial thickness, which has been shown in numerous studies to correlate with risk for cancer and atypical hyperplasia. Although the exact cutoff is a function of the sensitivity and specificity desired, most clinicians use a cutoff of 5 mm to categorize postmenopausal patients into a low-risk group with a combined risk for cancer and atypical hyperplasia from 2% to 3% (Granberg et al, 1991; Langer et al, 1997). In contrast, endometrial thickness greater than 5 mm suggests a greater than 5% risk for cancer and atypical hyperplasia. Not all studies of endometrial thickness look at symptomatic patients, that is, those who seek treatment for abnormal bleeding. The detection

rate for malignancies may be higher in symptomatic patients, and this factor should be kept in mind in overall patient assessment.

Alternatively, one may use a simple clinical prediction rule to assess risk. Using information from the clinical history on age, parity, menopausal status, and diabetes, one can stratify patients into risk groups. For instance, if a patient is younger than 70 years, is not nulliparous, is within 1 year of the cessation of menses, and does not have diabetes, she falls into a low-risk (<5%) group. Groups at successively higher risk can be determined by the addition of another risk factor. A woman who has all four risk factors is at approximately 80% risk for endometrial cancer or complex hyperplasia (Feldman et al, 1995).

In a study of 265 patients with postmenopausal or perimenopausal bleeding in whom initial biopsy specimens showed either benign or insufficient tissue, 2% were found within a 2-year period to have cancer and 3% were found to have atypical hyperplasia (Feldman et al, 1994). Thus, patients with persistent, unexplained bleeding need additional evaluation. Many of these patients have uterine fibroids,

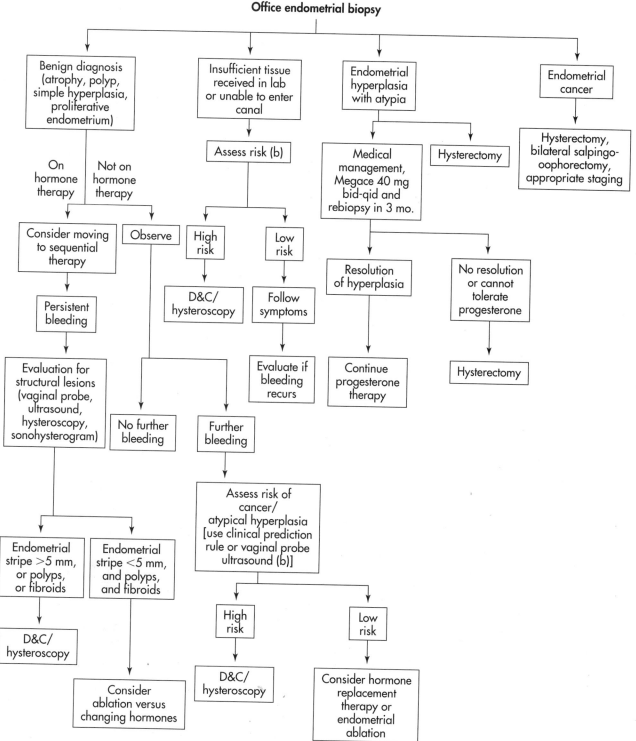

Fig. 7-5. Algorithm for the treatment of postmenopausal bleeding.

raising the concern that alterations to the endometrial cavity secondary to fibroids may increase sampling error.

PATHOLOGIC CONDITIONS OF THE UTERUS
Leiomyomas

Uterine leiomyomas, commonly known as fibroids or myomas, are well-circumscribed, benign tumors arising from the smooth muscle of the myometrium. They are composed of smooth muscle and extracellular matrix (collagen, proteoglycan, fibronectin).

Incidence and Etiology

Leiomyomas are the most common solid pelvic tumors in women. These are clinically apparent in 20% to 25% of women during the reproductive years, but careful pathologic inspection of the uterus reveals that they are present in more than 80% of women (Buttram and Reiter,1981; Cramer and Patel, 1990). It is accepted that leiomyomas are clonal in origin (Townsend et al, 1970; Mashel et al, 1994). Although the classic paradigm suggests that the gonadal steroids estrogen and progesterone are the only important modulators of leiomyoma growth and transformation, it is now clear that growth factors (particularly transforming growth factor-ß and basic fibroblast growth factor) and somatic mutations of genes such as HMGI-C play a role in the pathogenesis of these neoplasms (Stewart and Nowak, 1996; Schoenberg-Fejzo et al, 1996; Stewart and Nowak, 1998).

Leiomyomas are characterized by their location in the uterus (Fig. 7-6). Subserosal leiomyomas are located just under the uterine serosa and may be attached to the corpus by a narrow or a broad base. Intramural leiomyomas are found predominantly within the thick myometrium but may distort the cavity or cause an irregular external uterine contour. Submucous leiomyomas are located just under the uterine mucosa (endometrium); they also may be attached to the uterine corpus by a narrow or a broad base. Although this classification scheme is used widely, its limitation is that few leiomyomas are actually of a single "pure" type. Most leiomyomas are hybrids that span more than one anatomic location, such as a predominantly intramural leiomyoma with a submucous component.

There is an increased incidence of leiomyomas in women of color (RR = 1.82 to 3.25) (Marshall et al, 1997). Risk is increased in women with greater body mass index, but it is decreased in women who smoke or who have given birth (Ross et al, 1986; Parazzini et al, 1996). Although concern about the high estrogen levels in oral contraceptive pills has led some clinicians to consider leiomyomas a relative contraindication to their use, there is good epidemiologic evidence to suggest that use of oral contraceptive pills decreases the risk for leiomyomas (Ross et al, 1986).

Symptoms

It is estimated that between 20% and 50% of women with leiomyomas have tumor-related symptoms (Buttram and Reiter, 1981). The two most common symptoms of leiomyomas are abnormal uterine bleeding and pelvic pressure. Bleeding abnormalities are usually either prolonged or heavy menstrual flow (menorrhagia). Although menorrhagia can occur in any woman with myomas, women with submucous leiomyomas appear to be particularly prone to this complication. Pelvic pressure can result from an increase in uterine size or from the pressure of particular myomas on adjacent structures, including the colon or bladder, causing constipation or urinary frequency. Pressure of the myomatous uterus on the ureters causing hydronephrosis is a rare indication for surgical intervention.

Leiomyomas can also be associated with other kinds of reproductive dysfunction, including recurrent miscarriage,

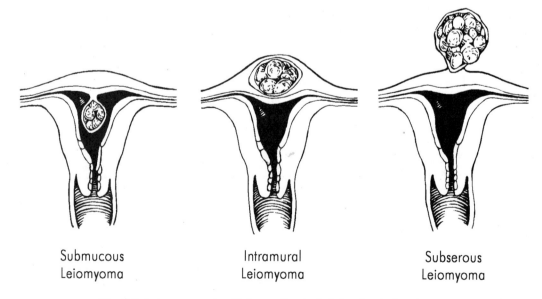

Submucous
Leiomyoma

Intramural
Leiomyoma

Subserous
Leiomyoma

Fig. 7-6. Leiomyomas classified according to their location in the uterus.

infertility, premature labor, fetal malpresentation, and complications of labor. Although good studies are unavailable, the common clinical perception is that these complications occur most often when there is distortion of the uterine cavity. Women with large or symptomatic fibroids may want to undergo assessment of the uterine cavity before attempting pregnancy. Sarcomatous transformation of uterine leiomyomas is thought not to occur. However, without pathologic examination of the uterus for abnormalities, differentiation is not possible. The clinical teaching has been that a rapidly enlarging fibroid may be a sign of sarcoma rather than leiomyoma, but there is no support for this in the literature.

Diagnosis

The diagnosis of leiomyoma is usually easily determined by bimanual examination. The uterus is enlarged, mobile, often irregular, and may be palpated abdominally above the symphysis. Ultrasonography is the most common method of confirming the diagnosis. Magnetic resonance imaging (MRI) may prove to be the most useful method because electron spin characteristics can often distinguish leiomyomas from other intramural lesions, including adenomyomas or leiomyosarcomas. For patients who experience menorrhagia or recurrent pregnancy loss, assessment of the uterine cavity after it is distended is important because a submucous fibroid can be missed on traditional ultrasonography (Cincinelli et al, 1995; Dijkhuizen et al, 1996). Hysterosalpingogram, sonohysterogram, or office hysteroscopy can all supply this information.

Treatment

The primary therapy for patients with large or symptomatic leiomyomas is surgery. Hysterectomy is the technique used most often to treat this disorder. In the United States more than 175,000 hysterectomies are performed yearly for leiomyomas, making the diagnosis of leiomyoma the most common indication for this procedure (Wilcox et al, 1994). Hysterectomy, the only true "cure" for leiomyoma, is a surgical option when women are no longer interested in future pregnancies.

When women want to preserve childbearing potential, a myomectomy may be performed. Approximately 18,000 myomectomies are performed yearly in the United States (National Center for Health Statistics, 1987). Myomectomy diminishes menorrhagia in roughly 80% of patients with this symptom (Buttram and Reiter, 1981). It is essential to inform patients about to undergo myomectomy that there is a significant risk for recurrence of leiomyomas after surgery. There is ultrasonographic evidence of recurrence in 25% to 51% of patients, and as many as 10% require a second major operative procedure (Buttram and Reiter, 1981; Fedelle et al, 1995).

GnRH agonists, which induce a hypoestrogenic pseudomenopausal state, represent a recent development in the medical treatment of leiomyomas. Because fibroids are dependent on estrogen for their development and growth, induction of a hypoestrogenic state causes shrinkage of these tumors and of myometrial mass. Uterine volume has been shown to decrease 40% to 60% after 3 months of GnRH agonist therapy (Stewart and Friedman, 1992). In addition, treatment with a GnRH agonist induces amenorrhea, allowing women with menorrhagia-induced anemia to increase iron stores and hemoglobin concentrations significantly. However, cessation of GnRH agonist treatment results in rapid regrowth of leiomyomas and of the uterus to pretreatment volume. Therefore, GnRH agonist treatment is primarily useful as a presurgical treatment, not as a long-term treatment option, in selected patients in whom uterine volume reduction or amenorrhea is an essential goal.

Combinations of GnRH agonists and low dosages of steroid hormones (that is, "add-back" regimens) have been administered in some clinical trials to extend the maximal duration of GnRH agonist therapy safely without sacrificing efficacy. However, before this medical strategy can be used to substitute for or to delay surgery, the optimal steroid add-back regimen and the most cost-effective way to monitor these patients must be defined.

Androgenic agents (danazol, gestrinone) and progestins (medroxyprogesterone acetate, depomedroxyprogesterone acetate, norethindrone) have also been used to control menorrhagia in women with leiomyomas (Coutinho and Goncalves, 1989). However, these medications do not consistently decrease uterine or fibroid volume, and their mechanism of action is thought to be the induction of endometrial atrophy. These agents are often not successful in controlling significant menorrhagia.

Adenomyosis

Adenomyosis is a benign uterine disease in which endometrial glands and stroma are found within the myometrium. Early authors sometimes referred to adenomyosis as endometriosis interna. The presence of endometrial tissue induces hypertrophy and hyperplasia of the surrounding myometrium and produces a diffusely enlarged uterus.

Incidence and Etiology

The diagnosis of adenomyosis can be made only by microscopic examination of a specimen, rarely from biopsy and most often from hysterectomy. For this reason, the exact incidence of the disease is unknown. It is generally estimated that 20% of women have adenomyosis. However, careful analysis of multiple myometrial sections may reveal an incidence as high as 65% (McElin and Bird, 1974).

Adenomyosis is associated with childbearing. It is estimated that at least 80% of women with this disorder are parous (McElin and Bird, 1974; Molitor, 1971). However, the incidence of adenomyosis is not correlated with increasing parity. Adenomyosis most often produces symptoms in women between the ages of 40 and 50 years.

More than 80% of women with adenomyosis have another uterine abnormality; 50% have associated leiomyomas, approximately 11% have endometriosis, and 7% have endometrial polyps (McElin and Bird, 1974). Symptoms of the associated condition often obscure the diagnosis of adenomyosis.

Pathology

The typical uterus with adenomyosis is boggy and uniformly enlarged. Approximately 80% of uteri with adenomyosis weigh more than 80 g, but it is unusual for a uterus with adenomyosis as the only abnormality to exceed 200 g. The disease may be suspected if a focal area of adenomyosis is mistaken for a leiomyoma and myomectomy is attempted. Areas of adenomyosis do not lend themselves to easy excision.

Microscopic Appearance

The pathognomonic feature of adenomyosis is the presence of endometrial tissue, glands, and stroma within the myometrium (Fig. 7-7), observed in at least one low-power field (some authorities insist on two) from the endomyometrial junction. Usually the myometrium is altered in uteri with extensive adenomyosis so that a surrounding zone of hypertrophy-hyperplasia is recognizable.

Symptoms

As mentioned earlier, adenomyosis most commonly produces symptoms in women between the ages of 40 and 50 years. Approximately 60% of them experience abnormal

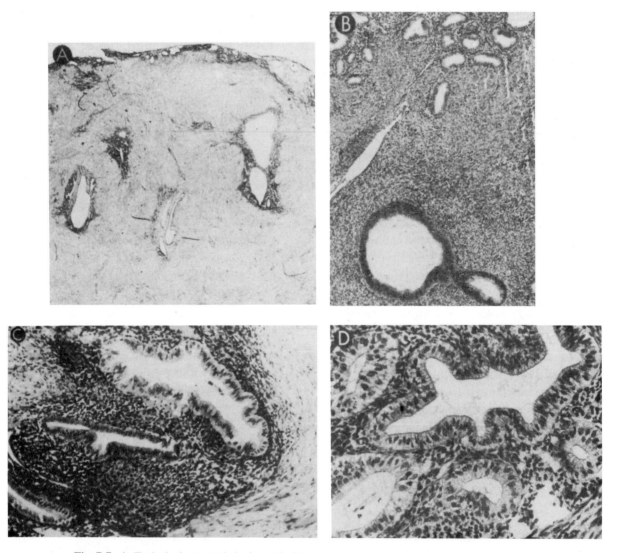

Fig. 7-7. A, Typical adenomyosis in the wall of the uterus. Foci of basal type of endometrium are located deep in the myometrium. The myometrium surrounding the areas of adenomyosis shows a whorled appearance similar to that seen in leiomyoma. **B,** High-power magnification of an area of adenomyosis showing cystic dilatation. The basal endometrium is at the top. **C,** Adenomyosis in which the glandular element at the top right has undergone anaplasia. The glands are surrounded by typical endometrial stroma. **D,** Adenomyosis showing secretory effect. (**A,** from Hertig AT, Gore HM: Tumors of the vulva, vagina and uterus. In *Tumors of the female sex organs*, part 2, section 9, fasc 33, *Atlas of tumor pathology*, Washington, DC, 1960, Armed Forces Institute of Pathology.)

uterine bleeding. Dysmenorrhea is the second most common symptom; it occurs in 25% of patients (McElin and Bird, 1974).

Treatment

The only definitive treatment for adenomyosis is total hysterectomy, with or without ovarian conservation. GnRH agonists have been used in a few patients. This treatment resulted in a transient decrease in uterine size and in amenorrhea, but regrowth of the uterus and recurrence of symptoms have usually been documented within 6 months of cessation of therapy.

Endometrial Polyps

Endometrial polyps are hyperplastic overgrowths of glands and stroma that are localized and that form a projection above the surface. Such polyps may be sessile or pedunculated and rarely include foci of neoplastic growth.

The prevalence of polyps has been estimated at 10% to 24% among women undergoing endometrial biopsy or hysterectomy (Van Bogaert, 1988). Endometrial polyps are rare among women younger than 20 years of age. The incidence of these polyps rises steadily with increasing age, peaks in the fifth decade of life, and gradually declines after menopause.

The most common symptom in women with endometrial polyps is metrorrhagia, or irregular bleeding; it is reported in 50% of symptomatic patients. Postmenstrual spotting is also common. Less common symptoms include menorrhagia, postmenopausal bleeding, and breakthrough bleeding during hormonal therapy. Overall, endometrial polyps account for 25% of abnormal bleeding in premenopausal and postmenopausal women (Van Bogaert, 1988).

Endometrial polyps can sometimes be seen prolapsing through the cervix. Often they are diagnosed by microscopic examination of a specimen obtained after dilatation and curettage (D & C) or after endometrial biopsy. As is the case with submucous fibroids, polyps can escape detection if the uterus is not distended. Increasingly these lesions are diagnosed by modalities such as ultrasonography and hysteroscopy.

Endometrial polyps usually are cured by thorough curettage. However, polyps or other structural abnormalities may be missed by blind curettage, and hysteroscopic-guided curettage is often useful (Brooks and Serden, 1988, Gimpelson and Rappold, 1988).

Uterine Anomalies

Uterine anomalies may be congenital or they may be acquired after infection or mechanical trauma, and they may lead to reproductive or menstrual dysfunction.

Congenital Anomalies

The uterus is formed from the paired müllerian ducts during embryogenesis. Uterine anomalies result from their defective migration, fusion, or absorption during embryonic life. The incidence of anomalies is difficult to estimate because many congenital anomalies do not result in clinical manifestations (Rock and Jones, 1977). Patients with symptomatic müllerian anomalies usually have signs of menstrual outflow obstruction or reproductive dysfunction. Diagnostic methods for determining the exact nature of a müllerian anomaly have evolved from bimanual examination, postpartum manual exploration, and D & C, to the more sophisticated techniques of hysterography, laparoscopy, hysteroscopy, ultrasonography, and MRI. Increased capacity of the latter techniques to yield complete information will undoubtedly be reflected in a higher reported incidence of the more subtle anomalies.

Retrospective studies reveal that approximately 25% of women with congenital uterine anomalies encounter reproductive difficulties, although conception rates are not different than they are among women in control groups (Abramovici et al, 1983; Harger, 1983). Spontaneous abortions, premature births, and fetal malpresentations are common in women with congenital uterine anomalies.

Anomalies can be classified as problems with hypoplasia or agenesis (American Fertility Society [AFS] class I) or as fusion defects (AFS classes II-V). Class I anomalies, also referred to as müllerian anomalies, usually are diagnosed in women who seek treatment for primary amenorrhea or for an inability to have vaginal intercourse. These defects are thought to occur developmentally when the müllerian structures fail to join with the structures arising from the vaginal bulb. There is a wide spectrum of defects ranging from isolated vaginal agenesis to hypoplasia of the vagina, cervix, ileus, and tubes. Clinically important points of these anomalies include:

1. In patients with complete müllerian agenesis, the possibility of complete androgen insensitivity (testicular feminization syndrome) should be considered because these women have Y chromosomes and must have their gonads removed because there is a high risk for neoplasia.
2. The patient with an absent vagina can have one that is adequate for intercourse created through the use of progressive dilators or surgery.

Fusion defects include unicornuate uterus (AFS class II), uterus didelphys (AFS class III), bicornuate uterus (AFS class IV), and septate uterus (class V). A unicornuate uterus has a single hemi-uterus that is attached to its fallopian tube. It may also be associated with a rudimentary cavity from the contralateral side. A didelphys uterus has two uterine cavities, and each has a separate cervix. The fundus of the uterus also has a deep cleft between the cavities. A bicornuate uterus has a single cervix, a heart-shaped fundus, and two uterine cavities separated by myometrium. Conversely, a septate uterus has a single cervix, a flat fundus, and two uterine cavities separated by relatively avascular scar tissue.

Two clinically relevant points for fusion defects are:

1. In a woman with a unicornuate uterus, a rudimentary horn can result in pain because of obstruction or retrograde flow, either of which may cause endometriosis or be a site of infection.

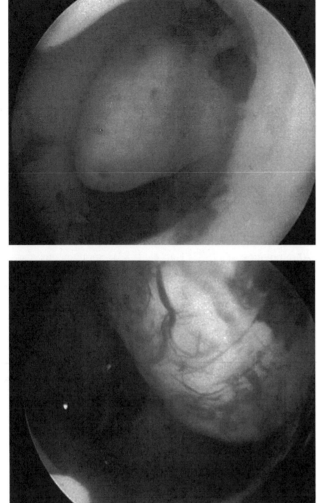

Fig. 7-8. Hysteroscopic views of intrauterine masses. **A,** An endometrial polyp is visualized. Although globular in shape, the fine vascular pattern and surface location suggest the histology. In contrast, **B,** a submucous fibroid has a much coarser vascular pattern and appears to be partially intramural.

2. Fusion defects may be associated with reproductive problems, from recurrent miscarriage to premature labor. The incidence of these problems is uncertain, however, because in women who have had only uncomplicated pregnancies, anomalies may never have been noted.

Among patients with AFS class I to IV uterine anomalies, there is an increased incidence of renal anomalies, usually renal agenesis ipsilateral to the associated hypoplastic müllerian defect. Therefore, a search for uterine anomalies should be conducted in patients with renal agenesis, and pelvic pain, or reproductive dysfunction.

Acquired Anomalies

The use of diethylstilbestrol (DES) between 1940 and 1970 created a special category of acquired congenital anomaly (class VII). It causes uterine abnormalities (primarily hypoplastic or T-shaped uteri) and cervical abnormalities. In a series of more than 250 patients, 69% had abnormalities of the uterus, and there was a significant relationship between uterine anomalies and cervical or vaginal anomalies. Women with antenatal DES exposure and abnormal uteri have higher rates of ectopic pregnancy, miscarriage, and premature delivery than do women with normal uteri.

Asherman Syndrome

Asherman syndrome is the partial or the complete obliteration of the uterine cavity by adherence of the uterine walls from scarring. It is often associated with menstrual or reproductive abnormalities, particularly amenorrhea or hypomenorrhea, dysmenorrhea, infertility, and recurrent abortion.

The incidence of Asherman syndrome is difficult to determine. It is estimated to be involved in 1.7% of all cases of secondary amenorrhea. (Jones, 1964) Historically, the diagnosis was based on hysterosalpingogram findings (Fig. 7-8), but hysteroscopy is the most accurate method of detection and is used more often.

Curettage of a gravid or recently gravid uterus is the most common cause of Asherman syndrome. In a combined series evaluating predisposing factors among patients with intrauterine adhesions, 91% were associated with pregnancy-related curettage (Schenker and Margalioth, 1982). Other rare causes of Asherman syndrome include infection (genital tuberculosis), myomectomy, metroplasty, and curettage of a nonpregnant uterus.

Approximately 14% of patients with Asherman syndrome have repeated pregnancy loss (Schenker and Margalioth, 1982). Among patients with Asherman syndrome who conceive, there is a high incidence of complications including premature labor, placenta accreta, placenta previa, and postpartum hemorrhage.

Treatment of Asherman syndrome requires the surgical removal of intrauterine adhesions with simultaneous prevention of the formation of new adhesions. Most patients with Asherman syndrome are treated by hysteroscopic lysis of adhesions, though occasionally laparotomy may be necessary if the endometrial cavity cannot be defined by the vaginal approach. Although many adjuncts—including postoperative use of an intrauterine stent (intrauterine device, Foley catheter) or postoperative treatment with high-dose estrogen, antibiotics, and steroids—aimed at minimizing the re-formation of adhesions have been used, the efficacy of these measures has not been evaluated in a randomized series.

Results of surgical therapy are excellent in terms of the restoration of normal menstrual function, and they are good in terms of reversing infertility. In a combined series that included 1586 patients treated for Asherman syndrome, normal menses was restored in 84%, and 51% of infertile patients conceived (Schenker and Margalioth, 1982). The prognosis for Asherman syndrome is related to the degree of endometrial obliteration. If there are extensive intrauterine synechiae, the restoration of fertility and normal menstrual function is more difficult.

Endometrial Hyperplasia

Endometrial hyperplasia is an overgrowth of endometrial glands and stroma, and it is characterized by a proliferative glandular pattern that has varying degrees of architectural and cytologic atypia (Fig. 7-9) (Welch and Scully, 1977). Some forms of endometrial hyperplasia have little or no malignant potential. Other forms, notably those demonstrating cytologic atypia, may develop into or coexist with invasive endometrial cancer (Kurman et al, 1985). All endometrial hyperplasias, regardless of their malignant potential, may cause significant blood loss through heavy and irregular vaginal bleeding. They are associated with chronic anovulatory states, estrogen-secreting ovarian tumors, and unopposed exogenous estrogen use. Appropriate medical or surgical management depends on the degree of hyperplasia, patient age, and patient preference concerning reproduction.

Etiology

Risk factors for endometrial hyperplasia are similar to those for endometrial cancer and include pathophysiologic states of relative estrogen excess despite relative progesterone deficiency. In premenopausal women, anovulatory states such as polycystic ovarian syndrome may result in continuous estrogen-induced endometrial proliferation.

In perimenopausal or postmenopausal women, continued though waning estrogen production in the absence of ovulation has the same effect. This estrogen-dominant state is particularly pronounced in obese women, who have higher circulating levels of the weak estrogen estrone, which is produced by the peripheral conversion of androstenedione in muscle and fat cells. Unopposed exogenous estrogens may cause iatrogenic hyperplasia. Tamoxifen, a mixed-estrogen agonist-antagonist, has also been associated with endometrial hyperplasia and adenocarcinoma in women treated for breast cancer (Cohen et al, 1993).

Estrogen-secreting ovarian tumors may induce endometrial hyperplasia. Although stromal tumors, such as granulosa cell tumors, are often estrogen secreting, it is important to keep in mind that any epithelial neoplasm may cause ovarian stromal hyperplasia and produce estrogen.

Malignant Potential

In classifying hyperplastic lesions, there are two histologic levels at which atypia can be described: the architectural and the cytologic. Architectural atypia is present when there is an abnormality in number, size, or complexity of the glandular elements in the lesion. Cytologic atypia refers to the abnormal morphology of the individual cells lining the glands. It is the degree of cytologic atypia that defines the malignant potential of endometrial hyperplasia. This was demonstrated by Kurman et al (1985), who showed that nonatypical hyperplasias with cytologic atypia progress to adenocarcinoma

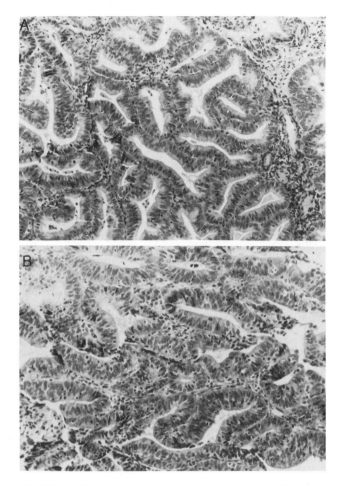

Fig. 7-9. A, Endometrial hyperplasia demonstrating architectural abnormalities without cytologic atypia. **B,** Endometrial hyperplasia with architectural and cytologic atypia. (Courtesy of Drs. W. Welch and J. Semple.)

29% of the time. In summary, the degree of cytologic atypia determines the malignant potential of the hyperplasia; hyperplasias in the absence of atypia do not represent premalignant lesions (Ferenczy and Gelfond, 1989).

Finally, as many as 25% of perimenopausal or postmenopausal women with atypical hyperplasia have coexisting endometrial cancer. Such information must be taken into account when designing an appropriate therapeutic approach for the patient with endometrial hyperplasia.

Diagnosis

The diagnosis of endometrial hyperplasia is made by endometrial biopsy. If an inadequate sample is obtained, D & C may be required.

Treatment

The treatment of endometrial hyperplasia must be tailored to the patient's age, wishes regarding reproduction, menopausal status, general medical health, and grade of hyperplasia. Treatment may be either medical or surgical. Medical therapy is directed toward reestablishing the equilibrium between estrogen and progesterone by stimulating the production of endogenous progestins through ovulation induction or by administering pharmacologic dosages of exogenous progestins.

Among premenopausal women who want immediate fertility, nonatypical hyperplasia may be treated with cyclic medroxyprogesterone for 3 months in dosages of 10 mg for 14 days per month. If a follow-up endometrial biopsy reveals a secretory endometrium without evidence of hyperplasia or neoplasia, ovulation induction may proceed. If atypical hyperplasia is present, continuous megestrol acetate, at dosages ranging from 40 mg twice daily to 80 mg three times daily, may be used for as long as 3 months (Gal, 1986). If a follow-up biopsy shows persistent atypical hyperplasia, an additional cycle of therapy may be warranted at a higher daily dosage. Because it is unusual for such lesions to persist after progestin therapy, patient compliance must be carefully assessed in all treatment failures. If there is a question of compliance, depot forms of progestin (depot medroxyprogesterone acetate) may be administered through intramuscular injection. In women who want to retain fertility but delay pregnancy, low-dose combination oral contraceptives are effective in preventing recurrent hyperplasia. Among premenopausal women with atypical hyperplasia who do not want to retain fertility, hysterectomy is a reasonable option. For the majority of premenopausal patients, medical management will effectively reverse atypical hyperplasia. However, continued cyclic progestin therapy may be required to prevent recurrences.

Among postmenopausal patients, hyperplasia without atypia should be treated with continuous progestin therapy for a period of 3 months. If the lesion persists, hysterectomy is advisable if concurrent medical conditions, such as diabetes, hypertension, or morbid obesity, do not preclude surgical management. Postmenopausal women with atypical hyperplasia have two options for treatment. If surgery is contraindicated because of medical reasons or patient preference, the patient may be offered medical management with continuous megestrol acetate at dosages ranging from 40 mg to 80 mg up to three times a day. A repeat endometrial biopsy is then obtained at 3 months. If atypical hyperplasia persists, the patient should be counseled to undergo hysterectomy. If there is regression of the hyperplasia, she should be put on a continuous maintenance dose of megestrol acetate and undergo follow-up biopsies at regular intervals (6 months to 1 year). Alternatively, because of the side effects of megestrol acetate and because of the possibility of coexisting cancer, she may opt for primary hysterectomy.

Continuous progestin therapy is generally well tolerated, but it may cause weight gain, mood swings, and depression (Wentz, 1985). There is no evidence to suggest that progestin therapy increases the likelihood of developing deep venous thrombosis, so progestins may be used in patients with a previous thrombotic event. A far more complex problem is the impact of long-term progestin therapy on the risk for cardiovascular disease. Synthetic progestins may have a deleterious effect on lipoprotein levels by decreasing cardioprotective high-density lipoprotein cholesterol concentrations. This may in turn increase the risk for coronary artery disease and cerebral vascular accidents. Alternatives to progestins include danazol and cyproterone acetate (Jasonni et al, 1986; Terakawa et al, 1988). Response rates are similar to those reported with progestins, but experience is limited.

Endometrial Cancer

Endometrial carcinoma is the most common gynecologic malignancy. The disease predominantly affects perimenopausal and postmenopausal women, whose median age at diagnosis is 61 years. Only 5% of patients are younger than 40 years. It is twice as common as ovarian cancer and three times more common than invasive carcinoma of the cervix. After a decade of increasing incidence, with a peak of 39,000 cases reported in 1979, the occurrence rate of endometrial cancer has gradually declined. Variations in the incidence of this malignancy have been attributed to the increasing age of the population, more refined histopathologic criteria for the diagnosis of the lesion, and a changing pattern in the use of hormone replacement therapy and the oral contraceptive pill.

Despite the transient increase in incidence through 1979, overall mortality from endometrial cancer has continued to decline, and the disease now accounts for fewer than 4000 cancer deaths per year. This has given the false impression that endometrial cancer is an indolent disease, whereas in fact, stage for stage, it is just as deadly as ovarian cancer. However, unlike ovarian cancer, endometrial cancer has a hallmark early symptom—perimenopausal or postmenopausal bleeding—which prompts the physician to take an endometrial biopsy. This biopsy leads to a diagnosis at a favorable stage in most patients.

Risk Factors

Most endometrial cancers arise from a background of endometrial hyperplasia and are the consequence of unopposed endogenous or exogenous estrogen on a hormonally responsive endometrium.

Obesity has been shown to be an important risk factor for endometrial cancer (Davies et al, 1981). Women who are overweight by up to 22.7 kg have a threefold increased risk for this malignancy. The risk jumps to ninefold for women overweight by more than 22.7 kg. Obesity increases the risk by increasing estrogen production and bioavailability. In postmenopausal women, the ovaries and adrenals secrete negligible amounts of estrogen. Most estrogen is in the form of estrone, which is produced in the peripheral conversion of androstenedione in muscle and adipose tissue. Increased production of estrone has been documented in obese women (Judd et al, 1980). In addition, obese women have lower levels of sex-hormone–binding globulin, which accounts for the increased bioavailability of circulating estrogen (Gambone et al, 1982).

Total intake of calories derived from saturated or unsaturated fats is a risk factor independent of body weight. Women reporting a high intake of animal fat and fried food have a 2.1-fold increased risk for endometrial carcinoma. Women with a high intake of complex carbohydrates, predominantly breads and cereals, have a decreased risk (RR = 0.6) after controlling for body mass (Potischman et al, 1993).

Other risk factors for endometrial cancer include a history of infertility, nulliparity, early menarche, and late menopause (Elwood et al, 1977; Kelsey et al, 1982). Hypertension and diabetes mellitus are often associated with obesity, but they may represent independent risk factors. Chronic anovulatory states, such as polycystic ovarian syndrome, substantially increase endometrial cancer risk. Functional ovarian neoplasms, such as certain epithelial ovarian cancers and granulosa cell tumors, may also increase risk by the endogenous production of unopposed estrogen. In women with postmenopausal bleeding, the most significant risk factor for endometrial cancer (and complex endometrial hyperplasia) is age. Patients who are older than 70 have a risk for endometrial cancer-complex atypical hyperplasia that is six to ten times higher than in younger women (Feldman et al, 1994).

Many studies demonstrate an association between unopposed estrogen replacement therapy and the development of endometrial cancer (Mack et al, 1976; Weiss et al, 1979). Risk increases with estrogen dose and duration of use. Widespread use of unopposed estrogen in the 1960s might have been responsible for the temporal rise in the endometrial cancer rate that peaked in 1979. The risk for endometrial cancer can be effectively eliminated with the addition of a progestin. Progesterone reduces estrogen-receptor synthesis and increases the conversion of estradiol to the less potent metabolite estrone. Women on combined estrogen and progestin replacement therapy actually have lower risk for endometrial cancer than do untreated patients.

Recent information regarding the negative impact of progestins on lipoprotein profiles has led to a resurgence of interest in the use of unopposed or minimally opposed estrogen replacement regimens. Patients on cyclic combined regimens of estrogen and progesterone should be administered progesterone at least 12 to 13 days each month (Paterson et al, 1980). The trend is to use continuous combined regimens because this eventually eliminates bleeding in most women. Given the indolent nature of "iatrogenic" endometrial cancer and improved biopsy and imaging techniques, the issue of low-dose estrogen replacement therapy deserves further study. The risk for endometrial cancer in a patient undergoing unopposed estrogen replacement therapy is two to four times the rate in women not on hormones, and it is related to duration of use (Weiss et al, 1979). Current recommendations suggest that patients on unopposed estrogen should undergo annual endometrial biopsy. In addition, women who have bleeding before day 11 of a cyclic progestin regimen should undergo endometrial biopsy (Padwick et al, 1986).

Tamoxifen has been used extensively in the treatment of estrogen receptor–positive breast cancer in postmenopausal women. While taking tamoxifen, these women had reductions in new malignancies forming in the contralateral breast. This observation resulted in the use of tamoxifen in a nationwide breast cancer chemoprevention trial (Kedar et al, 1994). Tamoxifen has antiestrogenic and estrogenic properties. It has been shown to reduce the risk for osteoporosis while increasing rates of endometrial hyperplasia and neoplasia. There is a trend toward more widespread use of this drug, so an increase in endometrial cancer may be anticipated.

The risk for endometrial cancer is reduced by half in patients taking the combination oral contraceptive pill. Most modern preparations are progestin dominant, and the degree of risk reduction is related to duration of use and total progestin dose. The protective effect may be greatest in nonobese, nulliparous women.

Women who smoke have a reduced risk for endometrial cancer. Smoking has been shown to increase concentrations of sex-hormone–binding globulin, thereby lowering levels of bioavailable estrogen. In addition, smoking has been linked to early menopause. Such benefits of smoking, however, are clearly outweighed by the marked increase in risk for lung cancer and cardiovascular disease (Friedman et al, 1987b).

An association between alcohol consumption and endometrial cancer is confusing, despite data from patients with breast cancer. These data suggest that alcohol consumption is an independent risk factor, perhaps mediated through altered estrogen metabolism (Gapstur et al, 1993).

Not all endometrial adenocarcinomas arise as a result of physiologic conditions of relative estrogen excess. There is a subset of adenocarcinomas that arise in women with no identifiable risk factors. These tumors may be of high grade and of unfavorable histologic type (for example, papillary serous, clear cell, or adenosquamous variants). They develop de novo, not in an environment of endometrial hyperplasia, and are often aggressive tumors. In addition, there are rare hereditary forms of endometrial cancer, including the Lynch II family cancer syndrome. This syndrome includes nonpolyposis colorectal cancer, ovarian, and endometrial cancer (Lynch et al, 1989). A careful family history should always be obtained from patients with cancer.

Diagnosis

The most common symptom of endometrial cancer, abnormal vaginal bleeding, occurs in more than 80% of patients. When this hallmark symptom occurs in postmenopausal women, it is dramatic, disturbing, and likely to prompt an immediate response from patient and physician. The amount of bleeding is not correlated with the likelihood of cancer because even a small amount of spotting may represent cancer (Fig. 7-5).

As many as 50% of patients with endometrial cancer have abnormal results on Papanicolaou smear. This makes the test unsatisfactory for screening. However, among postmenopausal women with normal endometrial cells on a routine smear, 6% have endometrial cancer and 13% have endometrial hyperplasia. If these endometrial cells are atypical, as many as 25% have endometrial cancer. Therefore, the detection of endometrial cells on a Papanicolaou smear in a postmenopausal woman indicates the need for endometrial biopsy (Zucker et al, 1985). Evaluation of endometrial cytologic preparations has not gained broad acceptance because of the difficulty in interpretation (Meisels and Jolicoeur, 1985).

Is the risk for endometrial hyperplasia or neoplasia so high in some patient groups that screening by ultrasonography or endometrial biopsy is warranted? Gronroos et al (1993) address this question by instituting mass screening of 597 women, 45 to 69 years of age, who have diabetes mellitus and hypertension. Among women with diabetes, 6.3% were found to have neoplasia. Among women with hypertension, 1.3% were found to have neoplasia. Eighty percent of women ultimately bleed, and 75% have highly curable stage 1 disease at this first sign of abnormality. Because of this, it is unclear how much benefit would be gained by screening women with diabetes mellitus and hypertension, especially in light of the costs of screening the 90% of patients who do not have cancer at the time of screening.

Women taking tamoxifen for breast cancer have an increased risk for endometrial neoplasms. This increased risk is partly a result of the estrogen agonist effects of tamoxifen on the endometrium. However, women with a history of breast cancer are also at increased risk for ovarian or endometrial cancer, regardless of tamoxifen use. In addition, some studies of women taking tamoxifen report an excess number of malignancies that carry poor prognoses, among them clear cell carcinoma and papillary serous carcinoma (Cohen et al, 1993; Magriples et al, 1993). Given these findings, yearly endometrial biopsies, or intermittent progesterone treatment of patients on long-term tamoxifen therapy, should be considered.

Pathology

Most forms of cancer arising in the endometrium are adenocarcinomas. There are distinct histopathologic types that evince very different biologic behaviors. Endometrioid adenocarcinomas are the most common. These lesions may be papillary, secretory, or ciliated. Squamous differentiation is a common feature. When the squamous tissue is anaplastic, it is designated as an adenosquamous variant. Variants that have been described are mucinous, clear cell, and pure squamous carcinoma.

The degree of carcinoma differentiation may be based on cytologic or architectural criteria. For endometrial carcinomas, the International Federation of Gynecologists and Obstetricians (FIGO) has established architectural criteria that may be applied to most cell types. A grade 1 tumor is de-

fined as a tumor that has less than 5% solid area. A grade 3 tumor is more than 50% solid. Tumor grade predicts the biologic behavior of endometrial cancer. Well-differentiated lesions tend to be associated with superficial invasion and have little propensity for nodal spread. Poorly differentiated lesions are often deeply invasive and metastatic. Clear cell carcinoma and papillary serous carcinoma are two particularly virulent forms of endometrial cancer. They represent less than 15% of all endometrial cancers combined, but they encompass a large proportion of the treatment failures (Kurman and Scully, 1976; Christopherson et al, 1982).

Pretreatment Evaluation

Once the diagnosis of endometrial cancer has been confirmed, a complete history and physical examination should be performed. Often, patients with endometrial cancer are obese and have hypertension or diabetes and possibly significant intercurrent medical problems. A complete blood count to rule out anemia secondary to vaginal bleeding should be performed. Abnormal liver function test results may suggest occult metastatic disease. A chest x-ray should be obtained to rule out pulmonary metastases. Intravenous pyelography, gastrointestinal series, and barium enema are not required in asymptomatic patients. A bone scan adds little to the initial evaluation.

Magnetic resonance imaging has proven to be accurate in the evaluation of myometrial invasion and lymph node involvement (Yazigi, 1989). Transvaginal sonography has been used to assess myometrial invasion but with less success (Yamashita, 1993). These modalities are expensive and less accurate than data derived from surgical staging. They may be helpful in evaluating patients in whom comorbid disease precludes surgical staging, but they are not required for surgical staging.

Although originally described as a tumor marker for ovarian cancer, serum levels of CA-125 have been shown to be elevated among patients with endometrial cancer (Niloff et al, 1994). It is unusual for early-stage disease to cause an abnormal level, and because most patients seek treatment at an early stage, it is not indicated as a routine test. In most studies, more than 80% of patients with elevated CA-125 levels are found to have extrauterine disease at the time of exploratory laparotomy (Pastner and Mann, 1988).

Endometrial cancer is a surgically staged disease. Therefore, imaging to assess the depth of myometrial invasion and tumor markers to suggest disseminated disease are not required before exploration.

Staging

The surgical staging of corpus uteri cancer is outlined in Table 7-1. In 1988 FIGO abandoned the clinical staging system after the completion of prospective surgical staging trials (Boronow et al, 1984; Creasman et al, 1987). These studies establish the importance of cell type, histologic grade, depth of myometrial invasion, and nodal, adnexal, or peritoneal spread as prognostic variables. The previous clinical staging system, which determined uterine size and endocervical involvement at a fractional D & C, is now used only for patients treated with primary radiation therapy.

Surgical staging begins with a vertical abdominal incision. Any collection of free pelvic fluid should be aspirated for cytologic evaluation. If no fluid is present, saline washings should be obtained. Thorough exploration of the abdomen, including palpation of the diaphragm, bowel mesentery, and para-aortic nodal groups, is essential. Biopsy specimens should be taken of suspicious areas. Total extrafascial hysterectomy and adnexectomy are then performed. In selected patients, para-aortic or pelvic lymph nodes may be sampled, and any enlarged lymph nodes must be removed. Omentectomy or omental biopsy is indicated for patients with the papillary serous variant.

Para-aortic or pelvic lymph node sampling may lead to morbidity and may be technically difficult in an obese patient. Nodal involvement risk is predictable based on histologic cell type, tumor grade, and depth of myometrial invasion. Stage I, grade 1 lesions with superficial invasion rarely metastasize to the pelvic or para-aortic nodes, whereas up to 45% of women with deeply invasive grade 3 lesions have nodal metastasis. Therefore, for patients with presumed stage I endometrial cancer, gross or frozen-section evaluation of the depth of myometrial invasion at the time of hysterectomy is invaluable in guiding intraoperative decision making. Lymph node sampling should be strongly considered for patients with presumed stage I, grade 3 lesions or for lesions of any grade with significant myometrial invasion. Patients with stage II or III disease or with disease of an unfavorable histologic type should also undergo paraaortic and pelvic lymph node sampling.

Vaginal hysterectomy remains an appropriate alternative to abdominal surgery for stage I, grade 1 endometrial cancer. Recent advances in operative laparoscopy have led to innovative approaches to the surgical staging of endometrial cancer. Childers and Surwitt (1993) report their experience with laparoscopically assisted surgical staging of endometrial cancer, including laparoscopic nodal sampling and vaginal hysterectomy. Preliminary data suggest that this investigational technique is well tolerated and that it significantly reduces hospital stays. Laparoscopy allows for upper abdominal exploration, node biopsy, and salpingooophorectomy. These procedures are not possible using a purely vaginal approach.

Postoperative Care

After primary therapy, patients with endometrial cancer should be examined at regular intervals with complete physicals and Papanicolaou smears. Frequency of visits and duration of follow-up must be based on the likelihood for disease recurrence in each patient. Among women with stage IA, grade 1 and stage IB endometrial cancer, hormone replacement therapy may be initiated after informed consent is obtained. In these patients, the risk for tumor recurrence is low and the benefits of replacement therapy far outweigh the risks (Lee et al, 1990). Estrogen replacement therapy may be contraindicated in advanced-stage, high-grade lesions.

Adjuvant Therapy

After surgical staging and treatment, adjuvant therapy may be required for patients at significant risk for disease recurrence in the pelvis or abdomen. Patients are at high risk if they have been found to have para-aortic lymph node metastasis or adnexal or peritoneal spread. Postoperative radiation to the pelvic and aortic areas may cure up to half the patients with advanced disease (Potish et al, 1985). Radiation treatment of the pelvis remains controversial. Most studies show a reduction in local recurrences but no significant impact on survival rates.

Prognosis

Overall, 72% of women with stage I adenocarcinoma of the endometrium survive at least 5 years. The 5-year survival rate falls to 56% for stage II disease and 30% for stage III disease. Unfortunately, only 10% of women with stage IV lesions survive at least 5 years (Pettersson, 1988).

Recurrence

Endometrial cancer may metastasize intraabdominally, hematologically, or through the lymphatics. The most common site of local recurrence is the vaginal cuff. Distant metastasis may be seen in lung, liver, or abdomen. Most recurrences develop within 3 years of initial diagnosis. Distant metastasis is associated with a grim prognosis because of a lack of effective systemic hormonal therapy or chemotherapy. However, an isolated vaginal recurrence, without pelvic extension, may be effectively treated with surgical excision or local irradiation. As many as 45% of women with this recurrence survive 10 years (Paulsen and Roberts, 1988).

Table 7-1	Staging of Cancer of the Uterine Corpus
Stage	**Description**
IA G123	Tumor limited to endometrium
IB G123	Invasion to 50% myometrium
IC G123	Invasion to 50% myometrium
IIA G123	Endocervical glandular involvement only
IIB G123	Cervical stromal invasion
IIIA G123	Tumor invades serosa and/or adnexa and/or there is positive peritoneal cytology
IIIB G123	Vaginal metastases
IIIC G123	Metastases to pelvic and/or paraaortic lymph nodes
IVA G123	Tumor invasion of bladder and/or bowel mucosa
IVB	Distant metastases including intraabdominal and/or inguinal nodes

Treatment of Recurrent Endometrial Cancer

Treatment of patients with distant recurrences of endometrial cancer is challenging and rarely results in cure. Local irradiation may control pain or disability from focal metastases. To control systemic disease, progestational agents or cytotoxic chemotherapy may be used. Response rates to progestin therapy may be as high as 15% to 20%, particularly in well-differentiated cancers that are more likely to be estrogen-receptor and progesterone-receptor positive.

The role of cytotoxic chemotherapy in the treatment of endometrial cancer is limited. The reported complete clinical response rate is only 15%. Regimens that contain platinum or doxorubicin hydrochloride have the highest overall response rates, but these responses tend to be short lived, and survival is not prolonged (Park et al, 1992).

Given the toxicity associated with cytotoxic chemotherapy, progestin treatment is a rational first step in treating recurrent disease. Progestins have some desirable secondary effects, particularly as appetite stimulants, and minimal toxicity. If progestin treatment fails, cytotoxin therapy may be considered.

Other Uterine Malignancies
Uterine Sarcomas

Uterine sarcomas represent only 2% of all uterine malignancies; the incidence is 2.3 in 100,000 in the United States (Harlow et al, 1986). Unlike endometrial adenocarcinoma, uterine sarcoma is more common among black women. The only known risk factor for gynecologic sarcoma is previous radiation therapy (Meredith et al, 1986). On average it occurs 16 years after radiation exposure (Doss et al, 1984).

Regardless of the histologic type, sarcomas of the uterus generally have the potential for aggressive biologic behavior. Low-grade leiomyosarcomas and endometrial stromal sarcomas, however, are indolent tumors associated with excellent long-term survival.

Leiomyosarcomas. Leiomyosarcomas represent 25% of all uterine sarcomas. Although they often arise in myomatous uteri, these sarcomas most likely develop de novo and are not the consequence of malignant degeneration of a leiomyoma. Rapid enlargement of a solitary uterine mass is a hallmark of leiomyosarcoma. This is particularly true when rapid growth occurs after menopause. These lesions are often found incidentally. Leiomyosarcomas may display a wide spectrum of biologic behaviors based on the number of mitoses per 10 high-power fields, the degree of cytologic atypia, and the extent of hypercellularity.

The treatment of leiomyosarcoma consists of total abdominal hysterectomy and bilateral salpingo-oophorectomy. A thorough staging procedure, including lymph node biopsies, is not necessary (Berchuk et al, 1988; O'Connor and Norris, 1990). Rarely, these tumors are detected at myomectomy.

Endometrial Stromal Sarcomas. Stromal tumors of the endometrium are divided into low-grade and high-grade lesions. A low-grade endometrial stromal sarcoma (for example, endometrial stromal myosis) is an indolent sarcoma that develops in younger women. Recurrences or metastases are uncommon and may occur many years after primary therapy. The lesion may be hormonally dependent; oophorectomy and progestin therapy may cause tumor regression (Gloor et al, 1982). High-grade endometrial stromal sarcoma, however, is a biologically virulent tumor with high mitotic counts (more than 10 mitoses per 10 high-power fields) that metastasizes quickly and is commonly fatal (Norris and Taylor, 1966a and 1966b).

Mixed Müllerian Sarcoma. Mixed müllerian sarcoma is the most common uterine sarcoma; it appears to arise from the endometrial stroma or from undifferentiated cell rests. Survival is related to the degree of invasion. Few survive if the tumor deeply invades the uterus or spreads outside the uterus (Antman, 1993). These tumors are composed of carcinomatous and sarcomatous elements, and the only proven therapy is hysterectomy and bilateral salpingo-oophorectomy.

Natural History

Sarcomas may recur locally or at distant sites, and patients should be carefully followed up. Uterine sarcomas tend to progress rapidly; 90% of recurrences occur within the first 2 years of diagnosis, and more than 90% develop outside the pelvis.

DIAGNOSTIC MODALITIES

Various diagnostic techniques are applicable to the diagnosis or management of uterine disease. A brief summary of techniques follows.

Endometrial Biopsy

Endometrial biopsy is a simple procedure that can be performed in the office, and it is the most cost-effective primary evaluation strategy for the assessment of abnormal uterine bleeding (Feldman et al, 1993). After placing a speculum in the vagina and preparing the cervix with iodine, a 3- to 5-mm flexible plastic tube is inserted in the cervix, and tissue is removed through capillary action and suction. Sensitivity and specificity of this method are high (Stovall et al, 1989). The main risk is patient discomfort (brief severe cramping), and there is a small risk for bleeding, infection, and uterine perforation. Administration of a nonsteroidal antiinflammatory agent or a local paracervical block before the procedure may decrease the discomfort.

Pelvic Ultrasonography

Pelvic ultrasonography can be performed either transabdominally using a full bladder as an acoustic window or transvaginally with a special probe. It is used to evaluate uterine size or to detect abnormal conditions within the uterus, such as leiomyoma, polyps, or a thickened endometrium suggestive of neoplasia. Ultrasonography may play a role in the diagnosis of endometrial cancer. In their study of 205 postmenopausal patients with vaginal bleeding, Granberg et al (1991) demonstrate through endometrial biopsy that mean endometrial thickness is 3.4 ± 1.2 mm in those with atrophic changes. Among women with endometrial cancer, the mean endometrial thickness is 18.2 ± 6.2 mm. Using a cutoff of 5 mm, they also report a positive predictive value for hyperplasia or neoplasia of 87.3%. These findings are reported by other investigators as well (Karlsson et al, 1993; Smith et al, 1991; Dijkhuizen et al, 1996). For premenopausal women or for postmenopausal women taking hormone therapy, a "normal" endometrial stripe has not been clearly determined.

Dilation and Curettage

Fractional D & C is a surgical procedure in which the cervix is dilated and the lining of the uterus and the cervix undergo manual curettage. It is indicated for the evaluation of abnormal bleeding when an office biopsy is technically impossible or when a specimen reveals insufficient tissue for diagnosis yet the clinical suspicion for cancer or atypical hyperplasia remains high. It is more costly, has a higher complication rate, and has lower sensitivity and specificity than office biopsy, so it should not be used in the primary evaluation of abnormal uterine bleeding.

Sonohysterography

Sonohysterography uses transvaginal ultrasonography after the placement of a small catheter (such as a pediatric-size Foley catheter) to allow for distention of the uterine cavity with saline. This approach is useful in identifying structural lesions of the endometrial cavity that can be hidden within the endometrial stripe of premenopausal women. It also allows simultaneous visualization of the myometrium and the ovaries.

Office Hysteroscopy

Flexible fiberoptic hysteroscopes (usually 3 mm) along with a medium for distending the uterus, such as saline or carbon dioxide, allow visualization of the intrauterine cavity without the need for anesthesia. Direct visualization of filling defects often provides information that is helpful in planning their removal. For example, a submucous fibroid and an endometrial polyp can often be differentiated by this method.

Hysterosalpingography

Hysterosalpingography uses iodinated contrast medium and fluoroscopic x-ray monitoring to define the intrauterine cavity and the fallopian tubes. Although it is the technique of choice for patients undergoing fertility evaluation, it has largely been replaced by the two preceding techniques for evaluation of the uterine cavity.

Magnetic Resonance Imaging

Magnetic resonance imaging is useful in the assessment of the uterus because structures that appear to have the same sonic density on ultrasonography can be differentiated by magnetic spin characteristics. Thus, MRI helps to delineate complex uterine anomalies. It is also better than ultrasonography at delineating intramyometrial lesions and it may help in the distinction between leiomyomas and adenomyomas. The cost of this technique limits its use, and ultrasonography is often ordered instead.

MANAGEMENT STRATEGIES

Management of abnormal uterine conditions depends on many factors, among them diagnosis, patient age, and desire for fertility. In addition, technical aspects of the examination, surgeon skill, and available technology affect the choice of procedure. In some situations, there are several acceptable alternatives. Patient and physician preference may then determine which procedure to use. Following is a summary of commonly used procedures.

Operative Hysteroscopy

By using conventional instruments such as scissors modified to fit through an operating channel or by using lasers or electrocautery, many techniques that previously required major abdominal surgery can now be performed through hysteroscopy as outpatient procedures. These include lysis of adhesions in Asherman syndrome and resection of submucous fibroids and intrauterine septa. Special surgical skills are often needed for these procedures, and the complications of surgery and the medium used to distend the uterus must be appreciated.

Endometrial Ablation

Endometrial ablation involves destruction of the endometrium so that menstruation results in decreased or absent bleeding. Conventional ablation involves use of a hysteroscope and electrocautery or laser resection. Recently, the Food and Drug Administration approved the use of a thermal balloon for this procedure, and this may make it more widely available. Before proceeding with the technique, the presence of a normal endometrium and the absence of structural lesions should be confirmed. Because destruction of the endometrium is incomplete with this technique, it should be used with caution in the patient at risk for endometrial hyperplasia. Desire for future pregnancies is a contraindication to endometrial ablation.

HYSTERECTOMY

Hysterectomy is the most common nonobstetric procedure performed on women in the United States (National Center for Health Statistics, 1992). Nonetheless, the annual number of hysterectomies has decreased significantly since the 1980s with the development of surgical and medical alternatives. Moreover, the development of laparoscopy-assisted vaginal hysterectomy, which aids in the removal of the ovaries and in evaluation of the upper abdomen, has resulted in an increase in the relative number of vaginal (as opposed to abdominal) hysterectomies. As discussed here, however, there still is an active role for each type of hysterectomy in the management of certain abnormalities of the uterus. Of note, laparoscopy-assisted vaginal hysterectomy costs more

(Dorsey et al, 1996; Weber and Lee, 1996) and entails higher complication rates than abdominal hysterectomy. The American College of Obstetrics and Gynecology has published guidelines for the appropriateness of hysterectomy for certain medical conditions (ACOG, 1997a and 1997b).

In one large prospective study, the Maine Women's Health Study (Carlson et al, 1994a and 1994b), two populations of patients were studied: those who underwent hysterectomy and those who elected nonsurgical management for leiomyomas, abnormal uterine bleeding, and chronic pelvic pain. Symptoms and quality of life were studied at 1 year. Of patients in the nonsurgical treatment arm, there were significant improvements in symptoms and quality of life. However, of the patients initially treated nonsurgically, approximately one fourth subsequently underwent hysterectomy. In multivariate logistic regression analysis, hysterectomy was the single factor most associated with a good outcome at 1 year. In a related study of patients who underwent hysterectomy for all benign diagnoses, significant improvement was found in symptoms and quality of life at 1 year (Carlson et al, 1994a and 1994b).

The most common indicator for hysterectomy remains uterine leiomyoma, followed by abnormal uterine bleeding, endometriosis, and uterine prolapse (Wilcox et al, 1994; Carlson et al, 1993). Cancer accounts for roughly 10% of the hysterectomies performed, and endometrial hyperplasia (a premalignant condition) accounts for 5%. The remaining 16% include a variety of conditions, including persistent cervical dysplasia, adenomyosis, infectious and peripartum bleeding or abnormal placenta-tion. There continues to be a fair amount of geographic variation across the United States as to the indications for and the incidences of hysterectomy (Haas et al, 1993; Roos, 1989).

Types of Hysterectomy and How to Choose
Vaginal Hysterectomy

Vaginal hysterectomy is performed entirely through the vagina. The most common indications include uterine prolapse or benign or premalignant conditions (such as endometrial hyperplasia or cervical dysplasia) that do not result in unusually large uteri and are not likely to result in significant intraabdominal adhesions and in which exploration of the upper abdomen is nonessential. Advantages of this procedure are the absence of an abdominal scar and the tendency for a quicker recovery and shorter hospital stay. Physical requirements for the procedure include the ability to lie on one's back with legs in stirrups for a prolonged time, a relatively small and mobile uterus, and adequate room in the vagina in which to operate. Thus, for women who have never had children or who are virginal, this option may not be possible. Experienced surgeons can sometimes remove larger uteri with this approach through coring or by removing the uterus in parts.

Laparoscopy-Assisted Vaginal Hysterectomy

Laparoscopy-assisted vaginal hysterectomy combines a vaginal approach with a laparoscopic abdominal approach.

This may be appropriate for patients in whom evaluation of the upper abdomen is indicated (for instance, for grade 1 endometrial cancer) or in whom removal of the ovaries is desired. Although this procedure has the advantages of smaller abdominal scars and shorter hospital stays, many studies (Dorsey et al, 1996; Weber and Lee, 1996) show it to have higher rates of complication, longer operative times, and higher costs than simple abdominal or simple vaginal hysterectomy. These disadvantages may be attributed, in part, to less experience on the part of the surgeons performing the procedure and inappropriate selection of patients. Another factor that determines high cost may be the greater use of disposable, expensive equipment. Appropriate case selection and high surgical volume are probably the two leading means of ensuring good outcomes. In general, patients should meet the same physical requirements as those for simple vaginal hysterectomy, and they should be at low risk for laparoscopic complication (no history suggestive of the formation of abdominal adhesions, normal weight range, and no large pelvic masses). If there is uncertainty about a patient but upper abdominal access is necessary, laparotomy with abdominal hysterectomy may be the procedure of choice.

Supracervical Hysterectomy

By definition, supracervical hysterectomy must be performed abdominally so that conservation of the cervix may be assured. The fundus of the uterus is removed to the level below the uterine vessels, and the cervix is conserved. Although it is rare, a small area of endometrium may be retained in the cervical stump, leading to monthly "menses," and there may be a long-term risk for endometrial cancer even after "hysterectomy." This procedure is indicated for the patient who desires to keep her cervix for its potential role in sexual function and who does not have a contraindication that would preclude her keeping it (such as cancer or a history of cervical dysplasia). It is also indicated for the patient in whom the surgical procedure would be made safer by the conservation of the cervix (such as with obliteration of the cul-de-sac because of advanced endometriosis) and in whom there is no contraindication to its retention. Advantages of this procedure include the greater ease and shorter time required for the procedure and the potential sexual benefits believed by some to be attributable to the cervix. Retention of the cervix may also result in less vaginal prolapse because of better vaginal support.

Total Abdominal Hysterectomy

Total abdominal hysterectomy (with or without salpingo-oophorectomy) is the most commonly performed hysterectomy. Both the uterine fundus and the cervix are removed at the cervico-vaginal junction. It may be performed through either a transverse or a vertical abdominal incision, depending on the indications for the procedure and the size of the uterus. This is the procedure of choice for most uterine and ovarian cancers, endometriosis, pelvic pain, large fibroid uteri (in which conservation of the cervix is not desired), and conditions in which evaluation of the full pelvis and abdomen is desirable (such as pelvic masses or adnexal masses of unknown diagnosis).

Radical Hysterectomy

Radical hysterectomy is a procedure in which the parametrial tissue and the upper vagina are removed in conjunction with the fundus and the cervix. It is primarily indicated in the treatment of early-stage cervical cancer. It carries with it a greater risk for bowel and bladder dysfunction, ureteral injury, and subsequent urinary fistula.

Preoperative Evaluation

Whatever method of hysterectomy is chosen, the preoperative evaluation consists of acquiring sufficient information to determine the appropriateness of the approach. For example, before performing a supracervical hysterectomy, a Papanicolaou smear and a record of previous normal smears should be documented. Before deciding on a vaginal hysterectomy, assessment of the adnexa and uterine size should be performed either through pelvic examination or pelvic ultrasonography. Any patient with unexplained abnormal bleeding should undergo endometrial biopsy to rule out cancer.

REFERENCES

Abramovici H, Faktor JH, Pascal B: Congenital uterine malformations as indication for cervical suture (cerclage) in habitual abortion and premature delivery. *Int J Fertil* 1983; 28:161-164.

Am Coll Obstet Gynecol Critical Set: *Hysterectomy, abdominal,* 1997 no. 28 and 29.

Akkad AA, Habiba MA, Ismail N, et al: Abnormal uterine bleeding on hormone replacement: The importance of intrauterine structural abnormalities. *Obstet Gynecol* 1995; 86:330-334.

Ambius JL, editor: *The Menopause and Post-Menopause,* Lancaster, UK, 1980, MTP Press.

American Fertility Society: Classifications of adnexal adhesions, distal robot occlusion, tubal occlusion secondary to robot ligation, robot pregnancies, müllerian anomalies and intrauterine adhesions. *Fertil Steril* 1988; 49:944-955.

Ansbacher R: Uterine anomalies and future pregnancies. *Clin Perinatol* 1983; 10:295-304.

Anson BJ, Curtis A: Anatomy of the female pelvis and perineum. In Curtis AH, editor: *Textbook of gynecology,* Philadelphia, 1946, WB Saunders.

Antman KH: Uterine sarcomas. In Knapp RC, Berkowitz RS, editors: *Gynecologic oncology,* New York, 1993, McGraw-Hill.

Antman KH, et al: Preliminary results of a randomized trial of adjuvant Adriamycin for sarcomas. *J Clin Oncol* 1984; 2:601.

Antunes CMF, et al: Endometrial cancer and estrogen use. *N Engl J Med* 1979; 300:9-13.

Asherman JG: Amenorrhoea traumatica (Atretica). *J Obstet Gynaecol Br Emp* 1948; 55:23-25.

Babaknia A, Rock JA, Jones HW Jr: Pregnancy-success following abdominal myomectomy for infertility. *Fertil Steril* 1978; 30:644-647.

Baggish MS: Mesenchymal tumors of the uterus. *Clin Obstet Gynecol* 1974; 17:51-88.

Bean HA, et al: Carcinoma of the endometrium in Saskatchewan: 1966-1971. *Gynecol Oncol* 1978; 6:503-514.

Berchuck A, et al: Treatment of uterine leiomyosarcoma. *Obstet Gynecol* 1988; 71:845-850.

Berkeley AS, DeCherney AB, Polan ML: Abdominal myomectomy and subsequent fertility. *Surg Gynecol Obstet* 1983; 156:319-322.

Bird CC, McElin TW, Manalo-Estrella P: The elusive adenomyosis of the uterus—revisited. *Am J Obstet Gynecol* 1972; 112:583-593.

Boronow RC, et al: Surgical staging in endometrial cancer: Clinical pathologic findings of a prospective study. *Obstet Gynecol* 1984; 63:825-832.

Brooks, PG, Serden SP: Hysteroscopic findings after unsuccessful dilatation and curettage for abnormal uterine bleeding. *Am J Obstet Gynecol* 1988; 158:1354-1357.

Brown JM, Malkasian GD Jr, Symmonds RE: Abdominal myomectomy. *Am J Obstet Gynecol* 1967; 99:126-129.

Bruckman JE, et al: Stage III adenocarcinoma of the endometrium: Two prognostic groups. *Gynecol Oncol* 1980; 9:12-17.

Burrell MO, Franklin EW II, Powell JL: Endometrial cancer: Evaluation of spread and follow-up in one hundred eighty-nine patients with stage I or stage II. *Am J Obstet Gynecol* 1982; 144:181-185.

Buttram VC Jr: Müllerian anomalies and their management. *Fertil Steril* 1983; 40:159-163.

Buttram VC Jr, Gibbons WE: Müllerian anomalies: A proposed classification (an analysis of 144 cases). *Fertil Steril* 1979; 32:40-46.

Buttram VC Jr, Reiter RC: Uterine leiomyomata: Etiology, symptomatology, and management. *Fertil Steril* 1981; 36:433-445.

Capraro VJ, Gallego MB: Vaginal agenesis. *Am J Obstet Gynecol* 1976; 124:98-107.

Chambers JT, et al: Uterine papillary serous carcinoma. *Obstet Gynecol* 1987; 69:109-113.

Carlson KJ, Miller BA, Fowler FJ Jr: The Maine women's health study, I: Outcomes of hysterectomy. *Obstet Gynecol* 1994; 83:556-565.

Carlson KJ, Miller BA, Fowler FJ: The Maine women's health study, II: Outcomes of nonsurgical management of leiomyomas, abnormal bleeding, and chronic pelvic pain. *Obstet Gynecol* 1994b; 83:566-572.

Carlson KJ, Nichols DH, Schiff I: Indications for hysterectomy. *N Engl J Med* 1993; 328:856-860.

Cheon HK: Prognosis of endometrial carcinoma. *Obstet Gynecol* 1969; 34:680-684.

Childers JM, et al: Laparoscopically assisted surgical staging (LASS). *J Endometr Cancer* 1993; 51:33.

Christopherson WM, Alberhasky RC, Connelly PJ: Carcinoma of the endometrium, II: Papillary adenocarcinoma–clinical pathological study of 46 cases. *Am J Clin Pathol* 1982; 77:534-540.

Chu J, Schweid AL, Weiss NS: Survival among women with endometrial cancer: A comparison of estrogen users and nonusers. *Am J Obstet Gynecol* 1982; 143:569-573.

Cicinelli E, Romano F, Anastasio PS, et al: Transabdominal sonohysterography, transvaginal sonography, and hysteroscopy in the evaluation of submucous myomas. *Obstet Gynecol* 1995; 85:42-47.

Claessens EA, Cowell CA: Acute adolescent menorrhagia. *Am J Obstet Gynecol* 1981; 139:277-280.

Cohen I, et al: Ultrasonographic evaluation of the endometrium and correlation with endometrial sampling in postmenopausal patients treated with tamoxifen. *J Ultrasound Med* 1993; 12:275-280.

Coulam CB, Annegers JF, Kranz JS: Chronic anovulation syndrome and associated neoplasia. *Obstet Gynecol* 1983; 61:403-407.

Counseller VS, Bedard RE: Uterine myomectomy. *JAMA* 1937; 111: 675-678.

Coutinho EM, Boulanger GA, Goncalves MT: Regression of uterine leiomyomas after treatment with gestrinone, an antiestrogen, antiprogesterone. *Am J Obstet Gynecol* 1986; 155:761-767.

Coutinho EM, Goncalves MT: Long-term treatment of leiomyomas with gestrinone. *Fertil Steril* 1989; 51:939-946.

Cramer DW, Cutler SJ, Christine B: Trends in the incidence of endometrial cancer in the United States. *Gynecol Oncol* 1974; 2:130-143.

Cramer DW, Knapp RC: Review of epidemiologic studies of endometrial cancer and exogenous estrogen. *Obstet Gynecol* 1979; 54:521-526.

Cramer SE, Patel D: The frequency of uterine leiomyomas. *Am J Clin Pathol* 1990; 94:435-438.

Creasman WT, et al: Prognostic significance of peritoneal cytology in patients with endometrial cancer and preliminary data concerning therapy with intraperitoneal radiopharmaceuticals. *Am J Obstet Gynecol* 1981; 141:921-929.

Creasman WT, et al: Clinical correlates of estrogen- and progesterone-binding proteins in human endometrial adenocarcinoma. *Obstet Gynecol* 1980; 55:363-370.

Creasman WT, et al: Surgical pathologic spread patterns of endmetrial cancer: A Gynecologic Oncology Group study. *Cancer* 1987; 60:2035-2041.

Daly DC, et al: Hysteroscopic metroplasty: Surgical technique and obstetric outcome. *Fertil Steril* 1983; 39:623-628.

Davies JL, et al: A review of the risk factors for endometrial carcinoma. *Obstet Gynecol Surv* 1981; 36:107-116.

Davis EW: Carcinoma of the corpus uteri: A study of 525 cases at the New York Hospital (1932-1961). *Am J Obstet Gynecol* 1964; 88:163.

DeCherney AH, et al: Resectoscopic management of müllerian fusion defects. *Fertil Steril* 1986; 45:726-728.

Deppe G, et al: Chemotherapy of advanced and recurrent endometrial carcinoma with cyclophosphamide, doxorubicin, 5-fluorouracil, and megestrol acetate. *Am J Obstet Gynecol* 1981; 140:313-316.

DeVore GR, Schwartz PE, Morris JM: Hysterography: A 5-year follow-up in patients with endometrial carcinoma. *Obstet Gynecol* 1982; 60:369-372.

Dijkhuizen FPHL, Brölmann HAM, Potters AG, et al: The accuracy of transvaginal ultrasonography in the diagnosis of endometrial abnormalities. *Obstet Gynecol* 1996; 87:345-349.

Dorsey JH, Holtz PM, Griffiths RI, et al: Costs and charges associated with three alternative techniques of hysterectomy. *N Engl J Med* 1996; 335:476-482.

Doss LL, Llorens AS, Henriquez FM: Carcinosarcoma of the uterus: A 40-year experience from the state of Missouri. *Gynecol Oncol* 1984; 18:43-53.

Ehrlich CE, et al: Steroid receptors and clinical outcome in patients with adenocarcinoma of the endometrium. *Am J Obstet Gynecol* 1988; 158:796-807.

Eifel PJ, et al: Adenocarcinoma of the endometrium: Analysis of 256 cases with disease limited to the uterine corpus: Treatment comparisons. *Cancer* 1983; 52:1026-1031.

Elwood JM, et al: Epidemiology of endometrial cancer. *J Natl Cancer Inst* 1977; 59:1055-1060.

Elwood JM, Boyes DA: Clinical and pathologic features and survival of endometrial cancer patients in relation to prior use of estrogens. *Gynecol Oncol* 1980; 10:173-187.

Farber M, et al: Estradiol binding by fibroid tumors and normal myometrium. *Obstet Gynecol* 1972; 40:479-486.

Fayez JA: Comparison between abdominal and hysteroscopic metroplasty. *Obstet Gynecol* 1986; 68:399-403.

Fedele L, et al: Magnetic resonance evaluation of double uteri. *Obstet Gynecol* 1989; 74:844-847.

Fedele L, et al: Transvaginal ultrasonography in the diagnosis of diffuse adenomyosis. *Fertil Steril* 1992; 58:94-97.

Fedele L, Parazzini F, Luchini L, et al: Recurrence of fibroids after myomectomy: A transvaginal ultrasonographic study. *Hum Reprod* 1995; 10:1795-1796.

Feldman S, Berkowitz RS, Tosteson AN: Cost-effectiveness of strategies to evaluate postmenopausal bleeding. *Obstet Gynecol* 1993; 81:968-975.

Feldman S, Cook EF, Harlow BL, et al: Predicting endometrial cancer among older women who present with abnormal vaginal bleeding. *Gynecol Oncol* 1995; 56:376-381.

Feldman S, Shapter A, Welch WR, et al: Two year follow-up of 263 patients with post/perimenopausal vaginal bleeding and negative initial biopsy. *Gynecol Oncol* 1994; 55:56-59.

Ferenczy A, Gelfand M: The biologic significance of cytologic atypia in progestogen-treated endometrial hyperplasia. *Am J Obstet Gynecol* 1989; 160:126-131.

Finn WF, Muller PE: Abdominal myomectomy: Special reference to subsequent pregnancy and to the reappearance of fibromyomas of the uterus. *Am J Obstet Gynecol* 1950; 60:109-114.

Forney JP, Buschbaum HJ: Classifying, staging, and treating uterine sarcomas. *Contemp Ob Gyn* 1981; 18:47-69.

Frank RT: The formation of an artificial vagina without operation. *Am J Obstet Gynecol* 1938; 35:1053-1059.

Friedman AJ, et al: Treatment of leiomyomata with intranasal or subcutaneous leaprolide, a gonadotropin-releasing hormone agonist. *Fertil Steril* 1987a; 48:560-564.

Friedman AJ, et al: A randomized double-blind trial of a gonadotropin-releasing hormone agonist (leuprolide) with or without medroxyprogesterone acetate in the treatment of leiomyomata uteri. *Fertil Steril* 1988; 49:404-409.

Friedman AJ, et al: A randomized, placebo-controlled, double-blind study evaluating the efficacy of leuprolide acetate depot in the treatment of uterine leiomyomata. *Fertil Steril* 1989; 51:251-256.

Friedman AJ, et al: Efficacy and safety considerations in women with uterine leiomyomata treated with gonadotropin-releasing hormone agonists: The estrogen threshold hypothesis. *Am J Obstet Gynecol* 1990; 163:1114-1119.

Friedman AJ, et al: Treatment of leiomyomata uteri with leuprolide acetate depot: A double-blind placebo-controlled multicenter study. *Obstet Gynecol* 1991; 77:720-725.

Friedman AJ, et al: Recurrence of myomas following myomectomy in women treated with a gonadotropin-releasing hormone agonist. *Fertil Steril* 1992; 58:205-208.

Friedman A, DeFazio J, DeCherney A: Severe obstetric complications after aggressive treatment of Asherman's syndrome. *Obstet Gynecol* 1986; 67:864-867.

Friedman AJ, Haas ST: Should uterine size be an indication for surgery for women with leiomyomas? *Am J Obstet Gynecol* 1993; 168:751-755.

Friedman AJ, Ravnikar VA, Barbieri RL: Serum steroid hormone profiles in postmenopausal smokers and nonsmokers. *Fertil Steril* 1987b; 47:398-401.

Fritsch H: Ein Fall von volligem Schwund der Gebarmutterhohle nach Auskratzung. *Zentralbl Gynaekol* 1984; 18:1337-1341.

Gal D: Hormonal therapy for lesions of the endometrium. *Semin Oncol* 1986; 13(suppl 4):33-36.

Gambone JC, et al: In vivo availability of circulating estradiol in postmenopausal women with and without endometrial cancer. *Obstet Gynecol* 1982; 59:416-421.

Gambrell RD Jr: The prevention of endometrial cancer in postmenopausal women with progestogens. *Maturitas* 1978; 1:107-112.

Gapstur SM, et al: Alcohol consumption and postmenopausal endometrial cancer: Results from the Iowa Women's Health Study. *Cancer Causes Control* 1993; 4:323-329.

Gimpelson RJ, Rappold HO: A comparative study between panoramic hysteroscopy with directed biopsies and dilatation and curettage: A review of 276 cases. *Am J Obstet Gynecol* 1988; 153:489-492.

Gloor E, et al: Endolymphatic stromal meiosis: Surgical and hormonal treatment of extensive abdominal recurrence 20 years after hysterectomy. *Cancer* 1982; 50:1889-1893.

Godsoe A, et al: Cardiopulmonary changes with intermittent endotoxin administration in sheep. *Circ Shock* 1988; 25:61-74.

Granberg S, et al: Endometrial thickness as measured by endovaginal ultrasonography for identifying endometrial abnormality. *Am J Obstet Gynecol* 1991; 164:47-52.

Graves EJ: National Center for Health Statistics: National hospital discharge survey; annual summary, 1990. *Vital and Health Statistics.* Series 13, No. 112, Washington, DC, 1992, Government Printing Office (DHHS publication no. 92-1773).

Gronroos M, et al: Mass screening for endometrial cancer directed in risk groups of patients with diabetes and patients with hypertension. *Cancer* 1993; 71:1279-1282.

Gros A, David A, Serr DM: Management of congenital malformations of the uterus: fetal salvage. *Acta Eur Fertil* 1974; 5:301-304.

Gurpide E: Hormone receptors in endometrial cancer. *Cancer* 1981; 48:638-641.

Haas S, Acker D, Donahue C, et al: Variation in hysterectomy rates across small geographic areas of Massachusetts. *Am J Obstet Gynecol* 1993; 169:150-154.

Hannigan EV, Gomez LG: Uterine leiomyosarcoma: A review of prognostic clinical and pathologic features. *Am J Obstet Gynecol* 1979; 134:557-564.

Harger JH, et al: Etiology of recurrent pregnancy losses and outcome of subsequent pregnancies. *Obstet Gynecol* 1983; 62:574-581.

Harlow BL, Weiss NS, Lofton S: The epidemiology of sarcomas of the uterus. *J Natl Cancer Inst* 1986; 76:399-402.

Hendrickson MR, et al: Adenocarcinoma of the endometrium: Analysis of 256 cases with carcinoma limited to the uterine corpus: Pathology review and analysis of prognostic variables. *Gynecol Oncol* 1982; 13: 373-392.

Hornback NB, Omura G, Major FJ: Observations on the use of adjuvant radiation therapy in patients with stage I and II uterine sarcoma. *Int J Radiat Oncol Biol Phys* 1986; 12:2127-2130.

Hulka BS, et al: Protection against endometrial carcinoma by combination-product oral contraceptives. *JAMA* 1982; 247:475.

Hunt JE, Wallach EE: Uterine factors in infertility–an overview. *Clin Obstet Gynecol* 1974; 17:44-64.

Imachi M, et al: Peritoneal cytology in patients with endometrial carcinoma. *Gynecol Oncol* 1988; 30:76-86.

Ingersoll FM: Fertility following myomectomy. *Fertil Steril* 1963; 14:596-601.

Israel SL, Woutersz TB: Adenomyosis: A neglected diagnosis. *Obstet Gynecol* 1959; 14:168-174.

Jasonni VM, et al: Treatment of endometrial hyperplasia with cyproterone acetate: Histological and hormonal aspects. *Acta Obstet Gynecol Scand* 1986; 65:685-687.

Jewelewicz R, et al: Obstetric complications after treatment of intrauterine synechiae (Asherman's syndrome). *Obstet Gynecol* 1976; 47:701-705.

Jick H, et al: Replacement estrogens and endometrial cancer. *N Engl J Med* 1979; 300:218-222.

Jones WE: Traumatic intrauterine adhesions: A report of 8 cases with emphasis on therapy. *Am J Obstet Gynecol* 1964; 89:304-309.

Judd HL, et al: Serum androgens and estrogens in postmenopausal women with and without endometrial cancer. *Am J Obstet Gynecol* 1980; 136:859-871.

Karlsson B, et al: Endovaginal scanning of the endometrium compared to cytology and histology in women with postmenopausal bleeding. *Gynecol Oncol* 1993; 50:173-178.

Kaufman RH, et al: Upper genital tract changes and pregnancy outcome in offspring exposed in utero to diethylstilbestrol. *Am J Obstet Gynecol* 1980; 137:299-308.

Kawaguchi K, et al: Mitotic activity in uterine leiomyomas during the menstrual cycle. *Am J Obstet Gynecol* 1989; 160:637-641.

Kedar RP, Bourne TH, Powles TJ, et al: Effects of tamoxifen on uterus and ovaries of postmenooausal women in a randomised brest cancer prevention trial. *Lancet* 1994; 343: 1318-1321.

Kelly HA. *Operative gynecology*, 2nd ed, New York, 1906, D Appleton.

Kelsey JL, et al: A case-control study of cancer of the endometrium. *Am J Epidemiol* 1982; 116:333-342.

Kempson RL, Bari W: Uterine sarcomas: Classification, diagnosis, and prognosis. *Hum Pathol* 1970; 1:331-349.

Kinsella TJ, et al: Stage II endometrial carcinoma: 10-year follow-up of combined radiation and surgical treatment. *Gynecol Oncol* 1980; 10:290-297.

Kurman RJ, Kaminski PF, Norris HJ: The behavior of endometrial hyperplasia: A longterm study of "untreated" hyperplasia in 170 patients. *Cancer* 1985; 56:403-412.

Kurman RJ, Scully RE: Clear cell carcinoma of the endometrium: An analysis of 21 cases. *Cancer* 1976; 37:872-882.

Langer RD, Pierce JJ, O'Hanlon KA, et al: Transvaginal ultrasonography compared with endometrial biopsy for the detection of endometrial disease: Postmenopausal Estrogen/Progestin Intervention Trial. *N Engl J Med* 1997; 337:1792-1798.

Lee RB, Burke TW, Park RC: Estrogen replacement therapy following treatment for stage I endometrial carcinoma. *Gynecol Oncol* 1990; 36:189-191.

Leibel SA, Wharam MD: Vaginal and paraaortic lymph node metastases in carcinoma of the endometrium. *Int J Radiat Oncol Biol Phys* 1980; 6:893-896.

Loeffler FE, Noble AD: Myomectomy at the Chelsea Hospital for Women. *J Obstet Gynaecol Br Commonw* 1970; 77:167-170.

Lucas WE, Yen SS: A study of endocrine and metabolic variables in postmenopausal women with endometrial carcinoma. *Am J Obstet Gynecol* 1979; 134:180-186.

Lynch HT, et al: Adenocarcinoma of the small bowel in Lynch syndrome II. *Cancer* 1989; 64:2178-2183.

Mack TM, et al: Estrogens and endometrial cancer in a retirement community. *N Engl J Med* 1976; 294:1262-1267.

MacMahon B: Risk factors for endometrial cancer. *Gynecol Oncol* 1974; 2:122-129.

Magriples U, et al: High-grade endometrial carcinoma in tamoxifen-treated breast cancer patients. *J Clin Oncol* 1993; 11:485-490.

Maheux R, et al: Luteinizing hormone-releasing hormone agonist and uterine leiomyoma: A pilot study. *Am J Obstet Gynecol* 1985; 152:1034-1038.

Malone LJ, Ingersoll FM: Myomectomy in infertility. In Behrman SJ, Kistner RW, editors: *Progress in infertility*, Boston, 1975, Little, Brown.

Malviya VK, et al: Reliability of frozen section examination in identifying poor prognostic indicators in stage I endometrial adenocarcinoma. *Gynecol Oncol* 1989; 34: 299-304.

March CM, Israel R, March AD: Hysteroscopic management of intrauterine adhesions. *Am J Obstet Gynecol* 1978; 130:653-657.

Marshall LM, Spiegelman D, Barbieri RL, et al: Variation in the incidence of uterine leiomyoma among premenopausal women by age and race. *Obstet Gynecol* 1997; 90: 967-973.

Mashal RD, Fejzo ML, Friedman AJ, et al: Analysis of androgen receptor DNA reveals the independent clonal origins of uterine leiomyomata and the secondary nature of cytogenetic aberrations in the development of leiomyomata. *Genes Chromosomes Cancer* 1994; 11:1-6.

McCausland AM: Hysteroscopic myometrial biopsy: Its use in diagnosing adenomyosis and its clinical application. *Am J Obstet Gynecol* 1991; 166:1619-1628.

McCormick TA: Myomectomy with subsequent pregnancy. *Am J Obstet Gynecol* 1958; 75:1128-1133.

McElin TW, Bird CC: Adenomyosis of the uterus. *Obstet Gynecol Anni* 1974; 3:425-441.

McIndoe AH: The treatment of congenital absence and obliterative conditions of the vagina. *Br J Plastic Surg* 1950; 2:254-263.

McShane PM, Reilly RJ, Schiff I: Pregnancy outcomes following Tompkins metroplasty. *Fertil Steril* 1983; 40:190-194.

Meisels A, Jolicoeur C: Criteria for the cytologic assessment of hyperplasia in endometrial samples obtained by the Endopap Endometrial Sampler. *Acta Cytol* 1985; 29:297-302.

Meredith RF, et al: An excess of uterine sarcomas after pelvic irradiation. *Cancer* 1986; 58:2003-2007.

Meyer R: Uber Drusen, Cyste und Adenom in Myometrium bei er Wachsen. *Z Geburtshilfe Gynaekol* 1900; 43:130-138.

Miller H, Tyrone C: A survey of a series of myomectomies with a follow-up. *Am J Obstet Gynecol* 1933; 26:575-581.

Misch KA, et al: Tuberculosis of the cervix: Cytology as an aid to diagnosis. *J Clin Pathol* 1976; 29:313-316.

Molitor JJ: Adenomyosis: A clinical and pathologic appraisal. *Am J Obstet Gynecol* 1971; 110:275-284.

Mortel R, Zaino R, Satyaswaroop PG: Modulation of growth and sex steroid receptor concentrations by tamoxifen in human endometrial carcinoma transplanted into nude mice. *Proc Soc Gynecol Oncol* 1983; 19:23.

Munnell EW, Martin FW: Abdominal myomectomy, advantages and disadvantages. *Am J Obstet Gynecol* 1951; 62:109-114.

Nasri MN, et al: The role of vaginal scan in measurement of endometrial thickness in postmenopausal women. *Br J Obstet Gynaecol* 1991; 98:470-475.

National Center for Health Statistics: Hysterectomies in the United States, 1965-84. *Vital and Health Statistics,* Series 13, No 92, Bethesda, 1987, Maryland Publishing.

Neuwirth RS, Friedman EA: Septic abortion: Changing concept of management. *Am J Obstet Gynecol* 1963; 85:24.

Ng AB, et al: Significance of endometrial cells in the detection of endometrial carcinoma and its precursors. *Acta Cytol* 1974; 18:356-361.

Niloff JM, et al: Elevation of serum CA-125 in carcinomas of the fallopian tube, endometrium, and endocervix. *Am J Obstet Gynecol* 1994; 148:1057-1058.

Nishida M: Relationship between the onset of dysmenorrhea and histologic findings in adenomyosis. *Am J Obstet Gynecol* 1991; 165:229-231.

Nishijima MK, et al: Effect of naloxone and ibuprofen on organ blood flow during endotoxic shock in pig. *Am J Physiol* 1988; 255:HI77-H184.

Norris HJ, Taylor HB: Mesenchymal tumors of the uterus, I: A clinical and pathologic study of 53 endometrial stromal tumors. *Cancer,* 1966a; 19:755-766.

Norris HJ, Taylor HB: Mesenchymal tumors of the uterus, III: A clinical and pathologic study of 31 carcinosarcomas. *Cancer* 1966b; 19:1459-1465.

Novak ER, Woodruff JD: Myoma and other benign tumors of the uterus. In *Gynecologic and obstetric pathology,* ed 8, Philadelphia, 1979, WB Saunders.

Nowak, RA, Stewart EA: New concepts in the treatment of uterine leiomyomas. *Obstet Gynecol* 1998; 92:624-627.

O'Connor DM, Norris HJ: Mitotically active leiomyomas of the uterus. *Hum Pathol* 1990; 21:223-227.

O'Leary JL, O'Leary JA: Rudimentary horn pregnancy. *Obstet Gynecol* 1963; 22:371-377.

Otubu JA, et al: Unconjugated steroids in leiomyomas and tumor-bearing myometrium. *Am J Obstet Gynecol* 1982; 143:130-133.

Padubidri V, et al: The detection of endometrial tuberculosis in cases of infertility by uterine aspiration cytology. *Acta Cytol* 1980. 24:319-324.

Padwick ML, Psryse-Davies J, Whitehead MI: A simple method for determining the optimal dosage of progestin in postmenopausal women receiving estrogens. *N Engl J Med* 1986; 315:930.

Parazzini, F, Negri E, LaVecchia C, et al: Reproductive factors and risk of uterine fibroids. *Epidemiology* 1996; 7:440-442.

Park RC, et al: Corpus: Epithelial tumors. In *Principles and practice of gynecologic oncology,* Philadelphia, 1992, JB Lippincott.

Parker WH, Fu YS, Berek JS: Uterine sarcoma in patients operated on for presumed leiomyoma and rapidly growing leiomyoma. *Obstet Gynecol* 1994; 83:414-8.

Paterson ME, Wade-Evans T, Sturdee DW, et al: Endometrial disease after treatment with oestrogens and progestogens in the climacteric. *Brit Med J* 1980; 280:822-824.

Patsner B, Mann WJ: Use of serum CA-125 in monitoring patients with uterine sarcoma: A preliminary report. *Cancer* 1988; 62:1355-1358.

Patsner B, Mann WJ, Cohen H, et al: Predictive value of preoperative serum CA- 125 levels in clinically localized and advanced endometrial carcinoma. *Am J Obstet Gynecol* 1988; 158:399-402.

Paulsen MG, Roberts SJ: The salvage of recurrent endometrial carcinoma in the vagina and pelvis. *Int J Radiat Oncol Biol Phys* 1988; 15:809-813.

Perino A, et al: Hysteroscopy for metroplasty of uterine septa: Report of 24 cases. *Fertil Steril* 1987; 48:321-323.

Pettersson F, editor: *Annual report on the results of treatment in gynecologic cancer,* vol 20, Stockholm, 1988, International Federation of Gynecology and Obstetrics.

Piver MS, et al: Para-aortic lymph node evaluation in stage I endometrial carcinoma. *Obstet Gynecol* 1982; 59:97-100.

Plentl AA, Friedman EA: Lymphatic system of the female genitalia. In *The morphologic basis of oncologic diagnosis and therapy,* Philadelphia, 1971, WB Saunders.

Pollow K, et al: In vitro conversion of estradiol-17 beta into estrone in normal human myometrium and leiomyoma. *J Clin Chem Clin Biochem* 1978; 16:493-502.

Potischman N, et al: Dietary associations in a case-control study of endometrial cancer. *Cancer Causes Control* 1993; 4:239-250.

Potish RA, et al: Paraaortic lymph node radiotherapy in cancer of the uterine corpus. *Obstet Gynecol* 1985; 65:251-256.

Ranney B, Frederick I: The occasional need for myomectomy. *Obstet Gynecol* 1979; 53:437-441.

Robbins SL, Cotran RS: Leiomyoma (fibromyoma). In *The pathogenic basis of disease,* ed 2, Philadelphia, 1979, WB Saunders.

Roberts DE, et al: Effects of prolonged naloxone infusion in septic shock. *Lancet* 1988; 2:699-702.

Rock JA, Jones HW Jr: The clinical management of the double uterus. *Fertil Steril* 1977; 28:798-806.

Roos NP: Hysterectomy: Variation in rates across small areas and across physician practices. *Am J Public Health* 1984; 74:327-335.

Ross RK, Pike MC, Vessey MP, et al: Risk factors for uterine fibroids: Reduced risk associated with oral contraceptives. *Br Med J* 1986; 293:359-362.

Rubin A, Ford JA: Uterine fibromyomata in urban Blacks: A preliminary survey of the relationship between symptomatology, blood pressure and haemoglobin levels. *S Afr Med J* 1974; 48:2060-2062.

Salazar OM, et al: Adenosquamous carcinoma of the endometrium: An entity with an inherent poor prognosis? *Cancer* 1977; 40:119-130.

Salazar OM, et al: Uterine sarcomas: Natural history, treatment and prognosis. *Cancer* 1978; 42:1152-1160.

Schenker JG, Margalioth EJ: Intrauterine adhesions: An updated appraisal. *Fertil Steril* 1982; 37:593-610.

Schoenberg Fejzo M, Ashar HR, Krauter KS, et al: Translocation breakpoints upstream of the HMGIC gene in uterine leiomyomata suggest dysregulation of this gene by a mechanism different from that in lipomas. *Genes Chromosomes Cancer* 1996; 17:1-6.

Schumer W: Steroids in the treatment of clinical septic shock. *Ann Surg* 1976; 184:333-341.

Shah CA, Green TH Jr: Evaluation of current management of endometrial carcinoma. *Obstet Gynecol* 1972; 39:500-509.

Silverberg E, Lubera JA: Cancer statistics, 1988. *CA Cancer J Clin* 1988; 38:5-22.

Skowronski GA: The pathophysiology of shock. *Med J Aust* 1988; 148:576-579, 582-593.

Smith DC, et al: Association of exogenous estrogen and endometrial carcinoma. *N Engl J Med* 1975; 293:1164-1167.

Smith P, et al: Transvaginal ultrasound for identifying endometrial abnormality. *Acta Obstet Gynecol Scand* 1991; 70:591-594.

Soper JT, et al: Cytoplasmic estrogen and progesterone receptor content of uterine sarcomas. *Am J Obstet Gynecol* 1984; 150:342-349.

Stewart EA, Friedman AJ, eds: Steroidal treatment of myomas: Preoperative and longterm medical therapy. In Barbieri RL, editor. *Seminars in reproductive endocrinology,* New York, 1992, Thieme.

Stewart EA, Nowak RA:. Leiomyoma-related bleeding: A classic hypothesis updated for the molecular era. *Hum Reprod Update* 1996; 2:295-306.

Stillman RJ: In utero exposure to diethylstilbestrol: Adverse effects on the reproductive tract and reproductive performance in male and female offspring. *Am J Obstet Gynecol* 1982; 142:905-921.

Stovall TG, Solomon SK, Ling FW: Endometrial sampling prior to hysterectomy. *Obstet Gynecol* 1989; 73:405-409.

Strassmann EO: Operations for double uterus and endometrial atresia. *Clin Obstet Gynecol* 1961; 4:240-251.

Strassmann EO: Fertility and unification of double uterus. *Fertil Steril* 1966; 17:165-176.

Sutherland AM: Gynaecologic tuberculosis: Analysis of a personal series of 710 cases. *Aust N Z J Obstet Gynaecol* 1985; 25:203-207.

Terakawa N, et al: Preliminary report on the use of danazol in the treatment of endometrial adenomatous hyperplasia. *Cancer* 1988; 62:2618-2621.

Thigpen JT, et al: Phase II trial of adriamycin in the treatment of advanced or recurrent endometrial carcinoma: A Gynecologic Oncology Group study. *Cancer Treat Rep* 1979; 63:21-27.

Tierney WM, et al: Intravenous leiomyomatosis of the uterus with extension into the heart. *Am J Med* 1980; 69:471-475.

Tiltman AJ: The effect of progestins on the mitotic activity of uterine fibromyomas. *Int J Gynecol Pathol* 1985; 4:89-96.

Townsend DE, et al: Unicellular histogenesis of uterine leiomyomas as determined by electrophoresis by glucose-6-phosphate dehydrogenase. *Am J Obstet Gynecol* 1970; 107:1168-1173.

Underwood PB, et al: Endometrial carcinoma the effect of estrogens. *Gynecol Oncol* 1979; 8:60-73.

Vadas P, et al: Pathogenesis of hypotension in septic shock correlation of circulating phospholipase A2 levels with circulatory collapse. *Crit Care Med* 1998; 16:1-7.

Valle RF, Sciarra JJ: Hysteroscopic treatment of the septate uterus. *Obstet Gynecol* 1986; 67:253-257.

Van Bogaert LJ: Clinicopathologic findings in endometrial polyps. *Obstet Gynecol* 1988; 71:771-773.

van Nagell JR Jr, et al: Adjuvant vincristine, dactinomycin and cyclophosphamide therapy in stage I uterine sarcomas: A pilot study. *Cancer* 1977; 57:1451-1457.

Velebil P, Wingo PA, Xia Z, et al: Rate of hospitalization for gynecologic disorders among reproductive-age women in the United States. *Obstet Gynecol* 1995; 86:764-769.

Weber AM, Lee J-C: Use of alternative technique of hysterectomy in Ohio, 1988-1994. *N Engl J Med* 1996; 335:483-489.

Weed JC, Bryan AC: Adenomyosis: Twenty years' experience. *J Med Assoc State Ala* 1963; 2:327-334.

Weiss DB, Alder A, Aboulafla Y: Erythrocytosis due to erythropoietin-producing uterine fibromyoma. *Am J Obstet Gynecol* 1975; 122:358-360.

Weiss NS, Sayvetz TA: Incidence of endometrial cancer in relation to the use of oral contraceptives. *N Engl J Med* 1980; 302:551-554.

Weiss NS, Szekely DR, English DR: Endometrial cancer in relation to patterns of menopausal estrogen use. *JAMA* 1979; 242:261-264.

Welch WR, Scully RE: Precancerous lesions of the endometrium. *Human Pathol* 1977; 8:503-512.

Wentz WB: Progestin therapy in endometrial hyperplasia. *Gynecol Oncol* 1974; 2:362-367.

Wentz WB: Progestin therapy in lesions of the endometrium. *Semin Oncol* 1985; 12:23-27.

Wilcox LS, Koonin LM, Pokras R, et al: Hysterectomy in the United States, 1988-1990. *Obstet Gynecol* 1994; 83:549-555.

Williams AJ, Powell WL, Collins T, Morton CC. HMGI(Y) expression in human uterine leiomyomata: Involvement of another high-mobility group architectural factor in a benign neoplasm. *Am J Pathol* 1997;150: 911-918.

Wilson EA, Yang F, Rees ED: Estradiol and progesterone binding in uterine leiomyomata and in normal uterine tissues. *Obstet Gynecol* 1980, 55:20-24.

Worthen NJ, Gonzalez F: Septate uterus: Monographic diagnosis and obstetric complications. *Obstet Gynecol* 1984; 64:34S-38S.

Yamashita Y, et al: Assessment of myometrial invasion by endometrial carcinoma: Transvaginal sonography vs contrast-enhanced MR imaging. *AJR Am J Roentgenol* 1993; 16:595-599.

Yazigi R, Cohen J, Munoz AK, et al: Magnetic resonance imaging determination of myometrial invasion in endometrial carcinoma. *Gynecol Oncol* 1989; 34:94-97.

Yazigi R, Piver MS, Blumenson L: Malignant peritoneal cytology as prognostic indicator in stage I endometrial cancer. *Obstet Gynecol* 1983; 62:359-362.

Zucker PK, Kasdon EJ, Feldstein ML: The validity of Pap smear parameters as predictors of endometrial pathology in menopausal women. *Cancer* 1985; 56:2256-2263.

CHAPTER

The Fallopian Tube and Ectopic Pregnancy

HELEN H. KIM
JANIS H. FOX

KEY ISSUES

1. The fallopian tube is a highly specialized structure that maintains and modulates a fluid-filled environment for the final maturation of gametes, for fertilization, and for early embryonic development.
2. The emergence, acceptance, and success of in vitro fertilization have dramatically changed the management of tubal disease.
3. Technologic advances have allowed for early diagnosis of unruptured ectopic pregnancy and shifted the prognosis from a grave, life-threatening disease to a more benign condition.
4. With early diagnosis of ectopic pregnancy, the treatment goal has also shifted from preventing mortality to reducing morbidity and preserving fertility.
5. Early diagnosis of unruptured ectopic pregnancy has dramatically expanded the available treatment options. Ectopic pregnancy is one of the few conditions that can be managed surgically, nonsurgically, or expectantly.
6. The ability to counsel patients regarding the most successful therapy for tubal pregnancy with the lowest associated morbidity and to counsel them regarding prospects for future fertility are limited by the lack of data from prospective, randomized studies that compare long- and short-term outcomes of various treatment modalities.

Fallopian tubes (oviducts) are paired muscular canals that are embryologically derived from the cephalic portion of the müllerian ducts (Kim and Laufer, 1994), providing a conduit between the ovary and the uterine cavity. Gabriele Fallopius published the first anatomic description of the oviduct in 1561 (Menezo and Guerin, 1997). The early concept was that the oviduct was merely a passive con-

duit, but now it is clear that the fallopian tube is a highly specialized structure with secretory and active transport functions. During the reproductive years, the tube maintains and modulates a fluid-filled environment in which the final maturation of gametes, fertilization, and early embryonic development occurs (Menezo and Guerin, 1997; Abe, 1996; Chegini, 1996).

ANATOMY, HISTOLOGY, AND PHYSIOLOGY
Anatomy

The normal fallopian tube extends from the uterus to its corresponding ovary and measures between 9 and 11 cm (Wheeler, 1994). Its arterial blood is supplied by tubal branches of the uterine and the ovarian arteries (Leese, 1988). Venous drainage parallels the arterial supply, and lymphatic drainage follows the ovarian vessels. The fallopian tube has sympathetic and parasympathetic innervation (Leese, 1988). Sensory fibers from the fallopian tube end in T9 to L1, and referred pain may be experienced in these dermatomes (Rapkin, 1990). There are four anatomic subdivisions of the tube—the interstitium, the isthmus, the ampulla, and the infundibulum—and they are described here (Fig. 8-1).

The interstitial portion refers to the intramural segment of the fallopian tube, which extends approximately 1 cm. It connects to the endometrial cavity by its ostium, traverses the thickness of the myometrium, and exits at the uterine cornua just superior to the round ligament, where it merges with the isthmic portion (Merchant et al, 1983).

The isthmic portion extends laterally for approximately 2 cm and is characterized by a relatively thick muscular wall (Wheeler, 1994). As it progresses laterally to merge with the ampullary portion, its luminal diameter gradually increases while the thickness of the muscular wall decreases.

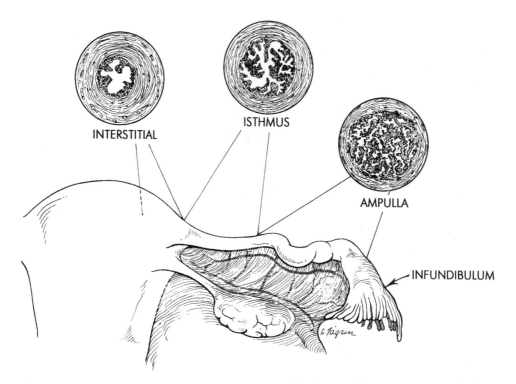

Fig. 8-1. Anatomic divisions of the fallopian tube.

The ampullary portion measures approximately 6 cm and has a luminal diameter of approximately 4 mm (Wheeler, 1994). It has a relatively thin muscular wall and extends anteriorly around the ovary, where it widens gradually to join the infundibulum.

The infundibular portion is the terminal portion of the fallopian tube that opens into the peritoneal cavity, near its corresponding ovary. It has a luminal diameter of approximately 1 cm and extends laterally for approximately 1 cm (Wheeler, 1994). At the ovarian end, the tube terminates in fimbriae, numerous finger-like extensions, that extend to the ovary (Wheeler, 1994).

Histology

The wall of the fallopian tube consists of three histologic layers: an external serous layer, an intermediate smooth muscle layer, and an internal mucosal layer, which are described here.

The external serosal layer is an extension of the broad ligament peritoneum that completely covers the extrauterine portion of the fallopian tube. It is lined by flattened mesothelial cells (Wheeler, 1994). Beneath the serosal layer, there is a thin connective tissue layer of blood vessels and nerves that intermingle with the intermediate muscular layer.

The intermediate smooth muscle layer consists of an outer longitudinal layer, an inner circular layer, and an additional inner longitudinal layer at the uterine end (Wheeler, 1994). The major muscle mass of the tube is formed by the inner circular layer, which ranges in thickness from 0.5 mm in the isthmus to 0.1 mm in the ampulla (Wheeler, 1994).

The internal mucosal layer lies directly on the inner, circular muscle layer. It has a characteristic folded pattern that becomes more complex as the tubal lumen enlarges from the uterine end to the ovarian end (Wheeler, 1994) (Fig. 8-1). It consists of a simple, columnar, epithelial lining that lines the tubal lumen and an underlying lamina propria that contains vessels and stromal cells (Wheeler, 1994). Scattered lymphocytes also may be seen above the basement membrane (Odor, 1974).

The tubal epithelium is composed of two histologic cell types: ciliated and secretory cells (Abe, 1996). Relative numbers of ciliated and secretory cells vary along the length of the tube; ciliated cells are more numerous in the fimbrial end and less common in the proximal portion. In the fimbriated portion, ciliated cells constitute 58.1% to 66.7% of the tubal epithelium, whereas in the isthmic portion, 26.7% to 33.9% of the cells are ciliated (Donnez et al, 1985). The highest percentage of ciliated cells is found around the time of ovulation in all regions of the tube (Donnez et al, 1985).

Surface morphology of the tubal epithelium also varies along the tube during the menstrual cycle (Donnez et al, 1985; Jansen, 1980; Verhage et al, 1979). During the proliferative phase, the ciliated cells are prominent, whereas the secretory cells are relatively inactive. As ovulation approaches, the secretory cells become distended and project beyond the ciliated cells. Shortly after ovulation, secretory activity decreases and cilia regain prominence. With menstruation, the epithelium appears relatively low, presumably because the secretory cells have depleted their cytoplasm. Maximal epithelial height is seen in the isthmus during each phase of the menstrual cycle. Changes in circulating estrogen and progesterone levels are probably responsible for the morphologic alterations during the menstrual cycle (Donnez et al, 1985; Verhage et al, 1979).

Characteristics of the tubal epithelium vary over the reproductive life span. Cilia appear during fetal life, and there is a gradual increase in the number of ciliated cells with advancing gestational age (Patek and Nilsson, 1973). After menopause, the epithelium is flat and the secretory cells appear inactive (Gaddum-Rosse et al, 1975). Cilia are lost as circulating estrogen levels decline, but they are restored with estrogen replacement therapy (Gaddum-Rosse et al, 1975).

Tubal Physiology

The fallopian tube has an essential role in several early events in reproduction. It captures the ovum at ovulation, transports sperm, and provides a suitable environment for fertilization and early embryo development. The developing embryo is transported through the tube and into the uterine cavity.

Many factors facilitate ovum pickup and transport. The fimbria reaches almost every portion of the ovary, and its numerous epithelial folds contain a predominance of ciliated cells (Donnez et al, 1985). At ovulation, the tubal epithelium is richly populated with cilia that beat in synchronized waves in the direction of the uterus (Critoph and Dennis, 1977). Increased tubal muscular activity is thought to aid ovum transport. During the periovulatory period, muscular contractions begin at the ampulla and proceed to the isthmus, whereas slower, more uniform contractions occur during the premenstrual phase (Talo and Pulkkinen, 1982). There appear to be redundant mechanisms for ovum pickup and transport because fertility may occur in the absence of fimbriae (Metz, 1977) and with disorders of ciliary motion (McComb et al, 1986).

It is unclear whether the tube has a role in sperm transport and function. Sperm can be found in the ampulla of the fallopian tube within minutes of insemination (Settlage et al, 1973). Intrinsic sperm motility probably plays the major role, but even inert, nonmotile particles deposited at the cervix can gain entry to the peritoneal cavity (Stone et al, 1985), which suggests that the uterus and the fallopian tubes participate in sperm transport. Evidence from animal studies suggests that the tube not only transports sperm, it may also serve to enhance sperm function (Abe, 1996). Secretions from the tubal isthmus appear to have a role in sperm capacitation, a process that enables the sperm to fertilize (Chang, 1951). Maintenance of sperm viability and motility may also be supported by tubal secretions (Abe, 1996).

The tubal environment also is essential for embryonic development. After ovulation, the ovum is retained within the fallopian tube for approximately 72 hours before it enters the uterine cavity (Croxatto et al, 1978). This delay in transit is necessary to allow time for fertilization and embryo maturation. Transfer of fertilized ova from the fallopian tube to the uterus before 72 hours leads to failure of implantation in rabbits (Chang, 1950). The mechanism by which the tube accomplishes this delay in transit has not been elucidated, but it may be related to the production of tenacious mucus by the isthmic epithelium at the time of ovulation (Jansen, 1980).

Fluid within the tubal lumen provides the necessary environment for the establishment and maintenance of early embryos. Composition and volume of this tubal fluid are under hormonal regulation. Tubal fluid volume increases with estrogen stimulation and decreases with progesterone stimulation (Leese, 1988). Tubal fluid is composed of a selective serum transudate and tubal epithelial secretions (Leese, 1988). The secretory products from the oviductal epithelia show segmental (Abe, 1996) and hormonal variation (Chegini, 1996). These growth factors, cytokines, and functional molecules act in an elaborate autocrine and paracrine fashion to enhance sperm function, modulate tubal muscle contractions, and promote early embryo development (Chegini, 1996).

Although most of the work on tubal physiology has focused on its role in reproduction, there is evidence of a tubal immune system that prevents infection. Immunologically competent cells are present in the fallopian tube and may have a role in providing mucosal immunity (Givan, 1997). It remains to be established whether the fallopian tube has a significant immunologic or antibacterial function.

DISORDERS OF THE FALLOPIAN TUBE
Salpingitis

Salpingitis may be classified into three major types—acute, chronic, and granulomatous (Wheeler, 1994). Acute salpingitis, or pelvic inflammatory disease, refers to infection of the uterus, tubes, and adjacent pelvic structures that usually results from the ascending passage of bacteria from the lower reproductive tract to the tubal lumen (McCormack, 1994).

After the inflammation subsides and the tube heals, chronic salpingitis may ensue and result in anatomic changes, such as tubal scarring or hydrosalpinx (Wheeler, 1994). Hydrosalpinx is characterized by obliteration of the fimbriated end of the tube, which results in obstructive tubal dilation. The endosalpinx becomes severely damaged from long-standing tubal dilation and scarring (Benadiva et al, 1995). The resultant tubal damage and occlusion increase the risk for tubal infertility and ectopic pregnancy (Westrom, 1980).

Mycoplasma tuberculosis is the predominant etiologic agent of granulomatous salpingitis, but a number of infectious and noninfectious processes may produce granulomatous lesions in the tube (Wheeler, 1994). Actinomycosis and granuloma-causing parasites such as pinworm, schistosomiasis, echinococccus, and cystocercosis, reportedly involve the tube. Systemic diseases, such as sarcoidosis and Crohn disease, may result in granulomatous lesions in the tube (Wheeler, 1994). Granulomatous salpingitis may be a sequela of foreign material introduced into the tube during pelvic surgery or during gynecologic procedures, such as hysterosalpingography performed with iodine oil preparations (Soules and Spadoni, 1982).

Salpingitis Isthmica Nodosa

Salpingitis isthmica nodosa is a well-described pathologic lesion of unknown cause. It consists of outpouchings or diverticula of tubal epithelium into the tubal musculature in the isthmic region. Invasion of the tubal epithelium into the isthmic muscularis appears to incite smooth muscle hypertrophy and result in nodularity (Jenkins et al, 1993). Tubal involvement is often bilateral (Benjamin and Beaver, 1951; Creasy et al, 1985). The external appearance is characterized by multiple, irregularly distributed, firm nodular swellings in the isthmus that vary in diameter from a few millimeters to 2.5 cm (Jenkins et al, 1993). Microscopically, salpingitis isthmica nodosa has a variable appearance. There may be simple outpouchings of the tubal mucosa into the tubal musculature, or diverticula may appear as dispersed glands of tubal epithelium surrounded by hyperplastic and hypertrophied muscle fibers (Wheeler, 1994).

Several theories about the pathogenesis of salpingitis isthmica nodosa have been proposed. The condition is thought to be acquired because salpingitis isthmica nodosa is not found at birth (Jenkins et al, 1993). It has been reported only once before adolescence (Shen et al, 1983), and its course is progressive (McComb and Rowe, 1989). Current theories of its etiology include postinflammatory distortion after salpingitis (Honore, 1978) and an adenomyosis-like process in the fallopian tube (Benjamin and Beaver, 1951; Wrork and Broders, 1942).

The most serious clinical sequelae of salpingitis isthmica nodosa are its association with infertility and ectopic pregnancy (Honore, 1978). In a healthy, fertile control group, the incidence of salpingitis isthmica nodosa has been reported to range from 0.6% to 11% (Jenkins et al, 1993). Incidence is reported as high as 50% in infertile women (Honore, 1978) and 57% in women with ectopic pregnancy (Majmudar et al, 1983).

Diagnosis is made most often in women between 25 and 50 years of age, usually during infertility investigation by hysterosalpingography or at the time of gynecologic surgery (Jenkins et al, 1993). On hysterosalpingogram (Fig. 8-2), salpingitis isthmica nodosa is characterized by punctate accumulations of contrast medium in close approximation to the isthmic portion of the oviducts bilaterally (Thomas and Rose, 1973). For infertile patients, the treatment options include tubal surgery, transcervical cannulation, or in vitro fertilization with embryo transfer (IVF-ET). Otherwise, the nodular lesions are innocuous and require no specific therapy.

Tubal Infertility

Tubal damange and dysfunction account for approximately 30% of infertility (Guzick, 1996). They may result from var-

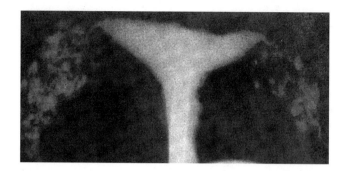

Fig. 8-2. Hysterosalpingogram demonstrating the characteristic lesions of salpingitis isthmica nodosa. (From Jenkins CS, Williams SR, Schmidt GE: Salpingitis isthmica nodosa: A review of the literature, discussion of clinical significance, and consideration of patient management. *Fertil Steril* 1993; 60:599-607.)

ious factors, such as infection, endometriosis, previous intraabdominal surgery, and previous ectopic pregnancy. Tubal obstruction may also result from salpingitis isthmica nodosa or previous tubal ligation.

Previous salpingitis is the cause for most incidences of tubal factor infertility. As many as 75% of infertile women with positive antichlamydial antibodies have tubal factor infertility, whereas only 28% of infertile women without chlamydial antibodies have tubal factor infertility (Jones et al, 1982). The risk for infertility increases with the number of episodes of pelvic inflammatory disease. Infertility develops in 11.4% of women after one episode, in 23.1% of women after two episodes, and in 54.3% of women after three episodes (Westrom, 1980).

Before the widespread availability of assisted reproductive technologies, tubal reconstructive surgery was the only option available for infertile patients with blocked fallopian tubes. Treatment emphasized the use of microsurgical techniques, microsurgical instruments, and surgical adjuvants to minimize postoperative adhesion formation and infection (Penzias and DeCherney, 1996). Historically, microsurgery was performed through laparotomy, but now procedures that previously required laparotomy can be performed on an outpatient basis with lower cost and faster recovery. Advances in reproductive surgery have made operative laparoscopy and transcervical tubal cannulation viable options for patients requiring tubal reconstructive surgery.

Tubal disease is classified by the anatomic location of the obstruction. Based on the site of obstruction, specific surgical procedures are used to restore tubal anatomy. Adnexal adhesions are treated with ovariolysis (lysis of adhesions around the ovary) and salpingolysis (lysis of peritubal adhesions). Proximal tubal disease has been treated with segmental resection and tubocornual anastomosis. Proximal obstruction has been successfully relieved by transcervical tubal cannulation with fluoroscopic, hysteroscopic, and ultrasonographic guidance (Flood and Grow, 1993). Midsegment tubal reconstruction (tubal reanastomosis) is usually performed for the reversal of elective tubal sterilization. Distal tubal disease may be treated with fimbrioplasty, which may include dilation of fimbrial phimosis and lysis of fimbrial adhesions. If a hydrosalpinx is present, neosalpingostomy (reopening and reconstruction of the terminal end of the tube) is required to relieve the obstruction.

The success of surgical treatments is difficult to assess accurately. Many studies report only tubal patency, but tubal patency does not predict the pregnancy potential of the tube. Pregnancy rates vary with the length of follow-up and the severity of tubal disease, as measured by the condition of the endosalpinx, the extent of pelvic adhesions, and the degree of fimbrial destruction (Benadiva et al, 1995). In 1988, the American Fertility Society published a staging system for adnexal adhesions, distal tubal occlusion, and tubal occlusion secondary to tubal ligation (Figs. 8-3, 8-4) with the hope of standardizing reports to allow for comparison of different studies (American Fertility Society, 1988). Staging systems also emphasize prognostic factors for successful tubal reconstruction, and they may facilitate the formation of prognosis for a particular patient.

Pregnancy rates, after surgical treatment of tubo-ovarian adhesions, are comparable with either laparotomy using microsurgical techniques or operative laparoscopy. Intrauterine pregnancy rates after salpingo-ovariolysis by either method range from 50% to 62% (Lavy et al, 1987). After salpingo-ovariolysis by laparotomy, the ectopic pregnancy rate is 1.8% (Lavy et al, 1987), and after operative laparoscopy, it is 5.4% to 8.3% (Fayez, 1983; Gomel, 1983). Fimbrioplasty, performed by microsurgical laparotomy, is associated with an intrauterine pregnancy rate of 59% and an ectopic pregnancy rate of 6% (Lavy et al, 1987). Laparoscopic fimbrioplasty is associated with an intrauterine pregnancy rate of 35% to 50% and an ectopic pregnancy rate of 0% to 14% (Fayez, 1983; Gomel, 1983).

Tubal reanastomosis for proximal tubal obstructions and reversal of tubal ligations is typically performed by laparotomy using microsurgical techniques, but successful laparoscopic tubal ligation reversals are reported. For proximal tubal obstructions, the reported intrauterine pregnancy rates after tubocornual anastomosis range from 37.5% to 57% (Lavy et al, 1986; Meldrum, 1981). The associated rate of ectopic pregnancy ranges from 0% to 25% (Gomel, 1977; Lavy et al, 1986). In preliminary studies, similar pregnancy rates of 30% to 57% are observed after transcervical tubal cannulation (Hepp et al, 1996).

Successful tubal ligation reversal depends on type of previous ligation procedure, tubal lengths after repair, and location of anastomosis (American Fertility Society, 1988; Benadiva et al, 1995). After tubal reanastomosis by laparotomy, intrauterine pregnancy rates are reported to be 62% to 63%, and ectopic pregnancy rates are reported to be 3.7% to 5% (Henderson, 1984; Lavy et al, 1987). The success of laparoscopic tubal ligation reversal is highly dependent on the surgeon's experience with the procedure. One group reports an intrauterine pregnancy rate of 75.5% and an ectopic pregnancy rate of 2% after a follow-up period of 12 months (Yoon et al, 1997).

Compared with other procedures for tubal reconstruction, surgical treatment for distal tubal disease is associated with lower pregnancy rates and higher rates of ectopic pregnancy (Benadiva et al, 1995; Penzias and DeCherney, 1996). Successful tubal reconstruction depends on the extent of tubal damage (Fig. 8-4). Poor prognosis after the repair of distal tubal disease is associated with numerous dense peritubal adhesions, ampullary distention with large hydrosalpinx diameter, poor condition of endosalpinx, thick edematous tubal wall, and absent fimbria (Nackley and Muasher, 1998). For patients with these poor prognostic factors, the intrauterine pregnancy rate is 3%; for patients without them, however, the intrauterine pregnancy rate is as high as 77% (Boer-Meisel et al, 1986). In patients who have severe distal tubal disease, the ectopic pregnancy rate is as high as 16.6% after surgical repair (Mage et al, 1986).

Counseling patients with tubal factor infertility has become complex since IVF-ET has become widely available and increasingly more successful. The rates of ectopic pregnancy are comparable after IVF-ET or tubal surgery. In 1995, the clinical pregnancy rate after one cycle of IVF-ET was 24.4% as reported in the annual report of the Society for Assisted Reproductive Technology (SART, 1997). This would predict a cumulative pregnancy rate of 56.8% after three cycles of IVF-ET. After tubal reconstructive surgery, the probability of achieving a pregnancy within one menstrual cycle is approximately 2% to 4%, which would predict a cumulative pregnancy rate of only 8.7% after 3 months but 52% after 24 months (Penzias and DeCherney, 1996). If successful, surgery provides the opportunity for multiple attempts at conception and the possibility of achieving more than one pregnancy. Furthermore, tubal reconstruction does not carry the complications of assisted reproductive techniques, such as ovarian hyperstimulation syndrome and multiple gestation (Schenker and Ezra, 1994).

Increasingly, IVF-ET has become the preferred option for many patients with tubal infertility. Compared with tubal surgery, IVF-ET offers a better chance of pregnancy per cycle for most women with tubal disease. Because fertility declines with age, IVF-ET is a better option than tubal reconstruction for older women. With continued advances in assisted reproductive technology, it is probable that tubal reconstructive surgery will have only a limited role in the treatment of infertility (Benadiva et al, 1995; Penzias and DeCherney, 1996). Pregnancy rates after IVF-ET have continued to increase each year as techniques improve. In addition, with the emergence of day 5 blastocyst transfer, a technique that allows for the selection of one to two high-quality embryos for transfer, the risk for high-order multiple gestations is almost eliminated without decreasing the pregnancy rate. Thus, the fear of high-order multiple gestations after IVF-ET may soon be a thing of the past.

Tubal and Paratubal Neoplasms

Tumors of the fallopian tube, whether benign or malignant, are uncommon. If they develop, they may be located in the

THE AMERICAN FERTILITY SOCIETY CLASSIFICATION OF ADNEXAL ADHESIONS

Patient's name_____ Date _____ Chart #_____

Age _____ G _____ P _____ Sp Ab _____ VTP _____ Ectopic _____ Infertile Yes _____ No _____

Other significant history (i.e. surgery, infection, etc.) _____

_____

HSG _____ Sonography _____ Photography _____ Laparoscopy _____ Laparotomy _____

	ADHESIONS		<1/3 Enclosure	1/3 - 2/3 Enclosure	>2/3 Enclosure
OVARY	R	Filmy	1	2	4
		Dense	4	8	16
	L	Filmy	1	2	4
		Dense	4	8	16
TUBE	R	Filmy	1	2	4
		Dense	4*	8*	16
	L	Filmy	1	2	4
		Dense	4*	8*	16

*If the fimbriated end of the fallopian tube is completely enclosed, change the point assignment to 16.

Prognostic classification for adnexal adhesions

	LEFT		RIGHT
A. Minimal	_____	0-5	_____
B. Mild	_____	6-10	_____
C. Moderate	_____	11-20	_____
D. Severe	_____	21-32	_____

Treatment (surgical procedures):_____

_____

_____

_____

Prognosis for conception & subsequent viable infant**

_____ Excellent (> 75%)

_____ Good   (50%-75%)

_____ Fair   (25%-50%)

_____ Poor   (< 25%)

**Physician's judgment based upon adnexa with least amount of pathology.

Recommended followup treatment:_____

_____

_____

Additional findings: _____

_____

_____

_____

_____

_____

_____

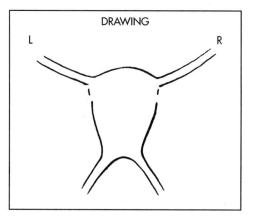

For additional supply write to:
The American Fertility Society
2140 11th Avenue, South
Suite 200
Birmingham, Alabama 35205

Property of
The American Fertility Society

Fig. 8-3. The American Fertility Society classification of adnexal adhesions. (From American Fertility Society: The American Fertility Society classification of adnexal adhesions, distal tubal occlusion, tubal occlusion secondary to tubal ligation, tubal pregnancies, müllerian anomalies and intrauterine adhesions. *Fertil Steril* 1988; 49:944-955.)

THE AMERICAN FERTILITY SOCIETY CLASSIFICATION OF DISTAL TUBAL OCCLUSION

Patient's name_____ Date _____ Chart #_____
Age _____ G _____ P _____ Sp Ab _____ VTP _____ Ectopic _____ Infertile Yes _____ No _____
Other significant history (i.e. surgery, infection, etc.) _____
_____

HSG _____ Sonography _____ Photography _____ Laparoscopy _____ Laparotomy _____

Distal ampullary diameter		<3 cm	3-5 cm	>5 cm
	L	1	4	6
	R	1	4	6
Tubal wall thickness		Normal/thin	Moderately thickened or edematous	Thick & rigid
	L	1	4	6
	R	1	4	6
Mucosal folds at neostomy site		Normal/ >75% preserved	35% to 75% Preserved	<35% Preserved adherent mucosal fold
	L	1	4	6
	R	1	4	6
Extent of adhesions		None/minimal/mild	Moderate	Extensive
	L	1	3	6
	R	1	3	6
Type of adhesions		None/filmy	Moderately dense (or vascular)	Dense
	L	1	2	4
	R	1	2	4

Prognostic classification for terminal
salpingostomy (salpingoneostomy)
              LEFT   RIGHT
A. Mild   _____   1-3   _____
B. Moderate _____   9-10 _____
C. Severe   _____   >10   _____
Treatment (surgical procedures):
     Salpingostomy   L   R
     A. Terminal   _____   _____
     B. Ampullary   _____   _____

Other: _____
_____
_____
_____

Prognosis for conception & subsequent viable infant*
_____ Excellent (> 75%)
_____ Good   (50%-75%)
_____ Fair   (25%-50%)
_____ Poor   (< 25%)
*Physician's judgment based upon adnexa with least amount of pathology.
Recommended followup treatment:_____
_____
_____

Additional findings: _____
_____
_____
_____
_____

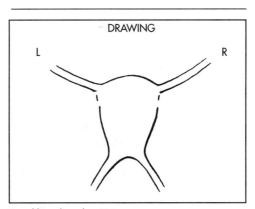

For additional supply write to:
The American Fertility Society
2140 11th Avenue, South
Suite 200
Birmingham, Alabama 35205

Property of
The American Fertility Society

Fig. 8-4. The American Fertility Society classification of distal tubal occlusion. (From American Fertility Society: The American Fertility Society classification of adnexal adhesions, distal tubal occlusion, tubal occlusion secondary to tubal ligation, tubal pregnancies, müllerian anomalies and intrauterine adhesions. *Fertil Steril* 1988; 49:944-955).

wall or within the lumen, or they may be pedunculated. Hydatids of Morgagni, paratubal cysts derived from müllerian structures, are commonly seen dangling from the tube and should not be considered abnormal (Wheeler, 1994).

Benign tumors are usually small and asymptomatic and are usually discovered incidentally at surgery that has been performed for another indication. Many benign neoplasms are reported to originate in the fallopian tube, among them inclusion cysts and Walthard rests, papilloma, leiomyoma, adenomyoma, and adenomatoid tumor (mesothelioma, lymphangioma). Hemangiomas, lipomas, angiomyolipomas, adenofibromas, neural tumors, and tubal teratomas are reported more rarely (Wheeler, 1994). At surgery, tumors of the fallopian tube are often mistaken for lesions of chronic salpingitis, pyosalpinx (Wheeler, 1994), and other benign abnormal conditions.

Primary malignant neoplasms of the fallopian tube are extremely uncommon and are rarely confirmed before surgery. Primary carcinoma of the fallopian tube is the rarest carcinoma of the female genital tract, and sarcomas are even less common (Podczaski and Herbst, 1993). Typically, tubal carcinomas and sarcomas develop after menopause. Patients usually have only subtle, nonspecific symptoms, and the classic triad of vaginal discharge (clear, serosanguineous, or bloody), pelvic pain, and pelvic mass, is not often seen (Podczaski and Herbst, 1993). Metastatic tumors account for 85% of fallopian tube malignancies (Podczaski and Herbst, 1993). Metastatic lesions usually are secondary to lymphatic spread from carcinoma of the ovary or the endometrium, but hematogenous spread of metastasis from extrapelvic tumors is also possible (Wheeler, 1994).

ECTOPIC PREGNANCY
Definition and Clinical Significance

Ectopic pregnancy is a potentially life-threatening condition in which the embryo implants outside the uterine endometrial cavity. Ectopic pregnancies have been described in all segments of the fallopian tube, uterine cornua (which includes the interstitial portion of the tube), cervix, ovary, and abdominal cavity (Fig. 8-5). In 96.5% of patients, the extrauterine implantation occurs in the fallopian tube, usually in the ampullary region where fertilization occurs (Breen, 1970).

The latter half of this century has brought dramatic advances in the diagnosis and treatment of this potentially fatal condition. As recently as the period between 1947 and 1967, only 8.45% of ectopic pregnancies were diagnosed before rupture (Breen, 1970). Sensitive blood pregnancy tests and transvaginal ultrasonography have enabled the earlier diagnosis of ectopic pregnancy. With this earlier diagnosis, the prognosis for ectopic pregnancy has shifted from a grave, life-threatening disease to a more benign condition. The treatment goal has also shifted from preventing mortality to reducing morbidity and preserving fertility. Technologic advances, such as improved transvaginal sonography,

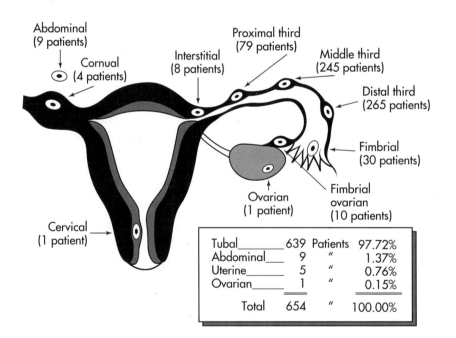

Fig. 8-5. Anatomic site of ectopic pregnancy: 96.5% (631/654) of extrauterine gestations are implanted in the extrauterine portion of the tube, and 3.5% of ectopic pregnancies are implanted outside the tube in the abdomen (1.37%), cervix (0.15%), ovary (0.15%), and cornu (1.83%). Today cornual and interstitial ectopic pregnancies are synonymous and refer to gestations that are implanted in the interstitial portion of the tube. (From Breen JL: A 21 year survey of 654 ectopic pregnancies. *Am J Obstet Gynecol* 1970; 106:1004-1019.)

laparoscopic equipment, and methotrexate chemotherapy, have also expanded the available treatment options for unruptured ectopic pregnancies.

Despite improved diagnostic capabilities, ectopic pregnancy remains a major health problem. In the United States, the number of patients admitted to the hospital for ectopic pregnancy suggests nearly a fourfold increase in incidence between 1970 and 1989. In 1992, ectopic pregnancies represented approximately 2% of pregnancies and accounted for 9% of all pregnancy-related deaths in the United States. Ectopic pregnancy is the leading cause of pregnancy-related death during the first trimester (Center for Disease Control, 1995). *To reduce maternal mortality and morbidity, early recognition of ectopic pregnancy is critical.*

Clinical Findings

A high index of suspicion is vital for the early diagnosis of ectopic pregnancy because the signs and symptoms of ectopic pregnancy overlap with many surgical and gynecologic conditions. Ectopic pregnancy must be considered in all sexually active women of reproductive age who have abdominal pain or abnormal vaginal bleeding. Contraceptive use does not rule out ectopic pregnancy because pregnancies that occur after contraceptive failures are very likely to be ectopic. After tubal sterilization failures, 32.9% of pregnancies are found to be extrauterine (Peterson, 1997). Failure of progestin-only oral contraception is associated with a 9.9% ectopic pregnancy rate, and as many as 16.3% of conceptions that result with a progestin intrauterine device (IUD) in place are ectopic gestations (Tatum and Schmidt, 1977).

History

Before rupture, women may remain asymptomatic. The classic triad of amenorrhea, irregular vaginal bleeding, and abdominal pain described in 1970 (Breen, 1970) is now absent in more than 50% of patients with proven ectopic pregnancies (Stovall et al, 1990). A history of amenorrhea or abnormal vaginal bleeding may not be readily revealed. An extremely detailed menstrual history is imperative because patients often mistake any vaginal bleeding for menses. Only careful questioning discerns that the recent bleeding episode was diminished in amount, occurred at an unusual time, or was otherwise uncharacteristic of menses. There is no characteristic pain associated with ectopic pregnancy. The nature and location of abdominal pain depends on the location, size, and bleeding status of the ectopic pregnancy.

History taking should also determine whether ectopic risk factors are present (Box 8-1). Theoretically, any structural or hormonal aberration that impairs the migration or implantation of the embryo increases the risk for ectopic pregnancy. A large case-control study identified four strong, independent risk factors for ectopic pregnancy: current IUD use, previous tubal surgery, history of pelvic inflammatory disease, and history of infertility (Marchbanks et al, 1988). Numerous studies consistently demonstrate an association between these four variables and ectopic pregnancy. A re-

cent meta-analysis finds that previous ectopic pregnancy, documented tubal disease, and in utero diethylstilbestrol exposure are also strongly associated with the occurrence of ectopic pregnancy (Ankum et al, 1996). Other commonly cited risks include a history of sexually transmitted disease, use of tobacco products, use of fertility drugs, and use of progestin-only contraceptives (Chow et al, 1987).

Although numerous risk factors are implicated in the development of ectopic pregnancy, it is important to remember that less than 50% of patients with proven ectopic pregnancy have an identifiable "ectopic risk factor" (Stovall et al, 1990). Therefore, even in the absence of risk factors, a high index of suspicion for ectopic pregnancy must be maintained in any sexually active women with a history of irregular vaginal bleeding or abdominal pain.

Physical Examination

Because there are no pathognomonic findings, the absence of physical findings does not exclude ectopic pregnancy. Before rupture, the physical findings are nonspecific. Pulse and blood pressure reflect the degree of blood loss and will be normal in unruptured ectopic pregnancies or in slowly leaking, ruptured ectopic pregnancies. If rupture and significant intraperitoneal bleeding have occurred, the patient may have orthostatic hypotension or may be in hypovolemic shock. The patient will also have peritoneal signs of guarding, diffuse abdominal tenderness, and rebound tenderness. On the other hand, the abdominal examination may be benign for

---

BOX 8-1
ECTOPIC RISK FACTORS*

Historical Factors

Pelvic inflammatory disease or previous sexually
   transmitted disease
Previous ectopic pregnancy
Previous tubal surgery
Known tubal disease
Infertility
In utero diethylstilbestrol exposure

Drug Exposures During Conception

Intrauterine device (especially in one containing progestin)
Progestin-only oral contraceptive pills
Ovulation induction drugs
Tobacco

Modified from Ankum WM, Mol BWJ, Van der Veen F, Bossuyt PMM: Risk factors for ectopic pregnancy: A meta-analysis. *Fertil Steril* 1996; 65:1093-1099; Chow WH, Daling JR, Cates W Jr, Greenberg RS: Epidemiology of ectopic pregnancy. *Epidemiol Rev* 1987; 9:70-94; Marchbanks PA, Annegers JF, Coulam CB, et al: Risk factors for ectopic pregnancy: A population based study. *JAMA* 1988; 259:1822-27.

*Theoretically, any hormonal or structural aberration that impairs embryo transport or implantation increases the risk for ectopic pregnancy. Numerous risk factors have been implicated.

patients with unruptured ectopic pregnancy or a locally confined process.

Pelvic examination findings are highly variable and are dependent on the duration of the pregnancy, degree of tubal distention, and presence, amount, and rate of intraperitoneal bleeding. A bulging cul-de-sac of Douglas may be seen with extensive intraperitoneal bleeding. The cervix and uterus may be of normal size and consistency, or they may have the appearance of early pregnancy. An adnexal mass may be present. In early, unruptured tubal pregnancy, however, the tubal enlargement may be too slight to be detected by bimanual examination. Adnexal masses are detected by examination in only 4% of unruptured ectopic pregnancies (Stovall et al, 1990). Patients with ruptured ectopic pregnancies have cervical motion tenderness and adnexal tenderness, whereas these symptoms are absent in 75% of patients with unruptured ectopic pregnancies (Stovall et al, 1990).

Diagnostic Testing
Human Chorionic Gonadotropin

Because the diagnosis of ectopic pregnancy is difficult to make by history and physical examination alone, it is essential to maintain a high index of suspicion. The initial step is to screen for the presence of pregnancy (even among patients using contraception). Human chorionic gonadotropin (hCG) is made by placental syncytiotrophoblast. It is composed of an α-subunit that is virtually identical to the α-subunits of other pituitary glycoprotein hormones and a β-subunit that is specific for hCG. In 1972, a sensitive and specific radioimmunoassay for hCG was developed; it allowed for a reliable diagnosis of early pregnancy (Vaitukaitis et al, 1972).

A test for urinary hCG levels can be performed in minutes and detects all but the earliest pregnancies. The urine pregnancy test detects hCG levels above 20 to 50 mIU/mL and is usually positive by the time menses are due. Radioimmunoassay can detect hCG in the maternal serum as early as 8 days after the luteinizing hormone surge, and it quantifies the hormone level (Wilcox et al, 1988). Depending on the laboratory, at least 1 hour is needed before a result is obtained.

Once the patient is determined to be pregnant, the absolute hCG level and its rate of rise over the next several days become important for the diagnosis of ectopic pregnancy. In normal pregnancies, the hCG level rises exponentially and peaks at 8 to 10 weeks' gestation (Braunstein et al, 1978). Although hCG levels are roughly correlated with gestational age, a single hCG value cannot distinguish between normal and abnormal pregnancies because there is a great range in normal hCG values for a given gestational age. Additionally, the dating of the pregnancy is often uncertain. Serial hCG measurements, however, can be useful for distinguishing between normal and abnormal gestations during the first trimester of pregnancy (Braunstein et al, 1978). Before 6 weeks' gestation, the mean doubling time for hCG is 1.98 days so that a minimum rise of 66% would be expected over 48 hours in normal pregnancies (Kadar et al, 1981a). Abnormal intrauterine and ectopic pregnancies produce less hCG, so the rate of rise of hCG will be slower (Kadar et al, 1981a).

This diagnostic method has several limitations. Most important, the rate of hCG rise only identifies abnormal gestations; it does not differentiate between abnormal intrauterine and ectopic pregnancies. As there are with all diagnostic tests, there is a false-positive and a false-negative rate (Kadar et al, 1981a). If a 66% rise in hCG is considered normal, 15% of normal pregnancies have an abnormally rising titer (false positive), whereas 13% of ectopic pregnancies have a normally rising hCG (false negative). Additionally, there is interassay variability even within a single laboratory, so caution should be used when interpreting rate of rise at low levels of hCG. Furthermore, hCG values cannot be compared between different laboratories because various assay methods are used.

The most significant drawback is that at least 2 days must elapse before the rate of hCG rise can be determined. Clearly, this is not an appropriate method to use in a symptomatic or an unstable patient. In the relatively asymptomatic patient with a low hCG titer, the risk for tubal rupture is low, but it is not zero. One third of women with a ruptured ectopic pregnancy had a serum hCG level below 100 mIU/mL (Hirata et al, 1991). All patients should be given careful instructions (ectopic precautions) to call if they experience any symptoms of concern while they await the results of their second hCG titers. Follow-up before 48 hours is warranted for increased abdominal-pelvic pain, heavy vaginal bleeding, or signs of hypovolemia such as lightheadedness.

Transvaginal Ultrasonography

Transvaginal ultrasonography has become an important modality for the diagnosis of ectopic pregnancy. Because of its higher resolution and closer proximity to the reproductive organs, it is superior to transabdominal ultrasonography in visualizing the uterus, the adnexa, and the cul-de-sac of Douglas. Transvaginal ultrasonography can detect normal pregnancies as early as 35 days from the last menstrual period, whereas the earliest transabdominal ultrasonography can detect pregnancy is at 42 days' gestation (Fossum et al, 1988). If an intrauterine pregnancy is found, it essentially excludes the diagnosis of ectopic pregnancy except in the rare patient with heterotopic pregnancy (the coexistence of intrauterine and extrauterine pregnancies).

In the absence of an intrauterine pregnancy, examination of the adnexa may be helpful in the diagnosis of ectopic pregnancy. Identification of an extrauterine gestational sac with the yolk sac or embryo is 100% specific for ectopic pregnancy, but sensitivity is low (37%) because finding an extrauterine pregnancy by ultrasonography is rare. In a woman whose pregnancy test was positive, any complex adnexal mass with an empty uterus is suspicious for an ectopic pregnancy; the sensitivity is 84.4%, and the specificity is

98.9% (positive and negative predictive values of 96.3% and 94.8%, respectively) (Brown and Doubilet, 1994).

Correlation with serum hCG levels is needed for the interpretation of ultrasound findings. *The minimal hCG level at which all viable intrauterine pregnancies should be seen is called the discriminatory zone.* The discriminatory zone was first described for transabdominal ultrasonography in 1981. All viable intrauterine pregnancies with hCG levels greater than 6500 mIU/mL were seen in this manner, whereas those with hCG levels below 6000 mIU/mL were not seen (Kadar et al, 1981b). The transvaginal probe detects the gestational sac at a lower hCG level of 1000 to 2000 mIU/mL. If an intrauterine pregnancy is not observed when the serum hCG level exceeds the discriminatory zone, it is diagnostic of ectopic pregnancy in 86% of patients (Romero et al, 1985b). The discriminatory zone is dependent on the type of hCG assay, the resolution of the ultrasonography imaging system, and the expertise of the sonographer. Each institution, therefore, must determine its own hCG discriminatory zone.

There are special situations in which correlation of ultrasonography findings with the discriminatory zone may lead to an incorrect diagnosis. Absence of an intrauterine gestational sac when the hCG concentration exceeds the discriminatory zone is not pathognomonic for ectopic pregnancy. Patients with multiple gestations have higher levels of hCG relative to identifying a gestational sac. In one study, sacs were always seen in singleton pregnancies with hCG levels greater than 1161 mIU/mL. However, in triplet pregnancies, the discriminatory hCG level was 3372 mIU/mL (Keith et al, 1993). The presence of fibroids, an IUD, and extreme retroversion may also obscure the sonographer's ability to visualize a sac even when the hCG titer is above the discriminatory zone. Finally, the presence of an intrauterine pregnancy does not exclude ectopic pregnancy in the rare case of heterotopic pregnancy. Because fertility treatment with ovulation in-duction medications increases the risk for multiple gesta-tion and heterotopic pregnancy (Tal et al, 1996), ultrasonography findings must be interpreted more cautiously in these patients.

Serum Progesterone

Serum progesterone levels are lower in nonviable pregnancies than in viable pregnancies. As pregnancy fails, progesterone levels decrease. Otherwise, progesterone levels remain fairly constant during the first 8 to 10 weeks of gestation (Buster and Carson, 1995). A single progesterone measurement may suggest the nonviability of a pregnancy without precise knowledge of gestational age, even when the serum hCG is below the discriminatory zone (Stovall et al, 1992). A progesterone concentration greater than or equal to 25 ng/mL is associated with a viable, intrauterine pregnancy in 97.5% of patients (Stovall et al, 1989). A progesterone level of 5 ng/mL or less indicates a nonviable pregnancy (either intrauterine or ectopic) in more than 99% of patients (McCord, 1996). *No viable pregnancy is seen when the pro-gesterone level is less than 2.5 ng/mL* (McCord et al, 1996). When the serum progesterone level is less than 2.5 ng/mL, uterine curettage may be performed to distinguish between nonviable intrauterine and extrauterine pregnancies; it is not necessary to wait 48 hours for a repeat hCG.

There are several problems with the use of a single progesterone measurement as a screening tool to differentiate between normal and abnormal pregnancies. There is no clear cutoff for progesterone levels between normal and abnormal pregnancies (McCord et al, 1996). In the 5- to 20-ng/mL range, there is a large overlap in progesterone levels between normal and abnormal pregnancies. Additionally, progesterone measurements may not be useful after ovulation induction cycles when multiple corpora lutea may be present or when supplemental progesterone is often used. Finally, not all laboratories are equipped to report serum progesterone levels in a timely fashion.

Uterine Curettage

When an nonviable pregnancy is identified by inappropriately rising hCG titers or by a progesterone level less than 2.5 ng/mL, uterine curettage can be used to distinguish between a failed abnormal intrauterine pregnancy and an ectopic pregnancy (Stovall et al, 1992). Histologic identification of chorionic villi or implantation site confirms the presence of intrauterine pregnancy and essentially eliminates the diagnosis of ectopic pregnancy, except in the rare patient with heterotopic pregnancy. A finding of only decidua or the Arias-Stella endometrial reaction (Arias-Stella, 1954) in the pathology specimen is suggestive of ectopic pregnancy.

A decline in hCG level can be diagnostic even before results from the pathology department are available. If the decline is 15% or more 12 to 24 hours after curettage, it suggests the evacuation of an intrauterine pregnancy (Stovall et al, 1992). A plateau or continued rise in hCG after curettage suggests the continued presence of pregnancy tissue and is suggestive of an ectopic pregnancy.

Because uterine curettage is an invasive procedure, it should be reserved for patients in whom noninvasive methods are insufficient for diagnosis. Uterine curettage may be particularly helpful with plateauing or abnormally rising hCG levels that persistently remain below the ultrasonography discriminatory zone. Additionally, before proceeding with uterine curettage, the nonviability of a pregnancy should be firmly established (evidenced by a progesterone level of less than 2.5 ng/mL and abnormally rising hCG levels).

Culdocentesis

Historically, culdocentesis was widely used as a rapid, inexpensive tool to aid in the diagnosis of ectopic pregnancy. It was performed at the time of pelvic examination by introducing an 18- to 20-gauge spinal needle attached to a syringe into the posterior cul-de-sac of Douglas and aspirating the contents of the peritoneal cavity.

A positive test result (nonclotting blood) in conjunction with a positive pregnancy test is associated with ectopic pregnancy in more than 99% of patients, but it is not necessarily predictive of rupture (Romero et al, 1985a). Of the ectopic pregnancies with positive culdocentesis, 62% are unruptured (Romero et al, 1985b). Negative test results (serous fluid) or nondiagnostic tests (clotting blood or no fluid) do not exclude the possibility of ectopic pregnancy. In one series, culdocentesis is nondiagnostic in 16% of ectopic pregnancies (Romero et al, 1985a). In another series, 76% of patients with negative or nondiagnostic culdocentesis are found to have ectopic pregnancies at surgery (Vermesh et al, 1990). Now that other noninvasive diagnostic modalities are available, culdocentesis is almost never indicated in the modern approach to diagnosing ectopic pregnancy.

Management

Modern management of ectopic pregnancy offers the physician and patient many options, if the diagnosis is made early. Technologic advances in diagnosis and treatment of ectopic pregnancy have dramatically expanded the range of available therapeutic options. Ectopic pregnancy is one of the few diseases in the whole of medical science that can be treated by either medical or surgical means. It can even be managed expectantly. The goal is to reduce disease and treatment-related morbidity while preserving the greatest potential for the patient's reproductive function (if she so desires). Therapeutic options for the management of ectopic pregnancy are summarized in Figure 8-6.

Surgical Management

History of Surgical Treatment. Before the twentieth century, ectopic pregnancy was nearly a universally fatal condition. When it was suspected, nonsurgical methods such as starvation, purging, bleeding, and administration of poisons were used in an attempt to end the extrauterine pregnancy. Despite these efforts, the fatality rate for ectopic

pregnancy was 72% to 99% at the end of nineteenth century (Lurie, 1992). In 1884, Robert Lawson Tait reported successful treatment of ectopic pregnancy with salpingectomy and demonstrated that timely surgical intervention could be lifesaving. In the mid-twentieth century, when the diagnosis of ectopic pregnancy before rupture was nearly impossible, the treatment for ectopic pregnancy was exclusively surgical and required removal of the ruptured tube to control hemorrhage. Mortality rates dropped as surgical techniques improved, and by 1947, mortality rates were 1.7% to 2.7% (Lurie, 1992).

In the latter part of the twentieth century, the ability to diagnose ectopic pregnancy before rupture shifted the goal of therapy from reducing mortality to preserving fertility. The first pregnancy to result after conservative, tube-sparing surgery for ectopic pregnancy was described in 1953 (Stromme, 1953). Several conservative operations now have been described for the treatment of unruptured tubal pregnancy: salpingotomy, salpingostomy, segmental resection, and fimbrial evacuation. The optimal surgical procedure is dictated by the location of the ectopic gestation.

Most studies focus on the treatment of ampullary tubal pregnancy because approximately 90% of ectopic gestations occur there (Breen, 1970). Because of the large lumen and the distensibility of the thin muscularis layer in the ampulla, trophoblastic spread is often predominantly intraluminal and the muscularis usually remains intact (Pauerstein et al, 1986). Given that there is little tubal destruction, tubal patency may be preserved after removal of the ectopic gestation. Ampullary ectopic pregnancy can be treated with either linear salpingotomy (tubal incision with reapproximation of tubal edges) or linear salpingostomy (tubal incision without closure of the incision site). Tubal suturing does not appear to affect subsequent fertility or adhesion formation (Tulandi and Guralnick, 1991).

Conversely, the isthmus is characterized by a narrow lumen and is surrounded by a thick muscularis. Ectopic preg-

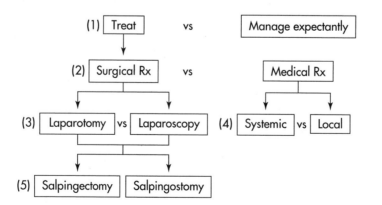

Fig. 8-6. Algorithm for the modern management of ectopic pregnancy. If diagnosed early, ectopic pregnancies may be treated or managed expectantly. Treatment may be surgical or nonsurgical. Surgery may be performed through laparotomy or laparoscopy, and both salpingectomy and salpingostomy can be performed by either modality. Medical treatment may be systemic or may involve the local administration of drugs into the ectopic gestational sac.

nancies may invade and destroy the surrounding muscula-ture (Budowick et al, 1980; Pauerstein et al, 1986), and some propose that isthmic gestations are treated optimally with segmental resection of the fallopian tube (DeCherney and Boyers, 1985). Segmental resection of the fallopian tube also may be necessary to treat large ampullary ectopic preg-nancies. Fimbrial evacuation of a distal ampullary preg-nancy has been found by some to be safe and effective (Sherman et al, 1987), whereas others have found the proce-dure to be associated with the incomplete removal of tro-phoblastic tissue (Bell et al, 1987).

Initially, ectopic pregnancies were treated by lapa-rotomy, but today laparoscopic procedures are standard. Laparoscopy, an endoscopic procedure that enables the di-rect visualization of the intraperitoneal structures, was first suggested as an aid in the diagnosis of ectopic pregnancy in 1937 (Hope, 1937). Since the 1970s, numerous technical improvements in laparoscopic equipment, along with im-provements in the ability to diagnose ectopic pregnancy, have shifted the role of laparoscopy from a diagnostic to a therapeutic procedure. The removal of an ectopic gestational sac solely through the laparoscope was first reported in 1973 (Shapiro and Adler, 1973). Laparoscopic linear salpin-gostomy with removal of the gestational tissue was first re-ported in 1980 (Bruhat et al, 1980). It is now the standard laparoscopic procedure because most ectopic pregnancies occur in the tubal ampulla.

Laparotomy versus Laparoscopy. Laparotomy is usu-ally reserved for patients with severe hemodynamic instabil-ity. Because salpingectomy and salpingostomy can be per-formed by laparoscopy or laparotomy, there are few indications for performing laparotomy in a stable patient. Laparotomy may be considered when the patient is a poor candidate for laparoscopic surgery because she is obese or she has an extensive surgical history and known dense ad-hesions. Laparotomy also may be indicated if the ectopic gestation is large or if it is implanted outside the tube. Cer-tainly, laparotomy should be performed if the surgeon is not trained in surgical laparoscopy or if the necessary laparo-scopic equipment is not available.

Laparoscopic salpingectomy and salpingostomy have largely replaced laparotomy and become the surgical stan-dard of care. Numerous studies demonstrate that laparo-scopic surgery is as effective as laparotomy for the treatment of ectopic pregnancy for patients who are hemodynamically stable. A comparison of results from 18 studies of salpin-gostomy by laparotomy with those from 12 studies of lap-aroscopic salpingostomy finds similar rates of subsequent intrauterine and ectopic pregnancy. Linear salpingostomy, performed by either technique, is associated with an in-trauterine pregnancy rate of 61% and a recurrent ectopic pregnancy rate of 15% (Yao and Tulandi, 1997). Prospective randomized trials comparing salpingostomy by laparotomy and laparoscopy also found similar reproductive outcomes (Lundorff et al, 1992; Murphy et al, 1992; Vermesh et al, 1989; Vermesh and Presser, 1992). Although both modali-ties are similarly effective, the laparoscopic approach is more economical, results in less morbidity, and is, therefore, thought to be superior. Women treated with laparoscopy have less intraoperative blood loss, reduced analgesia re-quirements, shorter hospital stays, and shorter periods of postoperative convalescence (Lundorff et al, 1991; Murphy et al, 1992; Vermesh et al, 1989).

Salpingectomy versus Salpingostomy. The patient's desire for future fertility plays a large role in the decision for conservative (salpingostomy) or radical (salpingectomy) surgery. Salpingectomy may be preferable for patients who have no desire for future pregnancies. In fact, bilateral salpingectomy may be considered for the patient who has had an ectopic pregnancy after a failed tubal ligation. For the patient who desires future pregnancy, on the other hand, it has generally been thought that salpingectomy re-sults in a significant reduction in fertility without a parallel decrease in the rate of recurrent ectopic pregnancy. This assumption, however, has recently been questioned and will be discussed later.

Conservative surgical management of ectopic pregnancy is usually attempted to preserve a fallopian tube that may be functional in the future. It is clear that tubal function can be preserved after the removal of an ectopic gestation. There are numerous reports of intrauterine pregnancies that occur after conservative tubal surgery in women who have only one tube (Yao and Tulandi, 1997). It is unclear, however, whether tubal preservation improves the reproductive out-come for women who have both tubes. A large retrospective study of 1025 patients suggests that most postoperative pregnancies occur through the contralateral tube (Korell et al, 1997). When both tubes are present, there is no difference in intrauterine and ectopic pregnancy rates after conserva-tive (35.6% and 8.2%, respectively) or radical (39.6% and 7.5%, respectively) surgery. On the other hand, when the contralateral tube is absent or blocked, the intrauterine preg-nancy rate is lower (17.6%) and the ectopic pregnancy rate is higher (16.0%).

Because there are no randomized controlled studies comparing reproductive outcomes after conservative and radical surgery, only data from retrospective comparisons are available for analysis. Combining the results of nine ret-rospective studies published between 1960 and 1993 re-vealed an overall intrauterine pregnancy rate of 49.3% after salpingectomy and 53% after conservative treatment. Re-peat ectopic pregnancy rates were 9.9% after salpingectomy and 14.8% after conservative treatment (Yao and Tulandi, 1997). Although these results cannot be compared directly given that patient selection criteria and follow-up periods are different in each study, they suggest that conservative treatment may offer a higher rate of intrauterine pregnancy but may also be associated with a higher rate of ectopic pregnancy. Conversely, recent retrospective (dela Cruz and Cumming, 1997) and cohort (Job-Spira et al, 1996) studies found no relationship between the surgical approach and rates of ectopic and intrauterine pregnancy.

Fertility after ectopic pregnancy may be more dependent on patient characteristics than on surgical approach. One cohort study finds higher subsequent fertility associated with young age, high educational level, and no previous tubal damage, but it finds no relationship between type of surgery and subsequent reproductive outcome (Job-Spira et al, 1996). A retrospective study identifies several factors that appear to influence future fertility after conservative surgery (Pouly et al, 1991). The presence of ipsilateral periadnexal adhesions and an abnormal contralateral tube and a history of infertility, salpingitis, previous ectopic pregnancy, or solitary tube are associated with a significantly lower rate of subsequent pregnancy and an increased rate of recurrent ectopic pregnancy.

Reproductive potential appears even more compromised after consecutive ectopic pregnancies (Pouly et al, 1991; Vermesh and Presser, 1992). In Pouly's series, treatment of a first ectopic gestation is associated with a 24% infertility rate, 54% intrauterine pregnancy rate, and 12% recurrent ectopic pregnancy rate. Treatment of a second ectopic pregnancy is associated with a 33% infertility rate, 21% intrauterine pregnancy rate, and 46% recurrent ectopic pregnancy rate. After three ectopic pregnancies, 82% of women are infertile, and the subsequent ectopic and intrauterine pregnancy rates are both 9% (Pouly et al, 1991). Similarly, Vermesh and Presser find a 20% intrauterine pregnancy rate and a 40% recurrent ectopic pregnancy rate after two consecutive ectopic pregnancies (Vermesh and Presser, 1992).

Now that IVF-ET is widely available and increasingly successful, salpingectomy may be the preferred surgical approach even for patients who desire future pregnancy. Attempts to preserve severely damaged tubes may increase a patient's chance for recurrent ectopic pregnancy (even as the result of an IVF-ET procedure) without improving her chance for successful pregnancy. Bilateral salpingectomy and referral for IVF-ET may be the best treatment option for patients with severely damaged tubes, history of tubal disease, infertility, or previous ectopic pregnancy. Because half of recurrent ectopic pregnancies occur in the contralateral tube (Hallatt, 1986), underlying tubal disease appears to play an important role in recurrent ectopic pregnancy. If the patient conceives through IVF but implants ectopically, bilateral salpingectomy may be warranted to prevent repeated ectopic pregnancies. Bilateral salpingectomy should also be considered if hydrosalpinges are encountered. The presence of hydrosalpinx makes successful tubal reconstruction unlikely and appears to have a negative impact on IVF-ET (Nackley and Muasher, 1998).

It is unlikely that a randomized controlled study comparing reproductive outcomes after conservative and radical surgery will be performed because such a trial would require nearly 1000 patients in each arm (dela Cruz and Cumming, 1997). At present, the choice of conservative versus radical surgery for ectopic pregnancy depends on many factors, including the patient's desire for future fertility, her medical history, and intraoperative findings. Certainly, salpingectomy should be performed if there is tubal rupture with uncontrollable bleeding. Until more definitive studies are performed, it seems prudent (provided the patient desires future fertility) to preserve the fallopian tube under most circumstances because it may be functional in the future. Salpingectomy should be reserved for the patient in whom the tube is severely damaged, for the patient committed to IVF-ET, or for the patient who does not desire future fertility.

Persistent Ectopic Pregnancy. The persistence of viable trophoblastic tissue is a particular risk inherent in conservative surgical treatment of ectopic pregnancy. If there is incomplete removal, the remaining trophoblastic tissue may continue to proliferate and lead to complications such as tubal rupture and intraabdominal hemorrhage. This clinical condition, referred to as persistent ectopic pregnancy, was first reported after a salpingotomy in 1979 (Kelly et al, 1979) and has increased in frequency with the shift in surgical treatment from salpingectomy to conservative procedures (Seifer, 1997). The frequency of persistent ectopic pregnancy after salpingostomy ranges from 3% to 29% (Yao and Tulandi, 1997).

Increased use of laparoscopy may slightly increase the incidence of persistent ectopic pregnancy. A compilation of data from 10 studies found persistent ectopic pregnancy in 8.3% of patients after laparoscopic salpingostomy and in 3.9% of patients after salpingostomy by laparotomy (Yao and Tulandi, 1997). Two randomized, prospective studies also reveal a trend toward slightly higher rates of persistent ectopic pregnancy in the laparoscopy group (12.7% to 17.6%) than in the laparotomy group (0% to 3.5%) (Lundorff et al, 1991; Murphy et al, 1992), but this was not statistically significant. On the other hand, one randomized, prospective study found the same rate of persistent ectopic pregnancy (3.3%) after linear salpingostomy by laparoscopy and laparotomy (Vermesh et al, 1989).

Risk factors that predispose a woman to persistent ectopic pregnancy have not been clearly identified. The risk for persistent ectopic pregnancy after conservative surgical treatment may be higher when the gestational age is less than 42 days and the diameter of the unruptured pregnancy is smaller than 2 cm (Seifer et al, 1990). The persistent trophoblast is usually found medial to the salpingostomy site (Stock, 1991). Fimbrial expression of trophoblastic tissue has been reported to be associated with a higher risk for persistent ectopic pregnancy (Bell et al, 1987). Persistent trophoblastic implants, however, have been reported not only in the fallopian tube but also on peritoneal surfaces (Cartwright, 1991; Reich et al, 1989; Thatcher et al, 1989). Presumably, viable trophoblast spilled during surgery may implant in the peritoneum.

Because of the risk for persistent ectopic pregnancy after conservative surgery, hCG titers should be observed until levels are undetectable, which takes approximately 18 days (Lundorff et al, 1991). Although weekly postoperative hCG titers have traditionally been recommended, the optimal follow-up interval has not been firmly established. A recent study found that the hCG level on the first postoperative day was predictive of persistent ectopic pregnancy (Spandorfer et al, 1997). A greater percentage of persistent ectopic pregnancies were seen when the decrease in hCG titer on the first postoperative day was less than 50% from the initial preoperative hCG level. In these patients, repeat hCG before 1 week may detect the early presence of persistent trophoblastic tissue and avoid possible tubal damage or rupture. As long as hCG levels continue to fall after surgery and the patient remains asymptomatic, expectant management with serial monitoring of hCG levels is sufficient. Intervention is certainly indicated if hCG levels plateau or increase or if symptoms develop that suggest persistent ectopic pregnancy or impending rupture. It is worth noting that ruptured ectopic pregnancies have been observed even when serum concentrations of hCG decline (Gertz and Quagliarello, 1987; Tulandi et al, 1991).

Treatment options for persistent ectopic pregnancy include salpingectomy, partial salpingectomy, and medical therapy with systemic methotrexate. One study uses a variety of modalities for the treatment of persistent ectopic pregnancy, and the intrauterine pregnancy rate is 59%, which is comparable with that observed after conservative surgical treatment (Seifer et al, 1994). Prophylactic medical treatment at the time of surgery has been proposed to decrease the risk for persistent trophoblastic tissue. One study demonstrates that a single dose of systemic methotrexate (1 mg/kg intramuscularly) within the first 24 hours after salpingostomy significantly reduces the rate of persistent ectopic pregnancy from 14.5% in the control group to 1.9% (Graczykowski and Mishell, 1997). Additional studies are needed to determine whether adjuvant medical therapy is necessary in all patients or whether it increases the effectiveness of conservative surgical management.

Nonsurgical Management

The medical treatment of ectopic pregnancy offers several advantages. Medical treatment is less invasive, eliminates the risks of surgery and anesthesia, reduces costs, and shortens recovery time. Furthermore, the use of medical therapy potentially eliminates the need for surgery in the treatment of ectopic pregnancy. Because ectopic pregnancy is now most often diagnosed before rupture, the disorder has become amenable to medical therapy. Nonsurgical management of ectopic pregnancy has become a popular option.

Methotrexate: Systemic Administration. Although various medical options have been investigated for the treatment of ectopic pregnancy, methotrexate has become the primary drug used for this purpose. Methotrexate is a folic acid analogue that interferes with the synthesis of DNA and the multiplication of cells by inhibiting the action of dihydrofolate reductase, an enzyme that converts dihydrofolate to tetrahydrofolate (American Medical Association, 1995). Methotrexate is effective in stopping trophoblastic prolifer-

ation (Berkowitz et al, 1986) and was first reported to be effective in the treatment of gestational trophoblastic disease in 1956 (Li et al, 1956). Extensive experience with methotrexate in gestational trophoblastic disease has diminished concern about the use of methotrexate in women of reproductive age. Methotrexate does not increase the risk for spontaneous abortion, subsequent neoplasia, or congenital anomalies (Ross, 1976; Berkowitz et al, 1998).

Methotrexate, however, has several dose-related side effects, some of which can be fatal. At high dosages, stomatitis and diarrhea are common and may result in hemorrhagic enteritis and intestinal perforation. Other dose-related effects of methotrexate include myelosuppression (leukopenia, thrombocytopenia, anemia), nephrotoxicity, hepatic dysfunction (which may be permanent), alopecia, dermatitis, pneumonitis, and acute hypersensitivity (American Medical Association, 1995). Even with the relatively lower dosages of methotrexate used for the treatment of ectopic pregnancy, 20% of patients treated with early protocols experienced side effects such as stomatitis, diarrhea, dermatitis, gastritis, pleuritis, reversible hepatic dysfunction, and transient bone marrow suppression (Pansky et al, 1991). Side effects are less common with the current protocols, which use even lower doses of methotrexate.

For the treatment of ectopic pregnancy, methotrexate has been administered systemically (intravenously, intramuscularly, orally) and by local injection into the ectopic gestation under ultrasonographic or laparoscopic guidance. In these protocols, folinic acid (leucovorin calcium or citrovorum factor) is often added. Folinic acid, a metabolically active form of tetrahydrofolate, is functionally identical to folic acid except that it does not require the action of dihydrofolate reductase (American Medical Association, 1995). The addition of folinic acid "rescues" normal cells and reduces the untoward effects of methotrexate.

The first successful use of methotrexate for ectopic pregnancy was reported in 1968 when systemic methotrexate (12.5 mg/day for 5 days) was used for the treatment of an abdominal pregnancy (Lathrop and Bowles, 1968). In 1982, normal tubal patency was reported after treatment of an interstitial gestation with systemic intramuscular methotrexate (210 mg over 15 days) (Tanaka, 1982). The first series of patients with ectopic pregnancy treated with systemic methotrexate was reported in the English literature in 1986 (Ory et al, 1986). This protocol uses a regimen similar to that used for the treatment of nonmetastatic gestational trophoblastic disease at that time: methotrexate (1 mg/kg/day for 4 days) and folinic acid (0.1 mg/kg/day for 4 days). These and other early protocols required inpatient hospital stays and multiple doses of methotrexate.

In time, outpatient methotrexate protocols were developed. Methotrexate (1 mg/kg/day) was administered along with folinic acid (0.1 mg/kg/day) for one to four doses, depending on patient's response to treatment. With these individualized regimens, only 20% of patients required four doses, and no major side effects to chemotherapy were observed. Only 5% of patients experienced minor side effects, such as transient elevation of liver enzymes and stomatitis (Stovall et al, 1991a).

Successful use of a single intramuscular dose of methotrexate (50 mg/m² body surface area) *without* folinic acid rescue was first reported in 1991 (Stovall et al, 1991b). This is now the most widely accepted methotrexate regimen for the treatment of unruptured or presumed ectopic pregnancy (Table 8-1). It has been evaluated in prospective studies (Glock et al, 1994; Gross et al, 1995; Stovall and Ling,

1993). Although Stovall and Gross find no significant side effects, Glock reports mild side effects (nausea, diarrhea, oral irritation, mild elevation in liver enzymes) in 34% of patients. Combining these studies, 92% (159 of 172) of the patients were treated successfully and did not need surgical intervention. To achieve resolution of the ectopic pregnancy as measured by an undetectable hCG level, a second dose of methotrexate was required in 3% to 6% of patients.

There is no consensus regarding proper patient selection criteria for single-dose intramuscular methotrexate (Table 8-2). It is generally agreed that absolute contraindications to methotrexate therapy include active liver or renal disease and tubal rupture. Abdominal pain and fetal cardiac activity are relative contraindications. The methotrexate failure rate is 14.3% when fetal cardiac activity is present and only 4.7% when it is absent (Stovall and Ling, 1993). Although it is recognized that higher failure rates are observed with higher serum hCG levels and larger ectopic gestations, there are no universally accepted absolute exclusion criteria for methotrexate treatment. By imposing strict criteria, the success rate may improve, but fewer patients would be eligible for treatment. For example, using relatively strict criteria, only 44.8% of patients with ectopic pregnancies in Stovall's series (Stovall and Ling, 1993) and 42.7% of patients with ectopic pregnancies in Glock's series (Glock et al, 1994) were considered eligible for treatment with methotrexate. With the increased use of single-dose methotrexate, more liberal inclusion criteria are used (Buster and Carson, 1995).

The clinical course after single-dose methotrexate treatment has been well described. Transient abdominal pain 6 to 7 days after therapy is common and can be difficult to distinguish from that of a rupturing ectopic gestation. The pain has been reported in 33.3% (Glock, 1994) to 59.2% (Stovall and Ling, 1993) of patients and is presumably caused by tubal abortion. Many physicians with limited experience

---

Table 8-1   Intramuscular Methotrexate (50 mg/m²) Protocol

Day	Laboratory Test, Therapy, or Both
0	hCG, CBC with differential and platelet count, AST, creatinine, blood type, Rh Uterine curettage if hCG < discriminatory zone
1	hCG, administer intramuscular methotrexate (50 mg/m²) (Administer rhogam, if indicated)
4	hCG
7	hCG a) If hCG titer is decreased <15% from day 4, administer second intramuscular methotrexate (50 mg/m²). b) If hCG titer is decreased >15% from day 4, check hCG weekly until undetectable. Administer additional methotrexate (50 mg/m²) if titer plateaus.

Modifed from Stovall TG, Ling FW: Single dose methotrexate: An expanded clinical trial. *Am J Obstet Gynecol* 1993; 168:1759-1765.

hCG, human chorionic gonadotropin; CBC, complete blood count; AST, aspartate aminotransferase.

Table 8-2   Exclusion Criteria for Intramuscular Methotrexate (50 mg/m²)*

	Stovall, 1993	Glock, 1994
Patient history	Future fertility not desired	Noncompliance
Physical examination	Hemodynamically unstable	Hemodynamically unstable
		Pelvic pain
hCG	Declining hCG titers	Declining hCG titers
Ultrasound (transvaginal)	Ectopic size >3.5 cm	Ectopic size >3.5 cm
		Fetal cardiac activity present
		Free fluid in cul-de-sac
Other laboratory values	AST >2 times normal	AST >50 IU/L
	Creatinine >1.5 mg/dL	Creatinine >1.3 mg/dL
	WBC <3000	WBC <3000
	Platelet count <100,000	Platelet count <100,000

Modified from Glock JL, Johnson JV, Brumsted JR: Efficacy and safety of single-dose systemic methotrexate in the treatment of ectopic pregnancy. *Fertil Steril* 1994; 62:716-721; Stovall TG, Ling FW: Single dose methotrexate: An expanded clinical trial. *Am J Obstet Gynecol* 1993; 168:1759-1765.

hCG, human chorionic gonadotropin; AST, aspartate aminotransferase; WBC, white blood cell.

*Imposing relatively conservative exclusion criteria would improve the success rate but limit the number of patients eligible for treatment. In Stovall's series, 44.8% of patients are eligible for treatment. In Glock's series, 42.7% of patients are eligible for treatment.

using methotrexate consider admitting patients to the hospital for observation and serial hematocrits until they are comfortable distinguishing the typical pain after methotrexate treatment from the pain of an impending rupture. Surgical intervention is not absolutely necessary unless the patient also has orthostatic tachycardia, hypotension, or a falling hematocrit value (Buster and Carson, 1995).

After the administration of systemic methotrexate, it is necessary to observe serial hCG levels to confirm successful treatment. Before treatment, it is essential to counsel patients that a prolonged follow-up period may be necessary (Box 8-2). The mean time to undetectable hCG levels ranges from 23.1 days (Glock et al, 1994) to 35.5 days (Stovall and Ling, 1993). After treatment, patients should be informed that an initial increase in serum hCG levels is common. A transient initial increase in serum hCG level was observed in 86% of patients between days 1 and 4 of treatment (Stovall and Ling, 1993).

Patients receiving methotrexate therapy should be given precautions about its side effects and about the natural history of ectopic pregnancy after treatment. Because methotrexate works as a folic acid antagonist, patients should not consume vitamins containing folic acid (Stovall and Ling, 1993). Abstinence from alcohol is recommended because alcohol can adversely affect liver function. To minimize the risk for tubal rupture, intercourse and bimanual pelvic examinations should be avoided until the pregnancy is resolved (Stovall and Ling, 1993). Because photosensitivity can be a complication, patients should avoid exposure to the sun and to sunlamps (Buster and Carson, 1995). Colicky abdominal pain is common during the first 2 or 3 days of therapy, and patients should be warned to avoid gas-producing

foods such as leeks and cabbage (Buster and Carson, 1995). Finally, it is important to inform patients about the expected pain that occurs 6 to 7 days after methotrexate treatment, but the possibility of tubal rupture should also be emphasized. Even with declining hCG levels, tubal rupture is described as late as 23 days after treatment with a methotrexate-folinic acid protocol (Stovall et al, 1991a).

To date, there has been no randomized trial directly comparing single-dose (50 mg/m^2) intramuscular methotrexate to laparoscopic salpingostomy. Based on existing reports, the reproductive outcomes after single-dose methotrexate and laparoscopic salpingostomy are comparable (Keefe et al, 1998). In Stovall's series, 69.4% of patients who wanted to conceive had intrauterine pregnancies, and 12.8% had recurrent ectopic pregnancies (Stovall and Ling, 1993). In Glock's smaller series of infertile patients, the intrauterine pregnancy rate was lower (20%), but no ectopic pregnancies resulted (Glock et al, 1994). The only randomized trial of methotrexate versus laparoscopic salpingostomy compares an older methotrexate protocol (1.0 mg/kg methotrexate alternating with citrovorum for 4 days) and finds no difference in tubal patency, but reproductive outcome has not yet been evaluated (Hajenius et al, 1997).

Now that laparoscopy is rarely used to diagnose ectopic pregnancy, single-dose intramuscular methotrexate has become an attractive treatment option. It appears to be safe and successful, and its long-term outcomes for reproduction are comparable to those of surgical treatment. Additionally, systemic methotrexate offers the potential for significant cost savings. Several studies have found methotrexate to be a more cost-effective alternative because it eliminates the need for surgery, anesthesia, laparoscopy equipment, and hospitalization (Alexander et al, 1996; Creinin and Washington, 1993; Yao et al, 1996).

Methotrexate: Local Injection. Technical improvements in laparoscopy, hysteroscopy, and transvaginal ultrasonography permit the direct injection of methotrexate into the ectopic gestational sac. Compared with systemic administration, direct administration can deliver much higher drug concentrations to the implantation site at dramatically reduced therapeutic dosages. With lower dosages, there should be less systemic distribution of the drug and, therefore, less toxicity (Buster and Carson, 1995). Local administration of methotrexate requires less surgical expertise than salpingostomy. The disadvantage of this approach is that the need for surgery and anesthesia may not be eliminated. Additionally, the question remains whether local methotrexate injection would be directly toxic to the fallopian tubes (Klinkert et al, 1993).

Successful treatment of ectopic pregnancy using methotrexate injection into the ectopic gestational sac was first reported using ultrasound guidance in 1987 (Feichtinger and Ketemer, 1987), laparoscopy in 1989 (Pansky et al, 1989), transcervical cannulation in 1990 (Risquez et al, 1990), and hysteroscopy in 1992 (Goldenberg et al, 1990). Many groups have since used both laparoscopic and transvaginal

---

BOX 8-2
PATIENT INSTRUCTIONS DURING TREATMENT WITH SINGLE-DOSE INTRAMUSCULAR METHOTREXATE (50 mg/m^2)

Until the Resolution of Pregnancy

Do not use multivitamins that contain folic acid.
Do not use alcohol.
Do not have intercourse.
Avoid pelvic examinations.
Avoid sun exposure.
Avoid gas-producing foods (leeks, cabbage).
Report any increases in abdominal and pelvic pain.

After Treatment Is Completed

Use contraception (barrier method or oral contraceptive pills) for at least 2 months.

Modified from Buster JE, Carson SA: Ectopic pregancy: New advances in diagnosis and treatment. *Curr Opin Obstet Gynecol* 1995; 7:168-176; Stovall TG, Ling FW: Single dose methotrexate: An expanded clinical trial. *Am J Obstet Gynecol* 1993; 168:1759-1765.

methotrexate administration for the reatment of early, unruptured tubal pregnancy. A compilation of data from four studies of ultrasound-guided intratubal methotrexate find an overall success rate of 81%, a subsequent intrauterine pregnancy rate of 48%, and a recurrent ectopic pregnancy rate of 6% (Yao and Tulandi, 1997). Six studies of laparoscopic methotrexate injection find an overall success rate of 79%, a subsequent intrauterine pregnancy rate of 58%, and a recurrent ectopic pregnancy rate of 10% (Yao and Tulandi, 1997).

Several groups have prospectively compared laparoscopic salpingostomy with laparoscopic intratubal methotrexate injection in a randomized fashion. One study reported similar success and tubal patency rates after salpingostomy (88% and 67%) and intratubal methotrexate injection (90% and 78%). Interestingly, patients in whom intratubal methotrexate failed required salpingectomy, whereas patients in whom salpingostomy failed were successfully treated with systemic methotrexate (O'Shea et al, 1994). Another trial comparing laparoscopic salpingostomy and intratubal methotrexate injection was terminated prematurely because of poor results in the intratubal methotrexate group (Mottla et al, 1992).

One prospective, *non*randomized study assigned patients to either laparoscopic salpingostomy or laparoscopic intratubal methotrexate based on a defined protocol (in which the presumed *poor* prognosis patients were assigned to salpingostomy), and found salpingostomy to be *more* successful. Laparoscopic salpingostomy is successful for 92.7% of patients who had a poor prognosis, whereas intratubal methotrexate is successful in 61.4% of patients with a better prognosis (Shalev et al, 1995). Although not statistically significant, subsequent salpingectomy was performed in 5.5% of patients after laparoscopic salpingostomy and in 13.6% of patients after intratubal methotrexate.

One prospective, randomized study compares ultrasound-guided intratubal injection and intramuscular systemic administration of methotrexate (Fernandez et al, 1995). The routes of administration are equivalent in terms of success of treatment (95%) and tubal patency (88%), but the follow-up period is too short to assess reproductive outcome.

Despite the theoretical advantages of local treatment, it seems to be less successful than systemic treatment with methotrexate or laparoscopic salpingostomy. The main advantage of medical treatment is its noninvasiveness. Hence, there appears to be little benefit in administering methotrexate laparoscopically because it entails exposing the patient to the risks of anesthesia and surgery. Although ultrasound-guided methotrexate administration does not require surgery, it is still more invasive and more operator dependent than intramuscular administration. Given the negligible rate of side effects, the apparent higher success rate, the noninvasive nature of single-dose intramuscular methotrexate therapy, and the fact that we cannot quantify the potential for tubal damage with intratubal injections, there is

no strong argument to favor local methotrexate injection over intramuscular systemic methotrexate.

Other Nonsurgical Therapies. Although systemic intramuscular methotrexate has become the most widely used nonsurgical treatment for unruptured ectopic pregnancy, numerous nonsurgical therapies have been used successfully and are worthy of mention. Systemic treatment with actinomycin D, a ribonucleic acid polymerase inhibitor, is successful for interstitial pregnancy (Altaras et al, 1988). Ultrasound-guided potassium chloride injections induce cardiac arrest and resorption of the ectopic fetus (Robertson et al, 1987; Timor-Tritsch et al, 1989). Because potassium chloride does not affect the trophoblast, trophoblastic tissue may continue to proliferate, and tubal rupture may occur (Pansky et al, 1991). Hyperosmolar glucose, injected laparoscopically, effectively treats ectopic pregnancy without side effects and appears to maintain tubal patency (Yeko et al, 1995). Prostaglandin $F_{2\alpha}$ causes tubal muscular contractions and local vasoconstriction and has been administered intratubally for the treatment of ectopic pregnancy. Although earlier studies report severe side effects, such as cardiac arrhythmia and cardiopulmonary edema (Egarter and Husslein, 1988), new protocols look promising (Lindblom et al, 1990; Paulsson et al, 1995). There are minimal data about subsequent tubal function and reproductive performance with these therapies, and none are in widespread use in the United States.

Expectant Management

It is well known that ectopic pregnancy can resolve spontaneously. The ability to diagnose ectopic pregnancy at an early stage has allowed for more treatment options but has also led to unnecessary treatment of ectopic pregnancies that would have resolved without any therapy. The first successful use of expectant management of ectopic pregnancy in hemodynamically stable patients was reported in 1955 (Lund, 1955). In this study, 57% of women randomized to expectant management had resolution of pregnancy without surgery. The subsequent rates of intrauterine pregnancy (46%) and recurrent ectopic pregnancy (15%) in the patients treated expectantly were similar to the rates found in the surgically treated group. When expectant management failed, however, the patients had had significant symptoms and often required emergency surgery for hemoperitoneum or rupture.

There are now many reports of successful expectant management of ectopic pregnancy in carefully selected patients. To minimize morbidity while awaiting resolution of the ectopic gestation, patients are monitored closely with serial hCG measurements and transvaginal ultrasound examinations. A review of 10 prospective studies found that 69.2% of hemodynamically stable patients with declining hCG levels were managed successfully without surgical or medical intervention (Yao and Tulandi, 1997). The time for the hCG level to become undetectable appears comparable to that for systemic methotrexate; it ranges from 21 days (Korhonen et al, 1994) to 31 days (Trio et al, 1995).

Nevertheless, data regarding reproductive potential after expectant management are limited. A compilation of data from six small case series found a subsequent tubal patency rate of 85% and a pregnancy rate of 52% in expectantly managed patients (Pansky et al, 1991). Another study found no difference in tubal patency or fertility between women who were successfully treated expectantly and those in whom expectant management failed (Shalev et al, 1995). A recent small study of 30 women successfully treated with expectant management found a 93% tubal patency rate, an 83.3% intrauterine pregnancy rate, and a 4.2% ectopic pregnancy rate (Rantala and Makinen, 1997).

A few investigators have attempted to identify prognostic factors that reliably predict success of expectant management. A lower initial hCG titer is clearly associated with a greater chance for success (Korhonen et al, 1994). If the initial hCG titer is less than 1000 mIU/mL, there is an 88% success rate for expectant management (Trio et al, 1995). Spontaneous resolution of the ectopic pregnancy is also associated with a rapidly decreasing hCG level, but it is not possible to define reliable criteria based on the rate of hCG decrease. Several patients with decreasing hCG levels ultimately require surgical intervention (Korhonen et al, 1994). Absence of a visible gestational sac on initial ultrasonography is also a predictor of success (Trio et al, 1995). A decrease in the size of the ectopic gestation on day 7 had a sensitivity of 84% and a specificity of 100% in predicting spontaneous resolution (Cacciatore et al, 1995). In general, the presence of abdominal pain, embryonic cardiac activity, adnexal mass larger than 4 cm, or intraperitoneal fluid are accepted as contraindications to expectant management.

Given the success rates of other treatment modalities, expectant management has a limited role in the treatment of ectopic pregnancy. The challenge in the modern management of ectopic pregnancy is to differentiate accurately those patients with abnormal pregnancies that will resolve spontaneously from patients with ectopic gestations that require therapeutic intervention. Increased use of expectant management could lower costs by reducing the need for surgery and for chemotherapy agents. With the identification of specific criteria that reliably predict spontaneous resolution of ectopic pregnancy, expectant management may become a safe alternative for carefully selected patients.

Special Situations

Extratubal Ectopic Gestation. Approximately 3.5% of ectopic pregnancies occur outside the fallopian tube (Fig. 8-5), as follows: uterine cornua (1.83%), ovarian (0.15%), cervical (0.15%), and abdominal (1.37%) (Breen, 1970). Although rare, these extratubal ectopic pregnancies represent some of the most serious complications of pregnancy. They are often diagnosed later in gestation than tubal pregnancies because these sites can accommodate an ex-

panding pregnancy better than the tube. Extratubal sites are also extremely well vascularized so that profuse hemorrhage may occur either as a result of rupture or of trophoblastic invasion into the vasculature.

Traditionally, the management of extratubal pregnancies has been surgical. Cornual (interstitial) pregnancies are gestations that implant in the interstitial portion of the tube. These pregnancies are treated with hysterectomy if bleeding is profuse or by cornual resection if damage to the cornua is minimal. Hysteroscopic removal of an unruptured interstitial gestation is also reported (Meyer and Mitchell, 1988). Hysterectomy used to be the only reliable modality to control the bleeding of cervical pregnancies. Now there are more conservative surgical options, such as cervical hysterotomy, internal iliac artery ligation, uterine artery ligation, and dilatation and evacuation, with adjuvant measures to achieve hemostasis (Foley catheter tamponade, uterine artery embolization, cerclage) (Ushakov et al, 1996). Although there are reports of ovarian and abdominal pregnancies that have produced living children, the prognosis for advanced pregnancies in these locations is thought to be poor (Strafford and Ragan, 1977; Rengachary et al, 1977). In the past, these pregnancies were managed by surgical removal with the preservation of intraabdominal organs or ovarian tissue.

As with tubal ectopic pregnancies, extratubal ectopic pregnancies have been treated successfully without surgery. In fact, the first attempts to treat ectopic pregnancies with methotrexate were in extratubal ectopic pregnancies. Systemic methotrexate was successfully administered in the 1960s to avoid complicated surgery in an abdominal ectopic pregnancy (Lathrop and Bowles, 1963) and in an interstitial pregnancy in the 1980s (Tanaka et al, 1982). The first attempt to treat cervical pregnancy with methotrexate failed (Farabow et al, 1983), but systemic methotrexate treatment of cervical pregnancy was later shown to be effective (Oyer et al, 1988). Ovarian pregnancy is also treated successfully with systemic methotrexate (Shamma and Schwartz, 1992; Chelmow et al, 1994) and local injection of prostaglandins (Koike et al, 1990). Local injection with potassium chloride has been used successfully to treat interstitial (Robertson et al, 1987; Oelsner et al, 1993) and cervical (Frates et al, 1994) pregnancies.

Experience with nonsurgical management of these unusual ectopic gestations is still limited, so it is difficult to make general recommendations. Treatment must be individualized based on the location and the size of the ectopic gestational sac.

Heterotopic Gestations. The incidence of heterotopic pregnancy (coexisting intrauterine and ectopic pregnancies) is dependent on the rate of ectopic pregnancy and the rate of multiple gestation. Fifty years ago, the incidence of spontaneous heterotopic pregnancy was estimated to occur in 1 in 30,000 pregnancies using an incidence of 0.37% for ectopic pregnancy and a dizygotic twin rate of 0.8% (DeVoe and

Pratt, 1948). The incidence of heterotopic pregnancy has dramatically increased with the use of ovulation induction and assisted reproductive technologies. These fertility treatments increase the risk for multiple gestation and ectopic pregnancy (Schenker and Ezra, 1994). After ovulation induction with menotropins or IVF-ET, both the observed and the calculated rates of heterotopic pregnancy are 1% (Tal et al, 1996).

Early diagnosis of heterotopic pregnancy is difficult. Serial hCG measurements and correlation with ultrasonography are not helpful in the diagnosis of heterotopic pregnancy. Normally rising hCG titers are often present because abnormal hormone production by the ectopic gestation is masked by the production of hCG from the normal intrauterine pregnancy. In heterotopic pregnancy, the detection of intrauterine pregnancy by ultrasonography may falsely rule out a coexisting ectopic pregnancy. Furthermore, 11% of the heterotopic pregnancies that occur after ovulation induction or assisted reproduction are located outside the tube, where they can grow to a larger size before symptoms develop (Tal et al, 1996; Rojansky and Schenker, 1996). Despite a high index of suspicion by the clinician and careful monitoring after fertility treatment, only 15.8% of heterotopic pregnancies are diagnosed prior to the development of symptoms (Tal et al, 1996). Symptoms and signs do not differ significantly between heterotopic pregnancies and sole ectopic pregnancies (Rojansky and Schenker, 1996).

Early diagnosis and treatment of heterotopic pregnancy increase the chance for survival of the intrauterine pregnancy (Tal et al, 1996). The goal of treatment for heterotopic pregnancies is to terminate the ectopic pregnancy while allowing the intrauterine pregnancy to continue. After treatment, approximately two thirds of the intrauterine pregnancies survive (Tal et al, 1996). Surgical management has been the most commonly used approach for removing the coexisting ectopic pregnancy. In a recent review, 92% of patients underwent surgical treatment (Tal et al, 1996). Nonsurgical management of heterotopic pregnancy with potassium chloride injection has been described, but experience is limited (Tal et al, 1996). For the treatment of cervical and cornual heterotopic pregnancies, conservative treatment with potassium chloride may be less traumatic to the intrauterine pregnancy than definitive surgical treatment because uterine manipulation is avoided. Systemic therapy

with methotrexate is contraindicated unless the intrauterine pregnancy is not viable.

CONCLUSIONS

Provided that the diagnosis of ectopic pregnancy is made early, the modern management of ectopic pregnancy offers the physician and the patient many therapeutic options, including surgical, nonsurgical, and expectant management (Table 8-3). As the management of ectopic pregnancy continues to evolve, it is likely that new treatment options will emerge. The selection of the optimal, appropriate therapy for a particular patient will be facilitated by evaluation of the various treatment modalities in a prospective, randomized fashion. Until more information is available, the physician and the patient must weigh the known and the unknown risks and benefits of the various available options and make the best attempt to maximize the potential for future fertility (if desired) while minimizing disease and treatment-related morbidity.

Table 8-3   Treatment Options for Unruptured Ectopic Pregnancy: Success Rates and Reproductive Outcomes*

	Success (%)	Intrauterine Pregnancy (%)	Ectopic Pregnancy (%)
Salpingostomy (laparotomy)	96	61	15
Salpingostomy (laparoscopy)	92	61	15
Methotrexate, systemic (IM, 50 mg/m²)	92	58	9
Methotrexate, intratubal (transvaginal ultrasound)	81	48	6
Methotrexate, intratubal (laparoscopic)	79	58	10
Expectant management	69	Unknown	Unknown

Modified from Yao M, Tulandi T: Current status of surgical and nonsurgical management of ectopic pregnancy. *Fertil Steril* 1997; 67:421-433.

*Results are compiled from several (predominantly retrospective) studies.

REFERENCES

Abe H: The mammalian oviductal epithelium: Regional variations in cytological and functional aspects of the oviductal secretory cells. *Histol Histopathol* 1996; 11:743-768.

Alexander JM, Rouse DJ, Varner E, et al: Treatment of the small unruptured ectopic pregnancy: A cost analysis of methotrexate versus laparoscopy. *Obstet Gynecol* 1996; 88:123-127.

Altaras M, Cohen I, Cordova M, et al: Treatment of an interstitial pregnancy with actinomycin-D. *Br J Obstet Gynaecol* 1988; 95:1321-1323.

American Fertility Society: The American Fertility Society classification of adnexal adhesions, distal tubal occlusion, tubal occlusion secondary to tubal ligation, tubal pregnancies, müllerian anomalies and intrauterine adhesions. *Fertil Steril* 1988; 49:944-955.

American Medical Association: *Drug evaluations annual 1995*, Chicago, 1995, American Medical Association.

Ankum WM, Mol BWJ, Van der Veen F, et al: Risk factors for ectopic pregnancy: A meta-analysis. *Fertil Steril* 1996; 65:1093-1099.

Arias-Stella J: Atypical endometrial changes associated with the presence of chorionic tissue. *Arch Pathol* 1954; 58:112-128.

Bell OR, Awadalla SG, Mattox JH: Persistent ectopic syndrome: A case report and literature review. *Obstet Gynecol* 1987; 69:521-523.

Benadiva CA, Kligman I, Davis O, et al: In vitro fertilization versus tubal surgery: Is pelvic reconstructive surgery obsolete? *Fertil Steril* 1995; 64:1051-1061.

Benjamin CL, Beaver DC: The pathogenesis of salpingitis isthmica nodosa. *Am J Clin Pathol* 1951; 21:212-222.

Berkowitz RS, Goldstein DP, Bernstein MR. Ten years' experience with methotrexate and folinic acid as primary therapy for gestational trophoblastic disease. *Gynecol Oncol* 1986; 23:111-118.

Berkowitz RS, Im SS, Bernstein MR, et al: Gestational trophoblastic disease: Subsequent pregnancy outcome, including repeat molar pregnancy. *J Reprod Med* 1998; 43:81-86.

Boer-Meisel ME, teVelde ER, Habbema JDF, et al: Predicting the pregnancy outcome in patients treated for hydrosalpinx: A prospective study. *Fertil Steril* 1986; 45:23-29.

Braunstein GD, Karow WG, Gentry WC, et al: First-trimester chorionic gonadotropin measurements as an aid in the diagnosis of early pregnancy disorders. *Am J Obstet Gynecol* 1978; 131:25-32.

Breen JL: A 21 year survey of 654 ectopic pregnancies. *Am J Obstet Gynecol* 1970; 106:1004-1019.

Brown DL, Doubilet PM: Transvaginal sonography for diagnosing ectopic pregnancy: Positivity criteria and performance characteristics. *J Ultrasound Med* 1994; 13:259-266.

Bruhat MA, Manhes H, Mage G, et al: Treatment of ectopic pregnancy by means of laparoscopy. *Fertil Steril* 1980; 33:411-414.

Budowick M, Johnson TR Jr, Genadry R, et al: The histopathology of the developing tubal ectopic pregnancy. *Fertil Steril* 1980; 34:169-171.

Buster JE, Carson SA: Ectopic pregancy: New advances in diagnosis and treatment. *Curr Opin Obstet Gynecol* 1995; 7:168-176.

Cacciatore B, Korhonen J, Stenman UH, et al: Transvaginal sonography and serum hCG in monitoring of presumed ectopic pregnancies selected for expectant management. *Ultrasound Obstet Gynecol* 1995; 5:297-300.

Cartwright PS: Peritoneal trophoblastic implants after surgical management of tubal pregnancy. *J Reprod Med* 1991; 36:523-524.

Centers for Disease Control: Ectopic pregnancy—United States 1990-1992. *MMWR Morb Mortal Wkly Rep* 1995; 44:46-48.

Chang MC: Development and fate of transferred rabbit ova or blastocysts in relation to the ovulation time of recipients. *J Exp Zool* 1950; 114:197-225.

Chang MC: Fertilizing capacity of spermatozoa deposited into the fallopian tube. *Nature* 1951; 168:697-698.

Chegini N: Oviductal-derived growth factors and cytokines: Implications in preimplantation. *Semin Reprod Endocrinol* 1996; 14:219-229.

Chelmow D, Gates E, Penzias AS: Laparoscopic diagnosis and methotrexate treatment of an ovarian pregnancy: A case report. *Fertil Steril* 1994; 62:879-881.

Chow WH, Daling JR, Cates W Jr, et al: Epidemiology of ectopic pregnancy. *Epidemiol Rev* 1987; 9:70-94.

Creinen MD, Washington AE: Cost of ectopic pregnancy management: Surgery versus methotrexate. *Fertil Steril* 1993; 60:963-969.

Creasy JL, Clark RL, Cuttino JT, et al: Salpingitis isthmica nodosa: Radiologic and clinical correlates. *Radiology* 1985; 154:597-600.

Critoph FN, Dennis KJ: Ciliary activity in the human oviduct. *Br J Obstet Gynaecol* 1977; 84:216-218.

Croxatto HB, Ortiz ME, Diaz S, et al: Studies on the duration of egg transport by the human oviduct: ovum location at various intervals following luteinizing hormone peak. *Am J Obstet Gynecol* 1978; 132:629-634.

DeCherney AH, Boyes SP: Isthmic ectopic pregnancy: Segmental resection as the treatment of choice. *Fertil Steril* 1985; 44:307-312.

Dela Cruz A, Cumming DC: Factors determining fertility after conservative or radical surgery treatment for ectopic pregnancy. *Fertil Steril* 1997; 68:871-874.

DeVoe RW, Pratt JH: Simultaneous intrauterine and extrauterine pregnancy. *Am J Obstet Gynecol* 1948; 56:1119-1123.

Donnez J, Casanas-Roux F, Caprasse J, et al: Cyclic changes in ciliation, cell height, and mitotic activity in human tubal epithelium during reproductive life. *Fertil Steril* 1985; 43:554-559.

Egarter C, Husslein P: Treatment of tubal pregnancy by prostaglandins. *Lancet* 1988; 1:1104-1105.

Farabow WS, Fulton JW, Fletcher V Jr, et al: Cervical pregnancy treated with methotrexate. *N C Med J* 1983; 44:91-93.

Fayez JA: An assessment of the role of operative laparoscopy in tuboplasty. *Fertil Steril* 1983; 39:476-479.

Feichtinger W, Kemeter P: Conservative treatment of ectopic pregnancy by transvaginal aspiration under sonographic control and injection of methotrexate. *Lancet* 1987; 1:381-382.

Fernandez H, Pauthier S, Doumerc S, et al: Ultrasound-guided injection of methotrexate versus laparoscopic salpingotomy in ectopic pregnancy. *Fertil Steril* 1995; 63:25-29.

Flood JT, Grow DR: Transcervial tubal cannulation: A review. *Obstet Gynecol Surv* 1993; 48:768-776.

Fossum GT, Davajan V, Kletzky OA: Early detection of pregnancy with transvaginal ultrasound. *Fertil Steril* 1988; 49: 788-791.

Frates MC, Benson CB, Doubilet PM, et al: Cervical ectopic pregnancy: Results of conservative treatment. *Radiology* 1994; 191:773-775.

Gaddum-Rosse P, Rumery RE, Blandau RJ, et al: Studies on the mucosa of postmenopausal oviducts: Surface appearance, ciliary activity, and the effect of estrogen treatment. *Fertil Steril* 1975; 26: 951-969.

Givan AL, White HD, Stern JE, et al: Flow cytometric analysis of leukocytes in the human female reproductive tract: Comparison of fallopian tube, uerus, cervix and vagina. *Am J Reprod Immunol* 1997; 38:350-359.

Glock JL, Johnson JV, Brumsted JR: Efficacy and safety of single-dose systemic methotrexate in the treatment of ectopic pregnancy. *Fertil Steril* 1994; 62:716-721.

Goldenberg M, Bider D, Oelsner G, et al: Treatment of interstitial pregnancy with methotrexate via hysteroscopy. *Fertil Steril* 1992; 58: 1234-1236.

Gomel V: Tubal reanastomosis by microsurgery. *Fertil Steril* 1977; 28:59-65.

Gomel V: Salpingo-ovariolysis by laparoscopy in infertility. *Fertil Steril* 1983; 40:607-611.

Graczykowski JW, Mishell DR Jr: Methotrexate prophylaxis of persistent ectopic pregnancy after conservative treatment by salpingostomy. *Obstet Gynecol* 1997; 89:118-122.

Gretz E, Quagliarello J: Declining serum concentrations of the β-subunit of human chorionic gonadotropin and ruptured ectopic pregnancy. *Am J Obstet Gynecol* 1987; 156:940-941.

Gross Z, Rodriguez JD, Stalnaker BL: Ectopic pregnancy: Nonsurgical, outpatient evaluation and single-dose methotrexate treatment. *J Reprod Med* 1995; 40:371-374.

Guzick DS: Human infertility: An introduction. In Adashi EY, Rock JA, Rosenwaks Z, editors: *Reproductive endocrinology, surgery, and technology*, Philadelphia, 1996, Lippincott-Raven.

Hajenious PJ, Engelsbel S, Mol BWJ, et al: Randomised trial of systemic methotrexate versus laparoscopic salpingostomy in tubal pregnancy. *Lancet* 1997; 350:774-779.

Hallatt JG: Tubal conservation in ectopic pregnancy: A study of 200 cases. *Am J Obstet Gynecol* 1986; 154:1216-1221.

Henderson SR: The reversibility of female sterilization with the use of microsurgery: A report of 102 patients with more than one year of follow-up. *Am J Obstet Gynecol* 1984; 149:57-65.

Hepp H, Korell M, Strowitzki T: Proximal tubal obstruction: Is there a best way to treat it? *Hum Reprod* 1996; 11:1828-1831.

Hirata AJ, Soper DE, Bump RC, et al: Ectopic pregnancy in an urban teaching hospital: Can tubal rupture be predicted? *South Med J* 1991; 84:1467-1469.

Honore LH: Salpingitis isthmica nodosa in female infertility and ectopic tubal pregnancy. *Fertil Steril* 1978; 29:164-168.

Hope RB: Differential diagnosis of ectopic gestation by peritonoscopy. *Surg Gynecol Obstet* 1937; 64:229-234.

Jansen RPS: Cyclic changes in the human fallopian tube isthmus and their functional importance. *Am J Obstet Gynecol* 1980; 136:292-308.

Jenkins CS, Williams SR, Schmidt GE: Salpingitis isthmica nodosa: A review of the literature, discussion of clinical significance, and consideration of patient management. *Fertil Steril* 1993; 60: 599-607.

Job-Spira N, Bouyer J, Pouly JL, et al: Fertility after ectopic pregnancy: First results of a population-based cohort study in France. *Hum Reprod* 1996; 11:99-104.

Jones RB, Ardery BR, Hui SL, et al: Correlation between serum antichlamydial antibodies and tubal factor as a cause of infertility. *Fertil Steril* 1982; 38:553-558.

Kadar N, Caldwell BV, Romero R: A method of screening for ectopic pregnancy and its indications. *Obstet Gynecol* 1981a; 58:162-166.

Kadar N, DeVore G, Romero R: The discriminatory zone: Its use in the sonographic evaluation of ectopic pregnancy. *Obstet Gynecol* 1981b; 58:156-161.

Keefe KA, Wald JS, Goldstein DP, et al: Reproductive outcome after methotrexate treatment of tubal pregnancies. *J Reprod Med* 1998; 43:28-32.

Keith SC, London SN, Weitzman GA, et al: Serial transvaginal ultrasound scans and beta-human chorionic gonadotropin levels in early singleton and multiple pregnancies. *Fertil Steril* 1993; 59:1007-1010.

Kelly RW, Martin SA, Strickler RC: Delayed hemorrhage in conservative surgery for ectopic pregnancy. *Am J Obstet Gynecol* 1979; 133:225-227.

Kim HH, Laufer MR: Developmental abnormalities of the female reproductive tract. *Curr Opin Obstet Gynecol* 1994; 6:518-525.

Klinkert J, van Geldorp HJ, Chadha-Ajwani H, et al: Tubal damage after intratubal methotrexate treatment. *Fertil Steril* 1993; 59:926-927.

Koike H, Chuganji Y, Watanabe H, et al: Conservative treatment of ovarian pregnancy by local prostaglandin F2-alpha injection [letter]. *Am J Obstet Gynecol* 1990; 163:696.

Korell M, Albrich W, Hepp H: Fertility after organ-preserving surgery of ectopic pregnancy: Results of a multicenter study. *Fertil Steril* 1997; 68:220-223.

Korhonen J, Stenman UH, Ylostalo P: Serum human chorionic gonadotropin dynamics during spontaneous resolution of ectopic pregnancy. *Fertil Steril* 1994; 61:632-636.

Lathrop JC, Bowles GE: Methotrexate in abdominal pregnancy: Report of a case. *Obstet Gynecol* 1968; 32:81-85.

Lavy G, Diamond MP, DeCherney AH: Pregnancy following tubocornual anastomosis. *Fertil Steril* 1986; 46:21-25.

Lavy G, Diamond MP, DeCherney AH: Ectopic pregnancy: Its relationship to tubal reconstructive surgery. *Fertil Steril* 1987; 47:543-556.

Leese HJ: The formation and function of oviduct fluid. *J Reprod Fertil* 1988; 82:843-856.

Li MC, Hertz A, Spencer DB: Effect of methotrexate therapy on choriocarcinoma and chorioadenoma. *Proc Soc Exp Biol Med* 1956; 93: 361-366.

Lindblom B, Hahlin M, Lundorff P, Thorburn J: Treatment of tubal pregnancy by laparoscope-guided injection of prostaglandin F2alpha. *Fertil Steril* 1990; 54:404-408.

Lund JJ: Early ectopic pregnancy. *J Obstet Gynaecol Br Empire*. 1955; 62:70-75.

Lundorff P, Thorburn J, Hahlin M, et al: Laparoscopic surgery in ectopic pregnancy: A randomized trial versus laparotomy. *Acta Obstet Gynecol Scand* 1991; 70:343-348.

Lundorff P, Thorburn J, Lindblom B: Fertility outcome after conservative surgical treatment of ectopic pregnancy evaluated in a randomized trial. *Fertil Steril* 1992; 57:998-1002.

Lurie S: The history of the diagnosis and treatment of ectopic pregnancy: A medical adventure. *Eur J Obstet Gynecol Reprod Biol* 1992; 43:1-7.

Mage G, Pouly JL, Bouquet de Joliniere J, et al: A preoperative classification to predict the intrauterine and ectopic pregnancy rates after distal tubal microsurgery. *Fertil Steril* 1986; 46:807-810.

Majmudar B, Henderson PH III, Semple E: Salpingitis isthmica nodosa: A high risk factor for tubal pregnancy. *Obstet Gynecol* 1983; 62: 73-78.

Marchbanks PA, Annegers JF, Coulam CB, et al: Risk factors for ectopic pregnancy: A population based study. *JAMA* 1988; 259:1822-1827.

McComb P, Langley L, Villalon M, et al: The oviductal cilia and Kartagener's syndrome. *Fertil Steril* 1986; 46:412-416.

McComb PF, Rowe TC: Salpingitis nodosa: Evidence it is a progressive disease. *Fertil Steril* 1989; 51: 542-545.

McCord ML, Muram D, Buster JE, et al: Single serum progesterone as a screen for ectopic pregnancy: Exchanging specificity and sensitivity to obtain optimal test performance. *Fertil Steril* 1996; 66:513-516.

McCormack WM: Pelvic inflammatory disease. *N Engl J Med* 1994; 330:115-119.

Meldrum DR: Microsurgical tubal reanastomosis—the role of splints. *Obstet Gynecol* 1981; 57:613-619.

Menezo Y, Guerin P: The mammalian oviduct: Biochemistry and physiology. *Eur J Obstet Gynecol Reprod Biol* 1997; 73:99-104.

Merchant RN, Prabhu SR, Chougale A: Uterotubal junction—morphology and clinical aspects. *Int J Fertil* 1983; 28:199-205.

Metz KGP: Failures following fimbriectomy. *Fertil Steril* 1977; 28:66-71.

Meyer WR, Mitchell DE: Hysteroscopic removal of an interstitial ectopic gestation: A case report. *J Reprod Med* 1989; 34:928-929.

Mottla GL, Rulin MC, Guzick DS: Lack of resolution of ectopic pregnancy by intratubal injection of methotrexate. *Fertil Steril* 1992; 57:685-687.

Murphy AA, Nager CW, Wujek JJ, et al: Operative laparoscopy versus laparotomy for the management of ectopic pregnancy: A prospective trial. *Fertil Steril* 1992; 57:1180-1185.

Nackley AC, Muasher SJ: The significance of hydrosalpinx in in vitro fertilization. *Fertil Steril* 1998; 69:373-384.

Odor DL: The question of "basal" cells in oviductal and endocervical epithelium. *Fertil Steril* 1974; 25:1047-1062.

Oelsner G, Admon D, Shaler E, et al: A new approach for the treatment of interstitial pregnancy. *Fertil Steril* 1993; 59:924-925.

Ory SJ, Villanueva AL, Sand PK, et al: Conservative treatment of ectopic pregnancy with methotrexate. *Am J Obstet Gynecol* 1986; 154:1299-1304.

O'Shea RT, Thompson GR, Harding A: Intraamniotic methotrexate versus CO_2 laser laparoscopic salpingotomy in the management of tubal ectopic pregnancy—a prospective randomized trial. *Fertil Steril* 1994; 62:876-878.

Oyer R, Tarakjian D, Friedman A, et al: Treatment of cervical pregnancy with methotrexate. *Obstet Gynecol* 1988; 71:469-471.

Pansky M, Bukovsky I, Golan A, et al: Local methotrexate injection: A nonsurgical treatment of ectopic pregnancy. *Am J Obstet Gynecol* 1989; 161:393-396.

Pansky M, Golan A, Bukovsky I, et al: Nonsurgical management of tubal pregnancy: Necessity in view of the changing clinical appearance. *Am J Obstet Gynecol* 1991; 164:888-895.

Patek E, Nilsson L: Scanning electron microscopic observations on the ciliogenesis of the infundibulum of the human fetal and adult fallopian tube epithelium. *Fertil Steril* 1973; 24: 819-831.

Pauerstein CJ, Croxatto B, Eddy CA, et al: Anatomy and pathology of tubal pregnancy. *Obstet Gynecol* 1986; 67:301-308.

Paulsson G, Kvint S, Labecker BM, et al: Laparoscopic prostaglandin injection in ectopic pregnancy: Success rates according to endocrine activity. *Fertil Steril* 1995; 63:473-477.

Penzias AS, DeCherney AH: Is there ever a role for tubal surgery? *Am J Obstet Gynecol* 1996; 174:1218-1221.

Peterson HB, Xia Z, Hughes JM, et al: The risk of ectopic pregnancy after tubal sterilization. *N Engl J Med* 1997; 336:762-767.

Podczaski E, Herbst AL: Cancer of the vagina and fallopian tube. In Knapp RC, Berkowitz RS, editors: *Gynecologic Oncology*, ed 2, New York, 1993, Macmillan.

Pouly JL, Chapron C, Manhes H, et al: Multifactorial analysis of fertility after conservative laparoscopic treatment of ectopic pregnancy in a series of 223 patients. *Fertil Steril* 1991; 56:453-460.

Rantala M, Makinen J: Tubal patency and fertility outcome after expectant management of ectopic pregnancy. *Fertil Steril* 1997; 68: 1043-1046.

Rapkin AJ: Neuroanatomy, neurophysiology, and neuropharmacology of pelvic pain. *Clin Obstet Gynecol* 1990; 33:119-129.

Reich H, DeCaprio J, McGlynn F, et al: Peritoneal trophoblastic tissue implants after laparoscopic treatment of tubal ectopic pregnancy. *Fert Steril* 1989; 52:337-339.

Rengachary D, Fayez JA, Jonas HS: Ovarian pregnancy. *Obstet Gynecol* 1977; 49(suppl): 76-78.

Risquez F, Mathieson J, Pariente D, et al: Diagnosis and treatment of ectopic pregnancy by retrograde selective salpingography and intraluminal methotrexate injection: Work in progress. *Hum Reprod* 1990; 5:759-762.

Robertson DE, Smith W, Moye MA, et al: Reduction of ectopic pregnancy by injection under ultrasound control. *Lancet* 1987; 1:974-975.

Rojansky N, Schenker JG: Heterotopic pregnancy and assisted reproduction—an update. *J Assist Reprod Genet* 1996; 13:594-601.

Romero R, Copel JA, Kadar N, et al: Value of culdocentesis in the diagnosis of ectopic pregnancy. *Obstet Gynecol* 1985a; 65:519-522.

Romero R, Kadar N, Jeanty P, et al: Diagnosis of ectopic pregnancy: Value of the discriminatory human chorionic gonadotropin zone. *Obstet Gynecol* 1985b; 66:357-360.

Ross GT: Congenital anomalies among children born of mothers receiving chemotherapy for gestational trophoblastic neoplasms. *Cancer* 1976; 37(suppl):1043-1047.

Schenker JG, Ezra Y: Complications of assisted reproductive techniques. *Fertil Steril* 1994; 61:411-422.

Seifer DB, Gutmann JN, Doyle MB, et al: Persistent ectopic pregnancy following laparoscopic linear salpingostomy. *Obstet Gynecol* 1990; 76:1121-1125.

Seifer DB: Persistent ectopic pregnancy: An argument for heightened vigilance and patient compliance. *Fertil Steril* 1997; 68:402-404.

Seifer DB, Silva PD, Grainger DA, et al: Reproductive potential after treatment for persistent ectopic pregnancy. *Fertil Steril* 1994; 62:194-196.

Settlage DSF, Motoshima M, Tredway DR: Sperm transport from the external cervical os to the fallopian tubes in women: A time and quantitation study. *Fertil Steril* 1973; 24: 655-661.

Shalev E, Peleg D, Bustan M, et al: Limited role for intratubal methotrexate treatment of ectopic pregnancy. *Fertil Steril* 1995a; 63:20-24.

Shalev E, Peleg D, Tsabari A, et al: Spontaneous resolution of ectopic tubal pregnancy: Natural history. *Fertil Steril* 1995b; 63:15-19.

Shamma FN, Schwartz LB: Primary ovarian pregnancy successfully treated with methotrexate. *Am J Obstet Gynecol* 1992; 167:1307-1308.

Shapiro HI, Adler DH: Excision of an ectopic pregnancy through the laparoscope. *Am J Obstet Gynecol* 1973; 117:290-291.

Shen SC, Bansal M, Purrazella R, et al: Benign and glandular inclusions in lymph nodes, endosalpingiosis, and salpingitis isthmica nodosa in a young girl with clear cell adenocarcinoma of the cervix. *Am J Surg Pathol* 1983; 7:293-300.

Sherman D, Langer R, Herman A, et al: Reproductive outcome after fimbrial evacuation of tubal pregnancy. *Fertil Steril* 1987; 47:420-424.

Society for Assisted Reproductive Technology, American Society for Reproductive Medicine. *1995 Assisted reproductive technology success rates: National summary and fertility clinic reports.* (Available from American Society for Reproductive Medicine)

Soules MR, Spadoni LR: Oil versus aqueous media for hysterosalpingography: A continuing debate based on many opinions and few facts. *Fertil Steril* 1982; 38:1-11.

Spandorfer SD, Sawin SW, Benjamin I, et al: Postoperative day 1 serum human chorionic gonadotropin level as a predictor of persistent ectopic pregnancy after conservative surgical management. *Fertil Steril* 1987; 68:430-434.

Stock RJ: Persistent tubal pregnancy. *Obstet Gynecol* 1991; 77:267-270.

Stone SC, McCalley M, Braunstein P, et al: Radionuclide evaluation of tubal function. *Fertil Steril* 1985; 43:757-760.

Stovall TG, Kellerman AL, Ling FW, et al: Emergency department diagnosis of ectopic pregnancy. *Ann Emer Med* 1990; 19:1098-1103.

Stovall TG, Ling FW: Single dose methotrexate: An expanded clinical trial. *Am J Obstet Gynecol* 1993; 168:1759-1765.

Stovall TG, Ling FW, Carson SA, et al: Serum progesterone and uterine curettage in differential diagnosis of ectopic pregnancy. *Fertil Steril* 1992; 57:456-458.

Stovall TG, Ling FW, Cope BJ, et al: Preventing ruptured ectopic pregnancy with a single serum progesterone. *Am J Obstet Gynecol* 1989; 160:1425-1428.

Stovall TG, Ling FW, Gray LA, et al: Methotrexate treatment of unruptured ectopic pregnancy: A report of 100 cases. *Obstet Gynecol* 1991a; 77:749-753.

Stovall TG, Ling FW, Gray LA: Single-dose methotrexate for treatment of ectopic pregnancy. *Obstet Gynecol* 1991b; 77:754-757.

Strafford JC, Ragan WD: Abdominal pregnancy: review of current management. *Obstet Gynecol* 1977; 50:548-552.

Stromme WB: Salpingotomy for tubal pregnancy: Report of a successful case. *Obstet Gynecol* 1953; 1:472-476.

Tal J, Haddad S, Gordon N, et al: Heterotopic pregnancy after ovulation induction and assisted reproductive technologies: A literature review from 1971 to 1993. *Fertil Steril* 1996; 66:1-12.

Talo A, Pulkkinen MO: Electrical activity in the human oviduct during the menstrual cycle. *Am J Obstet Gynecol* 1982; 142:135-147.

Tanaka T, Hayashi H, Kutsuzawa T, et al: Treatment of interstitial ectopic pregnancy with methotrexate: Report of a successful case. *Fertil Steril* 1982; 37:851-852.

Tatum HJ, Schmidt FH: Contraceptive and sterilization practices and extrauterine pregnancy: A realistic perspective. *Fertil Steril* 1077; 28:407-421.

Thatcher SS, Grainger DA, True LD, et al: Pelvic trophoblastic implants after laparoscopic removal of a tubal pregnancy. *Obstet Gynecol* 1989; 74:514-515.

Thomas ML, Rose DH. Salpingitis isthmica nodosa demonstrated by hysterosalpingogram. *Acta Radiol* 1973; 14:295-304.

Timor-Tritsch I, Baxi L, Peisner DB: Transvaginal salpingocentesis: A new technique for treating ectopic pregnancy. *Am J Obstet Gynecol* 1989; 160: 459-461.

Trio D, Strobelt N, Picciolo C, et al: Prognostic factors for successful expectant management of ectopic pregnancy. *Fertil Steril* 1995; 63:469-472.

Tulandi T, Guralnick M: Treatment of tubal ectopic pregnancy by salpingotomy with or without tubal suturing and salpingectomy. *Fertil Steril* 1991; 55:53-55.

Tulandi T, Hemmings R, Khalifa F: Rupture of ectopic pregnancy in women with low and declining serum B-human chorionic gonadotropin concentrations. *Fertil Steril* 1991; 56:786-787.

Ushakov FB, Elchalal U, Aceman PJ, et al: Cervical pregnancy: Past and future. *Obstet Gynecol Surv* 1996; 52:45-59.

Vaitukaitis JL, Braunstein GD, Ross GT: A radioimmunoassay which specifically measures human chorionic gonadotropin in the presence of luteinizing hormone. *Am J Obstet Gynecol* 1972; 113:751-758.

Verhage HG, Bareither ML, Jaffe RC, et al: Cyclic changes in ciliation, secretion and cell height of the oviductal epithelium in women. *Am J Anat* 1979; 156:505-521.

Vermesh M, Silva PD, Rosen GF, et al: Management of unruptured ectopic gestation by linear salpingostomy: A prospective, randomized clinical trail of laparoscopy versus laparotomy. *Obstet Gynecol* 1989; 73:400-404.

Vermesh M, Graczykowski JW, Sauer MV: Reevaluation of the role of culdocentesis in the management of ectopic pregnancy. *Am J Obstet Gynecol* 1990; 162:411-413.

Vermesh M, Presser SC: Reproductive outcome after linear salpingostomy for ectopic gestation: A prospective 3-year follow-up. *Fertil Steril* 1992; 57:682-684.

Westrom L: Incidence, prevalence, and trends of acute pelvic inflammatory disease and its consequences in industrialized countries. *Am J Obstet Gynecol* 1980; 138:880-892.

Wheeler JE: Pathology of the fallopian tube. In Kurman RJ, editor: *Blaustein's pathology of the female genital tract,* ed 4, New York, 1994, Springer-Verlag.

Wilcox AJ, Weinberg CR, O'Connor JF, et al: Incidence of early loss of pregnancy. *N Engl J Med* 1988; 319:189-194.

Wrork FH, Broders AC: Adenomyosis of the fallopian tube. *Am J Obstet Gynecol* 1942; 44:412-432.

Yao M, Tulandi T: Current status of surgical and nonsurgical management of ectopic pregnancy. *Fertil Steril* 1997; 67:421-433.

Yao M, Tulandi T, Kaplow M, et al: A comparison of methotrexate versus laparoscopic surgery for the treatment of ectopic pregnancy: A cost analysis. *Hum Reprod* 1996; 11:2762-2766.

Yeko TR, Mayer JC, Parsons AK, et al: A prospective series of unruptured ectopic pregnancies treated by tubal injection with hyperosmolar glucose. *Obstet Gynecol* 1995; 85:265-268.

Yoon TK, Sung HR, Cha SH, et al: Fertility outcome after laparoscopic microsurgical tubal anastomosis. *Fertil Steril* 1991; 67:18-22.

CHAPTER

9

The Ovary

LAUREL W. RICE

KEY ISSUES

1. Effective screening for ovarian cancer in the general population is not yet possible.
2. Genetic tests can be performed to detect hereditary ovarian cancer syndrome (BRCA1 and BRCA2). These tests identify patients more likely to benefit from ovarian cancer screening.
3. Decreasing a patient's risk for ovarian cancer is possible through the use of oral contraceptives, prophylactic oophorectomy, and possibly tubal ligation.
4. Follow-up observation for patients who have undergone surgery and chemotherapy for primary ovarian cancer includes rectovaginal pelvic examination and CA-125 testing every 3 to 4 months for the first 2 years, with a decrease in frequency in subsequent years.

The prevention, diagnosis, and management of ovarian neoplasms continue to challenge clinicians caring for women of all ages. The medical community and the public are well aware of the high mortality rate associated with the diagnosis of epithelial ovarian carcinoma and that it is responsible for approximately 15,000 deaths annually in the United States. Although there has been tremendous improvement in the survival rate of young women with germ cell ovarian malignancies, the same has not been true for women with epithelial ovarian carcinoma. The most important positive prognosticator for improved survival of patients with ovarian carcinoma is diagnosis at an early stage. Because of this, significant resources continue to be directed toward the prevention and the early diagnosis of ovarian cancer.

The technology associated with diagnosing and treating ovarian or adnexal disease is expanding exponentially. Radiographic examinations, including ultrasonography, computed tomography (CT), and magnetic resonance imaging, are used with increasing frequency. Laparoscopic surgery continues to evolve, and physicians not only must maintain the basic skills involved with the operative technique, they must stay abreast of new equipment and indications for its usage. It is essential that the clinician have a clear understanding of the wide range of disease processes that fall under the category of ovarian neoplasms. Developing and sustaining an understanding of the differential diagnoses of ovarian and adnexal diseases will allow the physician to process information as it becomes available and to put it into an appropriate framework.

EPIDEMIOLOGY
General

Histologic diversity complicates the determination of risk factors for benign and malignant ovarian neoplasms. Epithelial ovarian carcinoma is the second most common cancer of the female reproductive tract and the leading cause of death from gynecologic malignancies in the United States. Each year it is diagnosed in 25,000 to 30,000 women, and approximately 15,000 die of it in that time. In the United States, the annual lifetime risk for ovarian cancer is 1.4 per 100 women. There is wide variation in global incidence rates for ovarian carcinoma. The highest rates are observed in Scandinavia, Israel, and North America, whereas the lowest rates are observed in developing countries and Japan (Muir, 1987).

Factors Denoting Increased Ovarian Cancer Risk

Family History. Epithelial ovarian carcinoma develops sporadically in more than 95% of patients. However, when all risk factors are controlled for, the variable most strongly associated with it is family history. Three hereditary syndromes in which the familial aggregation of ovarian cancer occurs have been described: site-specific ovarian cancer syndrome, breast-ovarian cancer syndrome, and hereditary nonpolyposis colorectal cancer syndrome (Lynch syndrome II). Susceptibility to hereditary ovarian cancer appears to be transmitted as an autosomal dominant trait with incomplete penetrance and variable expression. Results of a population-based case-control study (Schildkraut and Thompson, 1989) indicate that among women with ovarian cancer but no family history, the odds ratios (OR) for its occurrence in first- and second-degree relatives are 3.6 (95% confidence interval [CI], 1.8 to 7.1) and 2.9 (95% CI, 1.6 to 5.3), respectively. Other authors have found similar results. A patient's risk for ovarian carcinoma can be as high as 50% if two first-degree relatives have had the disease. If ovarian carcinoma develops in the daughter of a woman with it, it is more likely to develop at a younger age (Amos et al, 1992).

In 1990, a susceptibility gene for inherited breast cancer was linked to the long arm of chromosome 17 (Hall et al, 1990). This gene, termed BRCA1, is also responsible for a 26% cumulative risk for ovarian cancer for most mutation carriers, with a small subset carrying a much higher risk of 85% (Easton et al, 1995; Easton et al, 1993; Ford et al, 1994; Ford and Easton, 1995). BRCA2, a second susceptibility gene, is located on chromosome 13q and increases the risk for ovarian cancer to a lesser degree (Ford and Easton, 1995). More precise estimates of ovarian cancer risk that consider heterogeneity of risk associated with particular classes of BRCA1 mutation will be available once the distribution of these mutations is described at a population-based level. As this type of genetic testing becomes available, persons carrying these mutations will need prophylactic oophorectomy and thoughtful counseling regarding the options available to them for cancer surveillance.

Infertility and Fertility Drugs. Including infertility and fertility drugs in a discussion such as this is controversial because the data are less consistent. Whittemore et al (1992) found a nonstatistically significant increased risk (OR, 1.4; 95% CI, 0.86 to 2.3) for ovarian cancer among nulliparous women with clinical diagnoses of infertility. Rossing et al (1994) also found an increase in ovarian cancer among a cohort of infertile women (standardized incidence ratio [SIR], 2.5; 95% CI, 1.3 to 4.5). Both studies suggest a higher risk for women with infertility that results from an ovulation-related cause.

Whittemore et al (1992) observe that infertile women treated with fertility drugs are at higher risk for ovarian cancer than women without a history of infertility (OR, 2.8; 95% CI, 1.3 to 6.1). They also observe that infertile women who do not use fertility drugs are not at a statistically significant increased risk. Rossing et al (1994) observe a statistically significant increased risk for ovarian tumors among women who use clomiphene (SIR, 11.1; 95% CI, 1.5 to 82.3). In contrast are the results of a Danish case-control study (Mosgaard et al, 1997) of 684 infertile case patients and 1721 infertile control patients with ovarian cancer. The authors compare treated nulliparous women with nontreated nulliparous women (OR, 0.8; CI, 0.4 to 2.0) and treated parous women with nontreated parous women (OR, 0.6; CI,

0.2 to 1.3) and find that treatment of parous and nulliparous women with fertility drugs does not increase the risk for ovarian cancer.

Several limitations should be taken into consideration when interpreting the results of all these studies, including the relatively small number of cases, potential recall, diagnosis and selection bias, and partial control of confounding factors. Larger epidemiologic studies are required to establish firmly the possible association between ovarian carcinoma and ovulation induction.

Other. It has been established that there is a relationship between exogenous substances, such as asbestos and talc, and the development of ovarian carcinoma. Pelvic irradiation and viruses (particularly mumps) have been associated with an increased risk for ovarian malignancy, presumably because of sustained elevations of gonadotropins.

Factors Associated with Decreased Ovarian Cancer Risk

Parity. Whittemore et al (1992) collected data from 12 case-control studies conducted in the United States between 1956 and 1986. Participants were 2197 white patients with ovarian cancer and 8893 white controls. They observe a significant risk reduction with any term pregnancy in population-based studies (OR, 0.47; 95% CI, 0.40 to 0.56) and in hospital-based studies (OR, 0.76; 95% CI, 0.63 to 0.93). The risk for ovarian cancer decreases with increasing numbers of pregnancies.

Oral Contraceptives. Numerous investigators have established that oral contraceptives reduce the risk for ovarian carcinoma (Centers for Disease Control, 1987; Cramer et al, 1982; Hankison et al, 1992; Prentice and Thomas, 1987; Rosenberg et al, 1994; Whittemore et al, 1992). Hankison et al (1992) estimate that ovarian cancer risk decreases by 11% with each year of oral contraceptive use and that it is decreased by 46% after 5 years of use. Little additional protection is observed after 6 or more years of use (Whittemore et al, 1992). The protective effect conferred by oral contraceptive use appears to be independent of parity, age at diagnosis, age at first oral contraceptive, or body mass index (CDC, 1987; Hankison et al, 1992; Rosenberg et al, 1982; World Health Organization, 1989).

Breast-Feeding. Women who have breast-fed are reported to have a lower risk for ovarian cancer than nulliparous women and parous women who have not breast-fed (Whittemore et al, 1992). The risk for ovarian cancer decreases with increasing duration of breast-feeding.

Tubal Ligation and Hysterectomy. Tubal ligation and hysterectomy with preservation of the ovaries have been associated with a decreased risk for ovarian cancer. Hankison et al (1993) observe a strong inverse association between tubal ligation and ovarian cancer, which persists after adjustment for age, oral contraceptive use, parity, and other ovarian cancer risk factors (multivariate relative risk, 0.33; 95% CI, 0.16 to 0.64). They note a weaker inverse association between simple hysterectomy and ovarian cancer.

Miracle-McMahill et al (1977) find the same protective effect of tubal ligation against ovarian cancer.

OVARIAN CANCER PREVENTION
Nonsurgical Prevention of Ovarian Cancer

Oral contraceptive use and possibly tubal ligation are the only reasonable options for the primary prevention of ovarian cancer because the other factors associated with altered risk are not routinely subject to modification. Hartge et al (1994) estimate that more than half the incidences of ovarian cancer in the United States might not have occurred if the patients had used oral contraceptives for at least 4 years. Thus, oral contraceptives appear to be a powerful primary preventive measure against ovarian cancer.

Surgical Prevention of Ovarian Cancer

Approximately 7% of patients with ovarian cancer have a positive family history for it, and 3% to 9% of that group may have a hereditary cancer syndrome. Women with hereditary cancer syndrome of germline BRCA1 mutation have as much as a 50% lifetime risk for ovarian cancer. Because of this high risk, prophylactic oophorectomy after childbearing or the age of 35 to 40 years is reasonable and indicated. In the group at moderate risk, which includes women with at least one affected first- or second-degree relative (without an autosomal dominant mode of transmission), the risk-benefit ratio is less clear. The morbidity and mortality associated with surgical intervention, castration, and hormone replacement therapy may or may not be justified, and patient-by-patient analysis is required.

CLASSIFICATION

The most useful classification system for ovarian neoplasms is based on the cell of origin (histology is the basis on which this chapter is organized). An abbreviated version of the World Health Organization's classification system for ovarian tumors is presented in Box 9-1. This system assigns ovarian neoplasm to one of five major categories:

I. *Epithelial tumors:* Serous, mucinous, endometrioid, clear cell, Brenner-transitional cell, mixed mesodermal, and undifferentiated tumors are considered epithelial tumors and account for approximately 70% of all ovarian neoplasms.

II. *Stromal tumors:* Approximately 5% to 10% of all ovarian neoplasms are derived from ovarian stromal cells. These include granulosa stromal cell tumor, Sertoli stromal cell tumor, sex cord tumor with annular tubules, Leydig cell tumor, lipid cell tumor, and gynandroblastoma.

III. *Germ cell tumors:* Approximately 15% to 20% of all ovarian neoplasms are of germ cell origin. This includes dysgerminoma, endodermal sinus tumor, embryonal carcinoma, polyembryoma, choriocarcinoma, teratoma, mixed forms, and gonadoblastoma.

BOX 9-1
MODIFIED WORLD HEALTH ORGANIZATION COMPREHENSIVE CLASSIFICATION OF OVARIAN TUMORS

I. Common "epithelial" tumors
  A. Serous
  B. Mucinous
  C. Endometrioid
  D. Clear cell
  E. Brenner
  F. Transitional
  G. Small cell
  H. Malignant mixed mesodermal
  I. Unclassified
II. Sex cord stromal tumors
  A. Granulosa stromal cell
    1. Granulosa cell
    2. Thecoma-fibroma
  B. Sertoli stromal cell
    1. Sertoli cell tumors
    2. Sertoli-Leydig cell tumors
      a. well differentiated
      b. intermediately differentiated
      c. poorly differentiated
      d. with heterologous elements
    3. Sex cord tumor with annular tubules (SCTAT)
    4. Leydig (hilus) cell tumors
  C. Lipid (lipoid) cell tumors
  D. Gynandroblastoma
III. Germ cell tumors
  A. Dysgerminoma
  B. Endodermal sinus tumor
  C. Embryonal carcinoma
  D. Polyembryoma
  E. Choriocarcinoma
  F. Teratomas
    1. Immature
    2. Mature (dermoid cyst)
    3. Monodermal (struma ovarii, carcinoid)
  G. Mixed forms
  H. Gonadoblastoma
IV. Metastatic
V. Other

IV. *Metastatic tumors:* Approximately 5% of ovarian malignancies are metastatic, most commonly from the breast or bowel.

V. *Other:* A small but significant number of ovarian "neoplasms" result from ovarian soft tissue or nonneoplastic processes.

SYMPTOMS

Irrespective of histology, most ovarian neoplasms cause symptoms by exerting pressure on the contiguous structures.

Table 9-1   Distribution of Symptoms in Women with Ovarian Carcinoma

Symptom	Symptom Noticed %	(N)	Symptom Convinced Patient to Seek Diagnosis %	(N)
Abdominal swelling	70.4	(38)	63.9	(23)
Fatigue	55.6	(30)	37.0	(11)
Abdominal pain	48.1	(26)	87.0	(20)
Urination problems	37.0	(20)	52.6	(10)
Indigestion	25.9	(14)	46.2	(6)
Irregular vaginal bleeding	22.2	(12)	66.7	(8)
Shortness of breath	22.2	(12)	45.5	(5)
Menorrhagia	18.9	(10)	50.0	(5)
Constipation/diarrhea	18.5	(10)	20.0	(2)
Appetite loss	18.5	(10)	30.0	(3)

From Smith EM, Andersen B: The effects of symptoms and delay in seeking diagnosis on stage of disease at diagnosis, among women with cancers of the ovary. *Cancer* 1985; 56:2727.

Pressure symptoms include urinary frequency, pelvic discomfort, and constipation. As the tumor enlarges, abdominal swelling is the most common symptom. Acute abdominal pain secondary to hemorrhage, rupture with leakage, or torsion can all result from tumor growth. Upper abdominal metastases or ascites cause nausea, heartburn, bloating, weight loss, and anorexia, symptoms usually associated with gastrointestinal processes. Irregular vaginal bleeding can accompany any type of ovarian neoplasm. Among patients with ascites or hydrothorax, shortness of breath can be the presenting symptom. Smith and Anderson (1985) review 83 patients with invasive epithelial ovarian carcinoma and find that the most common symptoms, regardless of stage, are abdominal swelling, fatigue, and abdominal pain (Table 9-1). Contrary to popular belief, the authors find that early-stage cancers do produce symptoms. Of the broad range of secondary symptoms, only menstrual irregularity is likely to convince patients with early-stage disease to see a physician. Late-stage disease is most often accompanied by abdominal pain and swelling, but only pain is likely to convince women to seek a diagnosis.

Biologically active hormones, including estrogen, progesterone, testosterone, corticosteroids, and human chorionic gonadotropin (hCG), may be produced by a variety of ovarian neoplasms and may cause the predicted symptoms associated with each compound. Teratomas may cause autoimmune hemolytic anemia by an unknown mechanism of action and may contain thyroid tissue, which may produce a hyperthyroid state. Hypercalcemia is a paraneoplastic syndrome associated with several gynecologic malignancies, including ovarian carcinoma.

PHYSICAL FINDINGS

A complete physical examination is imperative when evaluating a patient with a known or suspected pelvic mass, keeping in mind the differential diagnosis. Careful breast examination in the sitting and the supine positions is important. Abdominal examination, including palpation of all four quadrants, can diagnose ascites or an upper abdominal mass. All lymph node–bearing tissue, including axillary nodes, should be palpated carefully. Pleural effusions, a frequent finding among patients with ovarian cancer, are diagnosed with auscultation of both lungs. Examination of the lower extremities can reveal tenderness and a cord, indicating a deep vein thrombosis, which can be the presenting symptom in a patient with a pelvic mass.

Pelvic examination is the most important part of the physical diagnosis of a pelvic mass. Vulva, vagina, and cervix must be inspected first; any disease process or displacement secondary to a mass can then be sought. Rectal examination is an obligatory component of routine pelvic examination. Not only is it necessary to evaluate the posterior uterine surface, uterosacral ligaments, cul-de-sac of Douglas, and parametria, it is also necessary to screen for colorectal cancer. An occult stool guaiac should always be checked; if it is positive, the American Cancer Society recommends a screening flexible sigmoidoscopy or a full colonoscopy. Defining the size and the location of the uterus is important because adnexal masses often are enlarged uteri. Palpation of both adnexa should be carefully undertaken. In premenopausal women, the ovaries measure approximately 3 × 2 × 2 cm. In postmenopausal women, they should measure approximately 2 × 1 × 0.5 cm, the size of an almond. If no mass is palpated but the patient has symptoms, radiographic evaluation is appropriate (see below).

DIFFERENTIAL DIAGNOSIS OF ADNEXAL MASS
Nongynecologic
Diverticular Disease

Diverticulitis complicated by a sigmoid colon phlegmon or a pericolonic abscess may seem to be a pelvic mass, especially in postmenopausal women. The most common symptoms are left lower quadrant pain and obstipation. In addition to the mass, examination reveals toxicity, fever, localizing peritonitis, and leukocytosis. In patients with acute disease, this diagnosis is best confirmed by an abdominal-pelvic CT scan.

Appendiceal Abscess

Appendicitis complicated by an appendiceal abscess may appear as a right-sided pelvic mass. This is commonly found in women of childbearing age. Increasing right lower quadrant pain, anorexia, fever, tender right lower-quadrant mass, localizing peritonitis, fluctuant mass palpated on rectal examination, and leukocytosis all point to the diagnosis. An abdominal CT scan and a barium enema are often useful in confirming this diagnosis.

Crohn Disease

Regional enteritis, or Crohn disease, also may appear to be a pelvic or an abdominal mass. Because of the early age of onset of Crohn disease, secondary pelvic or abdominal masses are most common in women in the second and third decades of life. As in diverticular disease, a mass secondary to Crohn disease represents either a phlegmon or a perienteric abscess. The most common site of this disease is the terminal ileum, though any portion of the gastrointestinal tract may be involved. The patient with a Crohn-related abscess or a phlegmon often has had chronic diarrhea, weight loss, and abdominal pain and appears acutely ill with fever, localizing tenderness, and leukocytosis. Full gastrointestinal tract evaluation with a barium enema and an upper gastrointestinal series with a small bowel follow-through are essential for evaluating this disease. In addition, an abdominal CT scan may be helpful in the work-up of a patient with abscess or phlegmon secondary to Crohn disease (Schwartz, 1994).

Primary Nongynecologic Malignancy

Lymphomas, retroperitoneal tumors, small bowel tumors, and mesothelial tumors are rare pelvic malignancies that are easily confused with gynecologic neoplasms. Gynecologic neoplasms are almost always accurately diagnosed at laparotomy. Colorectal cancer is the second most commonly diagnosed visceral cancer in the United States and must always be kept in mind when evaluating a pelvic mass, especially in postmenopausal women. The American Cancer Society recommends that patients older than 50 years undergo screening flexible sigmoidoscopy every 3 to 5 years. Symptoms depend on tumor size and location and commonly include a change in bowel habits, pain, and hematochezia. On physical examination, rectal lesions and metastases to the ovaries can sometimes be palpated. If fecal occult blood is present, a screening evaluation for colorectal cancer should be undertaken before any other procedure.

Pelvic Kidney

In the general population, the incidence of pelvic kidney is 1:20,000. That rate increases to 7% to 15% in women with vaginal agenesis. With this in mind, any patient with a gynecologic malformation should undergo a complete urologic work-up that includes an intravenous pyelogram and, if indicated, cystoscopy and retrograde pyelography.

Gynecologic
Tuboovarian Abscess

Pelvic inflammatory disease followed by the development of a tuboovarian abscess almost always results from a sexually transmitted infectious disease, such as gonorrhea or chlamydia. Instrumentation (therapeutic abortion) can also be the initiating event. Symptoms usually are fever, bilateral pelvic pain, and vaginal discharge. On physical examination, cervi-

cal motion tenderness, bilateral adnexal tenderness, and cervical discharge are often found. Broad antibiotic coverage should be initiated and sometimes followed by exploration and removal of the abscess. Total abdominal hysterectomy/bilateral salpingo-oophorectomy (TAH/BSO) may be required. Drainage under CT guidance has been shown to be effective in some patients.

Ectopic Pregnancy

Ectopic pregnancy continues to be a major cause of maternal death in the United States. Its incidence has risen during the past decade. The triad of irregular menses, unilateral adnexal pain, and adnexal mass, combined with a positive urine or serum hCG level, signifies ectopic pregnancy unless proven otherwise.

Leiomyoma

A pedunculated uterine leiomyoma or a primary ovarian leiomyoma can appear as an adnexal mass.

Fallopian Tube "Neoplasia"

Benign and malignant processes of the fallopian tube appear as adnexal masses and can be confused with ovarian masses.

OVARIAN NEOPLASM
Differential Diagnoses of Ovarian Mass
Germ Cell Tumors

Germ cell tumors are principally diseases of young women. Among ovarian masses, they are second in frequency (15% to 20%) to epithelial tumors. Because the mean age of occurrence is 19 years, interest in improving survival rates and in maintaining childbearing potential is keen. The clinical presentation, histology, and biology are varied in this group of tumors; benign and malignant neoplasms are included. Figure 9-1 outlines the accepted derivation of germ cell tumors (Teilium, 1971). Gonadoblastoma is the benign tumor of greatest interest because of its frequent association with malignant germ cell tumors. Gonadoblastoma and dysgerminoma are most often associated with dysgenetic gonads and the presence of a Y chromosome.

The most common type of malignant germ cell tumor is dysgerminoma. In descending order of frequency, the other types are mixed carcinoma, endodermal sinus carcinoma, immature teratoma, embryonal carcinoma, and choriocarcinoma.

Benign Germ Cell Tumors

Gonadoblastoma. Gonadoblastoma is almost always found in patients with gonadal dysgenesis associated with a Y chromosome or Y-chromosome fragment. Although this tumor is benign, it is associated with a malignant germ cell tumor in approximately 40% of patients. Karyotyping should be undertaken in anyone with primary or secondary amenorrhea and abnormal sexual development (lack of secondary sexual characteristics, infantile external and internal genitalia, atrophic vaginal mucosa). Prompt bilateral go-

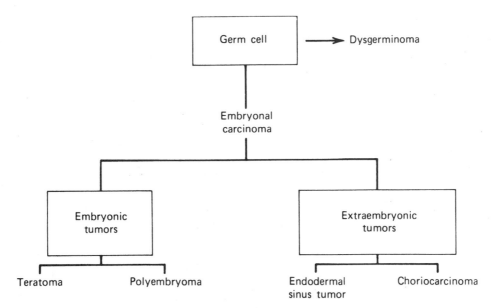

Fig. 9-1. Germ cell tumor derivation. (From Teilum G: *Special tumors of ovary and testis, and related extragonadal lesions: Comparative pathology and histologic identification,* ed 2, Philadelphia, 1977, JB Lippincott.)

nadectomy is indicated if a Y chromosome is present, except in patients with testicular feminization (androgen insensitivity syndrome) (Trochev and Hernandez, 1986). Among patients with testicular feminization, the removal of both gonads can be delayed up to age 30 years because the risk for cancer is low before that time.

Teratomas. A single totipotential germ cell gives rise to a teratoma. This neoplasm is characterized by the presence of all three germ cell layers: ectoderm, mesoderm, and endoderm. Teratomas can be malignant or benign, as determined by the presence of immature tissue.

The most common benign teratoma is the "cystic teratoma," or "dermoid cyst." This tumor accounts for 25% to 40% of all ovarian neoplasms. Most teratomas are diagnosed in premenopausal women, who will have no symptoms at the time of diagnosis. Torsion and rupture rarely occur, but they cause acute peritonitis and necessitate prompt exploratory laparotomy. Physical examination reveals an adnexal mass that is bilateral in approximately 12% to 15% of patients. Dermoids are often diagnosed by ultrasonography or plain abdominal radiography (Fig. 9-2). Gross examination usually reveals a prominent cavity with skin, teeth, bones, hair, and extremities. Rokitansky's protuberance is the part of the dermoid that contains the greatest variety of tissue. Histologic examination reveals only mature adult tissue (Fig. 9-3).

The risk for malignancy in a dermoid is small (approximately 1% to 2%) and usually occurs in postmenopausal women. Squamous cell carcinoma is the most common type of malignancy found in a dermoid; this is followed by carcinoid tumor.

Struma ovarii is a dermoid in which thyroid tissue comprises more than 50% of the teratoma. This is unusual oc-

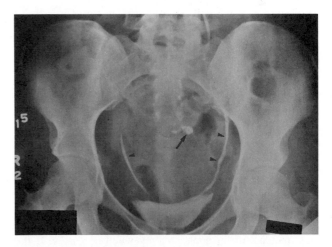

Fig. 9-2. Plain radiograph during intravenous pyelography demonstrates a calcific density overlying the sacrum *(arrow),* which represents a tooth formed within a dermoid tumor. Note also the ureters *(arrowheads).*

currence and accounts for only 2.7% of ovarian teratomas. On microscopic examination, mature thyroid tissue of any type can be found (Fig. 9-4). Rarely is there an associated hyperthyroidism.

Primary ovarian carcinoid is rare. When it does develop, it is usually unilateral; this is in contrast to metastatic carcinoid, which is almost always bilateral. Argentaffin cells, present in a dermoid, are usually the site of origin for ovarian carcinoid. Struma ovarii is a teratoma in which thyroid tissue develops in association with carcinoid, usually trabecular.

Management of benign teratomas. Laparoscopy or laparotomy can be used to remove dermoids by cystectomy in

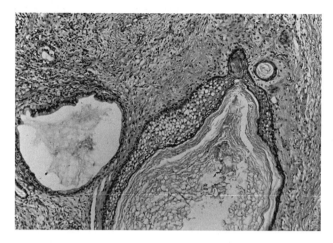

Fig. 9-3. Mature teratoma containing cysts lined by squamous and glandular epithelia of a mature adult type in a benign fibrous stroma.

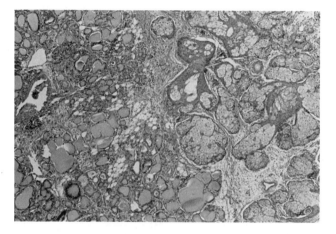

Fig. 9-4. Mature teratoma containing sebaceous epithelium and follicles of thyroid-type epithelium (struma ovarii).

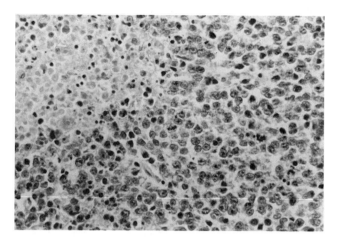

Fig. 9-5. Anaplastic dysgerminoma consisting of sheets of neoplastic cells with numerous mitotic figures and areas of necrosis but no evidence of differentiation. Lymphocytes are commonly seen with this tumor, but they are not obvious here.

most patients or by oophorectomy when necessary. If the dermoid is larger than 6 cm or the patient has undergone multiple surgical procedures with adhesions, laparotomy is the preferred treatment approach. A frozen section should be obtained in all patients. Although careful attention should be given to the other ovary because of the 12% rate for bilateral occurrence, routine bivalves for a normal-appearing ovary are not indicated.

Malignant Germ Cell Tumors

Dysgerminoma. Dysgerminoma is the most common germ cell malignancy; it accounts for 35% to 45% of all germ cell tumors. On gross examination, this tumor appears lobulated, solid, and fleshy, and it usually has a smooth external surface. Histologic examination reveals aggregates of large homogeneous polygonal cells that are its distinguishing features (Fig. 9-5). Lymphocyte infiltration and delicate fibrous septa are common.

This tumor is bilateral in approximately 10% to 15% of patients. Dysgerminomas metastasize lymphatically, not hematogenously, which makes them unique among ovarian tumors. The survival rate for patients with early stage disease is greater than 95% (Thomas et al, 1987). Even patients with advanced stage disease have favorable prognoses greater than 80% when appropriate adjuvant therapy is given.

Serum lactic dehydrogenase (LDH), specifically the fast fraction, can serve as a useful tumor marker. If it is a marker, it usually is greatly elevated (Awais, 1983). Serum hCG levels are elevated in a small number of patients as well.

Endodermal sinus tumors. Endodermal sinus tumor (EST), also known as yolk sac tumor, is an extremely aggressive malignancy, the histology of which previously predicted a uniformly poor outcome. Gross examination reveals that the external surface of this tumor is usually smooth and glistening; hemorrhage and necrosis are prominent features. Histologic examination reveals several distinguishing features, including intracellular and extracellular hyaline droplets (periodic acid-Schiff positive), a reticular growth pattern, and the famous Schiller-Duval bodies (a central capillary surrounded by simple papillae) (Fig. 9-6) (Teilum, 1959). This tumor is almost never bilateral. Intraperitoneal and hematogenous spread are common; lymph node metastasis is unusual. Commonly these patients present with an acute condition in the abdomen, secondary to spontaneous rupture and hemorrhage. Although the survival rate for patients with stage I or II endodermal sinus tumors ranges from 60% to 100%, patients with stage III or IV disease have a survival rate that ranges from 50% to 75% after appropriate chemotherapy. Platinum-based chemotherapy has significantly improved the survival rates of patients with EST.

Most ESTs secrete α-fetoprotein (AFP) and occasionally α_1-antitrypsin. Checking AFP serum levels can be useful when monitoring a patient's response to therapy and predicting a recurrence.

Immature teratomas. Immature teratomas comprise approximately 20% of all malignant germ cell tumors. Al-

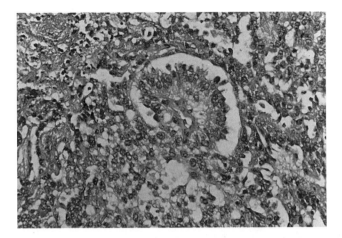

Fig. 9-6. Yolk sac tumor containing a well-formed Schiller-Duval body with a central papillary tuft surrounded by a glomerulus-like space.

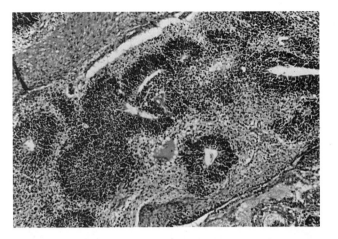

Fig. 9-7. Immature teratoma containing neural-type tissue forming primitive neural tubules.

though the three germ cell layers contain immature tissue, the amount of immature glial tissue is the most important for prognosis (Fig. 9-7). Grade 1 teratoma has no more than one focus of immature neuroepithelium per low-power (×40) field. Grade 2 teratoma has immature neuroepithelium, but not in excess of three low-power fields in any one slide. All grade 3 lesions have immature glial tissue in four or more low-power fields within individual sections. Spontaneous maturation of extraovarian glial implants is a unique feature of immature teratomas called gliomatosis peritonei, and it has been associated with a favorable outcome (Nielson et al, 1985). After grade, surgicopathologic stage is the most important prognostic factor. Although the survival rate for patients with stage I, grade 1 lesions is 100%, it falls to 50% for patients with stage III, grade 1 tumors. Fortunately, the disease is usually detected in the early stages. Occasionally, immature teratomas can produce AFP that can be used as a tumor marker, and the same is true for serum LDH and CA-125. Serum hCG is never produced by this tumor.

Embryonal carcinoma. Embryonal carcinoma is rare. On gross examination, it resembles a larger version of EST. Histologic examination reveals embryonal glands, glandlike clefts (embryoid bodies), and syntrophoblastic giant cells. The tumor is rarely bilateral, and it tends to spread intraperitoneally. Survival rates are slightly better than those for EST using the same platinum-based chemotherapy regimens. Both AFP and hCG can serve as tumor markers for this germ cell tumor.

Choriocarcinoma. Nongestational choriocarcinoma of the ovary is rare. It has the same histologic appearance as gestational choriocarcinoma. Approximately 50% of prepubertal girls with nongestational choriocarcinoma are isosexually precocious. Serum hCG is produced by this type of germ cell tumor, as it is in gestational choriocarcinoma, and can serve as a useful tumor marker. Although gestational choriocarcinoma is usually treated successfully by chemotherapy, remission is less common among patients with nongestational choriocar-

cinoma. Since the advent of platinum-based chemotherapy, there have been reports of sustained remission among patients with ovarian choriocarcinoma.

Mixed germ cell tumor. In 10% to 15% of germ cell tumors, more than one histologic type is present. The most commmon combination is dysgerminoma with EST, followed by immature teratomas with EST. Embryonal carcinoma and choriocarcinoma are found less often. The relative amount of the more malignant component and the stage will determine the prognosis. The prognosis for a mixed EST tumor is better than the prognosis for a pure EST tumor. Tumor marker or markers depend on the types of germ cell elements present.

Polyembryoma. Polyembryoma is another rare germ cell tumor. Histologically, it resembles embryoid bodies in different stages of presomite development. There are few reports of chemotherapy-induced remission.

Management of malignant germ cell tumors

Dysgerminomas. Fortunately, most patients with dysgerminoma have stage I disease. Unilateral oophorectomy alone is adequate for cure. Careful inspection of the opposite ovary, with biopsy specimens taken of any suspicious areas, is important because of the risk for overt and covert bilateralism. Because of its tendency for lymph node metastases, formal staging, including retroperitoneal lymphadenectomy, should be performed in every patient with dysgerminoma. All patients with disease advanced beyond stage I should undergo cytoreductive surgery and additional therapy (Thomas et al, 1987). Although it has been suggested that patients with stage I disease whose primary tumors are larger than 10 to 15 cm receive adjuvant therapy, this has not been supported in several large series. Dysgerminomas are exquisitely sensitive to radiation, and this has been a mainstay of therapy for patients with metastatic dysgerminoma (Bjorkholm et al, 1990). However, preservation of ovarian function and fertility is almost always of major importance in these primarily young patients. Because of this and the success of chemotherapy in treating men with seminomas (the male analogue to the female dysgerminoma), chemotherapy has replaced radiation therapy as the treatment of choice. Schwartz et al (1990) find advanced-stage dysgerminomas to be markedly sensitive to vincristine, dactinomycin, and cyclophosphamide (VAC). Other authors find that vinblastine, bleomycin, and cisplatin (VBP) or bleomycin, etoposide, and cisplatin (BEP) induce a complete response in a greater number of patients (Gershenson et al, 1990). Etoposide and cisplatin (EP) alone have been used with great success and is considered by many to be the regimen of choice (Bajorin et al, 1991).

Nondysgerminomatous malignancies. Unilateral tumors are the rule in nondysgerminomatous germ cell malignancies. Because of this, unilateral oophorectomy should be performed. This would preserve the contralateral ovary, as long as it appears normal, for hormone production and future childbearing potential. Staging is important and should include retroperitoneal lymph node dissection, intraperitoneal biopsy, and omentectomy. Although lymph node metastases are unusual, the possibility always exists that dysgerminomatous elements are present (mixed germ cell tumor) but were missed on frozen-section analysis. Cytoreductive surgery for advanced disease should be undertaken when possible.

As it has for patients with testicular germ cell tumors, platinum-based combination chemotherapy has had a significant impact on the survival rates of patients with nondysgerminomatous ovarian germ cell malignancies. The only patients who do not require postoperative chemotherapy are those with immature teratomas, stage IA, grade 1. All other patients, regardless of histology, undergo either adjuvant or curative chemotherapy. Although VAC used to be the combination of choice, platinum-based regimens consisting of VPB, BEP, or EP have shown superior results (Bajorin et al, 1991; Gershenson et al, 1990).

Maintaining future childbearing potential is a major issue for many of these young patients, as it is for patients with dysgerminoma. Gershenson et al (1998) find that the majority of women undergoing chemotherapy for ovarian germ cell tumors resume normal menses after successful chemotherapy. The benefit of oral contraceptives in preventing ovarian dysfunction for patients undergoing chemotherapy has not been established.

Second-look surgery for germ cell tumors is of limited value. Gershenson et al (1986) observe that 52 of 53 second-look surgeries were negative; only 1 of 52 patients had recurrent disease and died (Gershenson, 1986). With the useful tumor markers and radiographic examinations available, this type of surgery is rarely indicated.

Sex Cord Stromal Tumors

The gonadal stroma of the ovary gives rise to approximately 5% of all ovarian neoplasms. The primitive gonadal stroma has the potential to develop in either a male or a female direction. Although hormone production by stromal tumors is common and includes the production of estrogen, proges-

terone, testosterone, other androgenic compounds, and corticosteroids, it is not consistent and cannot be used as a means to classify this group of neoplasms. Most of these stromal tumors are granulosa-theca cell tumors, female directed.

Granulosa Stromal Tumor

Adult granulosa cell tumors. The presence of granulosa cells alone or in combination with theca elements defines adult granulosa cell tumor (GCT). The term *thecoma* or *theca cell tumor* should be used exclusively for tumors consisting only of theca cells. Excess estrogen production is often found in both tumor types, causing isosexual precocious puberty in young women and menometrorrhagia in menstruating and postmenopausal women. Endometrial hyperplasia or carcinoma rates are as high as 60% among patients with this tumor. More than 50% of GCTs develop in postmenopausal women; less than 5% develop in prepubertal girls. Rupture with intraabdominal bleeding is commonly the symptom that causes them to seek treatment. Different microscopic patterns have been described, including microfollicular, macrofollicular, trabecular, insular, and diffuse. Histologic features associated with a poor prognosis include diffuse growth pattern, increased mitotic figures, and cellular atypia. Call-Exner bodies are pathognomonic of this tumor type and are present in the microfollicular pattern (Fig. 9-8).

Granulosa cell tumors are indolent, and, if clinically confined to the ovary, they infrequently relapse and are rarely lethal (Stenwig et al, 1979). In one report of 118 patients, 10% have stage III disease, none have stage IV disease, and only 6.2% have stage IA1 disease and die of it (Evans et al, 1980). In contrast, 54% of patients with stage III disease die. The average time between the initial diagnosis and the first recurrence is 6 years, but one patient had a recurrence 23 years after diagnosis. Seventy-two percent of patients who have recurrences die of the disease. This tumor often produces estradiol or inhibin, which can serve as a useful tumor marker. Levels of estradiol greater than 30 pg in postmenopausal women are abnormal and represent exogenous tumor production.

Juvenile granulosa cell tumors. Juvenile GCT differs from the adult type in clinical and pathologic features (Table 9-2). As with adult GCTs, bilaterality is rare and most patients have stage IA disease. Young et al (1984) review 125 patients with juvenile GCT. The mortality rate is 1.5% for patients with stage IA disease, but there is a tenfold increase for the unusual patient whose disease has advanced beyond stage IA.

Fibromas. Fibromas are almost always unilateral and are often diagnosed in the fifth decade of life. Hormone production is unusual, but if it takes place, estrogen is the most common compound produced. Fibromas with ascites and hydrothorax signify Meigs syndrome, which can easily be mistaken for ovarian malignancy (Meigs et al, 1943).

Fibromas are benign tumors; less than 1% have increased mitotic activity. If there are fewer than three mitoses per high-power field, the tumor is considered low grade and is called a cellular fibroma. If there are more than three mitoses per high-power field, it is considered a fibrosarcoma.

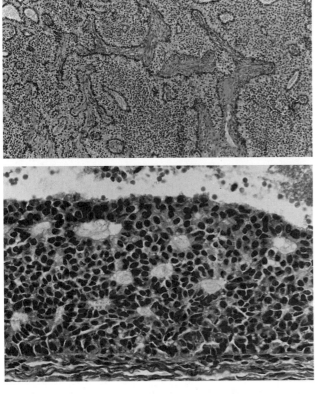

Fig. 9-8. A, Ovarian granulosa cell tumor consisting of well-differentiated granulosa cells with prominent cytoplasm. The complex cell nests show peripheral nuclear pallisading. **B,** Granulosa cell tumor containing multiple-cell Exner bodies consisting of extracellular spaces surrounded by neoplastic granulosa cells.

Table 9-2   Differences Between Adult and Juvenile Granulosa Cell Tumor

Adult	Juvenile
Less than 1% prepubertal	50% prepubertal
Usual after 30 years of age	Rare after 30 years of age
Follicles usually regular, without mucin; Call-Exner bodies common	Follicles often irregular, contain mucin; Call-Exner bodies rare
Nuclei pale, commonly grooved	Nuclei dark, rarely grooved
Luteinization infrequent	Luteinization frequent
Recurrence rarely early, often very late	Recurrence typically early

From Young RH, Dickersin GR, Scully RE: Juvenile granulosa cell tumor of the ovary: A clinicopathological anaylsis of 125 cases. *Am J Surg Pathol* 1984; 8:575.

In each case the tumor is usually larger than a benign fibroma and carries a worse prognosis.

Thecomas. Thecomas are similar to fibromas and often cannot be distinguished from them. The important clinical difference is that in general thecomas produce excess estrogen, which causes postmenopausal bleeding, menorrhagia, amenorrhea, and endometrial hyperplasia or cancer. Gross examination reveals that they are solid, yellow-orange tumors. It is unusual for a theca cell tumor to be malignant. The same criteria should be used to define malignant thecoma as are used to define ovarian fibrosarcoma.

Sertoli Stromal Cell Tumors. *Arrhenoblastoma* and *androblastoma* are dated terms to describe this group of neoplasms. They represent sex cord stromal tumors that exhibit a testicular or male direction of differentiation. This rare group of tumors represents less than 1% of all ovarian neoplasms. Although many of these neoplasms produce androgen, some are hormonally inert and produce estrogen only occasionally.

Sertoli cell tumors. A pure Sertoli cell tumor of the ovary is composed only of Sertoli cells in a tubular arrangement. Leydig cells produce androgens. This makes the diagnosis of a pure Sertoli cell tumor unlikely if there is virilization. This tumor is rarely malignant, but the associated features include large size, infiltration of the stroma with cells, increased mitotic activity, and hemorrhage with necrosis.

Sertoli-Leydig cell tumors. The Sertoli-Leydig cell tumors, also known as arrhenoblastoma, are the most common Sertoli stromal cell tumors. Both Sertoli and Leydig cells are present.

Approximately 40% of patients show evidence of excess androgen production, or virilization. There is excess estrogen production in a small percentage of patients, whereas some are hormonally inert. These tumors are almost always unilateral and occur most often in the third decade of life. The World Health Organization divides them into four microscopic categories: (1) well-differentiated (predominant tubular pattern); (2) intermediate differentiation (sheets of immature Sertoli cells with some stroma); (3) poor differentiation (immature Sertoli cells with little or no stroma); and (4) containing heterologous elements. Heterologous elements, which appear in 15% of patients, have a retiform pattern and connote a worse prognosis. Young and Scully (1985), in a review of 207 patients with Sertoli-Leydig cell tumors, found that 97.5% had a stage I tumor and only 2.5% had advanced-stage disease. Prognosis correlates most meaningfully with the stage and the degree of differentiation of the tumor. All well-differentiated tumors are benign, but 11% of those of intermediate differentiation, 59% of poor differentiation, and 19% of those with heterologous elements are malignant.

Conservative surgery with preservation of some ovarian tissue is appropriate for most patients with early-stage disease. In those patients with intermediate or poor differentiation or high-stage tumors, postoperative adjuvant therapy may be indicated.

Sex cord tumors with annular tubules. Histologic examination reveals that this tumor is characterized by simple and complex annular tubules. It is rarely associated with malignant adenoma of the cervix. In 30% of patients, it is associated with Peutz-Jeghers syndrome (gastrointestinal polyposis with oral mucocutaneous lesions). In spite of this,

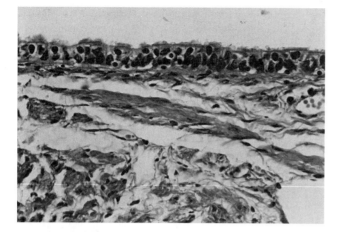

Fig. 9-9. High magnification shows that this serous cystadenoma is lined with ciliated tubal-type epithelium.

the tumor is usually bilateral, small, and benign. When not associated with this syndrome, it is usually unilateral and large, and it is malignant in 20% of patients. Young et al (1982), in a review of 74 patients with sex cord tumor with annular tubules, observe that 27 patients with this type of tumor have Peutz-Jeghers syndrome and small bilateral, benign tumors.

Leydig (hilus) cell tumors. Only Leydig cells coalesce in this tumor. When they are located exclusively in the hilus, the term *hilus cell tumor* is applied. This tumor develops in patients with a mean age of 50 years, and it almost always is benign. The presence of Reinke crystals differentiates this lesion histologically from lipid cell tumors. Most of these tumors produce testosterone, and patients have the associated features of virilization.

Lipid (Lipoid) Cell Tumors. Round Leydig-like cells, luteinized stroma, adrenocortical cells, and the absence of Reinke crystals points to the diagnosis of a lipid cell tumor. These tumors are typically virilizing. Occasionally, they produce such hormones as estradiol, estrone, and cortisol. Approximately 10% of patients have Cushing syndrome, which is clinically evident as obesity, hypertension, and glucose intolerance. In contrast to Leydig cell tumors, 20% of lipid cell tumors metastasize. No effective therapy is available to treat metastatic disease.

Gynandroblastoma. The diagnosis of gynandroblastoma should be limited to the rare ovarian tumors that contain significant components of granulosa stromal cells and Sertoli stromal cells. Androgen or estrogen may be produced, and the behavior of the tumor is dependent on the individual components.

Evaluation and management of sex cord stromal tumors. The preoperative evaluation of a pelvic mass thought to be a sex cord stromal tumor is similar to the evaluation of any type of ovarian mass, with two notable exceptions. First, if there is evidence of excess estrogen production, an endometrial biopsy specimen should be obtained before lap-

arotomy. In the event that endometrial carcinoma is found, consideration must be given to performing a TAH. Second, if androgen excess is evident, the differential diagnoses include adrenal tumor and ovarian tumor. This is particularly important if there is no ovarian enlargement. Generally, an elevated serum dehydroepiandrosterone level points to an adrenal source, whereas an elevated serum testosterone level most likely indicates an ovarian source. Radiographic evaluation of the adrenals and the ovaries is appropriate.

The surgical management of patients with sex cord stromal tumors is age dependent. For women beyond the childbearing years, TAH/BSO is appropriate. In younger women interested in preserving childbearing potential, unilateral oophorectomy should be performed. If the pathologist is confident of the diagnosis of a sex cord stromal tumor, peritoneal washings, selective biopsies, subtotal omentectomy, exploration for intraabdominal and retroperitoneal metastases, and careful inspection of the opposite ovary are indicated. In some patients, germ cell tumor cannot be ruled out after frozen-section analysis, and retroperitoneal lymphadenectomy should be performed.

Data are limited on treating patients with advanced or recurrent stromal tumors because of the rarity, multihistologic patterns, and indolent behavior of these tumors. Even less information is available regarding which patients should receive adjuvant therapy. Gershenson et al (1987) report on using cisplatin, doxorubicin, and cyclophosphamide to treat patients with metastatic stromal tumors, and they find a 63% overall response rate. Other combination chemotherapy regimens have been used and have yielded a small number of complete responses in each group. In several small series, pelvic radiation has been found helpful for patients with localized sex cord stromal tumors. Larger prospective studies are needed to assess fully the antitumor activity of chemotherapy against this group of tumors.

Although estradiol level has been a useful tumor marker in many patients with granulosa stromal cell tumors, testosterone level has been of benefit in some patients with Sertoli stromal cell tumors. Inhibin is reported to be a useful tumor marker in patients with granulosa cell tumors (Lappohn et al, 1989).

Epithelial Ovarian Neoplasia

Almost 85% of all ovarian malignancies are derived from ovarian epithelium, making epithelial malignancies the most commonly encountered ovarian cancer. Usually, each histologic subtype can be classified as benign, borderline, or malignant. Before discussing clinical features and management, each histologic subtype will be detailed.

Issues Specific to Histologic Type

Serous. Benign serous tumors are usually loculated, and they usually have a single layer of flattened or cuboidal epithelium (Fig. 9-9). Papillae may appear on the external and internal surfaces, making it difficult during gross examination to distinguish this benign tumor from malignant neoplasm. Mitoses are absent.

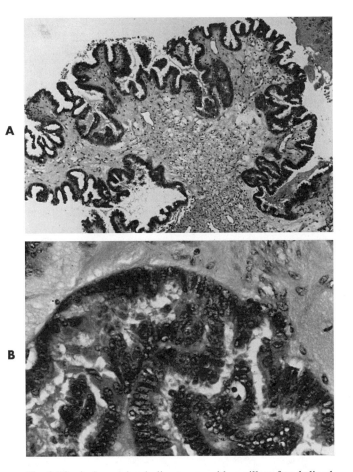

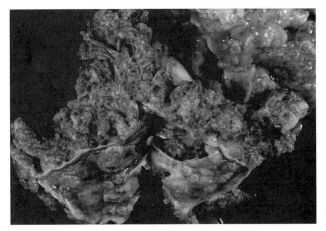

Fig. 9-11. Serous papillary adenocarcinoma produces a cauliflower-like exophytic mass that predominantly involves the surface of the bisected ovary.

Fig. 9-10. A, Serous borderline tumor with papillary fronds lined by mildly atypical serous-type epithelium. There is no stromal invasion. **B,** Borderline serous tumor lined with tubular-type epithelium showing nuclear pseudostratification and moderate nuclear pleomorphism, without invasion of the underlying stroma.

Borderline serous tumors account for 10% to 15% of all serous neoplasms. Histologic features that distinguish serous tumors of low malignant potential include papillary cystic pattern, stratification, tufting, increased mitotic figures, and cytologic atypia (Fig. 9-10). This tumor occurs bilaterally in approximately 15% to 25% of patients.

Malignant serous tumors of the ovary are the most common malignant ovarian tumors and account for more than 40% of all invasive epithelial carcinomas. As with borderline tumors, they are commonly bilateral. Gross examination reveals that they are cystic, multiloculated tumors with soft, friable papillae (Fig. 9-11). Microscopic examination confirms the grades noted here and reveals significant stromal invasion. Psammoma bodies (calcifications) develop in 32.5% of patients.

Approximately 9% of tumors classified as serous ovarian carcinoma are actually papillary serous carcinoma of the peritoneum. In the latter condition, often the ovaries are of normal size or are slightly enlarged and there is extensive intraabdominal carcinoma. Histologic examination shows that the tumors resemble malignant serous tumors of the ovary,

but only the ovary surface is involved (usually bilaterally). Treatment and prognosis are the same as for serous ovarian carcinoma.

Mucinous. Benign mucinous tumors have a single layer of tall, columnar epithelial cells and clear, mucin-containing cytoplasm (Fig. 9-12). They tend to be larger than serous tumors and are usually smooth.

Mucinous tumors that have low potential for malignancy, otherwise known as borderline tumors, are distinguished by complex patterns, two- to three-cell-layer stratification, cytologic atypia, and mitotic figures (Fig. 9-13). If stratification exceeds three cell layers or if there is significant stromal invasion, the diagnosis of carcinoma should be considered. In a study of 80 patients with borderline ovarian tumors, no tumor advanced beyond stage I disease and none recurred (Rice et al, 1990).

It is reasonable to remove the appendix when a mucinous tumor of the ovary is diagnosed. There is a strong association between appendiceal mucinous neoplasms and mucinous neoplasms of the ovary.

Pseudomyxoma peritonei, defined as the presence of mucinous ascites and peritoneal implants, is associated with appendiceal mucinous neoplasms and mucinous ovarian neoplasms, almost all of which are borderline tumors. The natural history of this clinical syndrome is characterized by persistent recurrences that require laparotomy or peritoneal lavage for the removal of gelatinous material.

Mucinous carcinomas are diagnosed at stage I in approximately 50% of patients. This is in contrast to serous tumors, which are usually diagnosed at advanced stages. On gross examination, mucinous adenocarcinomas are cystic, multiloculated tumors that can be as large as 50 cm in diameter. The differential diagnosis should always include a gastrointestinal malignancy that has metastasized to the ovary. Histologic features of mucinous ovarian adenocarcinomas are depicted

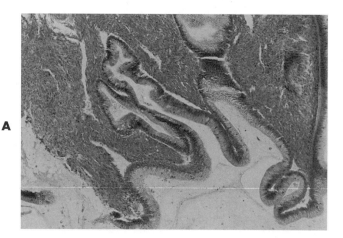

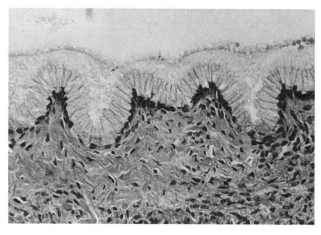

Fig. 9-12. A, Columnar cells with mucin-filled cytoplasm and partially stratified nuclei line this mucinous cystadenoma. B, At high magnification, this mucinous cystadenoma is lined with uniform, tall, columnar cells that resemble normal endocervical epithelium.

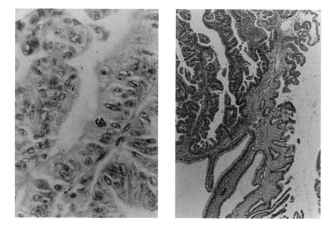

Fig. 9-13. (*left*) Low-power photomicrograph of a borderline mucinous tumor arises in association with a benign mucinous cystadenoma. (*right*) High-power photomicrograph demonstrates stratification, nuclear atypia, and mitotic activity.

in Fig. 9-14. Mucinous tumors of the ovary are the most heterogeneous of the epithelial tumors. Because of this, the pathologist must take a sufficient number of samples.

Endometrioid. Benign endometrioid cysts of the ovary are rare. The most common benign endometrial tumor of the ovary is the adenofibroma, or cystadenofibroma. This tends to develop in older women and can show evidence of epithelial atypia.

Endometrioid borderline tumors of the ovary are rarely reported, but endometrioid carcinoma of the ovary accounts for approximately 10% to 15% of all common epithelial ovarian malignancies. In approximately 20% of patients, there is concurrent endometrial carcinoma. Endometriosis is considered a risk factor for this epithelial type (Heaps et al, 1990). These tumors are usually unilateral, and the microscopic appearance is similar to that of endometrial carcinoma.

Clear cell. Benign or borderline clear cell tumors of the ovary are unusual and are almost always cystadenofibromas. Approximately 5% of ovarian epithelial malignancies are clear cell. An association with endometriosis is reported in

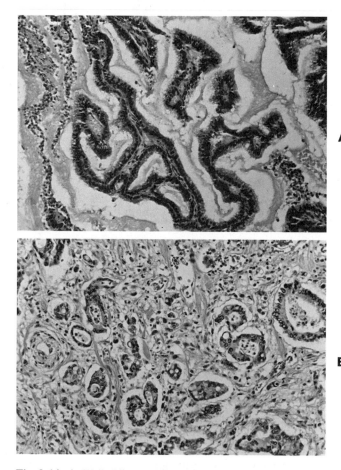

Fig. 9-14. A, Well-differentiated mucinous adenocarcinoma consisting of papillae lined with mucin-secreting cells. B, Mucinous adenocarcinoma consisting of well-formed glands, resembling those of colonic adenocarcinoma, and single malignant cells invading the desmoplastic stroma.

more than 25% of patients. These are large cystic tumors that are bilateral in a small but significant percentage of patients. The most common patterns are tubular glandular, papillary, and cystic. So-called hobnail cells appear in a significant number of patients, but not all. Jenison et al (1989) report on 44 patients with clear cell adenocarcinoma of the ovary (Jenison et al, 1989). Fifty percent of these patients sought treatment at stage I disease. When compared stage for stage with serous tumors, clear cell tumors are uniformly associated with poorer 5-year survival rates. The authors conclude that ovarian clear cell adenocarcinoma has a distinctly different clinical behavior than serous carcinoma and should be regarded as an aggressive epithelial histologic type.

Brenner tumor. Although the cell of origin of Brenner tumor was debated for years, it is now well accepted that it is derived from ovarian epithelium that undergoes metaplasia to assume the appearance of urothelial-like epithelium. This rare tumor is bilateral in only a small percentage of patients, and it tends to occur in premenopausal women. Gross examination reveals that it measures 2 to 8 cm, is solid, and has a white, whirled surface. It is associated with mucinous ovarian tumors in 33% of patients.

The cells resemble coffee beans and have a pronounced longitudinal groove in the nucleus. They form tight nests that are surrounded by bundles of tightly packed stroma. Although Brenner tumors were once considered to be benign, studies conducted in the past several decades establish the existence of proliferative and malignant Brenner tumors. Approximately 30% of patients have advanced-stage disease at diagnosis, and 60% die within 3 years.

Transitional cell carcinoma. The absence of a benign Brenner component separates transitional cell carcinoma (TCC) from malignant Brenner tumor (Austin and Norris, 1987). Both have similar malignant epithelial components that are usually transitional, squamous, or undifferentiated. Malignant Brenner tumors carry a more favorable prognosis than TCC. For patients with focal or predominant TCC, Silva et al (1990) demonstrate a 5-year survival rate of 37% after surgery. This survival rate is better than that reported for other epithelial ovarian carcinomas (26% to 29%). Positive prognostic factors include stage, minimal residual tumor, negative results on repeat laparotomy, TCC predominance in the primary tumor, and TCC predominance in the metastasis.

Small cell carcinoma. Small cell carcinoma of the ovary is a rare, poorly understood, aggressive tumor of young women and is associated with paraneoplastic hypercalcemia in two thirds of patients. Microscopic examination reveals that it is composed of small, closely packed epithelial cells with high mitotic activity. Some authors think this tumor is more likely to be of germ cell than epithelial origin, primarily because of the age distribution. The prognosis is uniformly poor.

Malignant mixed mesodermal tumors. Malignant mixed mesodermal tumors of the ovary are rare. They represent ap-proximately 1% of all forms of ovarian cancer. Gross examination reveals that these tumors are usually unilateral, cystic, and solid and that the median diameter measures 14 cm. They have malignant epithelial and stromal components. Management of this tumor before and after surgery is similar to that for other invasive epithelial ovarian carcinomas.

Issues Specific to Degree of Differentiation

Benign epithelial tumors. Conservative surgery with the preservation of some ovarian tissue is appropriate in young women with benign epithelial tumors. This usually includes ovarian cystectomy or oophorectomy. In postmenopausal women a TAH/BSO can be considered to avoid future cancer risk.

Epithelial ovarian tumors of low malignant potential (borderline tumors). Borderline tumors of the ovary were first described in 1929, but it was not until the mid-1970s that they were officially included in the World Health Organization and International Federation of Gynecology and Obstetrics (FIGO) classification systems. Histologically, borderline tumors of the ovary are defined as epithelial tumors in which there is stratification and increased atypia with intact basement membranes. However, in a subset of patients there is microscopic invasion, defined as small nests of cells just below the basement membrane. Bell and Scully (1990) and Tavassoli (1988) evaluate this group of patients and establish no adverse impact on recurrence or survival when this histologic feature is found.

The prognosis for patients with borderline ovarian tumors is better than for patients with invasive epithelial ovarian carcinomas. This is partly because only 20% to 25% of patients with borderline tumors have extraovarian disease at the time of diagnosis. In fact, the latter group has a better survival rate than do patients with epithelial ovarian carcinoma. The overall recurrence and death rate is 25%, with recurrence occurring up to 20 years after initial diagnosis. Type of extraovarian implant, whether endosalpingosis, noninvasive, or invasive, is thought to be important to the prognosis. According to Bell et al (1988), invasive implants are associated with poorer survival rates. In contrast, Gershenson and Silva (1990) report that survival is unaffected by type of extraovarian implant.

The mean age of patients with borderline tumors of the ovary is 39 years; for patients with invasive ovarian carcinoma, it is 52 years (Rice et al, 1990). Maintenance of future childbearing potential is an issue. Conservative surgery, with preservation of some ovarian tissue, is appropriate in many patients. Frozen-section analysis is extremely important to rule out the possibility of invasive carcinoma. If there is any question about the diagnosis, ovarian tissue should be preserved. A second operation may be necessary if invasive carcinoma is found. In women who have completed their childbearing, a TAH/BSO/omentectomy is appropriate. Surgical staging with retroperitoneal lymphadenectomy and omentectomy should be undertaken if invasive carcinoma cannot be ruled out by frozen-section analysis or by any other kind of investigation.

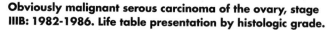

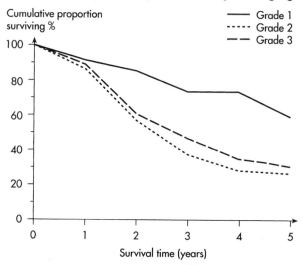

Fig. 9-15. Actuarial survival by year after treatment and by histologic grade for patients with stage IIIB disease. (From Pettersson F, editor: *Annual report of the results of treatment in gynecologic cancer,* vol 36 [suppl], Stockholm, 1990, FIGO.)

BOX 9-2
INTRAOPERATIVE FINDINGS CONSISTENT
WITH INVASIVE OVARIAN MALIGNANCY

Bilateral
Adherent to adjacent organs
Surface excrescences
Ruptured capsule
Ascites
Peritoneal implants
Hemorrhage and necrosis
Solid areas
Intracystic papillations

CA-125 can be a useful tumor marker for patients with serous borderline ovarian tumors of advanced stage. Rice et al (1992) report that 75% of patients with stage I serous tumors have normal preoperative CA-125 levels, whereas 92% of patients with stage II, III, or IV disease have elevated levels ($P < 0.001$).

Adjuvant or curative postoperative chemotherapy for patients with borderline tumors of the ovary is controversial. There are no prospective controlled studies establishing efficacy.

Malignant. Gross intraoperative features suggesting invasive epithelial ovarian carcinoma at the time of laparotomy are presented in Box 9-2. Histologic features of malignant epithelial ovarian carcinoma include increased mitotic activity, compromised basement membrane, and architectural dedifferentiation. These tumors are categorized as well differentiated, moderately differentiated, or poorly differentiated and as grades 1, 2, or 3. This grading system is based primarily on architectural pattern and not on nuclear characteristics. In a large retrospective review of more than 500 patients with ovarian carcinoma, Sorbe et al (1982) report that histologic grade is the most important prognostic indicator, followed by stage and histologic subtype. Figure 9-15 shows the influence of histologic grade on survival rates of patients with stage IIIB serous carcinoma of the ovary.

Stage. Invasive epithelial ovarian carcinoma can spread by local extension, lymphatic invasion, intraperitoneal implantation, hematogenous dissemination, and transdiaphragmatic passage, all of which have implications for staging. Ovarian carcinoma has a surgical-pathologic staging system (Box 9-3). Approximately 75% of patients with invasive epithelial ovarian carcinoma have disease that has advanced beyond stage I. Stage is a strong predictor of survival (Table 9-3).

Meticulous surgical staging is imperative for patients who have what appears to be early-stage epithelial ovarian carcinoma. Young et al (1983) report that 13% of patients referred for treatment of apparent stage I or II ovarian cancer have more advanced disease on further evaluation. If the tumor is mucinous, this includes methodical exploration of the entire peritoneal cavity, pelvic and para-aortic lymph node sampling, peritoneal cytologic sampling, subtotal omentectomy, and appendectomy (Hand et al, 1993; Young et al, 1999).

Cytoreductive surgery. Cytoreductive surgery is the removal of as much of the tumor and its metastases as possible. It includes TAH, BSO, and complete omentectomy with resection of any metastatic lesions. In some patients, bowel resection and retroperitoneal lymphadenopathy are necessary to obtain optimal cytoreduction. Optimal cytoreduction is achieved when the largest residual tumor mass measures less than 1.5 cm. In a review of 47 patients with stage III or IV invasive epithelial ovarian carcinoma who undergo cytoreductive surgery, Hacker et al (1983) report that the median survival time for the suboptimal group is 6 months. For patients whose largest residual tumor measures 0.5 to 1.5 cm, it is 6 months, and for patients whose residual nodules measure less than 0.5 cm, it is 40 months ($P < 0.001$). There appears to be a graded level of success from chemotherapy that is directly related to the size of residual disease at the initiation of chemotherapy. Neijt et al (1991) show that clinical outcomes become progressively worse as the size of the residual disease increases after surgery. However, Hunter et al (1992) raise the question of selection bias. Patients who can be adequately debulked may represent a group that is more sensitive to chemotherapy. In terms of secondary cytoreductive surgery, Eisenkop et al (1995) prospectively evaluate 36 patients with recurrent ovarian carcinoma. They report that 83% of patients are able to undergo complete surgical excision. The median survival time

---

BOX 9-3
STAGES OF OVARIAN CARCINOMA

Stage I   Growth limited to the ovaries
Stage IA   Growth limited to one ovary; no ascites
               No tumor on the external surfaces; capsules intact
Stage IB   Growth limited to both ovaries; no ascites
               No tumor on the external surfaces; capsules intact
Stage IC*   Tumor either stage IA or IB, but with tumor on surface of one or both ovaries; or with capsule ruptured; or with
               ascites containing malignant cells; or with positive peritoneal washings
Stage II   Growth involving one or both ovaries with pelvic extension
Stage IIA   Extension or metastases to the uterus or tubes
Stage IIB   Extension to other pelvic tissues
Stage IIC*   Tumor either IIA or IIB but on the surface of one or both ovaries; or with capsule(s) ruptured; or with ascites
               containing malignant cells; or with positive peritoneal washings
Stage III   Tumor involving one or both ovaries with peritoneal implants outside the pelvis or positive retroperitoneal or
               inguinal nodes; superficial liver metastasis equals stage III; tumor is limited to the true pelvis, but there is histolog-
               ically proven malignant extension to small bowel or omentum
Stage IIIA   Tumor grossly limited to the true pelvis with negative nodes but with histologically confirmed microscopic seeding
               of abdominal peritoneal surfaces
Stage IIIB   Tumor involving one or both ovaries with histologically confined implants of abdominal peritoneal surfaces, none
               exceeding 2 cm in diameter; nodes are negative
Stage IIIC   Abdominal implants larger than 2 cm in diameter or positive retroperitoneal or inguinal nodes
Stage IV   Growth involving one or both ovaries with distant metastases; if pleural effusion is present, there must be positive
               cytology to categorize as stage IV

*To evaluate the impact prognosis of the different criteria for categorizing carcinoma as stage IC or IIC, it is of value to know whether the source of the malignant cell
detected was peritoneal washings or ascites or whether the rupture of the capsule was spontaneous or caused by the surgeon.

Table 9-3   Five-Year Actuarial Survival Rates for Epithelial Ovarian Cancer (1982 to 1986)*

Stage	Survival Rate (%)
IA	82.3
IB	74.9
IC	67.7
IIA	60.6
IIB, IIC	53.8
III	22.7
IV	8.0

From Pettersson F, ed.: *Annual report of the results of treatment in gynecologic cancer,* vol 21, Stockholm, 1990, FIGO.
*Based on 10,912 cases.

is extended for patients who undergo complete resection before salvage chemotherapy or radiation, compared with those in whom macroscopic residual disease remains (43 versus 5 months; $P = 0.03$). If gross residual disease remains at the completion of a secondary cytoreductive procedure, it connotes a poor chance for survival and adds significantly to patient morbidity (Hoskins et al, 1989). Accurately assessing patients before surgery is clearly the way to avert operative procedures that do not help the patient and could certainly do harm.

Goodman et al (1992) report no improvement in survival for patients with stage IV disease who undergo cytoreductive surgery, either initially or on an interval basis, after several courses of chemotherapy.

Postoperative therapy. Postoperative treatment options for patients who have residual disease or who are at high risk for recurrence include radiation therapy and combination chemotherapy. Young et al (1990) identify a subset of patients who do not benefit from postoperative adjuvant therapy. This group includes patients with stage IA or IB tumors that are either grade 1 or 2. The 5-year disease-free interval is 91% to 98% with or without postoperative therapy. Patients with stage I, grade 3 tumors, all stage IC tumors, and all stage II tumors are at unacceptable risk for recurrence and should undergo postoperative adjuvant therapy, as should all patients with stage III and IV tumors regardless of whether they undergo optimal cytoreduction.

Radiation therapy. The role of radiotherapy in the management of epithelial ovarian cancer is unclear. In the Princess Margaret Hospital series (Dembo et al, 1979), whole abdomen and pelvic irradiation is as effective as chemotherapy in curing previously untreated patients with minimal residual disease. The radiation field extends 1 to 2 cm above the level of the diaphragm and includes the entire pelvis. Use of second-line radiotherapy after initial chemotherapy has not increased the progression-free interval or the cure but has been shown to increase toxicity levels significantly (Kucera et al, 1990).

Intraperitoneal therapy. Intraperitoneal (IP) chromic phosphate has been and continues to be investigated for the treatment of patients who have no residual disease but who are at high risk for recurrence. Intraperitoneal cisplatin is shown to induce a 20% to 30% response rate in patients with small-volume residual disease who previously responded to systemic platinum therapy (Howell et al, 1987). Bulky tumor masses do not respond to this type of administration because intraperitoneal cisplatin cannot penetrate more than 2 to 3 mm. Significant adhesions do not respond well either because of the poor distribution. In a recent SWOG-GOG-ECOG study of patients who underwent adequate cytoreduction, intravenous (IV) cyclophosphamide plus IP cisplatinum versus IV cyclophosphamide plus IV cisplatinum are compared in a prospective, randomized fashion. The IV-IP treatment arm is superior to the IV-IV arm regarding pathologically proven complete response rate, median survival time, and reduced incidence of clinical hearing loss and neutropenia (Alberts et al, 1995). Continued data collection in a prospective, randomized fashion is needed to elucidate fully the role of intraperitoneal therapy in the management of patients with ovarian carcinoma.

Systemic chemotherapy. Platinum-based combination chemotherapy is now the standard postoperative treatment for patients at high risk for recurrence (stage I, grade 3; all stage IC; and all stage II) or for residual disease (stage III or IV) (Louie et al, 1986; Piver et al, 1992). Multiagent therapy is associated with improved disease-response rates, enhanced survival times, and improved therapeutic indexes. A multiagent regimen generally includes either cisplatinum or carboplatinum and only one or two of the following three additional agents: cyclophosphamide, paclitaxel, and doxorubicin. Cisplatin-cyclophosphamide is compared with cisplatin-paclitaxel in a prospective, randomized study (McGuire et al, 1996) of patients who undergo suboptimal cytoreduction surgery. The paclitaxel combination is associated with a statistically significant improvement in median progression-free survival (18.1 months versus 13.6 months), and the survival curves continue to show an approximate 30% improvement for the paclitaxel combination at 2.5 years of follow-up observation. Thus, the Gynecologic Oncology Group has accepted this regimen as the standard of care for patients who undergo suboptimal cytoreduction (McGuire et al, 1993; McGuire et al, 1996). Although long-term survival data from several Gynecologic Oncology Group trials studying multiagent therapy directed at patients who are at high risk for recurrence or who undergo adequate cytoreduction are pending, it is reasonable to expect that these multiagent drugs are the most effective combinations in this patient population.

Because of the serious toxicity associated with cisplatin, namely gastrointestinal effects, neurotoxicity, and nephro-

toxicity, other platinum analogues have been developed. Carboplatinum is one such analogue. It has a different spectrum of toxicity and a less complicated administration protocol (Willemse, 1992). Carboplatinum-cyclophosphamide and cisplatin-cyclophosphamide are equally effective, but the latter has greater toxicity (Swenerton et al, 1992). At the molecular level and in the clinical arena, cisplatinum and carboplatinum appear to be equally efficacious in the treatment of ovarian cancer, and carboplatinum appears to be associated with decreased cost and toxicity (Alberts, 1994; Young et al, 1993).

Efforts to improve the survival rate in patients with advanced ovarian cancer have been directed at dosage intensification of platinum analogues and at the development of new chemotherapeutic agents (Hainsworth et al, 1990; Sutton et al, 1989). There are reports (Kaye et al, 1992) of significantly improved survival rates in patients treated with cisplatin 100 mg/m^2 compared with those treated with 50 mg/m^2, though these findings have not been confirmed by all investigators. Further investigation is needed to establish the effectiveness of dosage intensification. New chemotherapeutic agents directed primarily at recurrent disease, some of them platinum refractory, are continually investigated. Among them are topotecan, ifosfamide, etoposide, 5-fluorouracil with leucovorin, tamoxifen, and others of more investigational type.

Second-look procedure. Second-look surgery may be undertaken after the completion of chemotherapy to determine whether patients who have had complete clinical responses are free of disease. There is no evidence that patients who are in complete clinical remission after chemotherapy have improved survival after second-look surgery. The primary reason for performing second-look laparotomy after chemotherapy is to identify more precisely those patients with persistent disease. It provides patients the opportunity to prolong survival by continuing treatment. There are three essential considerations. First, a relapse rate of at least 25% can be expected if there are negative findings on second-look surgery (Gershenson et al, 1985). Second, limited salvage therapies are available if there is residual disease (Luesly et al, 1988). Third, secondary debulking that resects residual disease at the time of second-look surgery may be beneficial. Several small studies show a possible survival advantage to patients left with microscopic disease. Second-look laparotomy, with or without secondary cytoreduction, for the evaluation of experimental adjuvant or salvage therapy may be appropriate in a formal investigation if it takes into consideration the above-mentioned factors. Protocols should be developed to evaluate the benefits of consolidation therapy in the context of clinical trials.

Tumor marker CA-125. The role of the tumor marker CA-125 in the preoperative evaluation of a patient with a pelvic mass is discussed under the evaluation and management of the adnexal pelvic mass. The CA-125 antigen is elevated in 80% of patients with advanced ovarian carcinoma and in some patients with early-stage disease. However, it is not specific for ovarian cancer. Elevated levels have been found in various benign conditions, such as endometriosis, leiomyoma, pregnancy, pelvic inflammatory disease, and several other malignancies (Haliln et al, 1986; Malkassian et al, 1986; Pittaway et al, 1981). Lavin et al (1987) and Niloff et al (1986) demonstrate the usefulness of serial serum CA-125 assays in the follow-up observations of patients with confirmed ovarian carcinoma. CA-125 levels are elevated before clinical recurrence in 94% of patients, and the median lead time is 3 months (Niloff et al, 1986).

Guidelines for Follow-up of Patients with Ovarian Cancer. It is unclear what is the best follow-up for the asymptomatic patient who has undergone surgery and chemotherapy for primary ovarian cancer. Complete history and physical examination, rectovaginal pelvic examination, and CA-125 testing are recommended at 3- to 4-month intervals. After 2 years, longer intervals can be considered. The above-mentioned tests have been shown to detect disease progression in more than 90% of patients with recurrent epithelial ovarian cancer. Routine radiologic examination has not been shown to improve recurrence detection. Therefore, its use should be individualized (National Institutes of Health, 1995).

Metastatic Malignancy

Ovarian involvement from extragenital cancer is common. Approximately 5% of ovarian malignancies are metastases from other sites. The most frequent primary sites are colon (52%), breast (17%), stomach (10%), and pancreas (10%) (Yazigi and Sandstad, 1989). The classic Krukenberg tumor is one that metastasizes from the stomach and has the pathognomonic "signet-ring cells" (Fig. 9-16). Careful review of symptoms, physical examination, and appropriate radiographic studies can assist the clinician in making a diagnosis of the primary tumor before exploring for an ovarian mass. Generally, ovarian metastasis indicates poor prognosis.

Other

A miscellaneous group of ovarian lesions comprises less than 5% of the total number of neoplasms.

Nonneoplastic Tumorlike Conditions

Pregnancy luteoma. If a solid ovarian tumor develops during pregnancy, pregnancy luteoma must be kept in mind. It is established that this represents an exaggeration of the luteinization reaction of the ovary.

Ovarian hyperthecosis. Ovarian hyperthecosis is defined as a nonneoplastic proliferation of ovarian stromal cells that exhibit focal luteinization. Virilization is common and is secondary to the increased production of ovarian-derived testosterone and androstenedione.

Ovarian edema. Enlargement of the ovary by ovarian edema is rare. The most probable cause is intermittent torsion of the ovarian vessels. In many patients, a unilateral oophorectomy is necessary because of torsion-induced necrosis of the ovary.

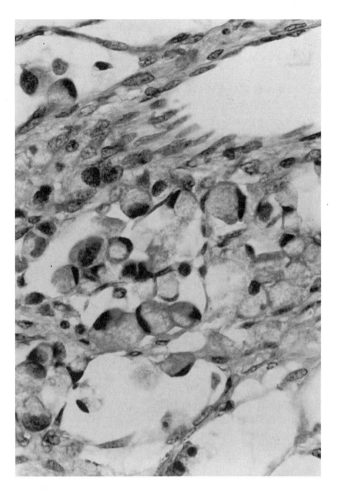

Fig. 9-16. Metastatic mucinous carcinoma (Krukenberg tumor) containing well-formed signet-ring cells with nuclei displaced by cytoplasmic mucin.

Follicular cyst/corpus luteal cyst. Follicular cysts and corpus luteal cysts represent the two possible causes of solitary functional cyst of the ovary. Follicular cysts are common during the reproductive years and are probably related to abnormalities in the release of anterior pituitary gonadotropins. Corpus luteal cysts, which also develop during the reproductive years, result from ovulation. Although most solitary functional cysts resolve spontaneously, oral contraceptives can be used to hasten the process.

Polycystic ovary syndrome. Polycystic ovary syndrome, also known as Stein-Leventhal syndrome, encompasses a spectrum of symptoms resulting from chronic anovulation and polycystic ovaries. Polycystic ovary syndrome typically develops in women in their 20s who have a history of premenarcheal obesity, postmenarcheal amenorrhea, infertility, and increased androgen production. Hyperestrogenism occurs less often and is manifested by menometrorrhagia with or without endometrial hyperplasia or endometrial carcinoma. Treatment is directed at normalizing cyclic pituitary gonadotropin levels and protecting the endometrium against the unopposed estrogen commonly seen in anovulatory women.

Theca-lutein cyst. Bilateral ovarian enlargement, secondary to numerous luteinized follicle cysts, is commonly seen in theca-lutein cysts. The conditions that often cause this disorder result from increased levels of circulating hCG, such as multiple gestations, gestational trophoblastic disease, and Rh sensitization with fetal hydrops.

Endometrioma. Endometriosis commonly occurs in the ovary; when cyclic bleeding occurs, an endometriotic cyst or endometrioma is formed. Accumulation of blood within this cavity results in the classic "chocolate cyst." The pain that is typically produced by endometriosis is similarly produced with endometriomas of the ovary. Physical examination reveals an adnexal and the typical findings of endometriosis, which include uterosacral nodularity and cul-de-sac of Douglas tenderness.

Germinal inclusion cyst. Germinal inclusion cysts of the ovary result from infolding of the surface epithelium after ovulation. There is no evidence to support a causal relationship between these germinal inclusions and the common benign and malignant epithelial neoplasms of the ovary.

Simple cyst. By definition, simple cysts have no identifiable epithelial lining. They are probably derived from follicular cysts, germinal inclusion cysts, or cystadenomas.

Evaluation and Management of the Pelvic-Adnexal Mass
Preoperative Evaluation

The complete differential diagnosis of a pelvic-adnexal mass must be kept in mind when evaluating a woman of any age with this finding. Killackey and Neuwirth (1988) review 540 patients with pelvic-adnexal masses. Of these patients, 291 undergo surgical evaluation for a pelvic mass of unknown cause, and 249 undergo surgical evaluation for suspected leiomyoma. Forty-four cancers are diagnosed, 10 of which are nongynecologic malignancies. This report emphasizes the importance of a complete differential diagnosis. As noted earlier, the importance of a complete history and physical examination cannot be emphasized enough.

The radiographic evaluation of a patient with a pelvic-adnexal mass must be tailored to the age of the patient and to the results of the history and physical examination. In a 4-year-old girl, a solid pelvic mass must raise the suspicion of germ cell malignancy, and ultrasonography is appropriate. A change in bowel habits in a 50-year-old woman necessitates evaluation for colon cancer, which includes a barium enema and colonoscopy. Hematuria and bladder symptoms would warrant an intravenous pyelogram with cystoscopy, urinalysis, and urine cytology.

Ultrasonography has assumed a major role in evaluating pelvic masses (Andolf et al, 1990). Using abdominal ultrasonography, Herrmann et al (1987) prospectively evaluated 404 women with suspected pelvic masses or a history suggesting ovarian cancer. Three hundred twelve patients underwent surgery and were evaluated within 3 weeks of sonography. The positive predictive value of the sonographic evidence of malignancy was 73% (38 of 52 patients), whereas the negative predictive value was 95.6% (117 of 185 patients). In a similar study of 102 postmenopausal women who underwent abdominal ultrasonography evaluation of adnexal masses before surgery, the positive predictive value for ovarian malignancy is 39% and the negative predictive value is 94% (Luxman et al, 1991). If a negative sonogram had been relied on, 6% of malignant ovarian tumors in these postmenopausal woman might have been overlooked.

In recent years, transvaginal ultrasonography has improved the ability to discern ovarian malignancy. Several authors substantiate the superiority of transvaginal (compared with abdominal) ultrasonography in diagnosing ovarian malignancies. Sassone et al (1991) correlate transvaginal sonographic pelvic images of 143 patients with surgical findings and histopathology. They devise a scoring system to delineate benign from malignant lesions, showing a specificity of 83%, a sensitivity of 100%, and positive and negative predictive values of 37% and 100%, respectively. Color Doppler imaging has been investigated as a means of increasing the specificity of transvaginal ultrasonography. This technique quantifies blood flow in the ovarian vessels. Impedance to blood flow in a malignant ovarian tumor is less than that found in a benign tumor. Additional investigations are needed to evaluate this technique fully.

Pelvic CT imaging is rarely used for primary evaluation of the adnexa because there is controversy regarding its ability to visualize normal ovaries. This radiographic technique can be useful in evaluating the extent of metastatic disease for patients with known or strongly suspected ovarian carcinoma.

Magnetic resonance imaging is another diagnostic modality that has recently been used with greater frequency.

Table 9-4 "Tumor Markers" Useful with Ovarian Neoplasms	
Substance/Marker	**Ovarian Tumor**
α-Fetoprotein	Endodermal sinus tumors; embryonal carcinomas; mixed germ cell tumors (rarely immature teratoma and polyembryoma)
CA-125	All epithelial tumors, especially serous (rarely immature teratoma)
Estradiol	Adult granulosa cell tumors; thecomas
Human chorionic cell gonadotropin	Choriocarcinoma; embryonal carcinoma; mixed germ tumors; thecomas
Lactic dehydrogenase	Dysgerminoma; mixed germ cell tumors
Testosterone	Sertoli cell tumors; Leydig (hilus) cell tumors

There are no useful prospective studies evaluating its ability to assess adnexal disease.

Special consideration must be given to the application of all radiographic techniques in diagnosing and following up on adnexal masses during pregnancy and childhood, specifically addressing the amount of radiation exposure. Ultrasonography and magnetic resonance imaging are superior in that there is no radiation exposure.

The age of the patient is extremely important in determining the appropriate laboratory test to conduct. Remembering to order the appropriate tumor marker before surgery is important (Table 9-4). In the patient younger than 20 years who has a solid adnexal pelvic mass, a malignant germ cell tumor of the ovary must be considered and serum AFP, serum hCG, and LDH should be ordered as potential tumor markers.

CA-125 is a tumor marker that deserves special attention. Although it is elevated in many patients with epithelial ovarian carcinoma, it is also elevated ($>$35 mIU/mL) in various benign and malignant conditions. In those conditions, the CA-125 level is usually below 200 mIU/mL. In a study evaluating 182 gynecology patients with pelvic masses, preoperative CA-125 levels are obtained for all (Vasilev et al, 1988). In 14 of 18 (77.8%) patients with malignant masses, the serum levels exceed 35 mIU/mL. However, only 14 of 51 patients (27.5%) with elevated CA-125 levels had malignant tumors. According to the authors, increasing the positive cut-off levels to 65 mIU/mL does not improve the results. The authors conclude that serum CA-125 levels alone do not sufficiently distinguish benign from malignant masses before surgery. It is important to recognize that if the preoperative CA-125 level is markedly elevated, ovarian carcinoma is more likely to be present.

Histologic confirmation, either by laparoscopy or laparotomy, is necessary to establish the diagnosis when a pelvic-adnexal mass is present and persistent. However, averting surgical intervention for common functional ovarian cysts is important. These functional cysts do not occur in postmenopausal women because corpus luteal and follicular cysts are caused by ovulation. For premenopausal women with simple cysts that measure less than 8 cm on transvaginal ultrasonography, a 6-week period of oral contraceptive suppression is appropriate. In a study by Spanos (1973), 81 of 286 premenopausal patients treated with oral contraceptives for cystic adnexal mass require laparotomy for mass persistence. None of these patients have functional cysts (Table 9-5).

Taking the above into consideration, Fig. 9-17 provides a framework for evaluating and treating premenopausal patients with adnexal masses; Fig. 9-18 provides the same for postmenopausal women.

Operative Management

A bowel preparation should always be given to patients thought to have malignancy or dense pelvic adhesions. This lowers the rate of infectious complications if colorectal surgery is necessary. It also reduces the need for colostomy if the colon or rectum is entered. One adequate mechanical bowel preparation is 4 L polyethylene glycol electrolyte solution, 8 oz of which should be given every 10 minutes the morning before surgery. This should be followed by 1 g neomycin and 1 g erythromycin given orally at 1:00, 2:00, and 11:00 PM the day before surgery. It is also important that the patient have clear liquids for 24 hours before surgery.

Laparoscopy. Laparoscopy is the most commonly performed gynecologic surgical procedure. It continues to be important for confirming the presence and establishing the types of various masses. Its value is not just in diagnosis; it is also used for treating ovarian masses. With the development of new technology, part or all of an ovarian mass can be removed through the laparoscope. Clinical judgment must be exercised. It is not always easy to distinguish a malignant ovarian tumor from a benign one. Laparoscopic removal of an ovarian lesion often results in upstaging if a tumor is malignant. Sainz de la Cuesta et al (1994) report that intraoperative rupture of malignant ovarian neoplasms worsens the prognosis for patients with stage I ovarian cancer. Dembo et al (1990) report different results in a similar study, but their inclusion criteria are also different. Both studies are too small to stratify for grade and treatment. Even in premenopausal women, in whom the risk is reduced, the risk for malignancy should be considered. Mecke et al (1992) report 773 patients younger than 45 who undergo pelviscopy. Only two patients (0.26%) have ovarian carcinoma and undergo pelviscopy before laparotomy. The authors state that sonography is extremely important in determining the appropriateness of pelviscopy. Patients with multilocular cysts that have echodense components and that are larger than 7 cm in diameter should not undergo pelviscopy. This is also true of cysts measuring more than 9 cm, regardless of their appearance on ultrasonography.

Table 9-5 Operative Findings with Persistent Adnexal Masses

Surgical exploration	81
Functional cysts	0
Neoplasm	81
Endometrioma	28
Simple serous cyst	18
Cystadenoma	
Serous	8
Pseudomucinous	6
Dermoid	9
Paraovarian cyst	4
Hydrosalpinx	3
Cystadenocarcinoma	
Serous	3
Pseudomucinous	1
Dysgerminoma	1

From Spanos WJ: Preoperative hormonal therapy of cystic adnexal masses. *Am J Obstet Gynecol* 1973; 116:551.

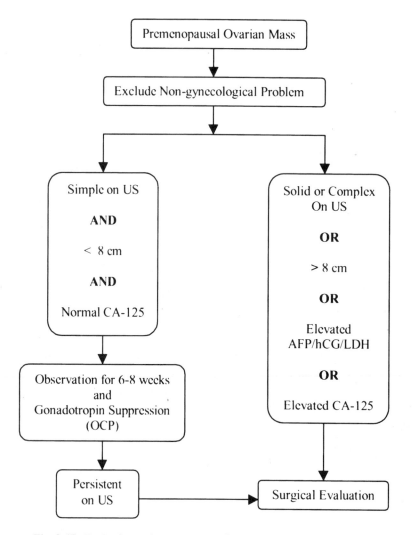

Fig. 9-17. Evaluation and management of a premenopausal ovarian mass.

Laparotomy. Laparotomy is the procedure of choice in many situations, as outlined in Figs. 9-17 and 9-18. The surgeon must exercise sound clinical judgment in determining the type of incision to be used. Although a vertical midline incision provides the best exposure, a low transverse incision can be used in premenopausal women ineligible for laparoscopic surgery who have uncomplicated-appearing ovarian cysts. The patient must understand clearly that if a malignancy is found, a second incision may be necessary for appropriate surgical management. Type of incision must not limit surgery. As discussed in the section on laparoscopic surgery, upstaging ovarian carcinoma by rupturing an ovarian cyst is undesirable. With that in mind, the surgeon should attempt to remove each ovarian cyst intact.

Conservative surgery with the preservation of reproductive function can be performed but is dependent on the malignant potential of the ovarian tumor. Frozen-section analysis can be extremely helpful, but patients must be informed that the final report may differ from the one given at the time of surgery. Ovarian neoplasms for which ovarian conservation may be considered include grade I, stage 1A invasive

epithelial tumors, borderline tumors, germ cell tumors, and stromal cell tumors. Extended surgical staging is imperative for all patients with suspected malignancy so that the patient can make an informed decision based on available information. The rate-limiting step should not be histologic information. A detailed discussion of the surgical management of ovarian carcinoma, including staging, cytoreductive surgery, and second-look surgery, is presented in the section on epithelial ovarian neoplasm.

Ovarian Cancer Screening

Because ovarian carcinoma is not usually diagnosed until its advanced stages, the professional and the public communities embrace the concept of "screening." Unfortunately, screening for ovarian cancer has not been effective. Programs designed to detect unsuspected ovarian cancer are more accurately described as "earlier detection programs."

Because the incidence of ovarian cancer is relatively low, methods used for detection must have stringent levels of specificity and sensitivity. The advent of the CA-125 serum tumor marker and improvements in pelvic ultrasonography,

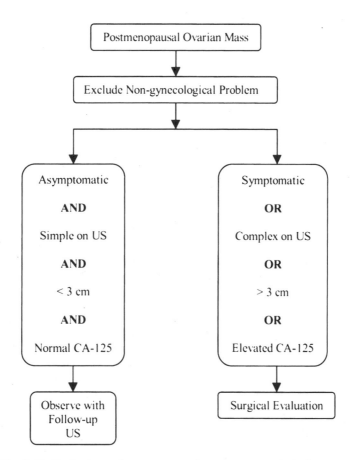

Fig. 9-18. Evaluation and management of a postmenopausal ovarian mass.

along with newer techniques for color Doppler imaging of ovarian vessels, have led some to advocate the use of these modalities to detect early-stage ovarian cancer. To satisfy the criteria for screening, a disease must have high prevalence and significant mortality rates. It must include a preclinical stage, and it must be amenable to treatment. The screening test itself must have adequate specificity, sensitivity, and positive predictive value to be effective. Furthermore, it must be cost-effective. If one assumes a prevalence for ovarian cancer of 50 patients per 100,000 population, a test with 99% specificity and 100% sensitivity would yield only 1 in 21 women with a positive screen (positive predictive value, 4.8%). Current screening tests do not attain this high level of sensitivity (National Institutes of Health, 1995). If the tests have low specificity, too many women will undergo unnecessary and potentially hazardous operations. If the sensitivity is low, affected women will pass through the screen undetected. The inability to perform screening in the classic sense does not, however, decrease the need to pursue methods for the detection of stage I cancer. Early detection favorably influences long-term prognosis and site-specific mortality from ovarian cancer. The three screening tests available for general use are bimanual rectovaginal pelvic examination, CA-125 testing, and transabdominal or transvaginal ultrasonography.

Pelvic Examination

Pelvic examination is a critical component of routine gynecologic care. However, it is well recognized that it lacks sensitivity and specificity as a screening test for ovarian carcinoma.

Transabdominal Ultrasonography

Transabdominal pelvic ultrasonography is effective in measuring the volume and the morphologic characteristics of ovaries in postmenopausal women (Campbell et al, 1989). In addition, ultrasonography is measurably more accurate than physical examination in detecting adnexal masses (Sparks and Varner, 1991). Unfortunately, the large prospective screening studies that use transabdominal ultrasonography have been hampered by its lack of reliability in distinguishing benign from malignant tissue, even though the practitioners performing the studies are among the most experienced in the world. Many of the thousands of women screened underwent surgery, but few—perhaps 1 in 1000—had ovarian cancer (Campbell et al, 1990). Transvaginal ultrasonography is the preferred approach.

Transvaginal Ultrasonography

Because the transducer is closer to the area of interest and the probes are of higher frequency, transvaginal ultrasonography produces images of better quality and perhaps greater accuracy. Although data regarding ovarian size and morphology are highly reproducible, transvaginal ultrasonography screening has the same limitations regarding tissue characterization that abdominal ultrasonography has (Higgins et al, 1990). Several authors have developed ultrasonographic morphology scoring systems to distinguish between benign and malignant lesions in a more reproducible manner (DePriest et al, 1993). Among the patients in these studies who underwent surgery because of abnormal results on transvaginal ultrasonography, few, approximately 1 per 1000, had ovarian cancer (Van Nagell Jr, 1991). Using color Doppler imaging to help differentiate between benign and malignant ovarian lesions has advocates, but there are no data regarding the impact on screening accuracy (Kawai et al, 1992). Transabdominal and transvaginal ultrasonography lack adequate specificity to be used alone as single screening modalities.

Serum CA-125

The serum marker CA-125 has been evaluated extensively as a screening test for ovarian cancer. In fact, the sensitivity of CA-125 before the diagnosis of ovarian cancer has been determined by the JANUS study (Zurawski et al, 1988). This seminal report involves the retrospective analysis of CA-125 levels in a serum bank of specimens taken from more than 100,000 persons between 1973 and 1986. Disappointingly, only 33% of women in whom ovarian cancer developed had elevated levels of CA-125 within 18 months before the diagnosis was made. Only approximately 20% had elevated levels of CA-125 18 to 60 months before the diagnosis was established.

Two large prospective studies confirm that serum CA-125 lacks satisfactory sensitivity to be used as an independent screening test for ovarian cancer, even when restricted to postmenopausal women (Einhorn et al, 1992; Jacobs et al, 1988). Furthermore, the specificity is low secondary to elevations seen in benign disease.

Carlson et al (1994) conduct a MEDLINE search of the English-language literature and the bibliographies of published studies that provide estimates of ovarian cancer risk and that test operating characteristics and treatment effectiveness according to disease stage. Death from ovarian cancer and morbidity from surgical procedures are the principal outcomes considered. Annual screening with CA-125 or ultrasonography in women older than 50 years who do not have family histories of ovarian cancer results in more than 30 false-positive results for every ovarian cancer detected

(Carlson et al, 1994). Either of these modalities alone is not useful for ovarian cancer screening.

Multimodality Screening

A combination of CA-125, ultrasonography, and physical examination is intellectually appealing. This combination has the potential advantage of improving the sensitivity and specificity of screening. Jacobs et al (1988) use vaginal examination with serum CA-125 as the initial examination (primary screen—higher sensitivity) and combine it with ultrasonography for those who have abnormalities (secondary screen—higher specificity). They screen 1010 apparently healthy postmenopausal volunteers. The only incidence of ovarian cancer to be detected involved a 10-cm mass found on initial pelvic examination. It is unclear how many women underwent a (potentially unnecessary) surgical procedure because of false results on the screening test. Screening for ovarian cancer using CA-125 and transvaginal ultrasonography significantly improves the specificity of screening and decreases the number of unnecessary operations. However, it is impossible to quantitate the morbidity, and even the mortality, associated with surgical procedures performed on women who have no disease. This approach has been applied to self-referred women who have a family history of ovarian cancer, and the results have been of mixed usefulness (Einhorn, 1992; Muto et al, 1993; Schwartz et al, 1991). It is difficult to demonstrate effectiveness because of the low prevalence of the disease and the lack of randomized, prospective screening trials.

Recommendations for Screening

The benefits of screening a woman who has one or no first-degree relative with ovarian cancer are unproven. The risks may outweigh the benefits, particularly in women with no family history or other high risk factors. Participating in clinical trials is a reasonable option. Women with two or more family members with ovarian cancer have a 3% chance of having a hereditary ovarian cancer syndrome and should be provided extensive counseling regarding their options (that is, genetic testing). For women with hereditary ovarian cancer syndrome, the lifetime risk for ovarian cancer approaches 50%. There are no data to prove that screening reduces the mortality from this disease. Nonetheless, the NIH Consensus Conference has recommended at least annual rectovaginal pelvic examinations, CA-125 testing, and transvaginal ultrasonography. After childbearing, or at least by age 35 years, prophylactic oophorectomy is recommended (NIH, 1995. Further prospective data are needed to alter the above recommendations.

REFERENCES

Alberts DS: Cisplatin versus carboplatin in advanced ovarian cancer: An economic analysis. *Pharmacol Ther* 1994; 19:692-706.

Alberts DS, Liu PY, Hannigan EV, et al: Phase III study of intraperitoneal cisplatinum/intravenous cyclophosphamide versus IV cisplatinum/IV cyclophosphamide, in patients with

optimal disease stage III ovarian cancer: A SWOG-GOG-ECOG intergroup study [abstr 760]. *Proc Am Soc Clin Oncol* 1995; 14:273.

Amos CI, Show GL, Tucker MA, et al: Age at onset for familial epithelial ovarian cancer. *JAMA* 1992; 268:1896-1899.

Andolf E, Jorgensen C, Astedt B: Ultrasound examination for detection of ovarian carcinoma in risk groups. *Obstet Gynecol* 1990; 75:106-109.

Austin RM, Norris HJ: Malignant Brenner tumor and transitional cell carcinoma of the ovary: A comparison. *Int J Gynecol Pathol* 1987; 6:29-39.

Awais GM: Dysgerminoma and serum lactic dehydrogenase levels. *Obstet Gynecol* 1983; 61:99-101.

Bajorin DF, Geller NL, Weisen SF, et al: Two-drug therapy in patients with metastatic germ cell tumors. *Cancer* 1991; 67:28-32.

Bell DA, Scully RE: Ovarian serous borderline tumors with stromal microinvasion: A report of 21 cases. *Hum Pathol* 1990; 21:397-403.

Bell DA, Weinstock MA, Scully RE: Peritoneal implants of ovarian serous borderline tumors: Histologic features and prognosis. *Cancer* 1988; 62:2212-2222.

Berek JS, Hacker NF: *Practical gynecologic oncology.* Baltimore, 1989, Williams & Wilkins.

Bjorkholm E, Lundell M, Gyftodimos A, et al: Dysgerminoma: The radiumhemmet series 1927-1984. *Cancer* 1990; 65:38-44.

Campbell S, Bhan V, Royston P, et al: Transabdominal ultrasound screening for early ovarian cancer. *Br Med J* 1989; 299:1363-1367.

Campbell S, Royston P, Vhan V, et al: Novel screening strategies for early ovarian cancer by transabdominal ultrasonography. *Br J Obstet Gynaecol* 1990; 97:304-311.

Carlson KJ, Skates SJ, Singer DE: Screening for ovarian cancer. *Ann Intern Med* 1994; 121:124-132.

Centers for Disease Control Cancer and Steroid Hormone Study: The reduction in risk of ovarian cancer associated with oral contraceptive use. *N Engl J Med* 1987; 316:650-655.

Cramer DW, Hutchinson GB, Welch WR, et al: Factors affecting the association of oral contraceptives and ovarian cancer. *N Engl J Med* 1982a; 307:1047-1051.

Dembo AJ, Bush RS, Beale FA, et al: Ovarian carcinoma: Improved survival following abdominopelvic irradiation in patients with completed pelvic operation. *Am J Obstet Gynecol* 1979; 134:793-800.

Dembo AJ, Davy M, Stenwig AE, et al: Prognostic factors in patients with stage I epithelial ovarian cancer. *Obstet Gynecol* 1990; 75:263-273.

DePriest PD, Shenson D, Fried A, et al: A morphology index based on monographic findings in ovarian cancer. *Gynecol Oncol* 1993; 51:7-11.

Easton DF, Bishop DT, Ford D, et al: Genetic linkage analysis in familial breast and ovarian cancer. *Am J Hum Genet* 1993; 52:678-701.

Easton DF, Ford D, Bishop DT, et al: Breast and ovarian cancer incidence in BRCA1-mutation carriers. *Am J Hum Genet* 1995; 56:265-271.

Einhorn N: Ovarian cancer: Early diagnosis and screening. *Hematol Oncol Clin North Am* 1992; 6:843-850.

Einhorn N, Siovail K, Knapp RC, et al: Prospective evaluation of serum CA-125 levels for early detection of ovarian cancer. *Obstet Gynecol* 1992; 80:14-18.

Eisenkop SM, Friedman RL, Wang H: Secondary cytoreductive surgery for recurrent ovarian cancer: A prospective study. *Cancer* 1995; 76:1606-1614.

Evans AT III, Gaffey TA, Malkaisan GD Jr, et al: Clinicopathologic review of 118 granulosa and 82 theca cell tumors. *Obstet Gynecol* 1980; 55:231-238.

Ford D, Easton DF: The genetics of breast and ovary cancer. *Br J Cancer* 1995; 72:805-812.

Ford D, Easton DF, Bishop DT, et al: Risks of cancer in BRCA1-mutation carriers. *Lancet* 1994; 343:692-695.

Gershenson DM: Menstrual and reproductive function after treatment with combination chemotherapy for malignant ovarian germ cell tumors. *J Clin Oncol* 1988; 6:270-275.

Gershenson DM, Copeland LJ, Whorton JT, et al: Prognosis of surgically determined complete responders in advanced ovarian carcinoma. *Cancer* 1985; 55:1129-1135.

Gershenson DM, Copeland LJ, del Junco G, et al: Second-look laparotomy in the management of malignant germ cell tumors of the ovary. *Obstet Gynecol* 1986; 67:789-793.

Gershenson DM, Copeland LJ, Kavanagh JJ, et al: Treatment of metastatic stromal tumors of the ovary with cisplatin, doxorubicin and cyclophosphamide. *Obstet Gynecol* 1987; 70:765-769.

Gershenson DM, Morris M, Congir A, et al: Treatment of malignant germ cell tumors of the ovary with bleomycin, etoposide, and cisplatin, *J Clin Oncol* 1990; 8:715-720.

Gershenson DM, Silva EG: Serous ovarian tumors of malignant potential with peritoneal implants. *Cancer* 1990; 65:578-585.

Goodman HM, Harlow BL, Sheets EE, et al: The role of cytoreductive surgery in the management of stage IV epithelial ovarian carcinoma. *Gynecol Oncol* 1992; 46:367-371.

Hacker NF, Berek JS, Lagasse LD, et al: Primary cytoreductive surgery for epithelial ovarian cancer. *Obstet Gynecol* 1983; 61:413-420.

Hainsworth JD, Burnett LS, Jones HW III, et al: High-dose cisplatin combination chemotherapy in the treatment of advanced epithelial ovarian carcinoma. *J Clin Oncol* 1990; 8:502-508.

Halila H, Stenman UH, Seppala M: Ovarian cancer antigen CA-125 levels in pelvic inflammatory disease and pregnancy. *Cancer* 1986; 57:1327-1329.

Hall JM, Lee MK, Newman B, et al: Linkage of early onset familial breast cancer to chromosome 17q21. *Science* 1990; 250:1684-1689.

Hand R, Fremgen A, Chmiel JS, et al: Staging procedures, clinical management, and survival outcome for ovarian carcinoma. *JAMA* 1993; 269:1119-1122.

Hankison SE, Colditz GA, Hunter DJ, et al: A quantitative assessment of oral contraceptive use and risk of ovarian cancer. *Obstet Gynecol* 1992; 80:708-714.

Hankison SE, Hunter DJ, Colditz GA, et al: Tubal ligation, hysterectomy and risk of ovarian cancer. *JAMA* 1993; 270:2813-1237.

Hartge P, Whittlemore AS, Itnyre J, et al: Rates and risks of ovarian cancer in subgroups of white women in the United States. *Obstet Gynecol* 1994; 84:760-764.

Heaps JM, Nieberg RK, Berek JS: Malignant neoplasms arising in endometriosis. *Obstet Gynecol* 1990; 75:1023-1028.

Herrmann UJ Jr, Locher GW, Goldhirsch A: Sonographic patterns of ovarian tumors: Prediction of malignancy. *Obstet Gynecol* 1987; 69:777-781.

Higgins RV, Rubin SC, Dulaney E, et al: Interobserver variation in ovarian measurements using transvaginal ultrasound. *Gynecol Oncol* 1990; 39:69-71.

Hoskins WJ, Rubin SC, Dulaney E, et al: Influence of secondary cytoreduction at the time of second-look laparotomy on the survival of patients with epithelial ovarian carcinoma. *Gynecol Oncol* 1989; 34:365-371.

Howell SB, Zimm S, Morkman M, et al: Long-term survival of advanced refractory ovarian carcinoma patients with small-volume disease treated with intraperitoneal chemotherapy. *J Clin Oncol* 1987; 5:1607-1612.

Hunter RW, Alexander NDE, Soutter WP: Meta-analysis of surgery in advanced ovarian carcinoma: Is maximum cytoreductive surgery an independent determinant of prognosis? *Am J Obstet Gynecol* 1992; 166:504-511.

Jacobs I, Stabile I, Bridges J, et al: Multimodal approach to screening for ovarian cancer. *Lancet* 1988; 1:268-271.

Jenison EL, Montag AG, Griffiths CT, et al: Clear cell adenocarcinoma of the ovary: Clinical analysis and comparison with serous carcinoma. *Gynecol Oncol* 1989; 32:65-71.

Kawai M, Kano T, Kikkawa F, et al: Transvaginal Doppler ultrasound with color-flow imaging in the diagnosis of ovarian cancer. *Obstet Gynecol* 1992; 79:163-167.

Kaye SB, Lewis CR, Poul J, et al: Randomized study of two doses of cisplatin with cyclophosphamide in epithelial ovarian cancer. *Lancet* 1992; 340:329-333.

Killackey MA, Neuwirth RS: Evaluation and management of the pelvic mass: A review of 540 cases. *Obstet Gynecol* 1988; 71:319-322.

Kucera PR, Berman ML, Treadwell P, et al: Whole abdominal radiotherapy for patients with minimal residual epithelial ovarian cancer. *Gynecol Oncol* 1990; 36:338-342.

Kurman RJ: *Blaustein's pathology of the female genital tract,* ed 3, New York, 1987, Springer-Verlag.

Lappohn RE, Burger HG, Bouma J, et al: Inhibin as a marker for granulosa cell tumors. *N Engl J Med* 1989; 321:790-793.

Lavin PT, Knapp RC, Malkasian G, et al: CA-125 for the monitoring of ovarian carcinoma during primary therapy. *Obstet Gynecol* 1987; 69:223-227.

Louie KG, Ozols RF, Meyers CE, et al: Long-term results of a cisplatin-containing combination chemotherapy regimen for the treatment of advanced ovarian carcinoma. *J Clin Oncol* 1986; 4:1579-1585.

Luesley D, Lawton F, Blackledge G, et al: Failure of second-look laparotomy to influence survival in epithelial ovarian cancer. *Lancet* 1988; 2:599-603.

Luxman D, Bergmon A, Sagi J, et al: The postmenopausal adnexal mass: Correlation between ultrasonic and pathological findings. *Obstet Gynecol* 1991; 77:726-728.

Malkasian GD Jr, Podratz KC, Stanhope CR, et al: CA-125 in gynecologic practice. *Am J Obstet Gynecol* 1986; 155:515-518.

McGuire WP, Hoskins, WJ, Brady MF, et al: A phase III trial comparing cisplatin/cytoxan and cisplatin/taxol (PT) in advanced ovarian cancer (AOC) [abstract]. *Proc Am Soc Clin Oncol* 1993; 12:255.

McGuire WP, Hoskins WJ, Brady MF, et al: Cyclophosphamide and cisplatin compared to paclitaxel and cisplatin in patients with stage III and stage IV ovarian cancer. *N Engl J Med* 1996; 334:1.

Mecke H, Lehmann-Willenbrock E, Ibrahim M, et al: Pelviscopic treatment of ovarian cysts in premenopausal women. *Gynecol Obstet Invest* 1992; 34:36-42.

Meigs JV, Armstrong SH, Hamilton HH: A further contribution to the syndrome of fibroma of the ovary with fluid in the abdomen and chest, Meigs syndrome. *Am J Obstet Gynecol* 1943; 46:19-37.

Miracle-McMahill HL, Calle EE, Kosinski AS, et al: Tubal ligation and fatal ovarian cancer in a large prospective cohort study. *Am J Epidemiol* 1997; 145:349-357.

Mosgaard BJ, Lidegaard O, Kjaer SK, et al: Infertility, fertility drugs, and invasive ovarian cancer: A case-control study. *Fertil Steril* 1997; 67:1005-1012.

Muir C: Cancer incidence in five continents. Vol. V. IARC, Lyon, France. *IARC Sci Publ* 1987; 88:892-893.

Muto M, Cramer DW, Brown DL, et al: Screening for ovarian cancer: The preliminary experience of a familial ovarian cancer center. *Gynecol Oncol* 1993; 51:12-20.

NIH Consensus Development Panel on Ovarian Cancer: Ovarian cancer: Screening, treatment, and follow-up. *JAMA* 1995; 273:491-497.

Neijt JP, Ten Bokkel Huinink WW, van der Burg ME, et al: Long-term survival in ovarian cancer: Mature data from the Netherlands Joint Study Group for ovarian cancer. *Eur J Cancer* 1991; 27:1367-1372.

Nielsen SN, Scheithauer BW, Gaffey TA: Gliomatosis peritonei. *Cancer* 1985; 56:2499-2503.

Niloff JM, Knapp RC, Lavin PT, et al: The CA-125 assay as a predictor of clinical recurrence in epithelial ovarian cancer. *Am J Obstet Gynecol* 1986; 155:56-60.

Pittaway DE, Fayez JA, Douglas JW: Serum CA-125 in the evaluation of benign adnexal cysts. *Am J Obstet Gynecol* 1981; 157:1426-1428.

Piver MS, Malfetano J, Baker TR, et al: Five year survival for stage IC or stage I/grade 3 epithelial ovarian cancer treated with cisplatin-based chemotherapy. *Gynecol Oncol* 1992; 46:357-360.

Prentice RL, Thomas DB: On the epidemiology of oral contraceptives and disease. *Adv Cancer Res* 1987; 49:285-401.

Rice LW, Berkowitz RS, Mark SD, et al: Epithelial ovarian tumors of borderline malignancy. *Gynecol Oncol* 1990; 39:195-198.

Rice LW, Lage JM, Berkowitz RS, et al: Preoperative serum CA-125 levels in borderline tumors of the ovary. *Gynecol Oncol* 1992; 46(2):226-229.

Rosenberg L, Shapiro S, Slone D, et al: Epithelial ovarian cancer and combination oral contraceptives. *JAMA* 1982; 247:3210-3212.

Rosenberg L, Palmer JR, Zauber AG, et al: A case-control study of oral contraceptive use

and invasive epithelial ovarian cancer. *Am J Epidemiol* 1994; 139:654-661.

Rossing MA, Daling JR, Weiss NS, et al: Ovarian tumors in a cohort of infertile women. *N Engl J Med* 1994; 331:771-776.

Sainz de la Cuesta R, Goff BA, Fuller AF Jr, et al: Prognostic importance of intraoperative rupture of malignant ovarian epithelial neoplasms. *Obstet Gynecol* 1994; 84:1-7.

Sassone AM, Timor-Tritsh IE, Artner A, et al: Transvaginal sonographic characterization of ovarian disease: Evaluation of a new scoring system to predict ovarian malignancy, *Obstet Gynecol* 1991; 78:70-76.

Schildkraut JM, Thompson WD: Familial ovarian cancer: A population-based case-control study. *Am J Epidemiol* 1989; 128:456-466.

Schwartz PE, Chambers JT, Taylor KJ, et al: Early detection of ovarian malignancy: Preliminary results of the Yale Early Detection Program. *Yale J Biol Med* 1991; 64:573-582.

Schwartz PE, Chambers SK, Chambers JT, et al: Ovarian germ cell malignancies: The Yale University experience. *Gynecol Oncol* 1992; 45:26-31.

Schwartz SI: *Principles of surgery,* ed 6, New York, 1994, McGraw-Hill.

Silva EG, Robey-Cafferty SS, Smith TL, et al: Ovarian carcinomas with transitional cell carcinoma pattern. *Am J Clin Pathol* 1990; 93:457-465.

Smith EM, Anderson B: The effects of symptoms and delay in seeking diagnosis on stage of disease at diagnosis, among women with cancers of the ovary. *Cancer* 1985; 56:2727-2732.

Sorbe B, Frankendal B, Veress B: Importance of histologic grading in the prognosis of epithelial ovarian carcinoma. *Obstet Gynecol* 1982; 59:576-582.

Spanos WJ: Preoperative hormonal therapy of cystic adnexal masses. *Am J Obstet Gynecol* 1973; 116:551-556.

Sparks JM, Varner RE: Ovarian cancer screening. *Obstet Gynecol* 1991; 77:787-792.

Stenwig JT, Hazekamp JT, Beecham JB: Granulosa cell tumors of the ovary: A clinicopathological study of 118 cases with long-term follow-up. *Gynecol Oncol* 1979; 7:136-152.

Sutton GP, Blessing JA, Homesley HD, et al: Phase II trial of ifosfamide and mesna in advanced ovarian carcinoma: A Gynecologic Oncology Group study. *J Clin Oncol* 1989; 7:1672-1676.

Swenerton K, Jeffrey J, Stuart G, et al: Cisplatin-cyclophosphamide versus carboplatinum-cyclophosphamide in advanced ovarian cancer: A randomized phase III study of the National Cancer Institute of Canada: Clinical Trials Group. *J Clin Oncol* 1992; 10:718-726.

Tavassoli FA: Serous tumors of low malignant potential with early stromal invasion (serous LMP with microinvasion). *Mod Pathol* 1988; 1:407-414.

Teilum G: Endometrial sinus tumors of the ovary and testes: Comparative morphogenesis of the so-called mesonephroma ovarii (Schiller) and extraembryonic (yolk sac allantoic) structures of the rat placenta. *Cancer* 1959; 12:1092-1105.

Teilum G: *Special tumors of ovary and testis, and related extragonadal lesions: Comparative pathology and histologic identification,* ed 2, Philadelphia, 1971, JB Lippincott.

Thomas GM, Dembo AJ, Hacker NF, et al: Current therapy for dysgerminoma of the ovary. *Obstet Gynecol* 1987; 70:268-275.

Troche V, Hernandez E: Neoplasia arising in dysgenetic gonads. *Obstet Gynecol Surv* 1986; 41:74-79.

Van Nagell JR Jr: Ovarian cancer screening. *Cancer* 1991; 68:679-680.

Vasilev SA, Schloerth JB, Campeau J, et al: Serum CA-125 levels in preoperative evaluation of pelvic masses. *Obstet Gynecol* 1988; 71:751-756.

Whittemore AS, Harris R, Itnyre J, et al: Characteristics relating to ovarian cancer risk: Collaborative analysis of 12 US case-control studies. *Am J Epidemiol* 1992; 136:1184-1203.

WHO Collaborative Study of Neoplasia and Steroid Contraceptives: Epithelial ovarian cancer and combined oral contraceptives. *Int J Epidemiol* 1989; 18:538-545.

Willemse PH: Carboplatinum with cyclophosphamide in patients with advanced ovarian cancer: An efficacy and quality-adjusted survival analysis. *Int J Gynecol Cancer* 1992; 2:236-243.

Yazigi R, Sandstad J: Ovarian involvement in extragenital cancer. *Gynecol Oncol* 1989; 34:84-87.

Young RC, Decker DG, Wharton JT, et al: Staging laparotomy in early ovarian cancer. *JAMA* 1983; 250:3072-3076.

Young RC, Walton LA, Ellenberg SS, et al: Adjuvant therapy in stage I and stage II epithelial ovarian cancer: Results of two prospective randomized trials. *N Engl J Med* 1990; 322:1021-1027.

Young RC, Perez CA, Hoskins WJ: Cancer of the ovary. In DeVita VT, Hellman S, Rosenberg SA, editors: *Cancer: Principles and practice of oncology,* ed 4, Philadelphia, 1993, JB Lippincott.

Young RH, Welch WR, Dickersin GR, et al: Ovarian sex cord tumor with annular tubules: Review of 74 cases including 27 with Peutz-Jeghers syndrome and four with adenoma malignum of the cervix. *Cancer* 1982; 50:1384-1402.

Young RH, Dickersin GR, Scully RE: Juvenile granulosa cell tumor of the ovary: A clinicopathological analysis of 125 cases. *Am J Surg Pathol* 1984; 8:575-596.

Young RH, Scully RE: Ovarian Sertoli-Leydig cell tumors: A clinicopathological analysis of 207 cases. *Am J Surg Pathol* 1985; 9:543-569.

Young RH, Gilks CB, Scully RE: Mucinous tumor of the appendix associated with mucinous tumors of the ovary and pseudomyxoma peritonei: A clinicopathologic analysis of 22 cases supporting an origin in the appendix. *Am J Surg Pathol* 1991; 15:415-429.

Zurawski VR Jr, Orjaseter H, Andersen A, et al: Elevated serum CA-125 levels prior to diagnosis of ovarian neoplasia: Revelance for early detection of ovarian cancer. *Int J Cancer* 1988; 42:677-680.

10

The Breast

BARBARA L. SMITH

KEY ISSUES

1. Genetic, hormonal, reproductive, and environmental factors may increase the risk for breast cancer. Careful surveillance and new chemoprevention options are appropriate for women at high risk.
2. Mammography screening clearly reduces breast cancer mortality rates for women older than 50 years of age and probably reduces mortality rates for women in their 40s.
3. All palpable solid breast masses require tissue diagnosis. For many women, fine-needle aspiration biopsy and core-needle biopsy are appropriate alternatives to open surgical biopsy.
4. For most women with invasive and noninvasive breast cancer, breast-conserving surgery results in survival rates equivalent to those of mastectomy.

ANATOMY AND DEVELOPMENT

During the fifth week of gestation, a milk streak develops and extends from the axilla to the groin. It progresses through the milk-ridge and milk-hill stages to form the early breast buds. During this time, mesenchymal cells form the smooth muscle of the nipple and areola while epithelial elements form buds that ultimately give rise to 15 to 25 future ducts and lobules. It is thought that phylogenetically the breast arises as a modified apocrine sweat gland. These early phases of breast development are independent of hormones and occur in fetuses of both sexes. During the third trimester of pregnancy, placental sex hormones cause the previously formed epithelial buds to be converted into hollow ducts. It is these structures that produce the colostrum or "witch's milk" of the newborn that may be observed 4 to 7 days after birth. These secretions cease over subsequent weeks as the effects of placental hormones wane.

The nipple itself protrudes from the center of the pigmented areola and contains 10 to 15 terminal duct openings. Within the areola are Montgomery's glands, the slightly raised, nodular apocrine glands.

As many as 2% to 6% of adult women have accessory nipples (polythelia) along the milk ridge, most commonly in the axilla or just inferior to the breast. Some have breast ductal tissue beneath the accessory nipple (polymastia). This breast tissue may enlarge and even lactate as the result of pregnancy, and must be distinguished from a breast mass appearing during pregnancy. In general, however, there is no need to remove this accessory nipple or breast tissue except for cosmetic purposes or if palpable abnormalities arise.

Asymmetry of the breasts is common and can range from slight asymmetry to dramatic hypoplasia on one side. Complete amastia is rare and is often accompanied by chest wall deformities. Poland syndrome produces absence of the breast with defects of varying severity in the underlying pectoralis major muscle and bony chest wall and is often associated with hand abnormalities.

Abnormalities of breast structure may also have iatrogenic sources. Overly extensive excision of the breast bud underneath the nipple and areola during biopsy of a subareolar lesion in a young child can result in removal of tissue critical for breast development and in gross asymmetry after puberty.

SURGICAL ANATOMY OF THE BREAST

The breast overlies ribs two through six and, for surgical purposes, extends medially to the sternum, superiorly to the clavicle, laterally to the latissimus dorsi muscle, and inferiorly below the inframammary fold for a variable distance down the costal margin. These structures serve as the borders of dissection during mastectomy. The blood supply to the breast comes primarily from perforating branches of the internal mammary artery to the medial and central portions of the breast. The lateral thoracic artery supplies blood to the upper and upper-outer portions of the breast, and there are additional minor contributions from the intercostal, subscapular, and thoracodorsal arteries. Venous drainage occurs through the veins accompanying these arteries.

The breast lies directly over the pectoralis major muscle, which serves as the deep margin of dissection medially and centrally during mastectomy. The rectus abdominis muscle lies under the most inferior portion of the breast, and the serratus anterior muscle lies beneath the most lateral portion of the breast. The latissimus dorsi muscle, as described above, defines the most lateral extension of breast tissue and may be used for breast reconstruction after mastectomy; it can be detached posteriorly and swung anteriorly based on the thoracodorsal vessels. Similarly, the rectus abdominis muscle is used for breast reconstruction after mastectomy. It can be detached from its inferior insertion and swung upward based on the vessels entering superiorly. In general, the contralateral rectus muscle is preferred for reconstruction, though it is possible to use the ipsilateral muscle.

Lymph from all parts of the breast drains to the axillary nodes, making the axillary nodes the most appropriate area of sampling for metastatic disease during breast cancer surgery. Studies with radiolabeled colloid demonstrate that approximately 97% of lymph from the breast drains to the axillary nodes, and only 3% drains to the internal mammary nodes (Hultborn et al, 1955).

Within the axilla, the pectoralis minor muscle and the axillary vein define the three surgical levels of dissection. Level I node dissection includes those lymph nodes below the axillary vein, and level II dissection includes nodes from the axillary vein medially behind the pectoralis minor muscle to its medial border. Level I dissection includes lymph nodes medial to the pectoralis minor muscle. Rotter's nodes are those lying between the pectoralis major and minor muscles.

Less than 2% of patients have "skip metastases" with positive nodes only in level III, though as many as 20% of women have positive nodes in level II but not in level I (Danforth et al, 1986; Pigott et al, 1984; Rosen et al, 1983; Veronesi et al, 1993). As a result, axillary staging generally includes levels I and II node dissection that can be expected to contain nearly all the relevant staging information and to reduce the risk for subsequent lymphedema. Axillary sentineal lymph node mapping with blue dye or radiolabeled sulfa colloid is potentially less invasive than axillary staging. The efficiency of this approach is under study.

A number of important structures are present within the axilla and must be preserved during the course of axillary dissection for breast cancer staging. The axillary artery lies superior and deep to the axillary vein. The brachial plexus lies just superior to the axillary vein. Parts of the brachial plexus may pass anterior to the vein as it courses laterally. The long thoracic nerve runs along the serratus anterior muscle and serves as its motor nerve. Dividing this nerve results in winging of the scapula. The thoracodorsal bundle,

including its artery, vein, and nerve, enters the latissimus dorsi muscle after coursing diagonally downward through the axilla in a medial to lateral direction. The thoracodorsal vein enters the axillary vein, and the thoracodorsal artery and thoracodorsal nerve pass posterior to the axillary vein to their origins from the axillary artery and brachial plexus, respectively. Injury to the thoracodorsal nerve results in weakness of the latissimus dorsi muscle but few clinically evident symptoms. The medial pectoral nerve enters the posterior surface of the lateral portion of the pectoralis major muscle just inferior to the point at which the axillary vein crosses the lateral border of the pectoralis major muscle. This confusing nomenclature—the *medial* pectoral nerve enters the *lateral* portion of the muscle—stems from the nerve being named for its origin at the medial cord of the brachial plexus. Dividing this nerve during axillary dissection results in partial atrophy of the pectoralis major muscle. The intercostal–brachial nerve runs medial to lateral across the axilla, more or less parallel to the axillary vein and 1 to 2 cm inferior to it. Division of this nerve during axillary dissection results in anesthesia of the medial portion of the upper arm.

Any of these structures may be involved by metastatic disease within the axilla, though symptoms are most likely to arise from compression of the axillary vein or from obstruction of lymphatics, either of which may result in swelling of the affected arm.

Lymphedema may also appear after surgical dissection or radiation of the axilla, presumably because of progressive scarring and obstruction of the lymphatics draining the arm. To reduce the possibility of this disabling complication, axillary dissection is generally limited to levels I and II, and axillary irradiation is combined with surgery only when specific clinical circumstances demand both modalities. Lymphedema may appear within the first year after surgery or radiation of the axilla, or it may have a delayed onset and appear 5 to 10 years after treatment of the axilla.

It has been postulated that lymphedema also may result from progressive scarring after repeated infection in the ipsilateral arm. Although these mechanisms are unclear, patients are admonished to avoid trauma to the ipsilateral arm after axillary dissection for breast cancer; this includes phlebotomy, intravenous lines, and other breaks in the skin.

RISK FACTORS FOR BREAST CANCER

Clinical observations have identified subgroups of women at increased risk for breast carcinoma (Henderson, 1993). Some known risk factors are:

- increasing age
- family history of breast cancer (Sellers et al, 1992; Slattery and Kerber, 1993)
- hormonal and reproductive factors, including early menarche, late menopause, late first pregnancy or nulliparity, and use of exogenous hormones (Colditz et al, 1990; Dupont and Page, 1991; Henderson, 1993;

Marchant, 1993; Newcomb et al, 1994; Squitieri et al, 1994; Steinberg et al, 1991; Willett et al, 1987)

- environmental factors, including diet and the lifestyle of developed Western nations (Armstrong and Doll, 1975; Hunter et al, 1993; Willett, 1992)
- pathologic features within breast tissue, including premalignant lesions or a prior breast cancer (Frykberg and Kirby, 1994; Page and Jensen, 1994)
- chest wall radiation, such as for Hodgkin's disease
- other malignancies associated with an increased risk of breast cancer, such as ovarian and endometrial carcinomas

Recognition of these risk factors allows for appropriate screening and clinical management of the individual woman.

Taking into account various combinations of risk factors for breast cancer, several mathematical models have been developed to quantify individual risk compared with the risk for the general population (Claus et al, 1994; Gail et al, 1989). These models may be useful for counseling a woman regarding her degree of risk and for determining the appropriate follow-up. It is important to recognize, however, that for many women in whom breast cancer develops, there are no known risk factors present. The absence of risk factors should not prevent full evaluation or biopsy of a suspicious breast lesion.

Age

The risk of developing breast cancer increases in a nearly linear fashion with increasing age. While a woman's annual risk of developing breast cancer is only 1 in 5900 at age 30, it rises to 1 in 590 by age 50 and 1 in 330 by age 70 (Public Health Services, 1984). Approximately 75% to 80% of breast cancers are diagnosed in women older than 50 (Osteen et al, 1994; Public Health Services, 1981).

Genetics and Family History

It has long been recognized that breast cancer clusters in some families. Relatives of women diagnosed with breast cancer have higher incidences of the disease than do women in the general population. Risk is highest when there is more than one affected relative, when the patient has a close biologic relationship to the relative (mother or sister versus aunt or grandmother), when the age of onset in the relative is young, and when the relative has bilateral breast cancer. Even if a third-degree relative has breast cancer, it can increase a patient's risk (Slattery and Kerber, 1993). In the past it was thought that maternal relatives contributed more significantly to genetic transmission of risk than did paternal relatives, but current understanding of breast cancer risk genes shows equal contribution to risk from both sets of relatives.

Mutations in breast cancer risk genes BRCA1 or BRCA2 may contribute to causing approximately 10% of breast cancers (Casey, 1997; Marcus et al, 1996). The BRCA1 gene, on chromosome 17, was first identified in families with clusters of breast and ovarian cancer (Hall et al, 1990; Narod et al, 1991). Data suggest that it confers a 55% to 85% lifetime risk for breast cancer and a 20% to 65% lifetime risk for ovarian cancer (Ford et al, 1994). The BRCA2 gene, on chromosome 13, is associated with increased risk for male and female breast cancer, with male lifetime breast cancer risk as high as 6% and female lifetime breast cancer risk as high as 50% to 85% (Wooster et al, 1995; Tavtigian et al, 1996). Certain populations, particularly Jewish women of Ashkenazi descent, are at increased risk for carrying mutations in the BRCA1 and BRCA2 genes (Strueing et al, 1995; Roa, 1996). Genetic testing is now commercially available for BRCA1 and BRCA2 mutations. Optimum screening and management options for patients with these mutations are under discussion (Cummings et al, 1998).

Several rare genetic syndromes have been identified that are associated with markedly increased risk for breast carcinoma. These include the Li-Fraumeni syndrome, in which breast and other malignancies, including brain, lung, lymphoma, and sarcoma, develop in young patients. It has been recognized that this syndrome is caused by germline mutations of the p53 tumor suppressor gene (Levine, 1992). Germline p53 mutations are thought to account for only 1% of all breast cancer, though somatic p53 mutations occur during tumor progression in many cases. Cowden's disease, a syndrome that produces multiple pathognomonic cutaneous trichilemmomas, is associated with an increased risk for breast cancer that is often bilateral (Brownstein et al, 1978). Cowden's disease appears to be inherited in an autosomal dominant pattern and probably accounts for less than 1% of breast carcinomas.

It is important to recognize that family history may interact with other risk factors and that family members share genetics and environment. There is an interaction between family history and risk factors such as body fat distribution, parity, and age at first pregnancy (Sellers et al, 1992), use of exogenous hormones (Steinberg et al, 1991), and histology (Page and Jensen, 1994).

Histopathologic Factors

Certain histopathologic findings are associated with increased risk for breast carcinoma. Women who have already had invasive or noninvasive breast cancer are at increased risk for development of additional breast cancers. There is an approximately 1% per year incidence of new cancers in the contralateral breast. If the initial breast cancer was treated with breast-conserving surgery, there is a risk of both true recurrence and new primary tumors, combining to give a 10% incidence of in-breast recurrence at 10 years follow-up. Women with a diagnosis of lobular carcinoma in situ (LCIS) have a 20% to 25% risk for developing invasive breast carcinoma, usually of ductal histology, in the next 20 to 30 years (Frykberg and Kirby, 1994; Page and Jensen, 1994). This risk is equally distributed across the breast with LCIS and the contralateral breast. An increased risk for breast cancer is also seen in women whose biopsies show either atypical ductal hyperplasia or atypical lobular hyperplasia. This risk is in the 15% range over the next 15 to 20 years, and, as in LCIS, it is equally distributed across both breasts. A small but measurable increase in breast cancer risk is seen in women with proliferative fibrocystic disease without atypia. Nonproliferative fibrocystic disease and simple cysts do not carry increased risk for breast cancer (Page and Jensen, 1994).

Dietary and Environmental Factors

Differences in breast cancer incidence in different countries have led to the speculation that dietary factors influence breast cancer risk. Some study results show a weak association between high intake of dietary fat and increased risk for breast cancer (Howe et al, 1991; Howe et al, 1990), but most show no association (Goodwin and Boyd, 1987; Jones et al, 1987; Knekt et al, 1990; Mills et al, 1989; Willett, 1992). These studies, however, do not rule out the possibility that the timing of fat intake, for example, fat intake early in life, may influence breast cancer risk or that extremely low-fat diets may reduce it. Women who continue to gain weight during mid-life (Huang et al, 1997) may be at increased risk for breast cancer. High dietary fiber intake does not appear to reduce breast cancer risk (Willett, 1992). Women whose diets are significantly deficient in vitamin A are found to have increased risk for breast cancer, but diets rich in vitamin A do not reduce the risk for breast cancer. No association is seen between vitamin E or vitamin C intake and breast cancer risk. There is clear-cut evidence of an increased risk in women who have two or more drinks of alcohol per day (Smith-Warner et al, 1998; Hunter et al, 1993). Although higher alcohol consumption has been associated with increased risk, the mechanism for this association is unclear (Howe et al, 1991; Willett et al, 1992). Higher levels of physical activity during work or leisure may lower risk (Thune et al, 1997). Recent reports raise the issue of increased risk for breast cancer among women exposed to electromagnetic fields (Loomis et al, 1994), but the methodology used in these studies has been severely criticized (Trichopoulos, 1994).

Hormonal and Reproductive Factors

Hormonal and reproductive factors are related to breast cancer risk (Henderson, 1993; Marchant, 1993; Newcomb et al, 1994). Women whose menarche occurred at or before age 11 have an increased risk for breast cancer compared to those whose menarche occurred at age 14 or later. Menopause after age 55 also is associated with increased breast cancer risk. Full-term pregnancy before age 30 reduces breast cancer risk, whereas nulliparity or first pregnancy after age 30 is associated with increased risk. The mechanism by which age at the birth of the first child influences risk is unknown, but there may be a differentiation of breast tissue at term that permanently reduces risk. There may be a slight reduction in breast cancer risk with increasing parity, though not all studies support this. Lactation for long periods may decrease risk, but this reduction may apply only to premenopausal breast cancer; it may have no effect on the risk for postmenopausal breast cancer (Newcomb et al, 1994).

Oral Contraceptives and Breast Cancer

Current data suggest that there is no significant increase in breast cancer risk among women who have used oral contraceptives. A recent meta-analysis of studies examining the possible influence of oral contraceptive use on breast cancer finds no increased risk (Romieu et al, 1990). However, this analysis finds a higher risk for premenopausal breast cancer among women who use oral contraceptives for a prolonged period of time before their first pregnancy (Romieu et al, 1990; Willett et al, 1987). Some of the increased risk observed with prolonged oral contraceptive use before the first pregnancy may actually reflect a delayed first pregnancy or an early menarche, both of which are known risk factors for breast carcinoma (Marchant, 1993). However, in view of this potentially increased risk, it is prudent to avoid early and prolonged oral contraceptive use in young nulliparous women unless they are sexually active and want to avoid pregnancy (Henderson, 1993).

Postmenopausal Hormone Replacement Therapy and Breast Cancer Risk

Hormone replacement therapy provides many benefits to postmenopausal women. Estrogens relieve many of the troubling symptoms of menopause and have a favorable effect on the cardiovascular system and on bone density. However, hormone replacement therapy carries with it an increased risk for other problems, among them thromboembolic disease, endometrial carcinoma, and breast carcinoma. The balance between risks and benefits for women as a group and for individual patients has been the source of much recent discussion.

A review of overall mortality rates among users and nonusers of postmenopausal hormone replacement therapy shows a statistically significant decrease in mortality from all causes (relative risk, 0.80; $p < 0.0001$). This benefit seems to derive mainly from a reduction in mortality rates from acute myocardial infarction (relative risk, 0.60; $p < 0.001$), but there is a trend toward decreased mortality from ischemic heart disease, stroke, and cancer of any type (Henderson et al, 1991). The Nurses' Health Study (Grodstein et al, 1997) also finds significantly decreased overall mortality rates among current users of hormone replacement compared with nonusers (relative risk: 0.63 overall, 0.51 for women with coronary risk factors, and 0.89 for women with low coronary risk factors). Risk for death from colon cancer is found to be lower in hormone users than in nonusers (Calle et al, 1995).

When breast cancer risk is analyzed separately from other causes of morbidity and mortality, an increased risk is seen among women who use hormone replacement therapy. Study results conflict concerning the degree and magnitude of breast cancer risk associated with hormone replacement therapy and whether subgroups of women at higher risk can be identified.

The Nurses' Health Study (Colditz et al, 1995) found a significant increase in breast cancer risk in current users of hormone replacement therapy, either as estrogen alone or as estrogen plus progestin, with a relative risk of 1.46 after 5 to 9 years of use. Relative risk for death from breast cancer was also increased to 1.45 among women who used hormone replacement therapy for more than 5 years. Interestingly, the increased risk related to hormone replacement therapy appeared to be temporary; it became comparable to that for nonusers within 2 to 3 years of discontinuation of hormone replacement (Colditz et al, 1990).

An older meta-analysis of breast cancer risk and hormone replacement therapy showed an approximately 10% overall increase in breast cancer risk among women using hormone replacement therapy relative to nonusers (Dupont and Page, 1991). Another meta-analysis that included only studies that met certain criteria found a relative risk of 1.3 for breast cancer among women using hormone replacement therapy for more than 15 years (Steinberg et al, 1991). A Swedish cohort study correlated increased risk with duration of use and showed an increased risk for breast cancer among women who used hormone replacement therapy for 9 years or more (Bergvist et al, 1989).

When estrogen use after menopause is combined with other risk factors for breast cancer, subsets of patients were identified whose risk was significantly increased (Steinberg et al, 1991). They are:
- women with a family history of breast cancer (relative risk, 3.4)
- nulliparous women who use hormone replacement therapy (relative risk, 1.5)
- women with benign breast disease (relative risk, 1.7)
- women whose first term pregnancy was after age 30 (relative risk, 1.7)

Some studies suggest that although the risk for breast cancer is higher among women who use hormone replacement therapy, when cancer does develop it is detected at an earlier stage and may have a more favorable prognosis (Gambrell, 1984; Gambrell, 1992; Squitieri et al, 1994). However, the Nurses' Health Study found a significant increase in breast cancer mortality rates among users of hormone replacement (Colditz et al, 1995). The early detection and more favorable outcomes observed in some series are attributed, at least in part, to increased patient and physician awareness of the risk for breast cancer and to increased access to medical care among hormone users.

Summary

For most postmenopausal women taking hormone replacement therapy, there appears to be a significant reduction in overall mortality rates, primarily from cardiovascular disease but also from colon cancer and osteoporosis-related problems. Conversely, evidence shows that there is a modest increase in the risk for breast cancer associated with postmenopausal hormone replacement therapy. This increase may be substantially higher for women with a family history of breast carcinoma or for those with other breast cancer risk factors. In clinical practice, it is prudent to weigh a woman's cardiovascular and perhaps osteoporosis risks against her risk for breast carcinoma before making a decision about the use of postmenopausal estrogen.

For postmenopausal women who have multiple risk factors for breast carcinoma or for those who are reluctant to increase their breast cancer risk in any way, it may be best to deal with cardiovascular and osteoporosis risks through exercise, diet, and other nonhormonal means rather than through hormone replacement therapy. It is hoped that selective estrogen receptor modulators (SERMs) will one day provide reliable cardiovascular and osteoporosis protection that does not increase, but perhaps reduces, breast cancer risk.

WORK-UP OF THE PATIENT WITH A BREAST PROBLEM

Benign breast disease is common among American women, and its symptoms are the chief complaint for many women seeking treatment from their gynecologists. Additional breast abnormalities are often discovered during the course of routine physical examination and mammography. The management of these benign problems can be difficult. More important, it may be difficult to distinguish benign breast lesions from malignant lesions. In evaluating breast problems it is critical to remember that mammography fails to detect 10% to 15% of all palpable malignant lesions.

Breast problems usually seen in clinical practice fall into several categories: discrete palpable masses; vague thickening or nodularity; breast pain; nipple discharge; abnormalities during pregnancy or lactation; abnormalities seen on mammography; and the persistently worried patient with a negative work-up. These will be addressed in the sections that follow. From a risk management perspective and for good medical practice, it is important to document any recommendations for mammography, ultrasonography, biopsy, referral, or follow-up interval in the patient's chart. It is also good practice to discuss these recommendations with the patient.

A proper evaluation of any breast problem requires a detailed history of the current breast problem, a review of previous breast problems, a review of risk factors for breast carcinoma, a thorough physical examination of the breasts, appropriate imaging studies, and an evaluation of the patient's general medical condition.

Pertinent History

A history should be taken that includes documentation of the current breast problem, documentation of risk factors for breast carcinoma, and any history of other breast diseases as listed in Box 10-1. The patient is asked to describe when the

---

BOX 10-1
BREAST-SPECIFIC MEDICAL HISTORY

Current age
Race
Age at menarche
Date of last menstrual period/age of menopause
Parity
Age at first pregnancy
Lactation history
Use of oral contraceptives and years of use before first
    pregnancy
Use of postmenopausal estrogen replacement
Use of other hormones, fertility regimens, diethylstilbestrol
Family history of breast cancer, age at diagnosis
Family history of ovarian cancer, age at diagnosis
Family history of other cancers, age at diagnosis
Dates of previous mammograms
Previous breast biopsies and abnormal findings
Previous other breast surgery
Personal history of cancer
Previous breast problems

---

problem was first identified and whether it was identified by self-examination, by a physician on routine examination, or by screening mammography. If there are any physical findings, the patient should be asked whether the area in question is tender to palpation. Changes in the size or tenderness of any palpable abnormalities since their initial discovery and any changes during the menstrual cycle should be recorded. The patient should also be asked whether she has had similar symptoms at any time in the past. Any previous breast problems or breast surgery should be documented, and pathology reports from previous breast surgery should be obtained. Earlier evaluation of the problem by another health care professional should be described, and, if possible, documentation of the visits should be obtained. Results of all imaging studies that have been performed to date should be obtained; the reports and the films themselves should be reviewed.

The next section of the history should detail portions of the medical history pertinent to breast cancer risk and include menstrual history, reproductive factors, and hormone exposures. Age at menarche, and if applicable, menopause is recorded. For menstruating women the date of the last menstrual period is recorded. The number of pregnancies and the age at first term pregnancy are determined. Any use of exogenous hormones is recorded and should include oral contraceptives and years of use before the first term pregnancy, postmenopausal estrogen replacement therapy, and use of any other sex hormones as part of a fertility program or for other purposes. Any family history of breast cancer should be detailed and include at least first-, second-, and third-

degree relatives, and the age at diagnosis of the family members. Ovarian cancer in the family should be recorded with age at diagnosis, as should other cancers, particularly those that affected family members at a young age. Any cancer syndromes affecting the family should be recorded. Any personal history of cancer should be recorded with particular attention to prior breast, ovarian, or endometrial cancers. Prior radiation exposures, especially to the chest wall, should be noted.

An overview of the general medical history should be obtained as for any surgical patient and should include current medications, allergies, tobacco and alcohol use, previous surgery of any type, any medical problems, and a brief social history.

Physical Examination

Physical examination of the breasts includes inspection of the skin, palpation of the breasts, examination of the nipples for discharge, and palpation of the axillary and supraclavicular node areas. The breasts should be inspected with the patient sitting with her hands behind her head and her elbows back to look for asymmetry, dimpling of the skin, and erythema or edema. Taking care to include the subareolar area, the breast should then be palpated and examined systematically from the clavicle to below the inframammary fold and from the sternum to the posterior axillary line. Examination should be performed first with the fingers flat and together using the region between the DIP and PIP joints of the examining hand to press breast tissue back against the ribs to look for masses or for areas of thickening or tenderness. Any questionable areas are then examined in more detail using the fingertips. Examination of both breasts is performed with the patient first supine and then sitting. If an abnormal area is identified, a careful description of its size, contour, texture, tenderness, and position should be recorded. A diagram of the lesion is extremely useful for future reference.

The nipples and the areolae are best examined with the patient supine. Any areas of skin breakdown should be noted. The nipples are then squeezed gently to check for discharge. The number and position of any ducts from which discharge arises should be documented. Color (milky, green, yellow, clear, brown, or bloody) and consistency (watery, sticky, or thick) of the discharge should be noted. Of most concern is spontaneous, single-duct discharge or any bloody discharge. If a discharge is identified on one side, a careful search for a discharge on the other side is important because unilateral, single-duct discharge is more likely to be pathologic, and bilateral, multiple-duct discharge is more likely to be physiologic. Any discharge should be tested for occult blood. Cytology of nipple discharge increases cost and only rarely changes management.

Axillary nodes are examined by using the examiner's left hand for the right axilla and the right hand for the left axilla. The fingers are pressed inward and upward to check for enlarged nodes. In the supine position, to facilitate the examination, the shoulder muscles may be relaxed by having the patient rest her elbow at her side, or the examiner may support the arm and have the patient reach her hand across her body toward the opposite shoulder. In the sitting position, the shoulder muscles may be relaxed if the examiner supports the patient's elbow with one hand while examining the axillary nodes with the other. Supraclavicular nodes may be examined with the patient supine or sitting. Should any enlarged nodes be discovered, their size, mobility, and number should be recorded. Any matting or fixation of nodes to the chest wall is significant and must be noted. Tenderness of enlarged nodes that may suggest a reactive process must be noted.

Imaging Studies
Mammography

Although current recommendations state that baseline screening mammography need not be performed until a woman is 40 and there is discussion about delaying this until she is 50, it is reasonable to perform mammography for any woman older than 35 who has a palpable breast mass or other specific symptoms. Approximately 4% to 5% of breast cancer occurs in women younger than 40, and 20% develops in women younger than 50 (Osteen et al, 1994; Public Health Services, 1981). By the time a woman is 35 and in the presence of a palpable lesion or other abnormality, there is a reasonable probability of finding additional abnormalities elsewhere in the symptomatic breast or in the opposite breast that would influence management of the presenting abnormality. However, it must be remembered that mammography fails to detect 10% to 15% of all malignant lesions. It is least accurate for lobular carcinoma and for women who have radiographically dense breast tissue.

It is, therefore, essential to emphasize that a negative mammogram should not influence the decision to biopsy a clinically palpable lesion. Mammography is performed to look for synchronous lesions or nonpalpable calcifications surrounding the palpable abnormality, not to rule out the need for biopsy of the palpable lesion.

Ultrasonography

The primary value of ultrasonography is to distinguish cystic from solid lesions. This distinction is best made for palpable lesions by needle aspiration, which is both diagnostic and therapeutic. For nonpalpable lesions, ultrasonography can prove the cystic nature of a lesion and can eliminate the need for additional work-up or treatment. Although it was initially hoped that ultrasonography would serve as a useful screening tool, it is inadequate for this purpose. Ultrasonography does not detect calcifications, and it fails to detect many malignancies. In addition, ultrasonography identifies a great deal of normal breast texture as potential nodules and produces false-positive readings.

However, advances in ultrasound technology have made it increasingly useful for characterizing lesions first identified by palpation or by mammography. Analysis of the contour and the internal echo texture of a solid lesion can be used to determine whether the lesion has a low or a high probability of malignancy.

Ultrasonography is also useful for directing fine-needle or core biopsy of lesions that are visualized because manipulation and positioning of the needle can be performed in real time and needle position can be directly confirmed.

MANAGEMENT OF SPECIFIC BREAST PROBLEMS
Discrete Palpable Masses

The management of the palpable breast mass is summarized in Fig. 10-1. Discrete masses, or those that are clearly different from surrounding normal breast tissue, may be solid or cystic. Distinguishing between these two possibilities is important (Donegan, 1992). Cysts are almost always benign and rarely require more than aspiration. Solid masses, on the other hand, require that a tissue diagnosis be obtained to rule out malignancy. Clinical examination is not accurate in distinguishing a cyst from a solid mass. Rosner and Baird (1985) found that physical examination correctly identified as cystic only 58% of 66 palpable cysts; the remaining cysts were incorrectly thought to represent solid masses.

Cysts

In general, a palpable mass thought to be a cyst should be confirmed as such by aspiration, even if ultrasonography suggests that it is a simple cyst. Aspiration confirms that the palpable mass corresponds to the lesion seen on ultrasonography. Additionally, removal of the mass by aspiration permits a more thorough examination of the surrounding breast tissue. Bloody cyst fluid or a persistent mass after aspiration may indicate malignancy, and the aspirated fluid should be sent for cytologic analysis (Hamed et al, 1989). In these circumstances, a biopsy should be performed even if the cytologic analysis is negative for malignancy. If the cyst fluid is not bloody and no mass remains after aspiration, there is little chance of malignancy, and the fluid need not be sent for cytology. Ciatto et al (1987a) found no malignancies among 6747 non-bloody cyst aspirations.

If a cyst is aspirated but there is no prior documentation by ultrasonography that it is a simple cyst, the patient should be reexamined in 4 to 8 weeks. Less than 20% of simple cysts recur after a single aspiration, and less than 9% recur after two or three aspirations (Leis, 1991). When the same cyst recurs rapidly after aspiration, it should be reaspirated and the cyst contents sent for cytological analysis. A biopsy should be performed if the results are atypical or suspicious or if the cyst recurs yet again. Appearance of a new cyst in a different area of breast tissue, however, does not require this additional work-up and should be evaluated and aspirated as a new problem. Additional cysts may be expected in more than half of patients (Hughes and Bundred, 1989).

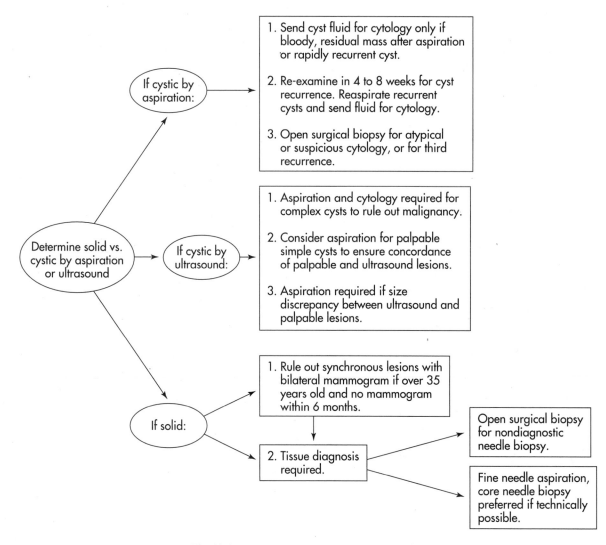

Fig. 10-1. Management of a palpable breast mass.

Solid Masses

Discrete masses within the breast that are solid by ultrasonography criteria or because they do not yield fluid on aspiration attempts must undergo needle or open surgical biopsy to exclude malignancy. Physical examination alone correctly identified a mass as malignant only 60% to 85% of the time in one series (Boyd et al, 1981; Layfield et al, 1989). Experienced examiners often disagree on the need for biopsy of a particular lesion. One study found that four surgeons uniformly agreed on the need for biopsy in only 73% of 15 palpable masses later shown on biopsy to be malignant (Boyd et al, 1981). Before a biopsy is performed, it is appropriate to order a mammogram for a woman older than 35 to look for synchronous lesions.

Vague Thickening or Nodularity

Normal breast texture is often heterogeneous, particularly in premenopausal women. These variations in texture may create areas that feel firmer than the surrounding tissue and may or may not be tender to the touch. These vague thickenings or areas of nodularity are common and must be distinguished from true masses.

In clinical practice, areas of nodularity or thickening should first be compared with the corresponding area of the opposite breast for symmetry. Symmetric areas of thickening are rarely pathologic. Asymmetric areas, particularly those that are tender, often represent fibrocystic disease and often resolve spontaneously. In premenopausal women, such vague areas should be reexamined after one or two menstrual cycles. If the asymmetry resolves, the finding was most likely a result of a benign process, and no further work-up is required. Areas of asymmetry that persist, however, must be viewed with some suspicion and the patient should be referred to a surgeon or a gynecologist who performs breast surgery for evaluation and potential biopsy. It is appropriate to order a mammogram to rule out synchronous lesions at this point for any woman older than 35 years of age who has not had a mammogram in the past 6 months. The value of a negative fine-needle aspiration biopsy of a vague thickening is unclear. Open biopsy is generally required for adequate sampling.

Breast Pain

Breast pain, also termed mastalgia, is one of the most common breast symptoms experienced by women of reproductive age, and it brings many to their physicians (Preece et al, 1976; Preece et al, 1978; Wingo et al, 1991). Often the concern is not about the severity of the pain but rather that the pain may indicate a serious condition such as breast cancer. Physiologic breast tenderness varies with the menstrual cycle; the breasts are most tender immediately before the menstrual period. In contrast, noncyclic pain bears no relationship to the menstrual cycle, and its cause is unknown. The pain may be intermittent or continuous and is often described by the patient as burning. Although breast pain is poorly understood, its cyclic nature and resolution at menopause suggest a hormonal cause. Results of several studies that measured estrogen levels in women with breast pain showed no difference in circulating hormone levels when they are compared with pain-free control subjects. On the other hand, it has been postulated that progesterone levels may be decreased in women with breast pain.

Although breast cancer rarely causes pain, evaluation of the patient with breast pain first requires that malignancy be ruled out. A careful physical examination should be performed, and any palpable masses should be evaluated as described earlier. A mammogram should be performed in any woman older than 35 years who has persistent, noncyclic breast pain. It is also important to rule out causes of pain that do not arise from the breast itself. This includes muscle strain, costochondritis, and pain of pleural or mediastinal origin. Once these less common causes of pain are excluded, the pain symptoms themselves are addressed.

For most women with breast pain, reassurance that the work-up shows no evidence of breast cancer or other serious abnormality is the only treatment necessary. The patient may also be reassured that breast pain is usually self-limited and resolves within a few months. During periods of more severe breast tenderness, symptomatic relief may be obtained with nonnarcotic analgesics, in particular nonsteroidal antiinflammatory agents. Maneuvers such as the elimination of caffeine, chocolate, or salt from the diet, though harmless, are of no proven benefit. It is often useful to reexamine the patient after one or two menstrual cycles to be sure that no palpable abnormality is evolving and to assess her response to conservative treatment.

Evening primrose oil resulted in significant or complete pain relief in 50% of women with cyclic mastalgia in one study (Pashby et al, 1981). The oil is obtained from the evening primrose flower and is extremely high in polyunsaturated oils. It is ingested orally and has few side effects. Vitamins E and B$_6$ may also reduce breast pain. For the rare patient whose breast pain is severe and unresponsive to conservative measures, pharmacologic therapy may be instituted. Danazol, a gonadotropin inhibitor, is the only drug approved in the United States by the Food and Drug Administration (FDA) for the treatment of breast pain (Baker and Snedecor, 1979; Lauerson and Wilson, 1976). It has androgenic effects that many patients find unacceptable. Other pharmacologic agents used to treat breast pain include bromocryptine (a prolactin antagonist) and tamoxifen (Fentiman et al, 1986; Mansel et al, 1978), but their use is rarely required.

Nipple Discharge and Other Nipple and Areola Abnormalities
Nipple Discharge

In as many as 60% to 70% of healthy women, a small amount of discharge, usually yellow to green, may be expressed from the nipples of both breasts (Petrakis, 1986). This is not spontaneous; it results only from attempts to express it. It is distinguished from galactorrhea, the bilateral, often spontaneous milky discharge that is almost never caused by breast malignancy. Microscopy shows that galactorrhea is different from physiologic discharge because there is fat in the secretions. As many as one third of women with galactorrhea have pituitary tumors, particularly if they also have amenorrhea. Hypothyroidism, chest-wall trauma, and certain pharmacologic agents may cause galactorrhea. The evaluation of galactorrhea includes measurement of serum prolactin concentration levels and thyroid function tests. If the prolactin level is elevated, magnetic resonance imaging of the head, with special attention paid the sella turcica, should be performed to rule out pituitary adenoma.

Unilateral nipple discharge or nipple discharge that is bloody, watery, or sticky may be an indicator of malignancy and should be evaluated further (Ciatto et al, 1987b; Devitt, 1985; Takeda et al, 1982). Careful physical examination should be performed to identify any palpable masses, and a mammogram should be ordered for women older than 35 years of age. Cytologic analysis is rarely useful because surgical evaluation is required whether the result is positive or negative. Ductograms are generally not useful for the same reason; they rarely provide data that change the need for surgery or the type of surgical procedure. Excision of the discharging duct is performed to rule out malignancy (Passaro et al, 1994; Urban, 1963).

Other Nipple and Areola Abnormalities

Erosion or chronic crusting of the nipple raises the suspicion of Paget's disease of the nipple, a variant of infiltrating or intraductal carcinoma arising in the terminal ducts and involving the surface of the nipple itself. A biopsy is required to distinguish Paget's disease from benign dermatologic conditions, such as eczema, that may also involve the nipple and areola. Subareolar infections are described in the next section.

Breast Infections

Infections of the breast fall into three general categories: lactational infections, chronic subareolar infections associated with duct ectasia, and nonlactational abscesses.

Infections and abscesses may occur during lactation and are often associated with weaning or with other times when engorgement occurs. Often this is accompanied by breakdown of the skin of the nipple. It is thought that the nursing infant may be the source of recurrent colonization of the nipple, and this may make weaning necessary. Early-stage infections are treated with oral antibiotics to cover gram-positive cocci including *Staphylococcus aureus*, with warm soaks, and with active attempts to keep the breast emptied, particularly the affected area of the breast. Weaning is unnecessary, and the infant is not adversely affected by nursing from the breast with the infection (Benson, 1989; Niebyl et al, 1978). Once an abscess forms, however, surgical drainage and weaning are usually required.

Abscesses of the lactating breast rarely form fluctuant masses because of the network of fibrous septae within the breast (Benson, 1989). This diagnosis is established by the features of fever, leukocytosis, and exquisite point tenderness in the breast. The abscesses that form are multiloculated, and all loculations must be broken up to ensure resolution of the infection. Needle aspiration of breast abscesses in lactating women, therefore, is inadequate. General anesthesia is almost always required for adequate pain relief during drainage of these abscesses because of the tenderness of the affected area and the amount of manipulation required to break up loculations within the abscess cavity. The cavity should be packed open, as for any abscess. Weaning is required.

In women who are not lactating, a chronic relapsing and remitting form of infection, variously known as periductal mastitis or duct ectasia, may develop in the subareolar ducts of the breast. The subareolar terminal duct walls become thin and fill with secretions. Series of infections with resultant inflammatory changes and scarring may ensue and may result in retraction or inversion of the nipple, masses in the subareolar area, recurrent periareolar abscesses, and occasionally chronic infectious fistulae from the subareolar ducts to the periareolar skin (Passaro et al, 1994; Smith, 1991). Palpable masses and mammographic changes that mimic carcinoma may result. It is unclear whether chronic infection causes the observed thinning and dilatation of the subareolar ducts or whether the dilatation and accumulation of secretions is the primary event and is followed by secondary bacterial infection of the accumulated secretions. The infection that results is most often a mixed infection and includes anaerobic skin flora (Brook, 1988; Veronesi et al, 1985).

Infection related to duct ectasia or periductal mastitis in the acute phase is treated by incision and drainage in combination with antibiotics directed against skin flora and anaerobes. Antibiotic treatment is often unsuccessful unless anaerobic coverage is included. Recurrent infection is treated by excision of the subareolar duct complex after the acute infection has completely resolved and by antibiotics during the perioperative period. The need for drain placement is debated. Even with wide excision of the subareolar duct complex and intravenous antibiotic coverage, some patients continue to have recurrent infections. Excision of the nipple and areola often resolves this (Hadfield, 1960; Urban, 1963).

Abscesses or cellulitis related to breaks in the skin or occasionally to a cyst that becomes infected may develop in the nonlactating breast. These infections are usually in peripheral rather than in subareolar breast tissue, and they are treated with antibiotics, warm soaks, and incision and drainage.

Breast Abnormalities in Pregnant or Lactating Women

Making the diagnosis of breast malignancy may be extremely difficult in pregnant or lactating women. Although engorgement and diffuse thickening of the breasts are expected with pregnancy and lactation, distinct masses, asymmetric tissue, or any area of persistent concern to the patient should be evaluated promptly without waiting for delivery or the elective cessation of lactation. Patients in this category should be referred promptly to a surgeon for evaluation and possible biopsy.

Mammography is generally not performed during pregnancy because of the density of breast tissue, which decreases mammographic sensitivity, and because of the potential effects of radiation on the fetus. Mammographic sensitivity is also poor during lactation and for 3 to 4 months after the cessation of breast-feeding. Ultrasonography may distinguish cystic from solid lesions, as it does in nonpregnant women, but it is not useful for screening.

Biopsy can be performed without difficulty during pregnancy, and fine-needle aspiration biopsy is the first step in many patients. Open biopsy with local anesthesia is well tolerated, and there are usually no difficulties with healing. Unless the lesion is immediately beneath the areola, subsequent breast-feeding is usually possible.

In women who are breast-feeding, transient plugging of the ducts must be distinguished from true masses. There is usually no difficulty distinguishing a mass from mastitis or from an abscess because tenderness and fever make the diagnosis of infection clear. Any persistent or residual mass after a plugged duct has been drained or following an episode of mastitis should be evaluated. As with any persistent breast mass, there should be a low threshold for obtaining a tissue diagnosis either with needle biopsy or open surgical biopsy. In approximately half of lactating women who undergo open biopsy, the incision heals without their having to discontinue breast-feeding. In the remaining half, however, milk fistulas develop at the incision sites, and it is necessary to stop breast-feeding to permit the incisions to heal.

The causes of breast masses in pregnant women are those common to premenopausal women, among them fibroadenoma, fibrocystic change, fibrosis, and occasionally breast cancer. Lactating adenomas are benign lesions of pregnancy and lactation that resemble fibroadenomas on gross examination.

Nonpalpable Mammographic Abnormalities

Widespread mammography screening has led to an increase in the identification of nonpalpable breast lesions. A survey by the American College of Surgeons' Commission on Cancer revealed that of women in whom breast cancer was detected in 1990, 56.1% had abnormal screening mammograms that prompted them to seek treatment, up from 29.6% in 1983 (Osteen et al, 1994). Two thirds of women who had positive mammograms in 1990 had no abnormalities on physical examination.

Most abnormal mammogram findings on mammography, however, are benign. Mammographers have developed a set of criteria by which they grade their suspicions for malignancy (Ciatto et al, 1987b; Hall et al, 1988; Moskowitz, 1983; Sickles, 1986). Recently, there have been attempts to standardize the terminology for reporting mammographic findings. In general, the practicing clinician relies on the recommendation of the mammographer regarding biopsy or follow-up.

Different mammographers set different thresholds for recommending biopsy of a lesion detected on mammography. On average in the United States, 15% to 30% of lesions observed by mammography for which biopsy is recommended prove to be malignant (Hall et al, 1988). Some authors, however, advocate a lower threshold for biopsy, one in which 10% of the lesions recommended for biopsy prove to be malignant, to minimize the chance of missing early-stage malignancy (Moskowitz, 1983; Wisbey et al, 1983).

Clearly, it is desirable to minimize the number of benign biopsies prompted by screening mammography while detecting as many early-stage malignancies as possible. Studies have been conducted to assess the effectiveness and safety of close mammographic follow-up of "probably benign" findings. Biopsy is then reserved for lesions that change and become suspicious during follow-up. The initial determination that the lesion is probably benign takes into account the patient's breast cancer risk factors, including personal history of breast cancer, family history, and current physical examination. Sickles (1991) reported the prospective follow-up of 3184 consecutive "probably benign" abnormalities detected on mammography in a protocol obtaining repeat mammograms at 6 months after the initial finding, 6 to 12 months after the initial finding, and then annually for two more examinations. Seventeen (0.5%) of these 3184 probably benign lesions subsequently proved malignant on biopsy: 15 were detected as changes in the mammographic appearance of the lesion, and two were detected as palpable findings. All malignancies were smaller than 2 cm, two were

purely in situ, and two had one positive lymph node each. Two smaller series reported 0.6% and 1.1% rates of malignancy in lesions detected on mammography and followed up as probably benign (Helvie et al, 1991; Wisbey et al, 1983). Using this policy of serial mammographic examination of probably benign findings, authors reported eliminating a number of benign biopsies; approximately 40% of lesions recommended for biopsy proved to be malignant (Helvie et al, 1991; Sickles, 1991).

These results support the balanced use of mammographic follow-up and biopsy to minimize morbidity rates, financial costs, and psychologic stress of benign biopsies prompted by mammography screening. The availability of stereotactic core-needle biopsy or ultrasonography-guided core-needle biopsy has reduced costs and morbidity rates associated with biopsy of nonpalpable lesions.

In general, if a mammographer recommends that a lesion identified by mammography be biopsied, biopsy should be performed. The decision for follow-up or biopsy of an equivocal mammographic finding should be made by the mammographer and the patient's clinician and should take the patient's overall situation, including breast cancer risk, into consideration. It is appropriate to refer such a patient to a surgeon for a second opinion. Nonpalpable cysts detected by mammography and ultrasonography and shown to be simple cysts (no debris or ragged walls) need not be aspirated except to relieve pain.

Management of Patients at High Risk

A woman's risk for breast cancer may be high because of family history, identification of a mutation in a breast cancer susceptibility gene, personal history of breast cancer, personal history of atypia on biopsy, or reasons described previously. There are three treatment options for such women: close surveillance, prophylactic mastectomy, or chemoprevention (Cummings et al, 1998).

Close surveillance is the option chosen most often. For women with a history of breast cancer, surveillance protocols are based on the stage of the initial tumor. For women with LCIS, atypical hyperplasia, or family history of breast carcinoma, surveillance should include semiannual physical examinations by a physician. Mammography should be performed annually if there is a diagnosis of LCIS or atypia. For women with a family history of breast cancer, annual mammography should begin at least 5 years before the age at diagnosis of the youngest affected relative and no later than age 35. For women from families with a proven or suspected breast cancer syndrome, annual screening should begin 10 years earlier than the age of the youngest affected relative (Lynch et al, 1991).

Data from the NSABP Tamoxifen Chemoprevention Trial (Fisher, 1998) suggest that tamoxifen can reduce the risk for breast cancer in women at increased risk. The option of participating in ongoing trials of tamoxifen or other agents to reduce breast cancer risk is now available to women at high risk (see Chemoprevention of Breast Cancer, later in this chapter).

The Persistently Worried Patient with a Negative Work-Up

Occasionally, a patient remains concerned about the possibility of breast cancer despite negative findings on physical examination and mammography. It is appropriate to refer such a patient to a surgeon for a second opinion.

BIOPSY TECHNIQUES

The methods for obtaining a tissue diagnosis of a palpable breast mass or an abnormality detected on mammography are fine-needle aspiration, core-needle biopsy, and open surgical biopsy.

Fine-Needle Aspiration

Fine-needle aspiration using a 22- to a 25-gauge needle may be performed with minimal patient discomfort at the time a palpable mass is identified on physical examination. Mammography- or ultrasonography-guided fine-needle aspiration also may be performed for nonpalpable lesions. The false-negative rate of fine-needle aspiration ranges from 1% to 35% for palpable lesions and is as high as 68% for non-palpable lesions (Dowlatshahi et al, 1991; Grant et al, 1986; Hammond et al, 1987; Layfield et al, 1989). The false-positive rate is generally in the 1% to 2% range but is reported to be as high as 18% in some series (Hammond et al, 1987; Layfield et al, 1989). The false-negative and false-positive rates at a given institution are clearly dependent on the technical quality of the aspiration itself and on the experience of the cytopathologist interpreting the slides. In view of this false-negative rate, any equivocal diagnosis, nonspecific findings such as normal or fibrocystic breast tissue, or atypical results of cytologic analysis should be evaluated further, usually through open surgical biopsy.

Core-Needle Biopsy

Another nonsurgical form of breast biopsy is core-needle biopsy. Through core-needle biopsy, an 11- to 14-gauge cylinder of tissue is obtained from a lesion and is analyzed by conventional pathology rather than by cytology. As a result, it is generally more accurate than fine-needle aspiration. In addition, because skilled pathology interpretation is available at most institutions, it is the technique of choice for image-guided biopsy (Ballo and Sneige, 1996). As with fine-needle aspiration, the false-positive rate is low. This technique is less comfortable for the patient than fine-needle aspiration because it entails the use of a much larger needle and requires that a small nick be made in the skin, but it is less invasive than open surgical biopsy.

Stereotactic core-needle biopsy and ultrasound-guided core-needle biopsy can now be used for most nonpalpable breast lesions (Parker et al, 1991), and it is usually the approach of choice. There is clearly a learning curve for oper-

ators of this technique (Elliott et al, 1992). Nondiagnostic and false-negative readings decrease with experience and with the use of 11-gauge biopsy needles and vacuum-assisted techniques (Meyer 1996, D'Angelo et al, 1997).

Sometimes the results of core-needle biopsy require a different management than when the same results are obtained in open surgical biopsy. If atypical ductal hyperplasia is observed on core-needle biopsy, additional tissue should be obtained through open surgical biopsy because nearly half of these patients are found to have ductal carcinoma in situ when additional tissue is examined. If core-needle biopsy results are discordant with mammographic or clinical interpretation of the lesion—for example, if a spiculated mass is seen on mammography but only normal breast tissue is seen on core biopsy—repeat core-needle biopsy or open-surgery biopsy should be considered.

Open Biopsy

Open surgical biopsy remains the standard for the diagnosis of breast lesions. Unlike fine-needle aspiration or core-needle biopsy, this procedure removes the entire lesion, enabling the pathologist to analyze it more completely, including the margins and the extent of intraductal disease if the lesion is malignant. Cost, time, and patient discomfort are highest with this approach. If the lesion is palpable, the surgeon should strive to excise it with only a narrow rim of normal-appearing breast tissue. Because most breast masses are benign, unnecessary distortion of the breast should be avoided.

Nonpalpable lesions require preoperative wire localization by the mammographer to direct the surgeon to the appropriate area. A specimen radiograph of the excised tissue should be obtained before surgery is completed to ensure that the lesion is contained within the specimen.

Most biopsies, including needle-localized biopsy of non-palpable lesions, are now performed with local anesthesia or local anesthesia with sedation; general anesthesia is reserved for special circumstances, among them the need for multiple biopsies. The former standard approach of biopsy under general anesthesia with frozen-section diagnosis and immediate definitive surgery if malignancy is identified has largely been abandoned. In addition to the logistic difficulties of this approach for the patient and the surgeon, it has been shown that there is no improvement in survival rates or reduction in recurrence rates by performing definitive surgery on the same day as biopsy. Because there are now multiple treatment options for breast cancer, a staged approach, allowing time for a discussion of treatment options and for decision making after a diagnosis of malignancy, is preferred.

Choice of Biopsy Technique

Once a decision has been made to obtain a biopsy of a breast abnormality, it must be determined whether fine-needle aspiration, core-needle biopsy, or open surgical biopsy is most appropriate. Little is lost by performing fine-needle aspiration or core biopsy in the office at the time of discovery of a palpable lesion. As discussed earlier, however, the decision to obtain a biopsy specimen of a nonpalpable lesion, detected on mammography, by stereotactic core-needle biopsy or needle-localized open biopsy is more complex and requires an understanding of the patient's risk for malignancy and a willingness to leave the lesion in place after sampling.

Analysis of Tissue Obtained at Biopsy

In addition to routine histologic analysis, additional tests that provide prognostic or therapeutic information are now routinely performed on malignant breast tissue.

Hormone Receptor Levels

Determination of estrogen and progesterone receptor levels in breast carcinomas is essential because these levels predict the patient's response to hormonal therapy. There has been some evidence that estrogen receptor-positive tumors have better prognoses than do receptor-negative tumors. Receptor levels are usually determined by immunohistochemical assays that use monoclonal antibodies to bind to receptors in fresh or fixed tissue samples.

DNA Ploidy and S-Phase Fraction

It has been observed that malignant cells often contain aberrant amounts of DNA. Such abnormal DNA levels are termed aneuploid in contrast to normal or diploid DNA levels. DNA content does not appear to be a good predictor of prognosis. *S-phase* refers to the fraction of cells within a population that synthesize DNA in preparation for cell division. This value is used to estimate the growth rate of a tumor. It has been suggested that a breast tumor with a high S-phase fraction has a poorer prognosis than a tumor with a low S-phase fraction. Both S-phase fraction and DNA content are weak prognostic factors, and many institutions no longer measure them (El-Ashry and Lippman, 1994).

Molecular Markers and Other Prognostic Factors

As molecular biology and immunology have increased our understanding of the properties of tumor cells, molecular markers have been identified that may have implications for prognosis or treatment. The true clinical value of these tumor markers remains to be determined, but a number of them have already been analyzed for their relevance to breast cancer (El-Ashry and Lippman, 1994; Gasparini et al, 1993).

At present the marker with the greatest clinical relevance is Her-2-neu. Her-2-neu, also called erbB-2, is an oncogene—a gene that when overexpressed contributes to malignant cell behavior. The Her-2-neu protein is a transmembrane protein thought to be involved in the control of cell growth. Studies suggest that Her-2-neu overexpression, observed in approximately 20% of breast cancers, is an independent predictor of poor prognosis (Gusterson et al, 1992; Slamon et al, 1989). Other studies suggest, however, that Her-2-neu overexpression is a predictor of poor response to chemotherapy in node-positive breast cancer (Gullick et al, 1991; Perren, 1991). Results of clinical trials suggest that antibodies to Her-2-neu, alone or in combination with chemotherapy, may be effective in tumors that overexpress Her-2-neu (Muss, 1994)

Measurements of the density of neovascularization (Weidner et al, 1993), cathepsin D, ki-67, myc, ras, and p53 have been performed on breast tumor specimens (El-Ashry and Lippman, 1994). These studies are investigational, however, and their impact on clinical practice remains undetermined.

BREAST CANCER SCREENING
Theory and Current Modalities

Breast cancer is a frightening disease that is prevalent in the Western world. Early detection remains the cornerstone of efforts to reduce breast cancer mortality rates. This has led to the development of screening programs designed to identify patients with breast cancer at the earliest stages, when treatment is thought to have the greatest impact on clinical outcome.

Most forms of breast cancer are thought to pass through a clinically occult phase during which the number of malignant cells is too few to be detected by imaging studies or by physical examination. As the tumor progresses, the lesion becomes large enough to be detected by mammography and by physical examination. Although it is possible for even a small tumor to metastasize, the chance that metastatic clones will emerge increases as the tumor becomes larger. Metastatic disease can sometimes be controlled, but few patients with metastatic disease are ever cured. Screening programs, therefore, are directed at detecting breast cancers at the smallest size possible, before metastasis.

Mammography can detect cancers smaller than those that can be detected by even the most skilled examiner, either as a calcification without an associated palpable mass or as a very small or deep mass. Mammography has, therefore, been a central component of screening programs.

Mammography and physical examination are complementary modalities for screening. As many as 10% to 15% of *palpable* breast malignancies are not visualized by mammography because they do not produce calcifications or a density radiologically distinguishable from surrounding breast tissue. A skilled examiner is able to detect smaller masses and to be more precise in identifying suspicious masses amid normal breast texture than the average woman performing breast self-examination. For this reason periodic physical examination by a skilled examiner, usually a physician or a specially trained nurse, is the second component of most screening programs.

Breast self-examination is the third component of breast cancer screening programs. It involves instructing the patient in systematic monthly self-examination to detect palpable abnormalities that may appear during intervals between mammograms and examinations by a health care professional. Patients are encouraged to report any abnormal findings to their physicians without delay. The efficacy of breast self-examination in reducing breast cancer mortality rates has been questioned by some studies (Thomas et al, 1997) but supported by others (Foster et al, 1992; Gastrin et al, 1994). Overall, breast self-examination is a low-cost, useful screening tool. Self-examination may generate anxiety in some women who become alarmed by the irregular or "lumpy" texture of normal breast tissue. However, because more than 40% of breast cancers are detected by the woman herself, self-examination remains an important component of any screening program (Osteen et al, 1994). Patient anxiety is best dealt with by education and reassurance that some nodularity is normal, and that cancer usually produces hard, distinct lumps that the patient will be able to distinguish from normal breast tissue.

Physical examination and mammography are the only accepted modalities for breast cancer screening. Ultrasonography is not a useful modality for screening because it detects many small irregularities in breast texture that raise concerns but are of no proven clinical significance. Ultrasonography should only be used to determine whether a palpable lesion or one found by mammography is cystic or solid. Magnetic resonance imaging, computed tomography, positron-emission tomography, thermography, and other imaging modalities are not appropriate for screening.

Current Issues in Breast Cancer Screening

Although there is general agreement about the importance of detecting breast cancer at the earliest possible stage, there has been a great deal of controversy about the ability of screening modalities to achieve this early detection in a cost-effective manner, particularly for women younger than 50. However, 20% to 25% of breast cancers are diagnosed in women younger than 50, which makes effective screening of this age group a serious concern (Osteen et al, 1994; Public Health Services, 1981).

Screening Issues in Women 40 to 49 Years of Age

Reexamination of the value and efficacy of screening mammography began in 1992 after the publication of 7-year results of the Canadian National Breast Cancer Screening Study (Miller et al, 1992a; Miller et al, 1992b). This study found no reduction in mortality rates in women 40 to 49 years of age who underwent annual screening mammography and physical examination when they were compared with women who conducted breast self-examination only.

These results prompted reappraisal of older screening data of women in their 40s (Chu et al, 1988; Nystrom et al, 1993; Smart et al, 1993; Tabar et al, 1993; Tabar et al, 1992) and critical appraisal of the design and methodology of the Canadian National Breast Cancer Screening Study. A 1993 National Cancer Institute (NCI) group's meta-analysis of randomized breast cancer screening studies concluded that there was no benefit to mammography for women 40 to 49 years of age at 5 to 7 years of follow-up (Fletcher et al,

1993). Based on this review, the NCI suggested that annual physical examination was recommended but that screening mammography was not recommended for 40- to 49-year-old women, except as dictated by risk factors.

There was considerable resistance from several fronts to eliminating screening mammography for women in this age group, and heated debate about the merits of screening continued (Baines, 1994; Berkell et al, 1992; Boyd et al, 1993; Eckhardt et al, 1994; Kopans and Feig, 1993; Mettlin and Smart, 1993; Moskowitz, 1992). A second National Institutes of Health Consensus Conference on screening mammography was called in early 1997 to assess new data from ongoing screening studies (NIH, 1997). Ten- to 12-year follow-up of ongoing Swedish studies was presented, with the Gothenborg study showing a statistically significant 44% reduction in breast cancer mortality rates and the Malmo study showing a 36% statistically significant reduction in mortality rates in women ages 40 to 49 who undergo mammographic screening. An overview combining these results with the results of other screening studies showed a 17% to 24% statistically significant reduction in mortality rates when women in their 40s undergo mammography.

Based on these data, the Consensus Conference suggested that women ages 40 to 49 decide for themselves whether to undergo screening mammography. However, the NCI broke ranks with the Consensus Panel and endorsed screening mammography for women ages 40 to 49. At nearly the same time, the American Cancer Society recommended that mammographic screening be performed every year rather than every other year for women older than 40.

Recommendations for Current Screening Practice

Even with the ongoing debate, there are areas of agreement about screening for breast cancer in current clinical practice. Monthly breast self-examination is encouraged for all women as a low-risk, low-cost, and potentially beneficial method to detect breast cancer. Annual physical examination by a health professional is recommended for women older than 40, though some groups recommend lowering the age to 35 or even younger. It is reasonable to include examination of the breasts in any general physical examination of a woman older than 30.

For women ages 40 to 49, the 1997 NCI recommendations suggest mammographic screening every 1 to 2 years, with the American Cancer Society recommending that mammograms be performed every year in this age group. It is likely that controversy will continue regarding screening guidelines for this age group.

Mammographic screening is recommended for women 50 and older, with nearly all analyses demonstrating a 30% reduction in breast cancer mortality rates in women who undergo screening (Farrow et al, 1992; Fletcher et al, 1993). Most groups that issue screening guidelines advocate annual mammography screening after age 50, though some state that every other year is sufficient.

An upper age limit for screening has not been defined. Few women older than 70 have been included in screening trials, but the annual incidence of breast cancer increases with increasing age, and breast tissue density decreases, reducing the number of false-negative and false-positive readings. It seems reasonable to continue physical examination and mammographic screening as long as a woman is in sufficiently good health to tolerate lumpectomy under local anesthesia.

CARCINOMA OF THE BREAST

Breast cancer develops in 10% to 12% of American women at some time in their lives. Treatment options are increasingly tailored to the specifics of an individual woman's situation, including the patient's preferences and the specific histopathology and other features of the tumor (Hortobagyi, 1998).

STAGING OF BREAST CANCER

Several staging systems have been used for breast cancer, and two are common. The first is the tumor node metastasis (TNM) staging system, which categorizes tumors according to primary tumor size, nodal disease, and distant metastases. Current TNM staging categories are shown in Table 10-1 (American Joint Committee on Cancer, 1989). Breast cancer is also characterized as stage I through stage IV based on specific combinations of tumor size, nodal status, and metastases. This staging system and its relation to the TNM staging system are presented in Table 10-2 (Wood et al, 1994).

EVOLUTION OF TREATMENT FOR BREAST CANCER

Breast cancer was recognized as a clinical entity in ancient times and was described, as were early attempts at treatment, in the records of ancient Egypt and Greece. The ability of physicians to improve the lives of women with breast cancer was extremely limited until late in the nineteenth century. Before the 1880s, breast cancer was almost always locally advanced at diagnosis and was generally viewed as a fatal disease. Attempts to perform local excision during these early years were met with local recurrence rates ranging from 50% to 100% and with high complication rates.

With improvements in anesthetic and aseptic techniques, larger surgical procedures for breast cancer were explored, including procedures to resect the entire breast and all or part of the pectoralis major muscle. Axillary lymph nodes began to be included in the dissection. Unfortunately, mortality rates after surgery were high, and there was little evidence of survival benefit from these larger procedures. Patients and physicians concluded that most women with breast cancer were better off without surgical treatment.

Table 10-1   Tumor Node Metastasis Clinical Classification

T—Tumor

TX   Primary tumor cannot be assessed
T0   No evidence of tumor
Tis Carcinoma in situ: intraductal carcinoma, or lobular carcinoma in situ, or Paget disease of the nipple with no invasive tumor
T1   Tumor <2 cm in greatest dimension
     T1mic: microinvasion 0.1 cm or less in greatest dimension
     T1a: Tumor >0.1 cm but <0.5 cm
     T1b: >0.5 but <1 cm
     T1c: >1 but <2 cm
T2   Tumor >2 but <5 cm in greatest dimension
T3   Tumor >5 cm in greatest dimension
T4   Tumor of any size with direct extension to chest wall or skin
T4a Extension to chest wall
T4b Edema (including peau d'orange), or ulceration of the skin of the breast, or satellite skin nodules confined to the same breast
T4c Both 4a and 4b
T4d Inflammatory carcinoma

N—Regional Lymph Nodes

NX   Regional lymph nodes cannot be assessed (e.g., previously removed)
N0   No regional lymph node metastasis
N1   Metastasis to movable ipsilateral axillary node(s)
N2   Metastasis to ipsilateral axillary node(s) fixed to one another or to other structures
N3   Metastasis to ipsilateral internal mammary lymph node(s)

M—Distant Metastasis

MX   Presence of distant metastasis cannot be assessed
M0   No distant metastasis
M1   Distant metastasis (includes metastasis to supraclavicular lymph nodes)

From the American Joint Committee on Cancer: *Manual for staging for breast carcinoma*, ed 5; Philadelphia: Lippincott, 1997.

This fatalistic era ended with the introduction of the Halsted radical mastectomy. Described in 1882, the Halsted radical mastectomy consisted of excision of the entire breast with all overlying skin and with complete level I-III axillary node dissection. The pectoralis major muscle and later the pectoralis minor muscle were included in the specimen. The amount of skin removed required a skin graft for closure. Halsted's 1894 series reported a local recurrence rate of only 6%, in contrast to the 50% to 100% local recurrence rates seen with earlier local excision attempts. This success gave physicians the opportunity to study the natural history of breast cancer in the absence of rapid local failure, and the significance of distant metastases was recognized.

Table 10-2 Staging Groups			
Stage	**Tumor**	**Node**	**Metastasis**
Stage 0	Tis	N0	M0
Stage I	T1	N0	M0
Stage IIA	T0	N1	M0
	T1	N1	M0
	T2	N0	M0
Stage IIB	T2	N1	M0
	T3	N0	M0
Stage IIIA	T0	N1	M0
	T1	N2	M0
	T2	N2	M0
	T3	N1, N2	M0
Stage IIIB	T4	Any N	M0
	Any T	N3	M0
Stage IV	Any T	Any N	M1

From Yeatman TJ, Bland KI: Staging of breast cancer. In Bland KI, Copeland EM, editors: *The breast: Comprehensive management of benign and malignant diseases,* Philadelphia, 1991, WB Saunders.

The Halsted radical mastectomy became the treatment of choice for breast cancer for more than 70 years. This success of a more extensive surgical precedure, where lesser procedures had failed, changed the way physicians viewed breast cancer. The favored biologic model became one that viewed breast cancer spread as centrifugal and extending outward in a "permeative" fashion from the primary tumor to reach other parts of the body. This led to progressively larger surgical procedures in the hope that a large enough procedure could encompass all cancer cells and eradicate the disease.

This model of breast cancer biology ushered in the surgical era of treatment that included trials of the supraradical mastectomy of Wangensteen, a procedure consisting of radical mastectomy, supraclavicular lymph node dissection, and median sternotomy taking bilateral internal mammary lymph node chains. Urban (1963) designed the extended radical mastectomy that included resection of the internal mammary nodes and the overlying ribs and sternum in continuity with the standard radical mastectomy resection. A fascia lata graft was used to close the pleural defect created by this procedure. As expected, both these ultraradical procedures increased morbidity and mortality but provided no significant improvement in survival.

The failure of increasingly radical surgical procedures to improve the survival of patients with breast cancer led to disillusionment with surgery and required a revision of the existing model of breast cancer progression. It became clear that breast cancer spread was not only centrifugal but also embolic through the bloodstream and the lymphatic system. It also became clear that micrometastases could arise early in a tumor's course. This led to the hypothesis that metastatic potential was biologically predetermined and unaffected by local control measures. This paradigm led to trials of lim-

ited surgery alone or radiation alone for the treatment of breast cancer. During the 1960s and 1970s, these efforts were organized into prospective randomized clinical trials to explore the use of smaller surgical procedures such as modified radical mastectomy, simple mastectomy, local excision alone, or radiation after incisional or excisional biopsy of the primary tumor.

The NSABP B-04 study and other trials showed that survival rates after modified radical mastectomy were equivalent to those after Halsted radical mastectomy, leading to the abandonment of radical mastectomy as a treatment option for breast cancer (Fisher et al, 1986; Maddox et al, 1987; Turner et al, 1981). The NSABP B-04 study also showed that simple mastectomy without axillary dissection resulted in a survival rate equivalent to that of radical or modified radical mastectomy but 18% of patients ultimately developed axilliary failures. Although this could be salvaged by delayed axillary dissection, this failure rate was generally considered unacceptable and axillary dissection remained an integral part of breast cancer surgery.

Trials of radiation alone for the treatment of breast cancer demonstrated its limited ability to control bulky disease but its effectiveness in providing local control of minimal residual disease (Calle et al, 1978). Trials of limited surgery plus radiation as an alternative to mastectomy were undertaken. Prospective randomized trials in the United States and Europe compared mastectomy with lumpectomy or with lumpectomy plus radiation (Fisher et al, 1985a; Fisher and Wolmark, 1985; Sarrazin et al, 1984; Veronesi et al, 1987). One of the most important of these trials was the NSAPB B-06 trial. It randomized 1843 women with stage I and stage II breast cancer and with primary tumors as large as 4 cm to treatment by modified radical mastectomy, segmental mastectomy with axillary dissection and no radiation, or segmental mastectomy with axillary dissection and 5000 cGy radiation to the entire breast. Clean margins were required, and patients were required to undergo mastectomy if the margins of resection on the partial mastectomy specimen were positive. Survival rates were equivalent in all three groups. Lumpectomy with radiation resulted in a local recurrence rate of 10% at 8 years. Without radiation, however, there was a 28% local recurrence rate at 5 years and a 39% recurrence rate at 8 years (Fisher et al, 1985a; Fisher and Wolmark, 1985).

Similar conclusions were drawn from the Milan trial, from 1973 to 1980, in which 701 patients younger than 70 who had tumors smaller than 2 cm were enrolled. Patients were randomized to treatment by radical mastectomy or quadrantectomy with axillary dissection and radiation consisting of 5000 cGy to the whole breast and a 1000 cGy boost to the tumor bed. Overall survival rates and disease-free survival rates are equivalent in the two treatment arms (Veronesi et al, 1986; Veronesi et al, 1987).

Another randomized trial of modified radical mastectomy versus local excision, axillary dissection, and 6000 cGy radiation also showed no difference in survival rates after breast-conserving surgery or mastectomy (Sarrazin et al, 1984). Other studies from the NCI, the EORTC, and the World Health Organization found no difference in survival rates after mastectomy alone compared with limited surgery plus radiation. However, the Guy's Hospital trial comparing radical mastectomy and local resection with only 3800 cGy of radiation showed both increased local recurrence rates and lower survival rates in the limited surgery plus radiation arm, which demonstrated the importance of adequate dosages of radiation (Hayward and Caleffi, 1987).

RADIATION THERAPY FOR BREAST CANCER

Current radiation therapy regimens consist of approximately 5000 cGy delivered in fractions of approximately 200 cGy per day to the whole breast and, in most patients, a boost of 1000 to 1500 cGy to the tumor bed. Axillary node fields are not treated unless axillary dissection findings suggest a high risk for axillary relapse. Combined surgery and radiation to the axilla increases the risk for lymphedema of the arm. Radiation to supraclavicular node fields is also generally restricted to those patients who have multiple positive axillary nodes and in whom the likelihood of occult supraclavicular disease is greater. Internal mammary nodes are not usually irradiated as a prophylactic measure.

Radiation is routinely delivered to the chest wall after mastectomy for T3 or T4 primary tumors, for inflammatory carcinomas, and when multiple axillary lymph nodes are positive. It is recognized that large primary tumors and significant axillary disease are predictive of higher rates of chest wall recurrence after mastectomy.

Results of two recent randomized trials of chest-wall and nodal radiation versus no radiation in premenopausal women treated with mastectomy and systemic chemotherapy suggest a significant survival advantage with the use of radiation after mastectomy. Overgaard et al (1998) randomized 1708 premenopausal women with stage II or stage III breast cancer to treatment by radiation to the chest wall and lymph nodes versus no radiation after mastectomy and eight cycles of cyclophosphamide, methotrexate, 5-fluorouracil chemotherapy. Radiation significantly reduced local recurrence and significantly improved survival rates. Overall survival at a median follow-up of 114 months was 48% in the radiated arm and only 32% in the nonradiated arm ($p < 0.001$). A smaller trial (Ragaz et al, 1998) randomized 318 women to treatment by chemotherapy alone or chemotherapy and radiation after mastectomy. At 15-year follow-up, there was a 33% reduction in recurrence and a 29% reduction in mortality among women who received radiation to the chest wall and nodes compared with those who did not. These data suggest that effective control of locoregional disease and the prevention of local recurrence can improve overall breast cancer survival rates (Hellman, 1998).

Radiation therapy to the breast or chest wall is generally well tolerated and results in only minor side effects in most

---

> **BOX 10-2**
> **PATIENT ELIGIBILITY CRITERIA FOR BREAST CONSERVATION AND RADIATION THERAPY**
>
> - Primary tumor size up to 5 cm
> - Lobular or ductal histology
> - Any location of primary tumor within breast; if acceptable, cosmetic result after lumpectomy to clean margins (including central lesions)
> - Clinically suspicious but mobile axillary nodes
> - Any estrogen receptor or progesterone receptor status
> - Any patient age

---

women. These include transient erythema or desquamation of the treated skin and mild fatigue. A small amount of lung volume is included in the fields, resulting in what is usually a clinically insignificant but measurable reduction in lung function. The heart receives some radiation during treatment to the left breast or left chest wall, and older studies showed a slightly increased risk for future myocardial infarction. Current techniques minimize this risk. There is also an approximately 1% risk for a second malignancy induced by the radiation, including sarcoma, leukemia, or breast carcinoma. These radiation-induced malignancies may appear after a long lag time of 7 to 15 years or more after treatment.

ELIGIBILITY FOR LUMPECTOMY AND RADIATION

As discussed earlier, clinical trials conducted in the 1970s and 1980s of stage I and II breast carcinoma clearly demonstrate that limited surgery with lumpectomy or quadrantectomy, axillary dissection, and radiation results in overall survival rates that are equivalent to survival rates after treatment with radical or modified radical mastectomy (Fisher et al, 1985a; Fisher and Wolmark, 1985; Sarrazin et al, 1984; Veronesi et al, 1987). Box 10-2 lists categories of patients who are eligible for breast conservation and radiation therapy. For these patients, the long-term survival after breast conservation and radiation is equivalent to that after modified radical mastectomy, and local recurrence rates are in the 5% to 10% range or lower. For women in these categories, the choice of mastectomy versus limited surgery and radiation is made on the basis of patient and physician choice, access to radiation therapy, or other contraindications to radiation. It has been estimated that although approximately two thirds of women with breast cancer are in these categories and are eligible for breast conservation, many women still undergo mastectomy (Farrow et al, 1992; Lazovich et al, 1991; Lee-Feldstein et al, 1994; Nattinger et al, 1992; Osteen et al, 1992).

Contraindications to Breast Conservation

There are groups of patients for whom mastectomy is clearly the preferred treatment. Indications for mastectomy fall into several broad categories, namely, contraindications to radiation therapy, technical and cosmetic limitations of lumpectomy, issues of local recurrence, and issues of prophylaxis for patients at high risk.

Contraindications to Radiation Therapy

There are some patients for whom radiation therapy is contraindicated. This group includes patients who choose not to undergo radiation therapy either because of the inconvenience of the treatment or because of concerns about potential complications and second malignancies. In addition, there are patients for whom access to radiation therapy is extremely difficult either because they live in rural areas or because of physical difficulties in making daily trips for therapy. There are also patients with psychiatric or other disorders who would find it difficult to comply with the daily treatment schedule for 6 or more weeks. Additional patients have other medical contraindications to radiation therapy and include women who are pregnant or those who have undergone previous radiation to the chest wall for other conditions, including prior breast cancer. Although some literature supports the use of repeat local excision without additional radiation therapy for local recurrence after radiation, most authors favor completion mastectomy (Haffty et al, 1989; Kurtz et al, 1989).

Technical and Cosmetic Issues Related to Lumpectomy

In some patients resection of the primary tumor to clean margins yields a cosmetically unacceptable result. For these patients, mastectomy with immediate reconstruction may be preferable to lumpectomy with radiation. This category includes patients whose primary tumors are large relative to their breast size where resection of the primary tumor would remove a significant portion of breast tissue. Also included in this category are patients with multiple primary tumors. In addition to having a higher local recurrence rate, removal of an unacceptable amount of breast tissue would be required to obtain adequate margins around all tumors. Patients with superficial central lesions that would necessitate excision of the nipple and areola for clean margins are, however, eligible for conservative surgery and radiation. It has been shown that for excision to clean margins that includes the nipple and the areola, survival and local recurrence rates are equivalent to those of other groups of patients undergoing lumpectomy and radiation (Clarke et al, 1985; Fisher and Fisher, 1977; Harris et al, 1985). For many women, the cosmetic result after this procedure is preferable to that obtained with immediate reconstruction. Some surgeons still favor mastectomy for patients with Paget's disease, though many now consider local excision with radiation appropriate treatment if negative margins can be obtained before radiation.

Local Recurrence

For most women with breast carcinoma, the appearance of distant metastases heralds incurable and ultimately fatal disease. In contrast, local recurrence after breast conservation appears to have little impact on overall survival. In prospective randomized trials, it has been difficult to show a statistically significant reduction in survival rates among women who have had local recurrences after limited surgery and radiation. It has been a concern that there is a decrement in survival among some patients who have local recurrences (Harris and Osteen, 1985). However, even without a large decrement in survival, there is a real cost in patient anxiety. Follow-up testing is required, and subsequent treatments must be taken into account when estimating the impact of local recurrence.

Therefore, it is worthwhile to identify those patients in whom local recurrence after breast conservation and radiation therapy is most likely to develop. These patients may choose primary mastectomy to avoid the potential problems of local recurrence. Several characteristics of primary tumors indicate a higher rate of local recurrence after limited surgery and radiation. They include gross residual disease after lumpectomy, multiple primary tumors within the breast, microscopically positive or close margins, and large tumor size.

Obtaining clean margins is probably the most critical factor in reducing the risk for local recurrence. The difficulty of obtaining microscopically clean margins in tumors with an extensive intraductal component and in lobular carcinomas may account for the higher local recurrence rates seen with these tumor types. Histologic analysis of mastectomy specimens from patients who have tumors with an extensive intraductal component has shown that these tumors have high rates of multifocality (Holland et al, 1990). It is likely that this residual disease is the cause of local recurrence.

BREAST RECONSTRUCTION AFTER MASTECTOMY

Breast reconstruction after mastectomy may provide cosmetic and psychological benefits. Reconstruction may be performed at any time after mastectomy. In the past, it was generally delayed for 1 to 2 years after mastectomy, but now it is often performed immediately as part of the initial surgical procedure. Immediate reconstruction has no significant impact on recurrence or survival and causes no significant delay in the detection of local recurrence or in the administration of adjuvant chemotherapy (Eberlein et al, 1993). Reconstruction options include the placement of subpectoral saline implants either immediately or after tissue expansion, latissimus dorsi myocutaneous flap reconstruction, or transverse rectus abdominus muscle (TRAM) flap reconstruction. Free flaps may be used under special circumstances. Mastectomies performed with reconstruction are performed employing a skin sparing technique, and involve excising only the nipple, areola, and tumor biopsy scar. The maximum amount of native breast skin is preserved for use in the reconstruction.

SYSTEMIC THERAPY FOR BREAST CANCER: CHEMOTHERAPY AND HORMONE THERAPY

Despite improvements in surgery and radiation therapy for local control of breast cancer, many patients still developed distant metastases and ultimately died of their disease. The ability to treat metastatic disease with cytotoxic chemotherapeutic drugs or hormones was explored. The superiority of multiple-agent combination chemotherapy versus single-agent chemotherapy was demonstrated in early trials (Bonadonna et al, 1986; Fisher et al, 1989c). It became clear that chemotherapy and hormone therapy were limited in their ability to control bulky distant metastases, although occasional patients had dramatic partial responses or even complete responses to therapy.

To treat micrometastases from breast cancer when they are thought to be most susceptible to treatment, systemic therapy is now administered on an adjuvant basis, when there is no evidence of distant metastases but only sufficient suspicion (Goldhirsch and Gelber, 1994). Until the late 1980s chemotherapy was given on this adjuvant basis primarily to women with axillary nodal metastases but with no other evidence of disease. Studies suggested that premenopausal women benefit most from adjuvant chemotherapy and benefit less from adjuvant hormone therapy. On the other hand, for postmenopausal women who have positive nodes, hormone therapy gave benefits equivalent to those of chemotherapy with less toxicity (Consensus Conferences, 1985).

This philosophy changed in 1988 when a clinical alert was issued by the NCI stating that there was sufficient evidence to recommend adjuvant chemotherapy or hormone therapy even for patients with node-negative breast cancer (National Cancer Institute, 1988). By this time results of numerous studies had shown a survival benefit with the use of adjuvant chemotherapy in node-negative breast cancer (National Cancer Institute, 1988; Fisher et al, 1989b; Fisher et al, 1985b; Mansur et al, 1989). A consensus conference of experts in the field suggested that this adjuvant therapy be offered to women with primary tumors larger than 1 cm (NIH Consensus Conference, 1991). In 1992 a meta-analysis was published reviewing the treatment of 75,000 women in 133 randomized clinical trials of adjuvant therapy for breast cancer (Early Breast Cancer Trialists' Collaborative Group, 1992). This study concluded that there was a 20% to 30% improvement in overall survival rates among premenopausal women with node-negative breast cancer who received chemotherapy compared with those who did not. This benefit also appeared to extend to postmenopausal women 50 to 60 years of age. For older postmenopausal women with node-negative breast cancer, tamoxifen conferred a similar 20% to 30% survival advantage over no adjuvant therapy. A recent update on the use of hormone therapy finds a significant benefit for women younger than 50 whose tumors are estrogen-receptor positive (Early Breast Cancer Trialists' Collaborative Group, 1998). Tamoxifen therapy is now recommended after chemotherapy in premenopausal women and is seen as a potential single agent for low-risk tumors.

CARCINOMA IN SITU
Ductal Carcinoma in Situ

With the wider use of mammography, ductal carcinoma in situ (DCIS) without invasion comprises an increasing proportion of breast cancer occurrences. It accounts for nearly 25% of all new breast cancers, and it is found in 6.6% of needle-localized breast biopsies, 30% of mammography-detected malignancies, and 1.4% of breast biopsies for palpable lesions (Frykberg and Kirby, 1994). It was recognized early that DCIS has a favorable prognosis compared with other forms of breast cancer; rates for long-term survival approach 100% after treatment with mastectomy. Axillary lymph nodes are positive in only 1% to 2% of patients, particularly those with large or palpable lesions or comedo histology.

DCIS is thought to be a true anatomic precursor of invasive breast cancer. Several lines of evidence support this conclusion. First, a review of patients with DCIS treated with biopsy alone (usually because the DCIS was missed at the initial biopsy and was found on review of the slides at a later date) shows a 25% to 50% rate of invasive carcinoma developing at the site of the initial biopsy. All these tumors appear within 10 years and are of ductal histology. Second, approximately 50% patients with local recurrence of DCIS after breast conservation have evidence of invasive ductal carcinoma in the recurrences. The true relationship between in situ and invasive ductal carcinoma awaits a better understanding of the molecular biology of breast cancer development.

Few clinical trials to date have been devoted exclusively to the management of DCIS. Results of the NSABP B-17 study, which tested the role of radiation for DCIS, are reported (Fisher et al, 1993). Data at the 43-month follow-up point suggested that the addition of radiation therapy decreases the recurrence rate by approximately half, from 16.4% with wide excision alone to 7% with wide excision and radiation. It appeared also that the addition of radiation therapy may result in fewer invasive recurrences than wide excision only.

Current Treatment of DCIS

Surgical treatment options for DCIS are similar to those used for invasive breast cancer. There is an increased risk for local recurrence after breast conservation with DCIS compared with mastectomy. The probability of metastatic disease is extremely low. With wide excision to clean margins microscopically, followed by radiation therapy, breast conservation has become an accepted alternative to mastectomy. If clean margins cannot be obtained or if the cosmetic result is expected to be poor after excision to clean margins, mastectomy should be performed.

Most patients whose DCIS is identified by mammography alone have the option of mastectomy or wide excision with or without radiation, each of which results in similar and excellent long-term survival rates. Although local recurrence rates are higher after wide excision and radiation and are highest with wide excision alone, most patients can be treated by mastectomy at the time of local recurrence. Axillary dissection is not usually performed with lumpectomy for DCIS without invasion because the probability of positive nodes is low. Low axillary dissection is often added to mastectomy for large lesions, particularly comedo DCIS lesions, because the risk for positive axillary nodes is higher and little morbidity is added.

For some patients with DCIS, mastectomy remains the preferred treatment. This category includes patients with lesions that measure more than 5 cm in greatest dimension, patients with large comedo lesions, and patients for whom poor cosmetic results are expected after wide excision to clean margins. These patients are at highest risk for positive axillary nodes, and level I axillary node dissection should be performed with the mastectomy.

Lobular Carcinoma in Situ

LCIS, also referred to as lobular neoplasia, does not have the same clinical implications as invasive ductal or invasive lobular carcinoma or DCIS (Haagensen et al, 1978). It is now generally accepted that LCIS is a marker of increased risk for subsequent breast carcinoma rather than a marker of the site at which future carcinoma will arise (Fisher et al, 1989a; Rosen, 1984). This increased risk is equally distributed between the affected and the contralateral breast. Unilateral mastectomy, therefore, is an inappropriate treatment because the contralateral breast is at equal risk for future carcinoma. Appropriate treatment options include careful observation by physical examination two or three times per year, annual mammograms, participation in chemoprevention trials, and prophylactic bilateral simple mastectomies with or without reconstruction. The risk contributed by LCIS may be additive with other risk factors, such as family history and reproductive and menstrual factors (Frykberg and Kirby, 1994; Page and Jensen, 1994). The overall risk for subsequent invasive carcinoma is thought to be 20% to 25%; most of these carcinomas show ductal histology (Frykberg and Kirby, 1994; Rosen et al, 1978). At present most patients choose careful follow-up rather than prophylactic mastectomy, and there is increasing interest in chemoprevention with tamoxifen or other agents. For some patients, however, prophylactic mastectomy is still a good option either because of patient anxiety or concurrent risk factors (Kinne, 1990).

TREATMENT OF EARLY INVASIVE BREAST CANCER

Although there continues to be active investigation of the optimum treatment of breast cancer, there is some consensus as to the currently favored treatment.

Local Treatment

For local treatment of stage I and stage II breast cancer, lumpectomy to microscopically clean margins with axillary dissection and radiation therapy continues to give long-term survival equivalent to that of mastectomy. Patients undergoing lumpectomy and radiation do, however, have a risk for local recurrence in the treated breast and a risk for new primary cancer in the remaining breast tissue. These local recurrences can generally be treated by mastectomy so that overall survival rates are essentially equivalent to those for women who undergo mastectomy at the time of initial diagnosis. Local recurrence, therefore, does not generally translate into significantly decreased overall survival, though there may be significant anxiety over recurrence, some morbidity, and potential mortality from a second surgical procedure. It is possible that in a small number of women, the chance for survival will decrease because of the local recurrence.

On the other hand, patients who choose mastectomy as their initial surgical treatment face the psychologic consequences of losing a breast. Although mastectomy entails a lower risk for local recurrence, overall survival rates are not significantly improved over those of lumpectomy, axillary node dissection, and radiation. Each physician and patient must weigh the inconvenience and potential complications of radiation therapy and the risk for local recurrence against the value of breast preservation, while knowing that the chance for survival does not appear to be significantly different with either option.

Adjuvant Therapy

The current consensus is that adjuvant chemotherapy, hormone therapy, or a combination of the two should be considered for all women with tumors larger than 1 cm in diameter. Very small tumors measuring less than 1 cm are already thought to have such a favorable prognosis that any potential benefit of adjuvant chemotherapy is outweighed by its risks. Hormone therapy with tamoxifen for the treatment of these small tumors and chemoprevention may be considered. For premenopausal women, adjuvant therapy should generally consist of combination chemotherapy, with hormone therapy added for hormone receptor–positive tumors. For postmenopausal women, hormone therapy, generally consisting of tamoxifen 20 mg/day, is the first line of treatment. There has been a reassessment of the concept of using menopause as the cut-off for consideration of chemotherapy. For healthy postmenopausal women, the decision to use hormonal therapy versus chemotherapy plus hormonal therapy is made on an individual basis and takes into account the woman's overall health and the specifics of her tumor.

If the axillary nodes are positive, combination chemotherapy is used for premenopausal women and for healthy postmenopausal women up to at least age 60. For postmenopausal women older than 60 with node-positive breast cancer or for women in poor health, hormone therapy is generally the treatment of choice, particularly if the tumor is estrogen–receptor positive. There is a renewed interest in other hormonal manipulations, such as oophorectomy and chemical castration, for premenopausal women at high risk for metastatic disease (Scottish Cancer Trials Breast Group, 1993). The use of chemotherapy after biopsy and before definitive surgery as neoadjuvant therapy is under investigation.

TREATMENT FOR ADVANCED BREAST CANCER

Patients with locally advanced breast cancer, including those with primary tumors larger than 5 cm, fixed or matted N2 axillary nodes, and inflammatory breast carcinoma, are generally treated with chemotherapy as the first treatment modality. This neoadjuvant chemotherapy serves to downstage local disease and, in some patients, makes inoperable tumors amenable to surgical resection. Patients with locally advanced disease are treated with needle or incisional biopsy to obtain a tissue diagnosis and hormone receptor data. These patients are also carefully staged to identify any distant metastases. Chemotherapy is administered first and is followed by surgery or radiation if the tumor responds to chemotherapy. Most patients require all three modalities.

PREGNANCY AND HORMONE REPLACEMENT AFTER BREAST CANCER
Pregnancy After Breast Cancer

There has been concern that the hormonal milieu of pregnancy would stimulate the growth of occult metastases and would have a negative impact on outcomes for women with a prior diagnosis of breast cancer. Available clinical data do not support this concern and suggest that women who become pregnant after treatment for breast cancer do as well as or better than those who do not become pregnant (Walker et al, 1988).

A number of studies report the outcomes of patients with breast cancer who subsequently became pregnant. White (1955) reported a 67% 5-year survival rate and a 58% 10-year survival rate. Rissanen (1968) recorded a 77% 5-year survival rate and a 69% 10-year survival rate in 53 patients. Another series of 52 patients showed a 5-year survival rate of 52% (Holleb and Farrow, 1962). Still other series reported 50% and 29% 5-year survival rates, respectively, in patients who become pregnant after treatment for breast cancer (Applewhite et al, 1973; Cheek, 1973).

There is probably some degree of selection bias in these figures—women with good prognoses are more likely to proceed with pregnancy than are those with poor prognoses. There may also be selection bias in tracking and reporting patients who become pregnant after treatment for breast cancer that favors reporting those patients who do well (Petrek, 1991). However, series that include controls matched for age and clinical stage also show equivalent or improved survival rates among those who become pregnant. Peters (1968) compareed 96 patients with breast cancer who subsequently became pregnant with age- and stage-matched controls who did not become pregnant and found the group that became pregnant had better overall and disease-free survival rates (Peters, 1968). Similarly, Cooper and Butterfield (1970) compared 40 patients with breast cancer who later became pregnant with 80 control subjects matched for age and disease stage, and they found greater 5-year survival rates (80%) among those who become pregnant.

Given the limitations of available data on the impact of subsequent pregnancy on survival rate after treatment for breast cancer, it has been standard practice to advise patients to wait several years after treatment before becoming pregnant. This waiting period is thought to allow aggressive, rapidly recurrent disease to declare itself. A frank discussion with the patient about her expected prognosis is also important to allow her to make an educated choice about pregnancy. Because of the increased use of adjuvant chemotherapy for premenopausal women and because of the premature ovarian failure rate commonly associated with this chemotherapy, pregnancy after treatment for breast cancer should be discussed early in the planning process to allow for consideration of embryo banking.

Hormone Replacement Therapy After Breast Cancer

Concerns about the possible stimulatory effects of exogenous estrogens on occult breast metastases leave many practitioners reluctant to prescribe hormone replacement therapy for women treated for breast cancer. There are few data on this.

There are some patients, such as those with DCIS treated by mastectomy, whose risk for local recurrence and occult metastasis is low. Although they are at increased risk for future contralateral breast cancer, their risk for morbidity and mortality from cardiovascular disease and osteoporosis may outweigh their risk for future breast cancer. For these women estrogen replacement therapy may reduce overall morbidity and mortality.

The situation is not as clear for the majority of women who have been treated for invasive breast cancer or for those who have had breast conservation after DCIS. These women are at some risk for local and distant recurrence, and it is unclear whether estrogen replacement therapy increases risk or whether any such increase would be offset by decreased cardiovascular and osteoporosis risk. There are no ongoing, large-scale clinical trials to test the risks and benefits of estrogen replacement therapy after treatment for breast cancer. Clarification of this issue, therefore, awaits better understanding of the biology of breast cancer. It is hoped that selective estrogen receptor modulators such as tamoxifen may safely provide protection from breast cancer as well as protection from cardiovascular disease and osteoporosis after treatment for breast cancer.

FUTURE DIRECTIONS IN THE TREATMENT OF BREAST CANCER
Surgery and Radiation

Exploration continues of the smallest possible treatment that will achieve the optimum control of breast cancer. Trials are under way to explore the need for radiation therapy in favorable small tumors or in tumors consisting of pure ductal carcinoma in situ.

Veronisi et al (1986) reported the results of wide excision of invasive tumors measuring less than 2.5 cm versus wide excision plus radiation therapy. Without radiation, there was a significantly higher rate of local recurrence, though it was only 3.3% in women older than 55; hence, it was suggested that there may be an age difference in the risk for recurrence without radiation.

At present it is not possible to identify these invasive tumors for which radiation therapy may be safely omitted. All patients undergoing lumpectomy for invasive tumors should receive radiation therapy other than in the setting of a clinical trial. For patients with areas of DCIS smaller than 2.5 cm in the greatest dimension, it may be possible to omit radiation. However, this is a complex decision that should be based on the patient's histology and other risk factors, and ideally it should be pursued in the setting of a clinical trial.

Trials also are under way to explore the possibility of wide excision plus tamoxifen as an alternative therapy to wide excision plus radiation for elderly women. Preliminary studies from Great Britain suggest that the local recurrence rate is higher with wide excision plus tamoxifen than it is with wide excision plus radiation, though other larger trials, as yet unpublished, are under way to test this hypothesis.

There is discussion of omitting axillary dissection in patients with clinically node-negative tumors and using features of the primary tumor alone to determine the need for adjuvant therapy. Newer data suggest decreased survival rates among women who do not undergo axillary dissection, possibly because more accurate staging allows more appropriate utilization of adjuvant therapies (Cabanes et al, 1992) or because of decreased survival rates resulting from local recurrence (Graverson et al, 1988; Harris and Osteen, 1985). Axillary lymph node mapping with selective sentinel lymph node mapping is being explored as a minimally invasive and increasingly accurate means of staging the axilla (Krag et al, 1998, Giuliano et al, 1997). Additional clinical trials to test the accuracy and applicability of sentinel node biopsy for breast cancer are planned. The appropriate follow-up testing regimen after treatment for breast cancer is also under discussion, and it includes issues of cost effectiveness and quality of life (Del Turco et al, 1994; GIVIO Investigators, 1994).

Systemic Therapy

Many chemotherapy trials for breast cancer focus on increasing the efficacy of treatment through dosage intensification (Wolfe et al, 1987). Trials of high-dose chemotherapy with growth-factor support or autologous bone marrow transplantation are under way with the hope that higher dosages of chemotherapy will result in improved response rates and improved duration of response. Early results of bone marrow transplantation have been disappointing; median survival rates are prolonged by only 7 to 10 months compared with standard chemotherapy. However, bone marrow transplantation has resulted in a small but significant number of long-term survivors who remain free of breast cancer for more than 5 years after treatment of women with 10 or more positive lymph nodes (Peters, 1991). It is hoped that a better understanding of breast cancer on the molecular level will lead to better selection of patients for aggressive chemotherapy and better identification of those patients who are equally well served by treatments with less morbidity (El-Ashry and Lippman, 1994; Gasparini et al, 1993). It is suggested that an elevated level of Her-2-neu predicts a more aggressive form of disease and a poorer response to standard chemotherapy (Allred et al, 1992; Gusterson et al, 1992; Muss et al, 1994) and that higher dose therapy and potentially anti–Her-2-neu antibody therapy may be more effective. It is hoped that a better understanding of the mechanisms of tumor growth will make it possible to design synergistic combination chemotherapy regimens and improved biologic therapies and immune therapies. These areas continue to be actively explored.

CHEMOPREVENTION OF BREAST CANCER

Efforts to reduce breast cancer mortality rates have been limited to attempts at early detection followed by aggressive treatment of the breast cancers that are discovered. Although continued attempts to achieve earlier detection and to improve therapy are important, it would be of great benefit to have interventions that prevent breast cancer from developing in the first place. This has become increasingly important as the understanding of breast cancer risk factors is refined and as persons carrying mutations in risk-conferring genes, such as BRCA1, BRCA2, and other risk-increasing genes, are identified. This concept of chemoprevention, using medication or other treatment to prevent the initiation or progression of breast cancer, is verified by data from the use of the selective estrogen receptor modulator (SERM), tamoxifen.

The first major national chemoprevention trial in the United States, the NSABP Tamoxifen Trial, was based on the observation that fewer contralateral cancers develop in women administered tamoxifen for node-positive breast cancer than in women in the control group not receiving tamoxifen (Fisher et al, 1989b). A 40% decrease was observed in the rate of contralateral cancers in the NSABP-B-14 study, and a 47% reduction was observed in contralateral breast cancers in the tamoxifen meta-analysis overview (Early Breast Cancer Trialists' Collaborative Group, 1998). In addition, data showed that tamoxifen reduced cardiovascular morbidity and improved lipid profile while it increased bone density. The NSABP tamoxifen trial began in 1992 and reported a 44% reduction in breast cancers in women at high risk who took 20 mg/day tamoxifen compared with those taking a placebo. To participate in the trial, a woman had to be older than 35 and to have a risk for breast cancer occurrence within 5 years equivalent to that of a 60-year-old woman. Risk was assessed using the Gail model that takes into account patient age, first-degree relatives with breast cancer, age at menarche, age at first pregnancy, and previous biopsies, particularly those showing atypical hyperplasia (Gail et al, 1989). Lobular carcinoma in situ was an automatic entry criterion. The tamoxifen arm demonstrated complications including increased rates of endometrial carcinoma, particularly in women older than 50, and increased thromboembolic disease, again primarily in women older than 50 and at rates similar to those seen in women taking estrogen replacement therapy.

Results of two other smaller trials that tested the efficacy of tamoxifen in the prevention of breast cancer have also been reported (Veronesi et al, 1998; Powles et al, 1998). Both these trials failed to show a significant reduction of breast cancer incidence in women taking tamoxifen compared with those taking a placebo. Absolute risk for breast cancer was lower in the participants in these trials than in those in the NSABP chemoprevention trial, and entry criteria were different. Overall compliance with the drug regimen, higher drop-out rates among participants, and concurrent use of hormone replacement therapy with tamoxifen in these trials may in part explain their negative results in comparison with NSABP trial results (Pritchard, 1998).

As a result of these data, the use of tamoxifen as a chemoprevention agent for breast cancer is expected to be under wide consideration in the United States, and guidelines for its use are under discussion. Other chemoprevention trials are under consideration or under development, including the recently opened NSABP STAR Trial, which will compare tamoxifen with another SERM, raloxifene, for chemoprevention of breast cancer (NSABP, 1998). Other potential chemoprevention agents include other SERMs, retinoids, protease inhibitors, and dietary modifications.

SILICONE BREAST IMPLANTS

Silicone gel–filled breast implants have been used for breast augmentation or reconstruction for nearly 30 years. These implants became the subject of controversy in 1991 when concerns were raised that silicone implants were contributing to or causing autoimmune disorders. These concerns led the FDA to institute a voluntary moratorium on the use of silicone breast implants in 1991. In 1992 it concluded that proof of the safety and efficacy of silicone breast implants had not been adequately established (AMA Council on Scientific Affairs, 1993; Kessler, 1992). It was recommended that additional controlled clinical trials be conducted to examine the safety of silicone implants for breast reconstruction and augmentation.

Based on the results of studies with more than 10 years of follow-up, there is no clinical evidence that silicone implants increase the incidence of breast carcinoma (Berkell et al, 1992; Deapen and Brody, 1992). On review of the data suggesting a link between silicone implants and collagen vascular disorders, a consensus review and an FDA advisory panel concluded that there was insufficient evidence to prove an association between silicone implants and any autoimmune disorder (Brody et al, 1992; Food and Drug Administration, 1992). For these reasons, it has not been recommended that women with silicone implants have their implants removed empirically.

Other reports raised the issue of a relationship between silicone implants and autoimmune disorders (Appleton and Lee, 1993; Kessler et al, 1993; Speira and Kerr, 1993). Some studies identified circulating autoantibodies to a variety of connective tissue–related peptides (Bridges et al, 1993), or types I and II collagen, or antinuclear antibodies in women with silicone implants (Press et al, 1992). These findings indicate the need for additional examination of the relationship between silicone and autoimmune disorders before the widespread use of silicone implants resumes.

A small study raised the possibility of a scleroderma-like esophageal motility disorder in breast-fed infants of mothers with silicone implants (Levine and Ilowite, 1994). It has been hypothesized that mother-to-child transmission of silicone or maternal antibodies may serve as an initiating event in this process (Flick, 1994). Further study of this issue has been recommended.

Although the moratorium on the use of silicone implants has been lifted and is replaced with specifically controlled use (Segal, 1992), nearly all breast reconstructions and augmentations are performed now with saline-filled implants. It is recommended that women with saline or silicone implants undergo routine breast examination and mammography as appropriate for age and risk profile. Some degree of capsule formation will be present with any breast implant. If it is severe, it may result in breast texture that is firm to hard. Capsule formation does not, however, create masses or nodularity. Any palpable mass in a woman with a breast implant should be evaluated by mammography, and a biopsy should be taken if the mass is persistent.

Leak or rupture of an implant may be identified as a change in the size or shape of the augmented or reconstructed breast through physical examination or, with variable success, by ultrasonography, mammography, or MRI. Gross rupture is generally treated with replacement of the implant.

REFERENCES

Allred DC et al: Her-2-neu in node-negative breast cancer: Prognostic significance of over expression influenced by the presence of in situ carcinoma. *J Clin Oncol* 1992; 10:599-605.

AMA Council on Scientific Affairs: Silicone gel breast implants. *JAMA* 1993; 270:2602-2606.

American Joint Committee on Cancer: *Manual for staging for breast carcinoma,* ed 5; Philadelphia: Lippincott-Raven, 1989.

Appleton BE, Lee P: The development of systemic sclerosis (scleroderma) following augmentation mammaplasty. *J Rheumatol* 1993; 20:1052-1054.

Applewhite RR, Smith LR, DeVicenti F: Carcinoma of the breast associated with pregnancy and lactation. *Am Surg* 1973; 39:101-l04.

Armstrong B, Doll R: Environmental factors and cancer incidence and mortality in different countries, with special reference to dietary practices. *Int J Cancer* 1975; 15:617-631.

Baker H, Snedecor P: Clinical trial of danazol for benign breast disease. *Am Surg* 1979; 45:727.

Baines CJ: The Canadian National Breast Screening Study: A perspective on criticisms. *Ann Intern Med* 1994; 120:326-334.

Ballo MS, Sneige N: Can core needle biopsy replace fine-needle aspiration cytology in the diagnosis of palpable breast carcinoma: A comparative study of 124 women. *Cancer* 1996; 78:773-777.

Benson EA: Management of breast abscesses. *World J Surg* 1989; 13:753-756.

Bergvist et al: The risk of breast cancer after estrogen and estrogen-progestin replacement. *N Engl J Med* 1989; 321:293-299.

Berkell H, Birdsell DC, Jenkins H: Breast augmentation: A risk factor for breast cancer? *N Engl J Med* 1992; 326:1649-1653.

Bonadonna G et al: Current status of Milan adjuvant chemotherapy trials for node-positive and node-negative breast cancer. *Natl Cancer Inst Monogr* 1986; 1:45-49.

Boyd NF et al: Prospective evaluation of physical examination of the breast. *Am J Surg* 1981; 142:331-334.

Boyd NF et al: A critical appraisal of the Canadian National Breast Cancer Screening Study. *Radiology* 1993; 189:661-663.

Bridges AJ et al: A clinical and immunological study of women with silicone breast implants and symptoms of rheumatic disease. *Ann Intern Med* 1993; 118:929-936.

Brody GS et al: Consensus statement on the relationship of breast implants to connective-tissue disorders. *Plast Reconstr Surg* 1992; 90:1102-1104.

Brook I: Microbiology of nonpuerperal breast abscesses. *J Infect Dis* 1988; 157:377-379.

Brownstein MH, Wolf M, Bikowski JB: Cowden's disease: A cutaneous marker of breast cancer. *Cancer* 1978; 41:2393-2398.

Cabanes et al: Value of axillary dissection in addition to lumpectomy and radiotherapy in early breast cancer: The Breast Carcinoma Collaborative Group of the Institut Curie. *Lancet* 1992; 339:1245-1248.

Calle EE, Miracle-McMahill HL, Thun, MJ, et al: Estrogen replacement therapy and risk of fatal colon cancer in a prospective cohort of postmenopausal women. *J Natl Cancer Inst* 1995; 87:7:517-522.

Calle R et al: Conservative management of operable breast cancer: Ten years experience at the Foundation Curie. *Cancer* 1978; 42:2045-2053.

Casey G: The BRCA1 and BRCA2 breast cancer genes. *Curr Opin Oncol* 1997; 9:88-93.

Chaudary M et al: Nipple discharge: The diagnostic value of testing for occult blood. *Am J Surg* 1982; 196:651.

Cheek JH: Cancer of the breast in pregnancy and lactation. *Am J Surg* 1973; 126:729-731.

Chu KC, Smart CR, Tarone RE: Analysis of breast cancer mortality and stage distribution by age for the Health Insurance Plan clinical trial. *J Natl Cancer Inst* 1988; 80:1125-1132.

Ciatto S, Cariaggi P, Bulgaresi P: The value of routine cytologic examination of breast cyst fluids. *Acta Cytol* 1987a; 31:301-304.

Ciatto S, Cataliotti L, Distante V: Nonpalpable lesions detected with mammography: Review of 512 consecutive cases. *Radiology* 1987b; 165:99-102.

Clarke DH et al: Analysis of local regional relapses in patients with early breast cancers treated by excision and radiotherapy: Experience of the Institut Gustave Roussy. *Int J Radiat Oncol Phys* 1985; 11:137.

Claus EB, Risch N, Thompson WD: Autosomal dominant inheritance of early-onset breast cancer: Implications for risk prediction. *Cancer* 1994; 73:643-651.

Colditz GA, Stampfer MJ, Willett WC: Prospective study of estrogen replacement therapy and risk of breast cancer in postmenopausal women. *JAMA* 1990; 264:2641-2653.

Colditz GA, Hankinson SE, Hunter DJ, et al: The use of estrogens and progestins and the risk of breast cancer in postmenopausal women. *N Engl J Med* 1995; 332:1589-1593.

Consensus Conferences: Adjuvant chemotherapy for breast cancer. *JAMA* 1985; 254:3461-3463.

Cooper DR, Butterfield J: Pregnancy subsequent to mastectomy for cancer of the breast. *Ann Surg* 1970; 171:429-433.

Cummings S, Olopade O: Predisposition testing for inherited breast cancer. *Oncology* 1998; 12:1227-1239.

Danforth DN et al: Complete axillary lymph node dissection for stage I-II carcinoma of the breast. *J Clin Oncol* 1986; 4:655.

D'Angelo PC, Galliano DE, Rosemurgy AS: Stereotactic excisional breast biopsies utilizing the advanced breast biopsy instrumentation system. *Am J Surg* 1997; 174:297-302.

Deapen DM, Brody GS: Augmentation mammaplasty and breast cancer: A 5-year update of the Los Angeles study. *Plast Reconstr Surg* 1992; 89:660-665.

Del Turco MR et al: Intensive diagnostic follow-up after treatment of primary breast cancer: A randomized trial. *JAMA* 1994; 271:1593-1597.

Devitt JE: Management of nipple discharge by clinical findings. *Am J Surg* 1985; 149:789-792.

Donegan WL: Evaluation of a palpable breast mass. *N Engl J Med* 1992; 327:937-942.

Dowlatshahi KD et al: Nonpalpable breast lesions: Findings of stereotaxic needle-core biopsy and fine-needle aspiration cytology. *Radiology* 1991; 181:745-750.

Dupont WD, Page DL: Menopausal estrogen-replacement therapy. *Arch Intern Med* 1991; 151:67-72.

Early Breast Cancer Trialists' Collaborative Group: Systemic treatment of early breast cancer by hormonal, cytotoxic, or immune therapy. *Lancet* 1992; 339:71-85.

Early Breast Cancer Trialists' Collaborative Group: Tamoxifen for early breast cancer: An overview of the randomised trials. *Lancet* 1998; 351:1451-1467.

Eberlein TJ et al: Prospective evaluation of immediate reconstruction following mastectomy. *Ann Surg* 1993; 218:29-36.

Eckhardt S, Badellino F, Murphy GP: UICC meeting on breast-cancer screening in premenopausal women in developed countries. *Int J Cancer* 1994; 56:1-5.

El-Ashry D, Lippman ME: Molecular biology of breast carcinoma. *World J Surg* 1994; 18: 12-20.

Elliott RL et al: Stereotaxic needle locationization and biopsy of occult breast lesions: First year's experience. *Am Surg* 1992; 58:126-131.

Elwood JM, Cox B, Richardson AK: The effectiveness of breast cancer screening by mammography in younger women. *Online J Curr Clin Trials* 1993; doc 32.

Farrow DC, Hunt WC, Samot JM: Geographic variation in the treatment of localized breast cancer. *N Engl J Med* 1992; 326:1097-2101.

Fentiman et al: Double-blind controlled trial of tamoxifen therapy for mastalgia. *Lancet* 1986; 1:287.

Fisher B et al: Five-year results of a randomized trial comparing total mastectomy and segmental mastectomy with or without radiation in the treatment of breast cancer. *N Engl J Med* 1985a; 312:665-673.

Fisher B et al: Ten-year results of a randomized clinical trial comparing radical mastectomy and total mastectomy with or without radiation. *N Engl J Med* 1985b; 312:674-681.

Fisher B, Wolmark N: Limited surgical management for primary breast: A commentary on the NSABP reports. *World J Surg* 1985; 9:682.

Fisher B et al: Systemic adjuvant therapy on treatment of previous operable breast career: NSABP experience. *Natl Cancer Inst Monogr* 1986; 1:35-43.

Fisher B et al: A randomized clinical trial evaluating sequential methotrexate and 5-fluorouracil in the treatment of patients with nodenegative breast cancer who have estrogen-receptor negative tumors. *N Engl J Med* 1989a; 320:473-478.

Fisher B et al: A randomized trial evaluating tamoxifen in the treatment of node-negative breast cancer women who have estrogen-receptor positive tumors. *N Engl J Med* 1989b; 320:479-484.

Fisher B et al: Eight-year results of a randomized trial comparing total mastectomy and lumpectomy without irradiation in the treatment of breast cancer. *N Engl J Med* 1989c; 320:822-828.

Fisher B et al: Lumpectomy compared with lumpectomy and radiation therapy for the treatment of intraductal breast cancer. *N Engl J Med* 1993; 328:1581-1586.

Fisher B et al: Tamoxifen for prevention of breast cancer: Report of the National Surgical Adjuvant Breast and Bowel Project P-1 Study, *J Natl Cancer Inst* 1998; 90:1371-1388.

Fisher ER, Fisher B: Lobular carcinoma of the breast: An overview. *Ann Surg* 1977; 195:377.

Fletcher SW et al: Report of the International Workshop on Screening for Breast Cancer. *J Natl Cancer Inst* 1993; 85:1644-1656.

Flick JA: Silicone implants and esophageal dysmotility: Are breastfed infants at risk? *JAMA* 1994; 271:240-241.

Food and Drug Administration: General and Plastic Surgery Devices Panel Meeting, February 18-20, 1992, Freedom of Information Services documents 100714, 107031, and 107032, Washington, DC, 1992, US Government Printing Office.

Ford D et al: Risks of cancer in BRCA 1-mutation carriers. *Lancet* 1994; 343:692-695.

Foster RS, Worden JK, Costanza MC, et al. Clinical breast examination and breast self-examination. *Cancer* 1992; 69:1992-1998.

Frykberg ER, Kirby IB: Management of in situ and minimally invasive breast carcinoma. *World J Surg* 1994; 18:45-57.

Gail MG et al: Projecting individualized probabilities of developing breast cancer for white females who are being examined annually. *J Natl Cancer Inst* 1989; 1:1879-1886.

Gambrell RD Jr: Proposal to decrease the risk and improve the prognosis of breast cancer. *Am J Obstet Gynecol* 1984; 150:119-128.

Gambrell RD Jr: Breast cancer: Improved prognosis in hormone users and decreased incidence in oestrogen-progestogen users. In Mann RD, editor: *Hormone replacement therapy and breast cancer risk,* Park Ridge, N.J., 1992, Parthenon Publishing.

Gasparini G, Pozza F, Harris AL: Evaluating the potential usefulness of new prognostic and predictive indicators in node-negative breast cancer patients. *J Natl Cancer Inst* 1993; 85:1206-1219.

Gastrin G, Miller AB, To T, et al: Incidence and mortality from breast cancer in the Mama Program for breast cancer screening in Finland, 1973-1986. *Cancer* 1994; 73:2168-2174.

Giuliano AE, Jones RC, Brennan MM, Statman R: Sentinel lymphadenectomy in breast cancer. *J Clin Oncol* 1997; 15:2345-2350.

GIVIO Investigators: Impact of follow-up testing on survival and health-related quality of life in breast cancer patients. *JAMA* 1994; 271:1587-1592.

Goldhirsch A, Gelber RD: Understanding adjuvant chemotherapy for breast cancer. *N Engl J Med* 1994; 330:1308-1309.

Goodwin PJ, Boyd NF: Critical appraisal of the evidence that dietary fat intake is related to breast cancer risk in humans. *J Natl Cancer Inst* 1987; 79:473-485.

Grant CS, et al: Fine-needle aspiration of the breast. *Mayo Clin Proc* 1986; 61:377-381.

Graverson HP, et al: Breast cancer: Risk of axillary recurrence in nodenegative patients following partial dissection of the axilla. *Eur J Surg Oncol* 1988; 14:407-412.

Grodstein F, Stampfer MJ, Colditz GA, et al: Postmenopausal hormone therapy and mortality. *N Engl J Med* 1997; 336:25:1769-1775.

Gullick WJ, et al: C-erbB-2 protein overexpression in breast cancer is a risk factor in patients with involved and uninvolved lymph nodes. *Br J Cancer* 1991; 63:434.

Gusterson BA, et al: Prognostic importance of c-erbB-2 expression in breast cancer: International (Ludwig) Breast Cancer Study Group. *J Clin Oncol* 1992; 10:1049.

Haagensen CD, et al: Lobular neoplasia (so-called lobular carcinoma in situ) of the breast. *Cancer* 1978; 42:737.

Hadfield J: Excision of the major duct system for benign disease of the breast. *Br J Surg* 1960; 47:472-477.

Haffty GB, et al: Conservative surgery with radiation therapy in clinical stage I and II breast cancer: Results of a 20-year experience. *Arch Surg* 1989; 124:1266.

Hall FM, et al: Nonpalpable breast lesions: Recommendations for biopsy based on suspicion of carcinoma at mammography. *Radiology* 1988; 167:353-358.

Hall JM, et al: Linkage of early-onset familial breast cancer to chromosome 17q21. *Science* 1990; 250:1684-1689.

Hamed H, et al: Follow-up of patients with aspirated breast cysts is necessary. *Arch Surg* 1989; 124:253-255.

Hammond S, et al: Statistical analysis of fine-needle aspiration cytology of the breast: A review of 678 cases plus 4265 cases from the literature. *Acta Cytol* 1987; 31:276-280.

Harris JR, Hellman S, Kinne DW: Limited surgery and radiotherapy for early breast cancer. *N Engl J Med* 1985; 313:1365.

Harris JR, Osteen RT: Patients with early breast cancer benefit from effective axillary treatment. *Breast Cancer Res Treat* 1985; 5:17-21.

Hayward J, Caleffi M: The significance of local control in the primary treatment of breast cancer. *Arch Surg* 1987; 122:1244-1247.

Hellman, S: Stopping metastases at their source. *N Engl J Med* 1997; 337:996-997.

Helvie MA, et al: Mammographic follow-up of low-suspicion lesions: Compliance rate and diagnostic yield. *Radiology* 1991; 178:155-158.

Henderson BE, Paganin-Hill A, Ross RK: Decreased mortality in users of estrogen replacement therapy. *Arch Intern Med* 1991; 151:75-78.

Henderson IC: Risk factors for breast cancer development. *Cancer* 1993; 71 (suppl):2127-2140.

Holland R, et al: The presence of an extensive intraductal component following a limited excision correlates with prominent residual disease in trial remainder of the breast. *J Clin Oncol* 1990; 8:113-118.

Holleb AI, Farrow JH: The relation of carcinoma of the breast and pregnancy in 283 patients. *Surg Gynecol Obstet* 1962; 115:65-71.

Hortobagyi GN: Treatment of breast cancer. *N Engl J Med* 1998; 339:974-982.

Howe GR, et al: Dietary factors and risk of breast cancer: Combined analysis of 12 case-control studies. *J Natl Cancer Inst* 1990; 82:561-569.

Howe G, et al: The association between alcohol and breast cancer risk: Evidence from the combined analysis of six dietary case-control studies. *Int J Cancer* 1991; 47:707-710.

Howe GR, et al: A cohort study of fat intake and risk of breast cancer. *J Natl Cancer Inst* 1991; 83:336-340.

Huang, Z, Hankinson, SE, Colditz, GA, et al: Dual effects of weight and weight gain on breast cancer risk. *JAMA* 1997; 278:17:1407-1411, 1448-1449.

Hughes LE, Bundred NJ: Breast macrocysts. *World J Surg* 1989; 13:711-714.

Hultborn KA, Larsen LG, Raghnult I: The lymph drainage from the breast to the axillary and parasternal lymph nodes: Studied with the aid of colloidal Au^{198}. *Acta Radiol* 1955; 43:52.

Hunter DJ, et al: A prospective study of the intake of vitamins C, E, and A and the risk of breast cancer. *N Engl J Med* 1993; 329:234-240.

Jones DY, et al: Dietary fat and breast cancer in the National Health and Nutrition Examination Survey, I: Epidemiologic follow-up study. *J Natl Cancer Inst* 1987; 79:465-471.

Kessler DA: The basis of the FDA's decision on breast implants. *N Engl J Med* 1992; 326:1713-1715.

Kessler DA, Merkata RB, Schapiro R: A call for higher standards for breast implants. *JAMA* 1993; 270:2607-2608.

Kinne D: Clinical management of lobular carcinoma in situ. In Harris JR, et al, editors: *Breast diseases,* Philadelphia, 1991, JB Lippincott.

Knekt P, et al: Dietary fat and risk of breast cancer. *Am J Clin Nutr* 1990; 52:903-908.

Kopans DB, Feig SA: The Canadian National Breast Screening Study: A critical review. *AJR Am J Roentgenol* 1993; 161:755-760.

Krag D, Weaver D, Ashikaga, et al: The sentinel node in breast cancer: A multicenter validation study. *N Engl J Med* 1998; 339:941-946.

Kurtz JM, et al: Results of wide excision for local recurrence after breast-conserving therapy. *Cancer* 1989; 61:1969.

Lauerson N, Wilson K: The effect of danazol in the treatment of chronic cystic mastitis. *Obstet Gynecol* 1976; 48:93.

Layfield LJ, Glasgow BJ, Cramer H: Fine-needle aspiration in the management of breast masses. *Pathol Annu* 1989; 24:23-62.

Lazovich D, et al: Underutilization of breast conserving surgery and radiation therapy among women with stage I or II breast cancer. *JAMA* 1991; 266:3433-3438.

Lee-Feldstein A, Anton-Calver H, Feldstein PJ: Treatment differences and other prognostic factors related to breast cancer survival delivery systems and medical outcomes. *JAMA* 1994; 271:1163-1168.

Leis HP Jr: Gross breast ovals: Significance and management. *Contemp Surg* 1991; 39:13-20.

Levine AJ: The p53 tumor-suppressor gene. *N Engl J Med* 1992; 326:1350-1351.

Levine JJ, Ilowite NT: Sclerodema-like esophageal disease in children breast-fed by mothers with silicone breast implants. *JAMA* 1994; 271:213-216.

Loomis DP, Savitz DA, Ananth CV: Breast cancer mortality among female electrical workers in the United States. *J Natl Cancer Inst* 1994; 86:921-925.

Love RR, et al: Effects of tamoxifen on bone mineral density in postmenopausal women with breast cancer. *N Engl J Med* 1992; 326:852-956.

Lynch HT, Marcus JN, Watson P: Familial breast cancer, family cancer syndromes, and predisposition to breast neoplasia. In Bland KI, Copeland EM III, editors: *The breast—comprehensive management of benign and malignant diseases,* Philadelphia, 1991, WB Saunders.

Maddox VA, et al: Does radical mastectomy still have a place in the treatment of primary operable breast cancer? *Arch Surg* 1987; 122:1317-1320.

Mansel R, Preece P, Hughes L: A double-blind trial of the prolactin inhibitor bromocriptine in painful benign breast disease. *Br J Surg* 1978; 65:724.

Mansur EG, et al: Efficacy of adjuvant chemotherapy in high-risk node-negative breast cancer. *N Engl J Med* 1989; 320:485-490.

Marchant DJ: Estrogen-replacement therapy after breast cancer. *Cancer* 1993; 71(suppl):2169-2176.

Marcus JN, Watson P, Page DL, et al: Hereditary breast cancer: Pathobiology, prognosis, and BRCA1 and BRCA2 gene linkage. *Cancer* 1996; 77:697-709.

Mettlin CJ, Smart CR: The Canadian National Breast Screening Study: An appraisal and implications for early-detection policy. *Cancer* 1993; 72(suppl):1461-1465.

Meyer JE, Christian RL, Lester SC, et al: Evaluation of non-palpable solid breast masses with stereotaxic large-needle core biopsy using a dedicated unit. *AJR Am J Roentgenol* 1996; 167:179-182.

Miller AB, et al: Canadian National Breast Screening Study, I: Breast cancer detection and death rates among women aged 40-49 years. *Can Med Assoc J* 1992a; 147:1459-1476.

Miller AB, et al: The Canadian National Breast Screening Study, II: Breast cancer detection and death rates among women aged 50-59 years. *Can Med Assoc J* 1992b; 147:1477-1488.

Mills PK, et al: Dietary habits and breast cancer incidence among Seventh-Day Adventists. *Cancer* 1989; 64:582-590.

Morehead JR: Anatomy and embryology of the breast. *Clin Obstet Gynecol* 1982; 25:353-357.

Moskowitz M: The predictive value of certain mammographic signs in screening for breast cancer. *Cancer* 1983; 51:1007-1011.

Moskowitz M: Guidelines for screening for breast cancer: Is a revision in order? *Radiol Clin North Am* 1992; 30:221-233.

Muss HB, et al: C-erB-2 expression and response to adjuvant therapy in women with node-positive early breast cancer. *N Engl J Med* 1994; 330:1260-1266.

Narod SA, et al: Familial breast-ovarian cancer locus on chromosome 17q2l-q23. *Lancet* 1991; 338:82-83.

National Cancer Institute, National Institutes of Health: *Clinical alert from the National Cancer Institute,* Department of Human Services, May 16, 1988. Washington, DC, US Government Printing Office.

Nattinger AB, et al: Geographic variation in the use of breast-conserving treatment for breast cancer. *N Engl Mled* 1992; 326:1102-1107.

Newcomb PA, et al: Lactation and a reduced risk of premenopausal breast cancer. *N Engl J Med* 1994; 330:81-87.

Niebyl JR, Spence MR, Parmley TH: Sporadic (nonepidemic) puerperal mastitis. *J Reprod Med* 1978; 20:97-100.

NIH Consensus Conference: Treatment of early-stage breast cancer. *JAMA* 1991; 265:391-397.

NIH Consensus Statement: Breast Cancer Screening for Women Ages 40-49, vol. 15, no. 1. Bethesda, Md. Office of Medical Application of Research 1997:1-35.

NSABP Researchers Report on the Tamoxifen Breast Cancer Prevention Trial. *Oncology* 1998; 12:1198.

Nystrom L, et al: Breast cancer screening with mammography: Overview of Swedish randomized trials. *Lancet* 1993; 341:973-978.

Osteen RT, et al: Regional differences in surgical management of breast cancer. *Cancer* 1992; 42:39-43.

Osteen RT, et al: 1991 National survey of carcinoma of the breast by the Commission on Cancer. *J Am Coll Surg* 1994; 178:213-219.

Overgaard, M, Hansen PS, Overgaard, J, et al: Postoperative radiotherapy in high-risk premenopausal women with breast cancer who receive adjuvant chemotherapy. *N Engl J Med* 1997; 337:14 949-954.

Page DL, Jensen RA: Evaluation and management of high risk and premalignant lesions of the breast. *World J Surg* 1994; 18:32-38.

Parker SH, et al: Stereotactic breast biopsy with a biopsy gun. *Radiology* 1990; 176:741-747.

Pashby NL, et al: A clinical trial of evening primrose oil in mastalgia. *Br J Surg* 1981; 68:801-805.

Passaro ME, et al: Lactiferous fistula. *J Am Coll Surg* 1994; 178:29-32.

Perren TJ: C-erbB-2 oncogene as a prognostic marker in breast cancer [editorial]. *Br J Cancer* 1991; 63:328.

Peters MV: The effect of pregnancy in breast cancer. In Forrest APM, Kunkler PB, editors: *Prognostic factors in breast cancer,* Baltimore, 1968, Williams & Wilkins.

Peters WP: High-dose chemotherapy and autologous bone marrow support for breast cancer. In DeVita VT Jr, Hellman S, Rosenberg SA, editors: *Important advances in oncology,* Philadelphia, 1991, JB Lippincott.

Petrakis NL: Physiologic, biochemical, and cytologic aspects of nipple aspirate fluid. *Breast Cancer Res Treat* 1986; 8:7-19.

Petrek JA: Incidence of pregnancy-associated breast cancer. In Harris JR, et al, editors, *Breast diseases,* Philadelphia, 1991, JB Lippincott.

Pigott J, et al: Metastases to the upper levels of the axillary nodes in carcinoma of the breast and its implications for nodal sampling procedure. *Surg Gynecol Obstet* 1984; 158:255.

Powles T, Eeles R, Ashley S, et al: Interim analysis of the incidence of breast cancer in the Royal Marsden Hospital tamoxifen randomised chemoprevention trial. *Lancet* 1998; 352:98-101.

Preece R, Mansel R, Bolton P: Clinical syndromes of mastalgia. *Lancet* 1976; 2:670.

Preece R, Mansel R, Hughes L: Mastalgia: Psychoneurosis or organic disease? *Br Med J* 1978; 1:29.

Press RI, et al: Antinuclear antibodies in women with silicone implants. *Lancet* 1992; 340:1304-1307.

Pritchard KI: Is tamoxifen effective in prevention of breast cancer? *Lancet* 1998; 352:80-81.

Public Health Services: Surveillance, epidemiology, and end results: Incidence and mortality data, 1973-1977, DHEW (NIH)81-2330,1981, Bethesda.

Public Health Services: Surveillance, epidemiology, and end results, DHEW (NIH)85-1837, 1984, Bethesda.

Ragaz J, Jackson SM, Le N, et al: Adjuvant radiotherapy and chemotherapy in node-positive premenopausal women with breast cancer. *N Engl J Med* 1997; 337:14:956-962.

Rissanen PM: Carcinoma of the breast during pregnancy and lactation. *Br J Cancer* 1968; 22:663-668.

Roa BB, Boyd AA, Volcik K, et al: Ashkenazi Jewish population frequencies for common mutations in BRCA1 and BRCA2. *Nat Genet* 1996; 14:185-187.

Romieu I, Berlin JA, Colditz GA: Oral contraceptives and breast cancer: Review and meta-analysis. *Cancer* 1990; 66:2253-2263.

Rosen PP: Lobular carcinoma in situ and intraductal carcinoma of the breast, *Monogr Pathol* 1984; 25:59.

Rosen PP, et al: Lobular carcinoma in situ of the breast: Detailed analysis of 99 patients with average follow-up of 24 years. *Am J Surg Pathol* 1978; 2:225.

Rosen PP, et al: Discontinuous or "skip" metastases in breast carcinoma: Analysis of 1228 axillary dissections. *Ann Surg* 1983; 197:276.

Rosner D, Baird D: What ultrasonography can tell in breast masses that mammography and physical examination cannot. *J Surg Oncol* 1985; 28:308-313.

Sarrazin D, et al: Conservative treatment versus mastectomy in breast cancer tumors with macroscopic diameter of 20 millimeters or less. *Cancer* 1984; 53:1209-1213.

Scottish Cancer Trials Breast Group: Adjuvant ovarian ablation versus CMF chemotherapy in premenopausal women with pathological stage II breast carcinoma: The Scottish trial. *Lancet* 1993; 341:1293-1298.

Segal M: Silicone breast implants: Available under tight controls. *FDA Consumer* June 1992.

Sellers TA, et al: Effect of family history, body-fat distribution, and reproductive factors on the risk of postmenopausal breast cancer. *N Engl J Med* 1992; 326:1323-1329.

Sickles EA: Mammographic features of 300 consecutive nonpalpable breast cancers. *AJR Am J Roentgenol* 1986; 146:661-663.

Sickles EA: Periodic mammographic follow-up of probably benign lesions: Results in 3184 consecutive cases. *Radiology* 1991; 179:463-468.

Slamon DJ, et al: Studies of the HER-2-neu proto-oncogene in human breast and ovarian cancer. *Science* 1989; 244:707.

Slattery ML, Kerber RA: A comprehensive evaluation of family history and breast cancer risk. *JAMA* 1993; 270:1563-1568.

Smart CR, et al: Insights into breast cancer screening of younger women: Evidence from the 14-year follow-up of the breast-cancer detection demonstration project. *Cancer* 1993; 72(suppl):1449-1456.

Smith BL: Duct ectasia, periductal mastitis, and breast infections. In Harris JR, et al, editors: *Breast diseases,* Philadelphia, 1991, JB Lippincott.

Smith-Warner SA, Spiegelman D, Yuan S-S, et al: Alcohol and breast cancer in women: A pooled analysis of cohort studies. *JAMA* 1998; 279:535-540.

Speira H, Kerr LD: Scleroderma following silicone implantation: A cumulative experience of 11 cases. *J Rheumatol* 1993; 20:958-961.

Squitieri R, et al: Carcinoma of the breast in postmenopausal hormone user and nonuser control groups. *J Am Coll Surg* 1994; 178:167-170.

Steinberg KK, et al: A meta-analysis of the effect of estrogen replacement therapy. *JAMA* 1991; 265:1985-1990.

Struewing JP, Abeliovich D, Peretz T, et al: The carrier frequency of the *BRCA1* 185delAG mutation is approximately 1% in Ashkenazi Jewish individuals. *Nat Genet* 1995; 11:198-200.

Tabar L, Duffy SW, Warren, Burhenne L: New Swedish breast cancer detection results for women aged 40-49. *Cancer* 1993; 72(suppl): 1437-1448.

Tabar L, et al: Update of the Swedish two-county trial of mammographic screening for breast cancer. *Radiol Clin North Am* 1992; 30:187-210.

Takeda T, et al: Cytologic studies of nipple discharge. *Acta Cytol* 1982; 26:35.

Tavtgian SV, Simard J, Rommens J, et al: The complete *BRAC2* gene and mutations in chromosome 13q-linked kindreds. *Nat Genet* 1996; 12:333-337.

Teuber SS, et al: Anticollagen autoantibodies are found in women with silicone breast implants. *J Autoimmun* 1993; 6:367-377.

Thomas DB, Gao DL, Self SG, et al: Randomized trial of breast self-examination in Shanghai: Methodology and preliminary results. *J Natl Cancer Inst* 1997; 89:355-365.

Thune I, Brenn T, Lund E, et al: Physical activity and the risk of breast cancer. *N Engl J Med* 1997; 336:18:1269-1274.

Trichopoulos D: Are electric or magnetic fields affecting mortality from breast cancer in women? *J Natl Cancer Inst* 1994; 86:885-986.

Turner L, et al: Radical versus modified radical mastectomy for breast cancer. *Ann R Coll Surg Engl* 1981; 63:239-243.

Urban J: Excision of the major duct system of the breast. *Cancer* 1963; 16:516-520.

Veronesi U, et al: Comparing radical mastectomy with quadrantectomy, axillary dissection, and radiotherapy in patients with small cancers of the breast. *N Engl J Med* 1985; 312:665-673.

Veronesi U, et al: Comparison of Halstead mastectomy with quadrantectomy, axillary dissection, and radiotherapy in early breast long term results. *Eur J Cancer Clin Oncol* 1986; 22:1085-1089.

Veronesi U, et al: Distribution of axillary node metastases by level of invasion: An analysis of 539 cases. *Cancer* 1987; 59:682.

Veronesi U, et al: Radiotherapy after breast-preserving surgery in women with localized cancer of the breast. *N Engl J Med* 1993; 328:1587-1591.

Veronesi U, Maisonneuve P, Costs A, et al: Prevention of breast cancer with tamoxifen: Preliminary findings from the Italian randomised trial among hysterectomised women. *Lancet* 1998; 352:93-97.

Walker AP, et al: A prospective study of the microflora of nonpuerperal breast abscess. *Arch Surg* 1988; 123:908-911.

Wallack MK, et al: Gestational carcinoma of the female breast. *Curr Probl Cancer* 1983; 7: 1-58.

Weidner N, et al: Tumor angiogenesis and metastasis—Correlation in invasive breast carcinoma. *N Engl J Med* 1991; 324:1-7.

Weidner N, et al: Tumor angiogenesis correlates with metastasis in invasive prostate carcinoma. *Am J Pathol* 1993; 143:401-409.

White TT: Carcinoma of the breast in the pregnant and the nursing patient. *Am J Obstet Gynecol* 1955; 69:1277-1286.

Willett WC, et al: Dietary fat and the risk of breast cancer. *N Engl J Med* 1987; 316:22-28.

Willett WC, et al: Dietary fat and fiber in relation to risk of breast cancer: An 8-year follow-up. *JAMA* 1992; 268:2037-2044.

Wingo PA, et al: Age-specific differences in the relationship between oral contraceptive use and breast cancer. *Obstet Gynecol* 1991; 78:161-170.

Wisbey J, Mansel R, Pye J: Natural history of breast pain. *Lancet* 1983; 2:672.

Wolfe JN, et al: Xeroradiography of the breast: Overview of 21,057 consecutive cases. *Radiology* 1987; 165:305-311.

Wood WC, et al: Dose and dose intensity of adjuvant chemotherapy for stage II, node-positive breast carcinoma. *N Engl J Med* 1994; 330:1253-1259.

Wooster R, Bignell G, Lancaster J, et al: Identification of the breast cancer susceptibility gene, *BRCA2. Nature* 1995; 378:789-792.

Yeatman TJ, Bland KI: Staging of breast cancer. In Bland KI, Copeland EM, editors: *Comprehensive management of benign and malignant diseases,* Philadelphia, 1991, WB Saunders.

11

Gestational Trophoblastic Disease

ROSS S. BERKOWITZ

DONALD P. GOLDSTEIN

KEY ISSUES

1. Complete moles commonly have a 46,XX karyotype, and all molar chromosomes are of paternal origin.
2. Partial moles usually have a triploid karyotype, and the extra haploid set of chromosomes is of paternal origin.
3. Because complete moles are now diagnosed earlier in gestation, few patients have the classic signs and symptoms of excessive uterine size, toxemia, or hyperemesis.
4. Gestational trophoblastic tumors are highly curable with chemotherapy even if they have metastasized.
5. After successful treatment with chemotherapy, patients who have had gestational trophoblastic tumors can generally expect normal reproductive outcomes in subsequent pregnancies.

MANAGEMENT OF MOLAR PREGNANCY AND GESTATIONAL TROPHOBLASTIC TUMORS

Gestational trophoblastic disease (GTD) includes a group of interrelated diseases, among them complete and partial molar pregnancy, invasive mole, placental-site trophoblastic tumor, and choriocarcinoma, all of which have varying propensities for invasion and spread. Gestational trophoblastic tumor (GTT) is one of the rare human malignancies that are highly curable even with widespread metastases (Goldstein and Berkowitz, 1982; Bagshawe, 1976). Although GTT commonly develops after molar pregnancy, it may ensue after any gestation. Important advances have been made in the diagnosis, treatment, and follow-up of patients with molar pregnancy and GTT. This chapter reviews these advances and discusses basic principles of management based on the clinical experience accumulated at the New England Trophoblastic Disease Center (NETDC).

Epidemiology

Reported incidences of gestational trophoblastic disease vary dramatically in different regions of the world. The frequency of molar pregnancy in Asian countries is 7 to 10 times greater that the reported incidence in North America or Europe (Bracken, 1987). Although hydatidiform mole occurs in 1 of 125 pregnancies in Taiwan, the incidence of molar gestation in the United States is approximately 1 in 1500 live births. Variations in the incidence rates of molar pregnancy partially result from differences between reporting hospital-based versus population-based data.

The high incidence of molar pregnancy in some populations has been attributed to socioeconomic and nutritional factors. It is observed in a case-control study that the risk for complete molar pregnancy progressively increases with decreasing levels of consumption of dietary carotene (vitamin A precursor) and animal fat (Berkowitz et al, 1985). Parazzini et al (1988) also report from Italy that low carotene consumption is associated with gestational trophoblastic disease. Global regions with high incidences of vitamin A deficiency correspond to areas with high frequencies of molar pregnancy. Dietary factors such as carotene may, therefore, partially explain regional variations in the incidence of complete molar pregnancy.

The risk for complete molar pregnancy also increases with advanced maternal age (Bracken, 1987). Women older than 40 years have a fivefold to tenfold greater risk. Ova from older women may be more susceptible to abnormal fertilization.

Certain epidemiologic features of complete and partial molar pregnancy differ markedly. Parazzini et al (1986) report that the risk for partial mole is not associated with maternal age. Additionally, the risk for partial mole is reported to be associated with the use of oral contraceptives and a history of irregular menstruation but not with dietary factors (Berkowitz et al, 1995). Hence, the risk for partial mole appears to be associated with reproductive history rather than with dietary factors.

MOLAR PREGNANCY
Complete versus Partial Molar Pregnancy
Pathologic and Chromosomal Features

Hydatidiform moles may be categorized as complete or partial based on gross morphology, histopathology, and karyotype (Table 11-1). Complete hydatidiform moles have no identifiable embryonic or fetal tissue. The chorionic villi have generalized swelling and diffuse trophoblastic hyperplasia, and the implantation-site trophoblast has diffuse, marked atypia (Fig. 11-1). Complete moles usually have a

Table 11-1   Complete and Partial Molar Pregnancy: Histopathologic and Chromosomal Features

	Complete Mole	Partial Mole
Fetal or embryonic tissue	Absent	Present
Hydatidiform swelling of chorionic villi	Diffuse	Focal
Trophoblastic hyperplasia	Diffuse	Focal
Scalloping of chorionic villi	Absent	Present
Trophoblastic stromal inclusions	Absent	Present
Karyotype	46,XX (mainly); 46,XY	Triploid (mainly); diploid

46,XX karyotype, and the molar chromosomes are derived entirely from paternal origin (Kajii and Ohama, 1977). Most complete moles appear to arise from an anuclear empty ovum fertilized by a haploid (23X) sperm that then duplicates its own chromosomes (Yamashita et al, 1979). Although most complete moles have a 46,XX chromosomal pattern, approximately 10% of complete moles have a 46,XY karyotype (Pattillo et al, 1981). The 46,XY complete mole arises from fertilization of an anuclear empty ovum by two sperm cells. Although chromosomes in the complete mole are entirely of paternal origin, the mitochondrial DNA is of maternal origin (Azuma et al, 1991).

Partial hydatidiform moles are characterized by the following abnormal features: chorionic villi of various sizes with focal swelling and focal trophoblastic hyperplasia (Fig. 11-2); focal, mild atypia of implantation-site trophoblast; marked villous scalloping and prominent stromal trophoblastic inclusions; and identifiable fetal or embryonic tissue (Szulman and Surti, 1978a). Partial moles generally have a triploid karyotype that results from the fertilization of an apparently normal ovum by two sperm (Szulman and Surti, 1978b). Lawler et al (1991) and Lage et al (1992) report that 93% and 90%, respectively, of partial moles are triploid. When fetuses are identified with partial moles, they generally have stigmata of triploidy, including growth retardation and multiple congenital anomalies.

Complete Molar Pregnancy
Signs and Symptoms

The clinical presentation of a complete molar pregnancy has changed dramatically over the past two decades. Vaginal bleeding occurred in 97% of our patients during the 1960s and 1970s (Berkowitz et al, 1991). Approximately half of our patients had anemia (hemoglobin, <10/dL) because bleeding was often heavy and prolonged. The uterus was palpably larger than it should have been for the

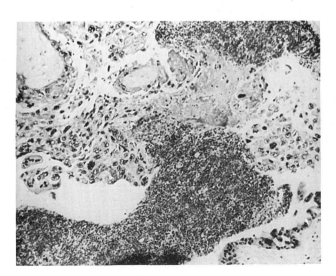

Fig. 11-1. Complete hydatidiform mole with marked trophoblastic hyperplasia and atypia. Note the syncytial border of villus (*lower right*) and the marked trophoblastic hyperplasia (*center*).

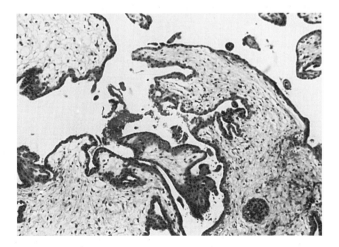

Fig. 11-2. Photomicrograph of partial mole demonstrating chorionic villi of various sizes with focal trophoblastic hyperplasia, villous scalloping, and stromal trophoblastic inclusions.

gestational age in half the patients, and it was commonly associated with markedly elevated human chorionic gonadotropin (hCG) levels. Prominent bilateral ovarian theca lutein cysts developed in half the patients as a result of ovarian hyperstimulation by high circulating blood levels of hCG (Osathanondh et al, 1986). Hyperemesis and preeclampsia were diagnosed in 26% and 27% of patients, respectively, and occurred almost exclusively among patients with excessive uterine size and markedly elevated hCG levels.

Respiratory insufficiency (2% of patients) and hyperthyroidism (7% of patients) were infrequent but medically important complications. Respiratory insufficiency infrequently developed from the cardiopulmonary complications of trophoblastic emboli, preeclampsia, massive fluid replacement, and thyroid storm. Respiratory distress generally resolved within 72 hours with appropriate cardiopulmonary support. Thyroid storm sometimes occurred at the time of molar evacuation in patients who had untreated hyperthyroidism.

During the 1960s and 1970s, complete molar pregnancy was usually diagnosed in the second trimester, but today the diagnosis of complete mole is generally made in the first trimester (Soto-Wright et al, 1995). Earlier diagnoses are possible because of the widespread use of ultrasonography and the availability of accurate and sensitive tests for hCG.

Complete mole is now often diagnosed before the classic clinical signs and symptoms develop. Vaginal bleeding, which occurs in 84% of patients, continues to be the most common symptom. Because of earlier detection, excessive uterine size, hyperemesis, anemia, and preeclampsia are now only observed in 28%, 8%, 5%, and 1% of patients, respectively (Soto-Wright et al, 1995). Neither hyperthyroidism nor respiratory distress developed in any of our 74 patients with complete mole between 1988 and 1993. However, before evacuation patients continue to have markedly elevated hCG levels.

Partial Molar Pregnancy
Signs and Symptoms

Patients with partial molar pregnancy usually do not have the classic clinical features characteristic of complete mole. Rather, they generally have the signs and symptoms of missed or incomplete abortion. Eighty-one patients with partial mole were followed up at the NETDC between January 1979 and August 1984 (Berkowitz et al, 1985). Excessive uterine size and preeclampsia was detected in only five patients. Szulman and Surti (1982) also report that 9 of 81 (11%) patients with partial mole had excessive uterine enlargement. None of our patients had prominent theca lutein ovarian cysts, hyperthyroidism, or hyperemesis. Preevacuation hCG values were measured in 30 patients and exceeded 100,000 mIU/mL in only two (7%). The diagnosis of partial mole is usually made after histologic review of curettage specimens.

Ultrasonography and Diagnosis of Hydatidiform Mole

Ultrasonography is a sensitive and reliable technique for detecting complete molar pregnancy. Because of marked swelling of the chorionic villi, complete mole produces a characteristic vesicular sonographic pattern. However, it may be difficult to distinguish an early complete mole from degenerative chorionic tissue because molar chorionic villi in the first trimester may be too small to visualize on ultrasonography. During ultrasonography, hCG measurements may help to differentiate an early, complete mole from a missed abortion.

Ultrasonography may also contribute to the diagnosis of partial molar pregnancy. Two sonographic findings are significantly associated with the diagnosis of partial mole: focal cystic changes in the placenta and a ratio greater than 3:2 of transverse-to-anteroposterior dimension of the gestational sac (Fine et al, 1989). When both findings are present, the positive predictive value for partial mole is 87%. On rare occasions, the sonogram shows the presence of a fetus with multiple congenital anomalies associated with a focally hydropic placenta.

Natural History of Molar Pregnancy and Prognostic Factors

Complete hydatidiform moles are known to have a potential for uterine invasion or distant spread. After molar evacuation, uterine invasion and metastasis occurs in 15% and 4% of patients, respectively (Berkowitz and Goldstein, 1993). Although complete moles are diagnosed earlier in pregnancy, the incidence of postmolar tumor has not been affected (Soto-Wright et al, 1995; Paradinas et al, 1996).

We reviewed 858 patients with complete mole to identify factors that predispose to postmolar tumor (Berkowitz and Goldstein, 1997). At the time of initial visit, 41% of the patients had the following signs of marked trophoblastic proliferation: hCG level >100,000 mIU/mL, uterine size greater than expected for gestational age, and theca lutein cysts >6 cm diameter. After evacuation, uterine invasion developed in 31% of these patients and metastases developed in 8.8%. The risk for persistent tumor is considerably less for patients who do not have signs of marked trophoblastic growth. After molar evacuation, invasion developed in only 3.4% and metastases developed in only 0.6%. Therefore, patients with complete moles, markedly elevated hCG levels, and excessive uterine size are at increased risk for postmolar tumor and are categorized as high risk.

An increased risk for postmolar GTT has been observed in women older than 40. Tow (1966) reports that persistent tumors develop in 37% of women older than 40 who have complete molar pregnancy. Complete moles in older women are more often aneuploid, and this may be related to their increased potential for local invasion and metastasis.

Nonmetastatic persistent GTT developed in 16 of 240 (6.6%) patients observed for partial mole at the New

England Trophoblastic Disease Center (Rice et al, 1990). Only one of these patients had the classic signs and symptoms of molar disease, which included excessive uterine enlargement, theca lutein ovarian cysts, and high hCG levels. Fifteen patients (94%) were thought to have missed abortions before evacuation. Patients with partial mole in whom persistent disease developed did not have clinical features that distinguished them from other patients with partial mole. Flow cytometric studies of partial moles that develop persistent tumors show a triploid pattern in 11 of 13 (85%) patients with interpretable histograms (Lage et al, 1991). In the remaining two patients there is a diploid pattern.

The risk for persistent GTT after partial mole has been reported to range from 0% to 11% (Table 11-2). A summary of data from nine centers showed that partial mole developed persistent GTT in 39 of 1125 (3.5%) patients and that only 7 (18%) of these patients had metastases.

Surgical Evacuation

After molar pregnancy is diagnosed, the patient should be evaluated carefully for the presence of medical complications such as preeclampsia, electrolyte imbalance, hyperthyroidism, and anemia, any of which could complicate surgical evacuation. The patient must first be stabilized, and then a decision must be made concerning the most appropriate method of evacuation.

If the patient no longer desires to preserve fertility, hysterectomy may be performed, and prominent theca lutein ovarian cysts may be aspirated at the time of surgery. Although hysterectomy eliminates the risk for local invasion, it does not prevent metastasis.

Suction curettage is the preferred method of evacuation, regardless of uterine size, for patients who desire to preserve fertility (Berkowitz and Goldstein , 1996). As the cervix is dilated, the surgeon may encounter brisk uterine bleeding caused by the passage of retained blood. Shortly after suction evacuation is begun, uterine bleeding is generally well controlled and the uterus rapidly regresses in size. If the uterus is larger than 14 weeks' size, one hand should be placed on top of the fundus and the uterus should be massaged to stimulate uterine contraction. When suction evacuation is thought to be complete, a sharp curettage should be performed to remove any residual chorionic tissue. Patients who are Rh negative should be given Rh-immune globulin at the time of evacuation because Rh D factor is expressed on trophoblast.

Role of Prophylactic Chemotherapy

The use of prophylactic chemotherapy at the time of molar evacuation remains controversial (Goldstein and Berkowitz, 1995). However, several investigators have reported that chemoprophylaxis reduces the risk for postmolar tumor.

Kim et al (1986) report a randomized, prospective trial of chemoprophylaxis in patients with complete mole. Chemoprophylaxis significantly reduces the incidence of postmolar tumor from 47% to 14% in patients with high-risk complete mole. However, chemoprophylaxis does not significantly influence the occurrence of persistent tumor in patients with low-risk complete mole.

We also report that prophylactic actinomycin D reduces the risk for persistent GTT among patients with high-risk complete mole (Berkowitz and Goldstein, 1993). Only 10 of 93 (11%) patients with high-risk complete mole have postmolar tumor after prophylactic therapy with actinomycin D. Chemoprophylaxis failure more commonly develops in patients with markedly elevated hCG values. Prophylactic chemotherapy may be of benefit for patients with high-risk complete moles, particularly when hormonal follow-up is unavailable or unreliable.

Hormonal Follow-up

After molar evacuation, all patients must have follow-up hCG measurements taken to ensure remission. This must continue on a weekly basis until hCG values are normal for 3 weeks and then on a monthly basis until they are normal for 6 months.

Patients are encouraged to use effective contraception during the entire follow-up interval. Intrauterine devices should not be inserted until the patient achieves normal hCG levels because of the risk for uterine perforation and infection if there is residual tumor. If the patient does not desire surgical sterilization, she must choose between hormonal contraceptives or barrier methods.

Postmolar tumor incidence is reportedly increased among patients who use oral contraceptives (Stone et al, 1976). However, data from our Center and the Gynecologic Oncology Group indicate that oral contraceptives do not increase the risk for postmolar trophoblastic disease (Berkowitz et al, 1981; Curry et al, 1989). Therefore, we believe that oral contraceptives may be safely prescribed after molar evacuation.

Table 11-2 Persistent Tumor After Partial Molar Pregnancy			
Series	Patients (No.)	Persistent Tumor (No.)	Metastases (No.)
Stone and Bagshawe, 1976	194	5	2
Vassilakos et al, 1977	56	0	0
Czernobilsky et al, 1982	25	1	0
Szulman and Surti, 1982	49	2	0
Wong and Ma, 1984	35	4	2
Ohama et al, 1986	56	0	0
Lawler et al, 1991	51	0	0
Lage et al, 1991	310	17	0
Goto et al, 1993	349	10	3
Total	1125	39 (3.5%)	7 (0.6%)

GESTATIONAL TROPHOBLASTIC TUMORS
Pathology Considerations

After a molar pregnancy, persistent GTT may have the histologic pattern of either molar tissue or choriocarcinoma. However, after a nonmolar gestation, persistent GTT may have the histologic features only of choriocarcinoma. Gestational choriocarcinoma does not contain chorionic villi; rather, it is composed of sheets of anaplastic cytotrophoblast and syncytiotrophoblast (Fig. 11-3).

Placental-site trophoblastic tumor (PSTT) is an uncommon variant of choriocarcinoma (Finkler et al, 1988). It is composed almost entirely of mononuclear intermediate trophoblast and does not contain chorionic villi. Because PSTT secretes small amounts of hCG, a large tumor may develop before hCG levels are detectable.

Natural History
Nonmetastatic Disease

Locally invasive GTT develops in 15% of patients after evacuation of a complete mole and less frequently after other types of gestation (Berkowitz and Goldstein, 1993). A trophoblastic tumor may perforate the myometrium and produce intraperitoneal bleeding, or it may erode the uterine vessels and cause vaginal hemorrhage. A bulky necrotic tumor may serve as a nidus for infection (Fig. 11-4).

Metastatic Disease

Metastatic GTT occurs in 4% of patients after evacuation of a complete mole and infrequently otherwise after pregnancy. Metastatic GTT is often associated with choriocarcinoma, which has a propensity for early vascular invasion with widespread dissemination. The most common metastatic sites are lung (80%), vagina (30%), brain (10%), and liver (10%). Because trophoblastic tumors are perfused with fragile vessels, metastases are often hemorrhagic. Patients may have signs and symptoms of bleeding from metastases such as hemoptysis or acute neurologic deficits. Cerebral and hepatic metastases are uncommon unless there is concurrent involvement of the lungs or the vagina.

Staging System

The International Federation of Gynecology and Obstetrics reports data on GTT using an anatomic staging system (Table 11-3). Stage I includes all patients with persistently elevated hCG levels and tumor confined to the uterus. Stage II comprises all patients with tumor outside of the uterus but localized to the vagina, pelvis, or both. Stage III includes all patients with pulmonary metastases with or without uterine, vaginal, or pelvic involvement. Stage IV indicates advanced disease with involvement of the brain, liver, kidneys, or gastrointestinal tract. Patients with stage IV disease are most likely to be resistant to chemotherapy. Stage IV tumors generally have the histologic pattern of choriocarcinoma and commonly develop after a nonmolar pregnancy.

It is helpful to use prognostic variables to predict the likelihood of drug resistance and to assist the selection of appropriate chemotherapy. The World Health Organization publishes a prognostic scoring system that reliably predicts the potential for chemotherapy resistance (Table 11-4). When the prognostic score is 8 or greater, the patient is considered at high risk and requires intensive combination chemotherapy to achieve remission. In general, patients with stage I disease have a low-risk score and patients with stage IV disease have a high-risk score. Therefore, the distinction between low risk and high risk primarily applies to stages II and III GTT.

Diagnostic Evaluation

The optimal management of GTT requires thorough evaluation of the extent of the disease before treatment. Each patient with a persistent tumor should undergo a thorough assessment that includes a complete history and physical

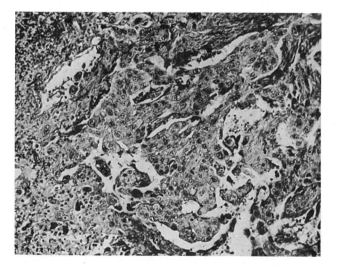

Fig. 11-3. Typical plexiform arrangement of trophoblastic cells in choriocarcinoma.

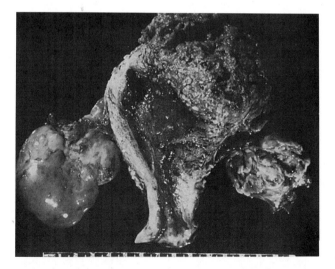

Fig. 11-4. Uterine choriocarcinoma with massive destruction of uterine wall.

Table 11-3　Staging of Gestational Trophoblastic Tumors

Stage	Description
I	Disease confined to uterus
IA	Disease confined to uterus with no risk factors
IB	Disease confined to uterus with one risk factor
IC	Disease confined to uterus with two risk factors
II	GTT extending outside uterus but limited to genital structures (adnexa, vagina, broad ligament)
IIA	GTT involving genital structures without risk factors
IIB	GTT extending outside uterus but limited to genital structures with one risk factor
IIC	GTT extending outside uterus but limited to genital structures with two risk factors
III	GTT extending to lungs with or without known genital tract involvement
IIIA	GTT extending to lungs with or without genital tract involvement and with no risk factors
IIIB	GTT extending to lungs with or without genital tract involvement and with one risk factor
IIIC	GTT extending to lungs with or without genital tract involvement and with two risk factors
IV	All other metastatic sites
IVA	All other metastatic sites without risk factors
IVB	All other metastatic sites with one risk factor
IVC	All other metastatic sites with two risk factors

Risk factors affecting staging include the following: (1) hCG >100,000 U/L and (2) duration of disease >6 months from termination of antecedent pregnancy.

The following factors should be considered and noted in reporting: (1) prior chemotherapy has been given for known GTT; (2) placental site tumors should be reported separately; (3) histological verification of disease is not required.

examination, determination of hCG levels, chest roentgenogram, and hepatic, thyroid, and renal function tests. It is unlikely that liver or brain metastases will be identified by additional radiographic studies in asymptomatic patients with normal results of pelvic examination and normal chest roentgenograms. Fig. 11-5 depicts an algorithm for the staging of patients with gestational trophoblastic tumors.

Management of Stage I Gestational Trophoblastic Tumor

Box 11-1 and Table 11-5 outline the NETDC protocol for the management of stage I disease and the results of therapy. The selection of treatment is based mainly on the patient's desire to preserve fertility.

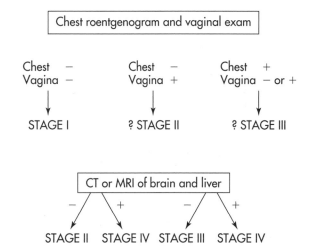

Fig. 11-5. Algorithm for staging of gestational trophoblastic tumor.

Table 11-4　Scoring System Based on Prognostic Factors

Prognostic Factors	Score* 0	Score* 1	Score* 2	Score* 4
Age (years)	≤38	>39		
Antecedent pregnancy	Hydatidiform mole	Abortion	Term	
Interval†	4	4-6	7-12	12
hCG (U/l)	10^3	10^3-10^4	10^4-10^5	10^5
ABO groups (female × male)		O × A A × O	B AB	
Largest tumor, including uterine tumor		3–5 cm	5 cm	
Site of metastases		Spleen Kidney	Gastrointestinal tract Liver	Brain
No. of metastases identified		1-4	4-8	8
Prior chemotherapy			Single drug	2 or more drugs

*The total score for a patient is obtained by adding the individual scores for each prognostic factor. Total score ≤4, low risk; 5-7, middle risk; ≥8, high risk.

†Interval time (months) between end of antecedent pregnancy and start of chemotherapy.

BOX 11-1
**TREATMENT PROTOCOL FOR STAGE I
GESTATIONAL TROPHOBLASTIC TUMOR
(NEW ENGLAND TROPHOBLASTIC
DISEASE CENTER)**

Initial

Single-agent chemotherapy or hysterectomy with adjunctive chemotherapy

Resistant

Combination chemotherapy
Hysterectomy with adjunctive chemotherapy
Local resection
Pelvic infusion

Follow-up

hCG   Weekly until normal ×3
        Monthly until normal ×12
        Contraception: 12 consecutive months of normal
            hCG levels

hCG, human chorionic gonadotropin.

BOX 11-2
**TREATMENT PROTOCOL FOR STAGE II
AND STAGE III GESTATIONAL
TROPHOBLASTIC TUMOR (NEW ENGLAND
TROPHOBLASTIC DISEASE CENTER)**

Low risk*
Initial   Single-agent chemotherapy
Resistant   Combination chemotherapy

High risk*
Initial   Combination chemotherapy
Resistant   Second-line combination chemotherapy

Follow-up
hCG   Weekly until normal × 3
                     Monthly until normal × 12
Contraception   12 consecutive months of normal
                         hCG levels

hCG, human chorionic gonadotropin.
*Local resection optional.

Table 11-5   New England Trophoblastic Disease Center: June 1965 to December 1995

Stage I: Confined to Uterine Corpus

Remission Therapy	No. of Patients	Remissions (%)
Initial	441 (93.5%)	
Sequential MTX/act-D		404 (91.6%)
Hysterectomy		29 (6.6%)
MAC		3 (0.7%)
EMA		5 (1.1%)
Resistant	35 (6.5%)	
MAC		10 (28.6%)
EMA		20 (57.1%)
Hysterectomy		2 (5.7%)
Local Uterine Resection		2 (5.7%)
Pelvic Infusion		1 (2.9%)
Totals	461	461 (100%)

MTX, methotrexate; act-D, actinomycin D; MAC, methotrexate, actinomycin D, cyclophosphamide; EMA, etoposide, methotrexate, actinomycin D.

If the patient no longer wants to retain fertility, hysterectomy with adjuvant single-agent chemotherapy may be performed as the primary treatment.

Adjuvant chemotherapy is administered to reduce the likelihood of disseminating viable tumor cells at surgery, to maintain cytotoxic levels of chemotherapy in the bloodstream and the tissues in case viable tumor cells are disseminated during surgery, and to treat occult metastases that may be present at the time of surgery. Occult pulmonary metastases may be detected by computed tomography imaging in approximately 40% of patients with presumed nonmetastatic disease (Mutch et al, 1986). Chemotherapy may be safely administered at the time of hysterectomy without increasing surgical complications. Twenty-nine patients were treated by primary hysterectomy and adjuvant chemotherapy at our Center, and all achieved complete remission with no additional therapy.

Nonmetastatic PSTT should be treated with hysterectomy because of its poor response to chemotherapy. Because PSTT is generally resistant to chemotherapy, there are few long-term survivors with metastases despite intensive multimodal therapy.

Single-agent chemotherapy is the preferred treatment for patients who have stage I disease and want to retain fertility. Primary single-agent chemotherapy induced complete remission in 404 of 439 (92.9%) patients who had stage I GTT. The 35 patients in whom there was resistance subsequently attained remission with either combination chemotherapy or surgical intervention. If the patient is resistant to chemotherapy and wants to preserve fertility, local uterine resection may be considered. When local resection is planned, ultrasonography, magnetic resonance imaging, or arteriography may identify the site of resistant tumor.

Management of Stages II and III Gestational Trophoblastic Tumor

The NETDC protocol for the management of stage II and stage III disease and the results of treatment are outlined in Box 11-2 and Tables 11-6 and 11-7. Although patients at low risk are treated with primary single-agent chemo-

Table 11-6   New England Trophoblastic Disease Center: June 1965 to December 1995

Stage II: Metastases to Pelvis and Vagina

Remission Therapy		No. of Patients	Remissions (%)
Low risk		19 (70.4%)	
Initial:	sequential MTX/act-D		16 (84.2%)
Resistant:	MAC		2 (10.5%)
	EMA-CO		1 (5.3%)
High risk		8 (29.6%)	
Initial:	sequential MTX/act-D		2 (25.0%)
	MAC		4 (50.0%)
Resistant:	MAC		1 (12.5%)
	CHAMOCA		1 (12.5%)
Totals		27	27 (100%)

MTX, methotrexate; act-D, actinomycin D; MAC, methotrexate, actinomycin D, cyclophosphamide; CHAMOCA, Bagshawe multi-agent regimen; EMA-CO, etoposide, methotrexate, actinomycin D-cyclophosphamide, oncovin.

Table 11-7   New England Trophoblastic Disease Center: June 1965 to December 1995

Stage III: Metastases to Lung

Remission Therapy		No. of Patients	Remissions (%)
Low risk		88 (65.7%)	
Initial:	sequential MTX/act-D		71 (80.7%)
Resistant:	MAC		12 (13.6%)
	EMA		5 (5.7%)
High risk		46 (34.3%)	
Initial:	sequential MTX/act-D		13 (28.3%)
	MAC		12 (26.1%)
	EMA		13 (28.3%)
Resistant:	MAC		2 (4.3%)
	CHAMOCA		1 (2.1%)
	5-FU-Adria		1 (2.1%)
	VPB		2 (4.3%)
	EMA		1 (2.1%)
Totals		134	133 (99.2%)

MTX, methotrexate; act-D, actinomycin-D; MAC, methotrexate, actinomycin D, cyclophosphamide; CHAMOCA, Bagshawe multi-agent regimen; 5-FU-Adria, 5-fluorouracil, adriamycin; VPB, vinblastine, cis-platinum, bleomycin; EMA, etoposide, methotrexate, actinomycin D.

therapy, patients at high risk are managed with primary combination chemotherapy.

Between June 1965 and December 1995, 27 patients with stage II disease were treated at the NETDC, and all achieved remission. Single-agent chemotherapy induced complete remission in 16 of 19 (84.2%) patients at low risk. In contrast,

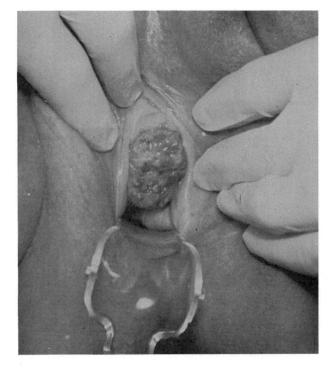

Fig. 11-6. Fungating suburethral metastasis of choriocarcinoma with necrosis and infection.

only 2 of 8 patients at high risk achieved remission with single-agent treatment.

Vaginal metastases may bleed profusely because they may be highly vascular and friable (Fig. 11-6). Bleeding may be controlled by packing the hemorrhagic lesion or by performing wide local excision. Occasionally, angiographic embolization of the hypogastric arteries may be required to control hemorrhage from vaginal metastases.

Between June 1965 and December 1995, 134 patients with stage III tumors were managed at the NETDC, and 133 (99.2%) attained complete remission. Single-agent chemotherapy induced complete remission in 71 of 88 (80.7%) patients with low-risk disease and in 13 of 46 (28.3%) patients with high-risk disease. All patients resistant to single-agent treatment achieved remission with combination chemotherapy.

Thoracotomy has a limited role in the management of stage III GTT. It should be performed if the diagnosis is seriously in doubt. Furthermore, if a patient has a persistent viable pulmonary nodule despite intensive chemotherapy, pulmonary resection may be performed. However, an extensive metastatic survey should be obtained to exclude other sites of persistent tumor. It is important to emphasize that fibrotic nodules may persist indefinitely on chest roentgenography after complete gonadotropin remission is achieved.

Hysterectomy may be required for patients with metastatic GTT to control uterine hemorrhage or sepsis. Additionally, for patients with bulky uterine tumor, hysterectomy may reduce the tumor burden and limit the need for chemotherapy.

BOX 11-3
TREATMENT PROTOCOL FOR STAGE IV
GESTATIONAL TROPHOBLASTIC TUMOR
(NEW ENGLAND TROPHOBLASTIC
DISEASE CENTER)

Initial

Combination chemotherapy
Brain—whole head irradiation (3000 cGy) craniotomy to
    manage complications
Liver—resection to manage complications

Resistant*

Second-line combination chemotherapy

Follow-up

hCG   Weekly until normal ×3
        Monthly until normal ×12

Contraception

12 consecutive months of normal hCG levels

hCG, human chorionic gonadotropin.
*Local resection optional.

Table 11-8   New England Trophoblastic Disease
Center: June 1965 to December 1995

Stage IV: Distant Metastases

Remission Therapy*	No. of Patients	Remissions (%)
Before 1975		
Initial: sequential MTX/act-D	5	
		6/20 (30%)
Resistant: MAC	1	
After 1975		
Initial: sequential MTX/act-D	2	
MAC	2	
Resistant: HD†MTX/act-D	4	14/18 (77.8%)
MAC	1	
CHAMOCA	1	
VPB	1	
EMA	3	

MTX, methotrexate; act-D, actinomycin D; MAC, methotrexate, actinomycin D,
cyclophosphamide; CHAMOCA, Bagshawe multi-agent regimen; VPB, vinblastine,
cis-platinum, bleomycin; EMA, etoposide, methotrexate, actinomycin D.

*Radiotherapy and surgery used when indicated.

†High dose.

Management of Stage IV Gestational Trophoblastic Tumor

Box 11-3 and Table 11-8 outline the NETDC protocol for
the management of stage IV disease and the results of treatment. These patients are at high risk for rapidly progressive
disease despite intensive therapy.

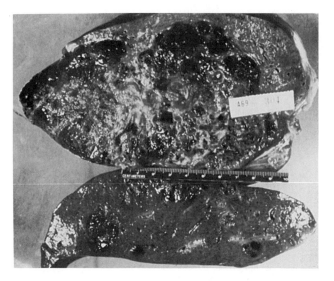

Fig. 11-7. Liver with diffuse choriocarcinoma involvement.

All patients with stage IV disease should be treated with
intensive combination chemotherapy and selective radiation
therapy and surgery (Lurain, 1998). Before 1975, only 6 of
20 (30%) patients with stage IV disease attained complete
remission. However, after 1975, 14 of 18 (77.8%) patients
with stage IV tumors achieved remission. This dramatic improvement in survival resulted from the introduction of intensive multimodal therapy early in the course of treatment.

The management of hepatic metastases is particularly
difficult and challenging. Hepatic resection may be required
to control bleeding or to excise resistant tumors (Fig. 11-7).

If cerebral metastases are detected, whole-brain irradiation is promptly instituted at our Center. The risk for spontaneous cerebral hemorrhage may be reduced by the concurrent use of chemotherapy and brain irradiation. Brain
irradiation may be hemostatic and tumoricidal. Yordan et al
(1987) report that deaths resulting from central nervous system involvement occur in 11 of 25 (44%) patients treated
with chemotherapy alone but in none of 18 patients treated
with brain irradiation and chemotherapy.

However, Rustin et al (1989) report excellent remission
rates in patients with cerebral metastases who are treated
with chemotherapy alone. Thirteen of 15 (86%) patients
with cerebral lesions achieve sustained remission with intensive combination chemotherapy, including high-dose
intravenous and intrathecal methotrexate.

Craniotomy should be performed to manage life-threatening complications, thereby providing the opportunity for
chemotherapy to induce complete remission. Craniotomy
may be necessary to provide acute decompression or to control bleeding (Fig. 11-8). Occasionally, cerebral metastases
that are resistant to chemotherapy may be amenable to resection. Fortunately, most patients with cerebral metastases
who achieve remission have no residual neurologic deficits.

Follow-up

All patients with stage I, stage II, and stage III GTT are followed up with weekly determinations of hCG values until

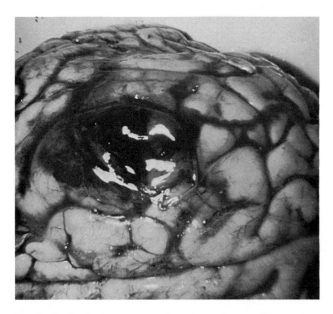

Fig. 11-8. Cerebral metastasis of choriocarcinoma with recent hemorrhage.

the values are normal for 3 weeks and then with monthly determinations of values until they are normal for 12 months. Patients are encouraged to use contraception during the entire follow-up interval.

Patients with stage IV disease are followed up with weekly determinations of hCG values until they are normal for 3 weeks and then with monthly determinations of values until they are normal for 24 months. These patients require prolonged follow-up because they are at increased risk for late recurrence.

CHEMOTHERAPY
Single-Agent Chemotherapy
Selection of Single-Agent Chemotherapy

Single-agent chemotherapy with either actinomycin D (act-D) or methotrexate (MTX) has induced comparable and excellent remission rates in nonmetastatic and metastatic GTT (Homesley, 1998). An optimal regimen should maximize the cure rate while it minimizes toxicity.

Methotrexate and folinic acid (MTX-FA) has been the preferred single-agent regimen for the treatment of GTT at the NETDC since 1974 (Berkowitz et al, 1986b). Between September 1974 and September 1984, 185 patients with GTT were treated with primary MTX-FA at the NETDC. Complete remission was induced with MTX-FA in 162 (87.6%) patients, and 132 (81.5%) of these patients required only one course of MTX-FA to achieve remission. MTX-FA induced remission in 147 of 163 (90.2%) patients with stage I GTT and in 15 of 22 (68.2%) patients with low-risk stages II and III GTT. After treatment with MTX-FA, thrombocytopenia, granulocytopenia, and hepatotoxicity occurred in only 11 (5.9%), 3 (1.6%), and 26 (14.1%) patients, respectively. No patient required platelet transfusion or had sepsis

because of myelosuppression. MTX-FA not only induces an excellent remission rate with minimal toxicity, it effectively limits chemotherapy exposure.

Combination Chemotherapy

Modified triple therapy with MTX-FA, act-D, and cyclophosphamide has been the preferred combination drug regimen at our Center (Berkowitz et al, 1984). However, triple therapy is inadequate as an initial treatment for patients with metastatic disease and a high-risk score (greater than 7) (DuBeshter et al, 1987). Triple therapy induced remission in only 5 of 11 (45%) patients with a high-risk score.

Etoposide (VP16) is a highly active antitumor agent in GTT. Primary oral etoposide induced complete sustained remission in 56 of 60 (93.3%) patients with nonmetastatic or low-risk metastatic GTT (Wong et al, 1986). Bagshawe (1984) reports an 83% remission rate in patients with metastatic disease and a high-risk score using a new combination regimen that includes etoposide. This new regimen (EMA-CO) includes etoposide, MTX, act-D, cyclophosphamide, and vincristine and is the preferred treatment for patients with metastatic GTT and high-risk scores. Bolis et al (1988) and Schink et al (1992) have similarly report that EMA-CO induces complete remission in 13 of 17 (76.4%) and in 5 of 5 (100%) patients with metastatic GTT and high-risk scores.

Unfortunately, the use of etoposide in GTT is reported to increase the risk for secondary tumors, among them myeloid leukemia, melanoma, colon cancer, and breast cancer (Rustin et al, 1996). Etoposide should be used only for patients who require it to achieve remission, particularly patients with metastatic GTT and high-risk scores.

Patients who require combination chemotherapy must be treated intensively to attain remission. We administer combination chemotherapy as frequently as toxicity permits until the patient attains three consecutive normal hCG values. After the patient achieves normal hCG levels, additional chemotherapy is administered to reduce the risk for relapse.

SUBSEQUENT PREGNANCIES
Pregnancy After Hydatidiform Mole

Patients with complete molar pregnancies can anticipate normal reproduction in the future (Berkowitz et al, 1998). Patients who were treated for complete mole at our center had 1234 later pregnancies between June 1965 and December 1996. These pregnancies resulted in 845 (68.5%) full-term live births, 93 (7.5%) premature deliveries, 11 (0.9%) ectopic pregnancies, and 7 (0.5%) stillbirths (Table 11-9). First-trimester spontaneous abortion occurred in 205 (16.5%) pregnancies, and major and minor congenital malformations were detected in 38 (4%) infants. Primary cesarean section was performed in 56 of 340 (16.5%) subsequent full-term and premature births between January 1979 and December 1996.

Table 11-9   Subsequent Pregnancies in Patients with Complete Mole (New England Trophoblastic Disease Center: June 1, 1965 to December 31, 1996)

Outcome	Number	Percentage
Term delivery	845	68.5
Stillbirth	7	0.5
Premature delivery	93	7.5
Spontaneous abortion		
1st trimester	205	16.5
2nd trimester	18	1.5
Therapeutic abortion	38	3.2
Ectopic	11	0.9
Repeat mole	17	1.4

Total number of pregnancies: 1234

Congenital malformations (major and minor): 38/945 (4.0%)
Primary cesarean section: 56/340 (16.5%)*

*January 1979 to December 1996.

Table 11-10   Subsequent Pregnancies in Patients with Partial Mole (New England Trophoblastic Disease Center: June 1, 1965 to December 31, 1996)

Outcome	Number	Percentage
Term delivery	144	73.8
Stillbirth	1	0.5
Premature delivery	4	2.2
Spontaneous abortion		
1st trimester	31	15.9
2nd trimester	1	0.5
Therapeutic abortion	10	5.1
Ectopic pregnancy	1	0.5
Repeat molar pregnancy	3	1.5

Total number of pregnancies: 195

Congenital malformations (major and minor): 3/149 (2.0%)
Primary cesarean section: 22/149 (14.8%)*

*January 1979 to December 1996.

Limited information is available regarding subsequent pregnancies among patients who had partial moles (Table 11-10). Patients who were treated for partial mole at our center had 195 later pregnancies between June 1965 and December 1996. These pregnancies resulted in 144 (73.8%) full-term live births, one (0.5%) stillbirth, one (0.5%) ectopic pregnancy, and four (2.2%) premature births. First-trimester spontaneous abortion occurred in 31 (15.9%) pregnancies, and major or minor congenital anomalies were detected in three (2%) infants. Preliminary data concerning subsequent conceptions after partial mole is, therefore, reassuring.

Table 11-11   Subsequent Pregnancies in Patients with Gestational Trophoblastic Tumors (New England Trophoblastic Disease Center: June 1, 1965 to December 31, 1996)

Outcome	Number	Percentage
Term delivery	348	69.0
Stillbirth	8	1.6
Premature delivery	27	5.4
Spontaneous abortion		
1st trimester	79	15.7
2nd trimester	7	1.4
Therapeutic abortion	25	4.9
Ectopic pregnancy	5	1.0
Repeat molar pregnancy	5	1.0

Total number of pregnancies: 504

Congenital malformations (major and minor): 10/383 (2.6%)
Primary cesarean section: 56/281 (19.9%)*

*January 1979 to December 1996.

When a patient has had a molar pregnancy, she is at increased risk for molar disease with later conceptions (Rice et al, 1989). Twenty-nine (0.7%) of our patients had at least two molar gestations between June 1965 and December 1996 (Berkowitz et al, 1998). Patients may have a complete or a partial mole with the first pregnancy and have the other type of molar disease with a later pregnancy. After two episodes of molar pregnancy, these 29 patients had 26 later conceptions that resulted in 14 (53.8%) full-term deliveries, 6 (23.1%) molar pregnancies (5 complete, 1 partial), 3 (11.6%) spontaneous abortions, one (3.8%) ectopic pregnancy, one intrauterine fetal death, and one therapeutic abortion.

It seems prudent to perform ultrasonography in the first trimester of any subsequent pregnancy to confirm normal gestational development. Furthermore, the placenta or the products of conception from later pregnancies should undergo pathologic review. Determination of hCG measurement should also be made 6 weeks after the completion of any future pregnancy to exclude occult trophoblastic disease.

Pregnancy After Gestational Trophoblastic Tumor

Patients with GTT who are successfully treated with chemotherapy can expect normal reproduction in the future (Walden and Bagshawe, 1976; Berkowitz et al, 1998). Patients with GTT who were treated with chemotherapy at our Center had 504 later pregnancies between June 1965 and December 1996. These later pregnancies resulted in 348 (69.0%) full-term live births, 27 (5.4%) premature deliveries, five (1%) ectopic pregnancies, and eight (1.6%) stillbirths (Table 11-11). First-trimester spontaneous abortion occurred in 79 (15.7%) pregnancies, and major and minor congenital anomalies were detected in 10 (2.6%) infants. It is particularly reassuring that the frequency of congenital malformations is not increased because chemotherapy may be teratogenic and mutagenic. Primary cesarean section was performed in only 56 (19.9%) of 281 subsequent full-term and premature deliveries between January 1979 and December 1996. Later pregnancies carry no increased risk for obstetric complications either prenatally or intrapartum.

REFERENCES

Azuma C, Saji F, Tokugawa Y, et al: Application of gene amplification by polymerase chain reaction to genetic analysis of molar mitochondrial DNA: The detection of anuclear empty ovum as the cause of complete mole. *Gynecol Oncol* 1991; 40:29-33.

Bagshawe KD: Risks and prognostic factors in trophoblastic neoplasia. *Cancer* 1976; 38: 1373-1385.

Bagshawe KD: Treatment of high-risk choriocarcinoma. *J Reprod Med* 1984; 29:813-820.

Berkowitz RS, Bernstein MR, Harlow BL, et al: Case-control study of risk factors for partial molar pregnancy. *AmJ Obstet Gynecol* 1995; 173:788-794.

Berkowitz RS, Cramer DW, Bernstein MR, Cassells S, Driscoll SG, Goldstein DG: Risk factors for complete molar pregnancy from a case-control study. *Am J Obstet Gynecol* 1985;152: 1016-1020.

Berkowitz RS, Goldstein DP: Management of molar pregnancy and gestational trophoblastic tumors. In Knapp RC, Berkowitz RS, editors: *Gynecologic oncology*, New York, 1993, McGraw-Hill.

Berkowitz RS, Goldstein DP: Chorionic tumors. *N Engl J Med* 1996; 335:1740-1748.

Berkowitz RS, Goldstein DP: Presentation and management of molar pregnancy. In Hancock BW, Newlands ES, Berkowitz RS, editors: *Gestational trophoblastic disease*, London, 1997, Chapman and Hall.

Berkowitz RS, Goldstein DP, Bernstein MR: Modified triple chemotherapy in the management of high-risk metastatic gestational trophoblastic tumors. *Gynecol Oncol* 1984; 19:173-181.

Berkowitz RS, Goldstein DP, Bernstein MR: Natural history of partial molar pregnancy. *Obstet Gynecol* 1986a; 66:677-681.

Berkowitz RS, Goldstein DP, Bernstein MR: Ten years experience with methotrexate and folinic acid as primary therapy for gestational trophoblastic disease. *Gynecol Oncol* 1986b; 23:111-118.

Berkowitz RS, Goldstein DP, Bernstein MR: Evolving concepts of molar pregnancy. *J Reprod Med* 1991; 36:40-44.

Berkowitz RS, Goldstein DP, Marean AR, Bernstein MR: Oral contraceptives and postmolar trophoblastic disease. *Obstet Gynecol* 1981; 58:474-478.

Berkowitz RS, Im SS, Bernstein MR, Goldstein DP: Gestational trophoblastic disease: Subsequent pregnancy outcome, including repeat molar pregnancy. *J Reprod Med* 1998; 43: 81-86.

Bolis G, Bonazzi C, Landoni F, et al: EMA/CO regimen in high-risk gestational trophoblastic tumor (GTT). *Gynecol Oncol* 1988; 31:439-444.

Bracken MB: Incidence and aetiology of hydatidiform mole: An epidemiologic review. *Br J Obstet Gynecol* 1987; 94:1123-1135.

Curry SL, Schlaerth JB, Kohorn EI, et al: Hormonal contraception and trophoblastic sequelae after hydatidiform mole (a Gynecologic Oncology Group study). *Am J Obstet Gynecol* 1989; 160:805-811.

Czernobilsky B, Barash A, Lancet M: Partial mole: A clinicopathologic study of 25 cases. *Obstet Gynecol* 1982; 59:75-77.

DuBeshter B, Berkowitz RS, Goldstein DP, Cramer DW, Bernstein MR: Metastatic gestational trophoblastic disease: Experience at the New England Trophoblastic Disease Center, 1965-1985. *Obstet Gynecol* 1987; 69:390-395.

Fine C, Bundy AL, Berkowitz RS, Boswell SB, Berezin AF, Doubilet PM: Sonographic diagnosis of partial hydatidiform mole. *Obstet Gynecol* 1989; 73:414-418.

Finkler NJ, Berkowitz RS, Driscoll SG, Goldstein DP, Bernstein MR: Clinical experience with placental site trophoblastic tumors at the New England Trophoblastic Disease Center. *Obstet Gynecol* 1988; 71: 854-857.

Goldstein DP, Berkowitz RS: *Gestational trophoblastic neoplasms—Clinical principles of diagnosis and management.* Philadelphia, 1982, WB Saunders.

Goldstein DP, Berkowitz RS: Prophylactic chemotherapy of complete molar pregnancy. *Semin Oncol* 1995; 22:157-160.

Goto S, Yamada A, Ishizuka T, Tomoda Y: Development of postmolar trophoblastic disease after partial molar pregnancy. *Gynecol Oncol* 1993; 48:165-170.

Homesley HD. Single-agent therapy for nonmetastatic and low-risk gestational trophoblastic disease. *J Reprod Med* 1998; 43:69-74.

Kajii T, Ohama K: Androgenetic origin of hydatidiform mole. *Nature* 1977; 268:633-634.

Kim DS, Moon H, Kim KT, Moon YJ, Hwang YY: Effects of prophylactic chemotherapy for persistent trophoblastic disease in patients with complete hydatidiform mole. *Obstet Gynecol* 1986; 67:690-694.

Lage JM, Berkowitz RS, Rice LW, Goldstein DP, Bernstein MR, Weinberg DS: Flow cytometric analysis of DNA content in partial hydatidiform moles with persistent gestational trophoblastic tumors. *Obstet Gynecol* 1991; 77:111-115.

Lage JM, Mark SD, Roberts D, Goldstein DP, Bernstein MR, Berkowitz RS: A flow cytometric study of 137 fresh hydropic placentas: Correlation between types of hydatidiform moles and nuclear DNA ploidy. *Obstet Gynecol* 1992; 79: 403-410.

Lawler SD, Fisher RA, Dent J: A prospective genetic study of complete and partial hydatidiform moles. *Am J Obstet Gynecol* 1991; 164: 1270-1277.

Lurain JR. Management of high-risk gestational trophoblastic disease. *J Reprod Med* 1998; 43:44-52.

Mutch DG, Soper JT, Baker ME, et al: Role of computed axial tomography of the chest in staging patients with nonmetastatic gestational trophoblastic disease. *Obstet Gynecol* 1986; 68: 348-352.

Ohama K, Katsunori U, Okamoto E, Takenaka M, Fujiwara A: Cytogenetic and clinicopathologic studies of partial moles. *Obstet Gynecol* 1986; 68:259-262.

Osathanondh R, Berkowitz RS, deCholnoky C, Smith BS, Goldstein DP, Tyson JE: Hormonal measurements in patients with theca lutein cysts and gestational trophoblastic disease. *J Reprod Med* 1986; 31:179-182.

Paradinas FJ, Browne P, Fisher RA, Foskett M, Bagshawe KD, Newlands E: A clinical, histopathological and flow cytometric study of 149 complete moles, 146 partial moles, 107 non-molar hydropic abortions. *Histopathology* 1996; 28:101-109.

Parazzini F, LaVecchia C, Mangili G, et al: Dietary factors and risk of trophoblastic disease. *Am J Obstet Gynecol* 1988; 158:93-100.

Pattillo RA, Sasaki S, Katayama KP, Roesler M, Mattingly RF: Genesis of 46, XY hydatidiform mole. *Am J Obstet Gynecol* 1981; 141:104-105.

Rice LW, Berkowitz RS, Lage JM, Goldstein DP, Bernstein MR: Persistent gestational trophoblastic tumor after partial hydatidiform mole. *Gynecol Oncol* 1990; 36:358-362.

Rice LW, Lage JM, Berkowitz RS, Goldstein DP, Bernstein MR: Repetitive complete and partial hydatidiform mole. *Obstet Gynecol* 1989; 74:217-221.

Rustin GJS, Newlands ES, Begent R, Dent J, Bagshawe KD: Weekly alternating etoposide, methotrexate, actinomycin-D/vincristin and cyclophosphamide chemotherapy for treatment of CNS metastases of choriocarcinoma. *J Clin Oncol* 1989; 7:900-903.

Rustin GJS, Newlands ES, Lutz JM, et al: Combination but not single-agent methotrexate chemotherapy for gestational trophoblastic tumors increases the incidence of second tumors. *J Clin Oncol* 1996; 14:2769-73.

Schink JC, Singh DK, Rademaker AW, Miller DS, Lurain JR: Etoposide, methotrexate, actinomycin D, cyclophosphamide and vincristine for the treatment of metastatic, high-risk gestational trophoblastic disease. *Obstet Gynecol* 1992; 80:817-820.

Soto-Wright V, Bernstein MR, Goldstein DP, Berkowitz R: The changing clinical presentation of complete molar pregnancy. *Obstet Gynecol* 1995; 86:775-779.

Stone M, Bagshawe KD: Hydatidiform mole: Two entities. *Lancet* 1976; 1:535-536.

Stone M, Dent J, Kardana A, Bagshawe KD: Relationship of oral contraception to development of trophoblastic tumour after evacuation of a hydatidiform mole. *Br J Obstet Gynaecol* 1976; 83:913-916.

Szulman AE, Surti U: The syndromes of hydatidiform mole, I: Cytogenetic and morphologic correlations. *Am J Obstet Gynecol* 1978a; 131:665-771.

Szulman AE, Surti U: The syndromes of hydatidiform mole, II: Morphologic evolution of the complete and partial mole. *Am J Obstet Gynecol* 1978b;132:20-27.

Szulman AE, Surti U: The clinicopathologic profile of the partial hydatidiform mole. *Obstet Gynecol* 1982; 59:597-602.

Tow WSH: The influence of the primary treatment of hydatidiform mole on its subsequent course. *J Obstet Gynaecol Br Commonw* 1966; 73:545-552.

Vassilakos P, Riotton G, Kajii T: Hydatidiform mole: Two entities. *Am J Obstet Gynecol* 1977; 127:167-170.

Walden PAM, Bagshawe KD: Reproductive performance of women successfully treated for gestational trophoblastic tumors. *Am J Obstet Gynecol* 1976; 125:1108-1114.

Wong LC, Choo YC, Ma HK: Primary oral etoposide therapy in gestational trophoblastic disease, an update. *Cancer* 1986; 58:14-17.

Wong LC, Ma HK: The syndrome of partial mole. *Arch Gynecol* 1984; 234:161-166.

Yamashita K, Wake N, Araki T, Ichinoe R, Makoto K: Human lymphocyte antigen expression in hydatidiform mole: Androgenesis following fertilization by a haploid sperm. *Am J Obstet Gynecol* 1979; 135:597-600.

Yordan EL Jr, Schlaerth J, Gaddis O, Morrow CP: Radiation therapy in the management of gestational choriocarcinoma metastatic to the central nervous system. *Obstet Gynecol* 1987; 69:627-630.

THE REPRODUCTIVE
LIFE CYCLE

CHAPTER

Pediatric and Adolescent Gynecology

MARC R. LAUFER
DONALD P. GOLDSTEIN

KEY ISSUES

1. The etiology of prepubertal vaginal bleeding is extensive, and the care provider must consider infection, foreign body, vaginal tumor, urethral prolapse, lichen sclerosis, hormonally active tumor, and trauma.
2. Sexual abuse in children is a disturbing and emotionally charged topic that must be addressed in girls with vaginal discharge, unexplained vaginal bleeding, or trauma. The most common physical finding in a person who has been sexually abused is a normal examination.
3. Pelvic pain in adolescents who do not respond to oral contraceptive pills and nonsteroidal agents should be evaluated by operative laparoscopy to rule out endometriosis because endometriosis does occur in adolescents.
4. Pelvic pain resulting from pelvic inflammatory disease in adolescents is particularly challenging because adolescents may not comply with medications and thus may require in-hospital intravenous antibiotic therapy.
5. Congenital anomalies of the reproductive tract must be completely evaluated to determine an appropriate medical and surgical approach; a recto-abdominal examination may be helpful if a vaginal examination cannot be performed. A magnetic resonance imaging study may be beneficial in documenting the müllerian structures.

Gynecologic treatment of the prepubertal and adolescent patient differs in many respects from the care of the adult woman. Unique problems are encountered in this population, especially in infants and young children, that are usu-

ally not seen by the practicing obstetrician-gynecologist. For this reason, it is appropriate that a chapter devoted to the gynecologic problems of this age group be included in a textbook of this scope. Fortunately, the evaluation and treatment of the most common conditions that affect these young patients requires minimal additional knowledge, equipment, and technical skill beyond the capabilities and resources of most gynecologists.

Gynecologic problems encountered in older adolescents are similar to those seen in adults. The distinction between these two groups is in the degree of emotional immaturity in the adolescents. The psychologic impact of the first gynecologic examination should not be underestimated. The outcome of this experience may have a profound influence on the care a patient seeks later.

Providing gynecologic treatment to adolescents undoubtedly is time consuming, and the physician with a busy practice may elect to avoid this population. Adolescents should be seen by a sensitive person who has time to listen to their needs, give satisfactory explanations, and answer questions in a way that is appropriate to their level of comprehension. These factors are essential to winning their confidence and, more important, to improving their compliance,

In this area of gynecologic practice, the attitude of the physician is also an important consideration. Children and adolescents are sensitive to adults' attitudes toward them. The gynecologist must, therefore, feel comfortable in communicating with these patients and their parents and should overcome any reticence about performing an adequate pelvic examination on young children and virginal adolescents. Maintaining a nonjudgmental attitude toward the patient's emerging sexuality is also of utmost importance.

In this chapter, the most commonly encountered gyneco-logic problems in the pediatric and adolescent populations are discussed. For the most part, conditions shared with the adult patient are discussed more comprehensively in other chapters. Material is organized according to developmental stages (prepubertal, pubertal, and postpubertal). Clinical signs and symptoms and management may differ depending on the age group.

OFFICE EVALUATION OF THE CHILD AND ADOLESCENT
Office Evaluation of the Child

Although gynecologic problems are uncommon among young girls, the physician should always include an inspec-tion of the external genitalia and palpation of the breast as part of the routine physical examination. If the child accepts a brief look at her genitalia as part of the normal physical ex-amination, she is less likely to feel embarrassed or upset by the same examination when she reaches adolescence. Errors in diagnosis often result from the lack of a simple inspec-tion. Furthermore, a healthy dialogue between parents and children on issues of sexuality should begin during the pre-pubertal years. Parents should be encouraged to answer their young children's questions with simple facts and correct ter-minology. Physicians should be knowledgeable about the books available at the local library and select appropriate pamphlets for the office.

Obtaining the History

The nature of the history depends on the presenting symp-tom. If the problem is vaginitis, questions should focus on perineal hygiene, antibiotic therapy, recent infections in the patient or other members of the family, and the possibility of sexual molestation. Behavioral changes and somatic symp-toms such as abdominal pain, headaches, and enuresis may suggest abuse. Information on the caretaker should always be elicited. If the problem is vaginal bleeding, the history should include information on recent growth and develop-ment, signs of puberty, use of hormonal creams or tablets (including maternal exposure), trauma, and foreign bodies previously found in the vagina. Although the history is usu-ally obtained from a parent, the child should be asked ques-tions not only about genital complaints but about toys or school to put her at ease. Eye contact should be maintained with the child, and it should be stressed that she is an im-portant part of the team. Questions focusing on what has bothered the child (such as itching or discharge) can help the child understand why the examination is important. She should be given the opportunity to ask questions. This time promotes the understanding that the physician is acting in her best interests.

Gynecologic Examination

The gynecologic examination should be explained carefully in advance to the parent and the child. It is extremely im-portant to tell the parent that the size of the vaginal opening is variable and that the examination will in no way alter the hymen. Often a diagram showing the introitus is helpful be-cause many parents still believe that the virginal introitus is totally covered by the hymen (Fig. 12-1).

Both parent and child should be told that instruments spe-cially designed for little girls will be used. The otoscope or hand lens to be used for external examination should be shown to the child with an emphasis that the physician will use these instruments "to look." If a colposcope will be used for a sexual abuse evaluation, the child should be given a chance to look at the instrument, turn the light on and off, and view fingers or jewelry through the binocular eyepieces to feel comfortable with the examination.

The child can then be offered the choice of having her parent lift her onto the table or climbing "up the big stairs." The parent or guardian typically stays in the room to talk with the young child and assist in the examination. Most children are comfortable on the examining tables with the mother, father, or guardian sitting close by or holding a hand. Some girls are fearful, especially if they have been sexually abused or have had a painful genital examination before. In this case, the mother (or the caretaker bringing the child) can sit on the table in the semi-reclined position with her feet in stirrups and have the child's legs straddle her thighs. The use of the hand mirror has been found helpful in allowing the child to relax and become an active participant in the examination. If the physician is confident and relaxed, the patient usually cooperates. An abrupt or hurried ap-proach precipitates anxiety and resistance in the child. Sometimes it is necessary to leave the room and return when the patient feels ready.

Examination of a child with gynecologic complaints should include a general pediatric assessment of the child's weight and height, head and neck, heart, lungs, and ab-domen. Abdominal examination is often easier if the child places her hand on the examiner's hand; she is less likely to tense her muscles or feel "tickled." Inguinal areas should be carefully palpated for a hernia or gonad. Breasts should be carefully inspected and palpated. The increasing diameter of the areola or a unilateral tender breast bud is often the first sign of puberty.

Gynecologic examination of the child includes inspec-tion of the external genitalia, visualization of the vagina and cervix, and rectoabdominal palpation (Emans, 1990a). This examination is usually possible without anesthetic if the child has not been traumatized by previous examinations and if the physician proceeds slowly. The child should be told explicitly that "the exam will not hurt." The young child should be examined supine with her knees apart and feet touching in the frog-leg position (Fig. 12-2), in the lithot-omy position with the use of adjustable stirrups or in the knee-chest position (Fig. 12-3). As the external genitalia are inspected, the young child may be less anxious if she assists the physician by holding the labia apart. The physician should note the presence of pubic hair, size of the clitoris, type of hymen, signs of estrogenization of the vaginal in-troitus, and perineal hygiene. Friability of the posterior

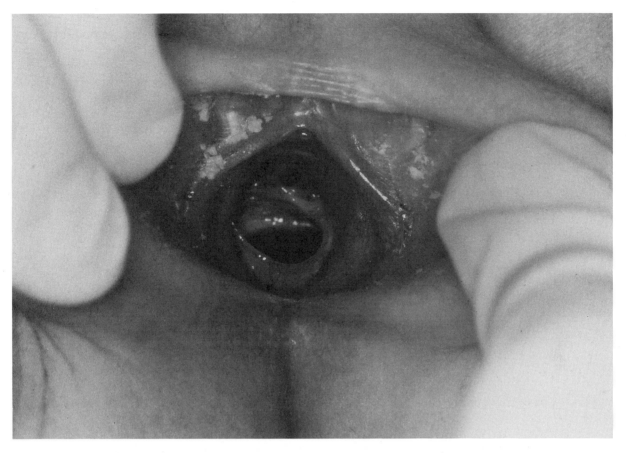

Fig. 12-1. External genitalia of the prepubertal child showing normal anatomy.

fourchette as the labia are separated can occur in children with vulvitis or a history of sexual abuse. If the hymenal orifice is still not visible, the labia can be gently gripped and pulled forward (traction maneuver) to view the anterior vagina (see Fig. 12-1). On average, a normal clitoral glans in the premenarchal child measures 3 mm in length and 3 mm in transverse diameter. Vaginal mucosa of the prepubertal child appears thin and red in contrast to the moist, dull pink, estrogenized mucosa of the pubertal child. Often, the perihymenal tissue is erythematous. The vaginal introitus often gapes open if the child takes a deep breath or coughs; if not, the labia should be pulled gently downward and laterally (Emans, 1990a).

Hymen type should be noted using a hand lens or an otoscope (without a speculum) for its light and magnification. Hymens can be classified as posterior rim (or crescent), annular, or redundant (Fig. 12-4) (Pokorny, 1987). The edges of a redundant hymen and of the orifice are often difficult to visualize. Congenital abnormalities of the hymen, especially microperforate and septate hymens, are not uncommon (Fig. 12-5). It may be difficult to establish that there is an opening in a microperforate hymen without probing with a nasopharyngeal Calgiswab (Spectrum Laboratories, Houston, Tx.) moistened with saline. Congenital absence of the hymen has not been documented. Acquired abnormalities of the hymen usually result from sexual abuse and only occasionally from accidental trauma.

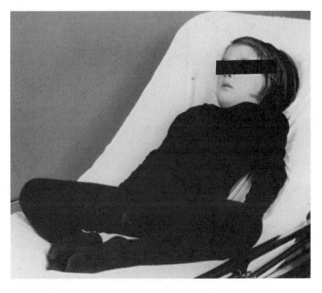

Fig. 12-2. Positioning of the prepubertal child in the frog-leg position. Child can lie flat, or the head of the examining table can be raised. (Courtesy Dr. Trina Anglin, Cleveland, Ohio.)

A physician performing an annual physical examination should visualize the genitalia and the hymen and make a drawing of its type in the office notes. (A change from previously noted anatomy may provide an important clue to ongoing sexual abuse.) The anus and labia should always be examined for cleanliness, excoriations, and erythema. Perianal excoriation often indicates the presence of pinworm infestation.

After the external genitalia have been fully examined, the physician should proceed with visualization of the vagina. In girls older than 2 years, the knee-chest position provides a particularly good view of the vagina and cervix without instrumentation. The patient is asked to "lie on her tummy with her bottom in the air." She should be reassured that the examiner plans to "take a look at her bottom" but "will not put anything inside her." In the knee-chest position (also used for sigmoidoscopy in older patients), the child rests her head to one side on her folded arms and supports her weight on bent knees (6 to 8 inches apart) (see Fig. 12-3). With her buttocks

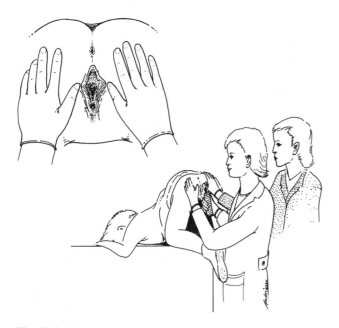

Fig. 12-3. Knee-chest position for visualization of the vagina. (From Emans SJ, Laufer MR, Goldstein DP: *Pediatric and adolescent gynecology,* 4th ed, Philadelphia, 1998, Lippincott-Raven.)

held up in the air, she is encouraged to let her spine and stomach sag downward. A pillow can be placed under her abdomen. An assistant or her mother helps to hold the buttocks apart, pressing laterally and slightly upward. As the child takes deep breaths, the vaginal orifice falls open for examination. In 80% to 90% of prepubertal girls, an ordinary otoscope head (without a speculum) provides the magnification and light necessary to visualize the cervix. Small talk about school, toys, and siblings often diverts the child's attention and helps her maintain this position for several minutes without moving or objecting. Because the vagina of the prepubertal child is short, the presence of a foreign body or a lesion is often easily ascertained (Emans and Goldstein, 1980).

An alternative method of visualization is the use of a small vaginoscope, cystoscope, hysteroscope, or flexible fiberopticscope with water insulation of the vagina. The child is examined supine with her knees held apart. Viscous xylocaine applied to the introitus makes insertion easier. Good visualization of the cervix and the vagina is thus possible without general anesthetic. Because it is unlikely that the general physician will have a vaginoscope or cystoscope in the office, examination with a narrow veterinary otoscope speculum with the child in the supine (lithotomy) position can be helpful. A narrow vaginal speculum may be useful in examining the older child only if insertion does not cause pain or trauma. For examinations with anesthesia, a Killian nasal speculum (Codman and Shurtlif, Randolph, Mass.) with light source can be used (Fig. 12-6).

If vaginal discharge is present, samples should be obtained for culture, Gram stain, saline, and potassium hydroxide preparations. Usually, the child prefers to lie on her back with her knees apart and feet together or in stirrups so that she can watch the procedure without becoming excessively anxious. The child should be allowed to feel a cotton-tipped applicator, Calgiswab, eyedropper, or catheter on her skin before the insertion of a sterile device into her vagina. For the prepubertal child, a nasopharyngeal Calgiswab moistened with nonbacteriostatic saline is appropriate. This can be inserted into the vagina painlessly by avoiding the hy-

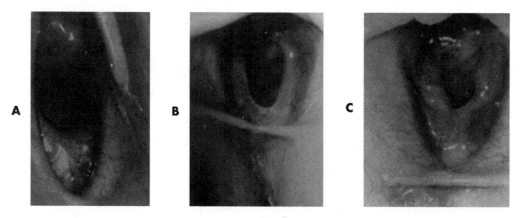

Fig. 12-4. Types of hymens in prepubertal girls. **A,** Posterior rim or crescent hymen. **B,** Circumferential or annular hymen. **C,** Fimbriated or redundant hymen.

menal edges. The child is asked to cough as the examiner inserts the swab. This action distracts the child and makes the hymen gape open. Several samples can be obtained in rapid succession without discomfort. If indicated, a chlamydia culture can be obtained by gently inserting a male urethral swab through the hymen and scraping the lateral vaginal wall. If multiple samples are needed, perhaps for a rape evaluation, a soft plastic eyedropper or a glass eyedropper with 4 to 5 cm of intravenous plastic tubing attached can be gently inserted through the hymen to aspirate secretions. Alternatively, a modified syringe and urethral catheter may be used. The proximal 4-inch end of an intravenous butterfly catheter is inserted into the 4-inch end piece of a #12 bladder catheter, and a syringe is attached. The catheter is slid into the vagina in an action similar to catheterizing the bladder. After that, 0.5 to 1 ml sterile saline is injected into the vagina and aspirated.

A culture for *Neisseria gonorrhoeae* should be grown on modified Thayer-Martin-Jembec media (Scott Laboratories, Fiskeville, R.I.) at the time of the examination. Cultures for other organisms are grown by placing the moistened Calgiswab in the transport Culturette II with medium (Marion Scientific, Kansas City, Mo.). The bacteriology laboratory should plate the swab in the standard genitourinary media, which usually include blood agar, MacConkey, and chocolate media. In addition, the laboratory should be notified that the Thayer-Martin-Jembec media being processed are from the vagina of a prepubertal child. In this way, if a *Neisseria* species grows, it will be properly and unequivocally identified as *N. gonorrhoeae* for medicolegal purposes (Murphy, 1990).

Cultures for *Chlamydia trachomatis* rather than indirect tests and slide immunofluorescent tests are recommended in the prepubertal child because of the possibility of false-positive resuls and the association of this organism with sexual abuse. For patients with itching or with a suspected yeast infection, a Biggy agar (Scott Laboratories, Fiskeville, R.I.) culture can be incubated and read in the office.

After the samples are obtained, a gentle rectoabdominal examination is performed with the patient in stirrups or supine with her legs apart. For bimanual palpation, the examiner places the index or little finger of one hand into the rectum and the other hand on the abdomen. The child can be reassured that this examination will feel similar to having her temperature taken rectally.

Except in the newborn period, when the uterus is enlarged secondary to maternal estrogen, the rectal examination in the prepubertal child reveals only the small "button" of the cervix. Because the ovaries are not palpable, adnexal masses should alert the physician to the possibility of a cyst or a tumor. As the finger is removed from the rectum, the vagina should be gently "milked" to promote the passage of polypoid tumors or discharge.

After assessing the patient's chief symptom and the results of the examination, the physician should spend time with parent and child discussing diagnosis, mode of therapy, and necessity of follow-up. Praising the young child for her cooperation and "bravery" helps establish the important doctor-patient relationship for future examinations.

Office Evaluation of the Adolescent

The evaluation of the adolescent requires additional technical skills, including speculum examination of the vagina and rectal-vaginal-abdominal palpation. More important, the physician needs the interpersonal skills, sensitivity, and time to establish a primary relationship with the adolescent. In

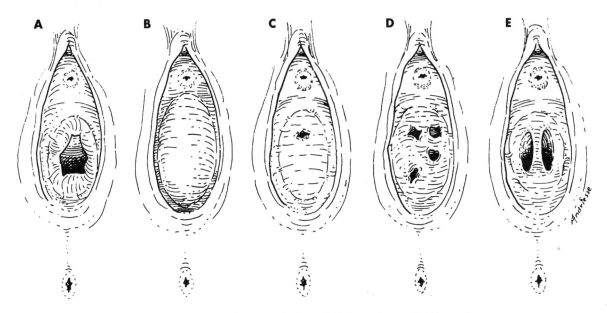

Fig. 12-5. Congenital variations of hymens. **A,** Normal. **B,** Imperforate. **C,** Microperforate. **D,** Cribiform. **E,** Septate.

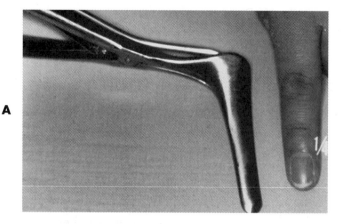

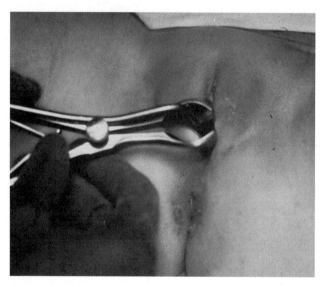

Fig. 12-6. A, Killian nasal speculum with fiberoptic light. **B,** Killian nasal speculum in use during anesthesia examination.

addition, the physician must be willing to see the teenager alone and listen to her concerns. It is helpful to discuss the special needs of adolescents with the pubescent girl when she reaches her eleventh or twelfth birthday. The parents also must understand that adolescents require special time to discuss their concerns about peer relations, school, family, drugs, alcohol, and sexuality.

Visits for the well teenager should be on at least an annual basis; a patient with medical or psychologic concerns should obviously be seen more often. Parents should be included as much as possible in important medical decisions, but the medical privacy of the adolescent should be respected. Parents should be encouraged to call in advance of an appointment if they have special concerns because an adolescent may be strikingly nonverbal about troubling issues at home or in school. At the same time, parents may need help communicating more effectively with their adolescent.

Body changes involved in the development of the prepubertal girl of 10 as she changes into the sexually mature woman of 20 underscore the many issues that arise in the medical care of adolescent girls. The appearance of pubic hair and the development of breasts, over which the girl has no control, can be distressing. The fact that these changes occur at the same rate within her peer group may offer some reassurance; however, early or late development can provoke considerable anxiety. A 12-year-old girl who looks 16 may be confronted with heterosexual demands that she is unable to cope with; a 16-year-old girl who looks 10 may be embarrassed to undress in physical education class or to interact with her peer group. Because the young adolescent has many fantasies about her body and its changes, she may ask the same questions at each visit. The older teenager is intellectually more capable of coping with a diagnosis and the physical examination. The physician must be sensitive to the different needs of each patient.

Obtaining the History

The source of the medical history depends on the medical setting and the age of the patient. Older adolescents tend to seek gynecologic care on their own initiative. In a clinic, the physician may see the mother (and father) first to ascertain the nature of the chief symptom and to ask about medical history, school problems, and psychosocial adjustment. More of the visit should be devoted to the teenager alone because her presenting complaint is often different from her mother's concerns.

In the private practice setting, the mother may make the appointment by telephone, and the teenager may arrive alone for the examination. A complete medical history should be obtained on the first visit and should always involve a carefully taken menstrual history and straightforward questions about sexual relations and birth control.

Physicians should explicitly state their approach toward confidentiality because few teenagers volunteer a need for birth control (Gidwani, 1993). Such discussions, however, must be skillfully handled because repeatedly offering birth control advice may push a young woman into premature sexual relations she may regret. Although the physician may have strong opinions regarding the morality of premarital intercourse, defining the issues under discussion and identifying alternatives may direct the adolescent to an acceptable solution. Concerned medical care sensitive to the patient's needs will assist her in the development of a healthy body image and responsible sexuality.

Gynecologic Examination

Once the history is obtained and the problems are identified, the patient should be given a thorough explanation of a pelvic examination. Diagrams or a plastic pelvic model are helpful. During the first examination, the feelings of the adolescent should be acknowledged. Providing her with adequate drapes and gowns and allowing her to control the tempo of the examination will alleviate her concerns. The patient should be given a gown and asked to remove all her clothes, including brassiere and underpants. If she is covered appropriately and approached in a relaxed manner, resistance is unlikely. The presence of a female nurse in the room is often reassuring, especially if the physician is a man. A young adolescent may request that her mother stay with her during a pelvic examination; however, most patients prefer the mother remain in the waiting room. The patient's wishes should be respected.

General physical examination of a teenage girl should always include a breast examination, inspection of the genitalia, and a careful notation of the Tanner stages of breast and pubic hair development. Demonstrating self-examination of the breast while performing the breast examination often puts the young woman at ease.

Bimanual rectoabdominal examination (in the lithotomy position) should be performed on any teenager with gynecologic complaints or unexplained abdominal pain. Vaginal examination is important to assess irregular bleeding, severe dysmenorrhea, vaginal discharge, sexually transmitted diseases, and amenorrhea. Ideally, sexually active patients should undergo routine vaginal examination every 6 to 12 months, including Papanicolaou smears and cultures for gonorrhea and chlamydia. A patient who is not sexually active can begin routine examinations at any age she feels comfortable initiating gynecologic care, hopefully by 17 or 18 years of age. Contrary to popular belief, rarely is a patient unable to cooperate fully during a pelvic examination if she has received a careful explanation about the procedure and its importance in evaluating her individual problem.

Pelvic examination is performed with the patient in the lithotomy position and with the use of stirrups. A mirror can be offered to the patient. External genitalia are inspected first; type of hymenal opening, estrogenization of the vaginal mucosa, distribution of pubic hair, and size of the clitoris are assessed. Pubic hair should be inspected for pediculosis pubis if the patient complains of itching. Inguinal areas should be palpated for evidence of lymphadenopathy. An estrogenized vagina has a moist or thick dull pink mucosa that is in contrast to the thin red mucosa of the prepubertal child. The normal clitoral glans measures 2 to 4 mm in width; a width of 10 mm is considered significant virilization. In the adolescent girl, the hymen is estrogenized and thickened. Minor changes resulting from sexual abuse or minor trauma that is easily seen in the thin, unestrogenized hymen of the prepubertal child may be impossible to visualize in the estrogenized adolescent. Because it is elastic, most adolescent girls can insert tampons without tearing the hymen. The hymenal opening in the virginal adolescent is usually large enough to allow insertion of a finger for palpation or a small speculum for visualization.

An adolescent who has been sexually active may have a hymen that does not show obvious trauma, or the hymen may have old or new lacerations (down to the base) or multiform caruncles (small bumps of residual hymen along the lower edge). During examination of the sexually abused adolescent, the hymenal ring can be examined carefully by running a saline-moistened, cotton-tipped applicator around the edges. Any hymenal abnormalities should be discussed with the patient. She should decide the need for, and the timing of, any intervention after discussion with her physician.

In the teenager who is not sexually active, a slow, one-finger examination will determine the size of the introitus and the location of the cervix and will allow easy insertion of the speculum. It is helpful to warm the speculum and then touch it to the patient's thigh to allow her to feel its temperature and quality. The speculum should be inserted posteriorly and downward to avoid the urethra. Applying pressure to the inner thigh while inserting the speculum or finger into the vagina is helpful. If the hymenal opening is small, a Hoffman-Graves adolescent vaginal speculum (11.5 × 1 cm) (V. Mueller, McGaw Park, Ill.) can be used to expose the cervix. In the virginal girl, a narrow speculum covered by a latex glove with the tip cut off keeps the vaginal walls from collapsing.

In the sexually active teenager, a Pederson vaginal speculum (7/8 × 4-1/2 inches) or occasionally (in the postpartum adolescent) a Graves (1-3/8 × 3-3/4 inches) speculum is appropriate. A child's speculum (5/8 × 3 inches or 7/8 × 3 inches) is rarely useful because of its inadequate length and excessive width.

A rectal-vaginal-abdominal examination performed with the index finger in the vagina, the middle finger in the rectum, and the other hand on the abdomen permits palpation of a retroverted uterus and assessment of the mobility of the adnexa and uterus. The patient is usually less anxious if she is told in advance that the rectal examination may produce the sensation that she is "moving her bowels" or "going to the bathroom." Allaying this fear usually elicits better relaxation and cooperation.

In a patient with a tight hymen, a single bimanual rectoabdominal examination, with the index finger pushing the cervix upward, allows palpation of the uterus and adnexa. In the relaxed patient, negative examination findings rule out the possibility of large ovarian masses or uterine enlargement.

After the examination is concluded and the patient has dressed, the physician should sit down and discuss in detail the patient's symptom and what was found on examination. It is essential that the adolescent be treated as an adult capable of understanding the explanation. If a parent has accompanied her, the patient should be asked whether she would like to tell her parent the findings herself or whether she would prefer to have the physician discuss the diagnosis with the parent in her presence. It is extremely important for the patient to know that the doctor and her parent will not have a "secret" about her and that confidential information will not be divulged to her parent.

GYNECOLOGIC PROBLEMS IN THE PEDIATRIC POPULATION
Congenital Malformations

Congenital malformations of the female genital tract are usually diagnosed at birth or during adolescence, when reproductive function begins and symptoms develop. Those that are recognized in the infant and young child are external and are usually noted either by a parent or the pediatrician. Anomalies diagnosed at menarche are usually those that result in an obstructive condition.

Normal Female Embryology

By the ninth week of gestation, the embryo has both male (wolffian) and female (müllerian) genital ducts that extend from the mesonephros cranially to the cloaca caudally. A cloaca exists in the human embryo for only a brief period; by the seventh week of gestation, it is divided into rectum and urogenital sinus by the descent of the urorectal septum. Normal female internal genitalia develop from the müllerian ductal system as the wolffian ducts regress.

Müllerian ducts develop from an invagination of the coelomic epithelium. Initially, these paired ducts are lateral. At the future pelvic brim, they turn medially and nearly touch in the midline before turning caudally to end on the posterior wall of the urogenital sinus, where the müllerian tubercle forms. Eventually the ducts fuse, forming the primitive uterovaginal canal (Fig. 12-7). The first and second portions of the müllerian ducts eventually form the fimbria and the fallopian tubes, and the distal segment forms the uterus and part of the vagina.

After the müllerian tubercle is formed, two solid evaginations grow from its distal aspect. These are the sinovaginal bulbs and they are of urogenital sinus origin. Slightly proximal to the sinovaginal bulbs, growth from the müllerian ducts results in the solid vaginal plate. Growth of the plate and the bulbs changes the urogenital sinus from a long, narrow tube to a broad, flat vestibule, bringing the urethra down to the future perineum.

Canalization of the vaginal plate starts caudally and continues in a cranial direction (Fig. 12-8). It is complete by the

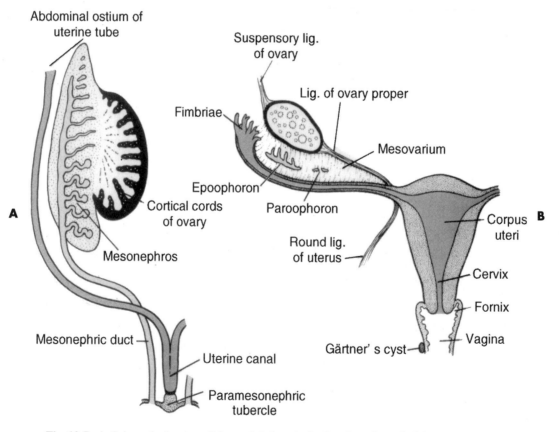

Fig. 12-7. A, Schematic drawing of the genital ducts in the female at the end of the second month of development. Note the paramesonephric or müllerian tubercle and the formation of the uterine canal. **B,** The genital ducts after descent of the ovary. The only parts remaining of the mesonephric system are the epoophoron, paroophoron, and Gärtner's cyst. Note the suspensory ligament of the ovary, the ligament of the ovary proper, and the round ligament of the uterus. (From Sadler TW: *Langman's medical embryology,* 6th ed, Baltimore, 1990, Williams & Wilkins.)

fifth month of intrauterine life. The distal portions of the sinovaginal bulbs coalesce to form the hymen. Shortly before birth, the central area of the hymen disintegrates so that it is normally perforate at birth.

The external genitalia form from structures that correlate with the development of the male (Fig. 12-9). They then differentiate to form normal female external genitalia (Fig. 12-10).

In summary, the uterus is of müllerian origin, as is the proximal four fifths of the vagina. The distal fifth of the vagina and the vaginal epithelium arise from the urogenital sinus.

Ambiguous Genitalia in the Newborn

Although most clinicians rarely see infants with ambiguous genitalia at birth, the need to assess the situation as quickly

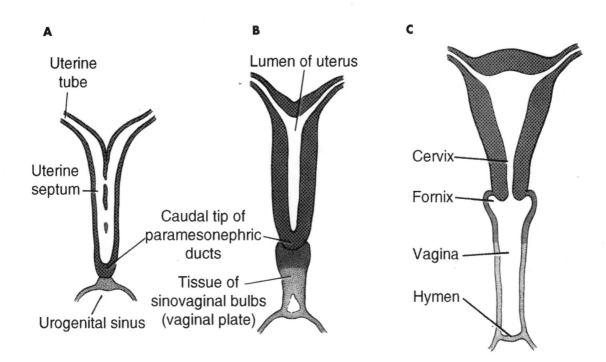

Fig. 12-8. Schematic drawing showing the formation of the uterus and vagina. **A,** At 9 weeks. Note the disappearance of the uterine septum. **B,** At the end of the third month. Note the tissue of the sinovaginal bulbs. **C,** Newborn. The upper portion of the vagina and the fornices are formed by vacuolization of the paramesonephric tissue and the lower portion by vacuolization of the sinovaginal bulbs. (From Sadler TW: *Langman's medical embryology,* 6th ed, Baltimore, 1990, Williams & Wilkins.)

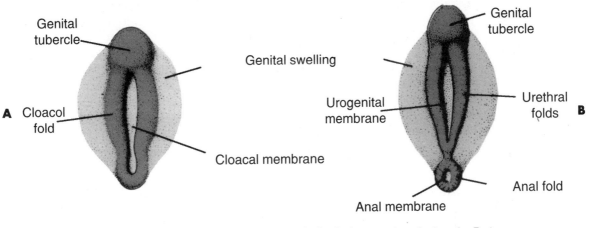

Fig. 12-9. The indifferent stage of the external genitalia. **A,** At approximately 4 weeks. **B,** At approximately 6 weeks. (From Sadler TW: *Langman's medical embryology*, 6th ed, Baltimore, 1990, Williams & Wilkins.)

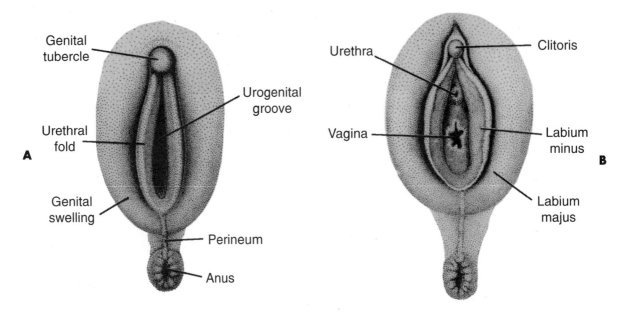

Fig. 12-10. Development of the external genitalia. **A,** In the female at 5 months. **B,** In the newborn. (From Sadler TW: *Langman's medical embryology,* 6th ed, Baltimore, 1990, Williams & Wilkins.)

as possible makes this subject essential for inclusion in this chapter. Any deviation from the normal appearance of male or female genitalia should prompt investigation. Incomplete or ambiguous male or female external genitals may be associated with the gonads and genotype of the opposite sex (e.g., the male with androgen insensitivity and the markedly virilized female with congenital adrenal hyperplasia [CAH]). Even a slight doubt that arises in the initial newborn examination should be pursued systematically to prevent a missed diagnosis. Bilateral cryptorchidism, unilateral cryptorchidism with incomplete scrotal fusion or hypospadias, labial fusion, and clitoromegaly require evaluation.

Determining Sex Assignment. If the physician finds that an infant has ambiguous genitalia, the parents should be reassured that they have a healthy infant but that because the external genital development is incomplete, tests are necessary to determine the sex. A straightforward explanation of the factors necessary for normal sexual development in utero may be helpful. Most parents will react with dismay and anxiety; they should be reassured that tests will show the cause of the problem and whether their baby is a girl or a boy. The possibility of an intersex disorder should not be raised at this time, and speculation about possible sex assignment should be kept to a minimum. Within a few days a definite answer will be possible. The physician should examine the baby in the presence of the parents and explain the common genital anlage for males and females. The concept of an "underdeveloped" boy or "overdeveloped" girl helps parents accept their baby's condition. Although a diagnosis of the patient's condition requires knowledge of the genotype, assignment of sex is based also on other criteria. The first issue is sexual function and fertility. A girl with CAH

may be virilized at birth, yet have normal ovaries and uterus, and is potentially capable of bearing children. Therefore management, including surgery, must aim for female gender identity. When fertility is not possible, as with mixed gonadal dysgenesis or male pseudohermaphroditism, decisions are based on surgical requirements for reconstruction of the external genitals. In general, surgical techniques are more suited to clitoral recession and later the creation of a vagina than to the construction of a normally functioning male phallus.

Once the sex is determined for rearing, the physician should help the parents accept their infant as a normal boy or girl. If attitudes toward the child's sex remain unequivocal, the child usually assumes his or her gender role without difficulty, regardless of the genotype.

The XX Newborn with Ambiguous Genitalia. The differential diagnosis of patients with XX chromosomes and ambiguous genitalia includes the following: (1) CAH; (2) female pseudohermaphroditism that results from maternal ingesting of drugs or from maternal CAH or maternal or fetal virilizing tumor or female pseudohermaphroditism that is idiopathic; and (3) true hermaphroditism.

Congenital Adrenal Hyperplasia. Congenital adrenal hyperplasia is the most common cause of ambiguous genitalia in the XX newborn. Because of the variability in enzymatic block, ambiguity ranges from labial fusion with or without slight clitoromegaly to a "male phallus" with labial fusion and rugae on the labioscrotal folds (Marshall and Lightner, 1980; Wolff et al, 1977).

21-hydroxylase deficiency. Most often, the enzyme involved in congenital adrenal hyperplasia is 21-hydroxylase, and the incidence is reported to be 1 in 5000 to 1 in 15,000

(Pang, 1988; Speiser, 1985). It converts 17-hydroxyprogesterone to 11-deoxycortisol and progesterone to deoxycorticosterone. Because of inadequate cortisol synthesis, ACTH increases, and there is a resultant increase in adrenal androgen production. Salt loss occurs in approximately 50% to 70% of patients with 21-hydroxylase deficiency because of the severity of the deficiency concomitant with decreased aldosterone antagonists.

11β-hydroxylase deficiency. A deficiency of 11β-hydroxylase interrupts the production of cortisol and aldosterone, resulting in an increase in the production of ACTH, 11-deoxycortisol, deoxycorticosterone, and adrenal androgens. This syndrome is usually associated with hypertension and with moderately increased urinary excretion of pregnanetriol and the metabolites for 11-deoxycortisol and deoxycorticosterone (tetrahydro-S and tetrahydro-DOC). An affected 46 XX fetus manifests similar ambiguity of the external genitals.

3β-hydroxysteroid dehydrogenase deficiency. The enzyme 3β-hydroxysteroid dehydrogenase promotes the conversion of pregnenolone to progesterone and 17-hydroxypregnenolone to 17-hydroxyprogesterone. A rare form of CAH, 3β-hydroxysteroid dehydrogenase deficiency, results in severe adrenal insufficiency and increased ACTH levels. This syndrome can result in ambiguous genitalia in both sexes. Virilization of an XX fetus is mild because the block occurs in the initial steps of hormone synthesis. Hence, only the weak androgen dehydroepiandrosterone (DHEA) can be produced in excess, whereas the more potent androgen testosterone is inadequately produced.

Clinical considerations in CAH. The diagnosis of CAH should be made as soon as possible after birth because of the need to prevent dehydration, hyponatremia, and hyperkalemia with glucocorticoid and mineralocorticoid replacement.

It should be emphasized that newborns with XX chromosomes and CAH are female and are potentially fertile. Thus, regardless of the appearance of the external genitalia, the sex assignment should be female. Surgery may be undertaken for recession of the clitoris, division of the labioscrotal folds, and creation of an adequate vagina. The buried clitoris can respond with painful erections to high levels of androgenism, which may result from medication noncompliance during adolescence. Therefore, recession is usually performed with resection of the corpora and preservation of the neurovascular bundle with reanastomosis of the glans (Donahoe and Hendren 1984; Hendren and Donahoe, 1980; Jones and Verkauf, 1970; Mininberg, 1981). Clitoral recession and vaginoplasty in infants whose vaginas enter distal to the external urethral sphincter are usually carried out within the first 6 months of life. For patients with high entry of the urethra into the vagina, vaginoplasty is delayed until 2 years of age. A second vaginoplasty, or the use of dilators, may be needed during adolescence; the age at which this is to take place should be discussed with the patient and depends on her readiness to undertake operative and postoperative care. If surgical construction is necessary, the postoperative use of dilators is usually necessary to keep the vagina patent until the patient has regular sexual relations.

Other Diagnoses of XX Neonates. If an infant has XX chromosomes and has no evidence of CAH, she either has a primary gonadal abnormality or has been exposed to exogenous hormones or to a virilizing lesion in her mother. If the mother has not ingested synthetic hormones, the patient should undergo careful physical examination and measurement of urinary and serum androgens.

If the mother has no virilization and has not ingested hormones, the infant's internal genital anatomy should be evaluated to determine the gonadal cause of the ambiguous genitalia: true hermaphroditism or idiopathic female pseudohermaphroditism.

The XY Newborn with Ambiguous Genitalia. The differential diagnosis of the infant with XY chromosomes includes: (1) male pseudohermaphroditism because of defects of testicular differentiation, deficient placental luteinizing hormone (LH) level, Leydig cell agenesis, defects in testosterone synthesis, 5-reductase deficiency, or receptor defects; and (2) hypogonadotropic hypogonadism (Kallmann syndrome).

Increased understanding of the differentiation of the fetal testis and the many steps involved in the development of the normal male has made it possible to diagnose more specifically the kind of syndrome seen in XY girls. The short arm of the Y chromosome is the region responsible for testicular determinants. The area of the Y chromosome that appears to be the most likely site of sex determination is the "sex-determining region Y." This region has been demonstrated in XX males and is absent in XY females (Berta et al, 1990; Jager et al, 1990; Sinclair et al, 1990).

In cases of pure gonadal dysgenesis or Swyer syndrome (streak gonads, normal stature), the XY female may be diagnosed during adolescence. If during development the human chorionic gonadotropin (hCG) level is deficient (because of a postulated placental insufficiency or an inadequate LH level), stimulation of testosterone secretion will be insufficient for complete masculinization. If the testis is unresponsive to hCG or lacks normal Leydig cells (Leydig cell agenesis), the infant will have abdominal testes, an elevated LH level, a female phenotype with a short vagina, and an absent uterus. Depending on when the testicular regression occurred during fetal life, patient phenotypes range from normal females to males with cryptorchidism.

Numerous defects in testosterone synthesis have been described. They include deficiencies of 20,22-desmolase; 3β-hydroxy-Δ5-steroid dehydrogenase; 17α-hydroxylase; 17,20-desmolase, and 17β-hydroxysteroid. The first three defects are also associated with adrenal insufficiency. Patients who have these deficiencies do not have müllerian structures, but the external genitalia are either female or ambiguous.

Failure to produce müllerian-inhibiting factor or the lack of müllerian-inhibiting factor receptors causes the persistence of müllerian structures and the presence of a uterus (hernia uteri inguinale) in a male who has unilateral or bilateral cryptorchidism. The development of the wolffian ducts varies; males are fertile.

The enzyme 5α-reductase is responsible for the conversion of testosterone to dihydrotestosterone, which results in the male differentiation of the external genitalia. Patients with 5α-reductase deficiency (so-called pseudovaginal perineoscrotal hypospadias), an autosomal recessive condition, have a cleft scrotum (hypospadias) and perineal invagination.

Ambiguous genitalia may also be caused by defects in receptor proteins or transcription mechanisms. Complete resistance to the action of testosterone results in the classic picture of androgen insensitivity (sometimes referred to as testicular feminization). The infant appears to be a phenotypic female, though occasionally testes are noted early in life. Partial androgen insensitivity results in a spectrum of ambiguous genitalia syndromes at birth and during adolescence; these include the Gilbert-Dreyfus, Reifenstein, Rosewater, and Lubs syndromes. These patients have partial wolffian development, some pubic hair, and partial labioscrotal fusion. Recent research in androgen insensitivity has delineated a number of different syndromes, some with an absence of receptors, some with an abnormal receptor structure, and some with presumed postreceptor defects. Errors in testosterone biosynthesis may produce a similar phenotype. The pattern of X-linked inheritance coupled with a high LH and testosterone level (especially before and after hCG stimulation) suggests androgen insensitivity.

Cytogenetic studies help distinguish between patients who have structural defects or dysgenetic testes and those who have structurally normal testes. Many patients in the former group have abnormal sex chromosomes with mosaicism; the patients in the latter group have XY karyotypes. Biochemical studies can pinpoint a diagnosis. Retrograde contrast x-ray studies, ultrasonography, magnetic resonance imaging (MRI), and possibly laparoscopy or laparotomy are necessary to establish the final diagnosis and to determine the chromatin-negative syndrome present.

Choice of gender identity depends on the external genitalia and the possibility of future coital adequacy. After the sex assignment is definitively made, the gonads that conflict with the assignment should be electively removed. For example, the patient with mixed gonadal dysgenesis and 45X/46XY who is given a female sex assignment should have her testis removed to prevent virilization at puberty. Intraabdominal testes should be removed prophylactically from patients with male pseudohermaphroditism and mixed gonadal dysgenesis because there is a substantial risk for malignancy, specifically dysgerminoma or gonadoblastoma, in approximately 20% to 30% of patients (Simpson, 1976). In addition, it should be noted that all patients with genital abnormalities should be carefully searched for associated anomalies, especially of the urinary tract.

Introital Abnormalities
Masses

The most common abnormality seen in the neonate and young child is a cystic mass at the introitus. It is first observed either in the delivery room by the obstetrician, during the neonatal examination by the pediatrician, or by the parent when changing diapers. Usually, the mass is cystic, enlarges during crying spells, and contains a clear or milky mucoid material. Differential diagnosis includes ectopic ureter, hymenal cyst, hymenal skin tag, periurethral cyst, vaginal cyst, or imperforate hymen with mucocolpos or hydrocolpos.

The child should be examined in the frog-leg position, ideally with magnification, using a moistened cotton-tipped applicator for retraction. The pull-down traction maneuver as shown in Fig. 12-1 opens the introitus so that the origin of the cyst can be ascertained.

Ectopic Ureter. If the cyst appears to rise from the periurethral area or the anterior vagina, an ectopic ureter should be suspected and pelvic and renal ultrasonography performed. If this confirms the diagnosis, consultation with a pediatric urologist is required. Intravenous pyelography (IVP) often determines the extent of the anomalous collecting system. High ligation of the ectopic ureter or partial nephrectomy is usually required.

Hymenal, Periurethral, and Vaginal Cysts. Most cysts that arise from the hymen or periurethral area are of the epidermal inclusion type. Spontaneous resolution is common. If regression does not occur within 3 months, simple marsupialization or fulguration is warranted. Before proceeding with surgery, however, urethroscopy should be performed to rule out the presence of a diverticulum of the distal urethra, which would require urologic treatment.

In the newborn, vaginal cysts can be located posterior to the urethral meatus at the vaginal introitus or arise from the anterior or lateral wall of the vagina, and they are lined by squamous epithelium. Abnormal manifestations are rare. Sometimes they rupture spontaneously, or they may disappear after surgical aspiration and removal of a milky white fluid. Occasionally, the cysts grow large enough to obstruct the urethra and cause urinary retention. Surgical removal is indicated in such patients. Cysts in the caudal portion of the vagina probably are derived from the epithelium of the urogenital sinus and are formed during the last months of gestation. In younger fetuses, multiple cysts can develop in proximal parts of the vagina. They are considered derivatives of epithelia of the müllerian or wolffian ducts.

Imperforate Hymen. When the cystic structure appears to obstruct the vaginal opening and no perforation can be identified, an imperforate hymen with mucocolpos/hydrocolpos is the most likely diagnosis. A mucocolpos/hydrocolpos is caused by distention of the vagina with retained secretions that are stimulated by maternal estrogens. Because of the ability of the vagina to distend, the uterus is rarely involved. Usual symptoms of a massive hydrocolpos in the neonate are midline lower abdominal mass, urinary retention resulting from bladder angulation, and occasionally respiratory distress. Bilateral hydroureter and hydronephrosis may be detected by antenatal ultrasonography. Ureters may be compressed at the pelvic brim. Respiratory distress may result from pressure on the diaphragm. Compression of the major abdominal veins may cause edema of the lower extremities. Retrograde flow of secretion through the fallopian tubes may cause intraperitoneal adhesions and subsequent partial bowel obstruction.

The treatment of mucocolpos/hydrocolpos depends on its cause. If significant mucocolpos/hydrocolpos is diagnosed, surgery is necessary to avert late complications of additional fluid accumulation and reflux. Simple hymenectomy with a scalpel or a needle-tip electrocautery is effective. Sutures may be required to maintain patency and to prevent recurrence of the obstruction because of scarring and reclosure of the hymenal orifice.

Other Hymenal Abnormalities. Hymenal tags can be congenital and appear as a fleshy mass protruding from the introitus. They often regress when the effects of maternal estrogen have diminished. These lesions may become inflamed and cause vaginal bleeding and discharge. If they are still present at 3 months, they can be removed through electrocautery or cold-knife excision.

Inadequate perforation of the hymen, such as septation, microperforation, or cribriform fenestration, is generally asymptomatic in the young child and does not require intervention until puberty, when it causes problems with tampon use or coitus. Surgical correction of the hymenal abnormality also is necessary if it appears to be the cause of recurrent vulvovaginitis and urinary tract infection brought on by the stagnation of urine within the partially obstructed vagina. Because most patients with this problem are between 3 and 6 years of age at diagnosis, either hymenectomy or hymenotomy and suture of the cut edges with absorbable sutures are satisfactory methods of treatment.

Perineal Fissure

A newborn may have a deep fissure of the median raphe. This area does not heal spontaneously. It remains open and granular, and there is purulent drainage because of fecal soiling. Perineorectal fistula must be ruled out, but the cause remains uncertain. Initial treatment is conservative and calls for topical antibiotic ointment, such as silver sulfadiazine, protective bland ointments, and silver nitrate applications. If healing does not occur in 2 to 3 months, laser vaporization or excision with primary closure is indicated.

Labia Minora Hypertrophy or Asymmetry

Sometimes one or both labia minora are unusually large, and the patient is brought for consultation because she notices the anomaly or because of irritation with exercise. Simple reassurance is usually all that is necessary. Comparison with asymmetry or hypertrophy of other parts of the body may help the patient to accept this peculiarity. Hygienic counseling and avoidance of tight clothes are sufficient to relieve discomfort for most patients. If these measures are ineffec-

tive, or if the patient also has a troublesome cosmetic problem, surgical reduction is in order. This can be accomplished in the ambulatory operating room by simple resection of the redundant labia so that they are symmetrical. Closure of the excised area is best accomplished with a running locking stitch of 3-0 chromic suture (Fig. 12-11). An alternative surgical approach involves identification of labial blood vessels, followed by a wedge resection and reanastomosis as shown in Fig. 12-12 (Laufer and Galvin, 1995).

Clitoromegaly

Clitoral reduction is accomplished surgically to gain a functional and cosmetically acceptable clitoris. The procedure for clitoral reduction is described in the section on the management of CAH.

Inguinal Ovary Syndrome

Inguinal hernias in infant girls are uncommon. The male-to-female ratio is approximately 6:1. A 1.5-cm firm mass palpated in the groin or the vulva usually indicates that it is a sliding-type hernia, in which a portion of the wall of the sac is composed of a tube and an ovary. It usually cannot be reduced, but the blood supply rarely is compromised.

Rarely, a girl with a palpable gonad in the labia is actually a male with testicular feminization syndrome. This represents less than 1% of hernias in girls. These patients can be identified by a 46 XY karyotype and by the discovery of testicles during surgery. Early identification is desirable, though no gender changes should be made because the genitalia are female. The identified testicles are removed.

Cloacal Anomalies

A cloaca is a common channel into which the products of the gastrointestinal, urinary, and genital tracts empty; cloacal anomalies are rare. The pathogenesis of faulty cloacal division is unknown, but it could result from arrest in the

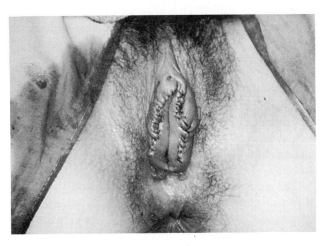

Fig. 12-11. Technique of labial reduction in a patient with symptomatic hypertrophy of labia minora.

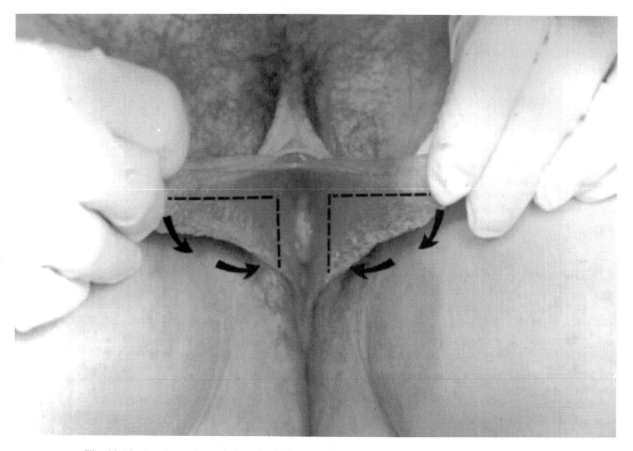

Fig. 12-12. An alternative technique for labial reduction in a patient with symptomatic hypertrophy of labia minora. (From Laufer MR, Galvin WJ: Labial hypertrophy: A new surgical approach. *Adolesc Pediatr Gynecol* 1995; 8:39-41.)

descent of the urorectal septum, preventing division of the cloaca into the rectum and urogenital sinus. It also stops approximation and fusion of the müllerian ducts, resulting in failure in the formation of the müllerian tubercle and duplication of the uterus and proximal vagina. Sinovaginal bulbs do not form, and the vaginal plate does not enlarge. The urogenital sinus remains in its primitive state as a long, narrow tube, and the urethra empties into the urogenital sinus, high on its anterior wall. There is no hymen.

Cloacal anomaly involves three major organ systems and complete or partial obstruction of the urinary, genital, or gastrointestinal tracts. In the absence of other lethal anomalies, urinary tract sepsis resulting from obstruction accounts for the majority of deaths. Other major system anomalies are common, particularly in the cardiovascular, genitourinary, gastrointestinal, central nervous, and respiratory systems. The most common anomalies are those of müllerian origin—septate vagina, duplication of the uterus, and bicornuate uterus.

The pathognomonic physical finding in cloacal dysgenesis is a single perineal orifice between the labia minora. This opening is the entrance to the cloaca. The urethral meatus and anus are not evident, and hydrometrocolpos is often present as an abdominal mass. Reconstruction is complex and best performed by a pediatric surgeon.

INFECTION
Vulvovaginitis
The Normal Vaginal Environment

The vagina undergoes constant change from birth, through childhood, menarche, reproductive years, menopause, and older ages. Consequently, the types and frequencies of inflammatory conditions of the vagina and vulva are different at various ages. At birth the mucous membranes of the vagina and vulva have an adult histologic appearance because of stimulation by circulating maternal estrogens. The cervical, paraurethral, and Bartholin's glands are large and secrete mucus during the immediate neonatal period. The pH is 5 to 7. Within a few weeks, however, the vaginal lining becomes thin and unestrogenized.

Throughout childhood until the immediate premenarchal period, the child is especially vulnerable to vulvovaginitis because of poor estrogenization of the vaginal epithelium. In addition, unsupervised and inadequate perineal hygiene contributes to the incidence of vulvovaginitis. Girls of this age lack the protection provided by pubic hair and the fat pads of the labia majora. Without these anatomic barriers, contaminants and irritants have free access to the sensitive vulvar and vaginal epithelia.

At puberty, estrogen stimulation changes the vaginal epithelium to a thick, stratified squamous epithelium. Subsequent normal flora establishment of Döderlein's bacillus causes the pH level to rise to the 6 to 8 range, which helps to maintain homeostasis and to decrease infection.

Vulvovaginitis. Vulvovaginitis is the most common reason for pediatric gynecologic examinations (Grunberger and Fisch, 1982). Symptoms differ but often consist of vaginal discharge that varies in quantity, color, and odor. Vulvar pruritus or burning and dysuria are also common. Whatever the underlying cause, the examination usually reveals edema, redness, discharge, excoriations, and secondary scratch lesions. The presence of fecal remnants and interlabial debris helps to confirm poor hygiene.

Physiologic Leukorrhea

Physiologic leukorrhea occurs at both extremes of childhood. During the neonatal period, maternal estrogens stimulate the newborn's endocervical glands and vaginal epithelium. Characteristically the discharge is grayish, gelatinous, and sticky. In the neonate, a small amount of blood may be present because of maternal hormonal withdrawal. This always provides the mother with some anxious moments, but normal examination results and lack of recurrence are reassuring.

During the 6 to 12 months preceding menarche, rising endogenous estrogen secretion is responsible for the appearance of a whitish discharge not associated with irritative symptoms. After appropriate evaluation, it is important to explain to these young women that this is part of the normal process of maturation. Breast development and growth acceleration usually begin at this time. The unjustified prescription of a vaginal cream or antibiotics serves only to make the patient think any vaginal discharge is abnormal, and it results in multiple unnecessary consultations.

Nonspecific Vulvovaginitis

Nonspecific or mixed vulvovaginitis accounts for approximately 70% of vulvovaginal infection in this age group. The cause can be traced to poor local hygiene and fecal contamination. Cultures predominantly grow *Escherichia coli* and other gastrointestinal organisms, such as enterococcus.

General hygienic measures are the first treatment step. Sitz baths in plain warm water should be taken two or three times daily, and the vulvar area should be dried with a hair dryer at the lowest speed and heat. A small amount of unscented cornstarch-based powder helps to keep the vulva dry. Only mild, nonperfumed soap should be used, and bubble bath should be avoided. Adequate counseling about clothing should also be provided (for instance, only white 100% cotton underpants should be worn; tight-fitting clothes, nonabsorbent fabrics, and wet bathing suits should be avoided). The importance of front-to-back wiping with soft, white unscented toilet tissue should also be stressed.

Specific Vulvovaginitis

Vulvovaginitis has various causes. Differential diagnoses, symptoms, and treatments of the various types are summarized in Table 12-1.

The character of the discharge and other clinical features vary according to the organism responsible; correct diagnosis depends on identification of the offending organism. The most common cause of vulvovaginitis is allergic, but bacterial or viral infections, parasitic infestation, and traumatic vulvovaginitis also occur.

Gonorrhea

Gonococcal infection in the prepubertal child is usually manifested as purulent vulvovaginitis rather than cervicitis. The infection may be asymptomatic or it may be evident as a thin, mucoid discharge. Gram stain and culture are important in the evaluation of vaginal discharge during prepuberty. Although the Gram stain is helpful, *Neisseria meningitidis* rarely causes vaginitis; therefore, it is essential that the diagnosis be proved by cultures.

After a diagnosis is made, the child should be interviewed by an experienced social worker, psychologist, or pediatrician to assess the possibility of sexual abuse. Play therapy and repeated interviews may be necessary to establish the history because the abuser is usually known to the child and is often a family member. Cultures may have to be taken from all family members and caretakers of the child. The source of infection is often a male relative, stepparent, or caretaker. In addition, the mother and sisters often are infected. Although it is theoretically possible that *N. gonorrhoeae* can be transmitted by sexual play between siblings and peers, the clinician must strongly suspect sexual abuse in all cases of prepubertal gonorrhea because almost 100% of the incidences result from sexual abuse. Often sexual abuse involves vulvar coitus or oral sex rather than penetration, so physical examination shows a normal hymen in many abused girls. Cultures should be obtained from oral, vaginal, and rectal orifices. Although contacts may be easier to culture and follow-up may be significantly improved if the child is hospitalized, this is usually treated on an outpatient basis. Suspected child sexual abuse must be reported to the mandated state agency.

Before treating a child with vaginal gonorrhea, rectal and pharyngeal cultures for *N. gonorrhoeae*, vaginal culture for *Chlamydia trachomatis,* and serology test results for syphilis should be obtained. For children who weigh more than 45 kg, adult schedules for treating cervicitis and urethritis are used. For children who weigh less than 45 kg, the recommended regimen is 125 mg ceftriaxone intramuscularly or spectinomycin 40 mg/kg (maximum 2 g) intramuscularly. Coinfection with *C. trachomatis* should be treated with 50 mg erythromycin/kg/day in four divided doses. In children older than 9 years, adult dosages of doxycycline or tetracycline can be used.

Follow-up cultures of the throat, rectum, and vagina should be taken 7 to 14 days after treatment. Reinfection is likely if the source is not identified and treated. Persistent vaginal discharge in a patient who has been adequately treated and has had negative cultures for gonorrhea may indicate coinfection with *C. trachomatis* that was not

Table 12-1   Differential Diagnosis of Specific Vulvovaginitis in Infancy and Childhood

Etiology	Clinical Signs	Discharge	Findings	Treatment
Dermatitis/allergy	Red, papular, pruritic vulvar rash	No discharge	Caused by bubble bath or laundry detergent	Discontinue bubble bath; symptomatic care with steroid or antihistaminic creams
Foreign body	Bloody discharge	Purulent, blood tinged, foul smelling	Foreign body identified on pelvic examination	Removal of foreign body
Bacterial				
Gonococcal	Neonate and premenarchal: Bartholin's, Skene's, and cervical glands involved	May have only scant vaginal discharge	Conjunctivitis (neonate), upper genital tract involvement, systemic symptoms, gram-negative intracellular diplococci in either type	Ceftriaxone, bacterial sensitivities for resistant gonococcus
	Postmenarchal: severe vulvar edema, purulent discharge	Profuse, yellow-green discharge, intense vulvovaginitis	Upper genital tract not involved	
Staphylococcus aureus	Labial abscesses	Thick, yellow	Abscesses present in other areas	Oxacillin, cephalosporins
Streptococcus pyogenes, β-hemolytic, group A	Systemic symptoms, vulvar pruritus and redness	Purulent, thin, yellow		Penicillin
Hemophilus influenzae, type B	May be associated with *H. influenzae* infections in more typical areas	Dark, yellow, purulent foul smelling	Rare in infancy and childhood	Ampicillin
Shigella	Reddened vulva, may be preceded by diarrhea	Severe, purulent vulvovaginitis	*Shigella* from stool and vaginal cultures	Ampicillin
Escherichia coli (enteropathic)	Preceded by diarrhea	Thin, watery, foul smelling	Culture *E. coli* from throat, stool, vagina	Local hygiene, amoxicillin
Fungal *Candida albicans*	Beefy red vulvovaginitis	Profuse, foul smelling, curdy	Budding yeast on wet preparation or Gram stain; search for systemic disease (diabetes) in preadolescent; rare in childhood	Topical nystatin
Viral Herpes simplex, type 2	Vulvovaginitis and herpetic stomatitis, perineal edema, painful vulvar eruption	Thin, watery	Tender, superficial labial ulcers; enlarged, tender inguinal lymph nodes; diagnosis by rising serum antibody titer or multinucleated giant cells on vaginal cytology; may be primary or recurrent	Symptomatic with local care
Parasitic Pinworm	Severe pruritus	Thin, colorless	Usually associated with enteric infestation; diagnosis by seeing worms or ova on fresh smear	Mebendazole
Trichomonas vaginalis	Moderate pruritus	Thin, malodorous	Rare before puberty	Metronidazole

adequately treated with single-dose therapy. The family may have been noncompliant with the 7-day course of tetracycline or erythromycin.

Only a few incidences of salpingitis secondary to *N. gonorrhoeae* have been reported in prepubertal girls; thus, no data exist on the best form of treatment. Antibiotics of a spectrum similar to that used in adolescents and adults with pelvic inflammatory disease (PID) are appropriate. (See Chapter 18.)

Candida Albicans

Monilial vulvovaginitis is uncommon in children and is usually associated with recent antibiotic therapy, diabetes mellitus, or human immunodeficiency virus. The clinical picture is characteristic; at the onset, it consists of an erythematous vulva with oozing granulomatous lesions that later become crusted. Satellite lesions are common, and the cottage-cheese appearance of the vaginal discharge is well known. Diagnosis is made by microscopic visualization of mycelia on a potassium hydroxide preparation of vulvar exudate or vaginal discharge, or by positive culture on appropriate medium (Biggy agar). Treatment consists of sitz baths three times daily followed by vulvar application of an antifungal preparation.

Trichomonas

Although the nonestrogenized vaginal epithelium of the prepubertal child is unfavorable to the growth of *Trichomonas,* this parasite is responsible occasionally for vulvovaginitis. This infection is acquired by direct contact, and the possibility of sexual abuse should be considered though nonsexual transmission is possible.

Vaginal discharge, characteristically greenish and malodorous, is associated with nonspecific signs of irritation. Treatment consists of the oral administration of 10 to 30 mg/kg/day metronidazole (maximum, 125 mg three times daily) for 7 days or 1 g in a single dose.

Pinworms

Enterobius vermicularis (pinworms), a common intestinal parasite in children, may infect the vagina and give rise to acute inflammatory symptoms and yellow mucopurulent discharge. Diagnosis is suggested by perianal scratching lesions and is confirmed by a positive result on the "Scotch-tape test," preferably performed in the morning. Because the treatment for pinworms is a single oral dose and side effects are minimal, some clinicians opt to treat without confirmation of a diagnosis by this test.

The parasite is usually eradicated by a single dose of 100 mg mebendazole. All family members should be treated. Pinworm vulvovaginitis is commonly associated with infection by other anal contaminants, which is treated as discussed earlier.

Condylomata Acuminata

Warty lesions associated with human papillomavirus (HPV) infection are found in infants and young children at increasing rates. This is of great concern. When HPV is present, the possibility of sexual molestation must be examined (Craighill, 1993). The incubation period for HPV is thought to be 4 to 12 weeks, but incubation periods as long as 20 months have been reported. In infants younger than 20 months, one must be suspicious of sexual abuse, but vertical transmission may be the cause.

DNA probes that identify viral types may be useful in documenting the HPV virus in cases that may involve legal matters. Types 1, 2, 4, 7, 26, 27, 28, and 29 are associated with the common hand wart. Types of genital DNA are 6, 11, 16, 18, 30 to 35, 39, 42 to 44, 48, and 51 to 55. Types 6 and 11, the most common, have a high rate of regression and a low rate of persistence. Types 16, 18, 31, 33, and 35 are associated with invasive cervical malignancies. Regression of these subtypes is rare; persistence and progression appear to be the rule.

It is important to obtain a definitive diagnosis and to provide treatment for the child in the least traumatic manner. For these reasons, children may be examined under anesthesia so that a biopsy can be obtained for pathologic documentation and DNA typing. At the same time, the condylomata are treated by excision or laser vaporization. Visualization of the urinary tract and anal canal is mandatory if recurrence is a problem. A serologic test for syphilis should be performed to exclude condyloma latum (secondary syphilis).

Long-term follow-up of children with HPV is important, but the long-term implications of this infection at such early ages are unknown. It is well documented that HPV infection is associated with an increased risk for neoplastic changes (Shiffman, 1992). Infections with more virulent DNA types pose greater clinical challenges because there are no accepted guidelines for monitoring these patients.

Molluscum Contagiosum

Molluscum contagiosum is usually evident as a small, fleshy papule with a central umbilication. The infectious agent is a poxvirus transmitted by autoinoculation or close contact with an infected person. Lesions are usually small (2 to 5 mm) and typically appear on the face, trunk, and extremities. The incubation period is 2 to 7 weeks. Definitive diagnosis is made by identification of viral inclusion bodies isolated from the central core of the lesion. The lesion is usually self-limited, but it can be treated with destructive procedures such as curettage of the central core, laser therapy, or cryotherapy.

Systemic Causes

Vulvovaginitis in children often follows an episode of infection in another part of the body, especially the upper respiratory tract. β-Hemolytic *Streptococcus pyogenes, Streptococcus pneumoniae, Staphylococcus aureus,* and *N. meningitidis* should be treated according to the sensitivity of each organism.

Systemic diseases such as measles, chicken pox, scarlet fever, and HIV may have vulvovaginal manifestations.

Symptoms usually follow the natural history of the primary disease. Because of scratching and fecal contamination, secondary bacterial infection may occur.

Dermatologic diseases such as *Herpes simplex* and *Herpes zoster,* eczema, psoriasis, molluscum contagiosum, and poison ivy may also involve the vulvar skin.

Anatomic Causes

In some instances, a microperforate hymen, especially when the opening lies high near the urethral meatus, may be responsible for the pooling of urine in the vagina. Constant maceration of the vulvovaginal tissue causes irritation and may cause secondary infection. Hymenotomy cures this.

Discharge from ectopic ureters can masquerade as chronic vulvovaginitis. Often these children are erroneously thought to be incontinent or to have enuresis. Workup should consist of pelvic ultrasonography, IVP, and cystoscopy. This can be treated by surgery and usually requires either high ligation or excision of the anomalous collecting system or nephrectomy.

Foreign Bodies

A greenish, bloody, foul-smelling discharge suggests the presence of an intravaginal foreign body. The most common finding is a small piece of toilet paper or stool. Cultures grow mixed flora. Any bloody or malodorous discharge should prompt a thorough vaginal examination, even if anesthesia or analgesia is required. Occasionally, a patient may have abdominal pain because of the retrograde flow of infected vaginal secretions into the fallopian tubes, which causes peritonitis.

A foreign body in the vagina may be a perplexing problem for the clinician because most are not visible on external examination. Reluctance to perform a pelvic examination in a child makes the diagnosis even more difficult. However, failure to diagnose and remove a foreign body can

result in severe PID, peritonitis, and migration of the foreign body to another area.

Vaginal foreign bodies are usually seen in children between 3 and 7 years of age. Usually there is no history of insertion, yet virtually any kind of object may be found within the vagina. A forgotten tampon may be the foreign body in a menarcheal girl.

Foreign bodies can sometimes be washed out by vaginal irrigation with room temperature saline through IV tubing. Initially, a rectal examination should be performed because it may reveal the presence of an intravaginal foreign body. If an object is felt, gentle attempts at milking it out may be successful. In girls younger than 6, general anesthesia may be necessary. Vaginoscopy may be performed in the young child with a Killian nasal speculum. Should vaginoscopy fail to reveal the foreign body, gentle probing of the vagina often reveals its presence. Once the object has been removed, the vaginal discharge ceases.

Although most foreign bodies are easily removed, the object occasionally erodes into the vaginal wall. An incision through the mucosa is necessary to remove it. If a vaginal foreign body remains for a long time, vaginal stricture may occur.

Labial Adhesions

Labial adhesions (synechiae vulvae), a complete or partial fusion of lower labia majora or labia minora in the midline, occur most commonly in girls 6 months to 6 years of age. The cause is unknown, but it may be related to low levels of circulating estrogen and to irritation that erodes the vulvar epithelium, making the labia stick together. This concept is supported by the observation that synechiae vulvae is not seen in neonates but is acquired within the first 2 years of life, when the level of circulating estrogen is extremely low and the use of estrogen creams causes synechiae to disappear.

Occasionally, the vaginal orifice is completely covered, resulting in poor drainage of vaginal secretions and sequestering of urine in the vagina. Parents often become alarmed because the vagina appears "absent."

Diagnosis is made by simple observation. The labia minora are fused, and the hymen is not visible. The line of fusion is a thin, transparent membrane that may involve the inner surfaces of the labia. Fusion often ends several millimeters behind the clitoris, anterior to the external urethral meatus. There may be several perforations in the membrane, or the adhesions may be partial either anteriorly or posteriorly (Fig. 12-13). Most cases are mild, and no treatment is necessary because the labia usually separate completely at puberty. If symptoms develop, they should be treated.

If a patient has complete synechia and vaginal or urinary drainage is impaired or the child complains of pain, an estrogen-containing cream should be applied twice daily for 3 weeks and then once daily for 3 weeks. After 2 weeks of therapy, the patient should be seen in follow-up. If the labial adhesion has resolved, treatment with premarin cream is

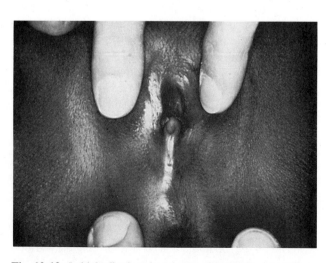

Fig. 12-13. Labial adhesions in a 4-year-old with almost totally fused labia. Note the small opening at the level of the urethra.

continued once daily for 1 week. After the discontinuation of the estrogen cream, the use of a bland ointment (Desitin or White's A & D) is helpful to keep labial adhesions from forming again. A repeat course of therapy may be necessary. Forceful separation without anesthesia is generally contraindicated because this is traumatic for the child, and it may cause the adhesions to form again. If estrogen therapy fails, separation is best performed under general anesthesia; this is followed by the application of a bland ointment and gentle separation by the parent at regular intervals. Separation may be accomplished in the examining room with the application of 5% lidocaine gel and manipulation with a cotton swab.

Regardless of the method of treatment, 10% to 15% of synechiae recur. Though spontaneous separation at puberty is the rule, sometimes patients in their mid-teens are referred because of hypoplastic labia. Once separation is accomplished under anesthesia, the vulva is found to be normal.

Vaginal Bleeding

Most girls have their first menstrual period between 9 and 16 years of age. Except for hormone withdrawal bleeding during the first or second week of life, genital bleeding before the age of 9 years is not normal and most likely results from organic causes. Therefore, vaginal bleeding in the prepubertal years should be taken seriously and should always be carefully assessed.

Classically, vaginal bleeding in childhood is classified as bleeding associated with signs of isosexual precocity and bleeding not associated with signs of isosexual precocity. However, we find it more useful to classify the problem on the basis of causal factors: infection, trauma, endocrine abnormalities, anatomic abnormalities, blood dyscrasia, neoplasm, or idiopathy (Box 12-1).

Vulvovaginitis

Vulvovaginitis with or without a foreign body is usually the cause of vaginal bleeding in patients younger than 9 years of age. When a young child has vaginal bleeding, a thorough investigation is mandatory to rule out the presence of malignancy. It is customary to perform the examination under anesthesia as part of the initial workup unless there is complete confidence that full visualization of the cervix and vagina is possible during the outpatient examination.

Coagulation Disorder

Hematologic evaluation to rule out coagulation disorders should be performed before surgery. However, patients with vaginal bleeding from blood dyscrasias usually have other signs of bleeding, such as epistaxis, petechiae, or hematomas.

Prolapse of the Urethra

Occasionally, vaginal bleeding is a sign of urethral prolapse. Examination reveals the characteristic friable, red-blue (doughnut-like) annular mass (Fig. 12-14). The patient may report dysuria, bleeding, and pain that develops after coughing, straining, or trauma. Diagnosis is based on the characteristic shape of the lesion and visualization of the vaginal orifice with the patient in the supine or knee-chest position. Urethral prolapse may resolve spontaneously with sitz baths, but it sometimes requires intervention. Because the distal urethra is estrogen dependent, twice-daily treatment with estrogen cream for 2 weeks usually results in resolution of the urethral prolapse. If the prolapse does not resolve, surgery may be needed. The carbon dioxide laser is ideally suited for this condition and is less traumatic than cold-knife excision. If prolapse is accompanied by necrosis of the distal urethra, surgery is the first line of therapy.

BOX 12-1
DIFFERENTIAL DIAGNOSIS OF VAGINAL BLEEDING IN PREPUBERTAL CHILDREN

Infection
　Primary
　　Bacterial
　　Fungal
　　Parasitic
　　Viral
　Secondary
　　Foreign body
　　Reflux of urine
　　Pelvic abscess
　　Fistula
Trauma
　Accidental
　Sexual abuse
Endocrine abnormalities
　Newborn bleeding resulting from maternal estrogen withdrawal
　Isosexual precocity
　Exogenous hormone ingestion
　Hypothyroidism
Anatomic abnormalities
　Prolapse of urethral mucosa
　Vaginal and/or uterine prolapse
　Cervical ectropion
　Ectopic ureter
Idiopathic
　Vulvar dystrophy
　Vulvitis secondary to irritants
　Premature endometrial activity
　Self-induced
Neoplasms
　Benign
　Malignant
Blood dyscrasias
　Coagulopathy
　Hematologic neoplasms

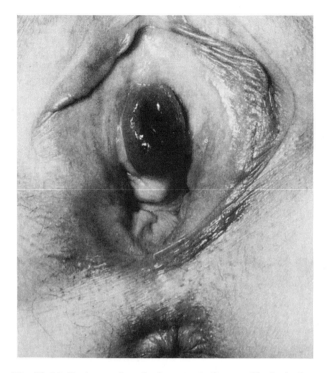

Fig. 12-14. Prolapse of urethral meatus in 9-year-old who had bloody discharge and dysuria.

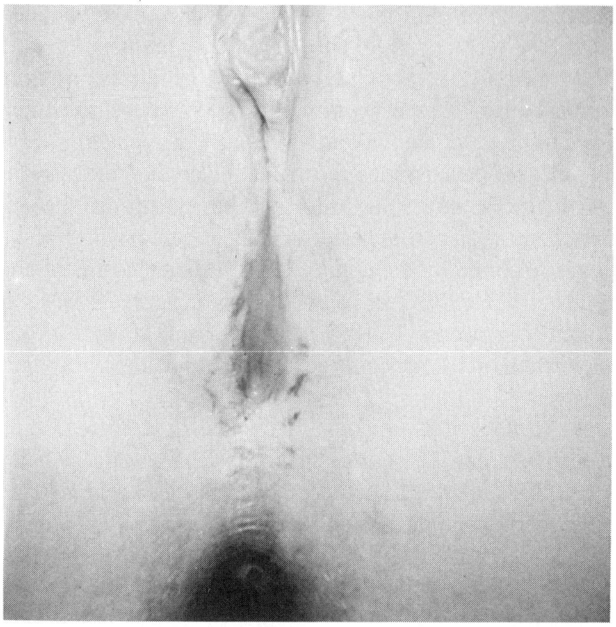

Fig. 12-15. Extensive lichen sclerosus et atrophicus in a prepubertal child with characteristic parchment-like skin, chronic ulceration, and secondary inflammation.

Premature Menarche

Cyclic vaginal bleeding without signs of pubertal development is rare. A full examination under anesthesia and an endometrial biopsy specimen are required to rule out endometrial disease. Results of the biopsy usually show only early proliferative endometrium despite the absence of sexual development. Although the etiology of precocious menarche is obscure, it probably can be attributed to the prolonged stimulation of unusually sensitive endometrium by weak extragonadal estrogens.

Lichen Sclerosis

Lichen sclerosus is an increasingly common disorder in prepubertal children. The reason is unknown. Patients usually report itching, irritation, soreness, and dysuria and, less commonly, constipation, vaginal discharge, and bleeding. The vulva characteristically has white, atrophic, parchment-like skin and shows evidence of chronic ulceration and inflammation from scratching. If the perianal area and the labia are involved, the affected area may have an hourglass configuration. Secondary infection often occurs. The condition should be distinguished from vitiligo, which causes loss of pigmentation but does not cause inflammation or atrophy.

The diagnosis of lichen sclerosus is made clinically; a biopsy specimen is almost never required in children (Fig. 12-15). Treatment aims at the elimination of local irritants and vaginitis, and improved hygiene is encouraged. Soaps should not be overused; the child should be encouraged to wear cotton underpants and loose-fitting pants or skirts to minimize local maceration and irritation. A short course of topical hydrocortisone ointment for a few weeks is used to bring the condition under control. At bedtime, oral medications such as hydroxyzine hydrochloride can be administered to children with intense pruritus. The use of 1% hydrocortisone cream applied one to three times daily is highly effective. If needed, clobetasol 2.5% gel can be applied twice daily. This medication has produced excellent responses in some patients. Topical testosterone is generally not administered to children.

Though it is rare, lichen sclerosus responds to superficial vaporization with the carbon dioxide laser, particularly if it is associated with extensive excoriation and debris. Dramatic results have been seen in a number of patients in whom conservative therapy has failed. Laser treatment may interrupt the scratch-itch cycle and allow healing. Most patients, but not all, see improvement or regression of lesions with puberty.

Clitoral Infection

Infection, with intense edema and erythema, may develop in the clitoral hood. Antibiotics such as dicloxacillin or cephalosporin should be given orally, and warm soaks should be applied. Surgical incision and drainage are necessary if an abscess becomes fluctuant.

Clitoral tourniquet syndrome, in which a hair wrapped around the clitoris resulted in edema and severe pain, has recently been described. After removal of the hair, the clitoris returned to normal size. This syndrome is similar to strangulation by hair of other parts of the body, such as fingers, toes, or penis.

Genital Trauma

Trauma to the External Genitalia

Female genital trauma is not unusual. The injury may be localized and relatively minor or may be accompanied by distant, life-threatening injuries.

In the child, the distance between the internal and the external genitalia makes a perineal injury potentially serious. The distance between the perineal skin and the peritoneal cavity is short in the young child. Thus, penetrating injuries can easily damage intraperitoneal organs. In the infant, the bladder is an intraperitoneal organ and is easily injured. The urogenital diaphragm, which contains the pudendal nerves and vessels, is superficial in infants and children. Therefore, a relatively superficial laceration can result in massive hemorrhage. Finally, the rectovaginal septum is thin and the perineal body is small; both can be torn easily.

Genital injuries may be accidental, self-induced, or result from assault. Straddle injury is responsible for 75% of genital injuries in girls and may be blunt or penetrating. Other common causes are stabbing and automobile accidents. Accidental genital trauma is most common between 4 and 12 years of age.

Because examination of the perineum is often difficult in a bleeding, distraught child, some sedation is advisable. The abdomen must be carefully examined for intraabdominal injury. Abdominal radiographs that include the pelvis may show free air from a perforated viscus, or a pelvic fracture may be evident. A urinalysis should be obtained and checked for blood; if hematuria is present, IVP and cystography are indicated. If there is no urine output, it may indicate a urethral or bladder laceration.

Treatment. Contusions of the perineum and vulva without laceration or bleeding are the most common injury. They may range from a mild ecchymotic area to a large vulvar hematoma requiring surgical intervention. In general, however, a conservative approach including the application of ice packs, analgesia, and bed rest is advocated. An indwelling Foley catheter or a suprapubic drain may be required, depending on the extent of the hematoma. Small lacerations of the labia and hymen usually require suturing. Bleeding can be profuse even though the laceration is small.

All lacerations require thorough examination of the vulva and vagina. This can be accomplished by the use of saline irrigation using intravenous tubing directed toward the perineum and into the vagina. Irrigating fluid washes out the vagina and permits the injection of local anesthesia with epinephrine to decrease the bleeding. Absorbable sutures can be inserted immediately. A laceration that does not extend through the hymen usually does not invade the vagina.

Extensive lacerations always require general anesthesia for evaluation and treatment. Thus, diagnosis and treatment often occur simultaneously. Endoscopic examination of the urethra, bladder, vagina, or rectum is indicated if injuries are adjacent. Most lacerations can be closed primarily, even if they are extensive, unless there is fecal contamination because of rectal injury. In that event, closure is delayed until appropriate antibiotic treatment and closure of the viscus is accomplished. Using absorbable sutures negates the need to remove them at a later date.

A particularly difficult injury occurs when the urogenital diaphragm is bluntly compressed against the pubic ramus. Tears in the periurethral structures bleed profusely and require deep mattress suture. Lacerations near or in the urethra require catheterization for 7 to 10 days.

Lacerations into the vaginal fornix may require laparotomy for closure because of the small size of the child's introitus.

A laceration extending in the posterior direction from the introitus should be evaluated for the possibility of sexual abuse, unless the child has had an accidental fall on a nail, picket fence, or some other penetrating object. Careful endoscopic examination for rectovaginal tears must be carried out before closure. Tetanus prophylaxis and antibiotics must be administered, and laparotomy is indicated for intraabdominal injury or for uncontrollable hemorrhage.

Most properly diagnosed and properly treated genital injuries heal quickly. However, inadequate treatment of lacerations may result in complications from infection. Urethral and vaginal strictures may develop, and an unrecognized rectovaginal tear will result in a rectovaginal fistula.

Frequent examinations must be performed until complete healing has occurred. Infection, stricture formation, and delayed hemorrhage develop even after adequate treatment in 11% to 25% of patients.

Sexual Abuse: The Gynecologist's Role

During the past 20 years the number of young girls referred for examination because of suspected sexual abuse has markedly increased. Although a child who has been sexually abused is treated most effectively by a team that includes a pediatrician, a clinical psychologist, a social worker, and a nurse practitioner, the gynecologist plays a vital role in the assessment, documentation, and treatment of sexually induced infection and trauma.

Great care must be exercised by the physician examining a child thought to have been sexually assaulted. Gentle questioning elicits enough information to evaluate the case gynecologically. Extensive questioning should be carried out by a qualified clinical psychologist or social worker. The gynecologist's goal is to perform the physical examination and collect the appropriate specimens for the forensic pathologist to evaluate.

The history of the assault is difficult to obtain from a very young child and usually must be obtained from relatives, police, or neighbors. A reliable history often can be obtained directly from a child 4 to 5 years of age. However, the physician must first determine the words used by the child to describe the genitals; this information is readily obtained from the child's parents.

The sex of the alleged assailant should be determined. *Rape* refers to the forced act of penetration or attempted penetration without consent of the victim. Penetration of the

---

BOX 12-2
EXAMINATION OF THE SEXUALLY ASSAULTED PATIENT

1. Obtain consent for examination from parent or guardian, preferably written.
2. Obtain detailed general history: past illnesses, accidents, operations.
3. Obtain detailed specific history: details of alleged incident.
4. Observe: manner, dress.
5. Examine all clothing: remove with physician present; inspect each item separately; retain each item in clean bag; note damage to clothes, staining, soiling, ultraviolet light on underpants, and so on.
6. Complete general clinical examination: examine entire body and record all findings; record all injuries, old and new, location, size, description.
7. Examine genitalia; swab vulva and vagina first without lubricant; note injury to labia, hymen, mucosa, thighs, signs of seminal fluid, blood, lubricant.
8. Obtain specimens: buccal swab; blood; saliva; hair; avulsed head hair, loose hairs, pubic hair combings; areas of soiling; fingernail scrapings, clippings; swabs from perineum; vaginal swabs; swabs of anal verge and anal canal.

---

vagina can be caused by a penis or another object, such as a finger, and thus may involve a male or a female assailant. In addition, penetration may involve the mouth or the anus.

The examination of the victim requires proper instrumentation; general anesthesia is necessary in infants and children. Box 12-2 outlines the examination of the pediatric patient who has been sexually assaulted.

Colposcopic Evaluation of the Hymen

Using the colposcope to document sexual trauma has increased (McCann et al, 1992; Muram and Elias, 1989; Slaughter and Brown, 1992; Teixeira, 1981). Advantages are that the hymen and the vulva can be greatly magnified to detect small changes not visible to the naked eye and that photographs are easily taken at the time of the examination to provide future documentation. The latter prevents the need for repeated examinations when physical findings are disputed. The problem with the use of colposcopy has been that, until recently, normal genital anatomy in prepubertal girls has not been well defined (Berenson et al, 1991a; Berenson et al, 1991b; Emans et al, 1987; Gardner, 1992; McCann et al, 1990). The problem has been compounded by these other factors: difficulty in assessing the strength of the association between a history of sexual abuse and variations in hymenal appearance; variations in state statutory definitions of sex crimes; and misunderstanding among professionals about the meaning of penetration.

An atlas of photographs to aid physicians in assessing their patients is of great benefit. One excellent example of such an atlas is *Evaluation of the Sexually Abused Child* (Heger and Emans, 1992). The use of the colposcope has greatly increased the physician's knowledge of normal anatomy and has fine-tuned the physician's visual skills. It is likely that a knowledgeable physician seeing a child for routine annual examination or assessing a genital problem will note changes suggestive of sexual abuse.

The value of the colposcopic examination in the determination of sexual abuse has been a subject of controversy. The percentage of children with "normal" examination results varies from 16% to 85% and depends on case mix, ages of patients, definition of normal, and examiners (Adams et al, 1988; Cantwell, 1983; Cantwell, 1987; Emans et al, 1987; Muram, 1988; Muram, 1989a; Muram, 1989b; White et al, 1989).

In a clinic survey, children who had been sexually abused were compared with children seen for either routine examination or genital problems. Girls with a history of sexual abuse were more likely to have scars, friability of the posterior fourchette because the labia were separate, synechiae, and attenuated hymens than girls seen for routine examinations. Hymenal transactions or tears, condylomata, and abrasions occurred only among the sexually abused girls. Girls with a history of genital problems often had findings similar to those of girls with a history of sexual abuse. Vulvar erythema and friability of the posterior fourchette probably develop secondary to inflammation; scars are probably the result of trauma. Because it may take months to years for girls to reveal that they were sexual abused, it is possible that some evaluated for vaginitis may have been abused. Narrow, thin, posterior hymenal rims in children with vaginitis may mean that these girls had been abused or that this particular anatomic variant may predispose a subset of girls to vaginal contamination and symptoms. In contrast, a narrow rim that has become rounded and scarred with attachment to the vagina probably results from sexual abuse.

The significance of a labial adhesion in a sexually abused child is controversial because many children who have not been abused have adhesions, yet it is possible that rubbing and irritation from abuse may cause agglutination to occur. These adhesions are sometimes mistaken for scars. The difference is usually evident after careful observation; if not, a short trial of estrogen-containing cream that lyses most labial adhesions (but not scars) can be used.

The white midline median raphe evident in some children is often confused with a scar in the posterior fourchette. Conditions such as lichen sclerosus, failure of midline fusion from the anus to the posterior fourchette, and ulcerating hemangioma have been confused with trauma from sexual abuse.

There are usually no abnormal findings in children who have been sodomized. Minor redness, hyperpigmentation, and reflex anal dilation are nonspecific findings that can stem from other causes. More specific findings include scars and distortion of the anus, though the latter can occur with inflammatory bowel disease. Fissures can result from abuse and from constipation.

Similarly, the significance of measurements of the hymenal orifice diameter is controversial (Emans et al, 1987; Heger and Emans, 1990; Paradise, 1989). Transverse and anteroposterior measurements are influenced by age, relaxation of the child, method of examination and measurement, and type of hymen. The older and the more relaxed the child, the larger the opening. The opening is larger with retraction on the labia and in the knee-chest position than it is with gentle separation alone in the supine position. The orifice of a posterior rim hymen appears larger than the opening of a redundant hymen. Because the hymen is distensible, vaginal penetration can have occurred even though the measurement is only 5 mm. In cases of sexual abuse, anteroposterior and transverse dimensions are measured using a Tine test 5-cm ruler. Some colposcopes have the markings in the eyepiece, and direct measurement can be made during the examination. More data on children with normal hymens are needed, but a study of 3- to 6-year-old girls found a mean transverse measurement of 2.9 ± 1.3 mm (range, 1 to 6 mm) and mean anteroposterior measurement of 3.3 ± 1.5 mm (range, 1 to 7 mm). A good rule of thumb is that 1 mm for each year of age comprises the upper limits of normal (8 mm for an 8-year-old child), remembering all the caveats of changes with relaxation and position. When the supine traction technique is used, mean horizontal diameters are 5.2 ± 1.4 mm (range, 2 to 8 mm) for girls aged 2 years to 4 years 11 months and 5.6 ± 1.8 mm (range, 1 to 9 mm) for girls aged 5 years to 7 years 11 months (McCann et al, 1990). A large hymenal orifice may be consistent with a history of sexual abuse, but it should be considered only a part of the evaluation, not the absolute criterion.

Gynecologic Findings During the Evaluation

Examination findings can be classified according to the system described by Muram (1988). They are normal, nonspecific (*e.g.*, inflammation, erythema), specific (*e.g.*, acute or healed laceration), and definitive (*e.g.*, presence of sperm). It has been shown, and must be remembered, that healing from vaginal and anal trauma is rapid (McCann and Voris, 1992; McCann and Voris, 1993); thus, by the time the examination is performed, the findings may be normal.

Repair of Sexual Trauma

Another important role for the gynecologist is the evaluation and repair of sexually induced trauma to the perineum in sexually abused children. The extent of the genital injury depends on the nature and size of the penetrating object, the size of the pelvic outlet and vagina, and the force with which penetration is attempted. Thus, injury may range from a simple vulvar or hymenal tear to a full-thickness laceration of the posterior fourchette with intraperitoneal involvement.

It is wise to postpone gynecologic examination until all appropriate cultures and specimens are obtained. Photo-graphic documentation of all traumatic injuries is essential. If adequate examination is not possible in the office, clinic, or emergency room, then an examination under anesthesia is mandatory.

In general, the younger and smaller the child, the more widespread the injuries produced by penile penetration because she is less able to resist assault. Thus, with the younger child, a lower threshold should be used to initiate an examination under anesthesia.

The only form of resistance to assault may be screaming, which may lead to attempts to silence her. The inner surfaces of the lips should be examined for abrasion or bruising from the lips being forced back against the teeth. Check for loose teeth and damage to the frenulum of the upper lip. Grasping injuries of the arms, thighs, wrists, legs, and ankles are common when the assailant is unknown to the child.

Anorectal injury must be evaluated by examination of the anal canal. Tearing in the anorectum is evidence of anal penetration. Bruising and swelling of the anal verge are common findings. Laxity of the anal sphincter is difficult to assess, especially under anesthesia.

After appropriate evaluation, injuries to the female genitalia from assault are treated in the same manner as accidental injuries. The full extent of the injury should be evaluated and then repaired, layer by layer, until the normal anatomy is restored.

TUMORS
Labial Masses

Gynecologic tumors are rare in childhood. They are usually benign and localized to the external genitalia. A few patients have fibromas, hemangiomas, lipomas, and myomas. In general, they should undergo surgical excision on an outpatient basis, unless they have hemangiomas. These should be allowed to involute spontaneously.

Abdominal/Pelvic Masses

Differential diagnosis of an abdominal/pelvic mass in this age group includes polycystic kidneys, pelvic kidneys, neuroblastomas, intussusception, rhabdomyosarcomas, congenital müllerian abnormalities, and ovarian neoplasms.

Benign Ovarian Masses

Congenital Ovarian Cysts. Because of the more widespread use of sonography in the third trimester, many newborn infants are referred for the management of cystic masses in the pelvis. These are characteristically single, fluid-filled structures that lack septation or solid components. Most of these are benign functional cysts thought to be the result of maternal estrogen and hCG stimulation of the fetal ovary. They usually resolve spontaneously within 2 to 3 months but may require a year to resolve fully. Generally, they are palpable on rectal examination. If they are large and persistent, they may become palpable abdominally. If the infant appears symptomatic and has difficulty feeding or has abdominal pain, it may be necessary to intervene. In these cases, aspiration under the guidance of ultrasonography has been successful. Caution should be exercised in transabdominal aspiration because a cystic structure in the pelvis may be the result of cysts in other organ systems, such as the urinary tract, mesentery, and paratubal or parovarian structures. Aspirated cyst fluid should be sent for cytologic evaluation. If the cyst is complex, unable to be aspirated, or recurs, laparoscopy or laparotomy may be required. Care should be taken to perform a procedure that maintains the pelvic anatomy. Whenever possible, ovarian cystectomy should be performed and normal ovarian tissue conserved. If torsion occurs in utero or goes unrecognized in the neonate, the ovary may atrophy and disappear.

Multiple small ovarian cysts may develop in children and are normal. They may be found incidentally on ultrasound evaluation for abdominal pain. They are simple (without septation, debris, or a thickened capsule) and usually resolve spontaneously.

Other benign masses of the ovary include simple serous or mucinous cysts. Solid tumors of the ovary may develop in children; these are usually mature cystic teratomas (dermoids).

Malignant Tumors

Ovarian cancer is the most common malignancy (60%) of the female genital tract in the pediatric population, and it accounts for 1% of all pediatric malignancies. The most common ovarian malignancy is a germ cell tumor. Germ cell tumors account for 20% of all ovarian malignancies, and they develop most often in the pediatric population.

Characteristically, germ cell tumors grow rapidly and are accompanied by pain or by a rapidly enlarging abdominal mass, or both. The most common germ cell tumors are immature teratoma and dysgerminoma. Among the other forms of germ cell tumor are endodermal sinus tumor, embryonal carcinoma, mixed germ cell tumor, and primary (nongestational) choriocarcinoma.

Other ovarian malignant tumors that develop in childhood include gonadoblastomas and sex cord tumors (granulosa-stromal cell tumors, Sertoli-Leydig cell tumors, gynandroblastoma, and nonspecific stromal tumors).

If a malignant tumor is suspected, tumor markers should be obtained. Common tumor markers and their associated tumors are discussed in detail in Chapter 9. The management of ovarian malignancies in the pediatric population is directed at conservative therapy with preservation of the pelvic anatomy and reproductive function. A staging laparotomy is performed according to International Federation of Gynecology and Obstetrics staging criteria for adult ovarian malignancies (Chapter 9). Unilateral salpingo-oophorectomy with adjuvant chemotherapy is the treatment of choice.

Vaginal Masses in the Pediatric Population
Benign

Hymenal tags and other hymenal abnormalities in children were discussed earlier, and those in adolescents are discussed later in this chapter. Benign vaginal polyps may also develop in the pediatric population.

Malignant

In young children, the most common malignant tumor that involves the vagina, uterus, bladder, and urethra is rhabdomyosarcoma (sarcoma botryoides). Symptoms include vaginal discharge, bleeding, abdominal pain or mass, and the passage of grapelike lesions. On examination, the tumors appear as grapelike masses protruding through the urethra or the vagina. A vaginal tag seen on examination should never be assumed to be benign. Growth of the tumor is rapid, and prognosis is poor unless the diagnosis is made early and prompt radical surgical excision is performed. Regardless of whether additional treatment is administered by radiotherapy or chemotherapy, prognosis depends on the extent of the disease.

Ovarian Transposition for Radiation Therapy

Radiation-induced gonadal dysfunction is dose dependent (Nicholson and Byrne, 1993). With improvements in long-term survival rates of patients with childhood malignancies, it is increasingly important for the pediatric gynecologist to offer options for gonadal protection.

Oophoropexy with repositioning of the ovaries out of the field of radiation has been well described. It can decrease the radiation dosage to the ovary and improve gonadal function (Damewood et al, 1990; LeFloch et al, 1976; Thibaud et al, 1992; Thomas et al, 1976). Historically, this procedure has been performed by laparotomy, but a new technique for laparoscopic ovarian transposition for young girls with medulloblastoma is reported (Laufer et al, 1995). With this procedure, it is shown that moving the ovary inferiorly and laterally out of the craniospinal irradiation field decreases the radiation exposure to the ovary that undergoes pexis to less than 5%. Future studies must be performed to document the beneficial effects on gonadal protection, though it is hypothesized that the beneficial effects will be similar to those of classic oophoropexy.

GYNECOLOGIC PROBLEMS AT PUBERTY
Normal Pubertal Development

Some conditions must exist for normal reproductive function to develop in girls. A normal hypothalamus must develop that is capable of responding to elevated levels of steroids by appropriate pulsatile secretion of GnRH. A normal pituitary must develop that is sensitive to GnRH and estrogen (or progesterone) and that contains a pool of releasable gonadotropins. Normal ovaries must develop that are capable of secreting steroids (estrogen and progesterone) in response to pituitary gonadotropins (LH and follicle-stimulating hormone [FSH]).

The harmony of the menstrual cycle is a product of an elaborate pubertal process in which the hypothalamic-pituitary-ovarian axis develops concomitant with noted physical changes in girls. It is after the completion of the pubertal process that a young woman is fully mature and able to reproduce. Onset of puberty is variable and is influenced profoundly by genetic and environmental factors (*e.g.,* chronic disease and nutrition). The average age of puberty onset in the United States is between ages 8 and 13 years, which is earlier than the average worldwide; better nutrition is one theory explaining this phenomenon (Frisch and McArthur, 1974; Frisch and Revelle, 1971). Because the age of puberty onset varies widely (8 to 18 years), bone age correlates best with pubertal age. Therefore, when a patient is evaluated for delayed or advanced puberty, it is important to obtain a bone age study.

To understand the hormone changes during puberty, we should review the changes in LH and FSH secretion from the time in utero to puberty. Gonadarche and adrenarche are separate events. It is thought that puberty is controlled by a GnRH sensitivity threshold in the hypothalamus that decreases with the increased maturity of the hypothalamic-pituitary axis. Therefore, the central nervous system (CNS) appears to control the onset of puberty and, thus, the secretion of steroid hormones. First signs of puberty include the commencement of sleep-associated pulsatile GnRH secretion. However, after normal pubertal development has been accomplished, the hypothalamic-pituitary axis becomes subservient to the positive and negative feedback signals from the ovary.

Adrenarche is not completely understood, but it appears to be under adrenal control. Adrenarche causes pubic and axillary hair growth. The rise in adrenal androgens precedes the growth spurt by 2 years and involves acceleration in the size of the zona reticularis. There is subsequent increased secretion of androgens (DHEA and DHEA sulfate [DHEAS]).

Pituitary secretion of gonadotropins decreases from approximately ages 4 to 11 years. This is thought to be the result of the development of an intrinsic CNS inhibitory mechanism that suppresses pulsatile GnRH release. Puberty is heralded by decreases in the CNS inhibitory restraint and in the negative feedback effect. An increase in GnRH secretion and pituitary responsiveness ensues.

This responsiveness is demonstrated by the LH response to exogenous GnRH administration (GnRH stimulation test). Before puberty, children show a minimal response to GnRH and secrete a small but significant LH peak. Pubertal children and adults have a much greater LH response to GnRH administration. This increase in pituitary reserve and in secretion of LH is the hallmark of puberty, and it is elicited before any physical evidence of secondary sexual development. As stated earlier, the maturational change seen in puberty is sleep-associated pulsatile LH secretion.

The final phase of the maturational changes that take place is cyclic release of LH in response to the positive feedback of estradiol. This elicits the midcycle surge in gonadotropins seen in the normal female menstrual cycle after puberty. A typical cyclic adult pattern is not achieved, however, until these are regular ovulatory events with resultant increased luteal progesterone concentrations (greater than 10 ng/ml).

Concomitant with these changes are differences in adrenocortical functioning and increases in adrenal androgen, namely DHEAS (adrenarche). Adrenal maturation, however, is a separate event. In agonadal children, a decrease in basal gonadotropins also occurs at ages 4 to 11 years, attesting to the isolated importance of a maturing CNS inhibitory influence during this period. Adrenarche also occurs among patients with hypergonadotropic and hypogonadotropic hypogonadism (not hypopituitarism).

Minimum weight is another criterion that appears to be associated with normal menstrual function. Losses as small as 10% to 15% of body weight affect the menstrual cycle; a relative degree of body fat is associated with sexual maturation. Table 12-2 contains a summary of normal pubertal developmental milestones.

Abnormal Pubertal Development

A thorough understanding of the normal progression of puberty is essential for the evaluation of patients with precocious puberty. Precocious puberty is defined as the development of secondary sexual characteristics before age 8. This represents 2.5 standard deviations from the norm.

In normal adolescence, estrogen is responsible for the development of breasts, the maturation of the external genitalia, vagina, and uterus, and the initiation of menses. An increase in adrenal androgens is associated with the appearance of pubic and axillary hair. Excess androgens of either ovarian or adrenal origin may cause acne, hirsutism, voice changes, increased muscle mass, and clitoromegaly.

Precocious puberty can be divided into three categories: complete or true precocious puberty (GnRH dependent), incomplete or pseudoprecocious puberty, and extrapituitary gonadotropin production (GnRH independent).

Premature Thelarche

Premature thelarche is seen among girls 1 to 4 years of age. Occasionally, neonatal breast hypertrophy fails to regress within 6 months after birth. This persistent breast development is characterized as premature thelarche. Typically, the child with premature thelarche has bilateral breast buds measuring 2 to 4 cm but little or no change in the nipple or areola. Breast tissue feels granular and may be slightly tender. Sometimes development is asymmetric; one side may develop 6 to 12 months before the other. Growth is not

Table 12-2   Normal Pubertal Development Milestones

	Age of Occurrence (Yrs)	
	Mean	Range
Thelarche	10.9	9.0-13.5
Adrenarche	11.2	9.5-14
Peak height velocity	11.5	9.0-14
Menarche	12.7	11.0-16

accelerated, and the bone age is normal for height age. No other evidence of puberty appears; the vulva and the vagina remain prepubertal and show no evidence of estrogen effect.

Although it was originally thought that premature thelarche was caused by increased end-organ sensitivity to low levels of endogenous estrogen, the fact that there are at least transiently elevated serum estrogen levels suggests that small luteinized or cystic graafian follicles may sometimes be responsible. The usual clinical course of regression or lack of progression of breast development correlates with waning estrogen levels as follicles become atretic. Treatment consists mainly of reassurance and careful follow-up to confirm that breast development does not represent the first sign of precocious puberty.

Premature Adrenarche

Most patients with premature adrenarche have slight increases in urinary 17-ketosteroid production and increased plasma DHEA and DHEAS levels, suggesting that hormone biosynthesis in the adrenal gland undergoes maturation prematurely to a pubertal pattern. Although production of these androgens can be suppressed by dexamethasone and, therefore, is dependent on ACTH, the mediator for change at puberty and in premature adrenarche is unknown.

The assessment of the patient with premature adrenarche is similar to that for the patient with heterosexual precocious puberty. Important physical findings are the presence of virilization (pubic hair), the absence of breast development, and estrogenization of the labia and vagina.

Laboratory tests should include radiologic examination of the nondominant wrist for bone age, vaginal smear (for maturational index), a 24-hour urine test for free cortisol, and serum DHEAS, testosterone, and 17-hydroxyprogesterone levels. Clinical studies should be directed at the differential diagnosis, which must exclude precocious puberty, congenital adrenal hyperplasia, and adrenal or ovarian tumor.

Treatment of premature adrenarche is reassurance and follow-up. The child should be examined every 6 months to confirm the original diagnosis. In general, pubertal development at adolescence can be expected to be normal, but follow-up is necessary to evaluate the progression of a hyperandrogenic state.

Precocious Puberty

Puberty is considered precocious if secondary sexual characteristics occur before the child is 8 years of age. In the general population of the United States this occurs at an incidence of 1 per 5000 to 1 per 10,000. The female-to-male ratio is between 4:1 and 8:1. This is usually a consequence of accelerated linear growth (advanced bone age). Precocity may be the result of constitutional or organic causes. Most incidences of isosexual precocious puberty are of a constitutional or idiopathic form (85% females), and it may be familial. It is, however, vital to distinguish these patients from those whose precocity is based on lesions of the brain,

ovary, or adrenal glands. Therefore, sexual precocity may stem from central or CNS causes (including constitutional) or extrapituitary causes (ovarian tumors, adrenal tumors).

Isosexual Precocious Puberty. In true isosexual precocity, the stimulus for development arises in the hypothalamus and pituitary gland. In response to rising LH and FSH levels, the ovaries produce estrogen. The young girl develops breasts and pubic and axillary hair and begins menstruation, sometimes not in the usual sequence. With the establishment of the cyclic midcycle LH peak, the child becomes potentially fertile.

In isosexual pseudoprecocity, an ovarian tumor or cyst or an adrenal adenoma produces estrogen autonomously. Fluctuating estrogen levels result in sexual development and anovulatory menses. In more than 80% of patients with isosexual precocious puberty, the hypothalamic-pituitary axis is activated prematurely for unknown reasons.

Despite the relatively high incidence of constitutional or idiopathic precocious puberty, this diagnosis cannot be made without a thorough evaluation and exclusion of some of the following organic causes:

1. Cerebral disorders (5% to 10% of patients)
2. Ovarian tumors (5% of patients)
3. Adrenal disorders (rare)
4. Gonadotropin-producing tumors (rare)
5. Hypothyroidism (rare)
6. Iatrogenic disorders (rare)

Patient assessment by the gynecologist or the reproductive endocrinologist should include a careful history and physical examination and a family history. It is important to perform appropriate studies to rule out cerebral disorders and ovarian tumors, which are the two most common organic causes of this condition.

The first crucial steps in an initial evaluation of precocious puberty are careful history taking (to rule out exogenous steroids, history of encephalitis, and cerebral trauma) and meticulous physical examination. Blood pressure, accelerated development of thelarche, pubarche, gonadarche, and growth spurts are noted. Skin changes and any café au lait spots are documented. Pelvic and abdominal examination may indicate the presence of an ovarian or adrenal mass, which is confirmed by ultrasonography. Bone radiography documents accelerated linear growth and epiphyseal closure (and excludes fibrous dysplasia). Skull radiography, computed tomography (CT) scan, or MRI rules out intracranial lesions. Chemical precocity is indicated by levels of FSH, LH, and estradiol equivalent to those found in adolescents. These may be elevated only on blood samples obtained at night. Thyroid function tests exclude hypothyroidism. Elevated DHEAS or 17-hydroxyprogesterone points to either late-onset CAH or adrenal neoplasm (especially if documented by imaging). In the patient with adrenal neoplasm, suppression does not occur with a dexamethasone suppression test, whereas suppression does in the patient with CAH. An increased urinary hCG level may indicate a rare trophoblastic tumor. Exogenous LH and GnRH administration can discriminate between extrapituitary causes of precocity (ovarian tumors) and central causes. The latter entails a pubertal LH response after such stimulation, whereas the former does not. Finally, if exogenous steroids, CNS disease, hypothyroidism, late-onset CAH, McCune-Albright syndrome, and adrenal or ovarian masses are excluded, idiopathic isosexual precocious puberty is the most likely diagnosis.

Treatment and follow-up depend on the diagnosis. Ovarian tumors and CNS tumors require surgical intervention. Idiopathic and CNS-induced precocity can be treated effectively with GnRH agonist therapy. The goals of treatment for precocious puberty are to halt the premature closure of the epiphyses and thus increase final adult height and to halt the precocious development of secondary sexual development so that the child is not at increased risk for sexual abuse or other emotionally scarring situations.

Despite the diagnosis of idiopathic precocious puberty, follow-up must continue at least every 6 months to exclude the possibility of organic disease not originally evident. Children with sexual precocity do not automatically manifest intellectual or psychosocial precocity; the degree of psychological maturity of a young girl is more likely to be related to the life experiences she encounters and transacts.

Heterosexual Precocious Puberty. Heterosexual precocity arises from excess androgen production from an adrenal or ovarian source, which results in acne, hirsutism, and virilization. Differential diagnosis includes CAH, Cushing syndrome, adrenal tumors, ovarian tumors such as Sertoli-Leydig cell, lipoid cell, and Sertoli cell tumors, and occasionally familial precocious puberty with isolated elevation of LH level.

As with isosexual precocity, patients should undergo careful history and physical examination. Laboratory tests should include determination of serum FSH, LH, estradiol, DHEA, DHEAS, testosterone, androstenedione, 17-hydroxyprogesterone, and 17-hydroxypregnenolone values. An ACTH stimulation test should be carried out. Additionally, 24-hour urinalysis should be performed to look for free cortisol.

Treatment and follow-up of heterosexual precocious puberty are based on the diagnosis. Ovarian and adrenal tumors should be surgically excised, if possible. Patients with CAH should undergo glucocorticoid replacement therapy. Follow-up should include careful monitoring of growth every 3 months. If the bone age is not too advanced in patients with CAH, breast development may regress with treatment.

GYNECOLOGIC PROBLEMS IN THE ADOLESCENT POPULATION
Infections

Most gynecologic infections in the adolescent are evaluated and treated as they are in the adult (Chapter 18). There are, however, certain aspects of these problems that are unique to the adolescent and deserve special emphasis.

Pelvic Inflammatory Disease

Pelvic inflammatory disease is addressed in great detail in Chapter 18. Adolescents are at especially high risk because they often have multiple sex partners and have high prevalence of infections with *N. gonorrhoeae* and *C. trachomatis*. Women with multiple partners have a 4.6-fold increased risk for PID. The use of nonbarrier methods of contraception makes adolescents more likely to acquire endocervical infections, and the immaturity of their immune systems appears to increase their susceptibility to ascending infection.

Oral contraceptive use appears to decrease the risk for gonococcal PID, perhaps because of changes in cervical mucus, lighter menstrual flow, diminished uterine contractions, less retrograde menstruation, and less canal dilation. Because most studies have been limited to hospital patients with PID (only 25% of all patients with PID), it is unclear whether protection from the pill can be generalized to other forms of PID. Because a history of PID is a risk factor for PID and because the sequelae of infertility, ectopic pregnancy, and pelvic pain are related to the number of episodes, it is clear that adolescents require prompt attention if they have symptoms suggestive of PID.

Although in the past PID has been divided into gonococcal and nongonococcal types based on the presence or absence of *N. gonorrhoeae* in the endocervical culture, the most appropriate designations are gonococcal chlamydial PID and nongonococcal nonchlamydial PID. A positive cervical culture for gonorrhea is found in 20% to 80% of patients with PID.

Chlamydial infection is found in 20% to 45% of patients with PID. Of great concern in the evaluation of adolescents is a study reporting that 40% of patients with asymptomatic endocervical chlamydial infection also have evidence of endometrial infection (Jones and Heller, 1986). The course of chlamydial PID can be subacute and indolent, and adolescents often delay seeking medical attention. Often, by the time they do, the sedimentation rate associated with chlamydial PID is elevated and the tubal damage significant.

Diagnosis. After the onset of a menses in a sexually active girl, the classic picture of acute salpingitis includes lower abdominal pain, vaginal discharge, and fever and chills. Symptoms may be less specific and may include menstrual irregularities, dyspareunia, vomiting, diarrhea, constipation, dysuria, and urinary frequency. The most recent CDC criteria for the diagnosis of PID are found in Chapter 18. The diagnosis of PID is sometimes difficult to make. Laparoscopic studies of patients with a presumptive diagnosis of acute salpingitis conclude that the clinical diagnosis is confirmed by visual inspection in only 60% to 70% of patients (Jacobson, 1980). An additional 5% of patients with negative examination results by laparoscopy do have gonococci in the cervical culture. Laparoscopy has proved invaluable in clarifying the etiologic agents and the clinical accuracy of PID diagnosis. Laparoscopy is indicated if the diagnosis is in doubt, especially for patients who seem to have recurrences of PID but in whom the criteria are never met. We recently showed that mini-laparoscopy (with a 2-mm scope) can be performed to assess adolescents for PID in an emergency room setting (Kahn et al, 1997).

Inpatient Therapy. Although antibiotic thereby resolves symptoms in most patients, the long-term results of treatment are still far from satisfactory. Given the frequency of noncompliance with medical therapy during adolescence and the risk for future reproductive problems, noncompliant adolescents should be considered a high priority for inpatient PID therapy. Some centers admit all adolescents routinely for parenteral therapy. In addition, any patient with PID in whom any of the following exists warrants inpatient therapy:

> questionable diagnosis
> suspected pelvic abscess
> upper quadrant pain
> signs of peritoneal infection
> temperature greater than 38°C
> vomiting
> prepuberty
> pregnancy
> noncompliance with outpatient treatment (including medication and follow-up appointments)

failure to respond to outpatient treatment within 48 hours Specific treatment regimens for outpatients and inpatients are provided in Chapter 18.

Sexual Assault

In contrast to the pattern of sexual abuse in prepubertal children, sexual abuse during adolescence is more likely to be a one-time assault by a stranger and to involve vaginal intercourse. However, even among adolescents, the rape may involve an acquaintance or someone the teenager sees in her neighborhood or school and whom she assumes is safe (Muram et al, 1993). In these cases, the adolescent may, for example, accept a ride with that person and then be forced into a sexual relationship, often involving intercourse. In other cases, the developmental changes that take place during adolescence may make a long-standing incestuous relationship intolerable. The adolescent may respond with a sudden disclosure, may seek medical care for somatic symptoms such as abdominal pain or headache, or may become involved in impulsive behavior such as running away. Pregnancy may be the first sign of a previous rape or chronic sexual abuse. Therefore, it is important to ask adolescents not only whether they have ever had sexual relations but also whether they have ever been forced into a sexual relationship.

In recording the history of the adolescent seeking treatment for alleged sexual assault, it is important to record the date of the visit, sources of the history, who transported the patient to the clinic or hospital, and who knows of the current situation. The date, time, and place of the sexual assault(s) should be recorded. In acute situations, the patient should be asked if she has bathed, douched, or urinated since the assault. Menstrual and contraceptive history should be

obtained. The physician should not try to decide whether rape or seduction has occurred on the basis of the patient's emotional response to the trauma, for clearly some patients will be tearful, tense, and hysterical and others will appear controlled or subdued. Questions in terms understood by the patient should focus on what happened and whether vaginal, rectal, or oral penetration occurred. These questions may have to be repeated during the examination when the adolescent is more familiar with the anatomic terms. The patient should be asked if she is aware of any other injuries or symptoms resulting from the attack. A rape protocol should be used to collect evidence. It is extremely helpful if a nurse, preferably an experienced rape victim counselor, can be assigned to the adolescent throughout the 2- to 4-hour stay in the emergency ward and can be present during the history taking and physical examination and be an ally to the patient. Some general hospitals now have a rotating system of nurses who have had special training in rape counseling and who are available on an on-call basis to provide such support for the victim. A police officer should not be present during the medical evaluation.

After the history is obtained, the need for a thorough physical examination to assess injury and to collect laboratory specimens should be explained to the patient. The assessment given here applies to the acute sexual assault. When there is a history of an ongoing incestuous relationship in which intercourse has occurred more than 5 days before the physical examination, the search for motile sperm is omitted.

The physical examination should include the following six steps:

1. A description of the patient's general appearance and emotional state, and especially of the condition of the clothing, should be recorded. Any clothing that may provide evidence in a legal case should be included in a bag containing evidence of the rape.

2. A general physical examination should note any evidence of bruises, scratches, or lacerations. As noted in the section on assessment of the prepubertal child, debris and dried secretions should be properly collected. The Tanner stage of sexual development should be noted. If the history indicates any attempt of the patient to scratch or fight her assailant, fingernail scrapings should be obtained with a wooden applicator stick and saved in an envelope.

3. The pelvic examination should include a careful inspection of the perineum, noting any evidence of bleeding or lacerations. A slightly moistened gauze pad should be used to swab any dried secretions, and the location of the dried secretions should be marked on a sketch. A collection paper should be placed under the buttocks of the patient and the pubic hair combed toward the paper to collect any debris. The comb and debris should be placed in the collection envelope. If any foreign hairs are noted, 6 to 12 pubic hairs of the patient should be included and

marked. The pubic hair can be cut near the surface to avoid discomfort. The size of the hymenal ring should be noted (*e.g.,* Cotton-tipped applicator size, one finger breadth, two finger breadths). Any evidence of a hymenal tear should be recorded. In most patients, a genital-vaginal examination can be performed with a water-moistened adolescent (Huffman) speculum. If the hymen is tight, samples may be obtained from the vagina with a saline-moistened cotton-tipped applicator a long eyedropper. It is extremely important to examine the teenager gently so that the examination does not represent additional trauma. The vagina is inspected for injury and the presence of semen or vaginal discharge. An endocervical culture should be obtained for gonorrhea and chlamydia. If a speculum examination is not performed, a vaginal culture for gonorrhea and chlamydia can be obtained by inserting a moistened cotton-tipped applicator well into the vagina. A cotton-tipped applicator should be swabbed into the posterior vaginal pool, and wet preparations should be made to look for the presence of motile sperm and trichomonads. Another swab from the vaginal pool should be smeared onto two dry slides (frosted at one end so that the patient's name and date can be recorded) and air dried. The swab should be placed in a test tube and saved for examination in a police forensic laboratory. If cervical smears also are taken to check for motile sperm, the wet and dry slides should be appropriately marked. A police laboratory can test for acid phosphatase and the blood group antigens of semen and can examine the dry slides for the presence of nonmotile perm. The anus should be inspected and cultures for gonorrhea and chlamydia obtained. Specimens for sperm and acid-phosphatase determinations should be obtained if there is a history of rectal assault. Anoscopy should be performed if there is rectal bleeding or if the rectal examination reveals guaiac-positive stool. A bimanual rectal-vaginal-abdominal examination should be performed gently to make sure there is no tenderness or enlargement of the uterus to suggest a preexisting pregnancy. Rectal sphincter tone should be assessed because patients subjected to chronic rectal abuse may have reflex relaxation.

4. If oral-genital contact has occurred, specimens from the girl's mouth should be obtained. A throat swab should be plated in modified Thayer-Martin-Jambee media.

5. Blood should be drawn for a serologic test for syphilis (rapid plasma reagin or Venereal Disease Research Laboratory), and a serum specimen should be frozen for future HIV and hepatitis B testing, if indicated.

6. A sensitive uterine pregnancy test should be performed to detect preexisting pregnancy, especially if the menses are late or irregular or the patient has had previous sexual exposure.

If the patient is unconscious, samples should be obtained from the vagina, rectum, and mouth.

All laboratory specimens to be given to the pathology laboratory or the police should be delivered personally by the doctor or the nurse involved in the case, and properly signed receipts should be obtained. Use of a rape evidence kit or rape protocol does not imply that the family or patient must push for prosecution; however, reporting the rape and using a protocol to collect the evidence ensures that the evidence has been appropriately handled and will be admissible in court if prosecution occurs. Under the stress of the crisis, many families may have difficulty deciding whether prosecution will be sought; therefore, it behooves the physician to obtain evidence that is medically and legally appropriate.

In cases of acute rape, the decision to prescribe antibiotics should be individualized and based on the risks. The benefits of prophylactic treatment for syphilis, gonorrhea, and chlamydia should be discussed with the patient. Current recommendations for prophylactic antibiotics in cases of sexual assault are provided in Chapter 18. In asymptomatic adolescents with long-standing incestuous relationships, the physician should wait for the results of the cultures and blood tests before initiating treatment, unless the perpetrator is known to be infected. Intramuscular ceftriaxone and oral metronidazole is the current treatment regimen of choice. The single-dose therapy should be followed by 14 days of tetracycline, doxycycline, or erythromycin. If the initial rapid plasma reagin is negative, a follow-up serologic test for syphilis is necessary whether spectinomycin is chosen for gonococcal prophylaxis or no prophylaxis is given. Tetanus toxoid should be administered according to standard pediatric guidelines for injuries.

The "morning-after pill" should be offered to the postpubertal adolescent who was raped less than 72 hours (preferably less than 48 hours) before treatment. It is important that the patient understand that the medicine should not be used if there is the possibility of a preexisting pregnancy. A sensitive pregnancy test should be conducted before medication is given.

A follow-up appointment should be made for 2 weeks later, during which a repeat pelvic examination should be performed to assess healing. The patient should be reassured that her genital anatomy is normal. Patients benefit greatly from drawings that show the range of hymenal size. The virginal adolescent who has had a forced episode of sexual intercourse may feel considerably relieved to understand that her introitus is not different from that of some adolescents who have not had intercourse. She must be reassured that the assault in no way changes her ability to have normal sexual intercourse in the future or to have normal, healthy children. Some older teenagers have unprotected intercourse because they feel that a rape that occurred when they were 12 or 13 years old markedly diminishes their reproductive potential.

The extent of the counseling in the aftermath of a sexual assault depends on the initial encounter. For example, if this is an isolated episode of exhibitionism or nonforceful genital fondling by a stranger or neighbor, counseling should help integrate the event with a strongly positive view of the future. A long-standing incestuous relationship requires proper reporting and a long-term treatment program. If the young adolescent has been trained to be a sexual object and to give and receive sexual pleasure to get approval, the outcome is often poor; such girls are often provocative in foster home settings. Cases of acute sexual assault during adolescence require that the physician discuss the possibility of prosecution and suggest the need for long-term counseling.

The availability of counseling should be stressed to the teenager. Even if she seems nonverbal or appears to be coping well, the counselor often can play an educational and supportive role in the initial interviews. The patient needs reassurance about her intactness and her femininity. She may need the opportunity to tell and retell her story to a caring, sympathetic person. Ideally, an experienced counselor should be available at the time the rape is reported and should be willing to follow up with the patient by telephone or home visits. It is not unusual for a patient to have somatic reactions such as muscle soreness, headache, fatigue, stomach pain, dysuria, sleep disturbances, and nightmares in the first several weeks following a rape. Most rape victims express an extreme fear of physical violence and death. Many older women move and change their telephone numbers.

In the course of counseling, it is important to acknowledge to the patient that she may feel vulnerable and helpless and that the rape may interfere with her ability to form trusting relationships in the future.

Menstrual Disorders

Abnormalities of the pubertal process involve isosexual or heterosexual precocity or delayed puberty. There may be variations in the pubertal process, with premature thelarche and premature adrenarche occurring in isolated form. The differential diagnosis of precocious development was discussed previously.

Delayed Menarche

Delayed menarche indicates the continued absence of menses in girls by the time they are 18 years of age. It may be classified as menarche of constitutional delay, hypogonadotrophic hypogonadism, or hypergonadotropic hypogonadism.

Most patients with delayed adolescent development have no abnormal organic conditions. The developmental retardation in these patients represents a normal variation in endocrine function that usually is rectified by time alone. For this reason, timing a diagnostic program is most perplexing. The answer lies in the individualization of each case, taking into account the history, the findings of physical examination, and the emotional attitudes of the patient and her family. Initiating therapy to promote sexual development is to be deplored unless adequate diagnostic studies have been undertaken.

The endocrine defect in delayed adolescent development and delayed menarche results from the lack of proper estrogenic stimulation necessary for maturation of the accessory sex organs and initiation of uterine bleeding. Estrogen secretion is dependent on the elaboration of gonadotropin hormones from the adenohypophysis. Gonadotropin secretion may be diminished or entirely lacking. It is assumed that, for reasons unknown, FSH and LH are held in abeyance.

Malnutrition resulting from starvation or chronic wasting disease may contribute to delayed development. Similarly, emotional or psychosomatic factors are known causes of secondary amenorrhea and may act to delay the onset of the puberty. Imbalances of other endocrine organs, such as the thyroid or adrenal glands, also may delay adolescent development and the menarche.

Clinical evaluation of patients with delayed adolescent development should begin with a thorough history and physical examination. Careful scrutiny of the accessory sex organs and the genitalia is mandatory. The internal genitalia may be examined rectally; mental trauma and physical discomfort are minimal if the examiner is reassuring and careful. Bone radiographs document bone age. Neurologic and ophthalmologic examinations are indicated if suspicious signs or symptoms, such as headaches, scotomata, or diplopia, are manifested.

Thorough rectovaginal examination is essential because delayed menarche is sometimes caused by a congenital mechanical obstruction in the vagina or cervix. This obstruction is usually an imperforate hymen, and rectal examination reveals accumulated menstrual discharge in the vagina. Normal menses immediately follow incision into the hymen and relief of the obstruction.

Gonadotropin assay distinguishes pituitary from ovarian failure. Elevated serum gonadotropin levels suggest ovarian failure (hypergonadotropic hypogonadism). Diminished levels focus attention on pituitary dysfunction (hypergonadotropic hypogonadism). Plasma FSH level is the single most reliable assay for ovarian failure. Estrogens measured in urine or blood are in the range found in prepubertal girls and postmenopausal women. Yet endometrial function is not altered because uterine bleeding may be induced by the administration of estrogens alone or by the combined administration of estrogens and progesterone. As previously stated, most patients with delayed adolescent development have no discernible abnormality. The prognosis for normal sexual development and reproductive function is excellent. If no lesions or hormonal deficiencies are observed, it is advisable to use endocrine preparations. Reassurance, explanation, and passage of time constitute the desired therapeutic regimen. Systemic abnormalities such as obesity, cachexia, infection, and diabetes should be appropriately treated. Adequate psychiatric therapy, if indicated, should be initiated.

Primary Amenorrhea

Primary amenorrhea denotes menarche that has not occurred by the time a girl is 16 years of age. It is part of normal pubertal development in patients who have vaginal or müllerian aplasia. Patients who have complete androgen insensitivity may have normal thelarche, but they do not have normal hair development and are amenorrheic. In deciphering the cause of primary amenorrhea, the patient's secondary sex characteristics should be examined; if there is good sexual development, the possibilities include testicular feminization, müllerian agenesis, vaginal atresia, and polycystic ovarian disease.

Most patients with primary amenorrhea have hypogonadotrophic hypogonadism or gonadal dysgenesis. Others have elevated plasma testosterone levels that indicate some form of polycystic ovary syndrome. Still others have elevated prolactin levels despite normal breast and uterine development. If the patient is normoprolactinemic, an intramuscular progesterone or oral medroxyprogesterone challenge test can be administered to determine estrogen status. If the patient is estrogenized, withdrawal bleeding occurs. If progesterone withdrawal test results are negative, additional FSH level testing rules out ovarian failure. This final diagnostic category is associated with secondary rather than primary amenorrhea.

Secondary Amenorrhea

Secondary amenorrhea denotes loss of menses for more than 6 months in a patient who has had normal cycles. Oligomenorrhea denotes irregular but consistent periods occurring at intervals of 2 to 5 months. Chronic anovulation usually accompanies secondary amenorrhea or oligomenorrhea. The most common causes for secondary amenorrhea or oligomenorrhea are hypothalamic dysfunction, hyperprolactinemia, and excess androgen production.

Anorexia nervosa or excessive weight loss, malnutrition, stress, sustained systemic illness, and certain levels of exercise are all possible causes for hypogonadism. This diagnosis is reached through exclusion, because pituitary, ovarian, and adrenal dysfunction must first be eliminated. Most patients with hypothalamic amenorrhea experience normal puberty. With the onset of amenorrhea, gonadotropins and estrogen levels decrease. Depending on the duration of their disorders and whether they have secondary amenorrhea, patients may be normoestrogenic or hypoestrogenic. Physical examination serves as a bioassay of estrogen status because a well-cornified, rugated, vaginal epithelium denotes normal estrogen status. Poorly cornified vaginal epithelium with scant cervical mucus denotes a low estrogen level. The progesterone challenge test produces withdrawal bleeding if the estrogen level is normal.

Three important factors to exclude are pregnancy, pituitary tumor, and premature menopause. Determination of β-hCG level precludes pregnancy; LH, FSH, and prolactin level assays and a MRI of the pituitary, if necessary, exclude hyperprolactinemia or hypergonadotropism. Other abnormal processes are, therefore, ruled out, and hypothalamic amenorrhea is indicated. Patients should be encouraged to gain weight or to decrease exercise activity if these are thought to be causative factors. Hormonal supplementation should be suggested to prevent osteoporosis.

Patients with hypothalamic amenorrhea should be counseled about its possible causes. If the cause is excessive dietary restriction, specifically from anorexia and bulemia, patients should be referred for psychiatric treatment; their care is founded on a multidisciplinary approach. There is no long-term effect on the uterus or the ovaries in these patients. This is an important point to make because many patients worry that they will be unable to maintain pregnancy if they have had prolonged amenorrhea from exercise or anorexia. However, they should be made aware of the long-term skeletal effects that result in osteoporosis from prolonged amenorrhea. Adequate diet, reasonable exercise, and exogenous calcium supplementation help to avert the premature onset of osteoporosis.

If amenorrhea or oligomenorrhea is caused by hyperprolactinemia, a careful evaluation of pituitary sellar contents is mandatory. A large pituitary adenoma may be treated medically or removed transsphenoidally by an experienced neurosurgeon. Hyperprolactinemia recurrence is high, and patients should be made aware of this. If a patient has microadenoma or if no tumor is visible on a sellar CT scan, bromocriptine therapy is indicated. Alternatively, cyclic oral contraceptive pills can be prescribed to regulate menses and avoid hypoestrogenism.

Abnormal Bleeding

Acute Adolescent Menorrhagia. Abnormal menstrual bleeding is one of the most common reasons for gynecologic consultation in adolescents. Symptoms range from minor deviations from the average menstrual pattern to life-threatening hemorrhage. Whatever the seriousness of symptoms, it is a subject of great concern for the patient and her parents, and it deserves attentive consideration.

Acute menorrhagia is dramatic and requires prompt treatment. The clinical picture is that of a pale, anxious teenager who is brought to the emergency ward because of heavy bleeding of several days' or weeks' duration. Dysfunctional uterine bleeding, by definition, occurs on the basis of anovulatory cycles. The adolescent in the first years of her menstrual life is the most susceptible candidate.

Differential diagnosis of acute adolescent vaginal hemorrhage is summarized in Box 12-3. Although dysfunctional (anovulatory) uterine bleeding accounts for the greatest number of incidences, other causes of abnormal genital bleeding should be ruled out systematically.

Pregnancy-related complications are common in adolescents and should be excluded even in the adolescent who denies sexual activity. These include spontaneous abortion, complications of elective abortion, ectopic pregnancy, and

---

BOX 12-3
DIFFERENTIAL DIAGNOSIS OF
ADOLESCENT MENORRHAGIA

Anovulatory uterine bleeding

Pregnancy-related complications
    Spontaneous abortion
    Complications of pregnancy termination procedures
    Ectopic pregnancy
    Gestational trophoblastic diseases
    Bleeding of the third trimester of pregnancy

Local genital tract conditions
    Benign and malignant tumors (vagina, cervix, uterus, ovary)
    Infection
    Intrauterine contraceptive devices
    Trauma
    Intravaginal foreign bodies

Systemic causes
    Coagulation disorders
    Thyroid dysfunction
    Diabetes mellitus
    Nutritional disorders, iron deficiency
    Hepatic diseases
    Renal diseases

Hormonal
    Oral contraceptives
    Intramuscular
    Subcutaneous

---

gestational trophoblastic disease. Occasionally, young patients seek treatment third-trimester bleeding in a previously undiagnosed pregnancy.

Though rare, benign and malignant conditions of the genital tract may be responsible for severe hemorrhage. Sarcoma botryoides, which most often occurs in young children, rarely develops in adolescents. Bleeding vaginal adenosis, clear-cell adenocarcinoma, extensive ectropion, and cervical or vaginal polyps or hemangiomas may be found on pelvic examination. Uterine neoplasms and endometrial polyps are rare in this age group. Estrogen-secreting ovarian tumors also can cause endometrial hyperplasia, which leads to heavy bleeding as it does in perimenopausal women. In association with endometritis and intrauterine contraceptive devices, PID may induce heavy vaginal bleeding. Postcoital or self-imposed traumatic conditions and intravaginal foreign bodies also should be considered.

Coagulation disorders are probably the most common systemic condition associated with acute menorrhagia. Idiopathic thrombocytopenic purpura, von Willebrand disease, Glanzmann disease, thalassemia major, Falconi anemia, leukemia, radiation and chemotherapy side effects, and some drugs (anticoagulants, aspirin, hepatotoxic drugs) are possi-

ble causes of deficient coagulation mechanisms (Claessons and Cowell, 1981). Other systemic conditions possibly associated with menorrhagia include thyroid dysfunction, diabetes mellitus, nutritional disorders, and hepatic and renal diseases. Older adolescents who have acute menstrual hemorrhage should be investigated for other causes of chronic anovulation.

A complete history of recent events and of premenarchal development should be obtained. It is difficult for the patient to assess the amount of blood loss. Questions about the number of perineal pads or tampons used, the degree of saturation, the quantity and size of blood clots, and the presence of orthostatic symptoms facilitate an estimation of blood loss. Normal menstrual volume averages 30 to 40 mL and corresponds to 10 to 15 moderately soaked pads or tampons. Information pertinent to all possible causes of vaginal hemorrhage should be obtained.

The patient must be given a complete physical examination, with special attention paid to signs of hypovolemia and anemia (namely pallor, low blood pressure, and orthostatic hypotension), tachycardia, and functional heart murmur. The abdomen should be carefully palpated for a mass, localized pain, or signs of peritoneal infection. Speculum examination is mandatory to evaluate the amount of bleeding, to rule out any vaginal abnormality, and to visualize the cervix. If the patient has a tight hymen, blood clots may accumulate and distend the vagina. It is not unusual to find as much as 500 mL of coagulated blood in the vagina. This retrograde accumulation of clots may also account for cervical dilation, which can be attributed erroneously to spontaneous abortion. Rectovaginal examination of internal genital structures discloses any uterine enlargement and adnexal masses or tenderness.

Laboratory evaluation should be conducted for hemoglobin and hematocrit levels, platelet count, blood type and cross-match, and basic clotting study results including prothrombin time, partial thromboplastin time, and bleeding time. These specimens should be drawn before hormonal or transfusion therapy is instituted. Serum β-hCG or another highly sensitive pregnancy test should be given, and cervical cultures for *N. gonorrhea* and *C. trachomatis* should be obtained for every patient. Blood sugar determination, thyroid function test results, and urinalysis are recommended but not essential before treatment is instituted. Pelvic sonography may be indicated for the evaluation of an enlarged uterus or adnexal mass. The need for additional diagnostic studies depends on the clinical assessment of each patient.

The aim of therapy for acute menorrhagia in the adolescent should be to control bleeding, restore adequate intravascular volume, correct anemia, treat any underlying conditions, and prevent recurrence. Method and intensity obviously depend on the severity of hemorrhage. The adolescent in whom bleeding is mild to moderate and in whom there is no sign of hypovolemia can be treated on an outpatient basis, provided close follow-up and good compliance are ensured. These patients often have moderate anemia caused by prolonged bleeding. For patients who have severe hemorrhage, anemia (hemoglobin less than 8 g/dL), or hypovolemia, hospital admission is strongly recommended.

Initial treatment is usually medical rather than surgical. Given that the primary cause of bleeding is instability in the endometrium caused by fluctuating levels of estrogen, the goal of therapy is to stop the hemorrhage with estrogen and to stabilize the endometrium with progestogens. Birth control pills may be effective. These are administered at the rate of one pill every 4 hours until the bleeding subsides. If bleeding does not stop within 24 to 36 hours, other causes should be considered. If hemorrhaging is acute and severe, some centers, in addition to giving oral progestogens, administer intravenous conjugated estrogens at a dosage of 25 mg every 4 hours for not more than three doses. The major side effect of this therapy is nausea and vomiting, for which antinausea medications may be administered prophylactically. Blood is replaced when necessary.

When the bleeding stops or decreases appreciably, oral contraceptives are tapered gradually for the next 7 days and then continued at a rate of one pill per day for 21 days. Withdrawal bleeding occurs after the discontinuation of treatment. The patient should be informed that this bleeding may be heavy but will be self-limited.

Dilation and curettage (D&C) is reserved for when medical treatment fails to control the bleeding within 24 to 36 hours. Because the incidence of intrauterine abnormality is small, this intervention is rarely required. If medical management fails, the patient usually has endometrial hyperplasia. Curettings may be scant after complete endometrial slough.

Two patients have been encountered who did not respond to D&C (Goldstein DP, personal observation). In both, uterine packing controlled the bleeding. Iodoform gauze was left in place for 24 hours and then withdrawn slowly. Prophylactic antibiotics should always be administered in this unusual situation. The only patient who has required hysterectomy for acute menorrhagia was a 20-year-old woman with artificial heart valves who was receiving anticoagulation therapy.

Close follow-up of patients with acute menorrhagia is essential to prevent recurrence and to provide adequate emotional support. After the initial phase of therapy, the patient may remain anovulatory. Therefore, it is advisable to continue therapy with low-dose birth control pills for at least 3 months. The adolescent in need of birth control can be continued on low-dose oral contraceptives. When the risk for unwanted pregnancy is not a concern, the best approach is to start the patient on basal body temperature charts and to administer oral progesterones cyclically if the temperature curve is monophasic. A rational regimen is to induce withdrawal bleeding every 6 weeks with a 10-day course of medroxyprogesterone acetate, 10 mg daily. This treatment is usually adequate to prevent endometrial hyperproliferation. Because it does not suppress the hypothalamic-pituitary-ovarian axis, it allows the development of regular ovulatory

cycles. However, the patient may menstruate spontaneously between courses.

Long-term follow-up includes correction of anemia with iron supplements and nutritional counseling and surveillance for spontaneous occurrence of ovulatory cycles. Patients with acute menorrhagia during the perimenarchal period are at greater risk for chronic anovulation, infertility, and endometrial carcinoma.

The emotional aspects of this problem cannot be underestimated. A hemorrhagic event is a sad way to begin active reproductive life. Adequate explanation, reassurance, and psychological support during the acute episode and the subsequent months guide these patients through their menstrual problems optimistically.

Chronic Anovulation

Persistent Hypermenorrhea. Cyclic heavy menses are common in adolescents. These patients usually have menstrual cycles that range from 4 to 6 weeks and that are characterized by excessive bleeding, either in amount or duration. Although anovulation is the leading cause of recurrent hypermenorrhea in this population, other causes such as uterine abnormalies, coagulation defects, and systemic diseases must be considered.

Besides a thorough history and physical examination, the basic workup of these patients should consist of hemoglobin, hematocrit, and platelet count determination, screening clotting studies, and thyroid function tests. Therapy depends on the degree of the bleeding abnormality. Patients who have mildly increased menstrual flow and no secondary anemia can be managed expectantly. Basal body temperature recordings confirm the diagnosis of anovulation. Prostaglandin inhibitors may decrease the amount of bleeding. Adolescents in need of birth control obviously benefit from oral contraception. When treatment is required because of the degree of flow or because of associated anemia, medroxyprogesterone acetate is prescribed to regulate cycles and to induce a progestational effect on the endometrium. For these patients, 10 mg daily is administered from the 6th to the 25th day of each cycle. For most of these young patients, a calendar-month schedule (treatment for the first 10 days of each month) is understood more easily. After 3 to 6 months, therapy is discontinued and the patient is observed for spontaneous occurrence of ovulatory cycles. Failure of hormonal therapy is an indication for D&C.

Persistent Polymenorrhea. Too-frequent menstruation is another common occurrence in this age group. Anovulation is the most common cause of polymenorrhea in adolescents. In some patients, this menstrual abnormality may originate from a short follicular phase or from corpus luteum dysfunction, which usually is self-limiting, until the hypothalamic-pituitary-ovarian axis matures.

Physicians should be aware that reports of polymenorrhea are often unjustified. A thorough history often reveals that the patient calculates her intermenstrual interval from the last day of a period to the first day of the next one.

Keeping a menstrual calendar and receiving information about normal physiology are usually sufficient to reassure these adolescents.

When cycles are shorter than 21 days, therapy with medroxyprogesterone acetate, administered as described earlier, is indicated. It may be necessary to start the treatment on the 10th day of the cycle for a period of 15 days.

Control of Abnormal Bleeding for Patients Receiving Chemotherapy

Abnormal bleeding may occur as a result of chemotherapy in the postmenarchal adolescent with leukemia and a low platelet count. The patient should be examined gently; ultrasonography may be helpful to exclude pelvic disease if adequate bimanual examination is difficult in the virginal girl. Hormonal therapy, such as continuous low-dose birth control pills, can be prescribed to induce amenorrhea and endometrial atrophy until the patient has normal platelet function and can cope with normal menses. An option is to use GnRH agonists such as those used for the induction of amenorrhea (Laufer and Rein, 1993; Laufer et al, 1997).

Dysmenorrhea

Dysmenorrhea is probably the most common gynecologic abnormality in adolescents. Usually it is primary (or functional), but it can be secondary to endometriosis, obstructing müllerian anomalies, and other pelvic disease.

Typically, the 14- or 15-year-old teenager, 1 to 3 years after menarche, has crampy lower abdominal pain with each menstrual period. The pain starts within 1 to 4 hours of the onset of the menses and lasts for 24 to 48 hours. Sometimes the pain starts 1 to 2 days before the menses and continues for 2 to 4 days into the menses. Nausea or vomiting (or both), diarrhea, lower backache, thigh pain, headache, fatigue, nervousness, dizziness, or syncope may accompany the cramps. Although dysmenorrhea is usually associated with the onset of ovulatory menses, some adolescents may experience cramps with the first few anovulatory cycles or during episodes of anovulatory dysfunctional bleeding associated with heavy menses and clots.

Nonsteroidal anti-inflammatory drugs (NSAIDs) have been most widely studied for the relief of pain in dysmenorrhea. Results of numerous clinical studies have found these agents to be effective in adults and in adolescents, with pain relief in 67% to 86% of patients. Oral contraceptives lessen the severity of dysmenorrhea, probably in part because of their antiovulatory actions and their ability to produce endometrial hypoplasia, reduced menstrual flow, and subsequently, fewer prostaglandins.

In assessing the adolescent with dysmenorrhea, the physician must know the patient's menstrual history, timing of cramps and her body's response to them, and premenstrual symptoms. Key questions are: Do the cramps cause her to miss school? If so, how many days? Does she miss other activities, such as parties? Does she have nausea and vomiting, diarrhea, or dizziness? What medications has she used before? Did her mother or sister have cramps? Is there a family history of endometriosis? The question about previous medications is particularly crucial because many adolescents have tried over-the-counter ibuprofen in subtherapeutic doses and have dismissed its usefulness.

For the virginal girl of 13 or 14 who has mild cramps the first day of her menses, a normal physical examination, including inspection of the genitalia to exclude an abnormality of the hymen, is reassuring. Speculum examination is not necessary. Treatment includes a careful explanation to the patient of the nature of the problem and a chance for her to ask questions regarding her anatomy. Mild analgesics, such as aspirin, acetaminophen, and especially over-the-counter ibuprofen (200 to 400 mg) usually give symptomatic relief.

Adolescent girls with moderate or severe dysmenorrhea should have a careful pelvic examination. For most adolescents who are carefully prepared, a vaginal examination is atraumatic. In some patients, a rectoabdominal examination in the lithotomy position is all that is possible, but even this excludes adnexal tenderness and masses. Ultrasonography is useful in defining uterine and vaginal anomalies with obstruction.

If examination results are normal, treatment should be directed at symptomatic relief. The most common approach is to prescribe one of the NSAID compounds. For most patients, effective relief can be obtained by taking the antiprostaglandin medicine at the onset of the menses and continuing for the first 1 to 2 days of the cycle (or for the usual duration of cramps). The patient should be told to start as soon as she knows her menses are coming (*i.e.*, at the first sign of cramps or bleeding). A loading dose is important for patients in whom symptoms are severe and occur rapidly. Generally, giving the medication at the onset of the menses prevents the inadvertent administration of the drug to a pregnant woman. However, a patient with severe cramps who is not sexually active may benefit from starting the drug 1 or 2 days before the onset of her menses. It is possible that a patient will respond to one of these drugs and not to another; each should be tried in increasing dosages before another drug is tried. Because life stresses may decrease a drug's effectiveness, dosage should be based on a patient's response in more than one cycle. Medication is customarily prescribed for two to three cycles before the type or the dosage is changed. Previous dosages, particularly of ibuprofen, may have been inadequate for pain relief.

The NSAID compounds should be avoided in patients with known or suspected ulcer, gastrointestinal bleeding, clotting disorders (because of effects on platelet aggregation), and renal disease. Similarly, they should be avoided in patients about to undergo surgery, in those allergic to aspirin and NSAIDs, and in those with aspirin-induced asthma. All these drugs should be taken with food, though some patients prefer liquids on the first day of the cycle. Side effects of these drugs are minimal with short-term use, but the possibility of allergy and gastrointestinal irritation and bleeding should be explained to the patient.

Some patients report fluid retention or fatigue while taking these agents.

If NSAIDs are contraindicated or produce undesirable side effects, acetaminophen, often in combination with 15 to 30 mg codeine, can be prescribed to some patients. Usually only a few pills are needed each month, but adolescents often experience dizziness and nausea with codeine-containing medications.

The patient should be seen every 3 or 4 months to evaluate the effectiveness of the medication. Such visits also facilitate the doctor-patient rapport essential for the treatment of this problem. Although a few adolescents use the excuse of cramps to stay out of school or to gain sympathy from their mothers, patients should not be made to feel emotionally unstable because they have cramps. Some girls can continue to exercise during their menses; others find the discomfort too great on the first day. Girls who are involved in competitive sports and have fewer ovulatory menses appear to have less dysmenorrhea.

If dysmenorrhea is relieved by oral contraception, medication is usually prescribed for 3 to 6 months and then discontinued (often during the summer when school attendance is not disrupted). Often the patient continues to have relief from cramps for several additional (commonly anovulatory) cycles before the severe dysmenorrhea recurs. When the cramps recur, a trial of other antiprostaglandin drugs should be undertaken before oral contraceptive therapy is reinstituted. Sexually active adolescents with severe dysmenorrhea usually prefer to continue long-term oral contraceptive therapy. The return of increasingly severe dysmenorrhea in spite of oral contraceptive use raises the possibility of organic disease such as endometriosis and calls for a reevaluation and the consideration of laparoscopy for diagnosis.

Pelvic Pain

If the patient does not respond to antiprostaglandin drugs and continues to have severe pain or vomiting, or if she needs birth control at the initial evaluation, a course of oral contraceptives should be tried. Pelvic examination is necessary before this medication is prescribed. Cramps are usually substantially, if not completely, relieved by anovulatory cycles and scantier flow. If severe cramps persist despite three to four cycles of ovulation suppression therapy, or if the examination reveals tenderness or modularity, laparoscopy is indicated to exclude endometriosis or other organic causes.

Acute Pelvic Pain

Acute pelvic pain necessitates aggressive management because of the intensity of symptoms and the possibility that a life-threatening condition exists. Differential diagnosis of acute pelvic pain in adolescents is summarized in Box 12-4. Gynecologic causes can be divided into three categories: infection, rupture, and torsion. In general, symptoms associated with infection usually develop progressively over a few days. If there is rupture or torsion, pain occurs suddenly, and

---

BOX 12-4
DIFFERENTIAL DIAGNOSIS OF ACUTE PELVIC PAIN IN ADOLESCENT GIRLS

Gynecologic Causes

Infection
Pelvic inflammatory disease

Rupture
Follicular cyst
Corpus luteum cyst
Ectopic pregnancy
Endometrioma
Tumor

Torsion
Ovarian cyst
Tube
Hydatid of Morgagni

Nongynecologic Causes

Gastrointestinal
Appendicitis
Meckel's diverticulitis
Gastroenteritis
Mesentery adenitis
Intestinal obstruction

Urinary
Cystitis
Pyelonephritis
Calculi

---

the patient often knows precisely at what time symptoms began. Nongynecologic causes primarily involve the digestive or the urinary tract.

Patient history should define the sequence of events, the location of pain and its radiation, and associated gastrointestinal, urinary tract, and systemic symptoms. Careful menstrual, contraceptive, and sexual history is mandatory.

Complete physical examination should be performed. Special attention should be given to the abdomen to localize the pain, to determine the presence and identity of signs of peritoneal infection, and to show evidence of bowel obstruction. Pelvic examination must be performed on each patient to determine the size, shape, and symmetry of the uterus and to identify adnexal or cervical tenderness and adnexal masses or thickening.

Basic laboratory workup should include complete blood count with differential diagnosis, erythrocyte sedimentation rate (ESR), complete urinalysis, urine culture, pregnancy test, and cervical culture for *N. gonorrhea* and *C. trachomatis.*

A high white blood cell count or a high ESR suggests either an infectious or an inflammatory process or ischemia secondary to adnexal torsion or bowel obstruction. Hemoglobin and hematocrit levels usually are poor indicators of bleeding because in acute hemorrhage, hemodilution may not have occurred. It should be remembered that negative pregnancy test results do not always rule out early intrauterine or ectopic pregnancy.

If pelvic examination results are not satisfactory, pelvic ultrasonography may confirm the presence of a mass, identify free fluid in the cul-de-sac of Douglas, or localize a suspected pregnancy.

At this point, laparoscopy becomes an invaluable diagnostic tool. The potential necessity of a surgical diagnostic procedure remains a concern for many physicians. Laparoscopy provides an immediate diagnosis that allows appropriate medical or surgical treatment. It is also more cost effective to perform immediate laparoscopy than to subject the patient to a long period of inpatient observation during which a surgical catastrophe, such as a ruptured appendix or an ectopic pregnancy, remains a possibility. If a patient has ruptured ovarian cysts or a hemorrhagic corpus luteum, in which there is no more active bleeding, it is possible to aspirate free blood and clots and to ensure hemostasis by fulguration of the bleeders. This technique may save the patient several days of agonizing pain and allow her to be discharged within 12 hours of the procedure. The advantages of laparoscopy outweigh the minimal surgical risks in these generally healthy teenagers, particularly if appendicitis is a real possibility (Goldstein et al, 1980b).

Table 12-3 summarizes the principal laparoscopic diagnoses in 121 patients, ages 11 to 17, treated for acute abdominal pain at Boston's Children's Hospital between 1980 and 1986. The most common cause of pain was complication from an ovarian cyst. Causes of acute abdominal pain in the adolescent do not appear to be age related (Table 12-4).

Chronic Pelvic Pain

Chronic pelvic pain (CPP) in adolescents is common and is a source of frustration for the patient, her parents, and her physician. It can be defined as 3 months or more of constant or intermittent, cyclic or acyclic pelvic pain that has neces-

sitated at least three separate visits to a physician and has not resulted in a definite diagnosis. Symptoms are dull or severe pain, dysmenorrhea, dyspareunia, or vaginal pain. Patients have been absent from school often, have seen a number of physicians, have undergone a number of radiologic examinations, and have tried a variety of analgesics without success. Many have already been referred for psychologic or psychiatric evaluation.

After having been told, often more than once, that nothing is wrong with her, the patient with CPP may feel a considerable amount of anger, frustration, or desperation. It is important to assure her that all efforts will be made to resolve her problem and that she will not be abandoned, nor her symptoms dismissed, as merely psychosomatic.

Box 12-5 summarizes the differential diagnosis of CPP in adolescent girls. It includes many organ systems that may be responsible for symptoms, either directly or by referred pain, and it includes symptoms of functional or psychogenic cause. An efficient approach to the problem involves taking a thorough history, performing an adequate physical examination, and judiciously using diagnostic studies.

It is essential to review the complete pain history, including the description, location, and radiation of the pain, exacerbating and relieving factors, association with the menstrual cycle, or association with gastrointestinal, urinary, and musculoskeletal symptoms. Medical and surgical history also may provide a clue. All previous diagnostic procedures and treatment trials should be recorded, and old medical records should be obtained if possible. Familial and social history and association of the pain episodes with stressful events should be detailed.

A complete physical examination should be performed and the abdomen carefully palpated to search for any masses, tender areas, or organomegaly. Special care should be taken

Table 12-3   Principal Laparoscopic Diagnoses in 121 Adolescent Girls, 11 to 17 Years Old, with Acute Pelvic Pain

Diagnosis	No. Patients (%)
Ovarian cyst	47 (39)
Acute pelvic inflammatory disease	21 (17)
Adnexal torsion	9 (8)
Endometriosis	6 (5)
Ectopic pregnancy	4 (3)
Appendicitis	13 (11)
No abnormality	21 (17)

From Emans SJ, Laufer MR, Goldstein DP: *Pediatric and adolescent gynecology,* 4th ed, Philadelphia, 1998, Lippincott-Raven.

Data are from Children's Hospital, Boston, 1980-1986.

Table 12-4   Age-Related Prevalence of Principal Laparoscopic Findings in 121 Adolescent Girls, 11 to 17 Years Old, with Acute Pelvic Pain

Diagnosis	No. Patients (%) Ages 11-13	Ages 14-15	Ages 16-17
Ovarian cyst	12 (50)	16 (35)	19 (37)
Acute pelvic inflammatory disease	4 (17)	7 (16)	10 (19)
Adnexal torsion	0 (0)	7 (16)	2 (4)
Endometriosis	0 (0)	2 (4)	4 (7)
Ectopic pregnancy	0 (0)	3 (7)	1 (2)
Appendicitis	3 (13)	4 (9)	6 (12)
No abnormality	5 (20)	6 (13)	10 (19)
Total	24 (20)	45 (37)	52 (43)

From Emans SJ, Laufer MR, Goldstein DP: *Pediatric and adolescent gynecology,* 4th ed, Philadelphia, 1998, Lippincott-Raven.

Data are from Children's Hospital, Boston, 1980-1986.

to differentiate deep pain from abdominal wall tenderness, especially among patients who have undergone previous surgery and who may have adhesions to the abdominal wall scar. It is also important to make a skeletal assessment to identify any orthopedic abnormality that may be the cause of referred pelvic pain or that may be associated with a congenital reproductive tract anomaly. Speculum examination should be performed to identify vaginal or cervical anomalies and to obtain cultures and specimens for cytologic analysis. Bimanual recto-vaginal-abdominal palpation allows evaluation of the pelvic structures and localization of tender areas. The posterior cul-de-sac of Douglas should also be assessed for pain and modularity.

Minimal laboratory workup in these patients consists of a complete blood count with differential white blood count and ESR, urinalysis, urine culture, and cervical cultures for *N. gonorrhea* and *C. trachomatis.* Other hematologic and biochemical studies are ordered depending on clinical indications.

Pelvic ultrasonography may be useful to define a mass, to provide information about a suspected genital tract malfor-

mation, and to screen patients in whom a satisfactory pelvic examination is impossible. Routine sonography in every patient is not advisable. A pelvic mass detected by ultrasonography often is not found during laparoscopy.

No specific rules can be given regarding radiologic examination. Submitting all these adolescents to pelvic radiation without clinical indication is not advisable. Gastrointestinal, urologic, and orthopedic studies should be ordered on the basis of the diagnosis made after thorough history, physical examination, and laboratory findings.

Laparoscopy is invaluable in the diagnosis of CPP. It can diagnose or confirm organic disease that cannot be demonstrated by physical, radiologic, and sonographic examinations. It allows the surgeon to obtain appropriate biopsies and to perform some primary therapy, such as fulguration of endometriosis, lysis of adhesions, and aspiration of ovarian cysts. Negative findings at laparoscopy may be equally valuable in that they reassure the patient that no organic disease is present, and they may help her accept the idea that she may have a functional problem that requires medical or psychological treatment.

Adolescents with CPP should undergo laparoscopy if the following are true:

- Dysmenorrhea is unresponsive to the usual therapy with prostaglandin inhibitors, ovulation suppression, or both.
- Clinically suspected endometriosis, chronic pelvic inflammatory disease, pelvic adhesions, appendiceal fecaliths, ovarian cysts, or pelvic serositis is confirmed or excluded.
- Undiagnosed pain must be evaluated after the appropriate workup.

At the Children's Hospital, 282 patients with CPP (age range, 9 to 21 years) underwent diagnostic laparoscopy between July 1974 and December 1983 because of chronic pelvic symptoms (Goldstein et al, 1980b). Most had been referred after negative findings on gastrointestinal and urinary tract workups or because of dysmenorrhea unresponsive to the usual therapy of prostaglandin inhibitors or oral contraceptives. Many had undergone psychiatric evaluation because of persistent and undiagnosed pain. Incidences of chronic PID were not included in the data because this condition is usually suspected because of the history and an elevated ESR. In these patients, laparoscopy is usually performed to confirm the diagnosis and to evaluate the severity rather than to establish the cause of CPP.

Table 12-5 summarizes the postoperative diagnosis in these patients. Three quarters of the patients had intrapelvic disease. Endometriosis, diagnosed in 45% of patients, was the most common finding. In most instances, the disease was mild to moderate, and implants were located in the posterior cul-de-sac of Douglas, on the ovaries, and on the lateral pelvic walls. The next most common finding was postoperative adhesions, which were found in 13% of patients and were, for the most part, secondary to appendectomy or ovarian cystectomy.

BOX 12-5
DIFFERENTIAL DIAGNOSIS OF CHRONIC PELVIC PAIN IN ADOLESCENT GIRLS

Gynecologic causes
    Dysmenorrhea (primary, secondary)
    Mittelschmerz
    Endometriosis
    Chronic pelvic inflammatory disease
    Ovarian cyst
    Genital tract malformations
    Pelvic congestion
    Pelvic serositis

Gastrointestinal causes
    Constipation, bowel spasms
    Appendiceal fecaliths
    Inflammatory bowel diseases
    Dietary intolerance (lactose)

Urinary causes
    Urinary tract infection
    Hydronephrosis
    Urethral stricture
    Urethral caruncle
    Urinary retention

Orthopedic causes
    Lordosis, kyphosis, scoliosis
    Herniation of intervertebral disk

Adhesions
    After surgery
    After pelvic infection

Psychogenic

One of the most puzzling laparoscopic findings was the presence of pelvic serositis in 5% of the patients. It is characterized by hyperemia and by granuloma-like lesions of the pelvic peritoneum and the uterine serosa. Peritoneal biopsies revealed the presence of mesothelial hyperplasia with hemosiderin deposits. Peritoneal culture and cytology findings were normal. The significance of these changes remains unclear. Pelvic peritoneal biopsies have demonstrated endosalpingiosis, which has symptoms similar to those for endometriosis and responds to medical therapy (Laufer et al, 1998). Identification of subtle endometriosis lesions can be facilitated by the use of a liquid distention medium in the pelvis that assists in the three-dimensional visualization of small, clear vesicles that could otherwise be confused as reflections of light on laparoscopic evaluation (Laufer, 1997). Other findings include ovarian cysts, obstructive uterine malformations, ileitis, infarcted hydatid of Morgagni, and pelvic congestion.

No organic disease was documented in 25% of the patients. In this group, pain was attributed to functional bowel disease or to psychogenic factors. Despite apparently normal bowel function, the condition of many teenagers with CPP improves when they are placed on a regimen of stool softeners and increased dietary fiber and fluid intake. The value of a negative laparoscopy should not be underestimated. In many instances the assurance that their pelvic structures are normal is sufficient to alleviate the symptoms in these adolescents. A significant number of these patients show symptomatic improvement after negative laparoscopy. In some, adjunctive psychological or behavioral modification therapy is necessary.

Results for patients treated between 1980 and 1983 are categorized by age group (Table 12-6). The incidence of endometriosis among adolescents with CPP increases progressively with age, from 12% in the 11- to 13-year-old group to 54% in the 20- to 21-year-old age group. Pelvic serositis was encountered mostly in the 11- to 15-year-old group. Other findings remained fairly constant in all age groups.

A more recent study at Children's Hospital, Boston evaluated patients between 13 to 21 years who had pelvic pain of more than 3 months' duration but who did not respond to NSAIDs or OCPs (Laufer et al, 1997). Approximately 70% women had endometriosis; all laparoscopic findings are shown in Table 12-7. Symptoms in patients with and without endometriosis are shown in Table 12-8.

Other series of laparoscopic findings in adolescents have found a higher proportion of patients with pelvic inflammatory disease. This may reflect the population studied (inner city versus suburban), the inclusion-exclusion criteria, the ability to recognize early or atypical endometriosis, and the distribution of the age of the study population. For example, in a study of 100 patients between the ages of 15 and 19 years, Strickland et al (1988) found that 46 had a normal pelvis, 29 had evidence of pelvic inflammatory disease, 12 had endometriosis, and 13 had another pelvic abnormality (including paratubal cysts, multicystic ovaries, and adhesions).

Table 12-5 Postoperative Diagnosis in 282 Adolescent Girls with Chronic Pelvic Pain

Diagnosis	No. Patients (%)
Endometriosis	126 (45)
Postoperative adhesions	37 (13)
Serositis	15 (5)
Ovarian cyst	14 (5)
Uterine malformation	15 (5)
Others*	4 (2)
No abnormality	71 (25)

From Emans SJ, Laufer MR, Goldstein DP: *Pediatric and adolescent gynecology,* 4th ed, Philadelphia, 1998, Lippincott-Raven.

*Ileitis, infarcted hydatid of Morgagni, pelvic congestion.

Data are from Children's Hospital, Boston, 1974-1983.

Table 12-6 Age-Related Incidence of Laparoscopic Findings in 129 Adolescent Girls and Young Women with Chronic Pelvic Pain

Diagnosis	No. Patients (%)				
	Ages 11-13	Ages 14-15	Ages 16-17	Ages 18-19	Ages 20-21
Endometriosis	2 (12)	9 (28)	21 (40)	17 (45)	7 (54)
Postoperative adhesions	1 (6)	4 (13)	7 (13)	5 (13)	2 (15)
Serositis	5 (29)	4 (13)	0 (0)	2 (5)	0 (0)
Ovarian cyst	2 (12)	2 (6)	3 (5)	2 (5)	0 (0)
Uterine malformation	1 (6)	0 (0)	1 (2)	0 (0)	1 (8)
Others	0 (0)	1 (3)	2 (4)	1 (3)	0 (0)
No abnormality	6 (35)	12 (37)	19 (36)	11 (29)	3 (23)

From Emans SJ, Laufer MR, Goldstein DP: *Pediatric and adolescent gynecology,* 4th ed, Philadelphia, 1998, Lippincott-Raven.

Data are from Children's Hospital, Boston, 1980-1983.

Acute and chronic pelvic pain in the adolescent patient must be taken seriously. In most an underlying cause can be identified. Under no circumstances should the label of psychogenic pain be proffered without negative laparoscopy results. Adequate diagnosis and early therapy are essential to improve the quality of life and to preserve reproductive capability of these young patients.

Treatment of Endometriosis in Adolescents

The importance of finding endometriosis early lies not only in the relief of symptoms but also, it is hoped, in the preservation of reproductive potential. Optimal therapy for adolescents and adult women with endometriosis is still debated. Patients must understand the advantages and disadvantages of each surgical and medical option and that endometriosis commonly recurs. Adolescents must know that studies in adult women have not shown increased infertility if endometriosis is minimal or mild.

Medical therapy for adolescents with pelvic pain from endometriosis is the same as that used for adults, as outlined in Chapter 19. GnRH agonists are used as a first-line therapy only in adolescents older than 16 because of concerns about the effects of permanent bone density; bone density modulation is an important event in adolescence. For adolescents younger than 16 who have endometriosis pain, continuous OCPs (pseudopregnancy) is the first line of medical therapy. After 6 months of GnRH agonist therapy for those older than 16 years, continuous OCPs or cyclic OCPs are initiated. If pelvic pain recurs, surgical resection of endometriosis may be necessitated. The use of a long-term GnRH agonist with hormonal "add-back" therapy may be appropriate for adolescents with persistent chronic endometriosis pain (Lubianca et al, 1998).

Obstructing and Nonobstructing Malformations of the Reproductive Tract

Many congenital abnormalities of the female genital tract are undiscovered until adolescence. These are usually diagnosed when symptoms occur, especially menstrual disorders and coital difficulties, or because most patients undergo their first pelvic examination at that time.

Although the diagnosis of some congenital malformations is obvious at first glance, the diagnosis of many of these defects requires a high index of suspicion. Thorough understanding of the nature of these anomalies is essential to the gynecologist who treats adolescents. Early diagnosis, adequate treatment, and appropriate psychologic support and counseling ensure the preservation of reproductive

Table 12-7   Laparoscopic Findings of Adolescent Patients with Chronic Pelvic Pain Who Do Not Respond to OCPs and NSAIDs

Laparoscopic Findings	Number (%)
Visible endometriosis	31/46 (67.4)
Adhesions	11/46 (23.9)
Prior surgery	8
With endometriosis	3
Without endometriosis	5
No prior surgery	3
With endometriosis	3
Without endometriosis	0
Grossly normal pelvis	5/46 (10.9)
Functional cysts	4/46 (8.7)
Paratubal cysts	4/46 (8.7)
Müllerian anomalies	3/46 (6.5)
With endometriosis	1
Without endometriosis	2

From Laufer MR, Goitein L, Bush M, et al: Prevalence of endometriosis in adolescent women with chronic pelvic pain not responding to conventional therapy. *J Pediatr Adolesc Gynecol* 1997; 10:199-202.

OCP, over-the-counter preparation; NSAID, nonsteroidal antiinflammatory agent.

Table 12-8   Characteristics of Subjects With and Without Endometriosis

Characteristics	Patients With Endometriosis	Patients Without Endometriosis
Age (years)		
≤14	7 (21.8)	1 (7.2)
15-17	20 (62.5)	10 (71.4)
≥18	5 (15.6)	3 (21.4)
Mean age (years) at menarche	12.3	12.3
Mean time (months) at menarche	3.7	3.9
Duration of over-the-counter preparations (months)		
≤3	17 (53.1)	5 (35.7)
4-11	9 (28.1)	6 (42.9)
≥12	6 (18.8)	3 (21.4)
Prior surgery	3 (9.4)	5 (35.7)
Presenting symptoms		
Acyclic and cyclic pain	20 (62.5)	8 (57.1)
Acyclic pain	9 (28.1)	3 (21.4)
Cyclic pain	3 (9.4)	3 (21.4)
Gastrointestinal pain	11 (34.3)	6 (42.9)
Urinary symptoms	4 (12.5)	4 (33.3)
Irregular menses	3 (9.4)	6 (42.9)*
Vaginal discharge	2 (6.3)	2 (14.3)

From Laufer MR, Goitein L, Bush M, et al: Prevalence of endometriosis in adolescent women with chronic pelvic pain not responding to conventional therapy. *J Pediatr Adolesc Gynecol* 1997; 10:199-202.

*$P < 0.05$.

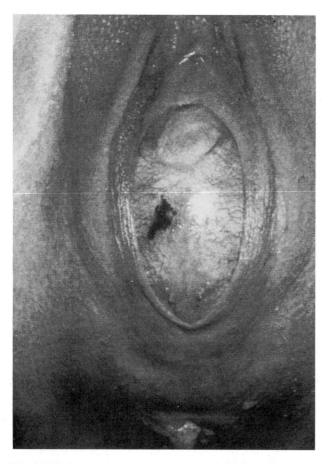

Fig. 12-16. Imperforate hymen in postpubertal patient who had abdominal pain, urinary retention, and a large pelvic mass, and from whose vagina 850 mL old blood was evacuated after hymenectomy.

function when feasible and allow these patients to develop serene attitudes toward their sexuality.

Obstructive defects require immediate attention to remove the obstruction and to stop retrograde menstruation. When there is no obstruction, medical attention is not mandated until reproductive and coital function is desired.

Classification of Uterovaginal Anomalies

The American Fertility Society (1988) has devised a classification scheme of müllerian anomalies based on the degree of failure of normal development. It separates anomalies into groups of similar clinical manifestation and prognosis for fetal salvage on treatment. This classification system does not include vaginal anomalies, but it does allow the health care provider to describe anomalies involving the vagina, tubes, or urinary tract as associated malformations. Drawings and classification of uterine, cervical, and vaginal anomalies are shown in detail in more recent publications (Laufer and Goldstein, 1998b; Banerjee and Laufer, 1998). Some prefer a simpler scheme based on the presence of an obstructed outflow tract (Pinsonneault and Goldstein, 1985).

Imperforate Hymen with Hematocolpos (or Hydrocolpos)

Although the diagnosis of an imperforate hymen should be made long before adolescence (and optimally during routine neonatal and pediatric examinations), it is not unusual for a teenager to have the typical picture of primary amenorrhea, cyclic or acyclic pelvic pain, bulging hymen, and hematocolpos. Hematometra does not usually develop with simple imperforate hymen because the vagina has great distensibility and can accommodate a large amount of blood. It is, however, commonly seen with a high transverse septum.

An imperforate hymen is usually a congenital condition that results from the failure of degeneration of the central epithelial cells of the hymenal membrane. If estrogen-induced secretions do not distend the vagina and the uterus at birth, the imperforate hymen may remain asymptomatic until after puberty. At that time, the accumulation of menstrual material engorges the vaginal tract, causing pelvic or abdominal pain. It is of historic interest that this condition was known to Aristotle and was mentioned in his treatise, the "Generation of Animals":

> We know of instances of women in whom the 'os uteri' was grown together and continued so until the time arrived for the menstrual discharge to begin and pain come on; in some, the passage burst open of its own accord, in others, it was separated by physicians; and in some cases, where the opening either was forcibly made or could not be made at all, the patients succumbed.

Imperforate hymen is usually diagnosed before a patient is 15 years of age. A cystic mass formed by the enlargement of the vagina and displacement of the uterus can extend above the symphysis and into the abdominal cavity. Abdominal pain is a regular symptom, and urinary difficulties, primarily acute retention, may develop. Many patients who have been inadequately examined undergo extensive radiologic evaluation before the correct diagnosis is made. Examination of the external genitalia reveals a mass protruding between the labia majora. The bulging mass varies in size, is bluish-red, and is continuous with the pelvic mass (Fig. 12-16). Constipation results in some patients because of pressure on the rectum from the distended vagina. Surgical therapy consists of hymenotomy, which often reveals a large accumulation of blood (hematocolpos), or secretion (hydrocolpos), depending on the age of the patient. The central part of the hymen should be excised to allow for further unobstructed menstrual flow. Needle-tip electrocautery facilitates hemostasis on the hymenal edge. This averts the need for multiple sutures and minimizes the stricture. The use of a Yankauer suction tip, inserted high into the vagina or through the dilated cervix into the uterus, facilitates evacuation. At times the wall suction becomes plugged, and a high-speed suction evacuator is required. Infection is rare once drainage is established, and prophylactic antibody therapy is not required. The distended vagina promptly regresses within days without long-term effects.

Uterine Duplication with Obstructed Hemivagina

In general, abnormalities of uterovaginal fusion diagnosed during adolescent years are obstructive. These anomalies can be divided into three categories, according to the site of obstruction. At The Children's Hospital, in a study of 28 uterine or vaginal obstructing duplications, the most commonly encountered anomaly was a didelphic uterus with unilateral vaginal obstruction secondary to a blind vagina (Pinsonneault and Goldstein, 1985). A unicornuate uterus with a contralateral blind horn, either rudimentary or of normal size, was second in frequency. Several patients had cervical obstruction of one horn of a bicornuate uterus associated with an ipsilateral blind vaginal pouch. Fistulous tracts of various types may connect the blind vagina to a septate cervix or to the main vaginal cavity. Intercervical fistulas also have been discovered.

Signs and symptoms depend on the type of the abnormality. Because the obstruction appeared only on one side in these patients, primary amenorrhea was not a feature.

By far the most common symptom is pelvic pain, either cyclic or acyclic, which is the consequence of unilaterally obstructed menstrual flow and secondary endometriosis. Other common symptoms include abnormal vaginal bleeding and purulent discharge usually associated with a fistulous tract connecting the obstructed to the unobstructed side. If a patient has a blind vagina, distention with menstrual blood may give rise to vaginal pain or to the sensation of pressure. During a physical examination, masses corresponding to distended pelvic structures, abnormal uterine shape, and discharge from possible fistulas usually can be visualized or palpated.

The minimal workup of these patients should include combined pelvic and renal sonography and IVP. In one series, unilateral renal agenesis and other urinary tract abnormalities were found in 75% of the patients. Renal tract abnormalities occur when factors affecting the development of the mesonephric duct or the paramesonephric duct lead to abnormal renal development. Mesonephric duct agenesis results not only in unilateral agenesis of the wolffian-derived genital structures but also unilateral renal agenesis. Laparoscopy and hysterosalpingography should be performed to determine the exact nature of the anomaly. Magnetic resonance imaging accurately assesses the anomaly without invasive procedures. Despite its cost, this technique should be seriously considered.

Treatment consists of surgical excision of the vaginal septum. Because the septum may be thick, surgery may be challenging. Generally, abdominal exploration is unnecessary and uterine reconstruction is not indicated. Reproductive potential is related to which category of double uterus a patient has, unless a delay in diagnosis has resulted in endometriosis or has destroyed tubal function.

Blind Uterine Horn

Asymmetric obstruction of the uterus, such as unicornuate uterus with a noncommunicating uterine anlagen and active endometrium, is rare and may pose a diagnostic dilemma.

Often, the patient is considered to have severe dysmenorrhea, and treatment with birth control pills or pain medication is instituted before an adequate workup is completed. With the advent of ultrasonography and MRI, this omission occurs less often and patients are investigated if their response medication is poor.

Dysmenorrhea or cyclic abdominal pain from cryptomenorrhea may be the only symptoms. The patient may have endometriosis from retrograde menstruation or a tender mass. Removal of the obstructed horn is the procedure of choice and should alleviate symptoms.

Transverse Vaginal Septum

A vaginal septum is a relatively uncommon anomaly. Septa can be congenital or acquired, they can occur in various positions, and they can be multiple. Transverse septa can occur at any level above the hymenal ring to the junction of the vagina and cervix. Vertical septa can be oriented in an anteroposterior plane (sagittal septum) or in the lateral plane (coronal septum). Finally, septa can be complete or partial, perforate or imperforate.

Transverse vaginal septa occur from lack of complete canalization of the solid primitive vaginal plate or the sinovaginal bulbs. Vertical vaginal septa occur in two ways. Failure of the müllerian ducts to fuse results in a duplication of the uterus and the vagina. What appears to be a vertical vaginal septum is in fact a duplicated vagina; two vaginal openings are found. Incomplete canalization of the vaginal plate in a longitudinal direction results in a septum that may be oriented in either the anteroposterior plane or the lateral plane. Symptoms produced by vaginal septa depend on the age of the patient, the degree of vaginal obstruction, and the amount of stimulation of the cervical mucous glands by circulating estrogen. The neonate with a completely obstructed vagina resulting from a transverse septum may have hydrometrocolpos. However, a transverse vaginal septum may not be recognized until the patient reaches menarche, when hematocolpos develops. The neonate or the older patient with a complete vertical septum may have a unilateral hydrocolpos or hematocolpos, whereas an older patient with an incomplete vertical septum may seek help for dyspareunia or, if pregnant, for difficulty in delivery.

Symptoms depend on the width and the location of the anomaly. A narrow annular septum usually is a fortuitous finding of no clinical significance and does not require any treatment. On the other hand, primary amenorrhea and early symptoms of obstruction develop in patients with complete septa, and surgical excision is imperative. When the upper and the lower vagina communicate only by a small fistulous tract through the septum, the clinical picture can be puzzling. These patients may have dysmenorrhea, irregular vaginal spotting, or purulent discharge because of partial obstruction and accumulation of infected blood above the defect. Secondary PID from ananaerobic infection may also be the initial symptom. A septum lying low in the vagina is often the cause of dyspareunia. Infertility and soft tissue dystocia are unusual symptoms of this malformation in adolescents.

Surgical correction consists of complete excision of the septum and anastomosis of the upper vagina to the lower vagina. This may prove difficult, depending on the thickness of the septum. Before surgery, MRI may help to define the thickness. A stent may be necessary if the septum involves a long vaginal segment and primary anastomosis is impossible. Care must be taken not to injure the urethra or the rectum. The use of a urinary catheter and a finger in the rectum can guide surgery.

After surgery, periodic vaginal examination at 6-week intervals should be performed with dilations as necessary. Recurrence is rare if the septum is entirely excised. Stricture may be encountered after surgery, and subsequent surgery may be required. A Z-plasty technique helps minimize the problem. In some patients, however, the fallopian tubes will have developed some degree of fibrosis from pyocolpos because of backflow before treatment,

Cervicovaginal Agenesis

Congenital absence of the cervix can occur in association with vaginal agenesis or with a normal vagina. This rare clinical entity causes early obstructive signs and symptoms characterized by hematometra, tubal regurgitation of menstrual blood with hematosalpingitis, and secondary endometriosis. In many patients, cyclic abdominal pain and amenorrhea are the presenting symptoms. The diagnosis is difficult to make before surgery, but ultrasonography and MRI have made this condition more recognizable. Attempts to preserve fertility by the creation of a fistulous tract between the endometrial cavity and the vagina have been disappointing (Casey and Laufer, 1997).

A conservative surgical approach usually leads to multiple operations, and only two successful pregnancies are reported in the literature. There have been reports of several deaths from sepsis after conservative surgery was attempted. The recommended therapy of cervical agenesis, therefore, remains hysterectomy with ovarian conservation, if possible.

Nonobstructive Malformations
Longitudinal Vaginal Septa

Longitudinal vaginal septa occur in association with abnormalities of uterine fusion, but they may be isolated malformations. Such septa divide the vagina sagittally into equal or unequal parts for its entire or partial length. Surgical excision is indicated when dyspareunia becomes a problem or when childbearing is anticipated.

Uterine Agenesis

Absence of the uterus is noted in some patients with male pseudohermaphrodism and testicular feminization. These apparently female patients are genetic males, and they have negative sex chromatin and XY karyotype. They do not menstruate and cannot bear children, but their external genitalia are those of a normal female. They feminize at puberty and have good breast development; in rare instances, they have rudimentary tubes and uteri. They also have intraabdominal or inguinal testes with nests of Leydig cells.

Similarly, the uterus is absent in most male pseudohermaphrodites with ambiguous genitalia. They may have testes situated intraabdominally, in the inguinal canal, or in the scrotum. The vagina can differ in size and length and often communicates with a hypospadiac urethra. Some male pseudohermaphrodites with ambiguous external genitalia have uteri and tubes. This can be of practical importance if, at laparotomy, gonads at the site of ovaries are seen in a child with tubes, uterus, and vagina; such gonads can be testes.

Vaginal Agenesis

Failure of development of the müllerian ducts at any time between origin and fusion with the urogenital sinus results in failure of development of the uterus and the vagina. The Mayer-Rokitansky-Küster-Hauser syndrome is the most common clinical example of this anomaly. In approximately 90% of patients, the uterus is rudimentary anlagen and the vagina is congenitally absent. Some series have included patients with uteri and absences of varying lengths of the vagina; however, these patients generally are not considered to have Mayer-Rokitansky-Küster-Hauser syndrome. They are more appropriately categorized as having defects in vertical fusion. The homogeneity and specificity of Mayer-Rokitansky-Küster-Hauser syndrome is the absence of a vagina and a uterus with a high incidence of urinary tract anomalies. Patients with disorders of vertical fusion have a low incidence of urinary tract anomalies.

Because these patients have a 46,XX karyotype and normal ovarian function with normal development of external genitalia and secondary sexual characteristics, they usually seek treatment for amenorrhea. Ovulation occurs normally, but because the uterus and vagina are missing, menstruation does not occur. An exact genetic etiologic diagnosis has not been elucidated.

A significant number of patients with müllerian agenesis have associated anomalies of the upper müllerian duct system and anomalies of other organ systems. In the classic form of the müllerian agenesis, the uterus is present only in the form of bilateral rudimentary uterine anlagen. These anlagen are located on the lateral pelvic sidewall adjacent to the ovaries, and they are usually connected to the fallopian tubes. However, they are usually not palpable on bimanual examination. The anlagen may or may not have endometrial tissue. Even if the endometrium is functional, the cavity of the anlagen may not communicate directly with the peritoneal cavity as often because of an obstruction located at the junction of the tube and the uterine bulb. Occasionally, anlagen communicate with the peritoneal cavity through the fallopian tubes, and active endometrium, if they are present, may regurgitate into the peritoneal cavity.

Renal anomalies are perhaps the most well-known anomalies associated with Mayer-Rokitansky-Küster-Hauser syndrome. They develop in approximately one third of patients. Abnormalities of the skeletal system are reported to occur in one tenth.

A serum testosterone level should be determined to rule out an androgen-insensitivity syndrome. Chromosomal analysis can confirm the androgen insensitivity or may be found to be 46,XX and, thus, an aberration of the Mayer-Rokitansky-Küster-Hauser syndrome. Renal sonography or IVP is mandatory to define the excretory system and to rule out anomalies. In addition, a radiograph can evaluate the lower spine for skeletal anomalies. If symptoms suggest active uterine anlagen or if a pelvic mass is present, appropriate studies such as ultrasonography or MRI can differentiate among hematometra, hematocolpos, endometriomas, or other cysts.

If functional endometrial tissue is present, symptoms of cryptomenorrhea will begin soon after secondary sexual characteristics start to develop. Surgical removal of the anlagen affords complete relief of symptoms. Occasionally, patients have dysmenorrhea, though most 15- to 16-year-old patients seek treatment for primary amenorrhea.

Vaginoplasty is usually performed on patients between the ages of 17 and 20, when they are emotionally mature and are intellectually capable of understanding the surgical procedure and of partaking in the postoperative care, which is extremely important for a favorable outcome. Psychological counseling is extremely important in the management of these patients. The single most important factor in determining the success of vaginoplasty is the psychological adjustment of the patient to her anomaly.

Surgical and nonsurgical methods for creating a vagina have been described and have been used with success. Nonsurgical methods use dilation of the vaginal dimple to create a functional vagina. The first method was described by Robert Frank in 1938 and involves active manipulation by the patient to dilate the neovaginal space. Ingram (1981) described a technique of creating a new vagina using dilators specially designed for use with a bicycle seat stool.

In younger, less motivated patients, the Frank dilation technique may be difficult. Several surgical methods of creating a vaginal space have been described. The McIndoe (1950) procedure or, more appropriately, the Abbe-Wharton-McIndoe procedure, is superior to all others. In essence, a skin graft taken from the buttock is placed around a plastic form molded in the shape of a vagina, which is then placed into a surgically created space between the vagina and the rectum (Counsellor and Davis, 1968). The form remains in place for 7 days (Fig. 12-17).

Serious complications associated with the McIndoe procedure have diminished significantly as techniques and experience have improved. Complications, however, still exist. These include morbidity and mortality from anesthesia, infection, and hemorrhage, failure of the graft to take, and formation of postoperative granulation tissues. Fistulas from the lower urinary tract or the rectum into the neovagina have

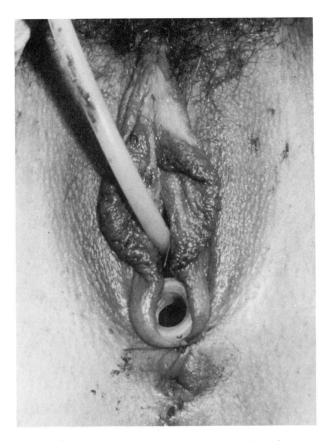

Fig. 12-17. Counsellor stent in place after the creation of a neovagina with a split-thickness skin graft (McIndoe procedure).

been reported in approximately 4% of patients. Malignancies have also been reported in the neovagina.

Other surgical procedures have been used and may sometimes be applicable. Under special circumstances, the vulvovaginal pouch of Williams (Fig. 12-18) or the sigmoid transplant of Pratt may be used.

Hymenal Anomalies

Incomplete fenestration of the hymenal opening is usually asymptomatic. Patients with this condition seek gynecologic treatment because of unsuccessful attempts at inserting tampons or because of coital difficulties. With a microperforate hymen, the adolescent may also report postmenstrual vaginal spotting or malodorous discharge secondary to incomplete obstruction and poor drainage. Hymenectomy should be performed in all patients.

If the diagnosis is made fortuitously, the patient should be told about this anatomic variant and informed of the necessity of surgical correction. Performing the procedure during early adolescence allows the patient to use tampons without problems and may avoid later embarrassment when the patient desires to become sexually active.

Vulvar Anomalies

In some instances, one or both labia minora are unusually large, and the patient consults because she notices this

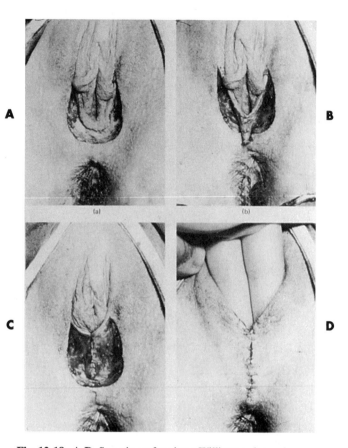

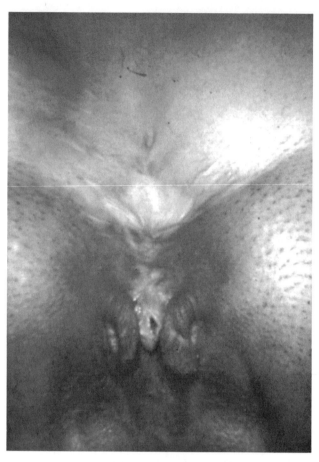

Fig. 12-18. **A-D,** Steps in performing a Williams vulvovaginoplasty, which creates a functional perineal pouch adequate for intercourse. Used primarily to augment a short vagina or a neovagina.

Fig. 12-19. Gynecologic features of bladder exstrophy in adolescent after successful bladder repair.

anomaly or because she experiences symptoms of irritation associated with exercise. Simple reassurance is usually all that is necessary. Comparison with asymmetry or hypertrophy of other parts of the body may help the patient to accept this peculiarity. Careful hygiene and the avoidance of tight clothing relieve discomfort. If these measures are ineffective, or if there is a troublesome cosmetic problem, surgical reduction is an option. This can be accomplished in the ambulatory operating room by resection of the redundant labia so that they are symmetrical (Laufer and Galvin, 1995). Closure of the excised area is best accomplished with a running locking stitch of 3-0 chromic. The results usually are excellent, and patients generally are pleased (see Fig. 12-11). An alternative method is shown in Fig. 12-12.

Gynecologic Sequelae of Bladder Exstrophy

Fortunately, exstrophy of the urinary bladder is an uncommon anomaly. It is distressing, frightening, and repulsive to the parents of a newborn. The term exstrophy comes from two Greek words; the prefix *exo* means "outside of" and the verb *strophe* means "to twist or turn about." The distraught parents see a child with a twisted, inside-out urinary bladder accompanied by abnormal genitalia.

Girls with this condition always have a bifid clitoris. Several series report a high incidence of myelomeningocele,

which is significant in terms of sphincter incontinence. The distance from the umbilicus to the anus is foreshortened. Often the umbilicus is just cephalad to the exotropic bladder, and sometimes it is associated with an omphalocele. The anal aperture is often close to the vagina (Chisholm, 1980).

Characteristically, the girl with bladder exstrophy requires gynecologic treatment after puberty because of abnormalities of the lower abdominal and vulvar areas that result from her urologic reconstruction (Fig. 12-19). Examination reveals scarring and deformity of the mons pubis, asymmetry of the labia, bifid clitoris, and introital stenosis. The upper tract is usually normal. Bladder exstrophy is one of the conditions that leads to congenital prolapse of the uterus; myelodysplasia and spinal bifida are the other two. From the psychological standpoint, these patients are distraught because of their strange appearance and often shun their emerging female sexuality. It is important, therefore, to assure them that total reconstruction can be accomplished.

Surgery corrects the anomalies. Usually it is necessary to perform a monsplasty, Williams vulvovaginoplasty, and Manchester-Fotnerquill procedure in a one-stage operation. The results usually are excellent, and full function is restored. Patients eventually can become pregnant, but deliv-

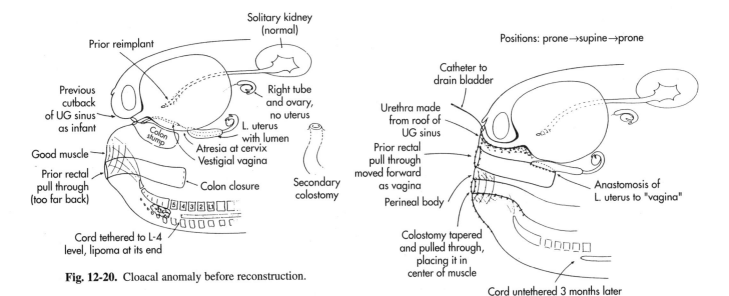

Fig. 12-20. Cloacal anomaly before reconstruction.

Fig. 12-21. Cloacal anomaly after reconstruction.

ery should be abdominal because of the abnormal configuration of the bony pelvis and fixation of the uterus.

Cloacal Anomalies

The remarkable similarity among otherwise normal persons with this bizarre defect suggests a similar mode of developmental disease. It has at its inception a single localized defect—theoretically in the early development of the mesoderm—that later contributes to the infraumbilical mesenchyme, cloacal septum, and caudal vertebrae. Consequences of this are as follows:

- failure of cloacal septation, with the persistence of a common cloaca into which the ureters, ileum, and a rudimentary hindgut open
- complete breakdown and exstrophy of the cloacal membrane with exstrophy of the cloaca, failure of fusion of the genital tubercles and pubic rami, and often omphalocele
- incomplete development of the lumbosacral vertebrae with herniation of a grossly dilated central canal of the spinal cord (hydromyelia), yielding a soft, cystic, skin-covered mass over the sacral area, sometimes asymmetric in its positioning (Fig. 12-20)

The rudimentary hindgut may contain two appendices, and no anal opening is evident. The small intestine may be relatively short. Cryptorchidism is a usual finding in males. Affected females have unfused müllerian elements with completely bifid uterine horns and short, duplicated, or atretic vaginas. Most patients have a single umbilical artery, and anomalies of the lower limbs are occasionally present. Surgical intervention should attempt to reestablish normal function of the urinary, gastrointestinal, and reproductive tracts (Fig. 12-21).

Gynecologic Problems in Chronic Diseases

Adolescents with chronic diseases and malignancies have benefited from improved medical management and now seek care for a number of gynecologic problems that were fatal in the past. Even the healthy adolescent girl may have difficulties as she experiences pubertal changes and new sexual feelings; the adolescent with a chronic disease has special needs that must be understood and must be given attention. Although only some of the common chronic diseases (cystic fibrosis, end-stage renal disease, diabetes mellitus, Crohn disease, sickle cell disease, and malignancy) are covered in this chapter, the physician must approach every adolescent with sensitivity to her unique concerns. This sensitivity will also enable the physician to treat patients with many chronic diseases not mentioned. Undoubtedly, an entire text could be devoted to the special gynecologic problems adolescents encounter in coping with chronic illness (Emans et al, 1990; Perlman et al, 1998).

Cystic Fibrosis

Cystic fibrosis is the most common lethal hereditary disease in the white population. Although in the past many children with cystic fibrosis died during infancy and early childhood, many patients with cystic fibrosis now live through their adolescence and into their reproductive years. Because these adolescents often have low weight for their height and chronic pulmonary infections, they often experience delays in pubertal development and menarchal age.

The adolescent with delayed menarche who was diagnosed with cystic fibrosis earlier in life has a lower weight-for-height index, a lower height, and a lower percentage of body fat than a postmenarchal girl. Because normal levels of sex steroids and gonadotropins usually are reached in late adolescence, the adolescent with cystic fibrosis and amenorrhea should receive good medical and gynecologic assessment and supportive counseling. Other causes of amenorrhea, especially pregnancy, should be excluded and reassurance should be given about the potential for normal menstruation.

Contraceptive choices for the patient with cystic fibrosis are not simple. Although oral contraceptives do not appear to alter pulmonary function, long-term safety data are unavailable. The risk for fluid retention and other side effects from high-estrogen pills necessitates the prescription of a low-dose pill. Weight, pulmonary and cardiac status, and liver function should be carefully monitored. Patients with preexisting chronic liver disease need careful assessment of the potential risks of pregnancy versus the unknown risk for potential hepatic effects. For most adolescents with cystic fibrosis, oral contraceptives are well tolerated and offer the many advantages of reliable contraception, diminished menstrual flow, and improved dysmenorrhea. Barrier forms of contraception can be used by the mature adolescent. An intrauterine device (IUD) is not recommended for most nulliparous adolescents, and it may be especially difficult to monitor in adolescents with recurrent abdominal pain and severe constipation. Medroxyprogesterone acetate and levonorgestrel are also alternatives for these young women. Tubal ligation is an option for the young adult with cystic fibrosis who has made a definitive choice to avoid pregnancy.

Chronic Renal Disease

Like many patients with other severe chronic diseases, adolescents with end-stage renal disease usually experience a delay in pubertal growth and development and in menarche. Postmenarchal patients with uremia who are on chronic dialysis rarely have regular menses.

Prolactin levels are often elevated in patients with uremia who are on hemodialysis. Hyperprolactinemia appears to be a direct consequence of impaired renal function. Associated with the chronic anovulation of uremia, ovarian cysts develop more often in patients on dialysis than in those not on it. Ovarian cysts may be asymptomatic or may cause acute symptoms because of torsion or hemorrhage into the cyst (perhaps related to anticoagulant therapy). These ovarian cysts usually respond to hormone suppression therapy or resolve promptly after successful transplantation.

Uremic patients on dialysis usually require no therapy for amenorrhea other than gynecologic assessment to exclude other causes. Although it is a rare occurrence, adolescents on dialysis can become pregnant. Adolescents with dysfunctional uterine bleeding require assessment and, depending on the patient, treatment with oral contraceptives or GnRH analogues.

It is extraordinarily important for the adolescent who has undergone successful renal transplantation to understand that ovulation usually returns between 1 and 12 months after renal function approaches normal. Adolescents may not appreciate the increase in fertility and may become pregnant after transplantation because of risk-taking behavior. Contraceptive counseling is paramount. If the adolescent has no contraindications (*e.g.,* hypertension) to the use of oral contraceptive pills, a low-dose formulation can be used. In addition, medroxy-progesterone acetate or levonorgestrel may

be an option. The IUD is not a good choice for the immunosuppressed nulliparous adolescent because of the potential risk for sepsis. Barrier contraception is an acceptable option for the mature adolescent. Patients should have good renal status for a minimum of 2 years after transplantation before becoming pregnant.

Diabetes Mellitus

Adolescents with diabetes mellitus are more likely than adolescents with other chronic illnesses to experience menarche at a normal age. Postmenarchal adolescents with diabetes may have irregular menses, dysfunctional uterine bleeding, or prolonged amenorrhea. Gonadotropin and prolactin levels in patients with amenorrhea and diabetes are usually in the low to normal range despite low estradiol levels, suggesting depression of the hypothalamic-pituitary axis.

Adolescents with diabetes are often troubled by recurrent and persistent monilial vulvovaginitis. Improved diabetic control and long-term antifungal vaginal medications can be helpful.

Surprisingly, some diabetics who have marked swelling and erythema of the vulva in association with chronic candidiasis have few or no symptoms. Condyloma acuminata can be a persistent problem, especially in poorly controlled diabetics. Treatment with 85% trichloroacetic acid may result in suboptimal results. Because extreme burning and irritation develop in some patients with diabetes who take this medication, the initial application should be limited to only a few warts. Other patients may have warts that are resistant to treatment and may require a combination of improved glucose control, antimonilial vaginal medications, and other medications such as Imiquimod 5% cream which can be applied by the patient. A carbon dioxide laser can vaporize extensive condyloma acuminata. In addition, the use of electric loop diathermy has been proposed.

Providing contraceptive services to adolescents with diabetes involves balancing the risks and benefits of each form of birth control. Oral contraceptives can alter glucose tolerance and lipoprotein levels, and they have been associated with increased vascular complications in patients with diabetes. Although optimally oral contraceptives should be avoided in adolescents with diabetes, barrier forms of contraception may not be acceptable to the young risk-taking adolescent. Oral contraceptives do not appear to be associated with proliferative retinopathy, but the potential for accelerating the progress of this disorder remains a concern. Thus, low-dose oral contraceptives with 20 to 35 μg ethinyl estradiol and a low-dose progestin with minimal impact on glucose tolerance can be considered for adolescents with diabetes, but medical status, blood glucose, and serum holds should be monitored. Adolescents should be counseled to avoid smoking.

Crohn Disease

Adolescents with Crohn disease may experience growth failure, pubertal delay, and menarchal delay. In fact, delayed growth may be the first manifestation of Crohn disease and may not at first be recognized as secondary to a gastrointestinal problem. Gonadotropins and estrogen levels are low and imply a depressed hypothalamic-pituitary axis. Nutritional and medical therapy, and sometimes surgery, to treat active Crohn disease are important to ensure normal pubertal growth and development. Although excess corticosteroids may impair growth, a patient with active Crohn disease who receives dosages that adequately treat the illness often has a growth spurt.

Adolescents with Crohn disease may experience vulvar and perianal symptoms. Perianal lesions may be the first sign leading to the diagnosis of Crohn disease. Characteristic vulvar lesions include edema of the labia majora and ulcerations in which skin granulomas are separated from the affected gastrointestinal tract by normal skin. These ulcerations, which may resemble small herpetic lesions, last for weeks to months. After proctocolectomy for Crohn disease, vaginal fistulas develop in some patients. A sinus tract may discharge onto the posterior wall of the vagina or directly onto the perineum. These fistulas have responded to long-term metronidazole therapy and to surgery.

Because of the treatment with corticosteroids and immunosuppressive drugs, young women with Crohn disease may experience recurrent monilial vulvovaginitis and condyloma acuminata. Adolescents can usually take oral contraceptives without difficulty, though an association between previous use of oral contraceptives and so-called Crohn disease of the colon (but not ulcerative colitis) has been suggested. Some cases of colitis associated with rectal sparing and segmental disease, but not with granulomas, have been attributed to the use of oral contraceptives and have improved after oral contraceptives were stopped. Thus, if colitis develops while a patient is using oral contraceptives, medication should be stopped to see whether remission occurs. True Crohn disease associated, on colonic biopsy, with granulomas does not improve with the cessation of oral contraceptives.

Sickle Cell Disease

Adolescents with sickle cell disease often have delays in growth and development and in menarche compared with their peers. Adolescents with hemoglobinopathies require contraceptive counseling. Because of the concern for potential thromboembolic phenomena, including nephropathies and strokes, among patients with vasoocclusive crises, combined oral contraceptives should be used with caution. Although the risks for the progesterone-only mini-pill are unknown, they appear to be well tolerated. Thus, levonorgestrel and medroxyprogesterone acetate are acceptable options. Other contraceptive choices include barrier contraception and, for some patients, the IUD.

Childhood Malignancy

Because many children with malignancies are now surviving into adulthood, it is important for physicians to be aware of the gynecologic problems that occur among these patients. Chemotherapy for leukemia appears to have a mini-

mal impact on later pubertal development and menses in girls diagnosed before puberty. In contrast, girls who are diagnosed with leukemia and treated with chemotherapy after the onset of puberty or menarche may experience a delay in menarche or secondary amenorrhea. In almost all patients, menses eventually become normal.

Radiation therapy for solid tumors and lymphomas often results in permanent ovarian damage and ovarian failure. Data on the long-term survivors of childhood malignancy show that ovarian failure occurred in 68% of patients whose ovaries were within abdominal radiotherapy fields, in 14% whose ovaries were at the edge of treatment fields, and in none of the patients whose ovaries were outside abdominal treatment fields (Emans, 1990). Adolescents with impaired ovarian function may experience either no adolescent sexual development or some estrogen effect at the normal pubertal age, accompanied by primary or secondary amenorrhea. Gonadotropin levels are elevated to the menopausal range, and estradiol levels are usually lower than 30 pg/ml. Replacement therapy with estrogen and medroxyprogesterone can provide normal sexual development and, in most patients, menses. Some adolescents also have vaginal adhesions that require dilators and hormonal therapy. Counseling should focus on the potential for normal development and sexual functioning.

Adnexal Masses

During the past decade, gynecologists have been consulted more frequently about the problem of ovarian masses during childhood and adolescence. The true incidence of this condition has probably not changed, but the increasing use of ultrasonography by pediatricians and family practitioners has led to the detection of many functional cysts that were previously undetected. Even though most of these masses are functional and require only reassurance, true ovarian neoplasms must receive immediate attention and therapy. It is, therefore, important that gynecologists feel comfortable in the evaluation of a child or a teenager with an adnexal mass. The differential diagnosis of adnexal masses includes the enlargement of other reproductive structures and masses of extragenital origin.

All types of ovarian tumors seen in the adult can also be encountered in children and adolescents. The relative incidence of each entity is different, however. For example, functional masses are more common in adolescents because of the high incidence of anovulatory cycles. In this age group, neoplastic tumors are more likely to be of germinal origin rather than of epithelial origin.

Fortunately, only 1 in 10 ovarian tumors is malignant in children and adolescents. It is difficult to obtain accurate statistics regarding the frequency of functional cysts given that most studies are based on surgical reviews. Because many patients with functional adnexal enlargement are treated expectantly and never undergo surgery, they are not included in published series.

Studies at the Children's Hospital of 242 children and adolescents who underwent surgery for ovarian masses

Table 12-9 Diagnosis of 242 Ovarian Tumors Treated Surgically at Children's Hospital Medical Center (Boston) 1928-1982

Tumor Type	No. Patients (%)
Tumorlike enlargements	76 (31)
Primary ovarian tumors	166 (69)
Germ cell tumors	118 (71)
Mature teratoma	78
Immature teratoma	17
Endodermal sinus tumor	14
Dysgerminoma	8
Choriocarcinoma	1
Epithelial tumors	27 (16)
Serous	14
Mucinous	12
Mixed	1
Sex cord stromal tumors	21 (13)
Granulosa	10
Sertoli-Leydig	7
Thecoma	2
Fibroma	1
Unclassified	1

From Lack EE, Goldstein DP: Primary ovarian tumors in childhood and adolescence. *Curr Probl Gynecol* 1984; 7.

revealed that 31% had a tumor-like condition including follicle, corpus luteum, and simple and endometriotic cysts (Table 12-9) (Lack and Goldstein, 1984). Of the 166 patients with primary ovarian tumors, there were 118 (71%) germ cell tumors, of which 78 (66%) consisted of benign mature teratoma. Of 27 epithelial tumors, 85% were benign. Twenty-one (13%) had a sex cord-stromal tumor, which is generally is considered a low-grade malignancy. These results are comparable to those of similar reports.

A considerable number of ovarian tumors are asymptomatic and are discovered fortuitously during a routine pelvic examination. Because most young patients do not consult for periodic pelvic examinations, ovarian masses are often detected only when they become large enough to cause symptoms or to be felt by abdominal palpation. Smaller ovarian enlargements are often incidental ultrasonographic findings at the time of an examination performed for an unrelated symptom such as pain. This accounts for a large number of consultations for masses that prove to be functional.

Symptoms are usually related to the size of the mass or to mechanical incidents, such as rupture, torsion, or hemorrhage. In the young prepubertal girl, pain occurs in the abdomen because of the reduced pelvic capacity and the fairly high position of the ovaries. In the older patient, symptoms occur more often in the pelvis. Bladder and ureteral compression may result from larger masses. Malignant tumors that infiltrate the surrounding tissue may induce bowel obstruction. In patients who have had mechanical ac-

cidents, symptoms develop acutely and usually are characterized by severe pain and peritoneal signs, including nausea and vomiting. In hormone-producing tumors, precocious puberty, menstrual irregularities, or virilization may lead to the diagnosis.

On pelvic examination, the mass usually can be palpated by rectoabdominal examination with the patient in the lithotomy position. As mentioned previously, ovarian tumors in children are often intraabdominal rather than pelvic and should be considered in the differential diagnosis of abdominal masses. Other physical findings depend on the degree of invasion of the tumor and its hormonal activity.

Ultrasonography is invaluable in the diagnosis of ovarian masses. It provides information about the size, location, and consistency of the tumor (*i.e.*, whether it is cystic, solid, or complex). Ultrasonography is also useful to determine the presence of free peritoneal fluid or ascites. Radiography of the abdomen reveals calcifications, which suggest a diagnosis of dermoid cyst. This information can, however, be obtained by ultrasonography. The remainder of the workup depends on the clinical picture. If there is a solid or hormonally active tumor, blood should be drawn for hCG, α-fetoprotein, CA-125, and estradiol. Determining FSH and LH levels may help to differentiate true precocious puberty responsible for a functional cyst from an estrogen-secreting tumor inducing pseudoprecocious puberty. If a patient has hirsutism or signs of virilization, the testosterone level should be obtained. If malignancy is suspected, a preoperative metastatic workup, including chest x-ray, CT scan of the abdomen, and liver function tests, should be performed.

Ovarian masses in the postmenarchal patient are approached as they are in the young adult. Ultrasonography should be performed on an ovarian mass to confirm the diagnosis and to define the tumor's characteristics. Because of the high incidence of functional masses, an asymptomatic, purely cystic tumor with a diameter of 6 cm or less is observed for two to three cycles for spontaneous regression. In these patients, the use of oral contraceptives or GnRH analogues to inhibit ovarian function may accelerate regression and may prevent the appearance of new functional enlargement. Cystic masses that do not decrease in size for 3 months, that enlarge, or that are larger than 6 cm initially, should be operated on. Laparoscopy may be performed before laparotomy to confirm the diagnosis. When the cyst appears to be functional and is smaller than 6 cm in diameter, puncture aspiration may be performed. All fluid obtained should be sent for cytologic examination. It is preferable, however, to remove the cyst entirely.

Solid and complex tumors should be removed without delay. Laparoscopy may be performed as the initial procedure to establish the diagnosis and to help in the decision for the optimal incision. If a patient has an unexpected malignancy, laparoscopy allows the surgeon to discuss the extensiveness of the proposed surgery with the patient.

Laparotomy should be performed through an incision large enough to allow excision of the tumor without rupture

Table 12-10   Review of the Literature: All Reported Breast Masses

	Year	N	Age (yrs)	Normal	Cyst	Fibro-adenoma	FC/Prolif	CP	Hyper-trophy	IP	Other Benign Lesion/Tumor	Infection	Malig-nancy
Daniel	1968	63	10-20	0	0	40	9	2	0	0	4	5	3
Simpson	1969	429	<21	0	0	338	76	0	0	2	2	10	1
Oberman	1971	118	10-20	0	0	0	118	0	0	0	0	0	0
Nichini	1972	59	8-20	2	2	41	4	0	0	1	3	0	0
Kern	1973	237	10-20	0	8	169	25	0	0	13	5	2	3
Seashore	1975	111	<16	2	1	84	2	0	4	1	7	9	1
Turbey	1975	42	12-18	—	—	30	—	—	—	—	—	8	0
Bower	1976	134	0-16	—	—	102	4	—	—	—	—	9	1
Ashikari	1977	145	<21	0	0	104	26	2	0	4	4	4	1
Stone	1977	143	11-20	—	—	103	9	—	—	—	—	4	1
Gogas	1979	63	10-20	—	—	42	9	—	—	—	—	5	3
Oberman	1979	40	12-22	0	0	19	11	1	5	0	2	0	2
Ligon	1980	249	11-30	—	—	167	37	—	—	—	—	—	5
Seltzer	1980	151	<21	0	0	119	7	0	0	0	5	20	0
Hammar	1981	5	10-16	0	0	5	0	0	0	0	0	0	0
Goldstein	1982	51	8-20	0	3	48	3	0	0	0	4	1	0
Ernster	1985	95	12-21	0	0	90	0	0	0	1	2	2	0
London	1985	30	<21	0	0	18	9	0	1	0	1	1	0
Lubin	1985	34	12-18	0	1	29	1	0	0	0	0	1	1
Raju	1985	95	12-21	0	9	71	0	2	0	0	2	11	0
Simmons	1989	185	<18	0	0	100	44	0	24	0	11	2	4
Totals	—	**2479**	—	**4**	**24**	**1719**	**394**	**7**	**34**	**22**	**52**	**94**	**26**
Percent	—	**100**	—	**0.16**	**0.97**	**69.34**	**15.89**	**0.28**	**1.37**	**0.89**	**2.10**	**3.79**	**1.05**

From: Goldstein DP, Emans SJ, Laufer MR. The breast examination and lesions. *In:* Emans SJ, Laufer MR, Goldstein DP. *Pediatric and Adolescent Gynecology* (4th edition), Philadelphia: Lippincott/Raven Publishing Company, 1998.

CP: Cystosarcoma phyllodes; FC/prolif: Fibrocystic/proliferative; IP: Intraductal papillomas.

and according to the principles of ovarian surgery (*i.e.,* peritoneal lavage, complete abdominal exploration, frozen-section analysis, and periaortic node dissection when indicated).

Uterine Myomas

Uterine myomas rarely develop in teenagers, but they have been reported in children as young as 10 years of age. They should be considered in the differential diagnosis of any solid pelvic mass. Ultrasonography is usually accurate. Treatment by myomectomy is recommended and is usually successful. Myoma can be encountered in the rudimentary muscular bud in patients with vaginal agenesis.

Sarcomas of the Uterus. Most of the reported malignancies of the uterine fundus in adolescents have been sarcomas; mixed mesodermal tumors are the most common. These are neoplasms that arise from malignant epithelial and mesenchymal stromal elements of the uterus. They are classified according to the nature of the sarcomatous component into homologous (tissue normally found in the uterus) or heterologous (tissue not normally found in the uterus, such as striated muscle or cartilage). The tumors are firm and sessile, and they fill the uterine cavity, unlike the grapelike sarcomas of the vagina. These tumors are usually found in postmenopausal women, but several mixed mülle-

rian tumors have been reported in children and adolescents from 4 to 19 years of age. Symptoms usually are vaginal bleeding and a pelvic mass. The treatment of the tumors requires early diagnosis and radical surgery followed by radiation and chemotherapy tailored to the patient.

Careful staging of the extent of the disease is essential to the treatment and prognosis of children with rhabdomyosarcoma. Pelvic ultrasound and CT can be useful in evaluating the extent of disease and in measuring tumor regression during chemotherapy.

Breast Mass

Most breast lumps in adolescents are normal physiologic breast tissue or are the result of fibrocystic changes (Hein et al, 1982). Adolescents typically have very dense breast tissue. Fibrocystic changes are characterized by diffuse cord-like thickening and by lumps that may become tender and enlarged before menses each month. Physical findings tend to change each month; suspected cysts can often be observed clinically.

In contrast, most breast masses that are excised in this age group are fibroadenomas (Goldstein and Pinsonneault, 1990). Table 12-10 consists of a recent review of the literature showing all reported breast masses (Goldstein, 1998). These lesions are typically firm or rubbery and mobile, and they have a clearly defined edge. They tend to be eccentric in position, and they occur more often in the lateral breast quadrants than in the medial quadrant. The breast mass may remain unchanged, or it may enlarge with subsequent menstrual cycles. Recurrent or multiple fibroadenomas may develop. Giant fibroadenomas may replace most of the breast tissue; in fact, initially they are often mistaken for normal tissue. A question that has often been raised is whether a patient with a history of fibroadenoma is at increased risk for breast cancer later. Dupont and Page (1994) report a retrospective cohort study of 1835 patients with fibroadenoma diagnosed between 1950 and 1968. The women in the study were compared with two control groups and with women chosen from among the patients' sisters-in-law. It was found that the risk for invasive breast cancer among patients with fibroadenoma was 2.15 times (95% confidence intervals, 1.5 and 3.2) greater than the risk for controls. Among patients with a family history of breast cancer and either complex fibroadenoma or proliferative disease, the incidence of breast cancer during the first 25 years after diagnosis of the fibroadenoma was found to be 20%.

Cancer of the breast is rare in children and adolescents. Primary lymphoma may appear as a breast mass in adolescents. Patients who have undergone previous radiation therapy to the chest have an increased risk for cancer of the breast at a young age and, therefore, require ongoing surveillance. Cystosarcoma phylloides is a rare primary tumor that is sometimes malignant.

A new entity, juvenile papillomatosis, is a rare breast tumor of young women first described by Boley in 1980. The tumor features atypical papillary duct hyperplasia and multiple cysts. The mean age of the patients is 23 years, and the range is 12 to 48 years. The localized tumor is often initially mistaken for a fibroadenoma. Twenty-eight percent of the patients have a relative with breast cancer, and 7% have a first-degree relative with breast cancer. In a small number of patients, breast cancer is diagnosed concurrently with juvenile papillomatosis, and it is diagnosed in several patients at follow-up. Bilateral juvenile papillomatosis may especially increase the risk for cancer at a later time. Thus, careful surveillance is indicated for patients with this diagnosis, found on excisional biopsy. Papillary hyperplasia without the cystic component of juvenile papillomatosis appears to be a more benign condition in young patients.

If the adolescent has a breast mass, palpation may make the diagnosis evident if there are accompanying symptoms such as fibrocystic changes or tenderness with overlying erythema consistent with a breast infection. Trauma may cause a breast mass, but examination immediately after a contusion may locate a preexisting lesion. If the differential diagnosis is a cyst or a fibroadenoma, the lesion can be measured and the patient should be instructed to return after her next menstrual period. If the lesion disappears, it was probably a cyst. If the lesion is still present and the patient is cooperative, a needle aspiration of the mass can be performed in the office using a 23-gauge needle on a 3-mL syringe. A small amount of lidocaine can be used to infiltrate the skin with a 25-gauge needle. In contrast, a fibroadenoma has a characteristic gritty, solid sensation. Any material obtained (even if just on the tip of the needle) should be smeared on a ground-glass slide, fixed, and sent for cytologic examination. If the mass collapses after aspiration, it is assumed to be a cyst and the mass is reevaluated in 3 months. A sonogram of the breast tissue can also help to delineate a fibroadenoma from a cyst and can be used to localize an abscess. Mammography should not be used to evaluate breast masses in adolescents because the breast tissue is dense, the chance that the patient has carcinoma is negligible, and radiographic features have not influenced clinical management.

When aspiration of a persistent, discrete mass is not feasible or is nonproductive, or when masses are nonmobile, enlarging, hard or tender, or when they are a source of considerable anxiety, the patient should undergo excisional biopsy. Unless there are underlying medical conditions, such as cardiac or pulmonary disease, an excisional biopsy can be performed in an ambulatory setting under general or local anesthesia, depending on technical considerations and on the patient's preference and ability to cooperate. Because breast scars can be cosmetically deforming, the optimal incision for a lesion near the center of the breast is a radial incision for better wound healing and cosmetic results. Periareolar ectopic lobules (Montgomery cysts), which often have clear or dark discharge from the areola (not the nipple), can be excised with a circumareolar incision.

A contusion to the breast may result in a poorly defined tender mass that resolves in several weeks. A mass from severe trauma may take several months to resolve; occasionally, scar tissue remains palpable indefinitely. Fat necrosis may also result from trauma, though the patient may not notice the growing lesion until several months later. A biopsy specimen should be obtained in such circumstances. It should be remembered that examination immediately after trauma to the breast may locate a preexisting lesion. A sharply delineated, nontender mass is probably unrelated to the recent injury.

REFERENCES

Adams J, Ahmad M, Phillips P: Anogenital findings and hymenal diameter in children referred for sexual abuse examination. *Adolesc Pediatr Gynecol* 1988; 1:123.

American Fertility Society: Classification of müllerian anomalies. *Fertil Steril* 1988; 49: 952.

Baker TG: Radiosensitivity of mammalian oocytes with particular reference to the human female. *Am J Obstet Gynecol* 1971; 110:746.

Banerjee R, Laufer MR: Reproductive disorders associated with pelvic pain. In Blythe MJ, Laufer MR, editors: *Seminars in pediatric surgery,* Philadelphia, 1998, WB Saunders.

Barbieri RL: Hormone treatment of endometriosis: The estrogen threshold hypothesis. *Am J Obstet Gynecol* 1992; 166:740.

Berenson A, Heger A, Andrews S: The appearance of the hymen in newborns. *Pediatrics* 1991; 87:458.

Berenson AB, Heger AH, Andrews SE: Morphology of the hymen in twins. *Adolesc Pediatr Gynecol* 1991; 4:82.

Berta R, Hawkins JR, Sinclair AH, et al: Genetic evidence equating SRY and the testis-determining factor. *Nature* 1990; 348:448.

Boley SJ: Lesions of the breast. InHolder TW, Ashcroft KW, editors: *Pediatric surgery,* Philadelphia, 1980, WB Saunders.

Bongiovanni AM, editor: *Adolescent gynecology: A guide for clinicians,* New York, 1982, Plenum Publishing

Cali RW, Pratt JH: Congenital absence of the vagina. *Am J Obstet Gynecol* 1968; 100:752.

Cantwell H: Vaginal inspection as it relates to child sexual abuse in girls under thirteen. *Child Abuse Negl* 1983; 7:171.

Cantwell H: Update on vaginal inspection as it relates to child sexual abuse in girls under thirteen. *Child Abuse Negl* 1987; 11:545.

Capraro VJ, Dillon WP, Gallego MB: Microperforate hymen: A distinct clinical entity. *Obstet Gynecol* 1974; 44:903.

Capraro VJ: Gynecologic examination in children and adolescents. *Pediatr Clin North Am* 1972; 19:511.

Carpenter SEK, Rock AJ: *Pediatric and adolescent gynecology,* New York, 1991, Raven Press.

Carson SA: Gynecologic problems of adolescence and puberty. In Sciarra JJ, editor: *Gynecology and obstetrics,* Philadelphia, 1984, JB Lippincott.

Casey AC, Laufer MR: Cervical agenesis: Septic death after surgery. *Obstet Gynecol* 1997; 90:706-707.

Chisholm TC: Exstrophy of the urinary bladder. In Holder TW, Ashcroft KW, editors: *Pediatric surgery,* Philadelphia, 1980, WB Saunders.

Christensen EH, Oster J: Adhesions of labia minora (synechia vulvae) in childhood: A review and report of fourteen cases. *Acta Paediatr Scand* 1971; 60:709.

Claessons EA, Cowell CA: Acute adolescent menorrhagia. *Am Obstet Gynecol* 1981; 193:377.

Counseller VS, Davis CE: Atresia of the vagina. *Obstet Gynecol* 1968; 32:528.

Craighill MC: Human papillomavirus infection in children and adolescents. *Semin Pediatr Infect Dis* 1993; 4:85.

Damewood MD, Hesla HS, Lowen M, Schultz MJ: Induction of ovulation and pregnancy following lateral oophoropexy for Hodgkin's disease. *Int J Gynecol Obstet* 1990; 33:369.

Dewhurst CJ: *Practical pediatric and adolescent gynecology,* New York, 1980, Marcel Dekker.

Donahoe PK, Hendren WH III: Perineal reconstruction in ambiguous genitalia infants raised as females. *Ann Surg* 1984; 200:363.

Donahue PK, Hendren WH: Intersex abnormalities in the newborn infant. In Holder TM, Ashcroft KW, editors: *Pediatric surgery,* Philadelphia, 1980, WB Saunders.

Dupont WD, Page DL: Long-term risk of breast cancer in women with fibroadenoma. *N Engl J Med* 1994; 331:10-15.

Emans SJ, Goldstein DP: The gynecologic examination of the prepubertal child with vulvovaginitis: Use of the knee-chest position. *Pediatrics* 1980; 65:758.

Emans SJ: Examination of the pediatric and adolescent female. *Clin Pract Gynecol* 1990a; 1:1.

Emans SJ: Gynecologic problems in adolescents with chronic diseases. *Clin Pract Gynecol* 1990b; 1:171.

Emans SJ, Woods ER, Flagg NT, Freeman A: Genital findings in sexual abuse: Symptomatic and asymptomatic girls. *Pediatrics* 1987; 79:778.

Emans SJ, Laufer MR, Goldstein DP: *Pediatric and adolescent gynecology,* 4th ed, Philadelphia, 1998, Lippincott-Raven.

Fiumara NJ, Rothman K, Tang S: Reemergence of chancroid as an important STD. *J Am Acad Dermatol* 1986; 15:939.

Frank RT: The formation of an artificial vagina without operation. *Am J Obstet Gynecol* 1938; 35:1035.

Frisch RE: Body weight, body fat, and ovulation. *Trends in Endocrine Metabolism* 1991; 2:191.

Frisch RE, Revelle R: Height and weight at menarche and a hypothesis of menarche. *Arch Dis Child* 1971; 46:695.

Frisch RE, McArthur JW: Menstrual cycles: Fatness as a determinant of minimum weight for height necessary for their maintenance or onset. *Science* 1974; 185:949.

Gantt PA, McDonough PG: Dysfunctional bleeding in adolescents. In Barwin BN, Belish S, editors: *Adolescent gynecology and sexuality,* New York, 1982, Masson.

Gardner JJ: Descriptive study of genital variation in healthy non-abused, premenarchal girls. *J Pediatr* 1992; 120:251.

Gidwani GP: Establishing a practice in pediatric and adolescent gynecology. *Female Patient* 1993; 18:33.

Goldstein DP: Female genital tract. In Welch KJ, editor: *Complications of pediatric surgery,* Philadelphia, 1982, WB Saunders.

Goldstein DP, DeCholnoky C, Emans SJ: Adolescent endometriosis. *J Adol Health Care,* 1980a; 1:37.

Goldstein DP, DeCholnoky C, Emans SJ, et al: Laparoscopy in the diagnosis and management of pelvic pain in adolescents. *J Reprod Med* 1980b; 24:251.

Goldstein DP, Emans SJ, Laufer MR: The breast: Examination and lesions. In Emans SJ, Laufer MR, Goldstein DP, editors: *Pediatric and adolescent gynecology,* 4th ed, Philadelphia, 1998, Lippincott-Raven.

Goldstein DP, Pinsonneault O: Management of breast masses in adolescent females. *Clin Pract Gynecol* 1990; 1:131.

Grunberger W, Fisch LF: Pediatric gynecological outpatient department: A report on 600 patients. *Wien Klin Wochenschr* 1982; 94:614.

Heald FP, editor: *Adolescent gynecology,* Baltimore, 1966, Williams & Wilkins.

Hebeler JR: The abused child. In Holder TW, Ashcroft KW, editors: *Pediatric surgery,* Philadelphia, 1980, WB Saunders.

Hein K, Dell R, Caten M: Self-detection of a breast mass in adolescent females. *J Adolesc Health Care* 1982; 3:15.

Heger A, Emans SJ: Introital diameter as the criterion for sexual abuse. *Pediatrics* 1990; 85:222.

Heger A, Emans SJ: *Evaluation of the sexually abused child.* New York, 1992, Oxford University Press.

Hendren WH III, Donahoe PK: Correction of congenital abnormalities of the vagina and perineum. *J Pediatr Surg* 1980; 15:751.

Huffman JW, Dewhurst CJ, Capraro VJ: *The gynecology of childhood and adolescence,* 2nd ed, Philadelphia, 1981, WB Saunders.

Ingram JM: The bicycle seat stool in the treatment of vaginal agenesis and stenosis: A preliminary report. *Am J Obstet Gynecol* 1981; 140:73.

Jacobson L: Differential diagnosis of acute PID. *Am J Obstet Gynecol* 1980; 138:124.

Jager RJ, Anvret M, Hall K, et al: A human XY female with a frame shift mutation in the candidate testis-determining-gene SRY. *Nature* 1990; 348:452.

Jirasek JE: Normal sex differentiation. In Sciarra JJ, editor: *Gynecology and obstetrics,* Philadelphia, 1991, JB Lippincott.

Jones HW Jr, Hellen RH: *Pediatric and adolescent gynecology,* Baltimore, 1966, Williams & Wilkins.

Jones HW Jr, Verkauf BS: Surgical treatment in congenital adrenal hyperplasia: Age at operation and other prognostic factors. *J Obstet Gynecol* 1970; 36:1.

Kahn JA, Chiang V, Shrier LA, et al: Microlaparoscopy with conscious sedation for the evaluation of suspected PID in adolescents: A preliminary report. *J Pediatr Adolesc Gynecol* 1997;10:163.

Kreutner AKK, Hollingsworth DR: *Adolescent obstetrics and gynecology,* Chicago, 1978, Year Book Medical Publishers.

Koff AK: Development of the vagina in the human fetus. *Contrib Embryol* 1933; 24:59.

Lack EE, Goldstein DP: Primary ovarian tumors in childhood and adolescence. *Curr Probl Obstet Gynecol,* 1984; 7; 8:1

Laufer MR: Endometriosis in adolescents. *Current Opin Pediatr* 1992; 4:582.

Laufer MR: Identification of clear vesicular lesions of atypical endometriosis: A new technique. *Fertil Steril* 1997; 68:739-740.

Laufer MR, Billett A, Diller L, et al: A new technique for laparoscopic prophylactic oophoropexy prior to cranioplasty irradiation in children with medulloblastoma. *Adolesc Pediatr Gynecol* 1995; 8:77-81.

Laufer MR, Galvin WJ: Labial hypertrophy: A new surgical approach. *Adolesc Pediatr Gynecol* 1995; 8:39-41.

Laufer MR, Goitein L, Bush M, et al: Prevalence of endometriosis in adolescent women with chronic pelvic pain not responding to conventional therapy. *J Pediatr Adolesc Gynecol* 1997; 10:199-202.

Laufer MR, Goldstein DP: Dysmenorrhea, pelvic pain, and the premenstrual syndrome. In Emans SJ, Laufer MR, Goldstein DP, editors: *Pediatric and adolescent gynecology,* 4th ed, Philadelphia, 1998a, Lippincott-Raven.

Laufer MR, Goldstein DP: Structural abnormalities of the female reproductive tract. In Emans SJ, Laufer MR, Goldstein DP: *Pediatric and adolescent gynecology,* 4th ed, Philadelphia, 1998b, Lippincott-Raven.

Laufer MR, Heerema AE, Parson KE, et al: Endosalpingiosis: Clinical presentation and follow-up. *Gynecol Obstet Invest* 1998; 46:195

Laufer MR, Rein MS: Treatment of abnormal uterine bleeding with gonadotropin-releasing hormone analogues. *Clin Obstet Gynecol* 1993; 36:668.

Laufer MR, Townsend NL, Parson KE, et al: Inducing amenorrhea during bone marrow transplantation: A pilot study of leuprolide acetate. *J Reprod Med* 1997; 42:537-541.

Lavery JP, Sanfilippo JS, editor: *Pediatric and adolescent obstetrics and gynecology*, New York, 1985, Springer-Verlag.

Le Floch O, Donaldson SS, Kaplan HS: Pregnancy following oophoropexy and total nodal irradiation in woman with Hodgkin's disease. *Cancer* 1976; 38:2263.

Lewis VG, Ehrhardt AA, Money J: Genital operations in girls with the adrenogenital syndrome. *Obstet Gynecol* 1970; 36:11.

Lubianca JN, Gordon CM, Laufer MR: Addback therapy for endometriosis in adolescents. *J Reprod Med* 1998; 43:164-172.

Mandl AM: A quantitative study of the sensitivity of oocytes to X-irradiation. *Proc R Soc Biol* 1958; 150:53.

Marshall WN, Lightner ES: Congenital adrenal hyperplasia presenting with labial fusion without clitoromegaly. *Pediatrics* 1980; 66:312.

McCann J: Use of the colposcope in childhood sexual abuse examinations. *Pediatr Clin North Am* 1990; 37:863.

McCann J, Wells R, Simon M, Voris J: Genital findings in prepubertal girls selected for nonabuse: A descriptive study. *Pediatrics* 1990; 86:428.

McCann J, Voris J, Simon M: Genital injuries resulting from sexual abuse. *Pediatrics* 1992; 89:307.

McCann J, Voris J: Perianal injuries resulting from sexual abuse: A longitudinal study. *Pediatrics* 1993; 91:390.

McIndoe A: Treatment of congenital absences and obliterative conditions of the vagina. *Br J Plast Surg* 1950; 2:254.

McIndoe AH, Banister JB: An operation for the cure of congenital absence of the vagina. *J Obstet Gynaecol Br Commonw* 1938; 45:490.

Mininberg DT: Phalloplasty in congenital adrenal hyperplasia. *J Urol* 1981; 128:355.

Morton KE, Dewhurst CJ: Human amnion in the treatment of vaginal malformations. *Br J Obstet Gynaecol* 1986; 93:50.

Muram D, Elias S: Child sexual abuse—genital tract findings in prepubertal girls, II: Comparison of colposcopic and unaided examinations. *Am J Obstet Gynecol* 1989; 160:333.

Muram D: Classification of genital findings in prepubertal girls who are victims of sexual abuse. *Adolesc Pediatr Gynecol* 1988a; 1:151.

Muram D: Classification of genital findings in prepubertal girls who are victims of sexual abuse. *Adolesc Pediatr Gynecol* 1988b; 2:149.

Muram D: Child sexual abuse—genital tract findings in prepubertal girls, I: The unaided medical examination. *Am J Obstet Gynecol* 1989; 160:328.

Muram D: Child sexual abuse: Relationship between sexual acts and genital findings. *Child Abuse Negl* 1989; 13:211.

Muram D, Hostetler BR, Jones CE: Adolescent victims of sexual assault. *Female Patient* 1993; 18:54.

Muckle CW: Developmental abnormalities of the female reproductive organs. In Sciarra JJ, editor: *Gynecology and obstetrics*, Philadelphia, 1988, JB Lippincott.

Murphy M: Sexual abuse in the pediatric and adolescent patient. *Clin Pract Gynecol* 1990; 1:31.

Nicholson HS, Byrne J: Fertility and pregnancy after treatment for cancer during childhood or adolescence. *Cancer* 1993; 71:3392.

Oberman HA: Breast lesions in the adolescent female. *Pathol Annu* 1979; 14:175.

Pang S, Wallace MA, Hofman L, et al: Worldwide experience in newborn screening for classical congenital adrenal hyperplasia due to 21-hydroxylase deficiency. *Pediatrics* 1988; 81:866.

Paradise JE: Predictive accuracy and the diagnosis of sexual abuse: A big issue about a little tissue. *Child Abuse Negl* 1989; 13:169.

Perlman SE, Emans SJ, Laufer MR: Gynecologic issues in young women with chronic diseases. In Emans SJ, Laufer MR, Goldstein DP. *Pediatric and adolescent gynecology*, 4th ed, Philadelphia, 1998, Lippincott-Raven.

Pinsonneault O, Goldstein DP: Obstructing malformations of the uterus and vagina. *Fertil Steril* 1985; 44:241.

Pokorny SF: Configuration of the prepubertal hymen. *Am J Obstet Gynecol* 1987; 157:157.

Ramenofsky ML: Vaginal lesions. In Holder TM, Ashcroft KW, editors: *Pediatric surgery*, Philadelphia, 1980, WB Saunders.

Ravnikar VA: Endocrine disorders. In Kistner RW, editor: *Gynecology—Principles and practice*, 4th ed, Chicago, 1985, Year Book Medical Publishers.

Reindollar RH, Byrd JR, McDonough PC: Delayed sexual development: A study of 252 patients. *Am J Obstet Gynecol* 1981; 140:371.

Rock JA: Surgical correction of uterovaginal anomalies. In Sciarra JJ, editor: *Gynecol-*

ogy and obstetrics, Philadelphia, 1984, JB Lippincott.

Sadler TW: *Langman's medical embryology*, 6th ed, Baltimore, 1990, Williams & Wilkins.

Sanfilippo JS: Dysmenorrhea in adolescents. *Female Patient* 1993; 18:29.

Sanfilippo JS, Muram D, Lee PA, Dewhurst J: *Pediatric and adolescent gynecology*, Philadelphia, 1994, WB Saunders.

Schiffman MH: Recent progress in defining the epidemiology of human papillomavirus infection and cervical neoplasia. *J Natl Cancer Inst* 1992; 84:394.

Simpson JL, Photopulos G: The relationship of neoplasia to disorders of abnormal sexual differentiation. *Birth Defects* 1976; 12:15.

Sinclair AH, Berta P, Palmer MS, et al: A gene from the human sex-determining region encodes a protein with homology to a conserved DNA-binding motif. *Nature* 1990; 346:240.

Slaughter L, Brown C: Colposcopy to establish physical findings in rape victims. *Am J Obstet Gynecol* 1992; 166:83.

Speiser PW, Dupont B, Rubenstein P, et al: High frequency of nonclassical steroid 21-hydroxylase deficiency. *Am J Hum Genet* 1985; 37:650.

Stone SC: Physiology of puberty. In Sciarra JJ, editor: *Gynecology and obstetrics*, Philadelphia, 1984, JB Lippincott.

Strickland DM, Hauth JC, Strickland KM: Laparoscopy for chronic pelvic pain in adolescent women. *Adolesc Pediatr Gynecol* 1988; 1:31.

Teixeira W: Hymenal colposcopic examination in sexual offenses. *Am J Forens Med Pathol* 1981; 2:209.

Thibaud E, Ramirez M, Brauner R, et al: Preservation of ovarian function by ovarian transposition performed before pelvic irradiation during childhood. *J Pediatr* 1992; 121:880.

Thomas PRM, Winstanly D, Peckham MJ, et al: Reproductive and endocrine function in patients with Hodgkin's disease: Effects of oophoropexy and irradiation. *Br J Cancer* 1976; 33:226.

White S, Ingram D, Lyna PR: Vaginal introital diameter in the evaluation of sexual abuse. *Child Abuse Negl* 1989; 13:217.

Williams EA: Congenital absence of the vagina, a simple operation for its relief. *J Obstet Gynecol Br Comm* 1964; 71:511.

Wolff PB, Wilbois RP, Weldon VV, et al: Posterior fusion without clitoromegaly in a female with partial 21-hydroxylase deficiency. *J Pediatr* 1977; 91:951.

CHAPTER

Conception Control

RAPIN OSATHANONDH

KEY ISSUES

1. There is no ideal contraceptive method, and the efficacy of most contraceptives is dependent on the motivation of the user.
2. Birth control pills are used by over 70 million women worldwide, and approximately 18 million women in the United States take birth control pills daily.
3. Most contraceptive methods do not protect against sexually transmitted infection, therefore condoms and counseling should also be offered.
4. High dosages of estrogen or progestins taken within two days of coitus (morning-after pills) can prevent pregnancy; they inhibit or delay ovulation, alter the endometrium and interfere with implantation, or interfere with tubal transport of fertilized egg.
5. Ninety-five percent of therapeutic abortions are safely performed in outpatient facilities or physician's offices using the dilatation and vacuum evacuation (D&E) method.
6. The most commonly used contraceptive methods are male and female sterilization.

The practice of birth control can be traced back to ancient societies of different racial and religious origins. Today voluntary prevention of pregnancy (contraception) and termination of unwanted pregnancy (therapeutic induced abortion) are widely accepted for medical (parental or fetal indications) and socioeconomic reasons. In spite of the rapid advancement in reproductive biology, there still exist four problems regarding birth control that may or may not be resolved in our time.

1. **There is no ideal method of contraception.** Each contraceptive method available in the United States is safer than carrying unwanted term pregnancy resulting from lack of contraception. However, it is impossible to make a contraceptive that is 100% effective, easy to use, reversible, and without side effects. For each woman, any method of contraception has advantages and disadvantages as well as relative and absolute contraindications. A suitable method means that its benefits far outweigh its risks. For example, statistical calculations by Tietze and Lewit (1979) suggested that the safest contraceptive practice for women of any age in the United States is the diaphragm or the condom. This practice can be backed by early, legal abortion should the method fail (Ory, 1983). Unfortunately, induced abortion may be costly or inaccessible in many localities. To guard against pregnancy and sexually transmitted diseases (STDs), a combination of the low-dose oral contraceptive pill and the use of a latex or polyurethane condom may represent the safest choice for women younger than 40 years of age who do not smoke cigarettes and have no other prothrombotic risks. Practitioners should always remind themselves and their patients that a relative risk is not an absolute risk. Risks and benefits should be viewed against unwanted pregnancy and other available contraceptive methods.
2. **Women who use contraceptives should see a gynecologist at least once a year.** Contraceptive-related problems may occur as a direct or indirect result of contraceptive use. Increased coital activity or an increased number of sexual partners may necessitate switching from one method of contraception to another. For example, studies before and after the use of the oral

contraceptive pill showed an increased incidence of bacteriuria in some women, with a tendency for recurrent bladder infections.

3. **The efficacy of most contraceptives is dependent on the motivation of the user.** The actual-use effectiveness may not be applicable in many circumstances. For some women, an intrauterine device may be more effective than the pill because of poor dosing compliance. For many women, the *natural family planning method* (abstinence or the rhythm method) is in fact unnatural and often results in high failure rates.

4. **There is an epidemic of unintended pregnancies among teenagers in the United States.** There has been a trend toward earlier and more frequent unprotected intercourse among teenagers. An annual occurrence of more than 1 million unintended teenage pregnancies in the United States is considered high when compared with those in other industrialized nations. Epidemiologic data reveal that adolescent marriages generally lead to eventual separation or divorce, less education, and low-paying jobs or no jobs. Recent national statistics revealed an average of one out-of-wedlock child for every five live births. Moreover, there are approximately 3 million women 15 to 44 years of age who do not want to conceive yet do not practice contraception. This is a serious public health problem and a great concern for society.

ORAL CONTRACEPTIVES

Birth control pills *(the pill)* represent the most studied class of medications since 1960. Worldwide, oral contraceptives (OCs) are taken daily by more than 70 million women, most of whom are not at risk for serious side effects. Approximately 18 million women in the United States take OCs daily. The pill is highly effective in preventing unwanted conception, with a crude contraceptive efficacy (Pearl Index) of less than two pregnancies per 100 women-years. Its effects are reversible, and there are many noncontraceptive health benefits (Box 13-1; Osathanondh, 1994), some of which last for years after use (Brenner, 1998; Connell, 1984; Cramer, 1982; del Junco, 1985; Franceschi, 1984; Hulka, 1982; Lines, 1983; Ostensen, 1983; Potts, 1983; Sturgis, 1940; Vandenbroucke, 1983). Most OCs contain ethinyl estradiol, a synthetic estrogen, and a progestin or progestogen (progesterone-like substance). These are called *combined* or *combination OCs*. Since October 1988 in the United States, each combined OC tablet contains 20 to 50 μg ethinyl estradiol or a pharmacologically similar steroid mestranol (Fig. 13-1) plus one of the six progestins: norgestrel, norethindrone, norethindrone acetate, ethynodiol diacetate, desogestrel, or norgestimate. A much less popular type of OC contains a small dose of progestin without estrogen and is known as the *minipill.* Unless the word *minipill* is specifically mentioned in this text, OC is generally understood to be the combined pill.

Administration and Types of Oral Contraceptives

The first OC tablet is usually taken on day 5 of menses, followed by one tablet per day for 21 days. For simplicity or better protection, some brands are begun either on the first day of bleeding or the first Sunday of the menstrual cycle. Anovulatory withdrawal bleeding generally occurs 3 to 5 days after the 21-day regimen, and the routine is begun again on day 5 of the new cycle. Thus there is 1 week off the routine with every 3 weeks on the routine. Most pharmaceutical manufacturers also provide a nonstop 28-day OC package in which the last seven tablets are hormonally inert placebos. The latter packaging system eliminates the need to remember the on-off intervals. Because each of the 21 hormonally active tablets contains the same amount of estrogen and progestin, this conventional OC is known as monophasic.

Because of continuous publicity regarding the metabolic side effects of the pill, the biphasic and triphasic types of OC have sporadically been introduced to lower the total amount of either the progestin or the estrogen component while mimicking the hormonal peak and trough levels within the physiologic menstrual cycles. Of the five types of multiphasic pills (Table 13-1), two formulations contain slightly varying amounts of estrogen, whereas three others put 35 μg estrogen in each hormonally active tablet. To date there are no well-controlled studies with solid clinical evidence for overall superiority of the multiphasic over the common monophasic low-dose pills. Theoretically, based primarily on laboratory data, these multiphasic formulations may represent a safer choice for certain pill users than others.

Mechanisms of Action

The low daily dosage of two synergistic steroids in the pill prevents ovulation by centrally inhibiting the midcycle pituitary gonadotropin surge (Orme, 1983; Rock, 1956). The pituitary gland may be unable to respond to the hypothalamic gonadotropin-releasing hormone while a woman is taking OCs (Dericks-Tan, 1983). This central effect consequently obliterates endogenous (ovarian) estrogen and progesterone production and commonly leads to diminished endometrial proliferation. In OCs with lesser amounts of estrogen, occasional small surges of gonadotropins may appear. However, such levels are usually insufficient to stimulate ovarian follicles (Grimes, 1994; Young, 1992). A much-debated report of ovarian retention cysts in the users of low-dose pills may challenge this general rule (Caillouette, 1987).

Peripherally, OCs exert antinidation effects involving decreased oviductal function, endometrial glycogen content, and cervical mucus (Liskin, 1983a; Liskin, 1987; Rock, 1956; Umapathysivam, 1980). These peripheral effects are probably responsible for the major contraceptive effect of the minipill. The scant, dry, cervical mucus renders the cervix impermeable to penetration by sperm. Furthermore, atrophic, out-of-phase endometrium with resultant amenorrhea is not an uncommon finding. The minipill regimen does not totally abolish surges of luteinizing hormone or

---

BOX 13-1
PATIENT CONSENT FORM FOR OBTAINING BIRTH CONTROL PILLS

Birth control pills (the pill), or oral contraceptives, are being used every day by more than 50 million women around the world for the prevention of unwanted pregnancy. There are many health benefits of taking birth control pills besides the prevention of pregnancy (noncontraceptive benefits). There are also risks associated with taking the pill. However, these risks (for stroke, blood clots, heart attack) are seen mostly among women over age 40 who smoke. The risk for younger women is very small. According to the U.S. Food and Drug Administration, an increased risk of breast cancer has not been demonstrated among pill users, but there may be a slight increase in the risk for cancer of the cervix. All women must have a Papanicolaou (Pap) test at least once every year. Also, be sure to read the package insert that comes with your birth control pills.

Noncontraceptive Benefits

1. The pill usually reduces menstrual cramps.
2. The pill generally protects women against having breast problems that are not cancer, cysts in the ovary, endometriosis (a disease that may cause severe menstrual cramps and infertility), and cancer of the ovary and the womb (uterus).
3. The pill decreases bleeding from the uterus and also reduces the risk of iron deficiency anemia in some women who bleed a lot during their periods and in those who bleed irregularly.
4. The pill may protect against rheumatoid arthritis.

Side Effects
Minor Side Effects

Stay on the pill through the third package cycle. Minor side effects, if they occur will usually go away by then. If not, consult a physician or a nurse. A different brand may agree with you better.
1. Bleeding or spotting between periods
2. Nausea (try taking the pill at bedtime to avoid feeling sick)
3. Weight gain from fluid retention
4. Weight gain or loss as a result of change in appetite (should not be more than 3 kg)
5. Breast tenderness, mild headaches, tiredness, or mood changes
6. Increased blood pressure
7. Enlargement of fibroid tumors in some women
8. Scant flow (less and less monthly bleeding) or missed periods
9. Decreased sex drive (however, most pill users report increased sex drive)
10. Facial complexion: Most pill users see a decrease in acne (pimple) problems. Some women who use the pill may develop redness or darkening of the skin over the cheeks
11. Eye irritation in some pill users who wear contact lenses

More Serious Side Effects

These are rare. Notify a physician immediately if they do occur.
1. Severe abdominal pain or discomfort (as a result of a gallbladder problem, a rare tumor in the liver, or blood clots in the bowel)
2. Severe chest pain or shortness of breath (as a result of blood clots in the heart or lungs)
3. Severe leg pain (as a result of stroke or other problems in the brain)
4. Severe headaches (as a result of stroke or other problems in the brain)
5. Eye problems such as blurred vision (as a result of blood clots or an inflamed nerve in the eye)

PATIENT'S STATEMENT

I have read the above and understand that there are benefits and risks associated with the use of birth control pills. I choose to take the pill because I believe that the benefits for me are greater than the risks.

_____   _____
Patient's Signature   Date

---

ovarian estrogens. However, it may partially block the central positive-feedback response to endogenous estrogens, resulting in inadequate amplitudes of pituitary luteinizing hormone surges (Liskin, 1983a). Nevertheless, the reported pregnancy rate of 2 to 7 per 100 women-years with this nonstop microdose progestin regimen is considerably higher than that observed with combination OC. Irregular vaginal bleeding and increased ectopic pregnancy rates among those in whom it fails further reduce the minipill's popularity. At present, the minipill may be appropriate for those few women with cardiovascular disease who cannot tolerate any estrogenic stimulation of their renin-angiotensin-aldosterone axis and those with known hypersensitivity to synthetic estrogens.

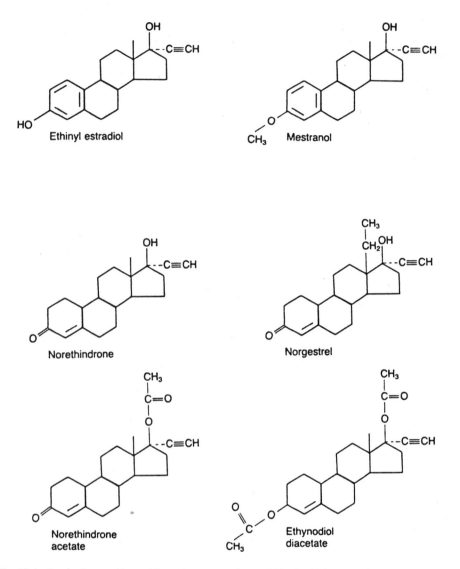

Fig. 13-1. Synthetic steroids used in oral contraceptives sold in the United States today. Estrogens: ethinyl estradiol and mestranol. Progestins: norethindrone, norethindrone acetate, norgestrel, and ethynodiol diacetate. (Courtesy Dr. P. G. Stubblefield.)

Advantages

Oral contraceptives provide noncontraceptive benefits to the appropriate user and to society. The pill protects the user from life-threatening ectopic pregnancy, reduces primary dysmenorrhea, and reduces the risks for benign and malignant gynecologic problems as listed in Box 13-1. Society also benefits from the annual reduction of more than 50,000 hospitalizations and office visits, according to studies in Britain and the United States (Brenner, 1988; Connell, 1984; Rubin, 1982). After only 1 year, pill users may be protected from the risk for endometrial and ovarian cancer for 10 years. In fact, recent data appear to suggest that pill use may even protect against hereditary forms of ovarian cancer (Narod, 1998). The progestin in OCs reduces the number of estrogen and progesterone receptors in the endometrium.

Furthermore, because ovulation does not occur, mitotic activity in the ovary, which is repeatedly high at the time of ovulation, is inhibited. There may be a delay in the return of ovulation after the cessation of OC use, with an initial prolongation of the follicular phase or a shortened luteal phase (Rice-Wray, 1967). Usually, menses resumes within 3 months and fertility returns to the preexisting rate by the end of 2 years. If regular menstruation does not return within 6 months after the cessation of OC, hormonal evaluation is indicated. These particular users may have preexisting, slow-growing, pituitary microadenomas that can be treated successfully. The pill itself does not cause pituitary tumors (Pituitary Adenoma Study Group, 1983; Shy, 1983). Weight change, stress, or undiagnosed pregnancy may explain postpill amenorrhea in other women.

Table 13-1   Some Steroidal Contraceptives in the United States

Brand Name in USA	Estrogen (μg)	Progestin (mg)	Cost ($)*
Monophasic Combination OC			
Alesse, Levlite	EE 20	D-Norgestrel 0.1	27
Loestrin 1/20	EE 20	Norethindrone acetate 1	28
Mircette	EE 20	Desogestrel 0.15	23
Desogen, Orthocept	EE 30	Desogestrel 0.15	23, 26
Loestrin 1.5/3.0	EE 30	Norethindrone acetate 1.5	28
Levlen, Levora, Nordette	EE 30	D-Norgestrel 0.15	26-27
Lo/Ovral	EE 30	DL-Norgestrel 0.3	28
Brevicon, Genora, Modicon, Necon, Nelova 0.5/35	EE 35	Norethindrone 0.5	12-29
Demulin, Zovia 1/35	EE 35	Ethynodiol diacetate 1	28, 25
Genora, Jenest, Necon, Nelova, Norethin, Norinyl, Ortho-Novum 1/35	EE 35	Norethindrone 1	15-26
Ovcon 35	EE 35	Norethindrone 0.4	28
Ortho-Cyclen	EE 35	Norgestimate 0.25	26
Ovral	EE 50	DL-Norgestrel 0.5	43
Demulen, Zovia 1/50	EE 50	Ethynodiol diacetate 1	31, 25
Ovcon 50	EE 50	Norethindrone 1	31
Genora, Necon, Norethin, Norinyl, Ortho-Novum 1/50	M 50	Norethindrone 1	15-26
Biphasic Combination OC			
Necon, Ortho-Novum 10/11	EE 35	Norethindrone 0.5 (days 1-10), 1 (days 11-21)	15, 28
Triphasic Combination OC			
Estrostep	EE 20-30-35	Norethindrone acetate 1 (days 1-5, 6-12, 13-21)	28
Tri-Levlen, Triphasil	EE 30-40-30	D-Norgestrel 0.05 (days 1-6), 0.075 (days 7-11), 0.125 (days 12-21)	25, 26
Ortho-Novum 7/7/7	EE 35	Norethindrone 0.5 (days 1-7), 0.75 (days 8-14), 1 (days 15-21)	26
Tri-Norinyl	EE 35	Norethindrone 0.5 (days 1-7), 1 (days 8-16), 0.5 (days 17-21)	25
Ortho Tri-Cyclen	EE 35	Norgestimate 0.18 (days 1-7), 0.215 (days 8-14), 0.25 (days 15-21)	26
Progestin-only OC (Minipill)			
Micronor, Nor-QD	none	Norethindrone 0.35	30
Ovrette	none	DL-Norgestrel 0.075	28
Time-Release Progestin			
Depo-Provera (injection q 3 months)	none	Medroxyprogesterone acetate 150 in aqueous suspension	8
Norplant (subdermal implant q 5 years)	none	D-Norgestrel 216 in 6 capsules	8

EE, ethinyl estradiol; M, mestranol, a methyl ester of EE that is converted by the liver into EE.

Cost to the pharmacist for 1 month's use, rounded to the nearest dollar, is based on the average wholesale price in the *1998 Drug Topics® Red Book.*

Disadvantages, Side Effects, and Contraindications

The pill must be taken daily and is considered a mild teratogen (Katz, 1985; Lammer, 1986; Linn, 1983a). Users must devise their own systems to ensure daily compliance. The pill should be taken at the same time every day. In addition, a backup method such as condoms should be used concomitantly during the first cycle, when low-estrogen OCs may not provide full protection. Lowering the content of ethinyl estradiol in each tablet from 50 μg to 20 μg increases the pregnancy rate in users (Lawson, 1979). The lower the hormonal content, the less danger there is from unwanted side effects but the higher the failure rate. Most gynecologists advise the user to take the previous day's pill if she forgets to take one pill and to take two pills each day for 2 days if she forgets to take her pill on two consecutive days. If the user forgets 3 days in a row during any given pill cycle, the pill may not be an appropriate contraceptive method. Inconsistent use or failure to establish a daily routine represents one aspect of poor compliance that may require better coaching by the health-care provider before switching methods. Other reasons leading to discontinuation are multiple side effects and unavailability of the product ("pills run out").

A disturbing side effect that can occur with or without missing the dose is intermittent or irregular breakthrough uterine bleeding (BTB). Most women do not mind having menses or amenorrhea as long as these symptoms are predictable. Therefore, careful precounseling on this possible side effect of OC is essential for successful therapy. During the first few months, BTB may resolve without treatment. Nonetheless, irregular bleeding could be a warning symptom that the efficacy of the OC may be compromised in a particular user. A thorough history should be obtained to rule out pregnancy, infection, or neoplastic bleeding. In many instances, watchful expectation may be preferred to the conventional methods of double dosing or adding more estrogen. Serious estrogen-related thromboembolic disorders appear to be dose dependent. If BTB develops or if it first occurs several months after the initiation of the pill, switching to a more progestogenic pill usually solves the problem. The use of norgestrel-containing OC may lessen the problem of irregular bleeding (Droegemueller, 1989; Ravenholt, 1987). The alternative of adding a low dose of estrogen or of switching to a more estrogenic pill should be tried only after other approaches fail (Wessler, 1976). The latter applies particularly to women committed to the daily use of OC who are not in a "prothrombotic" population, such as those with factor V Leiden Q506 mutation or prothrombin gene 20210A point mutation.

Other estrogen-induced side effects of OCs, listed on the patient consent form (Box 13-1), include nausea, vascular headache, elevated blood pressure, weight gain (from fluid retention), tender breasts (mastalgia), increased mucoid vaginal discharge, cervical erosion (ectropion), or polyposis (Goldzieher, 1971). A mild increase in blood pressure may occur because of the activation of the renin-angiotensin-aldosterone system, hypervolemia, and decreased prostacyclin (Petitti, 1983). If the diastolic blood pressure is elevated (greater than 90 mm Hg) in response to OC use, discontinuation should be considered. An undisputed pill-induced human tumor is hepatic adenoma. This tumor is related to the use of synthetic estrogens, and it develops in 3.4 of 100,000 women per year (Porter, 1981; Scott, 1984; Shar, 1982). Synthetic estrogens in the pill induce increased hepatic proteins (renin substrate, binding globulins, and most blood-clotting factors) and decreased antithrombin III, protein S, and plasminogen activators (Box 13-2) (Gaspard, 1987; Mammen, 1982; Seligsohn, 1984; von Kaulla, 1971). Hy-

---

BOX 13-2
SOME LABORATORY VALUES THAT ARE INFLUENCED BY COMBINATION ORAL CONTRACEPTIVE PILLS

Values That May Be Increased
Hematologic

Clotting factors (I, II, VII, VIII, IX, X, and XII)
Antiplasmins and antiactivators of fibrinolysis
Erythrocyte sedimentation rate
Red and white blood cells and platelets
Iron and iron-binding capacity

Hepatic Proteins and Related Tests

α_1-globulins, α_2-globulins, and various binding globulins
Renin, angiotensin, angiotensinogen, and aldosterone
Bromosulfophthalein, bilirubin, and alkaline phosphatase
Transaminases and transpeptidase
Coproporphyrin and porphobilinogen

Hormonal

Growth hormone and insulin (and blood glucose)
Urinary total estrogens

Sterol and Lipid

Vitamin A
Triglycerides and phospholipids
Low-density lipoprotein—cholesterol

Others

α_1-antitrypsin, C-reactive protein, serum copper, and ceruloplasmin
Urinary xanthuric acid
Positive results for antinuclear antibody and lupus erythematosus preparation

Values That May Be Decreased
Hematologic

Folate and vitamin B_{12}
Antithrombin III and fibrinolytic activity

Hormonal

Luteinizing and follicle-stimulating hormones
Urinary pregnanediol and 17-ketosteroids
Triiodothyronine resin uptake

Others

Glucose tolerance, zinc, magnesium, and ascorbic acid
High-density lipoprotein—cholesterol (HDL-C)
Hepatoglobulin and cholinesterase

---

percoagulability commonly occurs in pill users with an inherited resistance to activated protein C (factor V Leiden mutation) that can be specifically identified by a polymerase chain reaction probe. Prothrombotic women may be screened by blood coagulation testing on plasma (drawn in

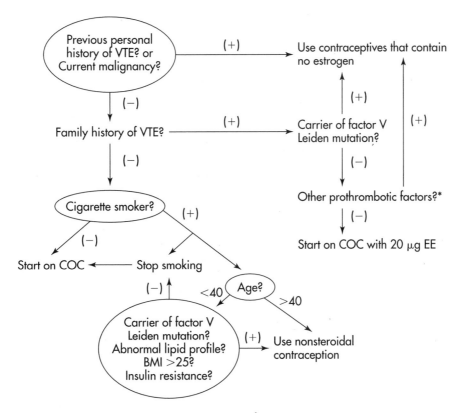

Fig. 13-2. Counseling steroidal contraceptors regarding risks for VTE. VTE, venous thromboembolism; BMI, body mass index; COC, combination oral contraceptive pills; EE, ethinyl estradiol. *Prothrombotic factors evaluation: tests of coagulation and anticoagulation, especially activities of antithrombin III, protein C, free protein S, fibrinolysis, antifibrinolysis, fibrin turnover, and prothrombin gene 20210A point mutation.

acid-citrate-dextrose), which can be performed at reputable commercial laboratories or tertiary hospitals. Activated protein C resistance can be acquired during pregnancy or OC use without the presence of factor V gene mutation. Thus, a positive finding on screening for reduced protein C activity could result from an undiagnosed pregnancy. At the current price of laboratory testing, it is controversial whether screening all prospective OC users would be cost effective. Two important points should be clarified in this regard. First, the strongest risk factor for venous thromboembolism (VTE) is a history of VTE. Another important risk factor is current or occult malignancy. Second, major advances in identifying women at high risk for VTE include the discovery of a familial thrombophilia related to factor V Leiden mutation (Dahlbäck, 1993; Bertina, 1994; Martinelli, 1998) and the fact that OC users born with this gene mutation are at extremely high risk for VTE (Vandenbroucke, 1994). Specifically, the risk for VTE among pill users with factor V Leiden mutation was increased eightfold when compared with pill users who were noncarriers and more than thirtyfold when compared with women who were neither pill users nor carriers of the mutation. Earlier epidemiologic studies also disclosed twofold to fourfold increases in the diagnoses of cholelithiasis, postoperative deep vein thrombosis, pulmonary embolism (1 of 30,000 women per year), and cerebral thrombosis (1 of 30,000 women per year) among

users of OCs that contained more than 50 μg synthetic estrogen in comparison with nonusers (Petitti, 1979; Porter, 1985; Ramcharan, 1980; Royal College of GP, 1982; Stadel, 1981; Vessey, 1977; Vessey, 1984). The overall annual risk for VTE may be 1 to 2 of 10,000 current users. Factors that affect risk are the estrogen content of the pill (and perhaps of certain progestins in the pill), blood type, race (more prevalent in white women of European descent), smoking, high body mass index, advanced age, and sedentary lifestyle. This risk is lower in women with type O blood (Jick, 1969). It disappears after cessation of the pill and is not related to the length of use of the pill. The effects of estrogen in reducing the activity of protein S and plasminogen activators are dose related (Mammen, 1982; Wessler, 1976; Lidegaard, 1993). Common sites of VTE are legs, lungs, brain, retina, liver, and mesentery. Figure 13-2 provides an algorithm for counseling prospective OC users to avoid or reduce the risk for VTE.

Untoward events related to progestins are decreased menses, reduced vaginal secretion, weight gain because of increased appetite, acne, leg cramps, fatigue, and sleepiness. In addition, BTB, chloasma, depression or mood change, and hypertension may be related to progestin use. Depression in some pill users may be result from pyridoxine deficiency with the concomitant increase in xanthurenic acid. Certain medications, including long-term antibiotics, anticonvulsants, and some sedatives, make OCs less effective (Editorial BMJ, 1980; Mattson, 1986; Orme, 1983; Potts, 1983; Szoka, 1988). The most notorious is the antituberculous drug rifampin. Increased hepatic microsomal activity results in increased OC metabolism and decreased contraceptive effectiveness. Additionally, a disturbed intestinal function (enterohepatic circulation) or a colonic bacterial milieu may lower the pill's efficacy. Commonly prescribed drugs that may decrease the contraceptive effect of the pill include barbiturates, carbamazepine, griseofulvin, primidone, phenytoin, long-term tetracycline, and troglitazone. Backup contraceptive methods and the use of a 50-μg estrogen pill may be required. Note also that the pill may delay the elimination of theophylline drugs, and it may decrease the efficacy of oral anticoagulant preparations.

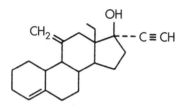

Desogestrel

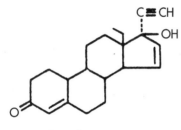

Gestodene

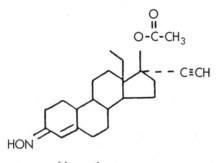

Norgestimate

Fig. 13-3. New progestins not yet available in the United States and Europe.

A recent subject of debate was the long-term metabolic effect of progestins if serum high-density lipoprotein (HDL) cholesterol levels are lowered (Arntzenius, 1978; Bradley, 1978; Burkman, 1988; Connell, 1984; Gaspard, 1987; Gordon, 1977; Kay, 1982; Lincoln, 1984; Mann, 1975; Meade, 1980; Mishell, 1988b; Petitti, 1979; Petitti, 1983; Porter; 1985; Royal College of GP, 1983; Stadel, 1981). One study revealed increased mortality rates among pill users 25 years of age and older because of circulatory diseases. Others showed an increased risk for coronary thrombosis and nonfatal myocardial infarction among pill users older than 30 years of age. However, close scrutiny later revealed that the risk was limited to those with hypertension, diabetes, and hyperlipidemia. The greatest risk, estimated to be 1 in 5000 women per year, was actually found among pill users older than 35 years of age who smoke. Interestingly, the risk for coronary heart disease is not increased in former pill users, and it is not correlated with the duration of OC use (Stampfer, 1988). The latter finding suggests that pill-induced coronary vascular changes may be thrombotic and not atherogenic in origin (Brenner, 1988). Progestins in the pill are associated with an increased risk for atherosclerosis because they tend to lower the levels of serum HDL and HDL$_2$ (Mishell, 1988b). In contrast, exogenous estrogens in the pill tend to raise HDL levels. Thus, the effects of a combination OC on the user's lipid profile may depend on the variable interactions between the relative estrogenicity of the estrogen versus the antiestrogenicity and androgenicity of the progestin and on the dosage of the two hormones. Note, however, that the potency of a progestin in terms of delayed menses, withdrawal bleeding, or endometrial glycogen vacuoles may not be applicable in different women (Goldzieher, 1984; Orme, 1983). Furthermore, some progestins display inherent estrogenic activity as they are converted in the body to estradiol. Norethynodrel, the first-generation progestin used in OCs, was highly estrogenic. All progestins in OC are synthetic derivatives of 19-nortestosterone (meaning no carbon 19). The addition of an ethinyl group to carbon 17 results in an orally active steroid, norethindrone, and in other estrane progestins that include norethynodrel, norethindrone acetate, ethynodiol diacetate, lynestrenol, norgestrienone, norgesterone, and quingestanol acetate. More potent progestins (the gonanes) contain an ethyl group at carbon 13 (e.g., norgestrel, norgestimate, and desogestrel). The active form of norgestrel is D-norgestrel (levonorgestrel). This 19-norsteroid stays in the body longer than other progestins. Unlike other progestins, levonorgestrel is unique in that its oral administration does not bring about any effects of first-pass hepatic metabolism. The third group of progestins (the pregnanes) are derivatives of 17-OH-progesterone such as chlormadinone acetate, medroxyprogesterone acetate, megestrol acetate, and cyproterone acetate. Thirteen progestins are used in more than 300 brand names of steroid contraceptives in various countries. Third-generation progestins such as desogestrel, gestodene, and norgestimate (Fig. 13-3) are less androgenic and may be associated with estrogen-induced side effects such as breast tenderness (Rakers, 1988). Oral contraceptives that contain desogestrel or norgestimate may be the most beneficial for women with idiopathic hirsutism or acne and for selected patients with polycystic ovary syndrome (Mall-Haefeli, 1982; Rojanasakul, 1987; Samsioe, 1982; Siegberg, 1984). Desogestrel lacks intrinsic androgenicity (Mall-Haefeli, 1982; Samsioe, 1982). It does not interfere with the estrogen's capacity to induce an increase in sex hormone–binding globulin. Consequently, combination OCs that contain desogestrel increase the binding capacity for androgens. This leads to a substantial decrease in free testosterone and free 5α-dihydrotestosterone (Rojanasakul, 1987). Other OCs also provide users with this beneficial effect. Active metabolites of desogestrel and norgestimate are 11-methylene-levonorgestrel (3-ketodesogestrel) and norgestrel-related compounds, respectively. A small risk for VTE, reported in some studies of third-generation pills, is the topic of debate in the United States. However, experts at the World Health Organization (WHO) meeting in November 1997 concluded that preparations containing desogestrel or gestodene probably carry a slightly higher risk for VTE than those with levonorgestrel (approximately 1 to 2 women per 10,000 pill users annually) (Farley, 1998). Data are insufficient to draw conclusions with regard to combined OCs containing norgestimate.

Although the use of OCs reduces the incidence of benign breast disease, limited epidemiologic and laboratory data emerge almost every year to suggest an increased risk for breast cancer in pill users. Specifically, worrisome findings with regard to breast cancer in pill users were disclosed after the 1984 exoneration of the pill by a U.S. Food and Drug Administration (FDA) panel of experts. Because OCs have been available since 1960 and because the peak incidence of female breast cancer occurs in women between 55 and 74 years of age, any long-term latency effects of early pill use may not show up until the millenium. Recently, WHO and World Bank scientists reviewed collaborative data from 25 countries (Meirik, 1996; Beral, 1996a; Beral, 1996b). These data suggest that current users of OCs are at slightly increased risk for breast cancer, that this relative risk (1.24) progressively declines toward baseline (1.0) or less 10 years after the cessation of OC use, and that cancers diagnosed in current or recent users of OCs appear to be clinically less advanced than those in women who never used OCs. Such data cannot explain whether this difference reflects early detection in the group that uses or has used the pill, a biologic effect of OCs, or a combination thereof. It appears that OC use does not influence breast cancer mortality rates among women in developed countries. Data implicating OC use with an increased risk for cervical cancer (Irwin, 1988; Lincoln, 1984; Royal College of GP, 1981; Vessey, 1983; WHO, 1985) and malignant melanoma have also been published (Stevens, 1980). Epithelial abnormalities of the uterine cervix in many OC users are a matter of concern among epidemiologists because of the transmission of the human papillomavirus, human immunodeficiency virus (HIV), and *Chlamydia trachomatis* (Louv, 1989; Piot, 1989; Washington, 1985; WHO, 1985). Definite conclusions on the risks for breast and cervical cancer and for malignant melanoma among pill users cannot be drawn based on the available data because study designs have not accounted for the presence and influence of important confounding factors (Swann, 1982). It is accepted, however, that breast cancer, some gynecologic tumors, and certain adenocarcinomas and adenomas may be stimulated by sex steroids. Therefore, women with a history of such tumors should not use the pill.

Absolute contraindications to OC use should include any history of thromboembolic disorder, chronic liver disease, undiagnosed uterine bleeding, pregnancy, breast cancer, and estrogen-dependent neoplasia. Other strong contraindications are coronary heart disease, unstable angina (unstable atheroma or other reactive lesions of the coronary artery), stroke, hypertension, dyslipidemia (especially type II hyperlipoproteinemia), smoking in women older than 40, cyanotic heart disease, sickle cell disease, severe headaches, active gallbladder disease, and conditions requiring total immobilization (Brennner, 1988; Freie, 1983; Mishell, 1988; Petitti, 1983; Porter, 1985; Vessey, 1984). A rare type of headache associated with papilledema (pseudotumor cerebri or idiopathic intracranial hypertension) contraindicates the use of any contraceptive steroid.

Relative contraindications include smoking in women older than 35, moderate or severe cervical intraepithelial neoplasia, migraines (especially with visual disturbance or additional neurologic symptoms), and certain types of diabetes mellitus. Women with diabetes and elevated blood pressure, nephropathy, or retinopathy must be discouraged from using the pill. Many women with well-controlled diabetes or migraines have tolerated OC use and are happy with it. The use of a low-dose OC does not appear to alter the pill user's tolerance to a 75-g oral glucose load (Kasdorf, 1988). Impaired carbohydrate metabolism occurs with a high-dose formulation that contains norgestrel (Diamond, 1988). Oral contraceptive-induced insulin resistance is manifested by reduced peripheral tissue insulin sensitivity and may ameliorate with time (Kasdorf, 1988).

BARRIER METHODS AND SPERMICIDES
Condoms (Prophylactics)

The condom is without doubt the most popular, yet underreported, mechanical contraceptive method, for various justifiable reasons. It is disposable, convenient to use, and sold over the counter, and it may help prevent the spread of STDs. It should be used by pregnant women who have or are at risk for STDs (Goldsmith, 1981). Its use may be indicated even though a couple is sterile. Regarding the feared viral transmission, latex appears to be superior to other materials for making condoms. However, the perfect barrier material has not yet been invented. An allergic reaction to latex is uncommon, but it can be life threatening. Furthermore, latex material can be destroyed by oil-based intravaginal medications. A newly approved condom made of polyurethane appears to be thinner and stronger than the latex rubber and may circumvent the allergy or incompatibility problem. The chance of failure may be further reduced when the condom is prelubricated with a spermicide. The failure rate was estimated to be 3 per 1000 with correct (perfect) use. Condoms cover the penis during coitus and serve as a reservoir to prevent the deposition of semen in the vagina. The prototype of a condom made of animal products, before the vulcanization of rubber, has been in use for centuries. Failures are related to the material itself or to the manufacturing process and to the user's technical or mental difficulties (*e.g.,* wearing the condom after some semen has been released into the vagina or after sperm has begun to escape as a result of failure to withdraw before detumescence). Besides improper technique, failure rates of barrier contraceptives are often influenced by inconsistent use.

Spermicidal Agents

Most vaginal spermicides contain nonoxynol-9, a surface-active, nontoxic detergent that immobilizes sperm. It is available as a cream, jelly, aerosol foam, foaming tablet, and suppository. Another formulation comes in the form of a semitransparent square of contraceptive film that dissolves at body temperature into a gel. Each product is available in 1% or 100-mg strength, but some contain as much as 5% to 28% nonoxynol-9. It is convenient and inexpensive, and it has a theoretical failure rate of 5 pregnancies per 100 women-years. No association has been established between the use of vaginal spermicides and birth defects (Harlap, 1985; Louik, 1987; Warburton, 1987). These agents are considered microbicidal and may lower the risk for most STDs. However, they disrupt the integrity of the mucosa's cell membrane, especially with repeated applications within a short period of time. Vaginal or penile irritation because of local hypersensitivity to nonoxynol-9 may occur in some users, but this adverse effect is not common.

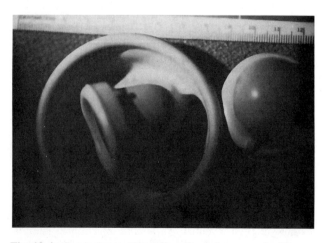

Fig. 13-4. Cervical caps (Prentiff cavity rim) compared with a diaphragm.

Another type of spermicide under investigation is a well-known drug, propranolol, which kills sperm on contact (Hong, 1982; Zipper, 1983). Its spermicidal property was first discovered in men with hypertension who became azoospermic after oral therapy. Among many β-sympathomimetic antagonists tested, propranolol showed the strongest spermicidal effect. The mechanism for this effect may be related to the drug's lipophilic activity (Peterson, 1973). National and international resources are now concentrated on research to find an ideal spermicide that can inactivate sexually transmitted microbes, especially immunodeficiency and oncogenic viruses.

Intravaginal Devices

The diaphragm is a barrier between the lower vaginal canal and the cervical canal. It is a circular patch made of latex rubber and held by a circular, collapsible metal frame that acts like a spring. The user must compress this circular spring rim to flatten and elongate it so that it can slip into the vagina while the user is in a squatting or one-thigh-up position. There are four types of rim: coil, flat, wide-seal, or arcing. The latter may be the easiest to insert correctly for full coverage of the cervical os. It comes in nine sizes based on the diameter of the circular rim (from 50 to 90 mm at 5-mm increments). The three sizes in the middle range (65, 70, and 75 mm) will fit most women. The proper size is determined after a vaginal examination and a trial with different-sized rings. The diaphragm should be adequately large but should not interfere with urination. It rests in place under the urethra. Women with frequent cystitis may not be good candidates for diaphragm use (Fihn, 1985). Anatomic changes, such as marked weight gain or loss or development of vaginismus, may require refitting. Proper retention of the device may not be possible in women with pelvic floor relaxation disorders and procidentia. If used correctly by women with high motivation and good compliance, its failure rate is theoretically less than 3 pregnancies per 100 women-years. Spermicidal jelly should be applied on each side of the diaphragm before its insertion, and the device should be left in place for at least 6 hours after intercourse. It is then removed, washed, dried, and put away until the next usage. It must not be dusted with talcum powder because talc may increase the risk for ovarian cancer. Diaphragm use may lower the risk for pelvic inflammatory disease (PID) and cervical epithelial neoplasia (Cramer, 1987; Kelaghan, 1982; Tatum, 1981). There is controversy regarding any association between toxic shock syndrome and diaphragm use.

The cervical cap is much smaller than the diaphragm (Fig. 13-4) and must fit tightly over the cervix. It has a soft, nonmetal rim with an external diameter that ranges from 22 to 35 mm. Its cuplike shape accommodates the body of the cervix, with the circular rim toward the fornix. The Prentiff cavity rim that is manufactured in England has gained acceptance in the United States. One active investigator advises the use of a spermicidal jelly with a high (3% to 5%) concentration of nonoxynol-9 on the cervical side for contraceptive efficacy and suction-cup effect (Koch, 1982). Such potent spermicides include Ramses (of Quality Health Products, Yaphank, N.Y.) (5%), Koromex (also of Quality Health Products) (3%), or K-Y Plus (of Ortho-McNeil, Raritan, N.J.) (2%). It can be left in place for several days and must be removed if vaginal or menstrual bleeding occurs. Each new user should have Papanicolaou smear taken before fitting and after the first 3 months. The increased risk for cervical erosion and neoplasia among cap users has been a concern. Other problems include the widely different sizes and shapes of the cervix and the difficulty in educating patients about the correct placement of the cap. Many women have trouble locating the cervix with their fingers. Other women, especially among certain cultures, do not like to touch their own genitals. If a user cannot remove the cap (a rare occurrence), a vaginal speculum is required; the cap will drop out of place once the speculum is opened inside the vagina. The cap's failure rate of 8 to 20 pregnancies per 100 women-years is higher than that of the diaphragm. Several designs of custom-fit caps are undergoing clinical trials. Such caps have a one-way valve to permit the outflow of uterine and cervical secretions while blocking sperm entrance.

The female condom is another type of mechanical barrier that has been used sporadically since the beginning of the twentieth century. The type that has received FDA approval is a disposable seamless polyurethane device that fits loosely inside the vagina and covers the perineum. It has flexible rings at both ends. At the closed end, the inner ring can be compressed and pushed into the vagina to cover the cervix. It is soft and prelubricated, and its aim is to prevent any contact with body secretions for both partners. However, additional lubrication may be required to prevent dislodgment and unpleasant noises during use. Its contraceptive efficacy is comparable to that of other barrier methods. The rebirth of the female condom reflects the need for more protection against viral transmission. In fact, barrier contraceptives have become immensely popular, even though some users consider them messy or inconvenient. Such methods require manipulation of the genitalia at or near the time of coitus and thus require serious motivation for successful use.

Intrauterine Devices

The intrauterine device (IUD) is a highly effective means of birth control for a well-selected group of women (Liskin, 1982). It is a small, plastic T-shaped rod or tiny circular ring made to fit easily inside the uterus. With an IUD in place, the uterus and oviducts become hostile to the sperm, oocyte, and fertilized ovum (WHO, 1987a). Consequently, 96% to 99% of women who wear an IUD for a year will not conceive. Use of an IUD is not associated with unwanted metabolic effects, and one device lasts a long time in comparison with other reversible contraceptive methods. It is appropriate for women at low risk for STD because its use is associated with an increased risk for PID and tubal infertility (Cramer,

1985; Daling, 1985). Because the IUD effectively prevents pregnancy, its use does not increase the overall incidence of tubal pregnancy. In fact, the incidence of ectopic pregnancy among 1000 women who use IUDs is significantly lower than it is among 1000 women who do not use contraceptives. However, a high incidence of ectopic pregnancy has been observed among women who conceive while using IUDs, particularly the type that releases progesterone or levonorgestrel (Diaz, 1980). This may be analogous to the increased risk for ectopic pregnancy among women in whom there is minipill failure. Any woman who has had an ectopic pregnancy or a venereal disease, such as gonorrhea or chlamydia, should not use an IUD (Box 13-3).

Of all the U.S. FDA-approved IUDs, only two kinds are available: the Copper T-380A, which lasts at least 10 years, and the Progestasert, which requires annual replacement. Both are T-shaped, radiopaque IUDs, but they differ in many aspects. The copper-containing device is superior to the non-copper device in contraceptive efficacy and perhaps carries lower relative risk for PID (Cramer, 1985; Sivin, 1981; Zipper, 1969). The worst record for PID risk in IUD devices was observed with the Dalkon shield, and it was attributed to poor design (Liskin, 1982). A significantly increased risk for PID in IUD wearers was observed during the first few months after insertion (Burkman, 1981). Women who have used a copper IUD for 6 months without adverse events tend to become successful, long-term users of this method. If salpingitis develops more than a few months after insertion, it is probably the result of an STD and not of the IUD (Liskin, 1982). Women at high risk for PID include, in order of significance, those with a history of PID or STD, those who have multiple sex partners, those who are nulliparous, and those younger than 25 years of age. (Mishell, 1988). They should be discouraged from using IUDs. Those at lowest risk for PID are parous women in a stable and mutually monogamous relationship. Because of its lack of metabolic effects, a copper-containing IUD may be ideal for an older parous woman who smokes and does not want permanent sterilization.

Mechanism of Action

The IUD prevents fertilization and implantation by several postulated mechanisms, all of which are promptly reversible on removal of the device. It alters the intrauterine environment by inducing a local, sterile, inflammatory response (foreign-body reaction) (Mishell, 1966). It is thought that leukocyte infiltration leads to an environment that is hostile to the oocyte, sperm, and fertilized ovum. Studies of daily serum human chorionic gonadotropin (hCG) levels in the luteal phase using highly sensitive assays led to the conclusion that implantation did not occur in IUD wearers (Segal, 1985; Sharpe, 1977; Wilcox, 1987). A controlled study of oocytes retrieved by tubal flushing strongly suggested that the IUD also inhibits fertilization (WHO, 1987a). Sperm may not reach the oocyte or may be unable to penetrate the oocyte coverings. Alternatively, an adverse tubal environment

---

BOX 13-3
PATIENT CONSENT FORM FOR INTRAUTERINE CONTRACEPTIVE DEVICE INSERTION

Intrauterine devices (IUDs) are effective means for birth control, especially for women older than 25 years of age who already have children. However, there are certain problems with IUDs that you must know about if you are considering having one inserted.

1. Sometimes women become pregnant, even with the IUD in place (2 to 4 pregnancies per 100 women per year). Women who become pregnant while using an IUD are more likely to have a miscarriage or a premature delivery if the pregnancy continues. Occasionally, a serious infection can develop in the uterus. Therefore, in the event you become pregnant with an IUD in place, termination of the pregnancy should be strongly considered.
2. Women who become pregnant while using an IUD have a slightly increased chance that the pregnancy may occur in the tube (ectopic pregnancy). Ectopic pregnancy is a serious condition that requires surgery or a toxic drug for its treatment. Therefore, if you think you are pregnant with an IUD in place, you must report to your doctor without undue delay.
3. Having an IUD slightly increases your risk for an infection in the fallopian tubes. Some of the infections can be serious and may result in infertility. Your risk for a tubal infection is greatly increased if you have more than one male partner. This risk for an IUD-related infection is low in women in a mutually monogamous relationship.
4. Many women with IUDs find that their menstrual patterns are changed and that they have bleeding between periods or that the menstrual period is heavier and more painful. You should consult your doctor if you have lower abdominal pain or abnormal vaginal discharge or bleeding, and if you think you are pregnant or have a sexually transmitted infection.
5. Sometimes the IUD can be expelled (it falls out).
6. Sometimes the IUD perforates the uterus (it makes a hole in your womb) at the time of insertion.

PATIENT'S STATEMENT

I have read the above and understand that there are risks associated with the use of an IUD. I have also read and signed the necessary form provided by the IUD manufacturer. I choose to use this method of contraception because I feel that the benefits for me are greater than the risks.

_____   _____
Patient's Signature   Date

---

may damage the oocyte. Macrophage destruction of oocytes was shown in copper IUD wearers. Copper may interfere with oocyte release or fimbria function, accelerate transport, or induce premature lysis of the ovum. In contrast to progesterone, copper inhibits the enzyme prostaglandin dehydrogenase in the local tissues (Kelly, 1983). The amount of copper absorbed in the systemic circulation is minute compared with the minimum daily dietary requirement. Rare incidences have been reported of allergic skin lesions with pruritus resulting from copper IUD use; these can be confirmed by standard skin tests (Ramaguero, 1981).

Insertion Technique

The optimal time to insert an IUD is during menses, when a woman is least likely to be pregnant. Before the day of insertion, the IUD user should have an opportunity to become acquainted with the instructions and the informed consent form. Some women may require local anesthesia (paracervical block), especially if the device is inserted on a day between menses. Bimanual pelvic examination determines uterine size and position. The cervix is exposed with a speculum and cleansed with a local antiseptic, and its anterior lip is grasped with a tenaculum. Gentle traction to straighten the angle between the cervical canal and the uterine cavity is followed by a probing of the uterine cavity with a uterine sound to determine the internal direction and depth. The short-bladed Moore-Graves speculum may be re-

quired if there is acute anteflexion. The device is loaded into its inserter and gently slipped through the cervical canal. It is then freed within the uterine cavity by withdrawing the inserter tube over the plunger. This withdrawal technique reduces the risk for uterine perforation. Women who use IUDs should report without delay any lower abdominal pain, fever, chills, unusual vaginal bleeding or spotting, pain during intercourse, or unpleasant vaginal discharge. A brief follow-up visit should be conducted 3 months after IUD insertion. Annual check-ups that include cytologic cervical smears should be performed after that.

Disadvantages, Adverse Effects, and Contraindications

Dysmenorrhea and increased menstrual flow are common IUD-related problems that may improve with the short-term intermittent use of a nonsteroidal anti-inflammatory drug (NSAID) such as ibuprofen or naproxen. These drugs (type 1 inhibitors) inhibit the biosynthesis of cyclic endoperoxides and prostaglandin E and F series. If the problems persist or worsen, the device should be removed and the patient should be offered another choice of contraceptive. A new IUD has been designed with side arms that open and close with uterine relaxation and contraction to decrease the incidence of IUD-related dysmenorrhea. Progestin-releasing IUDs were originally intended to alleviate bleeding and dysmenorrhea. Unfortunately, they have been shown to increase the number of days of bleeding and the incidence of midcycle spotting, even though the volume of monthly blood loss is actually reduced. A report by the WHO Task Force on Psychological Research in Family Planning indicated that an increase in the number of days of bleeding may be less acceptable to women than an increase in the volume of bleeding (WHO, 1987a). Another WHO study revealed no difference in dysmenorrhea symptoms induced by Progestasert and Copper-7 (Pizarro, 1979). Subsequently, those findings from WHO were confirmed by various independent investigators (Fylling, 1979; Nilsson, 1981), who reported similar removal rates for progestin-releasing IUDs and copper or nonmedicated devices.

Another IUD-related problem that received careful review concerned a unique organism, *Actinomyces* (Gupta and Woodruff, 1982). Reports have emerged on the frequent *Actinomyces*-positive Papanicolaou smears among users of nonmedicated IUDs. There was also a high degree of association between true pelvic actinomycosis and the use of multifilamented tailed IUDs (which have since been discontinued). Although uncommon, true pelvic actinomycosis is a serious disease. If a woman has PID and an *Actinomyces*-positive Papanicolaou smear, aggressive intravenous therapy with broad-spectrum antibiotics is required (Valicenti, 1982). Lack of prompt clinical improvement strongly indicates tuboovarian abscesses that generally require pelviscopic surgery. *Actinomyces*-positive Papanicolaou smears are less frequently found in conjunction with the use of a copper IUD than with a noncopper device (Duguid, 1980). It has been postulated that copper may adversely affect the microbes, the gametes, and the tubal mucosa.

In women older than 25, the reported failure rate of the Copper T-380A is only 1 in 100 users per year. However, 1 of 2 IUD users who conceives has a miscarriage, and 1 of 20 IUD users who conceives has an extrauterine pregnancy. With an IUD in place, there is high risk for sepsis among users who miscarry, particularly when the miscarriage occurs during the second trimester. Women who conceive while using an IUD should have the device removed or should consider a therapeutic induced abortion because the risks and consequences are serious. An important risk is prematurity with or without sepsis (Toth, 1988). If an unplanned pregnancy occurs after IUD use of more than 2 years, the risk for its being ectopic is high. Besides the IUD, contraceptive methods that predispose a user to ectopic pregnancy, should the method fail, include minipills and depot progestin injections, subdermal progestin implants, emergency postcoital steroid contraception, and most types of female sterilization.

Spontaneous expulsion of an IUD may occur in the first few months, especially during menses. The disappearance of the IUD string, which indicates that the patient should see her physician, may be the first sign of a lost IUD. Pregnancy must be ruled out, and pelvic ultrasonography can be helpful with this. High-resolution transabdominal and transvaginal ultrasound imaging by an experienced sonographer may reveal an abnormal position of the IUD in the uterine wall or

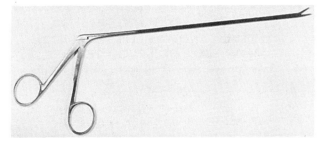

Fig. 13-5. Alligator forceps for IUD removal. (Courtesy Dr. P. G. Stubblefield.)

posterior wall of the cervix. Because most plastic devices are impregnated with barium sulfate, x-rays of the abdomen and pelvis confirm the absence or presence of the IUD in nonpregnant users who cannot find the IUD string. Ultrasound guidance and alligator forceps (Fig. 13-5) can facilitate the nontraumatic removal of an IUD when the string is not visible (Stubblefield, 1988). The failure of this method of removal usually suggests that part of the IUD has perforated the uterine wall, for which laparoscopy is indicated. Partial expulsion of the stem of the T-shaped device may occur through the cervical canal. This may result in cramps, vaginal or cervical erosion with spotting, lacerations of the penis, and reduced contraceptive efficacy. The device must be removed and replaced.

If the uterus becomes perforated from the intraperitoneal protrusion of a copper-containing IUD, the device must be removed without delay because tissue reactions will rapidly bring about severe adhesions and enclosure of the omentum. Downward displacement of the stem into the endocervix (usually posteriorly) may require slight upward dislocation before the whole device can be removed through the cervical canal.

Absolute contraindications for IUD use include a history of PID, STD, ectopic pregnancy, multiple male partners, purulent cervicitis, unresolved cervical neoplasia, undiagnosed genital bleeding, suspected pregnancy, Wilson's disease or known hypersensitivity to copper, valvular heart disease, genital actinomycosis, and any medical disorder that predisposes a patient to infection. Relative contraindications include nulliparity, age younger than 25 years, sexually active women who are not in a mutually monogamous relationship, recurrent vaginitis, anatomic derangement of the uterus (*e.g.,* congenital anomalies, leiomyoma, cervical stenosis), painful heavy menses, anemia, rheumatic heart disease, or mitral valve prolapse (WHO, 1987a).

POSTCOITAL CONTRACEPTION AND TREATMENT FOR SEXUAL ASSAULT

The morning-after pill or injection is the most practical way to terminate the natural development of the fertilized egg(s) after unprotected sexual intercourse. Initially, the hormonal way to prevent fertilization of an egg or implantation of a fer-

---

BOX 13-4
POSTCOITAL ANTIFERTILITY TREATMENT
FROM SELECTED CLINICAL TRIALS

Method	Regimen*
Alesse	5 tablets and 5 more 12 hrs later
Diethylstilbestrol†	50 mg daily for 5 days
Ethinyl estradiol	5 mg daily for 5 days
Conjugated estrogens	30 mg daily for 5 days or 50 mg daily injection for 2 days
Lo/Oral	4 tablets and 4 more 12 hrs later
Ovral	Two tablets and two more 12 hrs later
Danazol	400 mg and 400 mg 12 hrs later
D-norgestrel	0.4 mg within 3 hrs of coitus
RU486	Midluteal 50 or 100 mg daily for 4 days regardless of time of coitus
Copper-T IUD	Insertion within 5 days of coitus

*Starting as soon as possible and within 2 or 3 days of coitus unless otherwise stated.

†Not recommended by the manufacturer, according to the package insert.

---

tilized egg was the administration of high doses of a nonsteroidal estrogenic drug, diethylstilbestrol, within 3 days of unprotected coitus (Box 13-4). Morris and van Wagenen (1966) were among the first to demonstrate the effectiveness of the morning-after estrogenic pill for intercepting pregnancy in women who were raped. They reported that either diethylstilbestrol or ethinyl estradiol tablets could be administered for this purpose (Morris and van Wagenen, 1967). Other estrogens that have been effective are conjugated estrogens, estradiol benzoate, and stilbestrol diphosphate (Cook, 1986; Dickson, 1980; Morris and van Wagenen, 1973). Besides exogenous estrogens, a host of steroidal and nonsteroidal drugs, such as progesterone-receptor blockers, antimetabolites, alkaloids, and prostaglandins, have antifertility effects when administered after coitus (Shearman, 1973). They exert endocrine effects at local and possibly central levels, but the precise mode of action for each type of morning-after pill has not been conclusively demonstrated.

Postcoital estrogen may prevent pregnancy by several postulated mechanisms, depending on when it is administered in the cycle. A fertilized egg normally reaches the uterine wall in 4 or 5 days, after which implantation of the blastocyst may or may not take place (Croxatto, 1972). One of three midcycle exposures generally results in implantation of the blastocyst, which occurs on or after the sixth day of ovulation. Altered or asynchronic endometrial glandular and stromal development with resultant enzymatic and metabolic derangement, such as reduced cellular carbonic anhydrase, may render the secretory endometrium nonreceptive to implantation. Disturbances in the endogenous estrogen/progesterone ratio and decreased luteal progesterone may also be responsible for the drug's antifertility effects. A high

dose of estrogen administered late in the follicular phase may suppress ovulation and often prevents an elevation in basal body temperature (Gore, 1973; Johansson, 1973). Other hypotheses regarding its effectiveness include interferences with sperm or tubal motility, sperm capacitation, fertilization, and viability of the zygote. However, once implantation has taken place, the progression of pregnancy appears to be resistant to most steroids.

Birth defects may result if a woman is unknowingly pregnant and takes the morning-after pill. Controversy exists over whether such birth defects are directly related to the exposure to sex steroids during early pregnancy. Nevertheless, menstrual history must be carefully analyzed before administering any postcoital antifertility treatment. If pregnancy is possible, a rapid, specific, and sensitive pregnancy test should be performed and repeated at appropriate intervals. A signed informed consent form that addresses the immediate and late untoward effects of therapy and the recommendation of abortion in the case of treatment failure may be obtained before prescribing a specific postcoital antifertility therapy. Failure rates for most methods are generally less than 2 per 100 isolated courses of treatment. Rates of actual failure depend on the time of exposure in the cycle, factors inherent to each method, and the subject. However, a woman who requests postcoital antifertility therapy may choose to carry her unwanted pregnancy to term in the event of treatment failure. Interestingly, ectopic pregnancies were diagnosed in 10% of women whose postcoital estrogen therapy failed (Smythe, 1975)

High doses of estrogen often produce an uncomfortable bloated feeling, nausea, vomiting, and swelling of the hands and feet. Estrogen treatment may induce spotting or menstrual disturbances for several cycles (*i.e.,* shorter- or longer-than-expected cycles). An antiemetic pill or rectal suppository (*e.g.,* prochlorperazine) should be taken at least one half hour before therapy with high doses of estrogen. If vomiting occurs within 1 hour of a dose of estrogen, that dose should be repeated. Morris and van Wagenen (1973) reported one serious complication from such high dosages of estrogen. Acute pulmonary edema from diethylstilbestrol therapy developed in a woman who had a history of premenstrual fluid retention; it resolved after supportive treatment and discontinuation of the drug. A history of VTE, another possible complication of estrogen treatment, contraindicates the use of the estrogenic morning-after pill. Other contraindications to high dosages of estrogen include severe hypertension and hepatic impairment.

Routine use of high dosages of unopposed estrogen has been discouraged for the past decade not only because of its possible thromboembolic complications but also because of the recent awareness of its association with genital cancer. Consequently, the most popular morning-after pill is a combination of a potent progestin DL-norgestrel with 50 μg ethinyl estradiol (Ovral). Postcoital antifertility treatment with this commonly available contraceptive pill (the Yuzpe regimen) consists of two tablets followed by two more tablets 12 hours later (Yuzpe, 1982). As with conventional high-dose estrogens, therapy must be initiated within 2 or 3 days of unprotected coitus, preferably with an antiemetic prophylaxis. Two additional tablets should be provided in case one dose is not retained. Approximately half the women on this regimen experience the frequent side effects of nausea and vomiting unless time-release antiemetic pills have been prescribed. This method is highly effective, and it produces fewer side effects and has a shorter duration of therapy than the conventional high-dose estrogen regimens. Because of the high price of Ovral, practitioners have shifted to similar but lower-dose products, such as Lo/Ovral or Nordette or Alesse, by using more pills to retain the method's effectiveness while lowering the cost per patient.

A potent progestin alone, such as D-norgestrel (levonorgestrel), can also be used as a morning-after pill (Kesseru, 1974). Other successful progestins include clogestone, ethynodiol, norethindrone, norgestrienone, quingestanol acetate, and retroprogestagen. These progestins decidualize the endometrium, rendering it nonreceptive to implantation. Additionally, they alter the cervical mucus, making it hostile to sperm penetration. Other possible antifertility effects are reduced sperm and tubal motility, as well as reduced tubal secretions. Delayed ovulation and subsequent menstruation may occur with frequent isolated treatment (Craft, 1975). Increased intrauterine pH after the postcoital administration of D-norgestrel appears to be associated with a decreased number of motile sperm in the intrauterine fluid (Kesseru, 1974). It should be mentioned that besides progestins and estrogens, other steroids such as danazol and RU-486 have also been used for postcoital contraception (Kubba, 1986; Lahteenmaki, 1988; Schaison, 1985).

In many areas of the world outside the United States, the postcoital antifertility treatment of choice is the insertion of a copper IUD (preferably a small T-shaped device) (Lippes, 1975). The advantages of a copper IUD over steroidal drugs are in its longer, ongoing protection (up to several years if well tolerated) and the shorter duration of nausea or vagal reflex (usually less than 10 minutes). The latter can be blunted with premedication such as doxylamine, diphenhydramine, or other antihistamines with inherent anticholinergic effects. Local anesthesia (a paracervical block) may be required for the woman with a tight internal cervical os. Inert (unmedicated) IUDs are not recommended because they require several days for the achievement of the intended antifertility effects, whereas the released copper provides faster action after insertion. Women with a history of venous thromboembolism may be candidates for postcoital IUDs. A multiparous woman in a mutually monogamous relationship is the ideal candidate. Most pelvic infections that can be aggravated by IUDs are diagnosed within 6 months of the insertion, and a good number are evident shortly after the insertion (Burkman, 1981). A woman who has had unprotected coitus and opts for a "morning after" IUD should receive an adequate dose of broad-spectrum parenteral antibiotics before an IUD is inserted. The antibiotic spectrum should protect against gonorrheal and chlamydial infections. Undergoing clinical trial is an IUD impregnated with a chlorhexidine antiseptic that is slowly released and that may reduce insertion-related pelvic infections. Precautions, instructions, consent form, and follow-up for a postcoital IUD are similar to those for postcoital steroid therapy. Progestin-releasing IUDs should not be used for postcoital contraception in view of the increased risk for ectopic pregnancy and prolonged spotting associated with progestin treatment (Diaz, 1980; Nilsson, 1981).

Therapy for Sexual Assault

Sexual assault (rape) is usually committed against females, from the youngest to the oldest members of society. Rape is the most underreported violent crime. One third of all victims bear evidence of bodily harm besides genital trauma. A reported lifetime incidence of 1 in 10 females is rising annually at an alarming rate, especially among the older age groups. Rape is generally defined as any act of sexual intimacy or intercourse undertaken by force, threat of bodily injury, or the inability of the victim to give appropriate consent. This definition varies slightly from state to state.

Therapy for the girl or woman who has been raped reflects the interplay between the medical and the legal professions. It includes the diagnosis and treatment of physical and mental trauma, the objective documentation of the assault, and the collection and preservation of evidence; the prevention of pregnancy; and the prevention or treatment of an STD. Follow-up treatment and appropriate counseling are also important (Halbert, 1978; Hicks, 1980).

The victim should be isolated from the mainstream of medical activity but should not be left alone for a long period of time. She should receive high-priority, compassionate care and respect. Most victims feel helpless and degraded; hence, a nonjudgmental approach in obtaining a history and the details of the events is crucial. In Massachusetts, the victim (or the victim's guardian) must consent to a full-management protocol that includes appropriate diagnostic tests, medical treatment, and collection and release of evidence (*e.g.,* specimens, clothing, photographs) before the assault is reported (*i.e.,* the decision is the victim's). If possible, a brief description of the assault in the victim's own words should be recorded by only one clinician. Data may include:

Date of last menstrual period
Number of assailants
Lacerations on the victim or assailant that resulted in bleeding
Orifice of penetration, with or without ejaculation
Use of contraceptives
Victim's sexual activity in the 5 days before the assault
Victim's activities since the assault (*e.g.,* wiping, washing, bathing or showering, clenching, urinating, defecating, vomiting, brushing teeth, or change of clothing).

In addition to the physical findings on the victim's skin, hair, face, mouth, throat, breasts, abdomen, back, and extremities, the general physical and emotional status should be recorded. Symptoms and findings, including foreign matter, should be recorded or collected in a standard rape kit with meticulous labeling. Pertinent materials to be collected are fingernail scrapings (each in a separate test tube), foreign pubic hair (from combing), 10 of the victim's pubic hairs (from cutting), and instant or digital photographs. Data related to the assault are kept in a chain-of-evidence pattern.

The pelvic examination must be performed with a nonlubricated, warm, water-moistened speculum. Examination of the vagina and cervix should be concentrated toward signs of pregnancy, parity, menstruation, trauma, infection, foreign material, and nature of the fluid or discharge. The latter (from the vaginal pool) are smeared and dried on glass slides and preserved for evidence. Motile sperm can be identified within 4 to 6 hours in a saline preparation of vaginal fluid. However, acid phosphatase tablets are no longer used. Cellular antigen matching and modern DNA fingerprinting techniques are highly reliable and specific, even when applied years later on properly preserved specimens. Microbiologic cultures are obtained from each orifice involved in the assault. The risk for STD is associated with the degree of sexual contact and the number of assailants. The types of STDs associated with sexual assault (in respective order of frequency) are gonorrheal (up to 13%), trichomonal/monilial/gardnerella (more than 6%), chlamydial (more than 4%), herpetic (up to 4%), and treponemal (less than 1%) (Cates, 1984). Antibiotics of choice for prophylaxis are single-dose parenteral ceftriaxone and metronidazole (with trichomonads or a frothy and malodorous vaginal discharge) followed by 1 week of oral doxycycline (Dattel, 1988; Washington, 1987). If pregnancy is suspected, a highly sensitive (qualitative) urine pregnancy test that uses a specific antibody against β-hCG can be expediently obtained before quantitative serum testing. Pregnancy interception and its small or unknown risk for potential damage, if there is a retained embryo, should be made clear to the victim. Her willingness or unwillingness to abort a pregnancy should be ascertained. Finally, the victim should receive appropriate instructions concerning when and whom to contact for test results and whether to implement or cancel the postcoital antifertility hormone and antibiotic treatment. Long-term consequences or prognosis may depend on type and degree of assault (power rape, anger rape, sadistic rape), immediate and follow-up multilevel care, support from family and friends, and preexistent adaptive behavior pattern (Amir, 1971; Nadelson, 1982).

LONG-ACTING PROGESTINS AND OTHER AGENTS

Progestin in certain forms, with or without a synthetic estrogen, can be injected intramuscularly or subdermally to provide a prolonged contraceptive effect of several months to 5 years (Liskin, 1983; Liskin, 1987). Two long-acting injectables approved by the U.S. FDA are intramuscular depot medroxyprogesterone acetate (DMPA) in microcrystalline aqueous suspension and subdermal levonorgestrel (D-norgestrel). A single-capsule subdermal implant, Implanon, which releases etonogestrel, has also undergone extensive clinical testing. Etonogestrel (11-methylene-levonorgestrel), otherwise known as 3-keto-desogestrel, is the major active metabolite of desogestrel. Also undergoing clinical testing are biodegradable implants and new progestin contraceptives for women who are breast-feeding. Other long-acting steroid contraceptives contain norethindrone enanthate with estradiol valerate, dihydroxyprogesterone acetophenide with estradiol enanthate, or DMPA with estradiol cypionate (Cyclofem). The latter is entering phase 3 clinical testing in the United States as a once-a-month injectable contraceptive.

Medroxyprogesterone acetate (MPA) was synthesized for contraceptive purposes decades ago. It was used in the sequential type of combination OC, which had been discontinued along with other sequential pills. Today millions of women use intramuscular DMPA for either contraception or estrogen-induced neoplastic and proliferative disorders (Rosenfield, 1974). The contraceptive dosage is a 150-mg intramuscular injection every 12 weeks. The drug's aqueous solution (brand-named Depo-Provera) contains MPA with polyethylene glycol and many preservatives. The failure rate during the first year of use is less than 7 pregnancies per 1000 women (Kaunitz, 1993). Part of the reason that DMPA is so effective is that its effect may last slightly longer than 12 weeks. In fact, after a single 150-mg injection, it takes 8 to 9 months for the body to clear DMPA from the blood as a result of the slow release from the injection site (Mishell, 1972). Thus, users who delay receiving the next-scheduled injection are protected against accidental pregnancy for a few weeks. Its mechanisms of action are theoretically similar to those of the minipill. However, DMPA is more reliable in consistently inhibiting ovulation through its effect on the hypothalamus (Mishell, 1977). Mean serum estradiol levels during different periods of DMPA treatment are suppressed to those in the early follicular phase of the normal (untreated) cycle. The median estradiol level is slightly but notably lower than the mean (Mishell, 1972). Thus, decreased bone density has been observed in women who use it for 5 years compared with age-matched nonusers (Cundy, 1991). After several years of treatment, the resumption of ovulation and fertility may not occur for a year or even longer. Chronic intermenstrual spotting (from atrophic endometrium) may occur in some patients after prolonged use, and treatment is costly (Toppozada, 1977). Prolonged use of DMPA induces unfavorable changes in lipid metabolism, which varies among geographic sites (WHO, 1993). Additionally, a mild glucocorticoid effect in terms of weight gain is observed in most users. Thus, intramuscular DMPA may only be appropriate for thin, multiparous women. Other unwanted effects may include headache, decreased libido,

---

BOX 13-5
PATIENT CONSENT FORM FOR INJECTABLE MEANS OF CONTRACEPTION

The Food and Drug Administration has approved an intramuscular injection of Depo-Provera in the buttock for birth control. Each injection prevents pregnancy for 3 months. Every 3 months, another injection must be administered if you want to continue this method of birth control. This drug has been used for 3 decades in millions of women for other purposes. Pregnancy can be prevented if the injection is given within 5 days of the beginning of a normal period. If you are already pregnant when you receive the injection and your pregnancy is allowed to continue, your baby may have an increased chance (risk) of being smaller than usual (low birth weight). Babies who are born too small often have more health problems than those of normal weight. According to the manufacturer, there is a possible, but unproven, risk for birth defects. Additionally, if you are younger than 35 years of age and there is a history of breast cancer in your family, you many not want to use this drug. Short-term use may slightly increase the risk for breast cancer in young women, according to studies by the World Health Organization and in New Zealand. On the other hand, the use of Depo-Provera may protect you from cancer of the endometrium (uterine lining).

Common Side Effects

1. Depo-Provera frequently causes irregular periods (heavy bleeding, spotting, or no bleeding at all). Such problems usually stop after the drug clears the system. Estrogen pills can regulate abnormal bleeding.
2. Sometimes Depo-Provera causes weight gain, headaches, bloating of the abdomen or breast, nervousness, tiredness, or hair loss. It takes several months for these side effects to go away. There is no way to clear this drug quickly from your body.
3. If you use blood-thinning drugs such as coumadin and heparin or if you have prolonged bleeding times—for instance, from taking large amounts of aspirin or aspirin-like over-the-counter painkillers—you should not use Depo-Provera.
4. If you regularly take antiseizure drugs (carbamezepine, phenytoin) or certain antibiotics (rifamin, tetracycline), you should not use this method of contraception. If you take tetracycline, you should use a barrier method of contraception, such as a condom or a diaphragm.
5. Depo-Provera does not protect against sexually transmitted diseases. Therefore, you should always use condoms for this protection.
6. Repeated use of Depo-Provera for years may cause the uterine lining to thin, which may lead to difficulty in resuming periods or in conceiving. It could take 9 months or longer for you to get pregnant after using this drug.
7. Using birth control method for more than 5 years may make your bones slightly thinner. Whether the actual risk for fracture (broken bones) is increased is unclear because this effect on the bones seems to disappear after the drug is discontinued.

PATIENT'S STATEMENT

I have read the above information, and I understand that there are benefits and risks associated with the use of Depo-Provera. Additionally, I have read the manufacturer's package insert for patients. Any questions I had were answered. I choose to use Depo-Provera because I feel that the benefits for me are greater than the risks.

Patient's Signature   Date

---

tiredness, depression, and hair loss. Because each injection is irreversible for 8 months and in utero exposure may be associated with low-birthweight infants, this contraceptive method should be provided only during normal menses (Box 13-5). Undiagnosed genital bleeding and known or suspected breast cancer contraindicate the use of DMPA. Short-term use may slightly increase the risk for breast cancer in young women (WHO, 1991a). The use of DMPA may significantly reduce the risk for endometrial cancer (WHO, 1991b). Use of progestin-only contraceptives, particularly intramuscular DMPA, may increase a woman's risk for HIV-1 infection in a high-risk population (Ungchusak, 1996).

Controlled experiments on monkeys given progesterone (versus placebo) and exposed vaginally to simian immuno-deficiency virus (SIV) have revealed a greater than sevenfold increase in infection among the steroid-treated group (Marx, 1996). Subsequently, Depo-Provera and Norplant have been shown to reduce the thickness of the vaginal epithelium in rhesus monkeys (Hild-Petito, 1998). These reports raise serious concerns about whether women who use progestin-only contraceptives and are already at high risk for STDs would be at increased risk for HIV-1 seroconversion.

Subdermal Levonorgestrel Implant (Norplant)

The Population Council in New York developed a subdermal levonorgestrel implant, known as the Norplant system, for long-term contraception. Originally made and approved for use in Finland, the current system is composed of six subdermal capsules, each filled with 36-mg dry crystals of levonorgestrel. It releases the steroid at a rate decreasing from 80 μg/day during the first year of use to 30 μg/day after the third year, for an effective period of at least 5 years. Blood levels of levonorgestrel are comparable to those in minipill users or to one third of those using the combination OC. The Norplant system is as effective in the first 2 years as female sterilization (Gu, 1994). Duration of effectiveness may be inversely related to body weight but not to body mass index. The adverse influence of body weight on the method's duration of effectiveness appears minimal or nonexistent. Recently, the U.S. FDA and many other medical organizations reaffirmed the safety and effectiveness of Norplant, and more than 4 million women worldwide chose it as their long-term contraceptive. There are few contraindications to its use (Box 13-6). Patients should not undergo insertion if they have prolonged bleeding time from acute liver disease, heparin, coumadin, or aspirin, nor should they undergo insertion if they have undiagnosed genital bleeding. As with all progestins, a shift of glucose tolerance curves may be observed after use. Thus, brittle diabetics may not be ideal candidates for this method. Although the lipid profile remains intact with use, older women who smoke may not be ideal candidates either. A study also suggests that this method may not be effective if a woman is taking anticonvulsant drugs (Haukkamia, 1986). An implant user who conceives because of method failure should be evaluated for possible ectopic pregnancy. Note, however, that implants or other contraceptives actually reduce the risk for ectopic pregnancy. In fact, implant users have only one fifth (0.28/1000 women-years) the risk for ectopic pregnancy that women who do not use contraceptives have (1.5/1000). When compared with other reversible contraceptives, implants have the highest efficacy and continuation rates (Shoupe, 1989; Sivin, 1988). This is probably because the method is convenient (it requires no compliance) and users must return to the clinic to discontinue it. One third to three quarters of women continue the method after 5 years of use. Continuation rates after 1 year of use range from 76% to 99%. Proper preinsertion counseling is the key to high continuation rates. The failure rate during the first year of use is 6 pregnancies per 1000 women.

Mechanism of Action

Blood concentrations of 300 to 400 pg/mL levonorgestrel may centrally blunt the preovulatory surge of LH. Thus, 70% of the users' cycles are anovulatory. Remaining ovulatory cycles (as judged by vaginal ultrasonography) are usually associated with decreased peak serum progesterone levels (7 ng/mL versus 18 ng/mL) that indicate poor ovum or inadequate luteal support or luteinize unruptured follicles. Peripherally, sperm penetration may be inhibited by a local effect of progestin, which prevents midcycle thinning of the cervical mucus. This effect is seen with a levonorgestrel level as low as 200 pg/mL. Another progestational effect of levonorgestrel may render the endometrium unreceptive to implantation.

Side Effects

Irregular uterine bleeding in the form of frequent abnormal menses, spotting or staining, or amenorrhea is a common initial symptom. In the first year of use, the average number of days of bleeding is 129 (versus 70 among women who do not use contraceptives). Short-term oral therapy with ethinyl estradiol, norgestrel, or ibuprofen each day significantly reduces the number of days of abnormal bleeding (Diaz, 1990). One quarter of the users bleed every 3 to 5 weeks in the first year. By the fifth year, two thirds of the users have regular cycles. Generally, those who start out with amenorrhea or irregular bleeding patterns are not at risk for method failure. Users who have regular bleeding patterns and suddenly become amenorrheic should undergo pregnancy testing.

Less common side effects include headache, nausea, dizziness, nervousness, acne, and weight gain. Headache associated with papilledema may signal idiopathic intracranial hypertension (pseudotumor cerebri). This requires the cessation of steroid contraception and an appropriate neurologic examination. Intractable weight gain or classic migraine with an aura may also dictate method discontinuation. Acne may be relieved with proper dermatologic care. Because gonadotropin levels in users are not completely suppressed, follicular development still occurs and the resultant serum estradiol levels are indistinguishable from those of nonusers. As many as one third of users may have persistent follicles. Thus, simple follicular cysts are common and may reach 5 to 7 cm, but regression usually occurs spontaneously. Other problems reported are depression, irritation, and, in rare cases, hyperpigmentation and keloid at the insertion site.

Insertion and Removal Techniques

Insertion takes only 5 to 10 minutes but must be performed correctly to ensure easy removal. Capsules must be placed subdermally just below the skin on the inner surface of the upper arm. Use of a special template is strongly advised so that the six capsules are in a typical radial (fan-out) pattern and the infiltration of local anesthesia does not occur in excess. The manufacturer can provide videotapes to demonstrate insertion techniques and to answer questions that commonly arise. Insert the trocar with the skin tented up to ensure the superficial placement of the capsule. The beveled tip should be pointed upward so that its sharp end is pointed down. This keeps the advancing trocar from buttonholing the skin. Load the Norplant capsule into the barrel and push it gently in with the plunger until there is a slight resistance. Withdraw the barrel while the plunger is held stationary to facilitate the release of the capsule. The next step is to secure the capsule with digital pressure on the skin and withdraw the barrel together with the plunger set simultaneously to the incision site, but not beyond, for redirection and placement of the next capsule. This trocar withdrawal action causes the proximal tip of each capsule to pop down and out of the sharp bevel. Insertion should be performed during the normal menses or OC withdrawal bleeding. Insertion during the luteal phase or in the last half of the low-estrogen OC-induced cycle is not advised.

Removal takes 20 minutes or longer, depending on the skill and correct (or typical) alignment of the capsules placed years earlier. These removal techniques are based on

---

BOX 13-6
PATIENT CONSENT FORM FOR NORPLANT CONTRACEPTIVE IMPLANTS

Norplant (levonorgestrel subdermal implants), a long-acting and reversible birth control method, has been used by more than 1 million women worldwide for the prevention of unwanted pregnancy. Each of the six implants is made from a special silastic rubber commonly used in the body for other purposes. The drug used in Norplant has been used in birth control pills for the past three decades. These implants are inserted beneath the skin of the upper arm using a minor surgical technique. There have been no serious side effects reported from women who were appropriately selected to receive Norplant.

Advantages of Norplant over Other Birth Control Methods

1. Norplant lasts 5 years and is statistically more reliable than the pill. Unlike the pill, Norplant contains no estrogen and therefore has fewer side effects than the pill. The first-year discontinuation rate is lower than it is for the pill or an intrauterine device.
2. Norplant reduces the total monthly bleeding from the womb (uterus) and the risk for iron deficiency anemia in some women who have excessive menstrual bleeding. Using Norplant for more than 1 year generally leads to blood counts (hemoglobin and hematocrit) that are higher than they were before insertion.
3. Norplant may reduce menstrual cramps.
4. Norplant may protect against cancer of the endometrium (inside lining of the womb).
5. There is practically no age limit in using Norplant because the amount of drug that is released into the blood circulation is extremely low compared with the pill. Consequently, there are few unwanted metabolic effects in the body, except perhaps in cigarette smokers older than 45 years of age.

Disadvantages and Common Side Effects

1. Norplant must be surgically inserted (10-minute procedure) and removed (20-minute procedure) after 5 years. Thus the initial cost is higher than the pill or an intrauterine device. Although it is 99% effective, it must be removed if pregnancy occurs or if yellow jaundice develops.
2. Although Norplant can be removed whenever users want to discontinue contraception, removal usually takes longer than insertion. If Norplant was inserted too deeply under the skin, the user may have to undergo the removal procedure twice or undergo ultrasound-guided removal.
3. Some prospective candidates may require antibiotics before insertion and removal if they are at risk for heart valve infection.
4. Occasionally, an infection or a prolonged bruise may result from insertion or removal. Most users have a scar about the size of the tip of a pen, and it is unusual to for a keloid (excessive scarring) or darkening of the skin to occur. An allergic reaction to the antiseptic cleaning fluid or the local numbing medicine may occur.
5. Women who regularly take the following drugs may not be eligible for Norplant: blood-thinning drugs (heparin or coumadin), antiseizure drugs (phenytoin or carbamazepine), and some antibiotics (tetracycline or rifampicin). Norplant users who will take tetracycline for a long period of time must use a barrier method while on that antibiotic. Women with prolonged bleeding time, such as those who take a large amount of aspirin or aspirin-like over-the-counter painkillers, should not use Norplant until the disorder has been treated.
6. Because Norplant effectively prevents pregnancy, it automatically reduces the risk for ectopic tubal pregnancy. However, if this method of contraception fails and pregnancy results, 1of 5 pregnancies may develop in the tube (ectopic).
7. The use of Norplant may cause irregular staining or spotting between periods or it may cause periods to cease. Such problems may or may not go away with time. However, occasional blood pregnancy tests may be required. An additional drug or hormone may be used to reduce these irregular bleeding or menstrual problems.
8. Although Norplant theoretically prevents cancer of the endometrium, some users may have to undergo endometrial biopsy or other minor testing to detect cervical or endometrial cancer. Women with a history of breast cancer should not use Norplant.
9. Norplant is not a barrier contraceptive and so does not protect against sexually transmitted diseases.
10. Acne, headaches, and weight gain or loss (from a change in appetite) may develop in some Norplant users. Other minor side effects, listed in the manufacturer's package insert, are rare.
11. A Norplant user who has pain in the lower abdomen, pain during intercourse, fever and chills, unpleasant vaginal discharge, or a visual disturbance should contact her physician without delay.

PATIENT'S STATEMENT

I have read the above information, and I understand there are benefits and risks associated with the use of Norplant. Additionally, I have read the manufacturer's package insert for patients. Any questions I had were answered. I choose to use Norplant because I feel that the benefits for me are greater than the risks.

_____   _____
Patient's Signature   Date

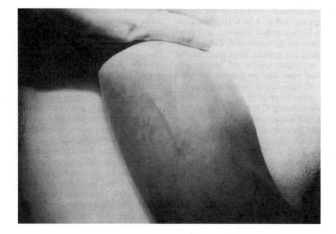

Fig. 13-6. Norplant-2 in situ (inner surface of the patient's upper arm). (Courtesy Dr. P. D. Darney.)

two decades of experience in other countries. Use of a waterproof surgical marker is strongly advised to mark on the skin the distal and proximal tips of each capsule that can be palpated digitally. An ample volume of local anesthetic solution (8 mL 1% lidocaine hydrochloride) is then infiltrated under the proximal tips of the implants. A 1-cm incision is made transversely over the proximal ends of all of the capsules, which are usually cephalad to the original insertion site. Pressure is applied at the distal end so that the capsule's proximal tip is pushed into the incision area. That tip is then grasped with a small hemostat or Kelly clamp. The fibrous tissue around the silastic tip is carefully scratched out with the tip of the knife blade or with dry surgical gauze until the shiny white implant is cleared of any attachment and can be slid out. Patients must be allowed to see and count all the removed capsules, and this should be recorded. If it takes too long to remove one capsule, the patient should be advised to return in 1 month for another attempt, after the bruising and swelling have disappeared. If difficulty in removal is anticipated, the patient should be referred to an experienced gynecologist. Ultrasonography can be used to locate any loose or broken capsule fragments. Insertion and removal of the two-capsule implants (Fig. 13-6), Norplant-2, which may become available in the United States, are easier to manage than in the six-capsule system. The FDA has approved Norplant-2, but its manufacturer is not marketing this product while it is contesting litigation against the original six-capsule Norplant system in the United States.

Other long-acting contraceptives undergoing testing include microcapsules, a progestin or a combined progestin-estrogen vaginal silastic ring, a once-a-month pill, and a skin patch (Ginsburg, 1988). The contraceptive vaginal ring (CVR) is interesting because the user can insert it and remove it by herself (Roy, 1983). The contraceptive steroid, which is easily absorbed by the vaginal mucosa into the systemic circulation, is released at a slow and relatively constant rate. It will not work if it is inserted just before coitus. However, after it has been used for one cycle, occasional re-moval of the vaginal ring for several hours will not decrease its contraceptive protection. In a way, the vaginal ring works in reverse of the barrier method because users can remove it in anticipation of sexual intercourse and reinsert it after coitus. A monthly schedule comprised of a 3-week period of wearing the CVR and 1 week free of it will bring about monthly withdrawal bleeding similar to that induced by combination OCs. Currently undergoing clinical trials are several CVRs that are used for 21 consecutive days per month and that contain ethinyl estradiol and one of the three progestins, etonogestrel, levonorgestrel, or norethindrone acetate (FemRing). FemRing (from Parke-Davis, a subsidiary of Warner-Lambert) has been undergoing phase 2 trials to define the appropriate amounts of ethinyl estradiol and norethindrone acetate needed to obtain the most metabolically neutral CVR with a favorable serum lipid profile.

A safe and practical contraceptive pill for men has not been invented. The suppression of spermatogenesis was demonstrated after treatment with exogenous testosterone or a combination of estrogen and testosterone. Unfortunately, the long-term use of testosterone leads to hepatic dysfunction. Chinese physicians used a cotton-plant pigment, gossypol, as an injectable or implantable contraceptive for men (Wu, 1986). Hypokalemia, hepatorenal dysfunction, irreversible azoospermia, and other toxicologic data from human trials prevent approval for its use in other countries. Another male contraceptive from the Chinese medicinal plant *Tripterygium wilfordii* was recently analyzed and found to be chlorohydrin. Its effects appear to be reversible (Matlin, 1993).

REVERSIBLE METHODS WITH HIGH FAILURE RATES

Coitus interruptus (withdrawal of the penis before ejaculation) is perhaps the oldest contraceptive practice, according to Catholic theologians and canonists (Noonan, 1986). Besides the demand for extreme self-control by the male, the method is ineffective in real practice because of the escape of seminal fluid before orgasm and, in many instances, the unavoidable deposition of semen near the vaginal orifice. In other instances, when the woman has not achieved orgasm before penile withdrawal, she may require further stimulation for gratification. Lovemaking modifications for contraceptive purposes include orogenital and anal intercourse. The latter is commonly practiced in certain parts of the world, but most cultures have long condemned anal intercourse as unhealthy.

The *postcoital douche,* also an ancient contraceptive method, is intended to flush the semen out of the vagina. Water, vinegar solution, and various over-the-counter products were used. Certain douching solutions may have a spermicidal effect. An example of a folk method is to douche with diet cola or bitter lemon. The carbonated drink actually has an in vitro spermicidal effect (Umpierre, 1985). Nevertheless, the effectiveness of a postcoital douche is probably low because sperm can find their way into the cervical mucus almost instantly after ejaculation, and minutes later they can be found in the oviducts (Settlage, 1973). Thus, post-coital douche is considered an unreliable contraceptive method.

The *rhythm method (periodic abstinence),* considered unnatural by many couples, is another ineffective way to prevent unwanted conception. A woman's fertile period within each cycle may be crudely estimated from the calendar, basal body temperature, or cervical mucus. Three factors that limit the method's effectiveness appear to be intraindividual variations in cycle length, variations in the length of survival of the sperm, and actual use compliance. Epidemiologic data at one time implied that an old sperm or an old egg could lead to an imperfect conceptus, but such fears were not borne out by results of the Walnut Creek Study (Ramcharan, 1980).

Prolonged nursing is an unreliable contraceptive method and perhaps is an unnatural way to nourish a well-grown child (McCann, 1981). The resumption of ovulation may occur before the first menstrual bleeding, and the antiovulatory effect of lactation varies from woman to woman. Breast-feeding mothers should always use a reliable contraceptive, such as a condom, diaphragm, or IUD. It should be mentioned, however, that postpartum breast-feeding for 3 to 6 months has been the only available contraceptive method for pregnancy spacing in many developing countries, and the method appears reasonably effective during the early postpartum period.

STERILIZATION

Sterilization generally refers to a surgical procedure that is aimed at permanently blocking or removing male or female genital tracts so that fertilization will not occur. The permanency of sterilization should be the main consideration for any user who contemplates undergoing it. The reversal of sterilization requires major surgery and is not always successful (Henry, 1980).

Among the effective methods for birth control, sterilization is the most frequently chosen by fertile men and multiparous women older than 30. In fact, the best contraception for an older multiparous woman in a stable, mutually monogamous relationship is male sterilization (vasectomy).

Vasectomy is an outpatient surgical procedure that occludes a portion of the vas deferens. It requires local anesthesia and usually takes an experienced person 15 minutes in a well-equipped facility. Complications, if they occur, are not serious. They include hematoma or sperm leakage, which leads to granulomatous reactions (sperm granulomas). Semen analysis is required 1 and 2 months after surgery because two sperm-free ejaculations are considered to be proof of sterility. However, it may take up to 20 ejaculations to determine sterility. Long-term deleterious effects of vasectomy have never been proven. The fear of decreased virility or atherosclerosis is unfounded (Campbell, 1988;

Goldacre, 1983; Liskin, 1983; Massey, 1984). However, several epidemiologic studies suggest that vasectomy may be associated with an elevated risk for prostate cancer (Cramer, 1993; Giovannucci, 1993).

Like vasectomy, most methods of female sterilization are outpatient or day surgery procedures. Nevertheless, female sterilization is not as simple to perform as vasectomy because the female genital tracts are located relatively deep in the pelvis. The risk for death (4 in 100,000) is lower than that from pregnancy and is primarily attributed to the complications of anesthesia (Liskin, 1985; Peterson, 1983). There is also an increased risk for extrauterine pregnancy should the procedure fail. Attempts at blocking the oviducts by transcervical (transvaginal) extraperitoneal procedures have been recorded for a century, but none is acceptable. Hysteroscopic methods for blocking the oviducts with silicone or caustic chemicals have been offered at some facilities. Such methods never gain popularity because of the high failure rates and the unacceptable risk for tubal pregnancy.

Female sterilization is commonly achieved by ligation or coagulation, with or without the segmental removal of both oviducts. This tubal sterilization can be performed through two main intraperitoneal routes—the abdominal approach through laparoscopy or minilaparotomy and the vaginal approach through colpotomy or culdoscopy.

Laparoscopic tubal sterilization with bipolar cautery has been the popular choice for interval sterilization in the United States. This method requires elaborate equipment, but the procedure is relatively short. Minilaparotomy has been an excellent choice for sterilization in the postpartum period, when the oviducts are located high in the abdomen. It is also a good way to perform interval sterilization using local anesthesia with the help of a uterine elevator device (Osathanondh, 1974). The latter technique is suitable in developing countries, where most multiparous women are thin. With a thin abdominal wall, the required amount of local anesthesia does not exceed the allowable limit. Vaginal tubal sterilization is not commonly performed. It requires considerable technical expertise because intraperitoneal visualization is limited compared with other interval sterilization methods. There is also an increased risk for ascending infection from the vagina than there is with abdominal incisions. Thus, broad-spectrum intravenous antibiotics should be given for prophylaxis in women who are undergoing vaginal tubal ligation.

Careful selection of candidates for tubal sterilization, with a discussion and a simplified consent form (Box 13-7), may obviate later regrets for the patient and the physician. Ideal candidates are multiparous women older than 35. Of women who undergo tubal ligation, 5% to 20% later regret having done so. Some risk factors for post-sterilization regret include young age, recent pregnancy, and black race. Nulliparous women and those younger than 25 may, with a legitimate medical indication, benefit from sterilization provided they have been counseled by another appropriate

---

BOX 13-7
PATIENT CONSENT FORM FOR TUBAL STERILIZATION

Tubal sterilization is a surgical procedure to block the fallopian tubes so that fertilization will not occur. This procedure is more effective than any other birth control method, but it should be chosen only if you are sure that you want no more children because your tubes will become permanently blocked. Occasionally, women who have had tubal sterilization change their minds and want more children. In vitro fertilization or major surgery to reconstruct the tubes is then necessary, but neither is successful all the time.

Tubal sterilization can be performed by a laparoscopic procedure that requires small punctures of the abdomen or by a minilaparotomy procedure that requires a small surgical opening of the abdomen. Methods of tubal sterilization are excision and ligation, surgical relocation, and constriction (each tube is constricted by tight band or by an electric current that passes through it). Complications of tubal sterilization may involve infection, bleeding, injuries to internal organs, or effects of anesthesia. Life-threatening complications requiring major surgery and blood transfusion, such as damage to the bowels or the blood vessels, are rare.

Your physician will discuss the choice of procedure most suitable for you based on its advantages and disadvantages. The possible risk for spontaneous healing that allows the tubes to reopen will be balanced against the complexity and complications of the various procedures. Spontaneous opening of the blocked tubes occurs after approximately 2 per 1000 operations. It is less likely to occur if the tubes are blocked immediately after childbirth or during cesarean section. If your tubes heal in such a way that an opening remains, pregnancy may take place months or even years later. This type of pregancy is called an ectopic pregnancy; it can develop outisde the womb and cause severe bleeding. It is difficult to predict who will have these complications; therefore, after tubal sterilization, you should report any menstrual irregularities or any signs of pregnancy immediately to your physician.

Some women are unknowingly pregnant at the time of tubal sterilization, especially if their periods have not been normal or if they undergo the procedure in the last 2 weeks of the menstrual cycle. Your physician may perform a blood pregnancy test around the time of the operation, but, again, you should report any irregular periods or signs of pregnancy to your physician after the tubal sterilization procedure.

Planned procedure:

Comments:

PATIENT'S STATEMENT

I have read this consent form and understand that there are failure rates and risks associated with tubal sterilization. My physician has discussed the advantages and disadvantages of tubal sterilization. I consent to the planned procedure.

_____   _____
Patient's Signature   Witness' Signature

_____   _____
Date   Date

---

authority besides the gynecologist performing the surgery (Harrison, 1988). Tubal ligation confers a one-third reduction in ovarian cancer risk (Miracle-McMahill, 1997.)

Laparoscopic Tubal Sterilization

Bipolar electrocoagulation is the method of choice using the two-puncture technique with general endotracheal anesthesia. It is safer than unipolar coagulation in averting accidental thermal injury to the bowel or neighboring structures because the electric current heats and coagulates only the oviductal tissues within the jaws of the electrocoagulation probe. Several contiguous fulgurations are preferred to the transaction or segmental removal. The two-puncture technique offers better visualization and easier manipulation of the intraabdominal organs. Immediate complications include anesthesia-related problems, damage to internal organs, and hemorrhage. Other problems that may occur after

discharge are infection, hematoma, adhesions, unrecognized bowel injury, luteal-phase pregnancy, and recanalization that results in intrauterine or ectopic pregnancy (Neil, 1975; Schiff, 1974). Suboptimal anesthetic techniques, such as mask inhalation, may result in fatal aspiration pneumonitis because pneumoperineum tends to induce the regurgitation and aspiration of gastric contents. Local bleeding may occur if tissue coagulation is inadequate. A major life-threatening hemorrhage is rare and requires immediate laparotomy to repair the lacerations of the blood vessels. Blood transfusion may be required. Unrecognized bowel burns may lead to symptoms analogous to a ruptured appendix. Bowel burns are rare with the use of regularly inspected and well-maintained bipolar instruments. Luteal-phase pregnancy may be averted if sterilization is performed during the first half of the cycle. The failure rate of most female sterilization methods is quoted as 2 per 1000 procedures in the first postoperative year, and it is higher if bipolar cautery is included (Peterson, 1996). Most failures result from recanalization of the oviduct or tuboperitoneal fistula. However, if the procedure is performed hastily and without identifying the entire length of the oviduct to its fimbriated end, a round ligament could be mistaken for an oviduct. A high incidence of ectopic pregnancy has been reported with failures of electrocoagulation, especially after the bipolar and the obsolete unipolar methods (Liskin, 1985). Nevertheless, the general safety of laparoscopic sterilization and the absence of sequelae in terms of menstrual or psychosocial problems have been amply documented (DeStefano, 1983).

In addition to electrocoagulation, mechanical constriction and obliteration of the oviduct can be accomplished with a silastic Yoon band (Falope ring), a spring-loaded Hulka clip, a Filshie clip, and various other radiopaque, non-electrical devices. Such devices may be unsuitable for use on swollen oviducts (such as in the puerperium) or in the presence of some pelvic adhesions. The Falope ring is suitable for the single-puncture technique most often used in outpatient laparoscopic sterilization with local anesthesia and monitored intravenous (conscious) sedation. However, several days of postoperative pain (more than that from electrocoagulation) may be expected after the Falope ring application. The Hulka clip is probably the least traumatic to the local tissues, but its failure rate is slightly higher than that with other methods. Major trauma to internal organs can be averted or substantially reduced with the open laparoscopy technique. This technique is also practical if the procedure has to be performed with local anesthesia. The peritoneum is identified and entered through a small infraumbilical incision using a blunt, funnel-shape Hasson cannula (Hasson, 1982). Blind stabbings of the abdominal wall with a Verres carbon dioxide needle and the sharp trocar of conventional laparoscopy are avoided in this open laparoscopy method.

Minilaparotomy

The ligation and transection, or resection, of a portion of the oviduct may be electively performed during the puerperium and in the nonpregnant interval. Electrocoagulation can also be used in the minilaparotomy method of tubal sterilization. The simple tie-and-cut technique is usually a modification of the Pomeroy method.

There are techniques to relocate and bury the proximal portion of the transected oviduct to minimize failure. The Uchida method calls for burying the ligated proximal stump of the tube retroperitoneally under the leaves of the broad ligament. The ligated distal stump remains intraperitoneal. The modified Irving method probably has the lowest failure rate, generally quoted as less than 0.1%. It is the sterilization method of choice immediately after cesarean delivery. The ligated proximal stump of the tube is buried in the uterine wall near the cornu. The original Irving method of burying the distal stump under the leaves of the broad ligament is not really necessary.

Together the obstetrician, the anesthesiologist, and the patient should determine the safe time for postpartum sterilization. Deferral until the patient is in optimal condition may be the best policy. Parturient and pregnant women in the second or third trimester are at increased risk for regurgitation and the aspiration of gastric contents. After natural childbirth, many anesthesiologists prefer a routine waiting period of 6 hours rather than immediate postpartum sterilization. Any medical, obstetric, neonatal survivability, or infectious problems should override the original plan for immediate or puerperal sterilization. With the advent of 24-hour broad-spectrum intravenous antibiotics for prophylaxis, there is no need for the patient to wait until 6 weeks after delivery to undergo tubal ligation. In the absence of intrapartum or puerperal infection, minilaparotomy can be performed safely with prophylactic intravenous antibiotics before the complete involution of the uterus. The advantages are easy access to the oviducts through a small abdominal incision and the patient's convenience in scheduling the surgery during allowable maternity leave. Postpartum sterilization has fewer failures than interval sterilization (Peterson, 1996).

Minilaparotomy can be performed with local anesthesia for interval sterilization or in conjunction with first-trimester induced abortion. A device such as the Hulka tenaculum or a uterine elevator designed by Osathanondh allows easy access to the oviduct through a small suprapubic incision (Osathanondh, 1974). Women who have successfully undergone natural childbirth or surgery with local anesthesia are good candidates. However, the patient should be of average body weight for her height and weigh less than 68 kg (<150 pounds). Hypertension, hyperthyroidism, cardiac arrhythmia, and hypersensitivity to local anesthesia or epinephrine are contraindications. A local anesthetic solution containing a minimal amount of epinephrine is injected into the abdominal wall and the oviducts before ligation or electrocoagulation. A paracervical block anesthetic should be given before applying the uterine elevator or Hulka tenaculum. Intravenous drugs that are helpful include a parasympatholytic agent (such as glycopyrrolate), a sedative (midazolam or droperidol) or an antihistamine (diphenhydramine), and a short-acting opioid (fentanyl citrate). The dosage of these combined medications may be clinically adjusted and should not exceed the maximum allowable limits.

A sterilized woman may undergo major surgery to reopen her fallopian tubes. The success rate of the tubal reanastomosis depends on the method of sterilization. The clip, the silastic band, and the modified Pomeroy method, in that order, are easier to reverse than the Irving, Uchida, and electrocoagulation methods. The most difficult to reverse is blockade after unipolar cautery because of the extensive tissue damage and the frequent postoperative adhesions. Besides complications inherent to laparotomy and anesthesia, tubal pregnancy occurs at very high rates, especially after the reversal of unipolar electrocoagulation (Henry, 1980).

Patients with major uterine or pelvic disease who request sterilization may benefit from hysterectomy. However, hysterectomy must not be viewed as a simple method of sterilization because it carries a higher complication rate than tubal sterilization.

PREGNANCY TERMINATION (THERAPEUTIC INDUCED ABORTION)
Pharmacotherapeutic Methods
Agents Disrupting Chorionic Villi

Progesterone-receptor blockers represent an important alternative in antifertility therapy. Such antiprogesterones are derivatives of norethindrone and are therefore within the class of 19-norsteroids.

A prototype of antiprogesterone, code-named RU38.486, was synthesized by the Roussel-Uclaf pharmaceutical company in Romainville, France. Specifically, the addition of a functional group dimethylaminophenyl ring to the norethindrone molecule at the 11β-carbon position resulted in a potent compound, RU486, that can displace progesterone from its receptors (Baulieu, 1984). This receptor blocker appears to have no direct effect on the ovarian production of progesterone. It was approved for use in China, France, and other European countries. In the United States, premarketing trials by the Population Council confirmed the drug's safety and efficacy, and the FDA Advisory Committee has recommended its approval (Bardin, 1997; Spitz, 1998). Nevertheless, this innovative drug of choice for medical abortion may be unavailable for women in many countries.

RU486 or mifepristone was used as an abortifacient in the first quarter of pregnancy, a morning-after pill, and in the treatment of Cushing syndrome and glaucoma. RU486 can also reduce the size of certain brain tumor cells, such as meningioma and meningioblastomas, probably through an obscure fluid exchange mechanism. Additionally, the drug is undergoing trials for the treatment of Alzheimer's disease, endometriosis, and leiomyomata. Although its contraceptive efficacy as a once-a-month pill is questionable, (Schaison, 1989), it has been successfully used for emergency contraception (Glaser, 1997).

RU486 effectively antagonizes progesterone actions on the gestational endometrium, which leads to the eventual detachment of the chorionic villi and a consequent decline in the peripheral blood levels of progesterone and hCG. When administered during the midluteal phase, it blocks the effects of progesterone by displacing the natural steroid from its receptors on the secretory endometrium, with the resultant induction of menses. With this method of administration, multiple sites of its action on the hypothalamic-hypophyseal-ovarian-endometrial axis have been proposed, based on dynamic hormonal studies (Garzo, 1988). In the absence of progesterone, RU486 exerts mild progesterone-like effects (in estrogen-treated postmenopausal women). This leads to a further decrease in the serum gonadotropin levels (Gravanis, 1985).

In addition to its action within the female reproductive tract, RU486 also binds to the glucocorticoid receptors and antagonizes the actions of cortisol. In high dosages, this drug may be beneficial in the treatment of Cushing syndrome. Small and transient compensatory rises in plasma adrenocorticotrophic hormone and cortisol levels were shown after the daily administration of 200 mg RU486 for 4 days. This course of treatment is required for early termination of pregnancy. More practically, a single oral dose of 600 mg was used with slightly less effectiveness but excellent patient acceptance and convenience, especially when it was followed by a prostaglandin. A continued search by German scientists for an ideal antiprogesterone that lacks antiglucocorticoid effects recently produced three other related compounds: ZK112.993, ZK98.734 (Lilopristone), and ZK98.299 (Onapristone) (Fig. 13-7). The latter appears to have less antiglucocorticoid activity while it is 10 times more effective than RU486 as an abortifacient in preliminary animal studies (Elger, 1987). In Europe, Onapristone and RU486 have undergone clinical trials for cervical ripening and as adjuncts to labor and delivery (Chwalisz, 1994).

The oral or, more effectively, parenteral administration of RU486 was shown to induce moderate uterine bleeding and a significant decrease in the hematocrit, followed by complete expulsion of early (first-quarter) gestational products in 80% of the patients. The remaining 20% of patients required dilation and curettage (D&C). Bleeding in many patients occurred before the decrease in serum progesterone levels. Successful therapy is associated with an increase in plasma levels of $PGF_{2\alpha}$, myometrial contraction, favorable changes in the uterine cervix, and, in some patients, hormonal evidence of luteolysis. However, the most effective

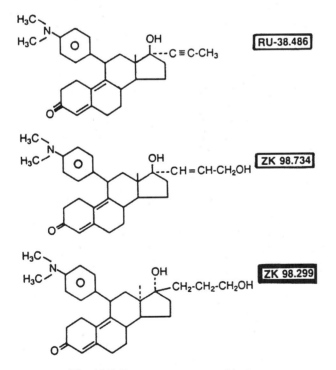

Fig. 13-7. Progesterone-receptor blockers.

pharmacotherapy to terminate an early gestation (and a later gestation with fetal demise) is the administration of RU486 in combination with an otherwise subtherapeutic dose of a uterotonic prostaglandin (Table 13-2) (Cabrol, 1985; Cameron, 1988). These two different classes of drugs are synergistic. One low dose of a prostaglandin administered toward the end of RU486 treatment ensures complete abortion without incurring the systemic side effects of that prostaglandin. The most common prostaglandin for this purpose is oral or vaginal PGE_1 methyl analogue (misoprostol), which induces uterine contraction at all stages of pregnancy (Margulies, 1992). RU486 was not beneficial for terminating ectopic tubal pregnancies in limited, unpublished clinical trials. Significant concentrations of this drug were experimentally demonstrated in the umbilical plasma during second-trimester therapeutic abortion, which indicates that it is effectively transferred across the placental barrier (Frydmann, 1995). It is unknown whether this steroid is teratogenic. Among the patients whose intrauterine pregnancies were not successfully terminated, there have been no fetal abnormalities reported to date. The plasma elimination half-life of RU486 is 10 to 25 hours. Data on long-term untoward effects from the repeated administration of RU486 are unavailable. Its prolonged use could hypothetically lead to unopposed estrogenic stimulation as a result of a blockage of progesterone action. The blood loss and time consumed in medical abortion appear greater than those found in surgical abortion. Furthermore, RU486 by itself is ineffective for abortion beyond the first quarter of a normal pregnancy. Another disadvantage of a drug-induced abortion (versus a surgical evacuation) may be the unavailability of placenta specimens, especially in Asian countries where trophoblastic disease is prevalent.

Inhibitors of progesterone biosynthesis, such as aminoglutethimide (Salhanick, 1982), epostane (Crooij, 1988), or trilostane (van der Spuy, 1983) have been moderately effective abortifacients until 50 days of pregnancy (from the last menstrual period). However, unwanted effects at the therapeutic antifertility dosage include adrenocortical suppression and, in many patients, significant uterine bleeding because of incomplete miscarriage.

Aminoglutethimide is a bicyclic chemical compound with two optically active isomers. It inhibits the major steroidogenic enzyme systems (cholesterol side-chain cleavage and aromatase) by blocking the terminal cytochrome P-450s. Besides its adrenal suppression effects, which can be used for medical adrenalectomy, this drug may depress the central nervous system and activate hepatic microsomal enzymes. Trilostane and epostane (Winthrop 24540 and 32729) are 4,5-epoxy steroids structurally related to testosterone and methyltestosterone, respectively. Each epoxy steroid blocks the biosynthesis of progesterone by inhibiting the enzyme 3β-hydroxysteroid dehydrogenase; epostane is less suppressive to the adrenals than trilostane. Nevertheless, a high dosage of epostane (800 mg/day for 1 week) is usually required for early pregnancy termination. Al-

though therapies with this class of drugs have not led to a subsequent menstrual or ovulational disorder, this group of antifertility agents does not appear as promising as the progesterone-receptor blockers.

Inhibitors of folate reductase were used as abortifacients. However, these antimetabolites should not be recommended as first-line drugs for terminating a normal intrauterine pregnancy. The required duration of therapy is lengthy. A prototype oral agent 4-aminopteroylglutamic acid was originally tried for this purpose almost half a century ago (Thiersch, 1952). All patients in that small series required either a D&C or a hysterotomy 5 to 47 days after the initiation of the therapy. Interestingly, one such case of a medically indicated therapeutic abortion for maternal tuberculosis resulted in a live fetus.

A common parenteral antimetabolite, methotrexate, was successfully used in the conservative treatment of placenta accreta. Blood transfusions, uterine packing, and antibiotics were also required. Stormy, intensive, and protracted hospitalization usually occurred before the patient recuperated with her uterus intact. The availability of sensitive and specific serum hCG measurements, together with high-resolution diagnostic ultrasonography, led investigators in Asia and, later on, a score of gynecologists in the United States to use methotrexate in the pharmacotherapy of a small tubal or cervical pregnancy (Farabow, 1983; Ory, 1986; Oyer, 1988). Methotrexate works well in destroying abnormal or ectopic trophoblastic cells, but it is ineffective against a large bulk of normal trophoblastic tissue, unless a prostaglandin drug, misoprostol, is given concomitantly (Creinin, 1993). This is unlike the action of RU486, which works better on normal intrauterine trophoblastic cells than on ectopic ones. The benefit of methotrexate for tubal pregnancy should be weighed against the as yet unknown long-term sequelae of elevated serum hepatic transaminases. Such increased liver enzymes appear reversible on cessation of the therapy. A fatal idiosyncratic reaction may occur when methotrexate is administered in conjunction with

Table 13-2   Therapeutic Abortion at 56 Days of Amenorrhea or Sooner

Method	Completion Rate
RU486 150 mg/day orally for 4 days	60% (12/20)
PGE$_1$ analogue 1 mg vaginal pessary every 3 hr up to five doses	97% (29/30)
Vacuum aspiration	96% (27/28)
RU486 as above protocol and one dose of PGE$_1$ on day 3	95% (18/19)

From Cameron IT, Baird DT: Early pregnancy termination: A comparison between vacuum aspiration and medical abortion using prostaglandin (16,16 dimethyl-trans-3D$_2$- PGE$_1$ methyl ester) or the antiprogestogen RU486. *Br J Obstet Gynaecol* 1988; 95:271-276.

PGE$_1$, prostaglandin E$_1$.

NSAIDs (Stockley, 1987). A combination of methotrexate ($50\ mg/m^2$) followed by vaginal misoprostol (0.8 mg) in 1 week has been used for medical abortions in several U.S. clinics with reasonable success rates (90% miscarriage within 7 weeks of the last menstrual period). There are some logistic problems with this medical abortion method, which may limit its popularity and practicality. First, the time interval between this antifolate-antitrophoblast and the prostaglandin misoprostol administration, the so-called "window" of 5 to 7 days, appears lengthy compared with the window of 36 to 60 hours with the more practical mifepristone-misoprostol regimen. Second, methotrexate-misoprostol abortion generally results in prolonged vaginal bleeding, spotting, and staining. Third, failure rates in as many as 1 in 5 patients may lead to D&C at a later stage in a lengthy abortion process.

Some patients with small tubal pregnancy do not require any treatment except careful monitoring until tubal abortion with resorption occurs. Such patients later conceive and give birth to normal live offspring (Carp, 1986). Therefore, it could be reasoned that some patients reported in those methotrexate-for-ectopic series might have done all right without any treatment at all. Opponents of the methotrexate-for-ectopic modality may label it a radical pharmacotherapy after considering the potential risks from this chemical agent when it is compared with conservative treatment by mini-laparotomy (salpingostomy) or pelviscopic surgery. Advocates, on the other hand, think that any toxic sequela, such as liver damage, should be negligible because of the long-term health of most patients with trophoblastic disease after they undergo oncolytic chemotherapy with methotrexate. The situation is different with cervical ectopic pregnancy because it may present increasing problems for infertile patients. An intrafetal injection of potassium chloride (KCl) may be the method of choice for nonsurgical ablation of the ectopic cervical or cornual pregnancy tissue (Frates, 1994). Unlike methotrexate, which disturbs the implantation site through the abrupt destruction of ectopic trophoblastic tissue, KCl intrafetal injection slowly disturbs the fetal hormonal factors, namely hCG, α-fetoprotein, estriol, and CA-125, as reflected by the changes in maternal serum levels. The end result is a gentle and complete involution of the placental bed within 2 months (Osathanondh, unpublished data, 1994).

Uterotonic Agents

Prostaglandins are long-chain 20-carbon derivatives of arachidonic acid that are naturally synthesized from tissue phospholipids. They bear a common chemical structure of the C20 prostanoic acid that contains a cyclopentane ring between C8 and C12. Biosynthesis of such compounds in the uterine tissue requires a lysosomal enzyme, phospholipase A_2, and a group of microsomal enzymes called prostaglandin synthetase (cyclooxygenase [COX], isomerase, and reductase). Some prostaglandin (PG) drugs that induce contractions of the gravid uterus include PGE_1 and its methyl analogue misoprostol; PGE_2 and its synthetic derivatives, such as meteneprost potassium and sulprostone; and $PGF_{2\alpha}$ and its 15-methyl analogue. They are extremely thermolabile in soluble form and must be kept at temperatures below $4°\ C$ until use.

PGE_2 (dinoprostone) is available in a suppository (wax) or gel base (Rakhshani, 1988). The FDA approved the vaginal suppository form of PGE_2 for labor induction if fetal demise occurred until 28 weeks of pregnancy. It is readily absorbed by the vaginal mucosa into the systemic circulation, with the resultant pharmacologic effects summarized in Box 13-8. The recommended dosage is 5 to 20 mg clinically adjusted (titrated) at safe intervals (usually every 3 or 4 hours) and based on the optimal uterotonic response versus its undesirable systemic effects. It stimulates the smooth muscles of the gravid uterus and gastrointestinal tract and disturbs the body's thermoregulatory center. Therefore, common side effects include nausea, vomiting, diarrhea, and fever. Gastrointestinal side effects can be reduced by pretreatment medications with oral diphenoxylate with atropine and an intramuscular antinauseant such as prochlorperazine or phenoxyzine hydrochloride. Fever can be reduced with rectal acetaminophen and a wet body sponge. Unlike $PGF_{2\alpha}$, PGE_2 dilates the bronchial and most vascular smooth mus-

---

BOX 13-8
SYSTEMIC EFFECTS OF PROSTAGLANDINS

Contraction of pregnant uterus
Fever
Nausea and vomiting
Diarrhea
Increased intraocular pressure
Increased histamine level
Increased platelet aggregation
Decreased noradrenaline level

Table 13-3   Differences Between Prostaglandin $F_{2\alpha}$ and Prostaglandin E_2

	$PGF_{2\alpha}$	PGE_2
Uterine muscle		
Pregnant	Contract	Contract
Nonpregnant	Contract	Inhibit
Bronchial smooth muscle	Constrict	Dilate
Arterial perfusion		
Coronary	Decreased	Increased
Regional	Decreased	Increased
Arterial pressure		
Systemic	Increased	Decreased
Pulmonary	Increased	Increased
Central venous pressure	Increased	Decreased
Cardiac output and heart rate	Increased	Increased

cles (Table 13-3), resulting in moderate peripheral vasodilation and lowered diastolic blood pressure when large doses are used (Shapiro, 1982). Patients with active asthma or compromised cardiopulmonary hemodynamics tolerate systemic PGE_2 better than they tolerate $PGF_{2\alpha}$.

Before the induction of labor with uterotonic PG, the degree of cervical effacement must be assessed. If the cervix is not well effaced, pretreatment with *Laminaria japoniea* is indicated regardless of cervical dilation. The induction-to-delivery period is much shorter with adequate laminaria pretreatment of the cervix. After the products of conception are expelled, a routine inspection and gentle exploration of the uterine cavity with a large curette is strongly advised before discharging the patient. This can be accomplished under minimal sedation with or without local anesthesia. Since 1981, multiple laminaria tents were routinely used during the overnight preparation of the cervix before PG induction. With this special pretreatment, there were no cervical lacerations or uterine ruptures in more than 7000 consecutive PG-induced midtrimester abortions. The use of a midtrimester dose of PGE_2 on pregnant women in the third trimester could lead to uterine rupture (Patterson, 1979; Valenzuela, 1980). Uterine rupture was also reported after an intraamniotic injection of $PGF_{2\alpha}$ or 15-methyl-$PGF_{2\alpha}$ (Cederqvist, 1980; Vergote, 1982). This complication tends to occur when a PG drug is administered in combination with oxytocin treatment. Near term the uterine muscle may be more sensitive to PG because of an increased number of oxytocin receptors. Prostaglandin and oxytocin are strongly synergistic, and PG itself may induce an increase in oxytocin receptors. Thus, oxytocin should not be administered within 2 hours of the last PG dose.

After an overnight laminaria preparation of the cervix, PGE_2 suppository can be inserted through the dilated cervical canal as the initial labor-inducing dose. This is done by compressing the PGE_2 wax onto the porous surface of the osmotic dilator Lamicel (Cooper Medical, Newtown, Pa.) at its distal, pointed end. To keep the drug inside the cervical canal, a large number of laminaria tents must be inserted snugly immediately after this intrauterine, extraamnionic, Lamicel and PGE_2 combination. The initial intrauterine dose may produce fewer systemic side effects than a vaginal application. This technique can also be used after rupture of the membranes, provided all amniotic fluid is manually expelled with suprapubic pressure.

15(S)-15-methyl-$PGF_{2\alpha}$ (carboprost tromethamine or Hemabate [Pharmacia-Upjohn, Kalamazoo, Mich.] has been used in combination with 64 to 100 ml hypertonic (23.4% or 4 mEq/mL) saline for intraamniotic abortion in an ambulatory service. This prostaglandin analogue was approved for intramuscular use to treat postpartum hemorrhage caused by an atonic uterus. However, parenteral administration may produce severe untoward events, including cardiac arrhythmia, bronchoconstriction, pulmonary hypertension, increased intrapulmonary shunting, and arterial oxygen desaturation (Hankins, 1988). Unlike $PGE_{2\alpha}$, $PGF_{2\alpha}$ and its synthetic derivatives stimulate uterine contractions even in

the nongravid state. Its efficacy after intraamniotic injection for labor induction was described more than two decades ago (Dingfelder, 1976; Karim, 1975). Using a strict protocol of active management, the interval from intraamniotic injection to abortion for midtrimester abortion averages 8 hours. Most patients who undergo prostaglandin abortion are safely discharged from the ambulatory unit within 12 hours. The free backflow of clear amniotic fluid must be seen at amniocentesis before the drug is injected into the amnionic sac. This caution is imperative because an accidental leakage of 15-methyl-$PGF_{2\alpha}$ into the systemic circulation may result in cardiopulmonary side effects that will not abate as quickly as those caused by $PGF_{2\alpha}$. A dose-response study revealed that 1.5 mg of 15-methyl-$PGF_{2\alpha}$ and 64 to 100 mL of 23.4% saline are optimal for a midtrimester intraamniotic labor-induction protocol. This protocol produces minimal or no systemic side effects when compared to the use of PGE_2 suppositories.

Misoprostol, a methyl analogue of PGE_1, was approved by the FDA for use in the treatment of peptic ulcer disease. This oral agent has antisecretory activity for as long as 5 hours at the usual recommended dose (Monk, 1987). However, it exerts a significant uterotonic effect at doses greater than 0.4 mg (Rabe, 1987). This drug has milder and fewer side effects than other available forms of prostaglandin. It is also the least expensive at present. When its use for therapeutic induced abortion during midtrimester is preceded by overnight laminaria preparation of the cervix, this drug has an excellent efficacy and safety profile. Conversely, the use of misoprostol without proper supervision often leads to tragic sequelae. Misoprostol has been a popular abortifacient in South America and Africa. The protocol requires adequate laminaria preparation of the cervix followed by intraamniotic injection of 64 to 100 ml of 23.4% saline and oral misoprostol 0.4 to 0.8 mg every 2 hours, based on each patient's uterine activity response. Fetal delivery is accomplished within 12 hours in 95% of patients.

Oxytocin, a neurohypophyseal hormone, was synthesized for the induction of labor beyond the second trimester of pregnancy. Unlike PG, oxytocin is uterotonic only in the presence of an adequate number of oxytocin receptors. It appears more potent than PG in causing the contraction of the myoepithelial cells of the mammary gland. This results in milk ejection. Thus, oxytocin nasal spray is available for stimulating initial milk letdown. Suckling is the only well-defined physiologic stimulus for oxytocin release. Cervical dilation is thought to be another stimulus for its release. Because of its similarity with vasopressin in amino acid sequence, oxytocin has 1/200 the antidiuretic potency of vasopressin. If a concentrated oxytocin solution is to be infused for a prolonged period of time, a limited volume of an electrolyte solution should be used instead of plain dextrose in water. This is to avoid water intoxication with the resultant hyponatremia and its consequences.

In midtrimester abortion, high-dose intravenous oxytocin is effective only when the patient's cervix is nearly fully (*i.e.,* 90%) effaced. Oxytocin exerts its uterotonic effect

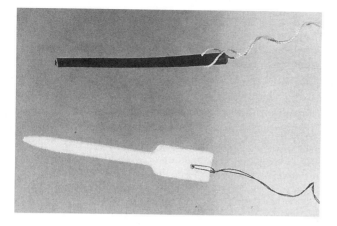

Fig. 13-8. A laminaria tent (dark) shown in comparison with a lamicel (white).

after the uterus has been adequately stimulated by an exogenous PG or by other factors. This leads to local endogenous PG production. For midtrimester labor induction of a nonviable fetus, the intravenous oxytocin augmentation protocol requires 60 U in 500 ml of an electrolyte solution at the initial rate of 10 ml/hr (equivalent to 20 mU/min) using an infusion pump. The rate is increased at intervals and in increments of 10 ml/hr up to the limit of 60 ml/hr (120 mU/min).

Two uterotonic agents that have fallen into disuse are buccal oxytocin citrate and an oxytocic alkaloid, sparteine sulfate, for intramuscular injection. The latter is potent, but its uterotonic effect is difficult to titrate. In fact, many ergot alkaloids are potent uterotonic agents. They were used in illegal abortions along with quinine tablets (Potts, 1983).

Hypertonic and locally toxic solutions were used for intraamniotic abortions long before the availability of PG drugs. They include 23.4% saline solution, 30% or 40% hyperosmolar urea, and an antiseptic acridine orange (acrinol) (Burkman, 1975; Kafrissen, 1984). Originally, hypertonic dextrose solution was also used, but it was associated with a high infection rate. An intraamniotic injection of hypertonic or hyperosmolar solutions induces a cascade of intrauterine events that lead to prostaglandin release in the local tissues. Effective uterine contractions occur within several hours. Many investigators have described the electrolyte and osmolar dynamics in these types of induced abortions (Anderson, 1968; Frigoletto, 1971; Goodlin, 1968). Too concentrated or too high a volume of saline solution may result in life-threatening, disseminated, intravascular coagulation or hypernatremia if accidentally injected into the uterine circulation.

Agents for Softening the Cervix

Hygroscopic devices are considered an integral part of therapeutic abortion after the twelfth week of pregnancy. They are placed in the cervical canal to induce gentle, nontraumatic dilation of the cervix. After adequate preparation of the cervix, the uterine evacuation procedure can be expediently accomplished by a trained physician, with mini-

mal risk for trauma or hemorrhage from the instrument (Blumenthal, 1988).

A laminaria tent (Fig. 13-8) is a dried stem of seaweed that feels like a wooden stick or a huge toothpick. It is 6 cm long and is available in sizes from 2 to 6 mm, based on the cross-section diameter at its tip. Large numbers of small-diameter (2 or 3 mm) laminaria tents are preferred to small numbers of large tents because of the greater ease of insertion and the greater surface area of exposure. Two small laminarias work better than a large one. They are left in the cervical canal for at least 4 hours, but preferably all night, before the uterine evacuation procedure is performed. The insertion technique is described in Box 13-9.

Laminaria was used in Europe before World War II. However, because it cannot be boiled, sepsis easily set in so it was quickly abandoned. Its rebirth in modern obstetrics and gynecology came after the availability of gas sterilization with ethylene oxide and broad-spectrum antibiotics (Eaton, 1972; Hale, 1972; Newton, 1972). The device swells to three to four times its original diameter (Fig. 13-9) and slowly dilates the cervix. After intracervical placement, the sonographic appearance of the laminaria varies with time because of its hygroscopic nature (Hirsch, 1988). While exerting its effect, the laminaria may produce moderate but tolerable crampy pain. Besides its hygroscopic (mechanical) action, laminaria significantly increases blood levels of PG metabolites (Ye, 1982). After overnight placement, each laminaria tent softens, becomes as large as a cigarette, and is easily removed. We prefer *L. japonica* to European types because of its uniform consistency and minimal hourglass (dumbbell) effect. Whenever this phenomenon occurs, removal may be difficult and may require paracervical block anesthesia. Each laminaria should be grasped with ring forceps, and the forceps should be rotated 360° before the incarcerated device can be pulled out.

Lamicel is a dried polyvinyl alcohol sponge stick impregnated with magnesium sulfate (Fig. 13-8). This scratchy, sharp stick becomes soft and immediately swells with a spongy consistency when placed in the cervical canal. Each stick contains 0.2 to 0.5 g magnesium sulfate, depending on its diameter. Minimal systemic absorption of magnesium sulfate may occur through the uterine tissue, but magnesium levels in the blood have not exceeded 4 mg/dL in a testing series. Through some histochemical and hygroscopic effects, the dilator softens the cervix within 2 hours, making it pliable to gradual dilation with conventional instruments or with multiple *L. japonica* tents. Overnight preparation of the cervix with this dilator, combined with three to five laminarias on the day before labor induction, significantly shortens the prostaglandin induction-to-delivery interval and has thus far eliminated the risk for cervical rupture or cervicovaginal fistula (*Fistula cervicovaginalis laqueatica*) (Ingvardsen, 1979). Paradoxical to its tocolytic effect, overnight preparation of the cervix with this magnesium sulfate device may enhance the effectiveness of PG-induced labor. Other investigators have effectively used this dilator before suction evacuation of the uterus.

BOX 13-9
LAMINARIA INSERTION TECHNIQUE

1. Make sure the patient understands that laminaria insertion is the beginning and most important part of the pregnancy termination procedure. If the patient is 18 weeks or more pregnant, ultrasound imaging should be performed to confirm the gestational age.
2. Conduct a pelvic examination to record the uterine size and axis, and then change gloves. Put on sterile gloves and insert the speculum.
3. Prepare the vagina and cervix with povidone-iodine (Betadine). Use diluted chlorhexidine gluconate (Hibiclens) if the patient is allergic to povidone-iodine.
4. Dip a small, long-stem cotton swab in povidone-iodine, and gently sound the endocervix with it. Do not go in far beyond the internal os. The brownish staining of the cotton swab stem indicates the length of cervical canal.
5. If necessary, grasp the cervix with a long Allis clamp or straight-ring forceps, taking care to grasp only a small fold of mucosa to minimize the patient's discomfort. Local (paracervical block) anesthesia may be required if the patient has cervical stenosis.
6. Grasp the laminaria at the string end with ring forceps and gently insert it until the tip with the string is flush with the external os. Always use the laminaria that has the smallest diameter. Up to 12 weeks of pregnancy, insert two laminarias; 13 to 17 weeks of pregnancy, insert three to five laminarias; 18 weeks of pregnancy and beyond, insert three to five laminarias, with one lamicel as tolerated by the patient.
7. Dip a folded 4 × 4-inch gauze in a small amount of povidone-iodine, lay it over the cervix, and tuck it gently into the fornices. Lay a second (dry) 4 × 4-inch gauze over the first one to pack the laminaria in place. Gently remove the speculum while holding the gauze sponges in place with the ring forceps.
8. Have the patient remain lying in the left lateral position for a few minutes to avoid syncope. Note in the chart the time of insertion and the number of laminarias and sponges inserted.
9. Be certain that the patient understands that she must return for the laminaria removal the next day. Severe infection may result if one set of laminaria is left in situ for more than 48 hours. Inform the patient that the cramping with insertion will subside in a few minutes. Tell her to come back to the hospital at once if the membranes rupture, if bleeding occurs, or if she has a fever. Forbid coitus (some patients have attempted coitus with laminarias in place; hence, give clear instructions against it). The patient may take one or two acetaminophen tablets as needed for cramping, but aspirin or other prostaglandin synthesis inhibitors should not be used. Give the patient an instruction card with the above advice and precautions in case she forgets the verbal information.

Dilapan (Gynotech, Lebanon, N.J.), another hygroscopic cervical dilator, is a synthetic polymer similar to a soft contact lens. The manufacturer recommends use within 4 hours of abortion on patients at or before 16 weeks of pregnancy. Compared with other hygroscopic dilators, this gluey and sticky device expands rapidly in and around the cervix. It may be difficult to remove the device within 2 hours of insertion.

In addition to hygroscopic devices, intracervical or vaginal PGE_2 and other PG derivatives were successfully used for softening the unfavorable (unripe) cervix. Meteneprost potassium, an analogue of PGE_2 in suppository form (10 mg), can induce adequate cervical softening within several hours of vaginal administration before a first-trimester induced abortion (Darney, 1987; Osathanondh, 1985; Shapiro, 1982). Preparing the cervix with a low dose of PGE_2 or one of its synthetic derivatives reduces the need for forceful instrument dilation of the cervix before uterine evacuation. Minimal but well-tolerated PG-induced side effects should be expected.

Conventional Methods of Induced Abortion

More than 1 million therapeutic abortions are reported in the United States each year, and there are probably as many unreported menstrual extraction or menstrual regulation procedures routinely performed in physicians' offices. In 1994

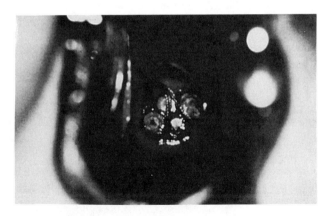

Fig. 13-9. Four laminaria tents that have been left in a cervix overnight. (Courtesy Dr. A. M. Altman.)

approximately one legal abortion was reported for every four live births in the United States (Henshaw, 1998). Ninety-five percent of therapeutic abortions are safely performed in an outpatient facility using the vacuum aspiration technique (Wu, 1958). It is not a good contraceptive choice, but it should be used as the last resort. Induced abortion is the best therapy to save the mother's life if she has severe cardiac, renal, metabolic, hepatic, hematologic, or cerebrovascular disease (Bowers, 1988). Appropriate fetal indications range from defects that are incompatible with extrauterine life, such as anencephaly, holoprosencephaly, and hypoplasia or agenesis of vital organs, to problems of chromosomal, metabolic, teratogenic, or infectious origin. Unique problems that combine maternal and fetal indications for terminating a pregnancy are maternal neoplastic disease requiring radiation or chemotherapy, fetal demise, and chorioamnionitis. With the latter diagnosis, the gravid uterus must be evacuated not only to save the mother but also to preserve her reproductive capability. Termination of a pregnancy beyond 24 weeks from the last menstrual period (LMP) is justified in cases of fetal demise or lethal malformation such as anencephaly (Chervenak, 1984; Osathanondh, 1980). Hysterotomy or gravid hysterectomy is rarely indicated when skilled physicians and modern techniques for uterine evacuation are readily available.

In general, complication rates from induced abortion increase with every advancing week of gestation (Grimes, 1988; Ory, 1983). As defined by the Centers for Disease Control's Joint Program for the Study of Abortion (JPSA), major complications include cardiac arrest, convulsions, death, endotoxic shock, fever for 3 days or more, hemorrhage necessitating transfusion, hypernatremia, injury to bladder, ureter, or intestine, pelvic infection with 2 or more days of fever and a peak of at least 40° C or with hospitalization for 11 days or more, pulmonary embolism or infarction, thrombophlebitis, major surgical treatment of complications, and wound disruption after hysterotomy or hysterectomy. Other complications not listed by the JPSA include retained pregnancy products or the continuation of pregnancy, hematometra, and coagulopathy (Osathanondh, 1981; White, 1983). Additionally, two or more induced abortions may increase the risk for subsequent first- and second-trimester loss (Hogue, 1981; Linn, 1983; Stubblefield, 1984).

Menstrual extraction (miniabortion, minisuction, or menstrual regulation) is usually performed in a physician's office with a soft, flexible, plastic cannula (sometimes referred to as a Karman cannula). The cannula is attached to a special self-locking syringe or a small suction pump operated electrically or hydrostatically (Vabra aspirator). An experienced operator can perform this miniabortion 6 to 7 weeks after the patient's LMP without anesthesia. Most of the time, a 4-mm or 3-mm cannula can be inserted into the gravid uterus without instrumental dilation of the cervix. The patient may receive preoperative medications, which consist of oral ibuprofen and sublingual lorazepam. An office pregnancy test using a rapid, specific, and sensitive assay is strongly advised before the minisuction to avoid unnecessary instrumentation of the uterine cavity. The minisuction evacuation can be accomplished within 5 minutes with an in-and-out movement of the canula while rotating it 360° around its long axis. After the procedure is complete, the aspirated products of conception (POC) must be carefully inspected for the presence of trophoblastic villous tissue (chorionic villi) (Fig. 13-10). If only the decidual (hypertrophic gestational endometrial) tissue is obtained but the villous structure cannot be identified, an ectopic pregnancy must be ruled out using an appropriate evaluation and treatment protocol. A bleeding (ruptured) tubal pregnancy with signs of peritoneal irritation may be observed shortly after minisuction of the uterine cavity of patients with unrecognized extrauterine gestation (Rubin, 1980). In spite of the obvious presence of villi, all patients should be reexamined several weeks thereafter because of the notoriously high incidence of retained POC or unrecognized continuation of an intrauterine pregnancy. Many authorities advise routine pregnancy testing at the postoperative follow-up visit if the soft plastic catheter was used for miniabortion.

Dilation and suction evacuation (D&E) is the most frequently used procedure for terminating a pregnancy up to 21 weeks from the LMP (Grimes, 1977). After 15 weeks of

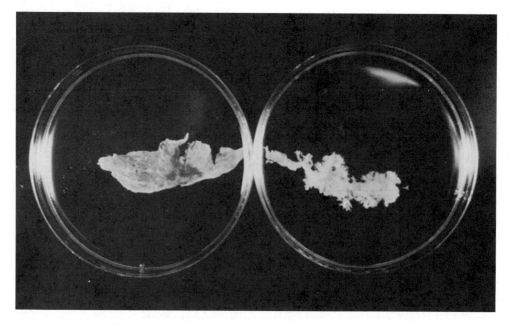

Fig. 13-10. Early pregnancy decidua *(left)* and trophoblastic villi *(right).*

pregnancy, however, only a qualified operator with a high degree of touch-and-feel ability should perform this procedure. Another important consideration is frequent exposure to late midtrimester D&E, which may cause undesirable stress among dedicated staff. This problem may be avoided if a labor induction method is routinely available as an alternative.

Ninety-nine percent of our D&E procedures are performed using local anesthesia with chloroprocaine hydrochloride instead of lidocaine. When injected into highly vascular tissue, chloroprocaine hydrochloride has a wider safety margin and a longer duration of action than lidocaine. Ideally, all D&E procedures should be performed with local anesthesia because blood loss and uterine perforation will be lower than they would be with general anesthesia. Discomfort can be ameliorated by appropriate intravenous medication and conversation with a nurse trained to coach the patient before and during the procedure. Simultaneously, the nurse monitors the patient's vital signs, respiration, and pulse-oxymeter oxygen saturation levels. Midazolam not exceeding 2 mg and fentanyl citrate 0.1 mg are used for monitored intravenous anesthesia or conscious intravenous sedation. Additionally, 25 mg diphenhydramine hydrochloride may be required for its mild anticholinergic effects. Vasoactive agents such as atropine or epinephrine or other pressor drugs such as pitressin are avoided. The cardiogenic risks of such vasoactive substances outweigh the claimed benefits of reducing blood loss or vagal reaction. In fact, many deaths from legal abortion in the United States are reportedly drug related (Cates, 1979; MMWR, 1986). Proper training of the operator with hands-on supervision and gentle manipulation with adequate dexterity contribute to the uneventful completion of the procedure with minimal blood loss. The patient must fast for at least 6 hours because of delayed gastrointestinal transit, especially during late midtrimester. She should not go home by herself after the procedure. An abortion after 12 weeks from the LMP should be preceded by adequate laminaria pretreatment of the cervix.

Blood type (ABO and Rh), serum antibody screening, and a hematocrit and platelets count are routinely obtained before laminaria insertion. Additionally, cervical cytology and screening for STDs may be indicated in some patients.

At the time of the procedure, an intravenous line is inserted and secured for monitored intravenous medications. The no-touch technique is used. This means that only the portion of the instrument that will be in the uterus is kept sterile throughout the procedure. The operator should wear protective goggles or eyeglasses and a mask. Bimanual palpation of the uterine cervix and fundus should be performed to ascertain the direction of the uterine axis. At this time the sponges and laminaria tents may be digitally removed. The short-blade (Moore-Graves) speculum is required for minimizing the angle between the cervical canal and the uterine axis (Fig. 13-11). The anterior lip of the cervix is cleansed with an antiseptic solution and then injected with 3 ml 1% chloroprocaine hydrochloride at the 12 o'clock position using a 22-gauge spinal needle. A single toothed tenaculum is

applied vertically with the inner jaw inside the cervical canal to include the whole thickness of the anterior lip of cervix within the bite. It is important to take a deep enough bite so that the tenaculum will not be inadvertently pulled out and tear the cervix during the procedure. The rest of the cervix and vaginal fornices are cleansed, and the paracervical tissue is injected with 3 ml of the same anesthesia at the 4, 8, 10, and 2 o'clock positions. The needle tip should reach the depth of only several millimeters within the submucosal (paracervical) tissue at or near the cervicovaginal junction. Preinjection aspiration is advised to avoid inadvertent leakage of the drug into a cervical tributary of the uterine vein. The uterine sound should not be inserted into any gravid uterus before the D&E procedure because the risk for perforating the thin, soft uterine wall outweighs any information to be gained. Depth and axis of the uterine cavity change rapidly during the suction evacuation, and they should be gently assessed with a large curette but not with the uterine sound. The direction of the already dilated cervical canal can be assessed with a large cotton swab (a scopette). Should there be a need to dilate the cervix forcefully after the retrieval of the laminarias, dilators with tapered ends, such as the Pratt dilator, are preferred. The optimal diameter of the cannula for uterine evacuation (Fig. 13-11) generally correlates with gestational age. For example, a 14-mm cannula is required for complete evacuation of a 13- to 15-week-old embryo. Five different sizes of rigid, clear, plastic cannula with internal diameters of 8, 10, 12, 14, and 16 mm are often used. The ability to insert a large-bore cannula through the laminaria-pretreated cervix greatly facilitates a safe and expedient D&E beyond the first trimester of pregnancy. However, when the uterus is larger than 16 gestational weeks, most solid POC must be extracted with the Sopher forceps (Fig. 13-12) because the parts are too large to be aspirated through the cannula. Membranes can often be easily ruptured with the use of sponge forceps, after which amniotic fluid is completely expelled to reduce the

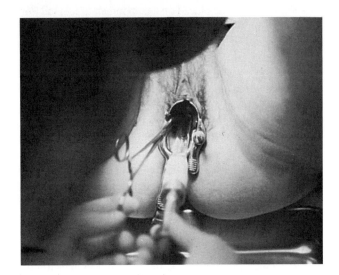

Fig. 13-11. A 16-mm rigid plastic cannula inserted through the cervical canal for suction evacuation of midtrimester uterus.

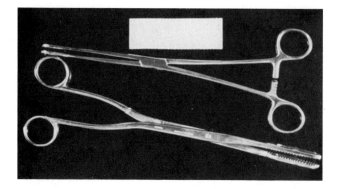

Fig. 13-12. Sopher forceps (with long jaws) compared with ordinary ring forceps.

uterine volume and the depth of uterine cavity. The large-bore cannula is required for the aspiration of the remaining amniotic fluid and for bringing the POC down to the lower uterine segment where the fetal parts can be safely extracted with the Sopher forceps. Ideally, the hinge of the Sopher forceps should be at the level of the cervical canal. Note that the cannula must be connected to the hose and vacuum jar through a specially designed handle. This special handle is the key to the D&E technique because it allows the cannula to be rotated 360° around its long axis while the hose remains immobile. The cannula is initially inserted just beyond the internal cervical os and rotated around the same cervicouterine axis while using a vacuum aspirating pressure of 50 to 60 cm Hg. Once the intrauterine volume is reduced after complete drainage of the amniotic fluid, this cervicouterine axis may change (*e.g.,* from midposition to anteflexed or retroflexed). In most instances, the uterine cavity eventually deviates toward the patient's right side and remains in its resting dextrorotational axis. Gentle exploration of the uterine cavity with a large curette is required before advancing the cannula slightly deeper (to bring down the parts) and before the use of the Sopher forceps. Only the large curette should be used for this exploration. The operator's left hand may be placed on the abdomen to feel the fundus and to apply suprapubic pressure. If the fetal calvarium cannot be easily brought down to the safe reach of the Sopher forceps, the patient should be given intravenous oxytocin using the high-dose protocol, and the procedure should be temporarily halted. The patient can be brought back to the procedure room in 1 or 2 hours when the fetal calvarium is seen or digitally felt at or above the internal cervical os. This second-stage uterine evacuation can be easily and rapidly accomplished without pain or discomfort to the patient. In general, however, a uterotonic agent is not administered during the D&E until after the fetal calvarium has been obtained for fear of trapping it up high or compressing it into the myometrium (Altman, 1985). The D&E procedure is considered complete after the identification of important fetal parts that include the calvarium, spine, and tips of the extremities. We routinely record the fetal foot length to corroborate the gestational age using Streeter's data as modified

by Moore (Moore, 1973). These data correlate well in the patient population. Fetal foot lengths at 10, 12, 14, 16, 18, 20, and 22 weeks from the LMP are 6, 9, 14, 20, 27, 33, and 39 mm, respectively. Induced abortions performed 8 to 10 weeks from the LMP should also yield a recognizable fetal part. Adding 6.5 to the crown-rump length in centimeters provides an estimation of the gestational age in weeks during the first trimester.

No descriptive text or manual on the D&E technique can replace proper training with hands-on instruction from a skillful physician. Resident physicians should receive daily D&E training by a small number of experienced attending faculty members (Altman, 1985). This training, a well-defined protocol, and a dedicated nursing staff facilitate the incorporation of the D&E procedure within emergency-room management of patients with incomplete miscarriage (Brennan, 1987). Such patients safely and expediently undergo D&E with local anesthesia in specially equipped emergency rooms.

When the fetal biparietal diameter measures 50 to 55 mm, the method of choice for abortion is the induction of labor after adequate preparation of the cervix with laminaria tents. (On average, fetal biparietal diameter increases by 0.43 mm per day or 3 mm per week during the second trimester of pregnancy.) This technique is also used if a patient requests an intact fetus, usually for personal reasons or reasons of genetic counseling. Several hours of effective labor in a patient whose cervix is not satisfactorily prepared by laminarias may lead to favorable changes in the cervix and lower uterine segment for a safe and easy D&E procedure. With a strict and active protocol for labor induction, the complication rate is much less than that reported by the Centers for Disease Control. This is in contradistinction to national statistics, which showed higher serious complication rates with intraamniotic prostaglandin. A complication rate of less than 2% (based on the JPSA criteria) is not higher than that of a late D&E and may be attributed to protocol variations. First, the patient must undergo a laminaria pretreatment of the cervix 20 hours before receiving prostaglandin. Second, ultrasound imaging (Hornstein, 1986), immediate coagulation screening tests, and blood products are available on site (Osathanondh, 1981). Third, a full-time director of the unit (or a designee) instantaneously evaluates and performs the late D&E in case of excessive bleeding or prolonged labor. No patient is allowed to labor longer than 20 hours. Fourth, membranes are artificially ruptured after 3 hours of prostaglandin-induced labor. Oral PGE$_1$ methyl analogue (misoprostol) 0.4 mg is used in the morning after at least 20 hours of laminaria preparation of the cervix. One hour after the administration of oral misoprostol, an intraamniotic injection of 64 to 100 ml of 23.4% hypertonic saline is made. The abdominal wall is infiltrated with local anesthesia, and then a large-bore needle in introduced to demonstrate the free backflow of clear amniotic fluid before the patient is injected with hypertonic saline. This procedure is immediately followed by the administration of 0.4 mg oral misoprostol every 2 hours based on uterine contraction response. Three hours after the hypertonic saline injection, osmotic dilators are removed and the membranes are artificially ruptured. After all the amniotic fluid has been expelled with suprapubic pressure, cervical effacement is reassessed. When the cervix is 80% to 90% effaced, high-dose intravenous oxytocin is administered through an infusion pump according to an intermittent regimen (10 minutes on, 10 minutes off). If the cervix is still thick and long, 0.4 mg vaginal misoprostol or 20 mg intracervical PGE_2 is administered with another insertion of multiple osmotic dilators. This is followed at 2-hour intervals by the administration of 0.4 mg vaginal misoprostol. Finally, uterine exploration and sharp curettage are performed after delivery of the placenta. Otherwise, the placenta must be removed using local anesthesia within 2 hours of fetal delivery.

The second prostaglandin of choice is an intraamnionic instillation of 1.5 mg of 15-methyl-$PGF_{2\alpha}$ (carboprost tromethamine) followed immediately by 64 to 100 mL of 23.4% saline (4 mEq/mL) using a three-way connecting tube. Again, free backflow of clear amniotic fluid must be demonstrated before any drug injection. Actually, prostaglandins are inactivated by normal amniotic fluid. However, the carefully selected pharmacologic dose is in excess and will set off an irreversible chain of intrauterine events leading to myometrial contractions within an hour of administration. The intraamnionic injection produces fewer side effects than the extraamnionic route. After artificial rupture of the membranes, pretreatment medications are given at least a half hour before the first dose of PGE_2 is administered, as described earlier. If the cervical effacement reaches 90%, the high-dose intravenous oxytocin infusion will be initiated as long as it is not within 2 hours of the last dose of PG. Prophylactic antibiotics are not routinely provided. However, broad-spectrum intravenous antibiotics are used liberally if the fetus has not been delivered after 6 hours of artificially or spontaneously ruptured membranes. Antibiotics are also prescribed if the procedure results in an excessive amount of blood loss, if a degree of myometrial injury is strongly suspected, or if a D&E procedure takes longer than 20 minutes to complete. Some well-controlled trials favored the routine use of a prophylactic antibiotic, but their small study populations limit any conclusive interpretation (Darj, 1988; Sonne-Holmes, 1981; Spence, 1982). Patients at high-risk are defined as those who may benefit from a course of antibiotic treatment from the time of laminaria insertion the day before the D&E or the induction of labor. High-risk conditions are fetal demise; placenta previa; previous miscarriage; Asherman syndrome; intrauterine device; orthopedic or cardiac prosthesis; trichomonads or koilocytosis revealed on cervical cytology; history of PID, STD, or tubal pregnancy; sickle-cell trait or disease; chronic hepatitis; intravenous drug abuse; tattoo; multiple male partners; and incarceration in a correctional institution.

Preoperative prophylaxis is administered for bacterial endocarditis not only to patients with cardiac abnormalities but also to intravenous drug abusers. Additionally, any patient with a dilated internal os from an incomplete, inevitable, or missed abortion accompanied by vaginal bleeding should receive prophylactic antibiotics. The spectrum of prescribed antibiotics should cover *C. trachomatis*. This organism is found in 12% of women who request legal abortion at our institution.

The complications of induced abortion are reportedly dependent on two main factors: the gestational age (too early or too advanced) and the operator's experience (or inexperience). Recent U.S. national statistics showed that induced abortions performed 7 to 12 weeks from the LMP were associated with fewer complications than those performed before or after this gestational age range (Ory, 1983). Increased risks for uterine trauma and hemorrhage are associated with D&E procedures performed by residents than with those performed by experienced attending physicians (Grimes, 1985). Other risk factors include general anesthesia, inadequate preparation of the cervix with laminarias, parity, previous abortion, and the woman's age (Grimes, 1979; Schutz, 1983). Conversely, the risk for cervical injury or related trauma is reduced if the patient has already had an abortion, if laminarias and local anesthesia are used, and if the D&E is performed by an attending physician. The risk for cervical injury or related trauma is increased, however, if the patient is 17 or younger, if general anesthesia is used, and if the D&E is performed by a physician-in-training. Risk factors for uterine perforation are similar to those for cervical injury except that multiparous women have three times the risk that nulliparous women have (Cates, 1983). Fortunately, two thirds of uterine perforations occur in the fundal region and are not associated with acute or uncontrollable hemorrhage. Obese patients and those with repeated cesarean scars may be at increased risk for uterine perforation. Prompt recognition of this complication is the key to minimizing the damage. Undetected uterine perforation may lead to devastating generalized peritonitis and death from bowel injury. Acute problems associated with uterine perforation include lacerations of the uterine vessels, which lead to severe hypovolemia or expanding broad-ligament hematoma, and injuries to intraperitoneal structures. Such problems dictate the need for a prompt laparotomy. A three-way indwelling catheter should be inserted into the urinary bladder before the laparotomy is performed. Thus, methylene blue or indigo carmine can be readily injected intravesically should a bladder injury arise during this lifesaving operation. Usually, bleeding vessels can be ligated, in which case the uterine trauma is repaired and hysterectomy is not required. If a suction or forceps was applied intraperitoneally, the entire length of bowel should be inspected for severe contusion or disruption of its blood supply. In the latter situation, the surgeon may decide to resect and reanastomose the damaged bowel. Most of the time, however, complete rest for bowel, with the help of intermittent nasogastric suction and broad-spectrum intravenous antibiotics, is sufficient. If the uterine perforation is promptly diagnosed before any intraperitoneal structure is damaged, the D&E procedure may be continued and readily accomplished by an experienced surgeon under laparoscopic or ultrasonographic visualization. Otherwise, the procedure may be postponed for one week to allow complete healing of the uterine wall before a repeat D&E is performed by an expert in a well-prepared setting. A delayed diagnosis of slowly expanding broad-ligament hematoma in a hemodynamically stable patient may require only intravenous antibiotics and ultrasound imaging at follow-up intervals. A liquefied infected hematoma can be successfully drained under competent ultrasound guidance to abolish the stormy, febrile course and to shorten the patient's period of incapacitation. Selective embolization of a damaged uterine vessel was successfully used in patients with broad-ligament hematoma and patients with pathology-proven focal placenta accreta after adequate uterine packing and intravenous antibiotic treatment. Such conservative therapies are best preserved for nulliparous patients who fully understand the inherent procedural risks and sign the informed consent form in the chart.

Another type of hemorrhagic complication of induced abortion is coagulopathy. It is not an uncommon problem after a fetal demise of long duration and a large uterus (beyond 13 weeks) or after an intraamniotic injection of high-volume hypertonic saline. Coagulopathy is a rare occurrence of an otherwise routine D&E beyond 13 weeks from the LMP (Osathanondh, 1981; White, 1983). It is advised that midtrimester abortion be performed near or within a facility in which blood products are readily available. Prolonged bleeding from the well-contracting, intact, empty uterus and from the tenaculum site should provoke a high index of suspicion. A tube of blood should be obtained to record the patient's clotting time, which may be prolonged, and abnormal clot retraction or lysis. At the same time, a profile of blood coagulation tests should be immediately obtained. Severe depletion of platelets and fibrinogen disproportionate to the minor decrease in hematocrit may promptly confirm this diagnosis. In general, coagulopathy in obstetric hemorrhage is associated with the severe depletion of circulating fibrinogen before the decline of other clotting factors. Significant leakage of the thromboplastic or trophoblastic fetal tissue into the maternal circulatory system may be responsible for this postulated consumptive coagulopathy. It is often associated with violent uterine contractions or prolonged intrauterine manipulation in D&E procedures performed because of fetal demise. The treatment requires an infusion of cryoprecipitate and fresh plasma.

Another enigmatic complication of D&E that may develop hours or days after surgery is hematometra. Some authorities call this complication the postabortal syndrome or the redo syndrome (Sands, 1974). It was first reported in 1974 as a unique type of uterine atony, and the incidence was one in several hundred D&E procedures. This syndrome is characterized by painful and acutely tender enlargement of a uterus filled with dark, clotted blood. Signs of general distress are usually evident on the patient's face; accompanying this are sweating and tachycardia, but vaginal bleeding is not excessive. Repeat suction evacuation of the uterine cavity promptly abolishes this puzzling phenomenon. Although the cause is unknown, the patient may be administered an ergot and an antibiotic for prophylaxis.

An acute drug reaction is a possible complication before or during D&E. If a toxic dose of the local anesthesia is inadvertently injected into the maternal circulatory system, convulsions, cardiac arrhythmias, and cardiovascular collapse may follow. Treatment consists of the establishment and maintenance of an airway by endotracheal intubation with adequate ventilation of the patient. Adequate blood pressure is maintained with intravenous fluids and an appropriate sympathomimetic agent, if necessary. However, this complication is preventable. Preinjection aspiration, as described earlier, must be a routine part of paracervical anesthesia. There should be a 3-minute interval between the injection of the paracervical anesthesia and the beginning of the D&E procedure. The use of chloroprocaine hydrochloride and the avoidance of epinephrine (or other pressor substances) in the highly vascular gravid tissues are also part of the protocol. Premedication with 2 mg intravenous midazolam, a short-acting anxiolytic benzodiazepine, may prevent chest wall stiffness, a rare syndrome caused by the intravenous injection of an opioid such as fentanyl citrate. High dosages of both drugs may lead to dose-related respiratory depression. Effective intravenous antidotes for fentanyl and midazolam are naloxone hydrochloride 0.4 mg and flumazenil 1 mg, respectively.

Occasionally, a respiratory complication may arise during a midtrimester D&E, especially with fetal demise of long duration. It is characterized by respiratory hypersecretion, coughing, and, if not promptly corrected, bronchospasm. This syndrome is not related to an amniotic fluid embolism because it is self-limited and often develops among patients with severe oligohydramnios or dry fetal demise. It is unlike a vasovagal reaction because of the presence of tachycardia and the borderline elevation of blood pressure. It has been observed in association with violent uterine contractions that produce features analogous to inadvertent intravenous infusion of $PGF_{2\alpha}$. In 1978 Kohorn, in collaboration with the New England Trophoblastic Disease Center, described a similar problem as a trophoblastic embolization after molar evacuation. The D&E procedure should be temporarily halted, and the patient should be turned on her side. Intravenous diphenhydramine (25 mg) is slowly administered to reduce the secretion. Epinephrine should not be used for this type of bronchospasm because the patient's blood pressure may become elevated and epinephrine may produce an adverse cardiac effect (Silva, 1987). In instances such as this, bronchospasm is better relieved with a rapidly acting intravenous glucocorticoid, (4 mg dexamethasone or betamethasone), than an aminophylline, which is slow-acting and produces tachycardia. With assurance and improved ventilation and respiration, the D&E procedure can proceed and be safely completed. Every once in a while an amniotic fluid embolism develops in a patient during a midtrimester abortion, either after the instrumental disruption of the placenta with a large volume of amniotic fluid in the uterine cavity or after abruptio placenta if labor has been induced. It is usually associated with the obvious signs of cardiopulmonary collapse and disseminated intravascular coagulation. Prompt arterial blood gas measurement, electrocardiography, and ventilation-perfusion radionuclide imaging confirm the diagnosis. Effective resuscitation and successful management require around-the-clock cardiopulmonary and hematologic care by a competent team (internist, gynecologist, anesthesiologist, hematologist or blood-bank specialist, nurses, and laboratory personnel) in a well-equipped intensive care facility. The patient's uterus must be emptied as soon as her cardiovascular status is reasonably stabilized.

Delayed complications of induced abortion include different degrees of postabortal infection, from endoparametritis to pelvic septic thrombophlebitis and thromboembolic abnormalities (Burkman, 1977). Infection is usually associated with retained POC. Common symptoms are crampy pain with prolonged vaginal bleeding and low-grade fever. The uterus is tender, slightly enlarged, and boggy. High-resolution ultrasound imaging may confirm or exclude the diagnosis of retained POC. Treatment consists of intravenous antibiotics, an ergot alkaloid, and repeated uterine evacuation if indicated. Patients with a retained pregnancy or with retained pregnancy products often have an unrecognized positional, anatomic, or congenital uterine anomaly. Such patients should undergo D&E under ultrasound guidance (Hornstein, 1986), a technique that is also useful during midtrimester for patients with known anatomic derangements and for patients with cervical stenosis.

Controversies exist about the possibility of late sequelae from repetitive induced abortions and their effect on premature delivery and low birth weight (Hogue, 1981). Most statistics are derived from patients who have undergone primitive abortion procedures. Increasing experience and opportunities for the proper training of physicians in the modern techniques of induced abortion may curtail those problems. Another controversy is related to intrauterine synechiae (Asherman syndrome), which may involve risk factors that include genetic predisposition and postoperative infection or hematometra. One late sequela that is theoretically possible is Rh isomune disease (Litvak, 1970). A fail-safe mechanism can be devised as part of the quality assurance program involving the nurse, physician, and patient to ensure that Rh-negative patients receive adequate dosages of Rh immunoglobulin for prophylaxis within 72 hours of induced abortion or miscarriage.

Multifetal Pregnancy Reduction

Successful techniques for "assisted reproduction" and aggressive pharmacotherapy of infertility have led to an increase in gestations with three or more fetuses. If there are several fetuses in one gestation, each fetus is at a significantly increased risk for premature birth and its serious sequelae. Procedures to reduce multiple fetuses to only two (twins) were performed with increasing experience and efficacy using ultrasonography. Early methods involved transcervical selective evacuation, transabdominal injection of air or hypertonic saline, needle disruption of a selected conceptus, and selective fetal exsanguination (Farguharson, 1987). The method of choice is an ultrasound-guided transabdominal percutaneous injection of 4 to 8 mEq KCl per embryo (intracardiac or intrathoracic) at the end of the first trimester. Selective reduction procedures were also performed in the second trimester for terminating a defective (anomalous) twin. The patient must be informed of the known and unknown risks of losing some of or all the fetuses. Such risks were described with and without the selective-reduction procedure. The risks vary at different gestational ages and increase with advanced maternal age. Fetal risks include the syndrome of a vanishing twin(s), trapped twin(s), twin-to-twin transfusion, and disseminated intravascular coagulation, which may lead to porencephaly. Maternal complications include bleeding, infection, leakage of amniotic fluid, need for a repeat procedure, risk for D&E, sterility, and hysterectomy. Any infertile woman who has already accepted the risks inherent in infertility treatment tends to accept any known or unknown risk associated with the selective reduction of her multifetal pregnancy. With triplets, however, the risk-benefit ratio of undergoing a selective-reduction procedure is unclear, especially at tertiary-care maternity centers in which triplets appear to do as well medically (physically) as twins do after birth. In this situation, each couple may take into account the quality of the offspring's life and perhaps the cost of upbringing. Complex ethical and legal ramifications of the selective-reduction procedure remain for future debate.

REFERENCES

Altman AM, Stubblefield PG, Schlam J, et al: Midtrimester abortion by laminaria and vacuum evacuation on a teaching service. *J Reprod Med* 1985; 30:601-606.

Amir M: *Patterns in forcible rape*, Chicago, 1971, University of Chicago Press.

Anderson ABM, Turnbull AC: Changes in amniotic fluid, serum, and urine following the in-traamniotic injection of hypertonic saline. *Acta Obstet Gynecol Scand* 1968; 47:1-21.

Arntzenius AC, et al: Reduced high-density lipoprotein in women aged 40-41 using oral contraceptives. *Lancet* 1978; 1:1221-1223.

Bardin CW, et al: Medical abortion. *Curr Ther Endocrinol Metab* 1997; 6:305-311.

Baulieu EE, Segal SJ, editors: *The antiprogestin steroid RU486 and human fertility control,* New York, 1985 Plenum Press.

Beaumont V, Lemort N, Beaumont JL: Evaluation of risk factors associated with vascular thrombosis in women on oral contraceptives: Possible role of anti-sex-steroid hormone antibodies. *Artery* 1983; 11:331-344.

Beral V, et al, and the Collaborative Group on Hormonal Factors in Breast Cancer: Breast cancer and hormonal contraceptives: Collaborative reanalysis of individual data on 53,297 women with breast cancer and 100,239 women without breast cancer from 54 epidemiological studies. *Lancet* 1996a; 347: 1713-1727.

Beral V, et al, and the Collaborative Group on Hormonal Factors in Breast Cancer. Breast cancer and hormonal contraceptives: Further results. *Contraception* 1996b; 54:1S-106S.

Bergink EW, et al: Binding of a contraceptive progestogen Org 2969 and its metabolites to receptor proteins and human sex hormone-binding globulin. *J Steroid Biochem* 1981; 14:175-183.

Bertina RM, et al: Mutation in blood coagulation factor V associated with resistance to activated protein C. *Nature* 1994; 369:64-67.

Blumenthal PD: Prospective comparison of dilapan and laminaria for pretreatment of the cervix in second-trimester induction abortion. *Obstet Gynecol* 1988; 72:243-246.

Bowers C, Devine PA, Chervenak FA: Dilation and evacuation during the second trimester of pregnancy in a woman with primary pulmonary hypertension. *J Reprod Med* 1988; 133:787-788.

Bradley DD, et al: Saturated high-density lipoprotein cholesterol in women using oral contraceptives, estrogens, and progestins. *N Engl J Med* 1978; 199:17-20.

Brennan DM, Caldwell M: Dilatation and evacuation performed in the emergency department for miscarriage. *J Emerg Nurs* 1987; 13:144-8.

Brenner PF: Oral combination contraceptives. In Bardin CW, editor: *Current therapy endocrinology metabolism,* ed 3, Toronto, 1988, BC Decker.

Bruce SC, Paul RH, Van Dorsten JP: Control of postpartum uterine atony by intramyometrial prostaglandin. *Obstet Gynecol* 1982; 59:47S-50S.

Burkman RT: Lipid and lipoprotein changes in relation to oral contraception and hormonal replacement therapy. *Fertil Steril* 1988; 49:39S-50S.

Burkman RT, Atienza ME, King TM: Culture and treatment results in endometritis following elective abortion. *Am J Obstet Gynecol* 1977; 129:556-559.

Burkman RT, et al: Intraamniotic urea as a midtrimester abortifacient: Clinical results and serum and urinary changes. *Am J Obstet Gynecol* 1975; 121:7-16.

Burkman RT and the Women's Health Study: Association between intrauterine device and pelvic inflammatory disease. *Obstet Gynecol* 1981; 57:269-276.

Cabrol D, et al: Induction of labor with mifepristone after intrauterine fetal death. *Lancet* 1985; 2:119.

Caillouette JC, Koehler AL: Phasic contraceptive pills and functional ovarian cysts. *Am J Obstet Gynecol* 1987; 156:1538-1542.

Cameron IT, Baird DT: Early prenancy termination: A comparison between vacuum aspiration and medical abortion using prostaglandin (16,16 dimethyl-trans-3D$_2$-PGE$_1$ methyl ester) or the antiprogestogen RU486. *Br J Obstet Gynaecol* 1988; 95:271-276.

Campbell WB: Vasectomy and arterial disease. *J R Soc Med* 1988; 81:682-695.

Carp HJ, et al: Fertility after nonsurgical treatment of ectopic pregnancy. *J Reprod Med* 1986; 31:119-122.

Cates W Jr, Blackmore CA: Sexual assault and sexually transmitted diseases. In Holmes KK, Märdh P-A, Sparling PF, et al, editors: *Sexually transmitted diseases,* New York, 1984, McGraw-Hill.

Cates W Jr, Jordaan HVF: Sudden collapse and death of women obtaining abortions induced with prostaglandin F$_{2\alpha}$. *Am J Obstet Gynecol* 1979; 133:398-400.

Cates W Jr, Schulz KF, Grimes DA: The risks associated with teenage abortion. *N Engl J Med* 1983; 309:621-624.

Cederqvist LL, Birnbaum SJ: Rupture of the uterus after midtrimester prostaglandin abortion. *J Reprod Med* 1980; 25:136-138.

Centers for Disease Control Epidemiologic Notes and Reports: Maternal deaths associated with barbiturate anesthetics— New York City. *MMWR Morb Mortal Wkly Rep* 1986; 35:579-587.

Chervenak EA, et al: When is termination of pregnancy during the third trimester morally justifiable? *N Engl J Med* 1984; 3l0:501-504.

Chwalisz K: The use of progesterone antagonists for cervical ripening and as anadjunct to labour and delivery. *Hum Reprod* 1994; 9(suppl 1):131-161.

Clarke EA , et al: Cervical dysplasia: Association with sexual behavior, smoking, and oral contraceptive use? *Am J Obstet Gynecol* 1985; 151:612-616.

Connell EB: Oral contraceptives: The current risk-benefit ratio. *J Reprod Med* 1984; 29:513-523.

Cook CL, Lance JW, Kraft SL: Pregnancy prophylaxis: Parenteral postcoital estrogen. *Obstet Gynecol* 1986; 67:331-333.

Craft I, et al: Effect of Norgestrel administered intermittently on pituitary ovarian function. *Contraception* 1975; 12:589-598.

Cramer DW: Vasectomy and increased risk of prostate cancer, possible hormonal mechanisms. *JAMA* 1993; 270:707.

Cramer DW, et al: Factors affecting the association of oral contraceptives and ovarian cancer. *N Engl J Med* 1982; 307:1047-1051.

Cramer DW, et al: The relationship of tubal infertility to barrier method and oral contraceptive use, *JAMA* 1987; 257:2446-2450.

Cramer DW, et al: Tubal infertility and intrauterine device. *N Engl J Med* 1985; 312:941-947.

Creinin MD, Darney PD: Methotrexate and misoprostol for early abortion. *Contraception* 1993; 48:339-348.

Crooij MJ, et al: Termination of early pregnancy by the 3β-hydroxysteroid dehydrogenase inhibitor epostane. *N Engl J Med* 1988; 319:813-817.

Croxatto HB, et al: Studies on the duration of egg transport in the human oviduct, I: The time interval between ovulation and egg recovery from the uterus in normal women. *Fertil Steril* 1972; 23:447-458.

Cundy T, et al: Bone density in women receiving depot medroxy-progesterone acetate for contraception. *Br Med J* 1991; 303:13-16.

Dahlbäck-B, Carlsson M, Svensson PJ: Familial thrombophilia due to a previously unrecognized mechanism characterized by poor anticoagulant response to activated protein C: Prediction of a cofactor to activated protein

C. *Proc Natl Acad Sci USA* 1993; 90: 1004-1008.

Daling JR, et al: Primary tubal infertility in relation to the use of an intrauterine device. *N Engl J Med* 1985; 312:937-941.

Darj E, Stralin EB, Nilsson S: The prophylactic effect of doxycycline on postoperative infection rate after first-trimester abortion. *Obstet Gynecol* 1988; 70:755-758.

Darney PD: Long-acting hormonal contraception. *Contemp Obstet Gynecol* 1988; 32: 90-100.

Darney PD, Dorward K: Cervical dilation before first-trimester elective abortion: A controlled comparison of meteneprost, laminaria, and dilapan. *Obstet Gynecol* 1987; 70:397-400.

Dattel BJ, et al: Isolation of *Chlamydia trachomatis* from sexually abused female adolescents. *Obstet Gynecol* 1988; 72:240-242.

del Junco DJ, Annegers JF, Luthra HS: Do oral contraceptives prevent rheumatoid arthritis? *JAMA* 1985; 254:1938-1941.

Dericks-Tan JSE, Kock P, Tauben HD: Synthesis and release of gonadotropins: Effect of an oral contraceptive. *Obstet Gynecol* 1983; 62:687-690.

DeStefano F, et al: Complications of interval laparoscopic tubal sterilization. *Obstet Gynecol* 1983; 61:153-158.

Diamond MP, Wentz AC, Cherrington AD: Alterations in carbohydrate metabolism as they apply to reproductive endocrinology. *Fertil Steril* 1988; 50:387-397.

Diaz S, Croxatto HB, Parez M, et al: Ectopic pregnancies associated with low-dose progestogen-releasing IUDS. *Contraception* 1980; 22:259-269.

Diaz S, et al: Clinical assessment of treatments for prolonged bleeding in users of Norplant implants. *Contraception* 1990; 42:97.

Dingfelder JR, et al: Intraamniotic administration of 15(S)-15-methyl-prostaglandin F$_{2\alpha}$ for the induction of midtrimester abortion. *Am J Obstet Gynecol* 1976; 125:821-826.

Dixon GW, et al: Ethinyl estradiol and conjugated estrogens as postcoital contraceptives. *JAMA* 1980; 244:1336.

Droegemueller W, et al: Triphasic randomized clinical trail comparative frequency of intermenstrual bleeding. *Am J Obstet Gynecol* 1989; 161:1407-1411.

Duguid HLD, Parratt D, Traynor R: Actinomyces-like organisms in cervical smears from women using intrauterine contraceptive devices. *Br Med J* 1980; 281:534-537.

Eaton CJ, Cohn F, Bollinger CC: Laminaria tent as a cervical dilator prior to aspiration type therapeutic abortion. *Obstet Gynecol* 1972; 39:533-536.

Editorial: Drug interaction with oral contraceptive steroids. *Br Med J* 1980; 281:93-94.

Elger W, et al: Endometrial and myometrial effect of progesterone antagonists in pregnant guinea pigs. *Am J Obstet Gynecol* 1987; 157:1065-1074.

Ellis JW: Multiphasic oral contraceptive efficacy and metabolic impact. *J Reprod Med* 1987; 32:28-36.

Farabow WS, Fulton JW, Fletcher V Jr: Cervical pregnancy treated with methotrexate. *N C Med J* 1983; 44:91.

Farley TMM, Collins J, Schlesselman JJ: Hormonal contraception and risk of cardiovascular disease: An international perspective. *Contraception* 1998; 57:211-230.

Farquharson D, et al: Management of quintuplet pregnancy by selective embryocide. Program of the 32nd Annual Convention of the American Institute of Ultrasound in Medicine, New Orleans, October 1987.

Fihn SD, et al: Association between diaphragm use and urinary tract infection. *JAMA* 1985; 254:240-245.

Franceschi S, et al: Oral contraceptives and benign breast disease: A case-control study. *Am J Obstet Gynecol* 1984; 149:602-606.

Frates MC, et al: The sonographic diagnosis and conservative treatment of cervical ectopic pregnancies. *Radiology* 1994; 191:773-775.

Freie HMP: Sickle cell diseases and hormonal contraception. *Acta Obstet Gynecol Scand* 1983; 62:211-217.

Frigoletto FD, Pokoly TB: Electrolyte dynamics in hypertonic saline-induced abortions. *Obstet Gynecol* 1971; 38:647-652.

Frydmann R, Taylor S, Ulmann A: Transplacentat passage of mifespristone. *Lancet* 1995; 2:1252.

Fylling P, Fagerhol M: Experience with two different medicated intrauterine devices: A comparative study of the Progestasert and Nova T. *Fertil Steril* 1979; 31:138-141.

Garzo VG, et al: Effects on an antiprogesterone (RU486) on the hepthalamic-hypophyseal-ovarian-endometrial axis during the luteal phase of the menstrual cycle. *J Clin Endocrinol Metab* 1988; 66:508-517.

Gaspard UJ: Metabolic effects of oral contraceptives. *Am J Obstet Gynecol* 1987; 157:1029-1041.

Ginsburg KA, Moghissi KS: Alternate delivery systems for contraceptive progestogens. *Fertil Steril* 1988; 49:16S-30S.

Giovannucci E, et al: A prospective cohort study of vasectomy and prostate cancer in U.S. men. *JAMA* 1993; 269:873-877.

Glasier A: Emergency postcoital contraception. *N Engl J Med* 1997; 337:1058-1064.

Goldacre MJ, Holford TR, Vessey MP: Cardiovascular disease and vasectomy. *N Engl J Med* 1983; 308:805-808.

Goldsmith MF: Pregnancy Dx? Rx may now include condoms. *JAMA* 1981; 261:678-679.

Goldzieher JW: Hormonal contraceptives: Past, present, future. *Horm Contrac* 1984; 75:75-86.

Goldzieher JW, et al: A placebo-controlled double-blind crossover investigation of the side effects attributed to oral contraceptives. *Fertil Steril* 1971; 22:609-623.

Goodlin RC, Kresch AD: Amniotic fluid osmolality following intraamniotic injection of saline. *Am J Obstet Gynecol* 1968; 100:839-842.

Gordon T, Castelli WP, Njortland M: HDL as a protective factor against coronary heart disease—the Framingham Study. *Am J Med* 1977; 62:707-714.

Gore BZ, Caldwell BV, Speroff L: Estrogen-induced human luteolysis. *J Clin Endocrinol Metab* 1973; 36:615.

Gravanis A, et al: Endometrial and pituitary responses to the steroidal antiprogestin RU486 in postmenopausal women. *J Clin Endocrinol Metab* 1985; 60:156-163.

Grimes DA, et al: Midtrimester abortion by dilatation and evacuation: A safe and practical alternative. *N Engl J Med* 1977; 296:1131-1145.

Grimes DA, et al: Local vs. general anesthesia: Which is safer for performing suction curettage abortions? *Am J Obstet Gynecol* 1979; 135:1030-1035.

Grimes DA, et al: Early abortion with a single dose of the antiprogestin RU-486. *Am J Obstet Gynecol* 1988; 158:1307-1312.

Grimes DA, et al: Ovulation and follicular development associated with three low-dose oral contraceptives: A randomized control trial. *Obstet Gynecol* 1994; 83:29.

Grimes DA, Scholz KF: Morbidity and mortality from second-trimester abortions. *J Reprod Med* 1985; 30:505-514.

Gu SJ, et al: A 5-year evaluation of norplant contraceptive implants in China. *Obstet Gynecol* 1994; 83:673-678.

Gupta PK, Woodruff ID: Actinomyces in vaginal smears. *JAMA* 1982; 247:1175-1176.

Halbert DR, Darnell-Jones DE: Medical management of the sexually assaulted woman. *J Reprod Med* 1978; 20:265-274.

Hale RW, Pion RJ: Laminaria: An underutilized clinical adjunct. *Clin Obstet Gynecol* 1972; 15:829-850.

Hankins GD, et al: Maternal arterial desaturation with 15-methyl prostaglandin $F_{2\alpha}$ for uterine atony. *Obstet Gynecol* 1988; 72:367-370.

Harlap S, Shiono PH, Ramcharan S: Congenital abnormalities in the offspring of women who used oral and other contraceptives around the time of conception. *Int J Fertil* 1985; 30:39-47.

Harrison DD, Cooke CW: An elucidation of factors influencing physicians' willingness to perform elective female sterilization. *Obstet Gynecol* 1988; 72:570.

Hasson HM: Open laparoscopy: In Zatuchni GI, Daly MJ, Sciarra JJ, editors: *Gynecology and obstetrics*, Philadelphia, 1982, Harper & Row.

Haukkamaa M: Contraception by Norplant® subdermal capsules is not reliable in epileptic patients on anticonvulsant treatment. *Contraception* 1986; 33:559.

Henry A, Rinehart W, Piotrow P: Reversing female sterilization. *Popul Rep* Ser G 1980; C8:97-123.

Henshaw SK: Unintended pregnancy in the United States. *Fam Plann Perspect* 1998; 30:24-29.

Hicks DJ: Rape: Sexual assault. *Am J Obstet Gynecol* 1980; 137:931-935.

Hild-Petito S, et al: Effects of two progestin-only contraceptives, depo-provera and norplant II, on the vaginal epithelium of rhesus monkeys: *AIDS Res Hum Retroviruses* 1998; 14:S125-S130.

Hirsh MP, Levy HM: The varied ultrasonographic appearance of laminaria. *J Ultrasound Med* 1988; 7:45-47.

Hogue CJR, Cates W Jr, Tietze C: The effects of induced abortion on subsequent reproduction. *Epidemiol Rev* 1981; 4:66-94.

Hong CY, Turner P: Influence of lipid solubility on the sperm immobilizing effect of 3-adrenoceptor blocking drugs. *Br J Clin Pharmacol* 1982; 14:269-272.

Hornstein MD, et al: Ultrasound guidance for selected dilatation and evactation procedures. *J Reprod Med* 1986; 31:947-950.

Hulka BS, Chambless LE, Kaufman DG: Protection against endometrial carcinoma by combination-product oral contraceptives. *JAMA* 1982; 247:475-477.

Ingvardsen A, Eriksen T: Cervical rapture following prostaglandin-induced midtrimester abortion. *Ugeskr Leeger* 1979; 141:3531-3532.

Irwin KL, et al: Oral contraceptives and cervical cancer risk in Costa Rica. *JAMA* 1988; 259:59-64.

Jick H, et al: Venous thromboembolic disease and ABO blood type. *Lancet* 1969; 1:539-542.

Johansson EDB: Inhibition of the corpus luteum function in women taking large doses of diethylstilbestrol. *Contraception* 1973; 8:27-35.

Kafrissen ME, et al: Midtrimester abortion: Intraamniotic instillation of hyperosmolar urea and prostaglandin $F_{2\alpha}$ vs dilation and evacuation. *JAMA* 1984; 251:916-919.

Karim SMM, Sivasamboo R: Termination of second trimester pregnancy with intraamniotic 15(S)-15-methyl prostaglandin $F_{2\alpha}$—a 2-dose schedule study. *Prostaglandins* 1975; 9:487-494.

Kasdorf G, Kalkhoff RK: Prospective studies of insulin sensitivity in normal women receiving oral contraceptive agents. *J Clin Endocrinol Metab* 1988; 66:846-852.

Katz Z, et al: Teratogenicity of progestogens given during the first trimester of pregnancy. *Obstet Gynecol* 1985; 65:775-780.

Kaunitz AM, Rosenfield A: Injectable contraception with depot medroxyprogesterone acetate. *Drugs* 1993; 45:857.

Kay CR: Progestogens and arterial disease—evidence from the Royal College of General Practitioner's Study. *Am J Obstet Gynecol* 1982; 142:762-760.

Kelaghan J, et al: Barrier method contraceptives and pelvic inflammatory disease. *JAMA* 1982; 248:184-187.

Kelly RW, Abel MH: Copper and zinc inhibit the metabolism of prostaglandin by the human uterus. *Biol Reprod* 1983; 28:883-889.

Kesseru E, et al: The hormonal and peripheral effects of D-norgestrel in postcoital contraception. *Contraception* 1974; 10:411-424.

Koch JP: The Prentiff contraceptive cervical cap: A contemporary study of its clinical safety and effectiveness. *Contraception* 1982; 25:135-159.

Kubba AA, et al: The biochemistry of human endometrium after two regimens of postcoital contraception: A DL-norgestrel/ethinylestradiol combination or danazol. *Fertil Steril* 1986; 45:512-516.

Lahteenmaki P, et al: Late postcoital treatment against pregnancy with antiprogesterone RU486. *Fertil Steril* 1988; 50:36-38.

Lammer EJ, Cordero JF: Exogenous sex hormone exposure and the risk of major malformations. *JAMA* 1986; 255:3128-3132.

Lawson JS, et al: Optimum dosage of an oral contraceptive. *Am J Obstet Gynecol* 1979; 134:315-320.

Lee NC, Rubin GL, Borucki R: The intrauterine device and pelvic inflammatory disease revisited: New results from the Women's Health Study. *Obstet Gynecol* 1988; 72:1-6.

Lidegaard O: Oral contraception and risk of a cerebral thromboembolic attack: Results of a case-control study. *BMJ* 1993; 306:956-963.

Lincoln P: The pill, breast, and cervical cancer, and the role of progestogens in arterial disease. *Fam Plann Perspect* 1984; 16:55-63.

Linn S, et al: Lack of association between contraceptive usage and congenital malformation in offspring. *Am J Obstet Gynecol* 1983a; 147:923-918.

Linn S, et al: The relationship between induced abortion and outcome of subsequent pregnancies. *Am J Obstet Gynecol* 1983b; 146:135-140.

Lines A, et al: Case-control study of rheumatoid arthritis and prior use of oral contraceptives. *Lancet* 1983; 1:1299-1300.

Lippes J, Malik T, Tatum HJ: *The postcoital Copper T.* Paper presented at the Thirteenth Annual Meeting of the Association of Planned Parenthood Physicians, Los Angeles, April 17, 1975.

Liskin LS: IUDS: An appropriate contraceptive for many women. *Popul Rep* Ser G 1982; 10(B4):101-135.

Liskin LS: Long-acting progestins—promise and prospects, injectable and implants. *Popul Rep K* 1983a; 11:17-55.

Liskin LS: Vasectomy—safe and simple. *Popul Rep D* 1983b; 11:61-100.

Liskin LS, Blackburn R: Hormonal contraception: New long-acting methods, injectables, and implants. *Popul Rep* Ser G, 1987; 15:K57-K87.

Liskin LS, Rinehart W: Minilaparotomy and laparoscopy: Safe, effective, and widely used. *Popul Rep C* 1985; 8:115-167.

Litvak O, et al: Fetal erythrocytes in maternal circulation after spontaneous abortion. *JAMA* 1970; 214:531-534.

Louik C, et al: Maternal exposure to spermicides in relation to certain birth defects. *N Engl J Med* 1987; 317:474-478.

Louv WC, et al: Oral contraceptive use and the risk of chlamydial and gonococcal infections. *Am J Obstet Gynecol* 1989; 160:396-402.

Mall-Haefeli M, et al: Klinische unit biochemische Resultate bei de Behandlung mit Marvelon-einem neuen steroidalen Ovulationishemmer. *Geburtshilfe Frauenheilkd* 1982; 42:215-222.

Mammen EF: Oral contraceptives and blood coagulation: A critical review. *Am J Obstet Gynecol* 1982; 142:781-790.

Mann JI, Inman WGW: Oral contraceptives and death from myocardial infarction, *BMJ* 1975; 2:245-248.

Margulies M, Perez GC, Veto LS: Misoprostol to induce labour. *Lancet* 1992; 339:64.

Martinelli I, et al: High risk of cerebral-vein thrombosis in carriers of a prothrombin-gene mutation and in users of oral contraceptives. *N Engl J Med* 1998; 338:1793-1797.

Massey FJ, et al: Vasectomy and health: Results from a large cohort study. *JAMA* 1984; 252:1023-1029.

Matlin SA, et al: Male antifertility compounds from *Tripterygium wilfordii. Contraception* 1993; 47:387-400.

Mattson RH, et al: Use of oral contraceptives by women with epilepsy. *JAMA* 1986; 256:238-240.

Marx PA, et al: Progesterone implants enhance SIV vaginal transmission and early virus load. *Nature Med* 1996; 2:1084-1089.

McCann MR, et al: Breast-feeding, fertility, and family planning. *Popul Rep J* 1981; 24:525-575.

Meade TW, Greenberg G, Thompson SG: Progestogens and cardiovascular reactions associated with oral contraceptives and a comparison of the safety of 50 and 30 mcg oestrogen preparations. *BMJ* 1980; 1:1157-1161.

Meirik O: The pill and breast cancer: New information. *Intl Planned Parenthood Fed Med Bull* 1996; 30:1-2.

Meirik O, et al: Oral contraceptive use and breast cancer in young women: A joint national case-control study in Sweden and Norway. *Lancet* 1986; 2:650-653.

Miracle-McMahill HL, Calle EE, Kosinski AS, et al: Tubal ligation and fatal ovarian cancer in a large prospective cohort study. *Am J Epidemiol* 1997; 145:349-357.

Mishell DR Jr: Contraception by intrauterine device. In Bardin CW, editor: *Current therapy endocrinology metabolism,* ed 3, Toronto, 1988a, BC Decker.

Mishell DR Jr: Use of oral contraceptives in women of older reproductive age. *Am J Obstet Gynecol* 1988b; 158:1652-1657.

Mishell DR Jr, et al: The intrauterine device: A bacteriologic study of the endometrial cavity. *Am J Obstet Gynecol* 1966; 96:119-126.

Mishell DR Jr, et al: Estrogenic activity in women receiving an injectable progestogen for contraception. *Am J Obstet Gynecol* 1972; 113:372.

Mishell DR Jr, et al: The effect of contraceptive steroids on hypothalamic pituitary function. *Am J Obstet Gynecol* 1977; 128:60.

Monk JP, Clissold SP: Misoprostol, a preliminary review of its pharmacodynamic and pharmacokinetic properties and therapeutic efficacy in the treatment of peptic ulcer disease. *Drugs* 1987; 33:1-30.

Moore KL: The developing human: Clinically oriented embryology. *The fetal period: The eighth week to birth,* Philadelphia, 1973, WB Saunders, p. 78.

Morris JM, van Wagenen G: Compounds interfering with ovum implantation and development, III: The role of estrogens. *Am J Obstet Gynecol* 1966; 96:804-815.

Morris JM, van Wagenen G: Postcoital oral contraception. In Hankinson RKB, Kleinman RL, Eckstein P, et al, editors: *Proceedings of the Eighth International Conference of the IPPF, Santiago, Chile, April 9-15, 1967* London, 1967, pp. 256-259, International Planned Parenthood Federation.

Morris JM, van Wagenen G: Interception: The use of postovulatory estrogens to prevent implantation. *Am J Obstet Gynecol* 1973; 115:101-106.

Nadelson CC, et al: A follow-up study of rape victims. *Am J Psychiatry* 1982; 139:1266-1270.

Narod SA, et al: Oral contraceptives and the risk of hereditary ovarian cancer. *N Engl J Med* 1998; 339:424-428.

Neil JR, et al: Late complications of sterilization by laparoscopy and tubal ligation: A controlled study. *Lancet* 1975; 2:669-671.

Newton BW: Laminaria tent: Relic of the past or modern medical device? *Am J Obstet Gyecol* 1972; 113:442-448.

Nilsson CG, et al: Intrauterine contraception with levonorgestrel: A comparative randomized clinical performance study. *Lancet* 1981; 1:577-580.

Noonan JT Jr: *Contraception, a history of its treatment by the Catholic theologians and canonists,* Cambridge, Mass., 1986, Harvard University Press.

Orme ML, Back DS, Breckenridge AM: Clinical pharmacokinetics of oral contraceptive steroids. *Clin Pharmacol* 1983; 8:95-136.

Ortiz A, et al: Serum medroxyprogesterone acetate concentrations and ovarian function following intramuscular injection of depot-MPA. *J Clin Endocrinol Metab* 1977; 43:32-38.

Ory HW: Mortality associated with fertility and fertility control. *Fam Plann Perspect* 1983; 15:57-63.

Ory SJ: Nonsurgical treatment of ectopic pregnancy (Editor's Corner). *Fertil Steril* 1986; 46:767-769.

Osathanondh R, et al: Induction of labor with anencephalic fetus. *Obstet Gynecol* 1980; 56:655-657.

Osathanondh R, et al: Coagulopathy associated with midtrimester D&E. *Adv Plann Parent* 1981; 16:30-33.

Osathanondh R, et al: Prostaglandins for cervical softening and dilatation: Recent experience with prostaglandins as dilators. Program of the Ninth Annual Meeting of National Abortion Federation (Advances in Cervical Dilatation), Boston, June 1985.

Osathanondh, R: Combination oral contraceptives. In Bardin CW, editor: *Current therapy in endocrinology and metabolism,* ed. 5. Toronto: BC Decker/Mosby, 1994, p. 252.

Osathanondh V: Suprapubic minilaparotomy, uterine elevation technique: Simple, inexpensive, and outpatient procedure for interval female sterilization. *Contraception* 1974; 10:251-262.

Ostensen M, Husby G: Pregnancy-associated 3α-glycoprotein, oral contraceptives, and rheumatoid arthritis. *Lancet* 1983; 1:1391.

Oyer R, et al: Treatment of cervical pregnancy with methotrexate. *Obstet Gynecol* 1988; 71:469-471.

Park T-K, et al: Preventing febrile complications of suction curettage abortion. *Am J Obstet Gynecol* 1985; 152:252-255.

Patterson SP, White JH, Reaves EM: A maternal death associated with prostaglandin E2. *Obstet Gynecol* 1979; 54:123-124.

Peterson HB, et al: Deaths attributable to tubal sterilization in the United States. *Am J Obstet Gynecol* 1983; 146:131-136.

Peterson HB, Xia Z, Hugh JM, et al: The risk of pregnancy after tubal sterilization: Findings from the U.S. Collaborative Review of Sterilization. *Am J Obstet Gynecol* 1996; 174:1161-1170.

Peterson RN, Freund M: Effects of (H+), (Na+), (K+), and certain membrane-active drugs on glycolysis, motility, and ATP synthesis by human spermatozoa. *Biol Reprod* 1973; 8:350-357.

Petitti DB, et al: Risk of vascular disease in women: Smoking, oral contraceptives, noncontraceptive estrogens, and other factors. *JAMA* 1979; 242:1150-1154.

Petitti DB, Klatsky AL: Malignant hypertension in women aged 15-44 years and its relation to cigarette smoking and oral contraceptives. *Am J Cardiol* 1983; 52:297-298.

Piot P, et al: AIDS: An international perspective. *Science* 1989; 239:573-579.

Pituitary Adenoma Study Group: Pituitary adenomas and oral contraceptives: A multicenter case-control study. *Fertil Steril* 1983; 39:753-760.

Pizarro E, Gomez-Rogers C, Rowe PJ: A comparative study of the effect of the Progestasert and Gravigard IUDs on dysmenorrhea. *Contraception* 1979; 20:455-466.

Porter JB, Jick H: Malignant liver minor associated with oral contraceptive use. *Pharmacotherapy* 1981; 1:160.

Porter JB, et al: Oral contraceptives and nonfatal vascular disease. *Obstet Gynecol* 1985; 66:1-8.

Potts M, Diggory P: *Textbook of contraceptive practice*, ed 2, London, 1983, Cambridge University Press.

Rabe T, et al: Effect of the PGE$_1$ methyl analog misoprostol on the pregnant uterus in the first trimester. *Geburtshilfe Frauenheilkd* 1987; 47:324-331.

Rakers H: Multicenter trial of a monophasic oral contraceptive containing ethinyl estradiol and desogestrel. *Acta Obstet Gynecol Seral* 1988; 67:171-174.

Rakhshani R, Grimes DA: Prostaglandin E$_2$ suppositories as a second-trimester abortifacient. *J Reprod Med* 1988; 33:817-820.

Ramcharan S, et al: The Walnut Creek Contraceptive Drug Study: A prospective study of the side effects of oral contraceptives. *J Reprod Med* 1980; 2(suppl 6):345-372.

Ravenholt RT, Kessell E, Speidel JJ: Comparison of the side effects of three oral contraceptives: A double-blind cross-over study of Ovral, Norinyl, and Norlestrin. A*dv Plann Parent* 1987; 12:222-239.

Rice-Wray E, et al: Return of ovulation after discontinuance of oral contraceptives. *Fertil Steril* 1967; 18:212-218.

Rock J, Pincus G, Garcia CR: Effects of certain 19-norsteroids on the normal human menstrual cycle. *Science* 1956; 124:891-893.

Rojanasakul A, et al: Effects of combined desogestrel-ethinylestradiol treatment on lipid profiles in women with polycystic ovarian disease. *Fertil Steril* 1987; 48:581-585.

Romaguero C, Grimalt F: Contact dematitis from a copper-containing intrauterine contraceptive device. *Contact Dermatitis* 1981; 73:163-164.

Rosenberg L, et al: Epithelial ovarian cancer and combination oral contraceptives. *JAMA* 1982; 247:3210-3212.

Rosenberg MJ, et al: Effect of the contraceptive sponge on chlamydial infection, gonorrhea, and candidiasis. *JAMA* 1987; 257:2308-2312.

Rosenfield AG: Injectable long-acting progestogen contraception a neglected modality. *Am J Obstet Gynecol* 1974; 120:537-548.

Roy S, Mishell DR: Current status of research and development of vaginal contraceptive rings as a fertility control method in the female. *Res Frontiers Fertil Regul* 1983; 2:1-10.

Royal College of General Practitioners' Oral Contraception Study: Further analysis of mortality in oral contraceptive users. *Lancet* 1981; 1:541-546.

Royal College of General Practitioners' Oral Contraception Study: Oral contraceptives and gall bladder disease. *Lancet* 1982; 2:957-959.

Royal College of General Practitioners' Oral Contraception Study: Incidence of arterial disease among oral contraceptive users. *Policy Statement* 1983; 33:75-82.

Rubin GE, et al: Fatal ectopic pregnancy after attempted legally induced abortion. *JAMA* 1980; 244:1705-1708.

Rubin GL, Ory HW, Layde PM: Oral contraceptives and pelvic inflammatory disease. *Am J Obstet Gynecol* 1982; 144:630-635.

Salhanick HA: Basic studies on aminoglutethimide. *Cancer Res* 1982; 42(suppl):3315-3321.

Samsioe G: Comparative effects of the oral contraceptive combinations 0.15 mg desogestrel + 0.030 mg ethinylestradiol and 0.150 mg levonorgestrel + 0.030 mg ethinylestradiol on lipid and lipoprotein metabolism in healthy female volunteers. *Contraception* 1982; 25:487-504.

Sands RX, Burnhill MS, Hakim-Elahi E: Postabortal uterine atony. *Obstet Gynecol* 1974; 43:595-598.

Schaison G: *RU486: Antiprogestin and antiglucocorticoid.* Program of the 70th Annual Meeting of the Endocrine Society (New Concept 1), New Orleans, June 1989.

Schaison G, et al: Effects of the antiprogesterone steroid RU486 during midluteal phase in normal women. *J Clin Endocrin Metab* 1985; 61:484-489.

Schiff I, Naftolin F: Small bowel incarceration after uncomplicated laparoscopy. *Obstet Gynecol* 1974; 43:674-675.

Schutz KF, Grimes DA, Cates W Jr: Measures to prevent cervical injury during suction curettage abortion. *Lancet* 1983; 1:1182-1184.

Scott LD, Katz AR, Duke JH: Oral contraceptives, pregnancy, and focal nodular hyperplasia of the liver. *JAMA* 1984; 251:1461-1463.

Segal SJ, et al: Absence of chorionic gonadotropin in sera of women who use intrauterine devices. *Fertil Steril* 1985; 44:214-218.

Seligsohn U, et al: Factor VII in plasma of women taking oral contraceptives. *Transfusion* 1984; 24:171-172.

Settlage DS, Motoshima M, Tredway DR: Sperm transport from the external cervical os to the fallopian tubes in women: A time and quantitation study. *Fertil Steril* 1973; 24:655-661.

Shapiro AG, et al: Intravaginal administration of 9-deoxo-9-methylene-16,16-dimethyl PGE$_2$ for cervical dilation prior to suction curettage. *Int J Gynaecol Obstet* 1982; 20:137-140.

Shar SR, Kew MC: Oral contraceptives and hepatocellular carcinoma. *Cancer* 1982; 49:407-410.

Sharpe RM, et al: Absence of hCG-like activity in the blood of women fitted with intrauterine contraceptive devices. *J Clin Endocrinol Metab* 1977; 45:496-499.

Shearman RP: Postcoital contraception: A review. *Contraception* 1973; 7:459-476.

Shoupe D, Mishell DR: Norplant: Subdermal implant system for long-term contraception. *Am J Obstet Gynecol* 1989; 160:1286-1292.

Shy KK, et al: Oral contraceptive use and occurrence of pituitary prolactinoma. *JAMA* 1983; 249:2204-2207.

Siegberg R, et al: Sex hormone profiles in oligomenorrheic adolescent girls and the effect of oral contraceptives. *Fertil Steril* 1984; 41:888-993.

Silva DA, et al: Acute hypertensive response to prostaglandin F$_{2\alpha}$ during anesthesia administration. *J Reprod Med* 1987; 32:700-702.

Sivin I: International experience with Norplant and Norplant-2 contraceptives. *Stud Fam Plann* 1988; 19:81.

Sivin I, Tatum HJ: Four years of experience with the TCU 380A intrauterine contraceptive device. *Fertil Steril* 1981; 36:159-163.

Smythe AR II, Underwood PB Jr: Ectopic pregnancy after postcoital diethylstilbestrol. *Am J Obstet Gynecol* 1975; 121:294.

Sonne-Holmes S, et al: Prophylactic antibiotics in first-trimester abortion: A clinical controlled trial. *Am J Obstet Gynecol* 1981; 139:693-696.

Spence MR, et al: Cephalothin prophylaxis for midtrimester abortion. *Obstet Gynecol* 1982; 60:502-505.

Spitz I, et al: Early pregnancy termination with mifepristone and misoprostol in the United States. *N Engl J Med* 1998; 338:1241-1247.

Stadel BV: Oral contraceptives and cardiovascular disease. *N Engl J Med* 1981; 305:612-618, 672-677.

Stampfer MJ, et al: A prospective study of past use of oral contraceptive agents and risk of cardiovascular diseases. *N Engl J Med* 1988; 319:1313-1317.

Stevens RG, Lee JAH, Moolgavkar SH: No association between oral contraceptives and malignant melanomas. *N Engl J Med* 1980; 302:966.

Stockley IH: Methotrexate-NSAID interactions. *Drug Intelligence Clin Pharmacol* 1987; 21:546.

Stubblefield PG, et al: Fertility after induced abortion: A prospective follow-up study. *Obstet Gynecol* 1984; 63:186-193.

Stubblefield PG, Fuller AF, Foster SC: Ultrasound-guided intrauterine removal of intrauterine contraceptive devices in pregnancy. *Obstet Gynecol* 1988; 72:961-964.

Sturgis SH, Albright F: The mechanism of estrin therapy in the relief of dysmenorrhea. *Endocrinology* 1940; 26:68-72.

Swann SH, Petitti DB: A review of problems of bias and confounding in epidemiologic studies of cervical neoplasia and oral contraceptive use. *Am J Epidemiol* 1982; 115:10-18.

Szoka PR, Edgren RA: Drug interactions with oral contraceptives: Compilation and analysis of an adverse experience report database. *Fertil Steril* 1988; 49(suppl):31-38.

Tatum HJ, Connell-Tatum EB: Barrier contraception: A comprehensive overview. *Fertil Steril* 1981; 36:1-12.

Thayssen P, Secher NJ, Arnsbo P: Systolic time intervals and hemodynamic changes during intravenous infusion of prostaglandins F$_{2\alpha}$ and E$_2$, *Br Heart J* 1981; 45:447-456.

Thiersch JB: Therapeutic abortions with a folic acid antagonist 4-aminopteroylglutamic acid administered by the oral route. *Am J Obstet Gynecol* 1952; 63:1298-1304.

Tietze C, Lewit S: Life risks associated with reversible methods of fertility regulation. *Int J Gynaecol Obstet* 1979; 16:456-459.

Toppozada M: The clinical use of monthly injectable contraceptive preparations. *Obstet Gynecol Surv* 1977; 32:335-347.

Toth M, et al: The role of infection in the etiology of preterm birth. *Obstet Gynecol* 1988; 71:723-726.

Umapathysivam K, Jones WR: Effects of contraceptive agents on the biochemical and protein composition of human endometrium. *Contraception* 1980; 22:425-440.

Umpierre SA, Hill JA, Anderson DJ: Effect of "Coke" on sperm motility. *N Engl J Med* 1985; 13:1351.

Ungchusak K, et al: Determinants of HIV infection among female commercial sex workers in northeastern Thailand: Results from a longitudinal study. *J AIDS Hum Retroviruses* 1996; 12:500-507.

Valenzuela G, et al: Uterine rupture at term with vaginal prostaglandin E$_2$. *Am J Obstet Gynecol* 1980; 139:1223-1224.

Valicenti JF, et al: Detection and prevalence of IUD-associated actinomyces colonization and related morbidity. *JAMA* 1982; 247:1149-1152.

Vandenbroucke JP: Oral contraceptives and rheumatoid arthritis. *Lancet* 1983; 2:228-229.

Vandenbroucke JP, et al: Oral contraceptives and rheumatoid arthritis: Further evidence for a preventive effect. *Lancet* 1983; 2:839-842.

Vandenbrouke JP, et al: Noncontraceptive hormones and rheumatoid arthritis in perimenopausal and postmenopausal women. *JAMA* 1986; 255:1299-1303.

Vandenbroucke JP, et al: Increased risk of venous thrombosis in oral-contraceptive users who are carriers of factor V Leiden mutation. *Lancet* 1994; 344:1453-1457.

van der Spuy ZM, et al: Inhibition of 3β-hydroxy-steroid dehydrogenase activity in first trimester human pregnancy with trilostane and WIN 32729. *Clin Endocrinol* 1983; 19:521-531.

Vergote I, et al: Uterine rupture due to 15-methylprostaglandin $F_{2\alpha}$. *Lancet* 1982; 2:1402.

Vessey M, Lawless M, Yeates D: Efficacy of different contraceptive methods. *Lancet* 1982; 1:841-843.

Vessey M, et al: Neoplasia of the cervix uteri and contraception: a possible adverse effect of the pill. *Lancet* 1983; 2:930-934.

Vessey ME, McPherson K, Johnson B: Mortality among women participating in the Oxford Family Planning Association Contraceptive Study. *Lancet* 1977; 2:731-733.

Vessey MP: Exogenous hormones in the aetiology of cancer in women. *J R Soc Med* 1984; 77:542-549.

Vessey MP, Lawless M: The Oxford Family Planning Association Contraceptive Study. *Clin Obstet Gynecol* 1984; 11:743-757.

von Kaulla E, et al: Antithrombin III depression and thrombin generation acceleration in women taking oral contraceptives. *Am J Obstet Gynecol* 1971; 109:868-873.

Warburton D, et al: Lack of association between spermicide use and trisomy. *N Engl J Med* 1987; 317:478-482.

Washington AE, et al: Oral contraceptives, *Chlamydia trachomatis* infection, and pelvic inflammatory disease. *JAMA* 1985; 233:2246-2150.

Washington AE, Browner WS, Korenbrof CC: Cost effectiveness of combined treatment for endocervical gonorrhea. *JAMA* 1987; 257:2056-2060.

Wessler S, et al: Estrogen-containing oral contraceptive agents: a basis for their thrombogenicity. *JAMA* 1976; 236:2179-2182.

White PE, et al: Disseminated intravascular coagulation following midtrimester abortions. *Anesthesiology* 1983; 58:99-101.

Wilcox AJ, et al: Urinary human chorionic gonadotropin among intrauterine device users: Detection with a highly specific and sensitive assay. *Fertil Steril* 1987; 47:265-269.

World Health Organization: Collaborative study of neoplasia and steroid contraceptive, invasive cervical cancer and combined oral contraceptives. *BMJ* 1985; 290:961-965.

World Health Organization: Mechanism of action, safety, and efficacy of intrauterine devices. *World Health Organ Tech Rep Ser* 1987a; 753:791.

World Health Organization: Special programme of research, development, and research taining in human reproduction and special programme on AIDS: Report of a meeting on contraceptive methods and HIV infections, Geneva, 1987b.

World Health Organization: Collaborative study of neoplasia and steroid contraceptives—breast cancer and depot medroxyprogesterone acetate: A multinational study. *Lancet* 1991a; 338:833.

World Health Organization: Collaborative study of neoplasia and steroid contraceptives: Depot medroxyprogesterone acetate (DMPA) and risk of endometrial cancer. *Int J Cancer* 1991b; 49:186.

World Health Organization: Task Force on Long-Acting Systemic Agents for Fertility Regulation: Special programme of research, development and research training in human reproduction: A multicentre comparative study of serum lipids and apolipoproteins in long-term users of DMPA and a control group of IUD users. *Contraception* 1993; 47:177.

Wu D-F, et al: Pharmacokinetics of ($\pm$)-, (+)-, and (-)- gossypol in humans and dogs. *Clin Pharmacol Ther* 1986; 39:613-618.

Wu YT: Suction in artificial abortion: 300 cases (Chinese). *Chung-Hua Fa Chan Ko Tsa Chih* 1958; 6:447-449.

Ye BL, Yamamoto K, Tyson JE: Functional and biochemical aspects of laminaria use in first-trimester pregnancy temination. *Am J Obstet Gynecol* 1982; 142:36-39.

Young RL, et al: A randomized double-blind placebo-controlled comparison of the impact of low-dose and triphasic oral contraceptives on follicular development. *Am J Obstet Gynecol* 1992; 167:678.

Yuzpe AA, Smith RP, Rademaker A W: A multicenter clinical investigation employing ethinyl estradiol combined with dl-norgestrel as a postcoital contraceptive agent. *Fertil Steril* 1982; 37:508-513.

Zipper J, et al: Propranolol as a novel, effective spermicide: Preliminary findings. *BMJ* 1983; 287:1245-1246.

Zipper JA, et al: Metallic copper as an intrauterine contraceptive adjunct to the "T" device. *Am J Obstet Gynecol* 1969; 105:1274-1278.

14

The Infertile Couple

MITCHELL S. REIN
ROBERT L. BARBIERI

KEY ISSUES

1. The initial approach to infertility should be limited to an evaluation of male, tubal, and ovulatory factors.
2. Fecundability, the probability of conceiving during a monthly cycle, is an important concept when discussing various treatment options.
3. The staircase approach to infertility treatment attempts to balance efficacy with risk, invasiveness, and cost.
4. Success rates with infertility treatment are dependent on the clinical characteristics of the couple, including the age of the woman and the cause of infertility.
5. Treating ovulatory disorders with a wide range of ovulation-induction agents results in an extremely favorable prognosis.
6. Tubal factor infertility is treated with surgical reconstruction or assisted reproduction.
7. Superovulation plus intrauterine insemination appears to be an efficacious therapy for unexplained infertility.
8. Assisted reproduction is indicated if infertility has not responded to simpler treatment options.
9. Intracytoplasmic sperm injection (ICSI) is a major advance in the treatment of male factor infertility.

Fertility is defined as the ability to produce offspring, and it requires the capacity to initiate and sustain a pregnancy. Infertility is defined as 1 year of frequent and unprotected coitus without conception, suggesting a diminished capacity to conceive and reproduce. In contrast to sterility, infertility is not an irreversible state. The term *primary infertility* is ap-

plied to the couple who has never achieved a pregnancy; *secondary infertility* implies that at least one previous conception has taken place.

This chapter reviews the evaluation and treatment of the infertile couple. An efficient and systematic evaluation is presented, and current knowledge of the predictive value of various traditional diagnostic tests is critically evaluated. A simplified approach to treatment options includes a review of the available randomized clinical trials. Clinical algorithms are based on a sequential approach to problems and diseases that cause or are associated with infertility.

Several factors contribute to patient satisfaction with infertility evaluation (Halman et al, 1993). The technical skill of the infertility specialist and the emotional support from the physician and staff are the most commonly cited. Other important factors include allowing women more control over their evaluation and treatment, explaining procedures, involving men more significantly, and discussing adoption as an alternative. Interestingly, according to Halman et al (1993), treatment cost and length of time a couple had been trying to conceive were not related to patient satisfaction.

The importance of a timely, cost-effective, and logical approach to infertility treatment cannot be overstated. Recently, there has been a conscientious effort to simplify the basic infertility evaluation. A thorough evaluation has four important goals:

To identify the cause(s) of the infertility
To provide a basis for potentially successful treatment options
To provide a realistic prognosis
To offer emotional support

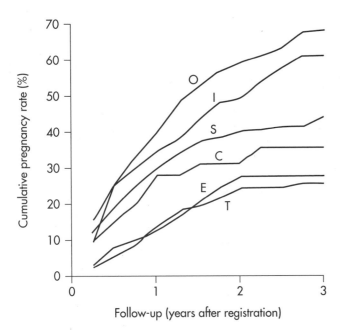

Fig. 14-1. Cumulative pregnancy rates and primary clinical diagnoses among infertile couples. O, ovulatory disorders; I, unexplained; S, male factor; C, cervical factor; E, endometriosis; T, tubal factor. (From Collins JA: A proportional hazards analysis of the clinical characteristics of infertile couples. *Am J Obstet Gynecol* 1984; 148:527.)

EPIDEMIOLOGY AND FECUNDABILITY

Fecundability is defined as the probability of conceiving during a monthly cycle, and it and provides the basis for estimating fertility over time. A related concept, fecundity, is the ability to achieve a pregnancy in one menstrual cycle that results in a live birth. Fecundability is a valuable concept because it creates a framework for the quantitative analysis of fertility potential. In addition, fecundability provides a convenient quantitative estimate of the efficiency of various fertility treatments and should assist patients and providers in choosing an optimal treatment plan.

The statistical model of Cramer et al (1979) encompasses a life-table method to express the cumulative probability of conception as a function of monthly fecundability. The authors estimated the fecundability of "normal" couples using no contraception to be 20% per cycle. Based on this estimate, 50% of couples with normal fecundability should conceive after 3 months, 75% should conceive after 6 months, and 95% should conceive after 13 months. However, several studies suggest that the observed fecundability of a population diminishes over time (Guttmacher, 1956; Zinaman et al, 1996; Wilcox et al, 1988). These studies suggest that larger populations consist of a heterogeneous mixture of couples with varying rates of fecundability. Couples with lower fecundability are less likely to conceive after 1 year than couples with normal fecundability, and they represent the cohort of couples who may seek infertility evaluation and treatment.

The National Survey of Family Growth estimates that 10% to 15% of couples may be classified as infertile (Mosher, 1988; Mosher, 1982; Mosher, 1985). Comparing 1982 and 1988 data, Mosher and Pratt (1990) reported that the annual number of women using infertility services increased by 25% but that the rate of impaired fecundability was unchanged. These authors suggested that the increase in the number of women seeking infertility services reflected delayed childbearing and the entry of baby boom cohorts to the reproductive age range of 25 to 44 years (Mosher and Pratt, 1991). In the last estimate, this represented approximately 5 million couples.

Unfortunately, a low percentage of couples with impaired fecundity seek medical assistance. Wilcox and Mosher (1993) reported that only 43% of all women with infertility obtained some form of infertility service and only 24% obtained specialized infertility treatment. Those most likely to have obtained specialized services were 30 years or older, nulliparous, married, white, and of higher socioeconomic status. Socioeconomic factors are also predictive of successful pregnancy outcomes (Collins et al, 1993).

Presumptive causes have been identified for some categories of infertility. Iatrogenic factors (cervical conization and cautery), sexually transmitted diseases, and smoking have been associated with the cervical factor (Phipps, 1987). Pelvic inflammatory disease (PID) has been strongly associated with the tubal factor (Westrom, 1983). The increasing incidence of ectopic pregnancy and infertility is largely attributed to the increasing incidence of PID. Other contributors to the tubal factor include endometriosis, diethylstilbestrol (DES) exposure, previous tubal surgery, appendicitis, intrauterine device (IUD) use, and smoking. Risk factors for endometriosis include menstrual irregularities, dysmenorrhea, and a family history of endometriosis (Cramer, 1986). Exercising and smoking appear to protect against the development of endometriosis. Factors associated with ovulatory dysfunction include smoking, exercise, body habitus, and genetics. Hereditary factors associated with premature ovarian failure include X chromosome deletions and errors of galactose metabolism. Multiple factors have been associated with male factor infertility; these will be discussed under the evaluation of the male factor.

The prognosis for the infertile couple appears to be strongly affected by the clinical characteristics of the couple, including the age of the woman and the cause of infertility (Collins, 1984). Cumulative probabilities of conception based on primary clinical diagnoses are shown in Fig. 14-1. Infertility caused by an ovulatory disorder carries the best prognosis. The relatively poor prognoses observed with tubal and male factor infertility have improved significantly as a result of in vitro fertilization. Duration of infertility is a predictor of subsequent pregnancies (Collins, 1984; Weir and Cicchinelli, 1964). Couples who have been infertile for less than 3 years are more likely to conceive. Prior pregnancy with the same partner may be the most powerful predictor of a subsequent pregnancy (Dor, 1977).

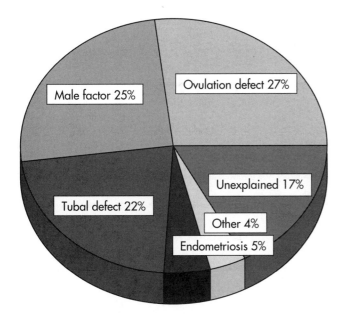

Fig. 14-2. Primary clinical diagnoses in infertile couples. (From Collins JA: Unexplained infertility; in Keyewe N, Chang RJ, Rebar RW, Soules MR: *Infertility: Evaluation and treatment.* Philadelphia, 1995, WB Saunders, p 250. Reprinted with permission.)

CAUSES OF INFERTILITY

It is important to categorize the nature of the fertility problem based on the underlying pathophysiological source in the man or the woman, or both. However, it is often difficult to distinguish disease conditions that cause underlying infertility from disease conditions associated with infertility. This is a major limitation of the current scientific literature, which includes descriptive observations and assumptions regarding which diseases *cause* or are *associated* with infertility. It is often preferable to state that there is an *association* between the disease condition and the infertile state and that *causality* has not been definitively established.

Realizing these limitations, the three major categories influencing fecundability are male factors, ovarian factors, and tubal factors. Other diseases or categories that may cause or be associated with difficulty conceiving include endometriosis, uterine factors, cervical factors, and immunologic factors. Finally, an idiopathic or unexplained category has also been recognized and widely accepted by the medical community. It has been estimated that 25% to 35% of all infertility problems are of multiple origin.

In a review of 21 published reports containing more than 14,000 infertile couples, Collins (1995) reported that the primary diagnoses among infertile couples were ovulatory factors (27%), male factors (25%), tubal factors (22%), endometriosis (5%), other (4%), and unexplained (17%; Fig. 14-2). Initial infertility evaluation focuses on these major categories.

Data from several sources also suggest that maternal age affects fecundability. The pathophysiology of female repro-

Table 14-1 Influence of Age on Cumulative Pregnancy Rate	
Age Group (Years)	**Conceiving in 12 Months (%)**
20-24	86
25-29	78
30-34	63
35-39	52

From Hendershot GE, Mosher WD, Pratt WF: Infertility and age: An unresolved issue. *Fam Plann Perspect* 1982; 14:287.

ductive aging clearly includes a well-established decline of oocyte quality with age. In contrast, the effect of aging on uterine receptivity remains less clear (Meldrum, 1993). A multicenter French study evaluated cumulative fertility rates in 2193 nulliparous women with azoospermic husbands who underwent artificial donor insemination (Schwartz and Mayhux, 1982). Cumulative fertility after 12 cycles of insemination declined after age 30. Cumulative probability of pregnancy after 12 cycles of insemination was 73% for women younger than 25 years, 74.1% for women 26 to 30 years of age, 61.5% for women 31 to 35 years of age, and 53.6% for women older than 35 years. Data extrapolated from the National Survey of Family Growth similarly suggest a decline in fecundity with increasing maternal age (Table 14-1; Hendershot, 1982). A substantial decline in fertility after age 30 has also been observed among Hutterite women (Tietze, 1957). Fecundity appears to be maximal in women at approximately the age of 25, and the incidence of infertility gradually increases after the age of 30.

THE INITIAL VISIT

A detailed interview is the critical first step in infertility evaluation. A major goal during the initial visit is to educate couples about reproductive physiology and the disease conditions that may contribute to infertility and to provide details of the subsequent infertility evaluation. This enables the couple to prepare adequately for what is often an emotionally and physically demanding evaluation. During the first visit both partners should be present and should be interviewed together. The male partner should always be encouraged to attend on the premise that infertility is a syndrome of multiple origin. An adequate investigation requires asking about all possible etiologies in both the man and the woman. In addition to obtaining complete medical, surgical, and gynecologic histories, the physician should elicit information regarding the psychological, emotional, and sexual behavior of each partner. This should include questions regarding sexual habits, frequency of intercourse, sexual dysfunction, and stability of the relationship. Certain couples may benefit from specific instructions regarding the timing and frequency of intercourse. Coital frequency of two to three times per week without the use of lubricants or douches is

---

BOX 14-1
IMPORTANT HISTORIC POINTS IN MALE FACTOR INFERTILITY

1. Duration of infertility
2. Fertility in other relationships
3. Medical and surgical history (childhood illnesses, venereal diseases, trauma)
4. Medications
5. Alcohol, cigarette, marijuana use
6. Occupational exposure (excessive heat, chemical, radiation)
7. Sexual dysfunction
8. Tight-fitting underwear, hot baths, saunas
9. Previous test and therapy for infertility

BOX 14-2
IMPORTANT HISTORIC POINTS IN THE FEMALE

1. Duration of infertility
2. Detailed menstrual history
3. Prior pregnancies
4. Fertility in other relationships
5. Prior contraceptive use (over-the-counter medication, intrauterine device)
6. Frequency of intercourse, sexual dysfunction
7. Gynecologic history (pelvic inflammatory disease, endometriosis, fibroids, cervical dysplasia)
8. Diethylstilbestrol exposure
9. Medical and surgical history
10. Medications
11. Previous tests and therapy for infertility

BOX 14-3
THE INFERTILITY EVALUATION: WHEN TO REFER OR INITIATE?*

<35 years of age: Begin evaluation after 12 months
35-40 years of age: Offer evaluation after 6 months
>40 years of age: Consider immediate evaluation

*Pertinent risk factors should prompt earlier evaluation.

BOX 14-4
INITIAL APPROACH TO THE INFERTILE COUPLE

Male factor
    Semen analysis
Tubal factor
    Document tubal patency
    Hysterosalpingogram
Ovarian factor
    Document ovulation
    Basal body temperature
    Midluteal progesterone
    Evaluate ovarian reserve if female partner >35 years old
    Day 3 FSH
    Clomiphene challenge test
Hormonal evaluation is not routine. Recommended tests are based on:
    Absent menses—FSH, prolactin, TSH, *progestin challenge
    Irregular menses—FSH, prolactin, TSH
    Galactorrhea—prolactin, TSH

FSH, follicle-stimulating hormone; TSH, thyroid-stimulating hormone.
*Oral medroxyprogesterone acetate 10 mg for 5 to 7 days.

---

usually adequate. The disruption of spontaneous sexuality should be discouraged. Coitus every 36 to 48 hours 3 to 4 days before and after the calculated day of ovulation is optimal. Wilcox et al (1995) reported that nearly all pregnancies are attributed to intercourse during a 6-day period ending on the day of ovulation.

The important historical points in the evaluation of both partners are outlined in Boxes 14-1 and 14-2. During the physical examination of the woman, particular attention should be given to height, weight, hair distribution, and presence of galactorrhea; the pelvic examination should be thorough. Examination of the male partner by a urologist is often recommended if there is a persistent abnormality in the semen analysis.

An explanation of the major categories of infertility provides an ideal introduction to the nature of the subsequent evaluation. The schedule for the planned investigation should be flexible. Most of the investigation, however, should be completed within 2 to 3 months. The sequence in which specific infertility tests should be offered depends on

the causative factors suggested by the history and physical examination. When to refer or to initiate infertility evaluation and treatment should be based on the woman's age and pertinent history. Guidelines for when to initiate an infertility evaluation are listed in Box 14-3. As a general rule, couples who have not conceived after 1 year of unprotected intercourse are reasonable candidates for infertility evaluation. Earlier investigation may be recommended based on the woman's age and pertinent risk factors such as irregular or absent periods, history of PID, endometriosis, IUD use, DES exposure, and previous ectopic pregnancy. In addition, patients planning chemotherapy should be offered an emergency evaluation.

The initial infertility evaluation should focus on the identification or exclusion of the major causes previously discussed. A modern cost-effective approach to infertility evaluation is presented in Box 14-4. Specific diagnostic tests will be discussed in the context of the disease conditions that cause or are associated with infertility.

THE OVARIAN FACTOR

Ovulatory disorders include anovulation, oligo-ovulation, and luteal phase defects. Regular menstrual cycles occurring at intervals of 25 to 35 days, particularly when associated with mittelschmerz, suggest ovulation. In contrast, ovulatory disorders are often associated with irregular menstrual cycles, oligomenorrhea, or amenorrhea. A history of obesity, excessive weight loss, galactorrhea, hirsutism, or acne is often associated with ovulatory disorders. Major clinical entities associated with anovulation and infertility are polycystic ovarian disease (PCOD), premature ovarian failure (POF), diminished ovarian reserve, hyperprolactinemia, and hypothalamic amenorrhea. Certain disorders of the adrenal and thyroid glands may be associated with ovulatory dysfunction. Luteal phase defects appear to be relatively uncommon causes of infertility. A comprehensive discussion of PCOD is presented in Chapter 15. After a discussion of the other major clinical diagnoses, the techniques for documenting ovulation and an adequate luteal phase will be presented. Treatment of a wide range of ovulatory disorders includes a practical approach to ovulation induction with many fertility medications and a balanced discussion of the potential risks and benefits.

Premature Ovarian Failure

Premature ovarian failure is defined as a failure of ovarian estrogen production in women younger than 35 who have hypergonadotropism. It may be the result of a reduced number of primordial follicles or an increased rate of atresia. The etiology of POF appears to be multifactorial. Most cases are idiopathic. Significant evidence suggests that specific genetic defects may cause POF (Krauss et al, 1987). Infectious and iatrogenic destruction of primordial follicles may occur as a result of mumps oophoritis, irradiation, or chemotherapy. Documentation of antiovarian antibodies and the association of POF with other immunologic endocrine disorders support the hypothesis that POF may be an autoimmune disease. An increased incidence of POF has also been associated with abnormal galactose metabolism (Kaufman et al, 1979).

The clinical presentation of POF is variable. Patients at varying ages may have symptoms of amenorrhea, infertility, or both. Symptoms suggestive of menopause, including hot flashes, vaginal dryness, sleep disturbances, and mood disturbances may be present. Ovarian failure may be temporary, and there may be a spontaneous return of menstrual function. Associated autoimmune disorders include Addison disease, thyroiditis, hypoparathyroidism, diabetes, pernicious anemia, myasthenia gravis, and vitiligo. Because of the associated polyendocrine autoimmune syndromes, patients should be screened for diabetes, anemia, thyroid, adrenal, and parathyroid insufficiency.

Table 14-2   Incidence of Abnormal CCCT

Age (Years)	Percentage
<30	3
30-34	7
35-39	10
>40	26

Diagnosis is confirmed by elevated gonadotropin levels, particularly FSH levels greater than 40 mIU/mL. All patients younger than 30 with POF should undergo chromosomal analysis to identify patients with Y chromosomes who are at risk for gonadal malignancy. The likelihood of achieving a successful pregnancy in the absence of in vitro fertilization (IVF) with donor eggs is poor.

Diminished Ovarian Reserve

Recently, a subgroup of patients with unexplained infertility has been described as having incipient ovarian failure or diminished ovarian reserve (Toner et al, 1991). These patients have elevated FSH levels on day 3 that are greater than 15 to 20 mIU/mL. They often have normal ovulation and menstrual cycles, but they respond poorly to human menopausal gonadotropins. As do patients with POF, these patients have an extremely poor chance for future fertility in the absence of IVF with donor oocytes.

In a recent review of the literature, Scott and Hoffman (1995) demonstrated the prognostic value of ovarian reserve testing. Day 3 FSH levels have become important predictors of successful pregnancy with infertility treatment, particularly assisted reproduction. Ovarian reserve testing also predicts the ovarian response to gonadotropin stimulation (Scott et al, 1989). Toner et al (1991) reported a 0% ongoing pregnancy rate for patients who undergo IVF and have a day 3 FSH level greater than 25 mIU/mL. Although false-positive test results are rare, day 3 FSH levels are limited by relatively poor negative predictive values (that is, false-negative results are common).

Several studies have demonstrated that the measurement of FSH levels before and after a course of clomiphene citrate is more sensitive than the day 3 FSH level alone (Scott et al, 1993; Sharara, 1994). The clomiphene citrate challenge test (CCCT) involves measuring FSH levels on cycle days 3 and 10. Clomiphene citrate is administered in a dosage of 100 mg daily from cycle day 5 to cycle day 9. An elevated FSH level on *either* cycle day 3 or 10 is associated with diminished ovarian reserve. The improved sensitivity of the CCCT is supported by the observation that 70% of patients with abnormal CCCT findings have normal day 3 FSH levels. It is not surprising that there is an association between advancing age of the woman and diminished ovarian reserve. Abnormal CCCT incidence increases with age among infertile couples (Table 14-2). However, it is important to note that the adverse influence of a woman's age on fecundability appears to be independent of ovarian reserve testing and should still be considered when counseling patients with normal day 3 FSH levels or CCCT findings. Ovarian reserve should be assessed in all couples with unexplained infertility and in women older 35 years, and it should be routine before assisted reproduction.

Hyperprolactinemia

The association between ovulatory dysfunction and hyperprolactinemia is well documented (Jacobs, 1976). Its primary mechanism appears to be the inhibition of pulsatile GnRH secretion that results in a hypoestrogenic state (Monroe et al, 1981). Elevated prolactin levels may cause the direct inhibition of steroidogenesis at the level of the ovary (McNatty et al, 1973). Numerous clinical conditions may cause elevated prolactin levels, among them pituitary tumors, certain medications, chest wall trauma, chronic renal insufficiency, hypothyroidism, empty sella syndrome, pituitary stalk transection, and occasionally nonpituitary tumors. Medications that commonly cause hyperprolactinemia include phenothiazines, tricyclic antidepressants, serotonergic agents, estrogens, oral contraceptive agents, butyrophenones, metoclopramide, reserpine, amphetamines, and methyldopa. Transient elevated levels of prolactin have been associated with beer and protein ingestion, *Herpes zoster*, nipple stimulation, stress, sexual intercourse, and hypoglycemia. Although associated galactorrhea is common, not all women with hyperprolactinemia have this symptom. Pituitary adenomas tend to be associated with high levels of prolactin, but they may be associated with any degree of hyperprolactinemia. Evaluation of the hypothalamus and pituitary with magnetic resonance imaging should be considered for all patients with persistent hyperprolactinemia.

Hypothalamic Amenorrhea

Hypothalamic amenorrhea is a diagnosis of exclusion. Despite multiple causative factors, the primary mechanism appears to be an alteration in GnRH secretion that results in decreased gonadotropin secretion, failure in the stimulation of follicular development, and diminution in gonadal steroidogenesis. Therefore, any process resulting in a disturbance of GnRH production may lead to hypothalamic amenorrhea. In contrast to polycystic ovarian syndrome (PCOS), hypothalamic amenorrhea is associated with a hypoestrogenic state. It must be distinguished from other forms of hypoestrogenic amenorrhea such as hyperprolactinemia, POF, and Asherman syndrome (see the section on uterine factors). Normal or low gonadotropin levels and the absence of progestin-induced bleeding confirm the diagnosis. Causes of hypothalamic amenorrhea include exercise, weight loss, and stress. Rare causes include anorexia nervosa, Kallmann syndrome, and nonfunctional hypothalamic pituitary tumors. In a large percentage of patients, there may be no obvious underlying cause. The most common clinical problem associated with hypothalamic amenorrhea is infertility. In contrast

to POF, symptoms of estrogen deficiency are relatively rare and the prognosis is favorable.

Luteal Phase Defect

Luteal phase defect (LPD) refers to a relative deficiency in the secretion of progesterone by the corpus luteum. Progesterone is important for the implantation of the embryo and the maintenance of early pregnancy. Any progesterone deficiency may occur in the amount or duration (or both) of secretion. *Short luteal phase* refers to a shortening of the interval between ovulation and the onset of menses to 10 days or less, and it may be associated with a normal peak value of progesterone. *Inadequate luteal phase* refers to a luteal phase of normal length with lower than normal progesterone secretion. Determining LPD as an abnormal condition is difficult, largely because of the lack of uniform diagnostic criteria in epidemiologic reports. In addition, there are limited data to address the incidence of LPD in the "normal" population. Davis et al (1989) reported that the incidence of LPD in normal fertile women was 6.6 %. Because the majority of reports estimate the incidence of LPD as a cause for infertility to be between 3% and 20% (Jones, 1976; Jones and Pourmand, 1962; Wentz, 1980), LPD may not represent a clinically significant cause of infertility. However, the frequency of LPD appears to be much higher in certain patients. For example, patients with recurrent miscarriage appear to have an incidence as high as 35% (Phung et al, 1979), and LPD appears to be more common in patients with hyperprolactinemia. It also appears to be more common at the extremes of reproductive life and with conditions such as strenuous exercise, significant weight loss, and hyperandrogenism. The patient who requires ovulation induction may have residual LPD; this appears to be particularly common among women treated with clomiphene citrate (Garcia et al, 1977).

The endometrial biopsy appears to be the most practical standard for diagnosing LPD. Not only does it identify inadequate progesterone production by the corpus luteum, it also identifies abnormal endometrial responsiveness. The usefulness of the endometrial biopsy is highlighted by Daly et al (1983), who demonstrate that the biopsy is predictive of the therapeutic outcome. As previously mentioned, the optimal criteria for diagnosing LPD remain controversial. The most widely accepted criterion is endometrial dating, which lags behind cycle time by more than 2 days when derived retrospectively in two separate cycles. Traditionally the biopsy is performed 2 to 3 days before the expected menses. If the biopsy is performed before the 25th day of the cycle, there is an increased rate of false-negative results. Accurately timing the endometrial biopsy for patients who have slightly irregular menstrual cycles is often difficult. Studies have focused on improving the timing and interpretation of the endometrial biopsy by determining the theoretical cycle day prospectively rather than retrospectively. Shoupe et al (1989) correlated endometrial maturation in fertile women with four methods for estimating the day of ovulation. An endometrial biopsy was performed in 13 women with normal cycles 8 to 11 days after the predicted day of ovulation. Determining the day of ovulation with ultrasonography, serum luteinizing hormone (LH) measurements, and basal body temperature (BBT) correlated well with the endometrial histology. In contrast, when the day of ovulation was determined retrospectively to be 14 days before the onset of the subsequent menses, the endometrial histology was in error more than 2 days in 35% of the specimens. The authors concluded that an accurate interpretation of the endometrial biopsy should be based on days since ovulation rather than days since onset of menses. Li et al (1987) similarly demonstrated improved accuracy for dating the endometrial biopsy based on serum LH determinations when compared with subsequent menses.

A sensitive serum pregnancy test should be offered to the patient to prevent the interruption of an early pregnancy. Pelvic examination should precede the biopsy so that the position and size of the uterus can be determined. The cervix is exposed with a speculum and cleansed with an antiseptic reagent. Premedication with a nonsteroidal anti-inflammatory agent and a paracervical block using 1% or 2% chloroprocaine may minimize patient discomfort. After a tenaculum is attached to the anterior cervix and a Pipelle curette is placed high in the anterior uterine fundus, the specimen is obtained by using a firm stroke extending from the fundus to the cervix. Biopsy tissue is immediately fixed in Bouin's solution.

Interpretation of the endometrial biopsy is based on the dating criteria set by Noyes et al (1950). The accuracy of the endometrial biopsy as a diagnostic test is highly dependent on the experience of the pathologist interpreting the histologic specimen. However, there appears to be significant intraobserver variability (Scott et al, 1993). Dated secretory endometrium secretions should be compared with the prospectively or retrospectively derived cycle day. The first day of bleeding is arbitrarily considered cycle day 28. A single normal endometrial biopsy is often termed *in phase* and is usually considered sufficient to exclude the diagnosis of LPD. An abnormal biopsy specimen is generally required in two separate cycles to make the diagnosis of LPD because an isolated out-of-phase biopsy is not uncommon in normally fertile women (Davis et al, 1989).

A midluteal serum progesterone level of greater than 10 ng/mL has been associated with adequate luteal function (Hall et al, 1982). Although a single midluteal progesterone determination offers a practical and cost-effective approach to the evaluation of LPD, there are limited data to support these recommendations. In fact, several investigators have demonstrated significant overlap between single serum progesterone levels obtained from patients with LPD and normal controls. The difficulty encountered in the interpretation of a single midluteal serum progesterone level may result from the pulsatile nature of progesterone secretion (Filcori et al, 1984; Soules et al, 1988). The BBT chart is notoriously inaccurate for detecting LPD. However, evidence of a luteal phase of less than 10 days on BBT charts does appear to correlate with the presence of a short luteal phase (Downs and Gibson, 1983). The importance of LPD as a significant cause of infertility remains to be proven. Therefore, the endometrial biopsy should not be recommended as a routine part of the infertility evaluation.

Thyroid Disease

Hyperthyroidism and hypothyroidism may be associated with menstrual irregularities and ovulatory dysfunction. The underlying mechanism appears to be related to alterations in the metabolism of androgens and estrogens. Thyroid disease may also be associated with abnormalities in gonadotropin secretion. Although many studies suggest a clear association between clinical hypothyroidism and ovulatory disorders, those demonstrating an association between hyperthyroidism and ovulatory disorders are lacking. Hypothyroidism and hyperthyroidism appear to be associated with decreased libido, and this may be another mechanism of thyroid-related infertility.

Despite its popularity, the efficacy of thyroid hormone therapy for euthyroid women remains unsubstantiated. Several well-controlled clinical studies have demonstrated no benefit from the use of thyroid-stimulating hormone (TSH) in euthyroid infertile women (Buxton and Herrman, 1954; Yen et al, 1970). The role of thyroid hormone therapy for patients with subclinical hypothyroidism (*i.e.*, elevated TSH level and normal thyroxine and triiodothyronine levels) remains unclear and warrants further investigation. In comparison, patients with clinical hypothyroidism may benefit from thyroid hormone replacement with a resumption of normal ovulatory function. For patients with panhypopituitarism, it is imperative that adrenal insufficiency be corrected before thyroid hormone replacement is initiated because the result may be fatal adrenal insufficiency.

Adrenal Disease

Certain disorders of the adrenal gland may be associated with ovulatory abnormalities. Autoimmune adrenal insufficiency (Addison disease) may be associated with POF as part of the syndromes of polyglandular failure (Neufeld et al, 1981). Cushing syndrome, characterized by an overproduction of glucocorticoids, may mimic PCOS by producing obesity, hirsutism, menstrual irregularities, and enlarged polycystic ovaries. Cushing syndrome may result from an overproduction of adrenocorticotrophic hormone (ACTH) or from the autonomous production of glucocorticoids. Clinical manifestations of Cushing syndrome are listed in Table 14-3, but the mechanisms by which it leads to ovulatory dysfunction are unclear. As in PCOS, there appears to be an increase in the peripheral production of estrogen that results in inappropriate acyclic feedback. In addition, there appears to be an abnormality in the pulsatile secretion of GnRH (Yen et al, 1970). Cushing syndrome may be distinguished from PCOS by a dexamethasone suppression test or by 24-hour urine collection for free cortisol. Dexamethasone

Table 14-3 Clinical Manifestations of Cushing Syndrome	
Symptom	%
Obesity	95
Moon facies	95
Hypertension	85
Glucose intolerance	80
Menstrual irregularities	75
Androgen excess	72
Striae	67
Proximal muscle weakness	65
Easy bruisability	55
Osteoporosis	55
Depression	50

(1 mg) is given at bedtime, and a fasting cortisol level is measured the next morning. If the plasma cortisol level is less than 5 μg/dL, the diagnosis of Cushing syndrome is excluded. Though an abnormal value greater than 5 μg/dL is not diagnostic, it does warrant further evaluation.

Adult-onset congenital adrenal hyperplasia (CAH) may also mimic PCOS; CAH was reviewed by White et al in 1987. Relative deficiencies of 21-hydroxylase and 11-hydroxylase may be associated with hirsutism, menstrual irregularities, and ovulatory dysfunction. As a result of these enzymatic defects, the normal biosynthetic pathways are interrupted and an accumulation of adrenal androgens develops. Because CAH appears to entail a strong genetic predisposition, a family history of hirsutism, menstrual disorders, and infertility may be suggestive of CAH. A fasting, morning 17-hydroxyprogesterone level is often obtained in the follicular phase as a screening test. If the concentration of 17-hydroxyprogesterone is greater than 2 ng/mL, the diagnosis of late-onset CAH should be pursued with an ACTH or cosyntropin (Cortrosyn) stimulation test (Azziz and Zacur, 1989; New et al, 1983).

TECHNIQUES FOR PREDICTING AND DETECTING OVULATION

Besides pregnancy, recovering an ovum from the female genital tract is the only direct evidence of ovulation. This is obviously impractical in clinical practice. Therefore, a variety of diagnostic tests that indirectly predict and detect ovulation are commonly used. Diagnostic tests commonly used to confirm ovulation include the BBT chart and midluteal serum progesterone levels. Diagnostic tests that predict the time of ovulation include the BBT chart, the serial assessment of plasma or urinary LH levels and ultrasonography.

Basal Body Temperature Chart

The BBT chart not only is able to provide indirect evidence of ovulation, it may aid in the timing of intercourse and in-

semination. Readings are taken each morning and are recorded on a chart, with day 1 corresponding to the first day of menses (Fig. 14-3). Basal body temperature thermometers show a range of only a few degrees and are easier to read. Readings are most accurate when they are taken immediately on awakening before any activity. During the follicular phase, the temperature is usually 97° F to 98° F. During the luteal phase, the temperature is generally greater than 98° F. The mechanism for temperature elevation appears to be related to the thermogenic properties of progesterone on the central nervous system. It is often difficult to pinpoint the exact day of ovulation. A significant rise in temperature is not noted until 2 days after the LH peak, and it coincides with a rise in the serum progesterone level to greater than 4 ng/mL (Moghissi et al, 1972). Ovulation probably occurs the day before the first temperature elevation, and it may be marked by a dip in the temperature to the lowest level of the cycle. This is supported by the observation that the most likely time for conception, based on a single artificial insemination, is the day before the temperature rise (Newill and Katz, 1982). The absence of a biphasic temperature pattern is suggestive but not diagnostic of anovulation. In approximately 75% of monophasic cycles, hormonal evidence of ovulation has been documented (Bauman, 1981; Moghissi, 1976a). A slow rise in a biphasic chart is not necessarily an indication of an ovulatory disorder. However, a temperature elevation of less than 10 days' duration is suggestive of a short luteal phase. In summary, the BBT chart is helpful when it is clearly biphasic. When the chart is monophasic or difficult to interpret, another diagnostic method should be used.

Midluteal Serum Progesterone

One midluteal serum progesterone level greater than 2 to 3 ng/mL is indirect evidence of ovulation. Although extremely accurate for confirming ovulation, one midluteal serum progesterone level is less reliable for evaluating the adequacy of the luteal phase.

Endometrial Biopsy

The finding of secretory endometrium on an endometrial biopsy is additional indirect evidence of ovulation. Although relatively safe and rarely uncomfortable, the endometrial biopsy should not be performed routinely for confirmation of ovulation because accurate, less invasive tests are available. The finding of a proliferative endometrium may suggest anovulation.

Ultrasound Monitoring

Serial ultrasound examinations can demonstrate the growth of a follicle. The disappearance of a dominant follicle, combined with the presence of free fluid in the cul-de-sac, suggests follicular rupture and is presumptive evidence of ovulation. Ultrasonography may be helpful in assessing corpus luteum formation. Because of the wide range of the preovulatory follicle's diameter (17 mm to 26 mm), ultrasonogra-

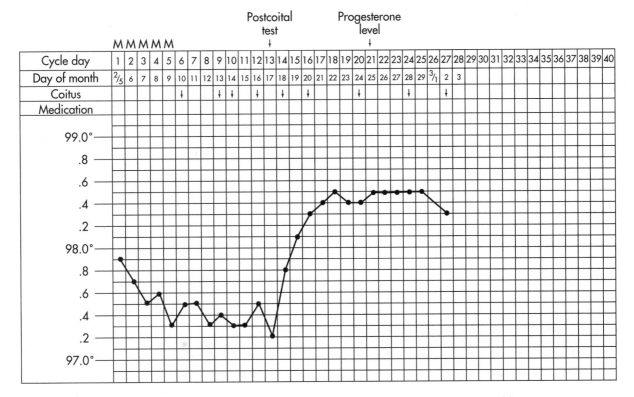

Fig. 14-3. This example of a basal body temperature chart indicates a biphasic pattern with notations for the days of menstruation (M) and the timing of coitus (*arrows*).

phy appears to be a less accurate predictor of ovulation, and it is rarely used as a primary diagnostic aid for confirming ovulation.

Ultrasound examination may be useful in the diagnosis of the luteinized unruptured follicle syndrome (LUFS), which is characterized by a normal pattern of gonadotropin secretion, regular menses, and no evidence of follicular rupture (Mareck and Hulka, 1978). The absence of follicular rupture is associated with entrapment of the oocyte and subsequent luteinization. The LUFS has been associated with unexplained infertility, endometriosis, and pelvic adhesions. Ultrasound criteria include the persistence of an echo-free dominant follicle beyond 36 hours after the LH peak (Ritchie, 1985). The absence of stigmata of ovulation at laparoscopy has also been suggestive of LUFS. There is no general agreement regarding the incidence of LUFS among the fertile or infertile patient population. A causal relationship between LUFS and infertility remains to be established because LUFS does not appear to be a recurrent problem. Routine ultrasound evaluation of infertile couples for LUFS is not recommended (Katz, 1988). Primarily, ultrasound monitoring appears to be useful for timing human chorionic gonadotropin (hCG) administration during ovulation induction protocols.

Luteinizing Hormone Monitoring

The measurement of daily preovulatory serum LH levels appears to be the optimal criterion for predicting ovulation.

Hoff et al (1983) found ovulation to occur approximately 34 to 36 hours after the onset of the LH surge. A twofold rise above the baseline serum LH level is suggestive of the onset of the LH surge. The accuracy of monitoring the serum LH level must be weighed against the relative inconvenience and significant cost of a daily blood test. Fortunately, simple urinary LH ovulation detection kits are readily available. In comparison with serum LH and BBT charts for timing intercourse and inseminations, the accuracy and reliability of these kits are good (Elkind-Hirsch et al, 1986; Vermesh et al, 1987).

TREATMENT OF OVULATORY DYSFUNCTION

Treatment of ovulatory disorders leads to extremely favorable prognoses. Rates of success with a wide range of ovulation induction agents are similar to fecundability rates observed among normal fertile couples. Treatment approach is strongly dependent on the underlying cause of the ovulatory dysfunction. The most common treatment options are clomiphene citrate, gonadotropin therapy, bromocriptine, and pulsatile GnRH.

Measuring serum FSH, TSH, and prolactin levels may help identify a specific cause of the ovulatory dysfunction. A progestin challenge test provides additional information regarding the presence or absence of ovarian estrogen production and should be recommended (after negative

PART III   The Reproductive Life Cycle

**CONTRAINDICATIONS TO
CLOMIPHENE CITRATE**

Moderate to large ovarian cysts
Pregnancy
Organic intracranial lesions
Pituitary macroadenomas
Liver disease
Uncontrolled thyroid or adrenal dysfunction
Visual disturbances
Undiagnosed abnormal uterine bleeding

---

pregnancy test results) to all women with amenorrhea. This simple evaluation (Box 14-4) should help guide treatment options. Most patients requiring ovulation induction can be broadly classified into one of four major clinical categories: those with polycystic ovary disease, those with hyperprolactinemia, those with hypothalamic amenorrhea, and those with premature ovarian failure or diminished ovarian reserve. The World Health Organization (WHO, 1976) published a simpler classification system that helps guide treatment options by dividing women with anovulation into two major groups (group 1 and group 2). This system is based on a combination of endogenous gonadotropin and estrogen secretion.

Clomiphene Citrate

Clomiphene citrate (CC) is a synthetic nonsteroidal estrogen agonist-antagonist, initially reported to be effective in the induction of ovulation (Greenblatt et al, 1961). It is produced as a mixture of *trans* (enclomiphene) and the more potent *cis* (zuclomiphene) isomers in a ratio of approximately 3 to 2. Clomiphene is metabolized by the liver and excreted in the feces, and it has a half-life of approximately 5 days. Its mechanism of action is complex; there are multiple target sites and variable degrees of estrogen agonist and antagonist activities at each. Clomiphene citrate has biologic effects on the hypothalamus, pituitary gland, ovary, endometrium, and cervix (Adashi, 1984). The preponderance of laboratory and clinical evidence suggests that the primary mechanism and site of action is an antiestrogenic effect at the level of the hypothalamus that results in an increase in GnRH pulse frequency and stimulates increased FSH and LH secretion. The clinical importance of the hypothalamic site of action is supported by the observation that the successful induction of ovulation with clomiphene citrate requires an intact hypothalamic-pituitary axis. This is in contrast to gonadotropin therapy, which is often successful if a patient lacks a functional hypothalamus or pituitary gland.

Successful ovulation induction with clomiphene citrate is strongly dependent on appropriate patient selection. Clomiphene citrate is most effective and should be considered the initial treatment of choice for women with anovula-

tion or oligo-ovulation associated with normal endogenous estrogen production and normal levels of FSH (WHO group 2). Clinically, this represents the large and heterogeneous group of women with polycystic ovary disease. Clomiphene is rarely effective and should not be recommended to women with hypothalamic anovulation (WHO group 1). These patients are excellent candidates for gonadotropin therapy or pulsatile GnRH. Patients with premature ovarian failure or diminished ovarian reserve are not only poor candidates for clomiphene citrate but for other ovulation induction agents as well. Patients with ovarian failure and diminished ovarian reserve are optimally treated with in vitro fertilization and donor eggs. Contraindications to clomiphene therapy are listed in Box 14-5. Although clomiphene citrate is relatively contraindicated in women with pituitary macroadenomas, it effectively induces ovulation in women with microprolactinomas or idiopathic hyperprolactinemia who do not ovulate after bromocriptine therapy (Turksoy et al, 1982). In the United States, clomiphene citrate is available as a 50-mg tablet. The initial recommended dosage is 50 mg once daily for 5 days, and it is usually initiated on the fifth day of a spontaneous or a progestin-induced menstrual period. In this regimen, the last day of treatment is cycle day 9. Several studies suggest that clomiphene citrate therapy can be initiated on cycle days 3, 4, or 5 with no significant impact on pregnancy outcome (Wu and Winkel, 1989). In properly selected patients, approximately 50% will ovulate after the initial 50-mg dosage. In the absence of documented ovulation, the clomiphene citrate dosage should be increased to 100 mg daily for 5 days. An additional 25% of patients will ovulate if the dosage of clomiphene citrate is increased to 100 mg daily for 5 days (Gysler et al, 1982). The maximum Food and Drug Administration (FDA)-approved dosage for clomiphene citrate is 100 mg daily for 5 days; as noted, approximately 75% of patients ovulate on these regimens.

Despite the FDA recommendations, experience with higher dosages of clomiphene is extensive. Gysler et al reported that 26% of patients who eventually ovulated required a daily dosage of 150 mg or more. Our standard approach to ovulation induction with clomiphene is listed in Box 14-6 and is generally limited to a maximum dosage of 150 mg daily. Once the minimal effective dose to induce ovulation has been determined, there is no advantage to increasing the dosage in subsequent cycles, even in the absence of pregnancy. Treatment with clomiphene citrate should be continued for three to six ovulatory cycles. Approximately 90% of clomiphene-induced pregnancies occur within four to six ovulatory cycles.

Detection of ovulation should be sought during each cycle. In most patients, ovulation takes place approximately 5 to 12 days after the last treatment dose. Different strategies may optimize the timing of intercourse or intrauterine inseminations. These include frequent intercourse after cycle day 10, BBT charting, measurement of urinary or serum LH, or serial ultrasound monitoring. Determining the midluteal serum progesterone level is often recommended during the initial cycle(s) to document the minimal ovulatory dose.

Various adjuvant treatment strategies should be considered when standard doses of clomiphene citrate are unable to induce ovulation. Extending the duration of therapy to 14 days may induce ovulation in a subgroup of patients unresponsive to the standard 5-day course (Drake et al, 1978; Adams et al, 1972). Combining clomiphene citrate with a single dose of hCG (5000 to 10,000 mIU) may trigger ovulation in some women who do not ovulate with standard doses (Swyer et al, 1975; O'Herlihy et al, 1982). Although rarely necessary, this approach includes the initiation of ultrasound monitoring at approximately cycle day 12 and the intramuscular injection of hCG if the mean follicular diameter exceeds 20 mm. This strategy also facilitates the timing of intercourse or inseminations.

Combining clomiphene citrate with glucocorticoids appears to increase the rate of successful ovulation and pregnancy in a subgroup of women with elevated levels of the adrenal androgen dehydroepiandrosterone sulfate (Lobo et al, 1982; Daly et al, 1984). The addition of dexamethasone 0.5 mg daily should be considered for patients with dehydroepiandrosterone sulfate levels greater than 2 μg/mL who do not ovulate after standard clomiphene citrate regimens.

Several studies have suggested a possible benefit of combining thyroid hormone replacement with clomiphene citrate for women with triiodothyronine levels below 80 ng/mL (Maruo et al, 1992). Combining clomiphene citrate with gonadotropin therapy reduces the quantity of gonadotropins needed to induce ovulation and may benefit a subgroup of patients who respond poorly to clomiphene citrate or gonadotropin therapy alone (Jarrel et al, 1981). Finally, the addition of bromocriptine to standard clomiphene citrate regimens for anovulatory women with normal prolactin levels is not supported by the current literature.

Another subgroup of patients treated with clomiphene citrate does not conceive despite the successful induction of ovulation. Besides possible coexisting infertility factors, such as male and tubal factor infertility, there are two major explanations for these failures to conceive. Antiestrogenic properties of clomiphene citrate have been associated with the inadequate stimulation of the endometrium (Garcia et al, 1977) and the inhibition of normal periovulatory cervical mucus (Von Campenhout al, 1968). Adverse effects on the endometrium have been characterized as a type of LPD. Some clinicians recommend performing an endometrial biopsy to rule out LPD and conducting a postcoital test to assess the possibility of a cervical infertility factor with clomiphene citrate therapy. Progesterone supplementation has been recommended after the diagnosis of clomiphene citrate–induced LPD, but it has not been shown to improve pregnancy outcome. Similarly, midcycle estrogen supplementation for inadequate hostile cervical mucus has not been shown to improve pregnancy outcome. The addition of intrauterine inseminations (IUI) should effectively bypass any issues related to hostile cervical mucus and will be discussed in the section on cervical factor and immunologic infertility.

BOX 14-6
STANDARD APPROACH TO OVULATION INDUCTION WITH CLOMIPHENE CITRATE

1. If necessary, induce menses with 10 mg medroxyprogesterone acetate for 5 days after negative pregnancy test results.
2. Initiate 50-mg of clomiphene citrate on days 5 to 9.
3. Initiate urine luteinizing hormone testing on cycle day 10 to time intercourse or inseminations.
4. Measure serum progesterone level on cycle day 21 to document ovulatory dose.
5. In the absence of ovulation, increase daily dose of clomiphene citrate by 50 mg to a maximum daily dose of 150 mg.
6. In the presence of ovulation, continue the ovulatory dose for 3 to 6 cycles.

Among properly selected patients, the probability of pregnancy is partially dependent on the presence of other infertility factors. The treatment-dependent fecundability of infertile couples with anovulation has been estimated to be between 0.20 and 0.25 (Hammond et al, 1983). There is a decline in monthly fecundability after 3 to 6 months of treatment. Failure to achieve pregnancy after six cycles of clomiphene citrate should prompt a review of the other potential causes of infertility and a consideration of alternative treatment options such as gonadotropin therapy. A specific advantage of clomiphene citrate therapy is the modest cost of approximately $100 per cycle, which is considerably less than all other fertility treatments.

The risks of clomiphene citrate therapy are small, and associated side effects are uncommon. Although some studies suggest an increased rate of spontaneous abortion after clomiphene citrate–induced pregnancy, most clinical studies suggest a 15% to 25% rate of spontaneous abortion. This is similar to the rates reported for all infertile couples (Adashi et al, 1979; Ahlgren et al, 1976; Jansen, 1982). The incidence of congenital birth defects in neonates conceived after clomiphene citrate treatment is 2.4%, which is no different than the incidence observed among the normal fertile population (2.7%) (Adashi et al, 1979; Ahlgren et al, 1976). The most common side effects associated with clomiphene citrate are hot flashes (20%), ovarian enlargement (15%), lower abdominal discomfort (5%), nausea (3%), general malaise (2%), and headache (1%). The rare but worrisome side effect of blurred vision or scotomata should prompt immediate discontinuation of clomiphene citrate therapy.

Major risks of clomiphene citrate therapy include ovarian hyperstimulation syndrome (OHSS) and multiple gestation. Both risks occur in approximately 5% to 10% of patients. Massive ovarian enlargement and other signs of moderate to severe OHSS are rarely associated with clomiphene citrate therapy. Evaluation and treatment of OHSS will be discussed in the section on gonadotropin therapy. The increased risk for multiple conception is largely limited to twin gestations. Merrell Dow Pharmaceuticals (1972) reported on the multiple conception rate from 2369 clomiphene-induced pregnancies with 7% twins, 0.5% triplets, 0.3% quadruplets, and 0.13% quintuplets.

Gonadotropin Therapy

In 1958, Gemzell extracted human FSH from pooled pituitary glands. Several years later, Lunenfeld (1960) reported the extraction of LH and FSH from menopausal urine to induce ovulation. The first pregnancies to result from exogenous gonadotropin therapy were reported by Gemzell (1960). During the next 35 years, human menopausal gonadotropin (hMG) extracted from postmenopausal urine became the standard for exogenous gonadotropin ovarian stimulation. Since the early 1990s, the pharmaceutical industry has committed significant research dollars toward the development of highly purified preparations of LH and FSH. Until recently, the urinary-derived gonadotropin therapies have been administered by intramuscular injections. However, the development of highly purified FSH preparations has led to the extremely rapid and popular transition to the subcutaneous administration of exogenous gonadotropin therapy. The recent introduction of FSH preparations derived from recombinant DNA technology provides better batch-to-batch consistency, steady supply amid increasing demand, and, most important, subcutaneous route of administration.

The most common indications for gonadotropin therapy include patients with hypothalamic amenorrhea (WHO group 1); patients with PCOD who do not conceive after clomiphene citrate therapy; patients with unexplained infertility or early-stage endometriosis; and patients undergoing assisted reproduction. Gonadotropin therapy is rarely successful and should not be encouraged in women with primary ovarian failure or diminished ovarian reserve.

FSH alone is clearly efficacious as a single agent in most patients who require gonadotropin therapy (Howles et al, 1994). Exogenous LH therapy is not required to stimulate optimal follicular growth or estradiol production because most anovulatory patients secrete adequate amounts of LH. There are case reports of inadequate stimulation of estradiol production with the highly purified FSH preparations in the rare patients with extremely low to undetectable levels of endogenous LH (Schoot, 1992). FSH preparations are theoretically well suited and often recommended to patients with PCOD who require gonadotropin therapy based on elevated levels of endogenous LH. The intramuscular injection of hCG is routinely required to complete the final maturation of the oocyte and to trigger ovulation. In this role, hCG mimics the activity of the LH surge and is preferred to exogenous LH as a result of its longer half-life.

In the United States, the commercially available gonadotropin medications include human menopausal gonadotropins (Pergonal, Humegon, Repronex) and FSH (Metrodin, Fertinex, Follistim, and Gonal-F). Pergonal, Humegon, and Repronex are hMGs derived from postmenopausal urine. These agents contain equal ratios of LH and FSH, with approximately 75 IU of FSH and 75 IU of LH per ampule. They must be administered by intramuscular injection. Metrodin was the first available preparation of purified FSH. Metrodin is derived from Pergonal, and it uses immunochromatography to absorb the less desirable LH. Although Metrodin contains 75 IU of FSH and less than 1 IU of LH per ampule, it still requires intramuscular administration. Fertinex is the second generation of purified FSH and is also derived from immunoaffinity chromatography. Fertinex is highly purified; it has less than 0.1 mIU/mL of LH activity for every 1000 IU of FSH activity. Fertinex was the first FSH preparation approved for subcutaneous administration.

Follistim and Gonal-F are the most recently available FSH products and are produced with recombinant DNA technology. Recombinant FSH preparations not only benefit from subcutaneous administration, they appear to be slightly more potent than urine-derived hMG and FSH (Out et al, 1996a). Recombinant LH preparations have been available for clinical trials since 1993, but they are not yet commercially available in the United States. The future of exogenous gonadotropin therapy will likely include an individual approach with varying combinations of recombinant LH and FSH. In addition, recombinant technology should enable the production of unique chimeric gonadotropin preparations with the potential for desirable properties such as oral or extended activity.

Gonadotropin therapies have been evaluated in numerous clinical studies (Howles et al, 1994; Daya et al, 1995; Out et al, 1996b; Larsen, 1990; McFaul, 1990; Sagle, 1991). Most studies demonstrate no significant differences in the major clinical outcomes. No randomized clinical trials demonstrate the superiority of purified preparations of FSH in comparison with hMG. However, in a metaanalysis of randomized clinical trials, Daya (1995) reported that the use of FSH rather than hMG in IVF treatment cycles was associated with a significantly higher clinical pregnancy rate. Although several studies suggest some differences in ovarian responsiveness, most studies have not been able to demonstrate clinically significant differences in pregnancy outcome, multiple conception, or risk for ovarian hyperstimulation. However, in a randomized clinical trial comparing recombinant and urinary FSH ($n = 1000$ cycles), Out et al (1995) reported a significantly higher ongoing pregnancy rate per cycle during IVF with recombinant FSH when subsequent cyroembryo transfer cycles were included in the analysis (25.6% versus 20.4%). In summary, the different gonadotropin therapies have favorable results with respect to efficacy and safety. Physician preference, cost, and route of administration often determine the choice of therapy.

As previously stated, patients with PCOD who require ovulation induction with gonadotropin therapy may benefit from low-dose, long-term FSH therapy. Homberg et al (1995) randomized 50 infertile women with PCOD who did not conceive after clomiphene therapy. They were given either conventional FSH treatment (75 IU daily, increased by 75 IU every 5 or 6 days until follicle maturation) or low-dose FSH treatment (75 IU daily for 14 days, increased by 37.5 IU every 7 days until follicle maturation). Pregnancy rates were higher in women who received low-dose, long-term FSH treatment than in women who received standard FSH treatment (40% versus 24%). Monofollicular development occurred more often in the group that received low-dose, long-term FSH than in those who received standard FSH treatment (74% versus 27%). There were also fewer incidences of high-order multiple gestation and ovarian hyperstimulation in the group that received low dosages of FSH. These results suggest that low-dose, long-term FSH may be the treatment of choice for women with PCOD who require ovulation induction and gonadotropin therapy.

The ovarian stimulation protocol is often determined after the underlying diagnosis is made and gonadotropin therapy is indicated. The initial dose should be individualized and should be based in part on the age and weight of the patient. Detailed patient education is required before the initiation of therapy; it includes information regarding injection techniques, serum estradiol administration, ultrasound monitoring, and potential risks inherent with treatment. Follicular development is determined by a combination of serum estradiol production and ultrasound measurement of follicular dimensions and growth. Estradiol and ultrasound monitoring should be available 7 days a week to minimize the risk for multiple gestation and ovarian hyperstimulation.

A comprehensive discussion of the management of gonadotropin stimulation is beyond the scope of this chapter. Therapy is usually started 2 to 3 days after the onset of a spontaneous or a progestin-induced menstrual flow. The usual starting dose for basic ovulation induction is one to two ampules of FSH or hMG and three to four ampules for protocols combined with assisted reproduction. This initial dosage is continued until cycle day 7, when serum estradiol is measured. If the estradiol level suggests an inadequate or low response, the dose of FSH or hMG can be increased on an individual basis. If the estradiol level on day 7 suggests a high response, the dose is often decreased. If the estradiol level rises appropriately, the initial dose is continued. Sequential serum estradiol and ultrasound measurements are performed until the maximum diameter of the two largest follicles are in the range of 18 to 22 mm and serum estradiol levels are between 500 to 2000 pg/mL. Once appropriate follicular development has been achieved, 5000 to 10,000 IU of hCG is administered to trigger ovulation. Ovulation is expected to occur approximately 36 hours after this final injection. The recommended timing of intercourse or inseminations is 24 to 48 hours after the injection of hCG. If estradiol levels are greater than 2000 pg/mL or if more than four follicles are larger than 18 mm, the administration of hCG may not be recommended and the cycle may be can-

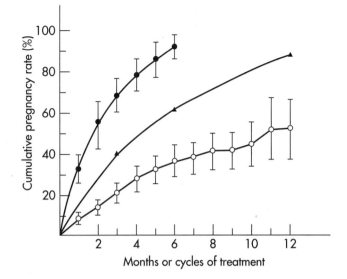

Fig. 14-4. Cumulative pregnancy rates for infertile and ovulatory women treated with gonadotropins for ovulation induction. Solid circles represent the cumulative pregnancy rate in women in WHO group 1. Open circles represent the cumulative pregnancy rate in women in WHO group 2 in whom induction of ovulation with clomiphene failed. For comparison, the triangles represent the cumulative pregnancy rate in normal women. (From Dor J, Itzkowitc DJ, Mashiach S: Cumulative pregnancy rates following gonadotropin therapy. *Am J Obstet Gynecol* 1980; 136:102-105. Reprinted with permission.)

celed because of the increased risk for high-order multiple gestation and ovarian hyperstimulation.

Success rates for ovulation and pregnancy after gonadotropin treatment are extremely high. Lunenfeld and Eshkol (1982) reported a 6-month cumulative probability of pregnancy of 91% in WHO group 1 women with hypothalamic amenorrhea. The average number of cycles required to achieve pregnancy is three. WHO group 1 patients with hypothalamic amenorrhea can expect an extremely high rate of ovulation and monthly fecundability that ranges between 10% and 40%. In contrast, WHO group 2 women with PCOD-related anovulation have lower fecundability rates after gonadotropin treatment (Fig. 14-4). Observed fecundability also depends on the age of the patient. The rate of spontaneous abortion is similar to that in the normal population, and there is no increased risk for congenital anomalies.

Major risks of gonadotropin therapy include multiple conception and ovarian hyperstimulation. The multiple conception rate is approximately 20%, with 15% twins and 5% high-order multiple conception (Dor, 1980).

Mild to moderate ovarian enlargement occurs in approximately 20% of women treated with gonadotropin therapy. OHSS refers to the development of increased vascular permeability, or leaky capillaries, in patients with enlarged ovaries. Symptoms of OHSS typically develop 5 to 7 days after the administration of hCG. They include abdominal pain, abdominal distention, nausea, vomiting, diarrhea, and dyspnea. Physical and laboratory findings may include

Table 14-4   Classification System for Ovarian Hyperstimulation Syndrome

Severity	Stage	Symptoms and Signs
Mild	A	Estradiol >2000 pg/mL
	B	Estradiol >2000 pg/mL plus enlargement of ovaries up to 6 cm in diameter
Moderate	A	Estradiol >4000 pg/mL plus enlargement of ovaries 6 to 12 cm
	B	Ascites by ultrasonography plus findings in stage A.
Severe	A	Estradiol >6000 pg/mL plus enlargement of ovaries >12 cm in diameter Ascites, liver function abnormalities
	B	Tension ascites, ARDS, shock, renal failure, thromboembolism

weight gain, ovarian enlargement, intravascular volume depletion, ascites, pleural effusions, hemoconcentration, electrolyte imbalances, renal dysfunction, and thrombosis (Schenker, 1978). An OHSS classification system is presented in Table 14-4.

Despite several decades of scientific investigation, the pathophysiology of OHSS remains poorly understood (Golan, 1989). Careful monitoring with serum estradiol and vaginal ultrasonography appears to decrease the incidence of OHSS because there is some correlation with peak estradiol levels and the number of intermediate-size follicles. Unfortunately, the predictive value of serum estradiol and the number of intermediate-size follicles are limited. Therefore, a high index of suspicion for the development of OHSS is recommended for all patients undergoing gonadotropin therapy.

The initial evaluation of OHSS includes an assessment of weight gain, serum electrolytes and hematocrit, and maximum ovarian dimensions by ultrasonography. Signs and symptoms of OHSS typically resolve within 1 to 2 weeks. In a woman with a successful pregnancy, OHSS may be more severe and have a longer course. There is no specific treatment to decrease the severity or shorten the course of OHSS. Several interesting strategies have been reported, including the prolonged administration of GnRH agonists (Forman, 1990). Supportive measures are often recommended to prevent serious complications, such as renal insufficiency and thromboembolic phenomena. Simple interventions include bed rest, pain medication, and maintenance of intravascular volume. Although patients with OHSS rarely require hospital admittance, those with severe hemoconcentration levels (hematocrit >45%), massive ascites, or renal insufficiency

or electrolyte imbalances should be considered candidates for more intensive inpatient observation. They should receive prophylaxis against thrombosis, and they often require intravenous fluid or colloid expanders to maintain intravascular volume. Paracentesis and pleuracentesis are generally limited to symptomatic relief but sometimes result in more rapid resolution of the disease. Although patients with OHSS appear to be at increased risk for ovarian torsion, surgical exploration generally should be avoided (Borenstein, 1959).

Bromocriptine

Bromocriptine (Parlodel) is the initial treatment for women with hyperprolactinemia and anovulation, oligo-ovulation, or luteal phase insufficiency. Bromocriptine is highly effective and rapidly restores ovulatory menstrual cycles in 90% of women with hyperprolactinemia. Women with hyperprolactinemia who already have ovulatory cycles are unlikely to benefit from bromocriptine therapy and often require an alternative approach to infertility treatment. Similarly, several studies have demonstrated no benefit from bromocriptine therapy for women with normoprolactinemic levels and anovulatory or ovulatory menstrual cycles (Harrison et al, 1979; Wright et al, 1979).

Bromocriptine is an oral dopamine agonist that directly inhibits pituitary prolactin production and secretion. Often the dosage range required to restore ovulation is 2.5 mg to 7.5 mg daily. Pills are available as 2.5-mg tablets and can be easily divided in half. The initial recommended dosage is 1.25 mg (half a tablet) at bedtime for 3 nights; this should be increased gradually because of the associated side effects, particularly orthostatic hypotension. Serum prolactin level should be redetermined after 3 to 4 weeks of treatment. The clinician should determine the minimum dose required to normalize serum prolactin levels. Most patients initially require the standard dosage of 2.5 mg twice a day. However, some patients can be maintained on dosages as low as 1.25 mg at bedtime. Although bromocriptine therapy usually restores ovulatory cycles after approximately 2 months, with or without the normalization of serum prolactin levels, alternative ovulation induction agents such as clomiphene citrate or gonadotropin therapy should be added if it does not. Alternative treatment options should also be considered after 4 to 6 months of ovulatory cycles without conception.

Bromocriptine therapy is often poorly tolerated despite careful efforts to titrate the dosage. Common side effects include lightheadedness, nausea, diarrhea, vomiting, fatigue, malaise, headache, runny nose, and watery eyes. There are several potential options to consider when associated side effects require the discontinuation of bromocriptine therapy. Vaginal administration of bromocriptine has been associated with fewer side effects in some but not all studies (Kletzky and Vermesh, 1989). The dopamine agonist Pergolide (Permax), approved for the treatment of Parkinson disease, has been shown to inhibit pituitary prolactin secretion and to restore ovulatory cycles in women with hyperprolactinemia (Kletsky et al, 1986). Unfortunately, Pergolide has side effects that are similar to those of bromocriptine. Cabergoline (Dostinex) is a relatively new agent recently approved for the treatment of hyperprolactinemia. Although it is centrally acting, Cabergoline is not a dopamine agonist, it only requires administration twice a week, and it appears to be associated with decreased gastrointestinal side effects (Webster et al, 1994).

Pregnancy rates of 80% have been reported in women with hyperprolactinemia, galactorrhea, and anovulation who were treated with bromocriptine. In the United States, bromocriptine administration is generally discontinued once pregnancy is confirmed. Bromocriptine does cross the placenta, and it has been shown to suppress fetal prolactin production. However, large retrospective studies in Europe on the continuation of bromocriptine during pregnancy show it to be safe. No increased risks for miscarriage, adverse obstetric outcomes, or congenital anomalies were reported (Krupp and Monka, 1987). The continuation of bromocriptine therapy during pregnancy should be strongly considered for patients with macroadenomas to minimize pregnancy-associated complications.

Pulsatile GnRH

Pulsatile administration of GnRH is an effective alternative to gonadotropin therapy, particularly for women with hypothalamic amenorrhea (WHO group 1). Successful induction of ovulation requires a normally responsive pituitary gland. Intravenous and subcutaneous administration with computerized pumps has been reported. Pumps, which are usually rented, often include a home maintenance service. Advantages of pulsatile GnRH therapy over gonadotropin therapy include minimal cycle monitoring and reduced risk for multiple conception and ovarian hyperstimulation.

Although the intravenous pump requires additional maintenance and is associated with an increased risk for superficial thrombophlebitis, it is generally more reliable and less expensive. Subcutaneous administration is simpler, but it is less reliable and it requires a higher total dose of medication (Jansen et al, 1987). Recommended dosages range from 2.5 to 5 μg per pulse for intravenous administration and 15 to 20 μg per pulse for subcutaneous administration. Recommended pulse frequency ranges from every 1 to 2 hours.

Spontaneous LH surge and subsequent ovulation usually occur by the second week of therapy; hence, more than 3 weeks of treatment is rarely necessary. The GnRH dose should be increased after 3 weeks if ovulation does not occur. Urine or serum LH tests are usually adequate to predict the day of ovulation for the timing of intercourse or inseminations. More extensive monitoring with serum estradiol levels and ultrasonography is usually unnecessary. However, some type of luteal phase support is routinely recommended to optimize the probability of a successful pregnancy. Physiological stimulation of the corpus luteum can be accomplished by continuing the pump therapy for 2 weeks after ovulation. Alternatively, supplemental doses of oral or vaginal progesterone (50 to 100 mg twice daily) or hCG (2500 mIU every 3 days for four doses) provide adequate luteal phase support.

Reported rates of ovulation with pulsatile GnRH range from 80% to 95%. The probability of conception among patients with hypothalamic amenorrhea is extremely high, with monthly fecundability rates of 30% and cumulative probability of pregnancy approaching 90% (Santoro et al, 1986). There is no increased risk for spontaneous abortion or congenital anomalies (Homberg et al, 1989). Martin et al (1993) compared gonadotropin with pulsatile GnRH therapy and reported similar rates of ovulation and pregnancy. However, the rate of multifollicular development with gonadotropin therapy was significantly higher. Pulsatile GnRH therapy is associated with a multiple gestation rate of 8%, which is comparable to that for clomiphene citrate therapy and significantly less than that for gonadotropin therapy. As with clomiphene citrate therapy, the risk for high-order multiple conception with pulsatile GnRH is extremely low.

Fertility Medications and the Risks for Ovarian Cancer

Since 1992, there has been a heightened awareness regarding the possible association between fertility medications and the subsequent development of ovarian cancer. It is important to emphasize that suggested association does not imply causality. Unfortunately, published studies supporting and refuting the association have limitations that prevent any definite conclusions. Nulliparity is clearly well established as a risk factor for ovarian cancer. However, Wittemore et al (1992) suggested that a small fraction of the excess ovarian cancer risk among nulliparous women is attributed to infertility and that any increased risk associated with infertility may result from the use of fertility drugs. The Wittemore study clearly generated significant concern, but it has been openly criticized because it was limited by small numbers of cases and controls, lack of detailed information regarding types of fertility medications, dosages, and duration of therapy, and failure to distinguish ovulatory from anovulatory patients. Rossing et al (1994) reported that more than 12 cycles of clomiphene therapy was associated with an increased risk for ovarian cancer (Rossing et al, 1994). Although this study describes a specific fertility medication and a threshold risk for duration of treatment, it is also limited by a small number of cases and by other problems with its design. In contrast to these earlier studies, Venn et al (1995) reported no increased incidence of breast or ovarian cancer in a cohort of 10,358 women observed for 1 to 15 years. Although reassuring, this study was limited by insufficient follow-up for the entire cohort of patients. Bristow and Karlan (1996) recently reviewed the current literature and concluded that long-standing primary infertility is more likely than treatment with ovulation induction agents to be a significant risk factor for ovarian cancer. The need for a properly designed long-term prospective study is clear. Until further data become available, women receiving fertility medications should be informed of the possible association with ovarian cancer. However, this potential association should be balanced against the benefit of a successful pregnancy, which is known to reduce the risk for ovarian cancer.

Surgical Treatment of Anovulation

Before the availability of fertility medications, ovarian wedge resection was recommended to anovulatory patients with PCOD. The efficacy, advantages, and disadvantages of ovarian wedge resection have been reviewed in multiple studies (Goldzieher and Green, 1962). It is limited by the temporary resumption of ovulation, and its other disadvantages include the administration of general anesthesia, recovery from surgery, and formation of subsequent adhesions. Greenblatt and Casper (1987) reported a minimally invasive laparoscopic approach termed ovarian drilling, the serial creation of millimeter cores of ovarian tissue through electrocautery or laser ablation (Daniell and Miller, 1989). Ovarian drilling is similar to ovarian wedge resection in that it is associated with the temporary inhibition of ovarian androgen production and the resumption of ovulation. Group pregnancy rates reportedly range from 25% to 65%. Laparoscopic ovarian drilling should be considered for patients who prefer to avoid gonadotropin therapy or who are unresponsive to treatment with clomiphene citrate. There is insufficient evidence to determine a difference in ovulation or pregnancy rates when ovarian drilling is compared with gonadotropin therapy (Abdel, 1990).

TUBAL AND PERITONEAL FACTOR INFERTILITY

Tubal disease is identified in approximately 30% of infertile couples. Causative factors that contribute to tubal disease include PID, appendicitis, endometriosis, pelvic adhesions, previous tubal surgery, and previous IUD use. Rates of tubal disease after one, two, or three episodes of PID have been reported to be 12%, 23%, and 54%, respectively (Westrom, 1980). Subclinical pelvic chlamydial infections appear to be a major cause of tubal factor infertility (Jones et al, 1982). A ruptured appendix is associated with risk that is increased fivefold (Mueller et al, 1986). Interestingly, there are no identifiable risk factors in approximately 50% of patients with documented tubal or peritoneal factor infertility (Rosenfeld et al, 1983). Routine infertility evaluation includes a test for tubal patency. The two most common tests for evaluating tubal patency are hysterosalpingography and laparoscopy. In certain situations, such as in the anovulatory patient undergoing ovulation induction or the infertile couple with moderate to severe male factor infertility, some clinicians recommend postponing the evaluation of tubal patency. Treatment of tubal factor infertility is generally limited to two options, surgical tubal reconstruction or in vitro fertilization. (The evaluation and treatment of endometriosis-associated infertility is discussed in this section as well.)

Hysterosalpingography

Hysterosalpingography (HSG) is the most commonly performed screening test for tubal patency. In addition to assessing tubal patency, HSG may provide useful information about the uterine cavity. An outpatient procedure, HSG is usually performed in conjunction with the department of radiology. To prevent the potential irradiation of a fertilized ovum, the procedure is scheduled before ovulation, usually between cycle days 5 and 11. The patient is placed in the dorsal lithotomy position, and a single-tooth tenaculum is placed on the anterior cervix. A cannula is snugly inserted into the cervical canal, and a sterile radiopaque contrast medium is slowly injected through the cannula. Various instruments are available to facilitate the injection of dye. The injection phase of the procedure is best visualized under fluoroscopy. If fluoroscopy is not possible, radiographs should be taken after the sequential injection of 3 to 5 mL. Depending on the size of the uterus, 10 to 20 mL contrast medium may be required.

A radiograph should be taken when the uterine cavity is filled. Many times HSG provides evidence suggesting proximal tubal obstruction. Several studies have demonstrated that the site of tubal obstruction is cornual in approximately half the patients with abnormal HSG findings (Rice et al, 1986). Salpingitis isthmic nodosa, first described in 1887, is a rare cause of proximal tubal obstruction (Chiari, 1887). It is characterized by numerous small diverticula involving the interstitial segment or isthmus (or both) of the fallopian tube, and it is often found in association with chronic inflammation or endometriosis.

Evaluation of the midportion and distal tube requires a second radiograph as the ampullae fill. Distal tubal occlusion is suggested when there is partial filling of the fallopian tube but no peritoneal spillage. This may occur in the isthmic, ampullary, or fimbrial portion of the fallopian tube, and it is often associated with radiographic evidence of hydrosalpinges. The presence of mucosal rugae appears to be a favorable prognostic factor for subsequent pregnancy, and the absence of rugae suggests a severely damaged tubal epithelium. Young et al (1970) demonstrated a 60.7% pregnancy rate in patients with rugal folds compared with a 7.3% pregnancy rate in patients without rugal folds. An irregular distribution of loculated contrast medium around the fimbriated end of the tube suggests periadnexal adhesions and emphasizes the importance of a final radiograph that demonstrates free intraperitoneal contrast material to document tubal patency. Fig. 14-5 shows the normal findings obtained by HSG and the findings seen with chronic PID. The accuracy of HSG will be discussed in the next section on laparoscopy.

The optimal contrast medium for HSG remains controversial (Soules and Spadoni, 1982). A water-soluble contrast medium may be used. It provides radiographs of excellent quality, but there may be a slight loss in image resolution

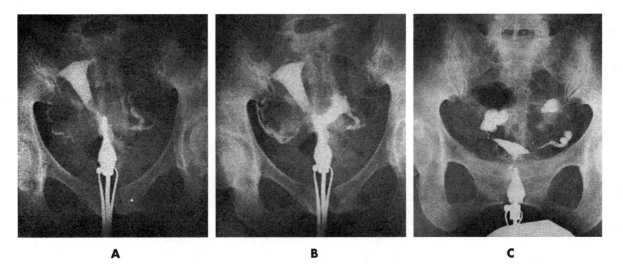

Fig. 14-5. Hysterosalpingograms. **A,** Visualization of uterus in both oviducts in a normal patient. **B,** Second film showing free passage of the dye from the oviduct into the peritoneal cavity. **C,** Patient with chronic pelvic inflammatory disease and bilateral hydrosalpinges.

and it may cause increased abdominal cramping. However, a water-soluble contrast medium averts the potential complications of lipid granulomas and lipid embolization found with an oil-based contrast medium. Lipid embolization is the result of the injection of contrast medium into the myometrium with subsequent intravasation into the venous or lymphatic system. Siegler (1974) reported nine deaths attributable to the intravasation of dye. According to Bateman et al (1980), there were 13 reports of intravasation in a series of 533 HSGs performed with an oil contrast medium. However, in only six of these patients was there embolization of dye, and there was no associated morbidity or mortality. The authors state that the use of fluoroscopy allows for early detection of intravasation and minimizes complications. Whenever there is evidence of intravasation, injection should be discontinued immediately, regardless of the contrast medium used. Intravasation includes a network of streaklike opacities adjacent to the uterine cavity that extend toward the pelvic side walls and subsequently migrate in a cephalad direction.

Ethiodized oil is popular in certain centers because of its possible value as a therapeutic agent. Despite anecdotal evidence, the therapeutic benefit of HSG remains controversial. Mechanisms by which HSG may enhance fertility include mechanical lavage of a partially obstructed tube, stimulation of the tubal cilia, and inhibition of hostile peritoneal fluid immune cells (Surrey and Meldrum, 1987; Goodman et al, 1993). Although results of several studies have suggested an increased pregnancy rate after HSG (Palmer, 1960), other studies have demonstrated no increase in the pregnancy rate (Alper et al, 1986; de Boer, 1988). Several studies have suggested an increased pregnancy rate with oil-based contrast compared with water-soluble contrast media (Rasmussen, 1991; Ogata, 1993; Lindequist, 1991). DeCherney et al (1980) studied 339 patients for 4 months and demonstrated a 29% pregnancy rate using an

oil-based medium compared with 13% with a water-soluble medium. In a well-designed study, de Boer et al (1988) randomized 175 women to undergo HSG with oil-based or water-soluble contrast agents. Oil-based contrast agents gave better resolution of the uterine cavity, but water-soluble agents gave better resolution of the tubal mucosa. Pregnancy rates were similar in the two groups.

Absolute contraindications for performing HSG include a possible pregnancy and a history of acute PID. Relative contraindications include a history suggestive of PID, recent uterine instrumentation, and iodine allergy. The risk for PID after HSG has been estimated to be 1% to 3% (Rice et al, 1986; Stumpf and March, 1980). Routine antibiotic prophylaxis has not been shown to be efficacious (Stumpf and March, 1980). However, patients at risk for acute PID may benefit from antibiotic therapy (Pitaway et al, 1983). Despite limited data, we recommend antibiotic prophylaxis with doxycycline 100 mg twice a day for 3 days for all patients. For patients at significant risk for acute PID, laparoscopy with tubal lavage is recommended in place of HSG.

Laparoscopy

Laparoscopy with tubal lavage is considered the criterion standard for evaluating tubal patency and other peritoneal factors. Its advantage is that it offers direct visualization of the pelvic anatomy. In addition to assessing tubal patency, laparoscopy helps to determine the appearance of the fimbria and the presence of periadnexal adhesions and endometriosis. Laparoscopy was thoroughly reviewed by Wheeless and Katayama (1985). It is usually performed as an outpatient procedure using general anesthesia.

The patient is placed in the lithotomy position, and a cannula is placed through the cervical canal for the injection of indigo carmine dye. A thin Verres needle is placed through an infraumbilical incision into the peritoneal cavity for the instillation of carbon dioxide. Approximately 2 to 3 L of

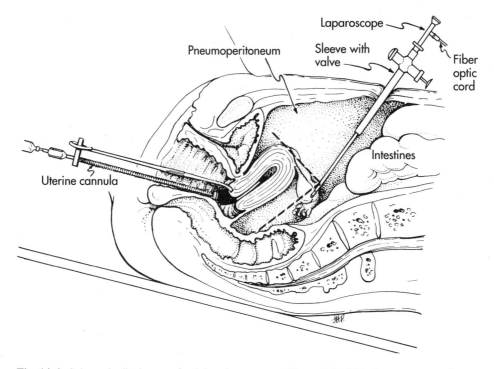

Fig. 14-6. Schematic diaphragm of pelvis at laparoscopy. (From Cohn MR: *Laparoscopy, culdoscopy, and gynecography.* Philadelphia, 1970, WB Saunders.)

carbon dioxide provides adequate preparation of the pneumoperitoneum so that the larger trochar may be inserted into peritoneal cavity. The laparoscope is inserted through this trochar (Fig. 14-6). A second suprapubic puncture is usually necessary to expose the pelvic anatomy adequately. Tubal lavage should be performed with indigo carmine dye to assess tubal patency.

Laparoscopy is often recommended when the HSG suggests a tubal factor. This is largely based on the potential for a therapeutic surgical intervention. However, it is important to note the relatively high incidence of false-positive HSGs, commonly caused by cornual spasm. To eliminate the complication of cornual spasm, Hutchins (1977) studied 62 patients under general anesthesia and found that 45 of 62 patients (73%) with proximal tubal occlusion on HSG had laparoscopic evidence of normal oviducts with evidence of tubal patency by methylene blue insufflation. Because of the high incidence of false cornual obstruction, two separate tubal studies should be performed before the diagnosis of proximal tubal obstruction is confirmed.

Among women whose HSGs reveal abnormalities, the most common laparoscopic finding is postinfection tubal disease (Collins, 1988). This may include pelvic adhesions, phimotic fimbria, hydrosalpinges, or tubal obstruction. The second most common laparoscopic finding is endometriosis. An extremely variable (range, 5% to 60%) prevalence of endometriosis among women undergoing laparoscopy for infertility has been reported (El Minawi et al, 1978). Laparoscopic visualization, biopsy, or both are required for the diagnosis of endometriosis because there are no specific screening tests. Surgical laparoscopy may include lysis of adhesions, fulguration or resection of endometriosis, and tubal reconstruction. The American Society of Reproductive Medicine's classifications of adnexal adhesions, distal tubal occlusion, and endometriosis is based on laparoscopic findings and provides a rational foundation for therapy (Buttram, 1985; American Fertility Society, 1988).

The value of performing laparoscopy after normal HSG findings has generated significant debate, largely supported by the diagnostic accuracy of HSG and the uncertain impact of surgical laparoscopy on subsequent fecundability. Although HSG is not a perfect predictor of tubal factor infertility, HSG is in agreement with the laparoscopic findings approximately two thirds of the time. Collins (1988) estimated the sensitivity and specificity of HSG to be 73% and 83%, respectively. Opsahl et al (1993) classified HSGs as normal, abnormal (bilateral, distal tubal obstruction), or suspicious (all others) and reported moderate to severe pelvic disease at laparoscopy in 62% of patients with normal, 53.9% of patients with suspicious, and 81.7% of patients with abnormal HSGs findings. In contrast, other studies have suggested less than 3% probability of identifying moderate to severe pelvic disease among infertile patients with normal HSG findings.

Marcoux et al (1997) recently reported that laparoscopic removal of stages I and II endometriosis is associated with significantly increased fecundability in comparison with diagnostic laparoscopy alone. Treatment of endometriosis-associated infertility will be discussed in the section on the treatment of tubal and peritoneal factor infertility. Although normal HSG findings have a high negative predictive value, laparoscopy should be considered if simple, nonsurgical infertility treatment is unsuccessful. Deciding when to proceed with laparoscopy, if at all, after a normal HSG finding should be individualized based on the patient's history and physical examination and on the remainder of the infertility evaluation.

Salpingoscopy

Salpingoscopy (falloposcopy) allows for the endoscopic evaluation of the endosalpinx and may help identify an abnormal mucosal pattern, intratubal adhesions, or both. It also may allow for a better understanding of tubal physiology, which includes the mechanisms of bidirectional tubal motility. There is no routine procedure to evaluate the functional integrity of the fallopian tube. Salpingoscopy may be performed at the time of laparoscopy or laparotomy. Kerin et al (1992) reported a diagnostic classification system for tubal lumen disease based on falloposcopy. They concluded that falloposcopy may be therapeutic because it dislodges intraluminal debris and breaks down filmy adhesions in minimally diseased tubes. Shapiro et al (1988) reported 17 patients who underwent salpingoscopy at the time of laparoscopy or laparotomy, and they found a 23.5% discordance rate between the fimbrial appearance at surgery and the salpingoscopic findings. Similarly, Marconi et al (1992) demonstrated abnormal endosalpingeal salpingoscopic findings in 37% of patients with normal findings on laparoscopy. In the future, salpingoscopy may aid in the difficult therapeutic decision between reconstructive tubal surgery and in vitro fertilization.

Future Diagnostic Procedures

Recent studies suggest a potential role for evaluating tubal patency with ultrasonography (Allahbadia, 1992). Tufekci et al (1992) compared transvaginal sonosalpingography with tubal lavage during laparoscopy in 42 patients. Ten to 40 mL of isotonic saline was injected into the uterine cavity through a semirigid Foley catheter. The authors demonstrated a 76% concordance rate by accurately revealing patency in 26 patients and bilateral nonpatency in 3 patients. The addition of pulsed wave or color Doppler imaging may improve the predictive value of transvaginal sonosalpingography (Stern et al, 1992; Deichert et al, 1992). Future studies will be necessary to confirm the clinical usefulness of ultrasonography in the evaluation of tubal patency.

TREATMENT OF TUBAL AND PERITONEAL FACTOR INFERTILITY
Tubal Reconstruction

Tubal reconstruction can generally be performed at the time of diagnostic laparoscopy. Neosalpingostomy and fimbrioplasty are the two most commonly performed procedures for distal tubal obstruction. Fimbrioplasty is the lysis of fimbrial adhesions or the dilation of fimbrial strictures. Neosalpingostomy is the creation of a new opening in a fallopian tube with a distal occlusion. The decision to proceed with surgical reconstruction is often based on various prognostic factors, including the severity of the tubal disease. In addition, the lack of third-party reimbursement for assisted reproduction often limits many couples to the option of surgical reconstruction. Schlaff et al (1990) evaluated the efficacy of neosalpingostomy for distal tubal obstruction in 95 patients. They identified the following poor prognostic factors after surgery for distal tubal obstruction: tubal diameter greater than 25 mm, absence of visible fimbria, dense pelvic adhesions, ovarian adhesions, advanced age of the woman, and duration of the infertility problem.

Dlugi et al (1994) compared the success of unilateral and bilateral distal tubal reconstruction in 113 women with tubal factor infertility. Overall, these procedures were associated with a fecundability of 0.026. Women who underwent bilateral procedures and had major adhesions had the lowest chance of achieving pregnancy. The cumulative probability of pregnancy was approximately 20%, with approximately 20% of the pregnancies ectopic, emphasizing the increased risk for ectopic pregnancy with tubal reconstruction. Repeat surgery is associated with even lower probabilities of success because of the high incidence of recurrent adhesions and tubal reocclusion.

Isolated proximal occlusion occurs in 10% to 20% of patients with tubal factor infertility. Surgical treatment for proximal tubal obstruction remains a formidable challenge for the reproductive surgeon. A major improvement in the surgical treatment of proximal tubal obstruction has been the introduction of minimally invasive transcervical procedures to restore tubal patency. Flexible tip guide-wire techniques have largely replaced the traditional cornual reimplantations. Transcervical cannulation of the proximal fallopian tube may be achieved through hysteroscopy (Novy et al, 1988), fluoroscopy (Platia and Krudy, 1985), or sonography (Leisse and Syndow, 1991). Risquez and Confino (1993) reported successful catheterization in 80% to 90% of patients whose cumulative probability of pregnancy ranged between 23% and 39% within the first 6 to 12 months. Ectopic pregnancy occurs in 5% to 13% of patients. Infertile women with bilateral proximal and distal tubal disease have low chances for conception after surgical intervention (Singhal et al, 1991). Treatment with in vitro fertilization is significantly more successful than any surgical approach to proximal tubal obstruction.

Patients who want to become pregnant after having undergone tubal sterilization may be candidates for tubal ligation reversal. This involves microsurgical reanastomosis of the fallopian tubes. Although tubal ligation reversal has traditionally been performed by laparotomy, recent studies suggest that laparoscopic surgical reanastomosis may be associated with comparable rates of success (Istre et al, 1993).

In properly selected patients, tubal ligation reversal can result in high pregnancy rates that exceed even those obtained through IVF. Prognostic factors associated with higher rates of success include maternal age younger than 40, tubal length greater than 4 cm, previous Falope ring, clip, or Pomeroy tubal ligation, absence of associated pelvic disease, and absence of male factor infertility. The site of reanastomosis (Silber and Cohen, 1980) is also predictive of subsequent pregnancy; isthmic-isthmic anastomoses have the best prognosis for normal pregnancy, and ampullary anastomoses have the highest risk for ectopic pregnancy. The 1-year cumulative pregnancy rates reported after tubal ligation reversal range from 35% to 80% (Boeckx et al, 1986; Henderson, 1984; Rock et al, 1987; Hulka and Halme, 1988).

Assisted Reproduction and In Vitro Fertilization

Assisted reproduction (AR) reinforces the value of basic science research. The rapid application of laboratory knowledge to clinical programs has led to the universal recognition of the accomplishments and controversies surrounding reproductive medicine and the assisted-reproductive technologies (ART). AR involves the direct handling and manipulation of the oocyte and sperm to enhance the probability of achieving a successful pregnancy. ART refers to an assortment of clinical and laboratory techniques, the most common of which are in vitro fertilization-embryo transfer (IVF-ET), gamete intrafallopian tube transfer (GIFT), intracytoplasmic sperm injection (ICSI), cyroembryo transfer (CET), and IVF-ET with donor eggs.

Rock and Menkin reported the first human IVF in 1944. However, the pioneering work of Edwards and Steptoe (1978) led to a birth after the first successful IVF-ET. During the past two decades, the rapid growth of AR includes more than 59,000 annual cycles of ART treatment in the United States and Canada alone (SART, 1998).

The field of ART is often criticized for a lack of randomized clinical trials demonstrating superior fecundability. In addition, new technologies are constantly introduced without appropriate clinical trials. Challenging ethical and societal questions are discussed on a regular basis. Despite these deficiencies, large descriptive studies demonstrate consistent improvement and strongly suggest superior rates of success with ART for most conditions associated with infertility. The following sections provide a brief overview of the current status of AR and focus on the most commonly performed procedure, IVF-ET.

Patient Selection and Indications for In Vitro Fertilization

Clinical characteristics of the male and female partners have a major impact on IVF outcome. Originally, the indication for IVF-ET was tubal factor infertility because IVF-ET is able to bypass the fallopian tubes completely. The most common indications for IVF are tubal factor infertility, male factor infertility, endometriosis, and unexplained infertility. However, IVF is recommended for essentially all conditions

that have not been successfully treated with other treatment strategies. Factors that influence the decision to proceed with tubal reconstruction versus IVF-ET have been discussed earlier. Standard IVF is less successful for couples with severe male factor infertility if the total motile sperm count is less than 1.5 million (van Uem, 1985).

A woman's age is strongly predictive of IVF success or failure. Multiple studies have confirmed the association between maternal age and IVF outcome (SART, 1998; Padilla and Garcia, 1989). This includes a decreased probability of conception and an increased probability of miscarriage with advancing maternal age. The association between maternal age and IVF outcome appears to be related to ovarian reserve. Ovarian reserve refers to available quantity and quality of mature, healthy oocytes during gonadotropin stimulation. As previously discussed, day 3 FSH level or the FSH response to clomiphene citrate is an accurate predictor of IVF outcome. Most successful ART programs require some assessment of ovarian reserve before IVF-ET to help counsel patients. In addition, most programs limit treatment with standard IVF-ET to women younger than 43 to 44 years of age. Patients older than 43 or patients with diminished ovarian reserve are poor candidates for standard IVF and should consider IVF with donor eggs.

Ovarian Stimulation

Although "natural" cycle IVF-ET avoids ovarian stimulation, it is limited by the harvest of only one to two oocytes. The natural cycle approach to IVF-ET has been largely abandoned by most programs because of low rates of success (Claman et al, 1993). Similarly, ovarian stimulation with clomiphene alone is associated with the harvest of one to two oocytes and low rates of success (MacDougall et al, 1994).

A contemporary cycle of IVF-ET usually begins with controlled ovarian hyperstimulation (COH) to stimulate numerous mature follicles to maximize the retrieval of multiple healthy oocytes. The number of ovarian stimulation protocols that have been combined with IVF-ET continues to expand. This is largely the result of ongoing efforts to define a satisfactory regimen for patients who respond poorly to gonadotropin therapy. The most common ovarian stimulation protocols associated with IVF-ET include a combination of GnRH-agonist and gonadotropin treatment.

Gonadotropin regimens may include hMG alone, FSH alone, or a combination of clomiphene citrate/hMG, clomiphene citrate/FSH, or hMG/FSH. The comparison of different gonadotropin protocols has been described earlier. Despite recent enthusiasm for recombinant FSH protocols, randomized clinical trials have failed to demonstrate a clearly superior approach to gonadotropin stimulation. The addition of GnRH-agonist therapy to COH for IVF-ET clearly increases the probability of a successful outcome.

Optimal timing of oocyte retrieval is determined by follicular monitoring with ultrasonography and estradiol measurements. Follicular monitoring is also intended to minimize the risk for severe OHSS. The criteria for hCG administration during cycles of IVF-ET are significantly more aggressive in comparison with routine ovulation induction protocols combined with intercourse or intrauterine insemination. The criteria for hCG administration vary between programs, but they often require estradiol levels greater than 600 pg/mL and at least two follicles larger than 20 mm. In contrast to ovarian stimulation with intercourse or intrauterine inseminations, estradiol levels greater than 2000 pg/mL are common. Although controversial, IVF-ET appears to be associated with a lower rate of OHSS when studies control for the estradiol level on the day of hCG (Rizk and Smitz, 1992).

The addition of a GnRH agonist to gonadotropin stimulation offers several benefits, among them decreased premature ovulation, decreased cycle cancellation, increased number of oocytes, increased number of embryos, and increased number of successful pregnancies per cycle. GnRH agonists have been used in several different protocols. The two most common protocols are mid-luteal initiation of GnRH-agonist therapy followed by the addition of gonadotropin stimulation once ovarian suppression has been achieved (downregulation or long protocol) and simultaneous initiation of GnRH-agonist and gonadotropin therapy during the early follicular phase (Flare or short protocol). Multiple studies including a metaanalysis comparing these two protocols have failed to demonstrate any significant differences in pregnancy outcome (Hughes et al, 1992). In addition, the type of GnRH analogue does not appear to be critical, though daily subcutaneous formulations are preferred over depot intramuscular formulations. A variation of the long protocol involves follicular-phase downregulation. Follicular-phase downregulation reduces the likelihood of early pregnancy at the time of GnRH-agonist initiation. The disadvantage of this protocol includes the need to administer GnRH-agonist therapy for a greater number of days (Kondaveeti-Gordon et al, 1996). More recent refinements in GnRH-agonist protocols include lower dosages (microdose) for women who respond poorly to conventional downregulation and discontinuation of the GnRH-agonist after ovarian suppression but before the initiation of gonadotropin stimulation (Scott and Navot, 1994).

Oocyte Retrieval and Fertilization

Oocyte retrieval is scheduled 34 to 36 hours after hCG administration and uses a transvaginal ultrasound-guidance technique. Timing of hCG administration should maximize oocyte maturation and minimize the risk for premature ovulation. The procedure is performed with a long 18-gauge needle that has an echogenic tip to facilitate ultrasound visualization. Individual follicles are serially punctured, and follicular fluid is aspirated and transferred to an adjacent embryology laboratory for oocyte identification. Typically, the procedure is completed in 15 to 30 minutes. Anesthesia

options vary from program to program but may include conscious sedation, spinal anesthesia, or light general anesthesia. The number of harvested oocytes is largely dependent on the number of follicles larger than 12 mm on the day of the retrieval (Wittmack et al, 1994).

Classification systems have been developed to grade oocytes and embryos based on morphologic appearance. Fig. 14-7 describes the Brigham and Women's Hospital oocyte classification system. Semen is collected the day of oocyte retrieval, usually by masturbation. Several sperm washing procedures have been described in combination with IVF-ET, including swim up and percoll gradient centrifugation techniques. The percoll gradient technique has become more popular for men with abnormal semen parameters because of increased fertilization rates (Sapienza et al, 1993; Van der Zwalmen et al, 1991). However, percoll has been routinely replaced with a synthetic equivalent, isolate, because of the manufacturer's theoretical concerns about viral contamination that could lead to Creutzfeldt-Jakob disease (Svalander et al, 1995). Sperm are incubated in a protein-supplemented medium for approximately 4 hours to initiate the process of capacitation. Oocytes are inseminated approximately 4 hours after their retrieval by coincubation with approximately 50,000 to 100,000 sperm per oocyte. Approximately 12 to 18 hours after insemination, oocytes are examined for fertilization. Mature oocytes have a fertilization rate that ranges between 50% to 70%. A zygote with two pronuclei and two polar bodies is morphologic evidence of fertilization (Fig 14-8).

Embryo Culture and Transfer

The fertilized oocytes are placed in growth medium and typically not examined until the day of embryo transfer. The meticulous handling of oocytes, sperm, and embryos is a major component of any successful AR program. In addition, ongoing refinements of the embryo culture medium have clearly contributed to consistent improvements in pregnancy outcome. Assessment of embryo quality is typically based on various morphologic characteristics such as number of blastomeres, degree of fragmentation, symmetry, granularity, vacuolation, membrane definition, and number of nuclei per blastomere. Although embryo quality is clearly associated with successful implantation, current classification systems remain subjective and suboptimal predictors of pregnancy and multiple gestation outcomes.

The major goal of all ART programs is to maximize the chance for successful pregnancy and to minimize the risk for high-order multiple gestation. Unfortunately, live birth pregnancy and multiple gestation rates per cycle are both strongly dependent on the number and the quality of embryos transferred (Svendsen et al, 1996). Deciding how many embryos to transfer is often based on individual program priorities and guidelines. Most guidelines consider several predictive factors including maternal age, embryo quality, number of previous treatment cycles, and the

OOCYTE CLASSIFICATION

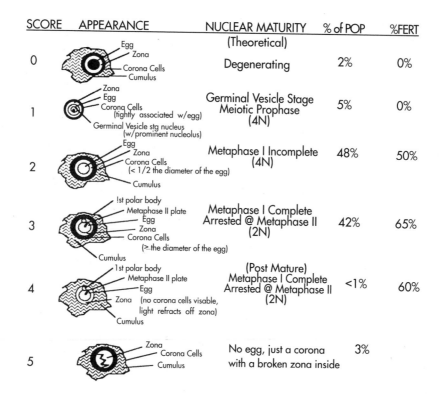

Fig. 14-7. Oocyte classification based on morphologic appearance. (From Brigham and Women's Hospital assisted reproductive technologies laboratory manual, 1993).

couple's concerns regarding high-order multiple gestation, including the acceptance of multifetal pregnancy reduction (Steer et al, 1992; Rosenbom et al, 1995).

Most programs transfer three to four embryos into the uterine cavity 3 days after oocyte retrieval. The Society for Assisted Reproductive Technology (SART) suggests the transfer of no more than three embryos to women younger than 35 years of age and four embryos to women older than 35 years of age during an initial cycle of IVF-ET. Transferring more than five embryos is uncommon. Several programs have reported the routine transfer of two embryos to eliminate the risk for high-order multiple conception. These programs reported minimal impact on their overall rates of live birth pregnancy, particularly when combined with cycles of CET (Staessen et al, 1993; Authier-Brouzes et al, 1994).

Recent advancements in embryo culture techniques have supported an increasing trend toward the transfer of blastocyst-stage embryos 5 days after oocyte retrieval (Templeton and Morris, 1998). Day 5 blastocyst transfer is associated with more stringent and predictive criteria for embryo selection. Blastocyst transfer may be associated with superior live birth pregnancy rates and is usually limited to the transfer of one or two embryos. Thus, blastocyst transfer eliminates the risk for high-order multiple concep-

tion and averts the transfer of unhealthy embryos that have discontinued the cell division required for normal development. The disadvantage of embryo transfer on day 5 is the possibility that none of the original cohort of fertilized oocytes will continue to develop in vitro for the entire 5 days. Day 5 blastocyst transfer may quickly become the standard of care for the ART based on the elimination of high-order multiple gestation without compromising the overall live birth pregnancy rate.

Embryo transfer is a simple procedure. The embryos are loaded into a flexible catheter with a small volume of culture medium, usually less than 25 μL. After a speculum is inserted into the vagina, the catheter is gently passed through the cervical canal into the uterine cavity. The catheter is placed in the fundal region of the uterine cavity at a distance predetermined either in the office or at the time of oocyte retrieval through a uterine sounding technique. Embryos are injected, and the catheter is slowly removed and passed to a member of the embryology staff. Then the catheter is carefully examined under the microscope for the possibility of a retained embryo. Although rare, this requires repeating the embryo transfer technique; both may contribute to the probability of a successful outcome. Preliminary studies have suggested that the Wallace catheter may be associated with an increased rate of success (Mayer et al, 1996). Recovery time after embryo transfer does not appear to affect pregnancy outcome, and patients are discharged home 30 to 60 minutes after embryo transfer. It is recommended that they limit their activities for 24 to 48 hours.

Luteal Phase Support

Adequate production of progesterone is critical during implantation and early pregnancy. A recent metaanalysis of randomized clinical trials suggests that luteal phase supplementation after oocyte retrieval improves pregnancy outcome (Soliman, 1994). Relative progesterone deficiency may be related to disruption of the granulosa-luteal cells at the time of oocyte retrieval and to GnRH-agonist suppression of endogenous LH stimulation of the corpora lutea. The two most common methods of providing luteal phase support are supplemental doses of progesterone and supplemental doses of hCG.

Progesterone is often administered as a daily 50-mg intramuscular injection. Severe myositis and the formation of welts have been associated with intramuscular progesterone (Phipps, 1988). Alternative routes of administration are intravaginal progesterone suppositories and oral micronized progesterone. Although randomized clinical trials are lacking, alternative routes of administration appear to be associated with comparable pregnancy outcomes (Smitz, 1992). Progesterone supplementation is generally initiated around the time of embryo transfer. When patients conceive, progesterone administration is typically continued until after the luteal-placental shift.

Supplemental hCG is administered at dosages ranging from 1500 to 10,000 IU intramuscularly once or more during the luteal phase (Hutchinson-Williams, 1990). Both hCG and progesterone are associated with increased pregnancy rates when compared to no luteal support (Soliman, 1994). Progesterone is associated with a higher pregnancy rate and a lower rate of OHSS than hCG (Morhtar et al, 1996). In the United States, progesterone supplementation remains the preferred method of luteal phase support.

Gamete Intrafallopian Transfer

Asch et al first described gamete intrafallopian transfer, or GIFT, in 1985. The GIFT procedure involves an initial approach to ovarian stimulation and oocyte retrieval identical to that for IVF-ET. In contrast to IVF-ET, GIFT requires general anesthesia and laparoscopy, which are performed immediately after transvaginal ultrasound-guided oocyte retrieval. Four to six unfertilized oocytes are combined with washed sperm and transferred into the ampullary portion of the fallopian tube, usually under laparoscopic visualization with a flexible catheter placed through the fimbriated end of the fallopian tube. Several programs have reported the successful transfer of gametes into the fallopian tube through a transcervical approach with hysteroscopy (Seracchioli, 1995) or ultrasonography (Bustillo, 1989).

GIFT requires a minimum of one easily accessible, normal-appearing, patent fallopian tube. The ideal candi-

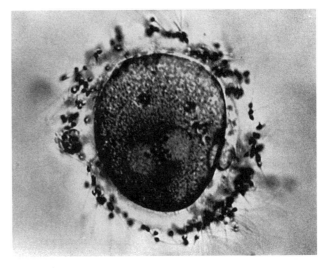

Fig. 14-8. Zygote with two pronuclei in the center of the figure and two polar bodies in the perivitelline space. (From Veeck LL: *Atlas of the human oocyte and early conceptus*, vol 2, Baltimore, 1991, Williams & Wilkins.)

dates for GIFT are couples with unexplained infertility, early-stage endometriosis, and mild male factor. GIFT offers the theoretical advantage of placing oocytes and sperm in proximity in their natural or physiological tubal environment. Unfortunately, there are no large-scale randomized trials comparing IVF-ET with GIFT. Leeton et al (1987) reported similar pregnancy rates for IVF-ET and GIFT in a small number of randomized patients. Several studies have also compared GIFT with gonadotropin stimulation and IUI and have reported similar monthly fecundity rates of 13% versus 9% (Hogerzeil, 1982). In recent years, the role of GIFT has been limited by ongoing improvements in embryo culture techniques and pregnancy outcome with IVF-ET. GIFT may be the treatment of choice for appropriate couples in programs that have relatively low pregnancy rates with IVF-ET.

Since the introduction of GIFT, other tubal transfer techniques have been described including zygote intrafallopian transfer (ZIFT; Homori et al, 1988), pronuclear stage tubal transfer (PROST; Yovich et al, 1987), tubal embryo transfer (TET) and tubal transfer of cryopreserved embryos (Van Voorhis et al, 1995). These procedures involve the tubal transfer of pronuclear (ZIFT and PROST) or cleavage-stage embryos (TET) and combine features of IVF and GIFT. These procedures have the hypothetical advantage of combining the confirmation of fertilization with incubation in the tubal environment. However, most clinical trials have failed to demonstrate any improvement in pregnancy outcome when comparing ZIFT, PROST, and TET to IVF-ET (Tournaye et al, 1992; Fluker, 1993; Preutthipan et al, 1994). In addition, each of these techniques requires two invasive procedures on separate days. Van Voorhis et al (1995) did report a significantly higher ongoing pregnancy rate per cycle

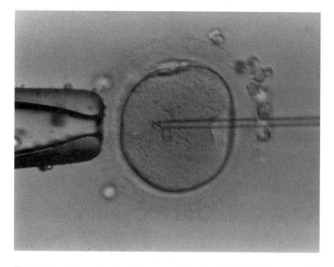

Fig. 14-9. Intracytoplasmic sperm injection (ICSI). (Courtesy of Katharine V. Jackson, Brigham and Women's Hospital Assisted Reproductive Technologies Embryology Laboratory.)

with tubal (58%) versus intrauterine transfer (19%) of cryopreserved embryos.

Intracytoplasmic Sperm Injection

Male partners with fewer than 1 million total motile sperm after sperm washing have a significantly lower probability of successful fertilization with standard in vitro fertilization (Ben-Chetrit, 1995). ICSI is the direct injection of a single sperm into the cytoplasm of the oocyte (Fig. 14-9). Before the clincial acceptance of ICSI, the treatment of male factor infertility had been associated with relatively lower rates of success than anovulatory or tubal factor infertility. Multiple studies have demonstrated superior success rates with ICSI than with earlier micromanulipation techniques such as partial zona drilling and subzonal sperm injection (Levran et al, 1995; Catt et al, 1995; Tarin, 1995).

A unique feature of IVF with ICSI is the small number of sperm required for a successful outcome. In fact, success with ICSI has been reported with immotile and immature sperm. Surprisingly, success with ICSI is strongly dependent on the number and quality of oocytes. Other strong predictors of ICSI success include the maternal age, sperm motility, and gonadal reserve testing (FSH levels) in both partners (Sherins, 1995). Indications for ICSI continue to evolve and now include severe male factor infertility and unexplained and oocyte-associated failed or poor fertilization.

A major advance during the past decade is the combination of sperm harvesting techniques with ICSI. Candidates for sperm harvest procedures include men with congential absence of the vas deferens, other causes of obstructive and nonobstructive azoospermia, and previous vasectomy. Sperm can be obtained from the epididymis using microsurgical or percutaneous techniques and from a testicular biopsy specimen (Verheyen, 1995). Sperm harvested from the epididymis or testis has been associated with live birth pregnancy rates in the range of 30% per cycle when com-

bined with IVF and ICSI (Silber, 1995). ICSI does not appear to improve the pregnancy rate with IVF if routinely offered to couples with normal semen parameters (Aboulghar, 1996). van Steirteghem (1998), considered one of the major pioneers in the development of ICSI technology, reported his experience with more than 48,000 oocytes from more than 4500 cycles. A fertilization rate of 70% was associated with live birth rate of 27% per embryo transfer. The rate of spontaneous pregnancy loss was 25%, and the rate of major congential malformations was 3.3%. These rates do not appear to be significantly different than those after spontaneous conception or standard IVF.

There is concern that genetic abnormalities associated with severe oligospermia or azoospermia may be transmitted to male offspring. Long-term follow-up of larger numbers of infants conceived with the help of ICSI technology will be necessary to understand fully any potential risks. Until more data are available, couples considering ICSI should be appropriately counseled about the uncertain risks of this relatively new technology. Men with severe oligospermia or azoospermia who plan IVF with ICSI should consider cytogenetic analysis. In addition, second-trimester ultrasonography and amniocentesis should be offered for all ICSI-conceived pregnancies, regardless of maternal age.

Cyroembryo Transfer

The application of basic cryobiology principles led to the development of successful embryo cryopreservation techniques (Zeilmaker, 1984). Cryopreservation of excess embryos enables indefinite storage for future transfer. Cyroembryo transfer involves the timed transfer of thawed embryos. This can be accomplished during a natural cycle or after artificial preparation of the endometrial lining with a combination of GnRH-agonist downregulation plus estrogen and progesterone hormone replacement. The major advantage of embryo cryopreservation is the ability to avoid ovarian stimulation and oocyte retrieval. Availability of successful embryo cryopreservation often supports the transfer of fewer embryos during the initial ovarian stimulation cycle. Transferring fewer embryos minimizes the risk for multiple gestation without compromising the overall pregnancy rate *per retrieval*.

The probability of surviving the freeze-thaw process and successfully implanting is strongly dependent on the quality of the embryo before freezing. Most programs set guidelines to define which excess embryos are suitable for freezing. Embryos that survive the freeze-thaw process and proceed with normal cleavage do not appear to be associated with an increased rate of chromosomal abnormalities (Shaw, 1991). Cryoprotectant used, stage of embryo development, and endometrial preparation (Schmidt et al, 1989) may also influence the probability of a successful CET. Van der Elst et al (1995) compared two different cryoprotectants in a prospective randomized clinical trial. The live birth rate per embryo thawed with dimethyl sulfoxide (DMSO; 3.5%) was significantly higher than with 1,2 propanediol (0.8%).

Reliable techniques and protocols for oocyte preservation would clearly have a major impact on ART, particularly in the area of donor oocytes. However, the ability to cryopreserve oocytes in a reproducible fashion remains a significant challenge. Advancements in oocyte cryopreservation have generated concerns about spindle disruption that could cause chromosomal abnormalities. Oocyte cryopreservation is only available under investigational protocols in a limited number of programs (Veeck, 1993). Refinements in oocyte cryopreservation will probably lead to the development of donor oocyte banks.

In Vitro Fertilization with Donor Oocytes

Treatment options available for women with ovarian failure or diminished ovarian reserve are limited. In the absence of IVF with donor oocytes, the remaining infertility treatments are associated with low probability of success. Initial indications for IVF with donor oocytes included the various causes of premature ovarian failure, such as Turner syndrome, bilateral salpingo-oophorectomy, chemotherapy or radiation therapy, and idiopathic premature failure. More recently, the indications for IVF with donor oocytes have been extended to perimenopausal and postmenopausal women, female carriers of genetic diseases, and infertile couples who cannot conceive after multiple cycles of traditional ART (Morris and Sauer, 1993).

IVF with donor oocytes raises serious ethical and social questions. For example, up to what age should women be candidates for IVF with donor oocytes? Some centers have treated women older than 60 years of age, whereas other centers limit IVF with donor oocytes to women younger than 50 years of age. Despite ongoing ethical and psychosocial controversy, IVF with donor oocytes can be performed with either known or anonymous oocyte donors. Most couples requiring IVF with donor oocytes are not interested in knowing the donor or lack an appropriate known candidate for oocyte donation. Unfortunately, the waiting times for anonymous donors are often long.

Using donor oocytes with IVF has shed important light on our understanding of the aging of the female reproductive system. Based on results from IVF with donor oocytes, the age of the oocyte appears to be significantly more important than the age of the uterus. IVF with donor oocytes requires the synchronization of the donor's and the recipient's reproductive cycles. This is typically accomplished with GnRH-agonist downregulation of the donor and, if necessary, the recipient and is followed by gonadotropin stimulation of the donor and artificial preparation of the recipient's endometrium with estrogen and progesterone hormone replacement. Recipients with premature ovarian failure do not require GnRH-agonist downregulation before uterine preparation with estrogen and progesterone.

Pregnancy Outcome

The live birth rate per cycle initiated provides the most consistent and realistic estimate of the probability of a success-

Table 14-5 Standard In Vitro Fertilization Outcomes as Reported by the Society for Assisted Reproductive Technology—American Society for Reproductive Medicine Registry 1986 and 1995

	1986	1995
Cycles initiated	4,867	36,035
Cancellations per cycle initiated	28%	16%
Oocyte retrievals	3,504	30,223
Embryo transfer per retrievals	85%	89.7%
Clinical pregnancies	485	8,299
Deliveries	NR	6,754
Deliveries per cycle initiated	<9%*	18.7%

Modified from Medical Research International, American Fertility Society Special Interest Group: *Fertil Steril* 1988; 49:212-215; and from Society for Assisted Reproductive Technology: *Fertil Steril* 1998; 69:389-398. With permission of the American Society for Reproductive Medicine.

NR, not reported.

*Assumes abortion and ectopic rates of at least 10%.

ful outcome. Unfortunately, many programs and authors have reported other numerators, such as pregnancy, clinical pregnancy, and ongoing pregnancy, and other denominators, such as per transfer and retrieval. These different estimates of pregnancy outcome often create unrealistic expectations and confuse the evaluation of ART outcome. The recent summary of 1995 ART activity was prepared by the Society of Assisted Reproductive Technologies, the American Society for Reproductive Medicine, and the Centers for Disease Control and Prevention (CDC). Voluntary reporting by 281 programs is potentially subject to validation and audit by these sponsoring agencies. Between 1986 and 1995, there was a significant increase in the live birth rate per cycle initiated, from less than 9% to almost 19% (Table 14-5) (Medical Research International, The American Society Special Interest Group, 1988; Society of Reproductive Technologies, 1995).

The impact of clinical characteristics and patient selection on ART outcome has been discussed earlier. Table 14-6 summarizes the influence of female age and the presence of a male factor on IVF outcome. The live birth rates per cycle initiated for IVF, ICSI, GIFT, ZIFT, and IVF with donor eggs and for CET are reported in Table 14-7. Differences in pregnancy outcomes resulting from various types of ART are probably dependent on clinical characteristics and patient selection.

Pregnancy aided by ART is strongly correlated with multiple gestation. In 1995, the rate of multiple conception associated with successful IVF included 29.6% twins, 6.4% triplets, and 0.6% high-order multiple gestations. Singleton pregnancies after IVF appear to have outcomes similar to spontaneously conceived singleton pregnancies when appropriately controlled for maternal age (Oliveness et al, 1997).

Table 14-6 Live Birth Rate Per Retrieval for Standard IVF In Vitro Fertilization Cycles as Influenced by the Age of the Female Partner and Status of Semen Factors.*

	Female Partner <35 Years	Female Partner 35-39 Years	Female Partner >39 Years
No male factor	27.5% (3,285/11,949)	21.7% (2,013/9,317)	10.6% (433/4,096)
Male factor	25.2% (660/2,615)	20.2% (319/1,583)	6.6% (44/663)

From Society for Assisted Reproductive Technology and American Society for Reproductive Medicine. Assisted reproductive technology in US and Canada: 1995 results. *Fertil Steril* 1998; 69:389-398. With permission of the American Society for Reproductive Medicine.

*Parentheses reflect the number of deliveries divided by the number of cycles initiated.

Table 14-7 Deliveries Per Cycle Initiated for Assisted Reproductive Technology Procedures: United States and Canada, 1995.

	Cycles Initiated	Deliveries per Cycle Initiated (%)
IVF	36,035	18.7
ICSI	5,052	23.5
GIFT	3,741	24.0
ZIFT	1,078	24.4
IVF with Donor oocyte	3,555	33.9
CET	8,453	13.4

From Society for Assisted Reproductive Technology and American Society for Reproductive Medicine. Assisted Reproductive Technology in United States and Canada 1995 results generated from the American Society for Reproductive Medicine/Society for Assisted Reproductive Technology Registry. *Fertil Steril* 1998; 69:389-398. With permission of the American Society for Reproductive Medicine.

IVF, in vitro fertilization; ICSI, intracytoplasmic sperm injection; GIFT, gamete intrafallopian tube transfer; ZIFT, zygote intrafallopian transfer; CET, cryoembryo transfer.

The rate of early miscarriage associated with IVF pregnancies is approximately 20%. Ectopic pregnancy is more common among women with tubal factor infertility; it accounted for approximately 3% of all IVF pregnancies in 1995. Overall incidences of poor obstetric outcomes, including stillbirths and birth defects, remains low. The incidence of congenital malformations reported in the 1995 data set was 0.7% of all neonates. However, not all outcomes among neonates were reported. More stringent requirements for follow-up and reporting will be included in future SART clinical outcome reports.

Risks with In Vitro Fertilization–Embryo Transfer

The major risks of ART are OHSS and multiple conception. The evaluation and treatment of OHSS were described earlier in the section on gonadotropin therapy. The potential association between gonadotropin stimulation and ovarian cancer was discussed earlier in the section on the treatment of ovulatory dysfunction.

During the past decade, the number of multiple pregnancies in the United States has steadily increased as a result of the increasing number of ART cycles. The economic impact of high-order multiple conception is enormous (Callahan et al, 1994). Wilcox et al (1996) reported that 22% of all triplet pregnancies result from treatment with IVF. Callahan (1994) reported that 77% of high-order multiple gestations (triplets or higher) resulted from ART-related pregnancies.

Recently reported rates of multiple conception with successful IVF cycles included 29.6% twins, 6.4% triplets, and 0.6% high-order multiple gestations. Couples with triplets and high-order multiple gestations are faced with the difficult considereration of multifetal pregnancy reduction. Usually, the procedure is performed with transabdominal ultrasound guidance at 12 to 13 weeks of gestation. Injecting potassium chloride into the fetal heart brings about rapid fetal demise. The risk for losing the entire pregnancy through spontaneous abortion after multifetal pregnancy reduction is estimated to be between 5% and 10%. Several studies suggest that multifetal pregnancy reduction is associated with improved pregnancy outcome because of the decrease in early preterm deliveries (Smith, 1996; Bollen et al, 1993; Berkowitz et al, 1996). It has been estimated that approximately 20% of couples offered selective reduction choose the procedure (Radestad, 1994).

New Frontiers in Assisted Reproduction

Since the birth of Louise Brown, new frontiers in assisted reproduction have continued to be explored. Assisted hatching is a micromanipulation technique proposed to improve embryo implantation. The embryologist performs assisted hatching on the day of embryo transfer. It involves the thinning or disruption of the *zona pellucida* by enzymatic or mechanical micromanipulation, which may allow the embryo to expand and "hatch" through the *zona pellucida,* facilitating a favorable interaction between the embryo and the endometrium. Assisted hatching may improve the probability of successful implantation in embryos with thickened *zona pellucida* and in women with elevated FSH levels (Cohen, 1992). Additional clinical trials are clearly needed to define the efficacy and indications for assisted hatching.

ART may be applied to preimplantation genetic diagnosis. In the human, removal of one blastomere from a six- to eight-cell embryo to provide useful genetic information has been associated with successful implantation and pregnancy (Handyside, 1990). Techniques such as fluorescent in situ hybridization and polymerase chain reaction are suitable for the genetic analyses because results can generally be obtained within less than 12 hours. A reasonable number of ge-

---

BOX 14-7
GENETIC DISORDERS THAT CAN BE DIAGNOSED BY BLASTOMERE BIOPSY

α-1 Antitrypsin deficiency
Cysic fibrosis
Tay-Sachs disease
Duchenne muscular dystrophy
Turner syndrome
Down syndrome
Hemophilia A
Fragile X syndrome
X-linked disorders

BOX 14-8
TREATMENT OF ENDOMETRIOSIS-ASSOCIATED INFERTILITY

Treatment of Early Stage I and II Endometriosis

Step 1 Identify and treat all reversible causes of infertility.

Step 2 Consider laparoscopic resection, vaporization, or fulguration of endometriosis implants.

Step 3 If the woman is younger than 32 years old, consider expectant management with timed intercourse using urine luteinizing hormone monitoring or basal body temperature charts.

Step 4 Consider empiric clomiphene with or without intrauterine insemination.

Step 5 Consider empiric gonadotropin therapy with intrauterine insemination.

Step 6 Consider assisted reproduction with in vitro fertilization or gamete intrafallopian tube transfer.

Treatment of Advanced Stage III and IV Endometriosis

Step 1 Identify and treat all reversible causes of infertility.

Step 2 If an endometrioma is suspected, consider surgical resection.

Step 3 If major pelvic adhesions are present and the patient has undergone no previous surgery for infertility, consider conservative surgery to restore normal pelvic anatomy with resection of endometriosis implants and lysis of adhesions.

Step 4 Consider empiric clomiphene with intrauterine insemination.

Step 5 Consider empiric gonadotropin therapy with intrauterine insemination.

Step 6 Consider in vitro fertilization.

---

netic diseases can be evaluated with preimplantation genetic diagnosis and blastomere biopsy (Box 14-7). In the future, ART may be used for a wider range of genetic disorders and could be combined with gene therapy.

Recently, the transfer of oocyte cytoplasm has been suggested as an alternative to IVF with donor oocytes for couples with severe oocyte abnormalities. In vitro oocyte maturation is another area of ongoing research, which, if properly developed, could be combined with the cryopreservation of ovarian biopsy specimens. At present, progress in this area remains exceedingly slow and clearly requires additional investigation.

Treatment of Endometriosis-Associated Infertility

The treatment of endometriosis-associated infertility is rarely limited to specific or definitive recommendations because of the lack of sufficient clinical trials. As a result, patients with endometriosis-associated infertility are potential candidates for a range of treatment options, among them conservative surgery, superovulation with fertility medications plus IUI, and assisted reproduction. The fecundability of women with endometriosis appears to be related to disease stage. The mechanism(s) that contribute to endometriosis-associated infertility are poorly understood. Women with advanced stages 3 and 4 endometriosis often have endometriomas or major pelvic adhesions, suggesting that distortion of the normal tubo-ovarian anatomy may contribute to their infertility. In contrast, women with early stages I and II endometriosis demonstrate relatively normal pelvic anatomy, suggesting a functional rather than an anatomic cause. Recent studies have documented the presence of a hostile immune environment as the most likely mechanism contributing to early-stage endometriosis-associated infertility (Hill, 1997). A stepwise approach to the treatment of endometriosis-associated infertility based on the severity of the disease is presented in Box 14-8.

Conservative surgical intervention refers to avoiding hysterectomy or oophorectomy, and it typically involves the restoration of normal pelvic anatomy with resection, ablation, or fulguration of endometriosis implants, excision of

endometriomas, lysis of adhesions, and occasional tubal reconstruction. Surgical treatment can usually be accomplished through a minimally invasive laparoscopic approach. Bowel preparation before surgery should be strongly recommended to patients with advanced stages of endometriosis, either known or suspected. It should include a liquid diet, cathartic agent, and possible antibiotic prophylaxis 24 hours before surgery.

Treatment of Advanced-Stage Endometriosis

Although there are limited data in humans, multiple animal studies suggest that stages III and IV endometriosis are associated with decreased fecundability (Schenken and Asch, 1980; Schenken et al, 1984; Vernon and Wilson, 1985). Results of several studies suggest that conservative surgical intervention for advanced stages of endometriosis results in improved rates of pregnancy. However, these studies are largely limited by their retrospective comparisons to expectant management. Olive and Lee (1986) reviewed 66 patients with advanced endometriosis treated with expectant management or surgery. Among 32 women treated with expectant management, none became pregnant during 231 months of cumulative follow-up. In contrast, among 34 women treated with conservative surgery, 10 (29%) became pregnant during 702 months of cumulative follow-up. Garcia and David (1977) have reported similar findings. Several investigators, including Telimaa (1988), have reported that deep endometriomas are associated with decreased fecundability, suggesting that surgical excision of an endometrioma may result in an improved rate of conception. Although limited, the current literature suggests that expectant management should not be recommended to women with advanced endometriosis-associated infertility.

There is some debate regarding the role of postoperative medical therapy after a conservative surgical procedure for endometriosis-associated infertility. This is partially related to the historical observation that the enhancement of fecundability peaks during the first 6 to 12 months after surgery. Once again, definitive recommendations are limited by the lack of clinical trials. Wheeler and Malinak (1981) reported crude pregnancy rates of 79% among women with advanced endometriosis treated with postoperative danazol therapy compared with crude pregnancy rates of 30% among women with advanced endometriosis treated with surgery alone. In contrast, Andrews and Larsen (1974) demonstrated a significantly decreased pregnancy rate when surgery was combined with postoperative hormonal therapy than when it was performed alone. The role of postoperative medical therapy in endometriosis-associated infertility clearly warrants additional investigation. Postoperative medical therapy with danazol or a GnRH-agonist is rarely recommended to couples after conservative surgery for endometriosis-associated infertility.

Similar to surgical tubal reconstruction, repeat conservative surgery does not appear to be associated with enhanced fecundability (Schenken and Malinak, 1978). Empiric ovarian stimulation with clomiphene citrate or gonadotropin therapy with intrauterine inseminations should be considered for patients who do not become pregnant after a conservative surgery. Candidates for ovarian stimulation plus IUI should have documented tubal patency and relatively normal tubal ovarian anatomy. Patients with advanced endometriosis and markedly distorted tubal anatomy should consider IVF the treatment of choice.

Recent studies suggest that treatment of advanced-stage endometriosis with in vitro fertilization and GIFT is associated with increased fecundability. IVF and GIFT are often recommended to women of advanced reproductive age who have not become pregnant after other treatments and who have prolonged or multifactor infertility. Large clinical trials evaluating the efficacy of assisted reproduction for the treatment of advanced endometriosis-associated infertility are lacking. Pal et al (1998) retrospectively evaluated the impact of endometriosis stage on IVF outcome. Sixty-one patients undergoing 85 cycles of IVF were studied. This study was controlled for maternal age, day 3 FSH level, male factor in-

fertility, and the ovulation induction regimen. The response to ovarian hyperstimulation and the number and quality of oocytes harvested were not affected by the severity of endometriosis. In contrast, fertilization rates for patients with advanced stages of endometriosis were significantly lower than for patients with early-stage endometriosis. In addition, implantation, clinical pregnancy, and miscarriage rates were not dependent on disease severity. The authors concluded that IVF outcome is unaffected by the severity of endometriosis and suggested that IVF may overcome the reduction in pregnancy potential of oocytes obtained from women with advanced disease.

In contrast, Damewood (1989) reported a compromise of oocyte recovery and fertilization rates among women with advanced endometriosis-associated infertility. Matson and Yovich (1986) also evaluated the impact of endometriosis on IVF outcome based on disease severity. Although number of oocytes and fertilization rates were similar in all groups, monthly fecundity was significantly reduced among women with stages III and IV endometriosis compared to patients with early-stage endometriosis and tubal factors.

The influence of advanced stages of endometriosis on IVF outcome may be related to the presence of ovarian endometriomas or diminished ovarian reserve. Previous ovarian surgery is associated with diminished ovarian reserve and poor response to gonadotropin stimulation with lower rates of pregnancy when compared with other infertility factors (Hornstein, 1989). In addition, several studies have suggested that the presence of endometriomas may be associated with alterations of oocyte and embryo quality (Pellicer et al, 1995). Yanushpolsky et al (1998) reported a significantly higher rate (47%) of early pregnancy loss among patients with endometriomas who undergo IVF than among controls (14%). These authors also demonstrated a trend toward fewer embryos reaching the four-cell stage 48 hours after egg retrieval in patients with endometriomas. In contrast, Isaacs et al (1997) reported that aspiration of an endometrioma at the time of oocyte harvest had no adverse effects on IVF outcome.

The IVF ovulation induction regimen may also influence IVF outcome in patients with advanced-stage endometriosis. Nakamura et al (1992) compared prolonged suppression with a GnRH-agonist for more than 60 days with standard midluteal downregulation before controlled ovarian stimulation. Among 33 patients with varying stages of endometriosis, the clinical pregnancy rate per transfer was superior with prolonged GnRH-agonist suppression (67% versus 27%). More recently, Fugii et al (1997) reported a prospective randomized comparison between long and discontinuous-long protocols of GnRH-agonist for IVF. These authors evaluated 137 IVF cycles in which patients were randomized to receive discontinuous GnRH-agonist luteal downregulation, which was discontinued on cycle day 7, or continuous GnRH-agonist luteal downregulation until the day before hCG administration. The authors reported that the number of embryos transferred was smaller and the cancellation rate was higher when the GnRH-agonist was discontinued on cycle day 7. Future clinical trials should improve our understanding of the apparent benefit of IVF for women with advanced endometriosis-associated infertility.

Treatment of Early-Stage Endometriosis

Treatment options available to women with early-stage endometriosis include expectant management; laparoscopic resection, vaporization, or fulguration of endometriosis implants; medical therapy with hormone suppression; empiric ovarian stimulation with clomiphene citrate or gonadotropins and IUI; and assisted reproduction with IVF or GIFT. Although most studies suggest that women with stages I and II endometriosis have reduced fecundability (range, 0.04 to 0.05), the number of randomized controlled clinical trials to guide definitive therapeutic recommendations is limited. In addition, interpretation of the current literature is limited by conflicting results. As with other infertility factors, the approach to couples with early-stage endometriosis often involves a stepwise staircase approach (Box 14-8).

There is no convincing evidence to suggest that hormone suppression medical therapy with progestins, danazol, or GnRH-agonists improves fecundability rates in women with early-stage endometriosis. Seibel et al (1982) randomized 73 patients with stage I or II endometriosis to receive either danazol or expectant management. Couples were observed for approximately 1 year. The authors reported no improvement in fecundability with danazol treatment; the monthly fecundity rate was 0.035 compared to 0.051 for the control group with expectant management. Fedele et al (1992a) randomized 71 patients with stage I or II endometriosis to receive either the GnRH-agonist Buserelin or expectant management. The couples were followed up for approximately 2 years. These authors reported no differences in the 2-year cumulative probability of pregnancy (60% versus 61%), suggesting that treatment with Buserelin does not improve fecundability in women with early-stage endometriosis.

The complex decision of when to proceed with laparoscopy, if at all, was discussed earlier. Previous studies of laparoscopic treatment of early-stage endometriosis have reported fecundability rates in the range of 0.03 to 0.05, which are similar to the reported rates for expectant management (Adamson, 1996; Adamson, 1993; Chong et al, 1990). A quantitative review of pooled data from laparoscopic surgery trials suggested a benefit for this procedure (Hughes, 1993). The conclusions of this metaanalysis were limited by the heterogeneity of the different study populations. However, recent data strongly suggest that laparoscopic removal of stages I and II endometriosis is associated with enhanced fecundability (Marcoux, 1997).

The Canadian collaborative group on endometriosis (Marcoux, 1997) reported a multicenter, prospective, randomized clinical trial during which 341 infertile women with stages I and II endometriosis were randomly assigned to undergo resection or ablation of visible endometriosis or diagnostic laparoscopy alone. Women were followed up for 36 weeks or, for those who conceived, up to 20 weeks of pregnancy. Laparoscopic removal of endometriosis was associated with a significantly increased cumulative probability of pregnancy of 30.7% compared to 17.7% for the women treated with diagnostic laparoscopy alone (Marcoux et al, 1997 [see Fig. 19-15 in Chapter 19]). The corresponding monthly fecundity rates were 0.047 and 0.024 respectively. This is the first well-designed clinical trial to demonstrate that laparoscopic resection or ablation of early-stage endometriosis improves fecundability.

Several studies suggest that treatment of early-stage endometriosis-associated infertility with empiric ovarian stimulation increases fecundability. Deaton et al (1990) randomized a subgroup of 24 patients with stages I and II endometriosis to receive empiric treatment with clomiphene citrate plus intrauterine inseminations versus expectant management. They reported a significant enhancement of monthly fecundability (0.092 versus 0.033) for women treated with empiric ovarian stimulation. This study included an identical number of women with unexplained infertility with similar results. However, the conclusions in this study relative to early-stage endometriosis may be partially confounded by the surgical correction of endometriosis at the time of laparoscopy.

Fedele et al (1992b) randomized 49 women with stages I and II endometriosis to either three cycles of hMG ovarian stimulation plus intrauterine insemination or expectant management. In women who received three cycles of hMG-IUI, the per-cycle pregnancy rate was 0.15 compared to 0.045 for the expectant management control group. The difference in monthly fecundability was statistically significant, suggesting that superovulation with hMG plus IUI enhances fecundability and is a reasonable treatment option for women with early-stage endometriosis.

Kemmann et al (1993) randomized women with infertility and early-stage endometriosis to one of four treatment groups—expectant management, clomiphene stimulation, clomiphene plus hMG stimulation, or IVF. Women treated with clomiphene plus hMG or IVF experienced a significantly increased monthly pregnancy rate of 0.114 and 0.22 compared with 0.028 for the untreated control group. Women who received clomiphene alone had a monthly pregnancy rate of 0.066, which was not significantly different than the rate for the untreated control group. This study suggests that superovulation with hMG increases the probability of achieving a pregnancy and that IVF is associated with the highest rate of fecundability.

Few randomized controlled trials have evaluated the efficacy of IVF and GIFT for women with early-stage endometriosis. Nevertheless, a large number of cohort studies involving women with stages I and II endometriosis reveal an extremely high pregnancy rate with assisted reproduction. Although they are age dependent, live birth pregnancy rates per cycle, ranging from 0.20 to 0.45, have been reported for women with early-stage endometriosis. The decision to proceed with assisted reproduction is part of our stepwise staircase approach and should be based on a balance between efficacy, cost, and risk for multiple conception.

**BOX 14-9
CAUSES OF MALE INFERTILITY**

Anatomic Factors

Varicocele
Cryptorchidism
Ductal obstruction (Young syndrome)
Congenital anomalies (hypospadias, epispadias, cystic fibrosis, testicular hypoplasia or aplasia, and partial or total absence of the vas deferens)

Endocrine Factors

Gonadotropin deficiency
Kallman syndrome
Pituitary tumors (Cushing disease, acromegaly)
Dwarfism
Hypothyroidism
Fertile eunuch syndrome
Enzymatic defects in testosterone synthesis
Androgen receptor deficiency
Congenital adrenal hyperplasia

Genetic Factors

Klinefelter syndrome
Down syndrome
47 XYY
Autosomal translocations

Inflammatory Factors

Orchitis
Epididymitis
Prostatitis
Urethritis

Immunologic Factors

Systemic
Local

Sexual Dysfunction/Faulty Coital Technique

Impotence
Retrograde ejaculation
Premature ejaculation
Spermicidal lubricants

Exogenous Factors

Medication (antihypertensives, antipsychotics, antidepressants, cimetidine, chemotherapy)
Radiation
Alcohol
Marijuana
Trauma
Excessive heat (hot tubs)
Cigarettes

THE MALE FACTOR

Although the male factor is often cited as a common cause of infertility, this is misleading because the tests available for the evaluation of men do not easily separate normal fertile men from those with reduced fertility. The evaluation of the male is limited not only by a large overlap in the semen parameters among fertile and subfertile men, it is limited by the wide fluctuations among sequential semen specimens from the same person. Some of the variation between ejaculates in the same man may be caused by environment exposures (season, illness, and stress) (Jequier and Ukombe, 1983). Because it is relatively rare to identify a male partner with azoospermia (no sperm in the ejaculate), it is often difficult to implicate the male factor as the principal cause of a couple's infertility. As in the other major categories, various factors are associated with male factor infertility. Different schemes to categorize the multiple causes of male infertility have been devised, one of which is outlined in Box 14-9.

Semen analysis remains the primary screening test for male factor infertility because of the general relationship between abnormal semen parameters and the relative risk for infertility (Table 14-8). If semen analysis results are persistently abnormal, the patient is referred to a urologist for examination and further evaluation. The importance of a thorough physical examination cannot be overstated. The most commonly identified conditions causing or associated with male factor infertility are varicocele (37%), testicular failure (9%), obstruction (6%), cryptorchidism (6%), low semen volume (5%), sperm agglutination (3%), and excessive semen viscosity (2%). A karyotype, vasography, and testicular biopsy may be recommended for patients with azoospermia or severe oligozoospermia. Endocrine studies measuring serum testosterone, LH, FSH, TSH, and prolactin should be considered for patients with azoospermia, oligozoospermia, or oligoasthenospermia (poor motility). Immunologic factors may be suggested if there is sperm agglutination, oligoasthenospermia, or poor cervical mucus penetrability. Immunologic infertility will be further discussed in the section on the cervical factor. Microbiologic studies should be considered if there is any suggestion of genital tract infections. Unfortunately, a specific cause for male factor infertility usually cannot be identified. However, it is useful to subcategorize male factor infertility as mild, moderate, or severe because the degree of severity determines the appropriate treatment options (Table 14-9).

Diagnostic Tests for the Evaluation of the Male
Semen Analysis

Basic semen analysis measures volume, pH, fructose, liquefaction, round cells, sperm density, motility, and morphology. Before obtaining the semen specimen, the patient is instructed to abstain from ejaculation for a minimum of 48 hours and no longer than 7 days. The method of choice for collection is masturbation with avoidance of potentially spermicidal lubricants. The specimen should be collected in a clean container and brought to the laboratory within 1 to 2 hours. Semen may be evaluated by an experienced technician or by semiautomated computers. Normal ranges for the major semen parameters are listed in Table 14-10.

The optimal period of sexual abstinence has not been determined. There are no scientific data to support the recommendation that having intercourse every other day is more likely to result in conception than having intercourse every day, and recent evidence suggests that the optimal period of abstinence may vary from person to person. Ejaculate volume, sperm concentrations, and sperm counts tend to rise continuously up to 10 days of abstinence (Blackwell and Zaneveld, 1992). In contrast, sperm motility does not appear to be affected by ejaculatory frequency (Sauer, 1988). Frequent ejaculation may be associated with decreased semen volume and decreased total motile sperm, whereas infrequent ejaculation has been associated with a decrease in normal morphology.

Normal semen volumes range from 2 to 6 mL. Small volume may be associated with retrograde ejaculation. Lack of fructose and acidic pH may suggest seminal vesicle dysfunction or ejaculatory duct obstruction. The absence of liquefaction may result in relatively immobilized spermatozoa. Leukocytospermia or an abnormal number of immature germ cells may be suggested by an abnormal number of round cells (greater than 1 million/mL). Unfortunately, total round cell counts are poorly predictive of leukocytospermia, and it is often difficult to distinguish white blood cells from immature germ cells by conventional microscopy (Politch, 1993).

An immunperoxidase staining technique (Endtz test) specific for white blood cells is primarily used and is recommended by the World Health Organization (Wolf and Anderson, 1988). Studies investigating the role of leukocytospermia and male factor infertility have yielded conflicting results. Tomlinson (1992) reported that leukocytes in the semen had no influence on fertilization. In contrast, other investigators have demonstrated a significant inverse relationship between fertilization rates and leukocyte numbers (Van de Ven, 1987). An abnormal number of immature germ cells, apparently associated with reduced fertilization, may be the result of a defect in spermatogenesis (Tomlinson, 1992).

Interpreting sperm density, motility, and morphology may be difficult for several reasons. As previously mentioned, there are wide fluctuations in sequential semen analyses from the same person, and there is significant overlap between fertile and subfertile men. There is additional difficulty correlating semen parameters with fertility potential because fertility is a function of both partners, not one. An additional drawback is that semen analysis does not measure the *functional* properties of spermatozoa. The predictive inadequacy of the seminal parameters is illustrated by the difficulty determining the lower limits of the fertile range. Nevertheless, among all the tests and parameters available, sperm density, motility, and morphology

Table 14-8   Relative Risk of Infertility Stratified by Sperm Count

Sperm Concentration (million/mL)	Relative Risk for Infertility	Statistical Significance Compared to Unit Risk
<10	10.3	P <0.000000001
10 to 20	5.2	P <0.00001
20 to 40	3.1	P <0.001
40 to 60	1.7	P <0.02
60 to 160	1.0	Unit risk
160 to 200	1.3	Not significant
>200	1.5	Not significant

From Jewelwicz R, Wallach EE. Evaluation of the infertile couple. In Wallach EE, Zacur HA, editors. *Reproductive medicine and surgery,* St. Louis, 1995, CV Mosby, p. 366. Adapted from Nelson CMK, Bunge R. *Fertil Steril* 1953; 4:10; DeCherney AH: In Kase NG, Weingold AB, editors. *Principles and practice of clinical gynecology,* New York, 1983, Churchill Livingstone.

Table 14-9   Subcategories of Male Factor Infertility

	Semen Parameters		
Subcategory	Sperm Concentration (10⁶/mL)	Motility (%)	Morphology* (% Normal)
Mild	15-20	40-50	30-40
Moderate	10-15	20-40	10-30
Severe	<10	<20	<10

*World Health Organization classification.

Table 14-10   Normal Semen Parameters

Volume	2 to 6 mL
Concentration	>20 million/mL
Motility	>50%
Morphology	>40%

have been most consistently correlated with fertility status.

Sperm density is a measure of the number of sperm in the ejaculate per milliliter. Based on studies of fertile men undergoing vasectomy and on follow-up studies of infertile groups (Bostofte et al, 1982; Smith et al, 1977), the lower limit for the number of sperm in the fertile range appears to be 5 million/mL. Despite these results, the most widely accepted lower limit of the normal range continues to be 20 million/mL, based on the landmark studies of MacLeod and Gold (1951). When a higher cutoff is applied, there is an increase in sensitivity at the expense of specificity. Patients whose sperm density is persistently less than 20 million/mL are considered to have male factor infertility and should be referred for additional urologic evaluation.

Assessing sperm motility is as important as determining sperm density. Sperm motility should be evaluated within 2 hours of delivery. It is generally expressed as the percentage of progressively motile sperm; however, as with sperm density, estimating the percentage of progressively motile sperm does not accurately identify subfertile men. Data obtained from IVF suggest that a cutoff of 50% motility has significant prognostic value (Mahadevan and Trounson, 1984). Sperm motility persistently less than that usually warrants additional urologic evaluation. To improve the predictive value of semen analysis, the analysis of sperm movement has expanded to include the evaluation of linear velocity and the amplitude of lateral head displacement. Mortimer (1988) has provided a detailed review of developments in the objective analysis of sperm movement characteristics. Various computer technologies have been developed for the evaluation of sperm movement, but the clinical usefulness of more complex motility data remains to be determined.

Sperm morphology is another semen parameter associated with fertility potential. All semen specimens contain a certain percentage of abnormal spermatozoa. Morphologic abnormalities may involve the sperm head, midpiece, or tail. Abnormalities of the head are often associated with infertility (Bostofte et al, 1985). Recommended cutoffs for normal sperm morphology range from 40% to 60% normal forms, according to a number of clinical studies (Bostofte et al, 1985). Patients with less than 40% morphologically normal spermatozoa are considered to have teratozoospermia and are referred for urologic evaluation. Although abnormal morphology is often associated with reduced sperm density and motility, isolated abnormalities of sperm morphology are not uncommon. Using strict criteria, Kruger et al (1986) suggested that sperm morphology is a powerful predictor of successful IVF. In vitro fertilization rates (below a critical threshold of 14%) were significantly reduced in men with normal sperm morphology. Impairment in fertilization was even more pronounced when the number of normal forms was below 5%. Based on these results, Kruger's morphology criteria have been adopted in many andrology laboratories.

Although separate evaluation of each semen variable is important, there may be advantages in combining them. Mathematical manipulations allow for the expression of the total number of motile sperm and the total number of morphologically normal motile sperm per ejaculate. Combining semen variables avoids the interpretation of several different "normal" standards. Although a total motile count of fewer than 20 million has been associated with lower pregnancy rates (Small et al, 1986), the prognostic superiority of combing semen variables remains to be established.

Testing Sperm Function

Although semen analysis remains the primary screening test for male factor infertility, additional diagnostic tests have been developed to define more precisely the reproductive potential of sperm. Most of these tests assess the functional properties of spermatozoa. The sperm penetration assay (SPA), also known as the zona-free hamster egg penetration test, provides more accurate evaluation of male factor infertility. This assay was designed to assess the ability of sperm to undergo capacitation and the acrosome reaction, to fuse with and penetrate the egg membrane, and to undergo chromosomal decondensation. Sperm are washed free of seminal plasma and incubated in a protein-enriched medium that promotes capacitation. After incubation, motile sperm are separated and used to inseminate hamster eggs that have been treated with enzymes to remove the cumulus and the zona pellucida. The SPA does not test the ability of sperm to penetrate the zona pellucida. Sperm from a donor of proven fertility is tested simultaneously as a positive control. Several hours after insemination, the hamster eggs are examined for sperm penetration. Penetration rates of less than 10% to 15% are considered abnormal. Although initial studies suggested a high degree of sensitivity and specificity (Rogers et al, 1979; Karp et al, 1981), subsequent studies have been unable to substantiate the excellent initial results (Margalioth et al, 1983; Wickings et al, 1983). After reviewing the world's literature, Mao and Grimes (1988) concluded that the validity, reproducibility, and usefulness of the SPA have not been established. They recommend the SPA not be used to evaluate infertile couples.

In vitro fertilization with human eggs has become the criterion by which to assess sperm function; the accuracy of the SPA in predicting success during IVF remains controversial. Although abnormal SPA results are not always associated with an inability to penetrate human eggs, there does appear to be a correlation between the SPA and IVF rates. The SPA is less predictive of fertilization success with abnormal semen parameters than with unexplained or tubal factor infertility (Margalioth et al, 1986). The long-term prognostic ability of the SPA is difficult to determine because prospective studies have yielded different results. Aitken et al (1984) found that 0% was the only SPA value diagnostic of infertility. It remains uncertain whether additional information is gained using the SPA rather than traditional semen analysis; therefore, the SPA is rarely recommended as part of modern infertility evaluation.

Additional methods have been described to evaluate sperm function. One of them, the hypoosmotic swelling test, measures the functional integrity of sperm membranes by placing specimens in hypoosmotic fluids (Jeyendran et al, 1984). This assay has been correlated with successful IVF (Van der Ven et al, 1986). Sperm nucleus maturation can be determined by staining a sperm specimen with acidic aniline blue (Terquem and Dadoune, 1983), acridine orange fluorescence (Tejada et al, 1984), or sodium dodecyl sulfate decondensation (Bedford et al, 1973). Several monoclonal antibodies can be used to detect the acrosome reaction (Wolf et al, 1985). These immunofluorescence assays determine whether a sperm population has the capacity to undergo acrosome reaction. Other simple techniques for assessing the acrosome include triple staining and fluorescein isothiocyanate labeling of lectins (Talbot and Chacon, 1981). The hemizona test assesses the ability of spermatozoa to bind the zona pellucida (Burkman et al, 1988). After the hemizona pellucida is bisected, half is incubated with donor sperm and the other half is incubated with sperm from an infertile patient. Liu et al (1988) established a similar sperm-zona pellucida-binding test using oocytes that failed to fertilize in vitro. They concluded that normal morphology using strict criteria such as linearity, acrosome status, and sperm-zona pellucida binding were the most important characteristics for predicting fertilization in vitro (Liu and Baker, 1992). Although newer sperm function tests appear to provide additional information, their clinical usefulness is unproven, and further studies are required to determine whether these tests predict fertility in vivo.

Varicocele

A dilatation of the pampiniform plexus of the scrotal veins, a varicocele is the most observed correctable cause of male infertility. Throughout the years, the role of varicoceles in male factor infertility has generated considerable debate. Varicoceles are present in 15% of the normal population, and they are estimated to be present in 25% to 40% of men with male factor infertility. They are thought to influence semen quality by increasing testicular temperature.

The World Health Organization recently evaluated 9034 infertile couples and concluded that the varicocele is clearly associated with impairment of testicular function and infertility (WHO, 1992b). Gorelick and Goldstein (1993) demonstrated that the incidence of varicocele is much higher in male factor *secondary* infertility than in primary infertility, suggesting that the varicocele causes progressive impairment in spermatogenesis. The clinical effect of the surgical treatment of varicocele has aroused controversy. Most authorities do not agree that treating small subclinical varicoceles improves fecundability (Yamamoto et al, 1996). In contrast, Madgar et al (1995) demonstrated that high spermatic vein ligation of clinically detectable varicoceles improves semen parameters and fecundability. In this prospective, randomized controlled clinical trial, varicocelectomy resulted in an average increase in sperm count of 20 million/mL. Motility also increased after varicocelectomy. In contrast, men with varicoceles randomized to no surgical treatment demonstrated no change in semen parameters. Although the effect of varicocele surgery on fecundability remains controversial, Madgar (1995) demonstrated a fourfold increase in fecundability among men who underwent high spermatic vein ligation. In the 12 months after randomization, fecundability in the men not surgically treated was approximately 0.01 compared to 0.04 in the men who underwent high spermatic vein ligation. In summary, repair of a varicocele should be considered if male factor infertility is documented, female infertility evaluation results are normal, and a varicocele is clinically detected on physical examination.

Gonadal Failure

The most common cause of gonadal failure in the male is Klinefelter syndrome (47, XXY). Other conditions associated with gonadal failure in the male include mumps orchi-tis, chemotherapy, and severe cryptorchidism. With an occurrence rate of 1 in 500 newborns, Klinefelter syndrome is relatively common. Its classic characteristics are small, firm testes, hyalinization of the seminiferous tubules, azoospermia, and gynecomastia. Its phenotypic appearance includes eunuchoid and tall stature, normal male external genitalia, and poorly developed facial hair. Mental retardation, learning disabilities, and other social impairments may be present. There is an increased incidence of major and minor congenital anomalies (Robinson et al, 1979). Variant and mosaic forms of Klinefelter syndrome exist and may be associated with testes of normal size and variable degrees of spermatogenesis. Treatment options for men with gonadal failure are largely limited to therapeutic donor insemination. The role of assisted reproduction in men with gonadal failure has not been defined, but it appears to be associated with a poor prognosis. Nevertheless, the successful extraction of viable sperm from testicular biopsy specimens among men with Klinefelter syndrome or other causes of gonadal failure have been reported. Successful fertilization has occurred with ICSI, and subsequent pregnancies have been normal.

Isolated Gonadotropin Deficiency

Isolated gonadotropin deficiency, or hypogonadotropic hypogonadism, may be associated with a number of different genetic disorders that result in the lack of adequate GnRH production by the hypothalamus. Patients with Kallman syndrome exhibit hyposmia or anosmia in addition to gonadotropin deficiency. Abnormal development of the olfactory bulbs and tracts results in the decreased sense of smell. The association between GnRH deficiency and anosmia appears to be related to the proximity of GnRH and olfactory neurons during embryologic development. Other abnormalities associated with Kallman syndrome include cryptorchidism, cleft lip, cleft palate, and congenital deafness (Lieblich et al, 1982). Phenotypic appearance includes eunuchoid stature and sexual infantilism or incomplete sexual development. Semen analyses to evaluate isolated gonadotropin deficiency reveal conditions ranging from azoospermia to severe oligoasthenospermia.

Hypogonadotropic hypogonadism is a rare cause of male infertility that usually can be successfully treated. Treatment goals include the stimulation of secondary sexual characteristics and of normal spermatogenesis. There are two approaches to the stimulation of spermatogenesis. One calls for the use of hCG and hMG. The other calls for the use of pulsatile GnRH. Finkel et al (1985) described a regimen that included hCG 2000 IU administered intramuscularly 3 times a week for 6 months, followed by the administration of 37.5 IU of either hMG or FSH intramuscularly 3 times a week. Schopohl et al (1991) compared pulsatile gonadotropin-releasing hormone with gonadotropin therapy in men with isolated gonadotropin deficiency. In this regimen, gonadotropin-releasing hormone is administered through a portable infusion pump at a dosage of approximately 4 μg every 3 hours. Although earlier studies demonstrated no differences between GnRH therapy and hCG/hMG (Liu et al, 1988), Schopohl et al (1991) demonstrated that GnRH leads to higher testicular volume and more rapid initiation of spermatogenesis than gonadotropin therapy. Treatment of these men is often associated with successful pregnancy despite extremely low sperm concentrations (fewer than 5 million/mL).

Obstructive Abnormalities of the Vas Deferens or Epididymis

Congenital absence of the vas deferens can be diagnosed by the absence of fructose in the semen and confirmed by vasography. Recent data suggest that many men with congenital absence of the vas deferens are carriers of mutations in the gene for cystic fibrosis (Chillon et al, 1995). The most common causes of obstruction in the male reproductive tract are previous vasectomy and accidental ligation during inguinal surgery.

Treatment options for men with obstructive abnormalities include microsurgical vasovasotomy or a sperm harvest procedure combined with assisted reproduction and ICSI. Sperm harvest procedures have been described for obstructive azoospermia. These include open and percutaneous epididymal aspiration and sperm extraction from testicular biopsy specimens (MarMar et al, 1993).

Among patients undergoing vasectomy, approximately 3% subsequently request reversal of the procedure. Pregnancy rates are widely variable and range from 15% to 75% (Sharlip, 1993). Pregnancy rates are high when reversals are performed within 3 years of vasectomy; the crude pregnancy rate is approximately 70%. This is in contrast to crude pregnancy rates of 30% among men who have undergone vasectomy reversal 15 years after vasectomy (Belker, 1991).

Retrograde Ejaculation

Retrograde ejaculation is caused by injury to the lumbar sympathetic nerves or by damage to the bladder neck. It is often associated with diabetic neuropathy. The diagnosis is suggested by low semen volume and is confirmed by a high number of sperm in the urine after ejaculation. Medical treatment with pseudoephedrine 60 mg four times a day is recommended to stimulate closure of the bladder neck sphincter. An alternative treatment is to collect and process sperm from a urine specimen immediately after ejaculation for intrauterine insemination or assisted reproduction. Urine should be alkalinized for optimal sperm function with 650-mg sodium bicarbonate tablets four times a day.

Spinal Cord Injury

Men with spinal cord injury often experience impotence, difficulty with ejaculation, reduction in testosterone production, and spermatogenesis (Claus-Walker, 1977). Electroejaculation can be used to obtain semen, but the semen often have abnormalities of sperm motility (Denil, 1992). As a result, electroejaculation may be combined with intrauterine insemination or assisted reproduction.

Idiopathic Oligoasthenospermia

In most infertile men with abnormal semen, there is no identifiable cause of the problem. Patients with idiopathic oligoasthenospermia have been treated with empiric hormonal regimens, most of which do not appear to be effective. Treatment with testosterone, hCG injections, clomiphene citrate, or testolactone have not been effective (Howards, 1995). Sokolrz et al (1988) reported a 12-month controlled comparison of clomiphene citrate and placebo that demonstrated significantly higher levels of serum LH, FSH, and testosterone with clomiphene citrate. However, there were no reported differences in sperm penetration assays or semen parameters between the treatment groups. In a multicenter, randomized double-blind study, the World Health Organization (1992a) reported no difference in cumulative fecundability between clomiphene citrate- and placebo-treated patients with male factor infertility. An efficacious, efficient approach to idiopathic oligoasthenospermia should be based on the severity of the male factor.

Treatment of idiopathic male factor infertility is ultimately dependent on the desires of the patient. However, the infertility specialist should discuss the limitations, including realistic expectations of specific treatment options. We prefer a simple staircase approach that is based on the severity of the semen abnormalities (see Table 14-9). Approaches to the treatment of mild, moderate, and severe male factor infertility are listed in Box 14-10. The approach to mild male factor infertility is similar to our empiric approach to early-stage endometriosis and unexplained infertility. In contrast, couples with severe male factor infertility generally require

---

BOX 14-10
TREATMENT OF MILD, MODERATE, AND SEVERE MALE FACTOR INFERTILITY

Mild Male Factor Infertility

Step 1   Expectant management (three cycles)
Step 2   Intrauterine insemination with or without clomiphene citrate (three cycles)
Step 3   Intrauterine insemination with injectable gonadotropin therapy (three cycles)
Step 4   In vitro fertilization with or without intracytoplasmic sperm injection (six-cycle maximum)

Moderate Male Factor Infertility

Step 1   Intrauterine insemination with or without ovulation induction (three cycles)
Step 2   In vitro fertilization with or without intracytoplasmic sperm injection (six-cycle maximum)

Severe Male Factor Infertility

Step 1a   Consider therapeutic donor inseminations
Step 1b   In vitro fertilization with intracytoplasmic sperm injection (six-cycle maximum)

the advanced reproductive technologies with IVF and often ICSI to achieve successful pregnancy. Specific treatment options may be modified based on the duration of infertility and maternal age.

Intrauterine Inseminations

Intrauterine insemination with or without ovarian stimulation is often recommended to couples with male factor infertility. Although IUI is simple, less invasive, and less expensive than alternative infertility treatments, the efficacy of IUI for male factor infertility remains a matter of debate. Most studies involve small treatment groups and lack life-table analysis and adequate controls for the other variables that influence the likelihood of pregnancy. When compared with timed intercourse, results of randomized controlled trials and large cohort studies do not support definitive conclusions regarding the ability of IUI to improve the probability of conception (Campana et al, 1996; Martinez et al, 1990; Cruz et al, 1986; Francavilla et al, 1990; Ho et al, 1989; Lalich et al, 1988; Kirby et al, 1991; Nan et al, 1994). Treatment of moderate to severe male factor infertility with IUI is associated with minimal improvement of fecundability. In contrast, patients with mild male factor infertility are considered better candidates for IUI. The reported fecundability rate of IUI among patients with male factor infertility ranges from 0.02 to 0.21. Treatment with ovarian stimulation and IUI appears to increase fecundability among patients with male factor infertility (Nulsen et al, 1993) and will be discussed in the section on unexplained infertility.

Therapeutic Donor Insemination

Donor insemination involves timed insemination with semen from an anonymous or a known donor. Indications for donor insemination include azoospermia, severe male factor infertility, women without partners, and lesbian couples. Both the FDA and the CDC recommend the use of frozen semen to prevent sexually transmitted diseases, including hepatitis and human immunodeficiency virus. Using thawed sperm allows for an appropriate quarantine period to exclude infectious disease. Anonymous sperm is commercially available through sperm banks. Recently, "yes" donor sperm has become available through banks that allow disclosure of the donor at some future date. Couples are able to choose from detailed donor biographies that include physical and personal characteristics, medical history, ethnic background, and education. Intrauterine insemination significantly increases monthly fecundability compared with intracervical insemination (4% versus 18%) (Hurd et al, 1993). Therapeutic donor insemination should be continued for at least three to six cycles before consideration of additional fertility evaluation or treatment.

In Vitro Fertilization and Intracytoplasmic Sperm Injection

IVF and ICSI revolutionized the treatment of male factor infertility and have been discussed earlier in the section on assisted reproduction.

THE CERVICAL FACTOR AND IMMUNOLOGIC INFERTILITY

The uterine cervix has several important roles in reproduction and is often considered the gateway to the upper reproductive tract. During midcycle, cervical mucus facilitates the transport of spermatozoa. At other times during the menstrual cycle, cervical mucus functions as a barrier by preventing the passage of foreign material into the upper reproductive tract. The cervical factor is best defined as the midcycle interaction of spermatozoa and cervical mucus. Intrauterine insemination is the initial treatment for most couples with cervical factor infertility.

The Postcoital Test

The postcoital test (PCT) remains the standard for assessing the cervical factor and is often recommended early in the evaluation of infertility. However, there has been a recent, gradual elimination of the PCT from the routine evaluation of the infertile couple primarily because it lacks standardization and reproducibility, which has resulted in considerable disagreement regarding timing and interpretation. In addition, the increasing popularity of superovulation with intrauterine insemination has limited the usefulness of the PCT in guiding treatment options.

The PCT should be conducted as close to the time of ovulation as possible. The couple is instructed to abstain from intercourse for 2 days before the test. Douches or intravaginal medications should not be used during those 48 hours.

A nonlubricated speculum is inserted into the vagina, and a sample of cervical mucus is obtained. Techniques for collecting cervical mucus have been described. A long, narrow dressing forceps with a small oval aperture at the tip is often used. Alternatively, if the cervical os is too small to admit a metal instrument, an angiocatheter and a syringe may be used to aspirate a sample of cervical mucus. A flexible suction device called a mucus sampler has become available (Cheshire Medical Specialties, Cheshire, CT). The cervical mucus should be placed on a glass slide, covered with a coverslip, and examined under the microscope. Number of spermatozoa per high-power field, percentage of motility, and quality of forward progression should be noted. Whenever possible, the quality of the cervical mucus should be described.

The controversy regarding the timing of the PCT in relation to coitus has been addressed (Taymor and Overstreet, 1988). Several authors have recommended conducting the test 2 to 3 hours after coitus because this is when sperm concentration is highest (Davajan, 1985; Young et al, 1970). In contrast, many authors have recommended delaying the PCT until at least 6 hours after coitus, emphasizing the role of the cervix as a reservoir for spermatozoa. Moghissi (1976b) recommended performing the PCT initially at 6 to 8 hours after coitus. Taymor and Overstreet (1988) emphasize the importance of sperm longevity and the impracticality of having intercourse several hours before going to the physician's office. They recommend having intercourse "at bedtime" and performing the PCT 10 to 16 hours after

---

BOX 14-11
CAUSES OF ABNORMAL POSTCOITAL
TEST RESULTS

Male Factors

Oligospermia
Oligoasthenospermia
Sexual dysfunction

Abnormal Cervical Mucus

Poor timing
Hypoestrogenism
Cervical stenosis
Cervical varicosities
Cauterization or cryotherapy
Cervicitis
Cervical prolapse
Clomiphene citrate

Abnormal Sperm–Cervical Mucus Interaction

Idiopathic
Immunologic

---

coitus. Performing the PCT 10 to 16 hours after coitus allows greater flexibility in the timing of intercourse. If the initial PCT results are abnormal, earlier timing should be considered.

The clinical value of the PCT in predicting subsequent fertility is highly controversial. Well-designed prospective studies that demonstrate significant prognostic value for the PCT are balanced by equally well-designed studies that demonstrate no predictive value (Collins et al, 1984b; Hall et al, 1982; Jette and Glass, 1972). Lack of predictive value has been further supported by several laparoscopic studies in which peritoneal fluid was recovered at approximately the time of ovulation and examined for spermatozoa (Asch, 1976). Stone (1983) observed numerous motile sperm in the peritoneal fluid in 56% of patients with poor to absent cervical mucus and repetitively poor PCT results (fewer than five sperm per HPF). In contrast, sperm was recovered from only 53% of control subjects with normal PCT results. Thus, several studies highlight the limitations of the PCT in the evaluation of sperm migration and sperm longevity.

There is also debate about what constitutes a normal PCT result. Moghissi's (1976b) criterion for a normal PCT result is 10 or more sperm with directional motility per high-power field. Several other investigators contend that five or more actively motile sperm per high-power field may be considered satisfactory (Davajan and Kunitake, 1969; Treadway et al, 1975). Jette and Glass (1972) have observed that a PCT result with more than 20 motile sperm per high-power field is associated with an increased likelihood of pregnancy and an analysis that reveals normal semen. Although often quoted, these authors have emphasized that no specific num-

ber of motile spermatozoa in the PCT result should be judged as normal. Interpretation of the PCT result is further complicated by the difficulty in determining the day of ovulation. So-called abnormal cervical mucus is often the result of inaccurate timing with respect to ovulation.

The multiple causes of an abnormal PCT result are listed in Box 14-11. Persistently abnormal PCT results suggest oligoasthenospermia, abnormal cervical mucus, faulty coital technique, or abnormal cervical mucus–spermatozoa interaction. Male factor infertility is often suggested when multiple abnormal PCT results are associated with persistently abnormal semen analysis results.

Abnormal cervical mucus may have hormonal, anatomic, or infectious causes. Any hypoestrogenic state may be associated with unfavorable cervical mucus. Subtle abnormalities in follicular maturation may lead to a relatively low level of preovulatory estradiol and abnormal cervical mucus. Clomiphene citrate has been clearly associated with poor PCT results (Graff, 1971; Maxson et al, 1984). The mechanism may be related to an antiestrogen effect at the level of the cervix. Anatomic defects that may contribute to abnormal cervical mucus include the hypoplastic cervix and cervical stenosis. Anatomic variations in the position of the cervix are unlikely to contribute to a poor PCT result. Varicosities of the hypoplastic endocervical canal have been associated with extreme friability and scant cervical mucus (Scott et al, 1977). Cervical stenosis may be associated with scant cervical mucus and is often the result of previous cervical conization. Extensive cauterization or cryotherapy of the endocervix, significant cervical prolapse, and acute and chronic cervicitis may also be associated with abnormal cervical mucus. Faulty coital technique may be suspected when semen analysis results and cervical mucus are relatively normal and there are no spermatozoa seen on the PCT. This may be the result of male or female sexual dysfunction such as impotence, premature or retrograde ejaculation, or vaginismus. In addition, the partners of extremely obese women may not be able to penetrate the vagina fully and deposit their semen in the posterior fornix.

Abnormal cervical mucus sperm interaction is often suggested when the PCT result is poor and the cervical mucus and semen analysis results are normal. In most cases no specific cause can be identified. However, an immunologic cause should be suspected when spermatozoa are immotile, shake, or display poor forward progression.

The immunology of the male and female reproductive tract has been reviewed (Alexander and Anderson, 1987; Hill and Anderson, 1988). Cellular and humoral immunity appear to contribute to reproductive failure. Soluble products of macrophages and lymphocytes inhibit sperm motility and penetrability in vitro (Hill et al, 1989; Hill et al, 1987). Clinically there appears to be a relationship between immunity to sperm and infertility (Bronson et al, 1984; Haas et al, 1980; Menge et al, 1982).

Antisperm antibodies have been isolated from semen, cervical mucus, and male and female serum. These antibod-

---

BOX 14-12
TESTS FOR DETECTING SPERM IMMUNITY

Isojima Immobilization Test (Complement-Dependent Cytotoxity)

Measures the ratio of motile sperm in control and test serum
Test of IgG, IgM (IgAs do not fix complement)
Highly specific; lacks sensitivity (false-negative results common)

Kibrick, Friberg-Trey Agglutination Test (Sperm Agglutination)

Classic serum test measures agglutinating antibodies
False-positives results from nonspecific binding

Enzyme-Linked Immunosorbent Assay

Antiglobulin binds to human immunoglobulin on sperm surface
False positives and false negatives result from fixation process and membrane damage (*i.e.,* membrane extracts may not contain relevant antigens)

Fluorescein-Conjugated Antiglobulins

False-positive results common

Radiolabeled Antiglobulin Assay

High specificity and sensitivity when used with living sperm
Does not determine regional specificity of binding
Does not determine proportion of antibody-bound sperm

Mixed Agglutination Reaction

Uses sensitized Rh-positive red blood cells and IgG antiglobulin
Limitations similar to those of radiolabeled antiglobulin assay

Immunobead Test

Detects sperm coating immunoglobulins in seminal plasma and cervical mucus
Subclass specific (IgM, IgG, IgA)
Can determine regional specificity
Can determine proportion of antibody-bound sperm

From Bronson R, Cooper G, Rosenfeld D, et al: Sperm antibodies: Their role in infertility. *Fertil Steril* 1984; 42:171.

---

ies may be secreted locally within the reproductive tract or they may be associated with circulating serum antibodies (Hall et al, 1982; Uehling, 1971). The presence of sperm antibodies in semen and cervical mucus is more strongly associated with reproductive impairment than their presence in serum. There is also a lack of correlation between the levels of antisperm antibodies in serum and cervical mucus (Stern, 1992b). Precisely how antisperm antibodies contribute to in-

fertility remains to be elucidated, but they may interfere with sperm transport, gamete interaction, and macrophage phagocytosis (Bronson et al, 1981; London et al, 1984).

Bronson et al (1984) have emphasized that immunity to sperm is not an all-or-nothing phenomenon. The extent to which antisperm antibodies are present in the reproductive tract appears to influence the degree of fertility impairment. For example, when less than 50% of sperm is antibody bound, the number of motile sperm in the PCT is no different from that in antibody-negative couples (Bronson et al, 1984). In addition, spontaneous remission of immunity to sperm has been reported (Bronson et al, 1984). The etiology of antisperm antibodies appears to be multifactorial. An increased incidence has been associated with vasectomy (Shulman et al, 1972), genital tract infections (Witkins and Toth, 1983), and gastrointestinal exposure to sperm (Bronson et al, 1984).

A relationship between decreased fertility and antisperm antibodies has been more clearly established in men than in women. In a study of 254 infertile men, Rumke et al (1974) demonstrated that the prognosis for future pregnancy was inversely correlated with antibody titers. Ayvaliotis et al (1985) have shown that when more than 50% of the spermatozoa in the ejaculate are found to have surface-bound immunoglobulins, the pregnancy rate is 15%; in comparison, the rate is 67% when less than 50% of the sperm are antibody bound. The role of immunologic factors in the cervical mucus and upper reproductive tract remains unclear.

Several different assays for the detection of antisperm antibodies have been described. The incidence of abnormal test results varies according to the patient population, the test, and the titer that is considered abnormal. The Isojima immobilization test result is abnormal in 5% to 10% of women with unexplained infertility (Isojima et al, 1968). Although no single assay has proved to be superior, the immunobead assay is the most popular because it determines the proportion of antibody-bound sperm, immunoglobin subclass specificity, and localization of sperm attachment.

A brief description and the relative advantages and disadvantages of several of the tests for antisperm antibodies are outlined in Box 14-12. As with the postcoital test, the clinical usefulness of measuring antisperm antibodies is often challenged. Although the presence of antisperm antibodies may influence physician counseling, antibody testing continues to lack any clear predictive value and rarely has an impact on subsequent treatment options.

TREATMENT OF CERVICAL FACTOR AND IMMUNOLOGIC INFERTILITY
Intrauterine Insemination

Intrauterine insemination (IUI) with or without ovulation induction agents is the initial treatment for most couples with cervical factor infertility. This technique is more successful in the treatment of cervical factor infertility than in the treatment of male factor infertility and unexplained infertility.

BOX 14-13
TREATMENT OF UNEXPLAINED AND CERVICAL FACTOR INFERTILITY

Step 1　Consider expectant management with timed intercourse in female patients younger than 32 years old.
Step 2　Consider empiric clomiphene with or without intrauterine inseminations.
or
Consider intrauterine inseminations with or without clomiphene.
Step 3　Consider empiric gonadotropin therapy with intrauterine insemination.
Step 4　Consider assisted reproduction with in vitro fertilization or gamete intrafallopian tube transfer.

However, studies reveal conflicting data and are generally limited by poor study designs. Treatment with IUI with or without ovulation induction agents is usually recommended for three to six cycles before consideration of alternative treatment options. Our approach to cervical factor infertility is identical to our empiric approach to unexplained infertility (Box 14-13) largely because of our abandonment of the PCT. The reported fecundability for IUI among patients with cervical factor infertility ranges from 0.05 to more than 0.20. Combination treatment with ovarian stimulation and IUI increases fecundability with cervical factor infertility and immunologic infertility (Nulsen et al, 1993). This will be further discussed in the section on unexplained infertility.

Treatment of Antisperm Antibodies

A variety of treatments have been proposed for couples with antisperm antibodies. These include condom use in an attempt to reduce antigenic stimuli (Franklin and Dukes, 1964); immunosuppressive glucocorticoid therapy (Alexander et al, 1983); sperm washing and intrauterine inseminations (Haas et al, 1988; Margalioth et al, 1988); and assisted reproduction. In the absence of assisted reproduction, there are limited data to support the efficacy and safety of the remainder of these treatment options. Both IVF and GIFT appear to be effective approaches to immunologic infertility. Acosta et al (1989) reported an overall fertilization rate of 82% and an ongoing pregnancy rate per cycle of 22% among patients with antisperm antibodies. Van der Merwe et al (1990) reported a 43% ongoing pregnancy rate with GIFT among 16 couples with immunologic infertility.

UTERINE FACTORS

Although uterine abnormalities are often associated with recurrent pregnancy loss, they are not generally considered a cause of infertility. The association between uterine factors

and infertility remains unclear because the hormonal and immunologic prerequisites for normal implantation and early embryo development are poorly understood.

Transvaginal ultrasonography is an excellent method for identifying uterine abnormalities. Unfortunately, ultrasound evaluation of the uterine cavity is limited. Several studies have demonstrated the superior diagnostic capability of hysteroscopy in detecting intracavitary disease compared with standard transvaginal ultrasonography. However, the accuracy of transvaginal ultrasonography can be dramatically improved with the instillation of saline into the uterine cavity. This relatively new diagnostic modality is referred to as sonohysterography (SHSG).

Sonohysterography is generally performed in the middle to late follicular phase. Saline solution is injected into the uterine cavity and provides a negative contrast during transvaginal ultrasonography. Various techniques have been described, usually involving the placement of an intrauterine catheter for saline infusion. Between 3 and 10 mL of slowly infused saline is generally required for uterine distention. After adequate distention, the cavity is examined in the sagittal and the coronal views. SHSG appears to be more accurate than HSG, and its sensitivity and specificity are comparable to those of hysteroscopy. Additionally, it provides information regarding the relative proportions and locations of the intracavitary abnormalities. Cincinelli et al (1995) reported that SHSG measured myoma size more accurately than hysteroscopy. Another suggested benefit of SHSG is the precise estimation of the percentage of intracavitary versus intramural myoma extension. Magnetic resonance imaging may be used to diagnose uterine abnormalities accurately (Woodward, 1993). The preferred approach to the evaluation of a suspected uterine factor depends on the physician and is often determined by the availability of the necessary equipment and by convenience and cost.

Any association between DES exposure and infertility may be partially the result of uterine factors and impaired implantation (Ayvaliotis et al, 1985). The relationship between DES and infertility remains controversial. Several investigators have reported an increased incidence of infertility in DES-exposed women (Berger and Alper, 1986; Bibbo et al, 1977; Herbst et al, 1980; Kaufman et al, 1986). In contrast, other investigators have reported no significant difference (Barnes et al, 1980; Cousins et al, 1980). These conflicting results probably are related to confounding factors and inadequate control groups. Nevertheless, many DES-exposed women have associated abnormalities that are presumed to be the cause of their infertility. DES exposure is not only associated with abnormal uterine contours but with an increased incidence of tubal disease, endometriosis, and cervical factor infertility (Cramer et al, 1986; Stillman and Hershlag, 1987).

Uterine leiomyomas or myomas are often implicated as a cause of infertility, even though well-controlled epidemiologic and clinical studies are lacking. A review of the literature suggests that by themselves myomas rarely cause infertility. In fact, Buttram and Reiter (1981) estimated that myomas alone were responsible for difficulties in conception in only approximately 2% of infertile couples.

There are several mechanisms, however, by which myomas may cause infertility (Buttram and Reiter, 1981). Myomas located within the uterine cavity (submucous myomas) may reduce the likelihood of successful implantation. Myomas located near the uterotubal junction may cause tubal obstruction. Large myomas may distort the normal anatomic relationship between the fallopian tube and the ovary. Some investigators have suggested that myomas interfere with sperm transport. Regardless of the mechanism, the anatomic location and the individual size of myomas appear critical when evaluating the potential relationship between uterine myomas and infertility.

Counseling patients with uterine myomas and infertility remains a major challenge because of the paucity of well-designed clinical trials. Our approach to patients with uterine myomas and infertility is to exclude the common causes of infertility, such as ovulatory, tubal, and male factor infertility. All patients with myomas should be educated about specific risks during pregnancy, including miscarriage, pelvic pain, premature labor, and postpartum hemorrhage. In the absence of other causes of infertility or after the unsuccessful treatment of other infertility factors, it is reasonable to suggest myomectomy as an option. Most patients can be treated without surgery.

Several investigators have suggested that anatomic location may be more important than myoma size. Farhi et al (1995) suggested that myomas that distort the uterine cavity are associated with decreased fecundability. Conventional sonography, sonohysterography, magnetic resonance imaging, and hysteroscopy may be helpful in identifying the specific location of individual myomas. Widely ranging crude pregnancy rates have been reported after myomectomy. Term pregnancy rates ranging from 16% to 60% appear to be partially influenced by patient age, number and size of myomas removed, and uterine size before surgery (Buttram and Reiter, 1981; Babakina, 1978; Rosenfeld, 1986; Berkeley et al, 1983; Corsonn and Brooks, 1991).

Congenital uterine anomalies such as uterus didelphys and septate uterus are also more commonly associated with mid-trimester pregnancy loss and early fetal wastage than infertility. HSG or hysteroscopy alone cannot accurately differentiate between bicornuate and septate uteri (Fig. 14-10). Concomitant laparoscopy and hysteroscopy should be recommended to patients with suspected müllerian anomalies on HSG. Kidney evaluation with either ultrasonography or intravenous pyelography should be performed because of the association with renal tract abnormalities.

Asherman syndrome (intrauterine synechiae) is associated with amenorrhea, menstrual irregularities, habitual abortion, and poor obstetric outcome. It also may be associated with infertility. Patients with severe intrauterine adhesions may have mechanical obstruction of sperm migration and an unfavorable endometrial environment for implanta-

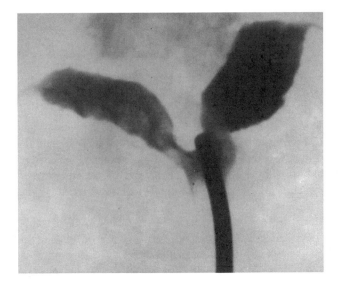

Fig. 14-10. Hysterosalpingogram demonstrates a congenital uterine anomaly. This may represent a bicornuate uterus or a uterine septum. Laparoscopy and hysteroscopic visualization of the external and internal uterine surface are required to distinguish these two entities.

tion (Sohenker and Margalioth, 1982). The reproductive outcome after hysteroscopic adhesiolysis appears to be dependent on the severity of the adhesions; live birth rates range between 25% and 50% (Valle and Sciarra, 1988; March et al, 1978).

Although the significance of uterine factors may be difficult to determine, women at high risk for intrauterine disease require further evaluation. HSG is considered an excellent screening test for uterine factors because false-negative diagnoses are uncommon. The diagnostic accuracy of HSG for the evaluation of uterine factors has been evaluated in many studies that compare HSG and hysteroscopy (Fayez et al, 1987; Taylor, 1977; Valle, 1980). Hysteroscopy remains the criterion for evaluating the uterine cavity, and it is required to confirm and treat suspicious diagnoses. However, hysteroscopy should not be recommended routinely as part of the infertility evaluation.

UNEXPLAINED INFERTILITY

Perhaps the most frustrated patients, and the most frustrating to take care of, are couples with unexplained infertility. Moghissi and Wallach (1983) defined unexplained infertility as occurring in "any couple who has failed to establish a pregnancy despite an evaluation that uncovers no obvious reason for infertility or after correction of the factor(s) identified as responsible for the infertility." The incidence of unexplained infertility appears to be decreasing, and it is estimated to be approximately 15% (Collins and Crosignani, 1992; Templeton and Penny, 1982). Although unexplained infertility may represent the inability of diagnostic tests to identify a potential cause, alternatively it may represent a lack of understanding of some aspect of the reproductive process.

Coulam et al (1988) suggested that additional tests may reduce the incidence of unexplained infertility. If the initial evaluation is normal, additional testing may be considered. However, when the infertility evaluation fails to identify a particular cause, empiric therapy should be considered. Studies evaluating the efficacy of ovarian stimulation and IUI for unexplained infertility have revealed conflicting results. Compared to the literature on cervical and male factor infertility, there is a reasonable number of randomized controlled trials evaluating the efficacy of superovulation and IUI for unexplained infertility.

Glazener (1990) performed a randomized placebo-controlled trial of clomiphene in 118 women with unexplained infertility. Although the difference in monthly fecundability was small (0.07 versus 0.05 for the placebo group), the 3-month cumulative probability of pregnancy was significantly higher with clomiphene treatment (22% versus 15%). Deaton (1990) reported a placebo-controlled trial of clomiphene citrate plus IUI in 67 couples with unexplained infertility or early-stage endometriosis. Patients treated with clomiphene citrate plus IUI experienced significantly higher fecundability (0.095) than did placebo-treated controls (0.033). In a large cohort study, Dicky reported a similar fecundability (0.072) with 1974 cycles of clomiphene citrate plus IUI among 849 women with various diagnoses.

Serhal (1988) published one of the first randomized controlled trials of empiric treatment for unexplained infertility. In this study, 62 women were randomized to IUI alone, hMG alone, or the combination of hMG plus IUI. Although this trial was limited by a small number of patients in each treatment group, the monthly fecundability rates were 0.022, 0.061, and 0.264 respectively, suggesting that the combination of hMG plus IUI is associated with a superior rate of success. Similar results have been reported by others (Sher et al, 1984; Dodson et al, 1987).

Several other investigators reported that treatment of unexplained infertility with ovarian stimulation and IUI is superior to treatment with IUI alone. The randomized controlled trial by Arcaini (1996) suggests the addition of IUI to hMG treatment improves the probability of success. Arici et al (1994) reported a higher pregnancy rate per cycle with clomiphene citrate plus IUI versus IUI alone (0.26 versus 0.05). In contrast, Melis et al (1995) and Karlstrom et al (1993) reported that IUI did not increase fecundability in couples with unexplained infertility treated with ovarian stimulation. The frequency of IUI (*i.e.,* one versus two per cycle) during treatment with superovulation has also generated some debate based on conflicting studies (Ransom et al, 1994; Silverburg, 1992).

Our empiric staircase approach to unexplained infertility is similar to our approach to mild male factor infertility, cervical factor infertility, and early-stage endometriosis (Box 14-13). Individual treatments should be recommended for no more than three to six cycles. Our approach attempts to balance efficacy, safety, and risk with the cost of individual treatment options. The literature suggests that the efficacy of IVF and GIFT is superior to ovarian stimulation plus IUI, which is superior to ovarian stimulation or IUI alone (Peterson et al, 1994).

SUMMARY

A modern approach to the infertile couple is quite simple. An efficient and systematic evaluation should begin with an assessment of male, tubal, and ovulatory factors. This most commonly involves a semen analysis and hysterosalpingogram. A hormonal evaluation including day 3 FSH, TSH, and prolactin levels should be recommended to patients with irregular or absent menstrual cycles suggestive of oligo- or anovulation. Ovarian reserve testing should also be considered, particularly in women older than 35 years of age. The role of laparoscopy continues to evolve and should be considered after the initial evaluation to rule out endometriosis-associated infertility. In the majority of cases, the probable cause or causes of infertility can be determined.

Fecundability, the probability of conceiving during a monthly cycle, provides an estimate of the efficacy of various fertility treatments. Combined with a consideration of clinical characteristics and maternal age, the fecundability of various treatment options should assist both patients and providers in choosing an optimal treatment plan. Our staircase approach to infertility treatment attempts to balance the probability of success with risk, invasiveness, and cost. The staircase approach requires regular follow-up visits to provide couples with updated treatment options and realistic prognoses. A comprehensive approach to the infertile couple should also include emotional support.

REFERENCES

Abdel GA, Mowafi R, Alnase J, et al: Ovarian electrocautery versus human menopausal gonadotropins and pure follicle stimulating hormone therapy in the treatment of patients with polycystic ovarian disease. *Clin Endocrinol* 1990; 33:585-592.

Aboulghar MA, Mansour RT, Serour GI, et al: Prospective controlled randomized study of in vitro fertilization versus intracytoplasmic sperm injection in the treatment of tubal factor infertility with normal semen parameters. *Fertil Steril* 1996; 66:753-756.

Acosta AA, Oehninger S, Morshed M, et al: Assisted reproduction and the diagnosis and treatment of the male factor. *Obstet Gynecol Surv* 1989; 44:1.

Adams R, Mishell DR Jr, Israel R: Treatment of refractory anovulation with increased dosage and prolonged duration of cyclic clomiphene citrate. *Obstet Gynecol* 1972; 39:562.

Adamson GD: Laparoscopic treatment is better than medical treatment for minimal or mild endometriosis. *Int J Fertil* 1996; 41:396-399.

Adamson GD, Hurd SJ, Pasta DJ: Laparoscopic endometriosis treatment: Is it better? *Fertil Steril* 1993; 59:35-44.

Adashi EY: Clomiphene citrate mechanism(s) and site(s) of action: A hypothesis revisited. *Fertil Steril* 1984; 42:331.

Adashi EY, et al : Gestational outcome of clomiphene-related conceptions. *Fertil Steril* 1979; 31:620.

Ahlgren M, Källen B, Rannevik G: Outcome of pregnancy after Clomid therapy. *Acta Obstet Gynecol Scand* 1976; 53:671.

Aitken RJ, et al: A prospective study of the relationship between semen quality and fertility in cases of unexplained infertility. *J Androl* 1984; 5:297.

Alexander NJ, Sampson JH, Fulgham DL: Pregnancy rates in patients treated for antisperm antibodies with prednisone. *Int J Fertil* 1983; 28:63-67.

Alexander NT, Anderson DJ: Immunology of semen. *Fertil Steril* 1987; 47:192.

Allahbadia GN: Fallopian tubes and ultrasonography: The Sion experience. *Fertil Steril* 1992; 58:901.

Alper MA, et al: Pregnancy rates after hysterosalpingography with oil and water-soluble contrast media. *Obstet Gynecol* 1986; 68:6.

American Fertility Society: The American Fertility Society classifications of adnexal adhesions, distal tubal occlusion, robot occlusion secondary to tubal ligation, tubal pregnancies, muellerian anomalies and intrauterine adhesions. *Fertil Steril* 1988; 49:944.

Andrews WC, Larsen GD: Endometriosis: Treatment with hormonal pseudopregnancy and/or operation. *Am J Obstet Gynecol* 1974; 118:643.

Arcaini L, Bianchi S, Baglioni A, et al: Superovulation and intrauterine insemination vs superovulation alone in the treatment of unexplained infertility *J Reprod Med* 1996; 41:614-618.

Arici A, Byrd W, Bradshaw K, et al: Evaluation of clomiphene citrate and human chorionic gonadotropin treatment: A prospective randomized crossover study during intrauterine insemination cycles. *Fertil Steril* 1994; 61: 314-318.

Asch RH: Laparoscopic recovery of sperm from peritoneal fluid in patients with negative or poor Sims-Huhner test. *Fertil Steril* 1976; 27:1111.

Asch RH, et al: Gamete intrafallopian transfer (GIFT): A new treatment for infertility. *Int J Fertil* 1985; 30:41-45.

Ayvaliotis B, et al: Conception rates in couples where autoimmunity to sperm is detected. *Fertil Steril* 1985; 43:739.

Azziz R, Zacur HA: 21-Hydroxylase deficiency in female hyperandrogenism: Screening and diagnosis. *J Clin Endocrinol Metab* 1989; 69:577.

Babaknia A, Rock JA, Jones WH Jr: Pregnancy success following abdominal myomectomy for infertility. *Fertil Steril* 1978; 30:644-647.

Barnes AB, Colton T, Gundersen J, et al: Fertility and outcome of pregnancy in women exposed in utero to diethylstilbestrol. *N Engl J Med* 1980; 302:609.

Bateman BG, Nunley WC Jr, Kitchin JD: Intravasation during hysterosalpingography using oil-base contrast media. *Fertil Steril.*, 1980; 34:439.

Batista MC, et al: Midluteal phase endometrial biopsy does not accurately predict luteal function. *Fertil Steril* 1993; 59:294.

Battin DA, et al: In vitro fertilization rates of male factor patients. *Fertil Steril* 1984; 41:42S.

Bauman JE: Basal body temperature: Unreliable method of ovulation detection. *Fertil Steril* 1981; 36:729.

Bedford JM, Best MJ, Calvin H: Variations in the structural character and stability of nuclear chromatic in morphologically normal human spermatozoa. *J Reprod Fertil* 1973; 33:19.

Belker AM, Thomas AJ, Fuchs EF, et al: Results of 1469 microsurgical vasectomy reversals by the vasovasostomy study group. *J Urol* 1991; 145:505-511.

Bell SC, et al: Protein synthesis and secretion by the human endometrium during the menstrual cycle and effect of progesterone in vitro. *J Reprod Fertil* 1986; 77:221.

Ben-Chetrit A, Senoz S, Greenblatt EM, Casper RF: In vitro fertilization outcome in the presence of severe male factor infertility. *Fertil Steril* 1995; 63:1032-1037.

Berger M, Alper M: Intractable primary infertility in women exposed to diethylstilbestrol in utero. *J Reprod Med* 1986; 31:231.

Berkeley AS, DeCherney AH, Polan ML: Abdominal myomectomy and subsequent fertility. *Surg Gynecol Obstet* 1983; 156:319-322.

Berkowitz RL, Lynch L, Stone J, Alvarez M: The current status of multifetal pregnancy reduction. *Am J Obstet Gynecol* 1996; 174:1265-1272.

Bibbo M, et al: Follow-up study of male and female offspring of DES exposed mothers. *Obstet Gynecol* 1977; 49:1.

Blackwell JM, Zaneveld LJD: Effect of abstinence on sperm acrosin, hypoosmotic swelling, and other semen variables. *Fertil Steril* 1992; 58:798.

Boeckx W, et al: Reversibility after female sterilization. *Br J Obstet Gynecol* 1986; 93:839-842.

Bollen N, Camus M, Tournaye H, et al: Embryo reduction in triplet pregnancies after assisted procreation: A comparative study. *Fertil Steril* 1993; 60:504-509.

Borenstein R, Elhalah U, Luenfeld B, Schwartz ZS: Severe ovarian hyperstimulation syndrome: A reevaluated therapeutic approach. *Fertil Steril* 1989; 51:791-795.

Bostofte E, Serup J, Rebbe H: The clinical value of morphological rating of human spermatozoa. *Int J Fertil* 1985; 30:31.

Bostofte E, Serup J, Rebbe H: Relation between sperm count and semen volume, and pregnancies obtained during a 20-year follow-up period. *Int J Androl* 1982; 5:267.

Bristow RE, Karlan BY: Ovulation induction, infertility, and ovarian cancer risk. *Fertil Steril* 1996; 66:507.

Bronson R, Cooper G, Rosenfeld D: Ability of antibody-bound human sperm to penetrate zona-free hamster ova in vitro. *Fertil Steril* 1981; 36:778.

Bronson R, Cooper G, Rosenfeld D: Sperm antibodies: Their role in infertility. *Fertil Steril* 1984; 42:171.

Burkman LJ, et al: The hemizona assay (HZA): Development of a diagnostic test for the binding of human spermatozoa to the hemizona pellucida to predict fertilization potential. *Fertil Steril* 1985; 43:739.

Bustillo M, Schulman JD: Transcervical ultrasound-guided intrafallopian replacement of gametes, zygotes, and embryos. *J In Vitro Fert Embryo Transf* 1989; 6:321.

Buttram VC: Evolution of the revised American Fertility Society's classification of endometriosis. *Fertil Steril*, 1985; 43:347.

Buttram VC, Reiter RC: Uterine leiomyomata: Etiology, symptomatology, and management. *Fertil Steril* 1981; 36:433-445.

Buxton CL, Herrman WL: Effect of thyroid hormone on menstrual disorders and sterility. *JAMA* 1954; 155:1035.

Campana A, Sakkas D, Stalberg A, et al: Intrauterine insemination: Evaluation of the results according to the woman's age, sperm quality, total sperm count per insemination and life table analysis. *Hum Reprod* 1996; 11:732-736.

Catt J, Ryan J, Pike I, O'Neil C: Fertilization rates using intracytoplasmic sperm injection are greater than subzonal insemination but are dependent on prior treatmenet of sperm. *Fertil Steril* 1995; 64:764-769.

Chiari H: zur Pathologischen Anatomie des Eileitercatarrha. *A Heilkunde* 1887; 8:457.

Chillon M, Casals T, Mercier B, et al: Mutations in the cystic fibrosis gene in patients with congenital absence of the vas deferens. *N Engl J Med* 1995; 332:1475-1480.

Chong AP, Keene ME, Thorton NL: Comparison of three modes of treatment for infertility patients with minimal pelvic endometriosis. *Fertil Steril* 1990; 53:407-410.

Chopra IJ, Tulchinsky D: Status of estrogen-androgen balance in hyperthyroid men with Grave's disease. *J Clin Endocrinol Metab* 1974; 38:269.

Cicinelli E, et al: Transabdominal sonohysterography, transvaginal sonography, and hysteroscopy in the evaluation of submucous myomas. *Obstet Gynecol* 1995; 85:42-47.

Claman P, Domingo M, Garner P, et al: Natural cycle in vitro fertilization embryo transfer at the University of Ottawa: An inefficient therapy for tubal infertility. *Fertil Steril* 1993; 60:298-302.

Claus-Walker J, Scurry M, Carter RE, Campos RJ: Steady state hormonal secretion in traumatic quadriplegia. *J Clin Endocrinal Metab* 1977; 44:530.

Cohen J, Alikani M, Trowbridge J, Rosenwaks Z: Implantation enhancement by selective assisted hatching using zona drilling of embryos with poor prognosis. *Human Reprod* 1992; 7:685-691.

Collins, JA: Diagnostic assessment of infertile female partner. *Curr Probl Obstet Gynecol Fertil* 1988b; 11:27.

Collins JA: Unexplained infertility. In Keye WR, Chang RJ, Rebar RW, Soules MR, editors. *Infertility: Evaluation and treatment,* Philadelphia, 1995, WB Saunders.

Collins JA, et al: A proportional hazards analysis of the clinical characteristics of infertile couples. *Am J Obstet Gynecol* 1984a; 148:527.

Collins JA, et al: The postcoital test as a predictor of pregnancy among 355 infertile couples. *Fertil Steril* 1984b; 41:703.

Collins JA, Burrows EA, Willan AR: Occupation and the follow-up of infertile couples. *Fertil Steril* 1993; 60:477.

Collins JA, Crosignani PG: Unexplained infertility: A review of diagnosis, prognosis, treatment efficacy, and management. *Int J Gynecol Obstet* 1992; 39:267.

Corson SL, Brooks PG: Resectoscopic myomectomy. *Fertil Steril* 1991; 55:1041.

Coulam CB, Moore SB, O'Fallon W: Investigating unexplained infertility. *Am J Obstet Gynecol* 1988; 158:1374.

Cousins L, et al: Reproductive outcome of women exposed to diethylstilbestrol in utero. *Obstet Gynecol* 1980; 56:70.

Cramer DW, Walker AN, Schiff I: Statistical methods in evaluating the outcome of infertility therapy. *Fertil Steril* 1979; 32:80.

Cramer DW, et al: Association of endometriosis with maternal diethylstilbestrol (DES) exposure. *Fertil Steril* 1986; 65:185.

Cramer DW, et al: The relation of endometriosis to menstrual characteristics, smoking, and exercise. *JAMA* 1986; 255:1904.

Cruz RI, Kemmann E, Brandeis VT, et al: A prospective study of intrauterine insemination of processed sperm from men with oligoasthenospermia in superovulated women. *Fertil Steril* 1986; 46:673-677.

Daly DC, et al: Endometrial biopsy during treatment of luteal phase defects is predictive of therapeutic outcome. *Fertil Steril* 1983; 40:305.

Daly DC, Walters CA, Soto-Albors CE, et al: A randomized study of dexamethasone in ovulation induction with clomiphene citrate. *Fertil Steril* 1984; 41:844-848.

Damewood MD: The role of new reproductive technologies including IVF and GIFT in endometriosis. *Obstet Gynecol Clin North Am* 1989; 16:179-191.

Daniell JF, Miller W: Polycystic ovaries treated by laparoscopic laser vaporization. *Fertil Steril* 1989; 51:232-233.

Davajan V: Postcoital testing. In Mishell DR, Davajan V, editors: *Infertility, contraception, and reproductive endocrinology*, Oradell, N.J., 1985, Medical Economics.

Davajan V, Kunitake GM: Fractional in vitro and in vitro examination of postcoital cervical mucus in the human. *Fertil Steril* 1969; 20:197.

Davis OK, et al: The incidence of luteal phase defect in normal fertile women, determined by serial endometrial biopsies. *Fertil Steril* 1989; 51:582.

Daya S, Gunby J, Hughes EG, et al: Follicle-stimulating hormone versus human menopausal gonadotropin for in vitro fertilization cycles: A meta-analysis. *Fertil Steril* 1995; 64:347-354.

Daya S, Ward S, Burrows E: Progesterone profiles in luteal phase deficient cycles and outcome of progesterone treatment in patients with recurrent spontaneous abortion. *Am J Obstet Gynecol* 1988; 158:225.

Deaton JL, Gibson M, Blackmer KM, et al: A randomized controlled trial of clomiphene citrate and intrauterine insemination in couples with unexplained infertility or surgically corrected endometriosis. *Fertil Steril* 1990; 54:1083-1088.

De Boer AD, Vemer HN, Willemsen WN, Sanders FB: Oil or aqueous contrast media for hysterosalpingography: A prospective randomized clinical study. *Eur J Obstet Gynecol Reprod Biol* 1988; 28:65-68.

DeCherney AH, et al: Increased pregnancy rate with oil soluble hysterosalpingography dye. *Fertil Steril* 1980; 33:407.

Deichert U, et al: Transvaginal hysterosalpingo-contrast sonography for the assessment of tubal patency with gray scale imaging and additional use of pulsed wave Doppler. *Fertil Steril* 1992; 57:62-67.

Denil J, Ohl DA, McGuire EJ, Jonas U: Treatment of an ejaculation with electroejaculation. *Acta Urol Belg* 1992; 60:15-25.

Dlugi AM, Reddy S, Saleh WA, et al: Pregnancy rates after operative endoscopic treatment of total or near total distal tubal occlusion. *Fertil Steril* 1994; 62:913-920.

Dodson WC, Whiteside DB, Hughes CL, et al: Superovulation with intrauterine insemination in the treatment of infertility: A possible alternative to gamete intrafallopian transfer and in vitro fertilization. *Fertil Steril* 1987; 48:441-445.

Dor J, et al: Cumulative conception rates following gonadotroopin therapy. *Am J Obstet Gynecol* 1980; 136:102.

Dor J, Homburg R, Rabau E: An evaluation of etiologic factors and therapy in 665 infertile couples. *Fertil Steril* 1977; 28:718.

Downs KA, Gibson M: Basal body temperature graph and the luteal phase defect. *Fertil Steril* 1983; 40:446.

Drake TS, Tredway DR, Buchanan GC: Continued clinical experience with an increasing dosage regimen of clomiphene citrate administration. *Fertil Steril* 1978; 30:274.

Elkind-Hirsch K, et al: Evaluation of the Ovu-Stick urinary luteinizing hormone kit in normal and stimulated menstrual cycles. *Obstet Gynecol* 1986; 67:450.

El Minawi ME, et al: Comparative evaluation of laparoscopy and hysterosalpingography in infertile patients. *Obstet Gynecol* 1978; 51:29.

Farhi J, Ashkenazi J, Feldberg D, et al: Effect of uterine leiomyomata on results of IVF treatment. *Hum Reprod*, 1995; 10:2576-2578.

Fayez JA, Mutie G, Schneider PJ: The diagnostic value of hysterosalpingography and hysteroscopy in infertility investigation. *Am J Obstet Gynecol* 1987; 156:558.

Fedele L, Bianchi S, Marchini M, et al: Superovulation with human menopausal gonadotropins in the treatment of infertility associated with minimal or mild endometriosis. *Fertil Steril* 1992; 58:28-31.

Fedele L, Parazzini F, Radici E: Buserelin acetate versus expectant management in the treatment of infertility associated with minimal or mild endometriosis: A randomized clincal trial. *Am J Obstet Gynecol* 1992b; 166:1345-1350.

Fernando RS, Regas J, Betz G: Prediction of ovulation with the use of oral and vaginal electrical measurements during treatment with clomiphene citrate. *Fertil Steril* 1987; 47:409.

Filcori M, Butler JP, Crowley WF: Neuroendocrine regulation of the corpus luteum in the human: Evidence for pulsatile progesterone secretion. *J Clin Invest* 1984; 73:1638.

Finkel DM, Phillips JL, Synder PJ: Stimulation of spermatogenesis by gonadotropins in men with hypogonadotropic hypogonadism. *N Engl J Med* 1985; 313:651-655.

Fishman J, et al: Effect of thyroid on hydroxylation of estrogen in man. *J Clin Endocrinol Metab* 1965; 25:365.

Fishman J, Jellman L, Zumoff B: Influence of thyroid hormone on estrogen metabolism in man. *J Clin Endocrinol Metab* 1962; 22:389.

Fluker MR, Zouves CG, Bebbington MW: A prospective randomized comparison of zygote intrafallopian transfer and in vitro fertilization—embryo transfer for non-tubal factor infertility *Fertil Steril* 1993; 60:515-9.

Forman RG, Frydman R, Egan D, et al: Severe ovarian hyperstimulation syndrome using agonists of gonadotropin-releasing hormone for in vitro fertilization: A European series and a proposal for prevention. *Fertil Steril* 1990; 53:502-509.

Francavilla F, Romano R, Santucci R, Pocia G: Effect of sperm morphology and motile sperm count on outcome of intrauterine insemination in oligozoospermia and/or asthenozoospermia. *Fertil Steril* 1990; 53:892-897.

Franklin RR, Dukes CD: Antispermatozoal antibody and unexplained infertility. *Am J Obstet Gynecol* 1964; 89:6.

Fujii S, Sagara M, Kudo H, et al: A prospective randomized comparison between long and discontinuous-long protocols of gonadotropin-releasing hormone agonist for in vitro fertilization. *Fertil Steril* 1997; 67:1166-1168.

Garcia J, Jones GS, Wentz AC: The use of clomiphene citrate. *Fertil Steril* 1977; 28:707.

Gemzell CA, Diczfalusy E, Tillinger KG: Clinical effect of human pituitary follicle stimulating hormone. *J Clin Endocrinol Metab* 1958; 18:1333-1339.

Gemzell CA, Dicfaluzy E, Tillinger KG: Human pituatary follicle-simulating hormone, I: Clinical effect of a partly purified preparation. *CIBA Found Colloq Endocrinol* 1960; 13:191-200.

Glazener CM, Coulson C, Lambert PA, et al: Clomiphene treatment for women with unexplained infertility: Placebo-controlled study of hormonal responses and conception rates. *Gynecol Endocrinol* 1990; 4:75-83.

Golan A, Ron-EL R, Herman A, et al: Ovarian hyperstimulation syndrome: An update review. *Obstet Gynecol Surv* 1989; 44:430.

Goldzieher JW, Green JA: The polycystic ovary: Clinical and histological features. *J Clin Endocrinol Metab* 1962; 22:325.

Goodman SB, Rein MS, Hill JA: Hysterosalpingography contrast media and chromotubation dye inhibit peritoneal lymphocyte and macrophage function in vitro: A potential mechanism for fertility enhancement. *Fertil Steril* 1993; 59:1022.

Gordon GG, et al: Effect of hyperthyroidism and hypothyroidism on the metabolism of testosterone and androstenedione in man. *J Clin Endocrinol Metab.* 1969; 29:164.

Gorelick JI, Goldstein M: Loss of fertility in men with varicocele. *Fertil Steril* 1993; 59:613-616.

Graff G: Suppression of cervical mucus during clomiphene therapy. *Fertil Steril* 1971; 22:209.

Greenblatt E, Casper R: Endocrine changes after laparoscopic ovarian cautery in polycystic ovarian syndrome. *Am J Obstet Gynecol* 1987; 156:279-285.

Greenblatt RB, Barfield WE, Jungck EC, Ray AW: Induction of ovulation with MRL-41. *JAMA* 1961; 178:101-106.

Guttmacher AF: Factors affecting normal expectancy of conception. *JAMA* 1956; 161:855-860.

Gysler M, March CM, Mishell DR, Bailey EJ: A decade's experience with an individualized clomiphene treatment regimen including its effect on the postcoital test. *Fertil Steril* 1982; 37:161-167.

Haas GG, Cines DB, Schreiber AD: Immunologic infertility: Identification of patients with antisperm antibody. *N Engl J Med* 1980; 180:303.

Haas GG Jr, D'Cruz OJ, Denum B: Effect of repeated washing on sperm-bound immunoglobulin G. *J Androl* 1988; 9:190.

Hall MG, Savage PE, Bromham DR: Prognostic value of the postcoital test: Prospective study based on time-specific conception rates. *Br J Obstet Gynecol* 1982; 89:299.

Halman LJ, Abbey A, Andrews FM: Why are couples satisfied with infertility treatment? *Fertil Steril* 1993; 59:1046.

Hammond MG, Halme JK, Talbert LM: Factors affecting the pregnancy rate in clomiphene citrate induction in ovulation. *Obstet Gynecol* 1983; 62:196-202.

Hamori M, et al: Zygote intrafallopian transfer (ZIFT): Evaluation of 42 cases. *Fertil Steril* 1988; 50:519.

Handyside AH, Kontogianni EH, Hardy K, Winston RM: Pregnancies from biopsied human preimplantation embryos sexed by Y-specific DNA amplification. *Nature* 1990; 344:768-770.

Harrison R, O'Moore R, McSweeny J: Idiopathic infertility: A trial of bromocriptine versus placebo. *Journal of the Irish Medical Association* 1979; 72:479-82.

Hendershot GE, Mosher WD, Pratt WE: Infertility and age: An unresolved issue. *Fam Plann Perspect* 1982; 14:287.

Henderson SR: The reversibility of female sterilization with the use of microsurgery: A report on 102 patients with more than one year of follow-up. *Am J Obstet Gynecol* 1984; 149:57-65.

Hensleigh PA, Fainstat T: Corpus luteum dysfunction: Serum progesterone levels in diagnosis and assessment of therapy for recurrent and threatened abortion. *Fertil Steril* 1979; 32:396.

Herbst AL, et al: A comparison of pregnancy experience in DES-exposed and DES-unexposed daughters. *J Reprod Med* 1980; 24:62.

Hill JA. Immunology and endometriosis: Fact, artifact, or epiphenomenon? *Obstet Gynecol Clin North Am* 1997; 24:291-306.

Hill JA, Anderson DJ: Immunological mechanisms of female infertility. In Johnson PM, editor: *Bailliere's clinical immunology and allergy: Immunologic disease in pregnancy*, London 1988, Bailliere Tindall.

Hill JA, Cohen J, Anderson DJ: The effects of lymphokines and monokines on human sperm fertilizing ability in the hamster egg penetration test. *Am J Obstet Gynecol* 1989; 160:1154.

Hill JA, Haimovici F, Anderson DJ: Effects of soluble products of activated lymphocytes and macrophages (lymphokines and monokines)

on human sperm motion parameters. *Fertil Steril* 1987; 47:460.

Ho PC, Poon IML, Chan SYW, Wang C: Intrauterine insemination is not useful in oligoasthenospermia. *Fertil Steril* 1989; 51:682-684.

Hodges RE, Hamilton AG, Keetel WC: Pregnancy in myxedema. *Arch Intern Med* 1952; 90:863.

Hoff JD, Quigley ME, Yen SS: Hormonal dynamics at midcycle: A re-evaluation. *J Clin Edoncrinol Metab* 1983; 57:792.

Hogerzeil HV, Spiekerman JC, de Vries JW, de Schepper G: A randomized trial between GIFT and ovarian stimulation for the treatment of unexplained infertility and failed artifical insemination by donor. *Hum Reprod* 1992; 7:1235-1239.

Homburg R, et al: One hundred pregnancies after treatment with pulsatile luteinizing hormone-releasing hormone to induce ovulation. *BMJ* 1989; 2998:809.

Homburg R, Levy T, Ben Rafael Z: A comparative study of conventional regimen with low dose FSH for ovulation in PCOS. *Fertil Steril* 1995; 63:729-733.

Hornstein MH, Barbieri RL, McShane PM: The effects of previous ovarian surgery on the follicular response to ovulation induction in an in vitro fertilization program. *J Reprod Med* 1989; 34:277-281.

Howards SS: Treatment of male infertility. *N Engl J Med* 1995; 332:312-317.

Howles CM, Loumaye E, Giroud D, Luyet G: Multiple follicular development and ovarian steroidogenesis following subcutaneous administration of a highly purified urinary FSH preparation in pituitary desensitized women undergoing IVF: A multicentre European phase III study. *Hum Reprod* 1994; 9:424-430.

Hughes EG, Fedorkow DM, Collins JA: A quantitative overview of controlled trials in endometriosis-associated infertility. *Fertil Steril* 1993; 59:963-970.

Hughes EG, Fedorkow DM, Daya S, et al: The routine use of gonadotropin releasing hormone agonists prior to in vitro fertilization and gamete intrafallopian tube transfer: A meta analysis of randomized controlled trials. *Fertil Steril* 1992; 58:888-896.

Hulka JF, Halme J: Sterilization reversal: results of 101 attempts. *Am J Obstet Gynecol* 1988; 159:767-774.

Hurd WW, et al: Comparison of intracervical, intrauterine, and intratubal techniques for donor inseminations. *Fertil Steril* 1993; 59:339-342.

Hutchins CJ: Laparoscopy and hysterosalpingography in the assessment of tubal potency. *Obstet Gynecol* 1977; 49:325.

Hutchinson-Williams KA, DeCherney AH, Lavy G, et al: Luteal research in in vitro fertilization embryo transfer. *Fertil Steril* 1990; 53:459-501.

Isojima S, Li T, Ashitaka Y: Immunologic analysis of sperm-immobilizing factor found in sera of women with unexplained sterility. *Am J Obstet Gynecol* 1968; 101:677.

Issacs JD, Hines RS, Sopelak VM, et al: Ovarian endometriomas do not adversely effect pregnancy success following treatment with in vitro fertilization. *J Assist Reprod Genet* 1997; 14:551-553.

Istre O, Olsboe F, Trolle B: Laparoscopic tubal anastomosis: Reversal of sterilization. *Acta Obstet Gynecol Scand* 1993; 72:680-681.

Jacobs HS: Prolactin and amenorrhea. *N Engl J Med* 1976; 295:954.

Jansen PPS, et al: Pulsatile intravenous gonadotropin-releasing hormone for ovulation induction, I: Safety and effectiveness with outpatient therapy. *Fertil Steril* 1987; 48:33.

Jansen RP: Spontaneous abortion incidence in the treatment of infertility. *Am J Obstet Gynecol* 1982; 143:451-456.

Jarrell J, McInnes R, Crooke R: Observations on the combination of clomiphene citrate-hMG-hCG in the management of anovulation. *Fertil Steril* 1981; 35:634-639.

Jequier AM, Ukombe EB: Errors inherent in the performance of a routine semen analysis. *Br J Urol* 1983; 55:434-436.

Jette NT, Glass RH: Prognostic value of the postcoital test. *Fertil Steril* 1972; 23:29.

Jeyendran RS, et al: Development of an assay to assess the functional integrity of the human sperm membrane and its relationship to other semen characteristics. *J Reprod Fertil* 1984; 70:219.

Jones GES: The luteal phase defect. *Fertil Steril* 1976; 27:351.

Jones GES, Pourmand K: An evaluation of etiologic factors and therapy in 555 private patients with primary infertility. *Fertil Steril* 1962; 13:389.

Jones RH, et al: Correlation between serum antichlamydial antibodies and tubal factor as a cause of infertility. *Fertil Steril* 1982; 38:553.

Karlstrom PO, Bergh T, Lundkvist O: A prospective randomized trial of artificial treatment versus intercourse in cycles stimulated with human menopausal gonadotropin or clomiphene citrate. *Fertil Steril* 1993; 59:554-559.

Karp LE, Williamson RA, Moore DE, et al: Sperm penetration assay: Useful test in evaluation of male fertility. *Obstet Gynecol* 1981; 57:620.

Katz E: The luteinized unruptured follicles and other ovulatory disorders. *Fertil Steril* 1988; 50:839.

Kaufman F, et al: Ovarian failure in galactosemia. *Lancet* 1979; 2:737.

Kaufman RH, et al: Upper genital tract changes and infertility in diethylstilbestrol-exposed women. *Am J Obstet Gynecol* 1986; 154:1312.

Kemmann E, Chazi D, Corsan G: Does ovulation stimulation improve fertility in women with minimal/mild endometriosis after laser laparoscopy. *Int J Fertil* 1993; 38:16-21.

Kerin JF, et al: Falloposcopic classification and treatment of fallopian tube lumen disease. *Fertil Steril* 1992; 57:731.

Kirby CA, Flaherty SP, Godfrey BM, et al: A prospective trial of intrauterine insemination of motile spermatozoa versus timed intercourse. *Fertil Steril* 1991; 56:102-107.

Kletsky OA, Borenstein R, Mileikowsky GN: Pergolide and bromocriptine for the treatment of patients with hyperprolactinemia. *Am J Obstet Gynecol* 1986; 154:431-43

Kletzky OA, Vermesh M: Effectiveness of vaginal bromocriptine in treating women with hyperprolactinemia. *Fertil Steril* 1989; 51:269-272.

Kondaveeti-Gordon U, Harrison RF, Barry-Kinsella C, et al: A randomized prospective study of early follicular or midluteal initiation of long protocol gonadotropin releasing hormone in an in vitro fertilization program. *Fertil Steril* 1996; 66:582-586.

Krauss CM, et al: Familial premature ovarian failure due to an interstitial deletion of the long arm of the X chromosome. *N Engl J Med* 1987; 317:125.

Kruger TF, et al: Sperm morphologic features as a prognostic factor in in vitro fertilization. *Fertil Steril* 1986; 46:1118.

Krupp P, Monka C: Bromocriptine in pregnancy: Safety aspects. *Klin Wochenschr* 1987; 65: 823-827.

Lalich RA, Marut EL, Prins GS, Scommegna A: Lifetable analysis of intrauterine insemination pregnancy rates. *Am J Obstet Gynecol* 1988; 4:980-984.

Larsen T, Larsen JF, Schioler V, et al: Comparison of urinary human follicle-stimulating hormone and human menopausal gonadotropin for ovarian stimulation in polycystic ovarian syndrome. *Fertil Steril* 1990; 53:426-431.

Leeton J, Rogers P, Caro C, et al: A controlled study between the use of gamete intrafallopian transfer and in vitro fertilization and embryo transfer in the management of idiopathic and male infertility. *Fertil Steril* 1987; 48:605-607.

Levran D, Bider D, Yonesh M, et al: A randomized study of intracytoplasmic sperm injection (ICSI) versus subzonal insemination (SUZI) for the management of severe male factor infertility. *J Assist Reprod Genet* 1995; 12:319-321.

Li T-C, et al: A comparison between two methods of chronological dating of human endometrial biopsies during the luteal phase, and their correlation with histologic dating. *Fertil Steril* 1987; 48:928.

Lieblich JM, Rogol AD, White BJ, Rosen SW: Syndrome of anosmia with hypogonadotropic hypogonadism (Kallman syndrome): Clinical and laboratory studies in 23 cases. *Am J Med* 1982; 73:506.

Lindequist S, Justesen P, Larsen C, Rasmussen F: Diagnostic quality and complications of hysterosalpingography: Oil- versus water-soluble contrast media: A randomized prospective study. *Radiology* 1991; 179:69-74.

Lisse K, Syndow P: Fallopian tube catheterization recanalization under ultrasonic observation: A simplified technique to evaluate tubal patency and open proximally obstructed tubes. *Fertil Steril* 1991; 56:198-201.

Liu DY, Baker WHG: Tests of human sperm function and fertilization in vitro. *Fertil Steril* 1992; 58:465.

Liu DY, et al: A human sperm-zona pellucida binding test using oocytes that failed to fertilize in vitro. *Fertil Steril* 1988; 50:782.

Liu L, Banks SM, Barnes KM, Sherins RJ: Two year comparison of testicular responses to pulsatile gonadotropin releasing hormone and exogenous gonadotropins from the inception of therapy in men with isolated hypogonadotropic hypogonadism. *J Clin Endcrinol Metab* 1988; 67:1140.

Lobo RA, Paul W, March CM, et al: Clomiphene and dexamethasone in women unresponsive to clomiphene alone. *Obstet Gynecol* 1982; 60:497.

London SN, Haney AF, Weinberg JB: Diverse humoral and cell-mediated effects of antisperm antibodies on reproduction. *Fertil Steril* 1984; 41:907.

Lunenfeld B, Eshkol A: Induction of ovulation with gonadotropin. In Rolland R, van Hall EV, Hillier SG, editors: *Follicular maturation and ovulation,* Amsterdam, 1982, Excerpta Medica.

Lunenfeld B, Sulimovici S, Rabau E, Eshkol A: L'induction de l'ovulation dans les amenorrhees hypophysaires par un traitement de gonadotrophines urinaires menopausiques et de gonadotrophines chorioniques. *Comptes Rendus de la Societe Francaise de Gynecologie* 1962; 32:346-351.

MacDougall MJ, Tan SL, Hall V, et al: Comparison of natural with clomiphene citrate stimulated cycles in in vitro fertilization: A prospective randomized trial. *Fertil Steril* 1994; 61:1052-1057.

MacLeod J, Gold PZ: The male factor in fertility and infertility, II: Spermatozoan counts in 1000 men of known fertility and in 1000 cases of infertile marriages. *J Urol* 1951a; 66:436.

Madgar I, Weissenberg R, Lunefeld B, et al: Controlled trial of high spermatic vein ligation for varicocele in infertile men. *Fertil Steril* 1995; 63:120-124.

Mahadevan MM, Trounson AO: The influence of seminal characteristics on the success rate of human in vitro fertilization. *Fertil Steril* 1984; 42:400.

Mao C, Grimes DA: The sperm penetration assay: Can it discriminate between fertile and infertile men? *Am J Obstet Gynecol* 1988; 159:279.

March CM: Update: Luteal phase defects. *Endocr Fertil Forum* 1987; 10:3.

March CM, Israel R, March AD: Hysteroscopic management of intrauterine adhesions. *Am J Obstet Gynecol* 1978; 130:653-657.

Marconi G, et al: Salpingoscopy: Systematic use in diagnostic laparoscopy. *Fertil Steril* 1992; 57:742.

Marcoux S, Marcoux R, Berube S: Laparoscopic surgery in infertile women with minimal or mild endometriosis. *N Engl J Med* 1997; 337:217-222.

Mareck J, Hulka JF: Luteinized unruptured follicle syndrome: A subtle cause of infertility. *Fertil Steril* 1978; 29:270.

Margalioth EJ, et al: Correlation between the zona-free hamster egg sperm penetration assay and human in vitro fertilization. *Fertil Steril* 1986; 45:665.

Margalioth EJ, et al: Intrauterine insemination as treatment for antisperm antibodies in the female. *Fertil Steril* 1988; 50:441-446.

Margalioth EJ et al: Reduced fertilization ability of zona-free hamster ova by spermatozoa from male partners of normal infertile couples. *Arch Androl* 1983; 10:67.

MarMar JL, et al: Microsurgical aspiration of sperm from the epididymis: A mobile program. *J Urol* 1993; 149:1368-1373.

Martin KA, Hall JE, Adams JM, Crowley WF: Comparison of exogenous gonadotropins and pulsatile gonadotropin releasing hormone for induction of ovulation in hypogonadotropic amenorrhea. *J Clin Endocrinol Metab* 1993; 77:125-129.

Martinez AR, Bernadus RE, Voorhorst FJ, et al: Intrauterine insemination does and clomiphene citrate does not improve fecundity in couples with infertility due to a male or idiopathic factor: A prospective randomized, controlled study. *Fertil Steril,* 1990; 53:847-853.

Maruo T, Katayama K, Barnea ER, Mochizuki M: A role for thyroid hormone in the induction of ovulation and corpus luteum function. *Horm Res* 1992; 37(suppl):12-18.

Matson PL, Yovich JL: The treatment of infertility associated with endometriosis by in vitro fertilization. *Fertil Steril* 1986; 46:432.

Maxson WS, et al: Antiestrogenic effect of clomiphene citrate: Correlation with serum estradiol concentrations. *Fertil Steril* 1984; 42:356.

Mayer J, Walker D, Jones E, et al: Significantly different pregnancy rates in a randomized study of two different transfer catheters and procedures. *Am Soc Reprod Med Prog* 1996; (suppl):S211 (abstract P-253).

McFaul P, Traub A, Thompson W: Treatment of clomiphene citrate-resistant polycystic ovarian syndrome with pure follicle-stimulating hormone or human menopausal gonadotropin. *Fertil Steril* 1990; 53:792-797.

McNatty KP, Sawers RS, McNeilly AS: A possible role for prolactin in control of steroid secretion by the human graafian follicle. *Nature* 1973; 250:653.

Medical Research International, The American Fertility Society Special Interest Group: In vitro fertilization/embryo transfer in the United States 1985 and 1986 results from the National IVF/ET registry. *Fertil Steril* 1988; 49:212-215.

Meldrum DR: Female reproductive aging—ovarian and uterine factors. *Fertil Steril* 1993; 59:1-5.

Melis GB, Paoletti AM, Ajossa S, et al: Ovulation induction with gonadotropins as sole treatment in infertile couples with open tubes: A randomized prospective comparison between intrauterine insemination and timed vaginal intercourse. *Fertil Steril* 1995; 64: 1088-1093.

Menge AC, et al: The incidence and influence of antisperm antibodies in infertile human couples on sperm-cervical mucus interactions and subsequent fertility. *Fertil Steril* 1982; 38:439.

Merrell Dow Pharmaceuticals National Laboratories: *Product information bulletin,* Cincinnati, Ohio, 1972, Author.

Mochtar MH, Hogarzeil HU, Mol BW: Progesterone alone vs progesterone combined with hCG as luteal support in GnRH-a/HMG induced IVF cycles: A randomized clinical trial. *Hum Reprod* 1996; 11:1602-1605.

Moghissi KS: Accuracy of basal body temperature for ovulation detection. *Fertil Steril* 1976a; 27:1415.

Moghissi KS: Postcoital test: Physiologic basis, technique, and interpretation. *Fertil Steril* 1976b; 27:117.

Moghissi KS, Sacco AJ, Borin K: Immunologic infertility, I: Cervical mucus antibodies and postcoital tests. *Am J Obstet Gynecol* 1980; 136:941.

Moghissi KS, Syner FN, Evans TN: A composite picture of the menstrual cycle. *Am J Obstet Gynecol* 1972; 114:405.

Moghissi KS, Wallach EE: Unexplained infertility. *Fertil Steril* 1983; 39:5.

Monroe SE, et al: Prolactin-secreting pituitary adenomas, V Increased gonadotropin responsivity in hyperprolactinemic women with pituitary adenomas. *J Clin Endocrinol Metab* 1981; 52:1171.

Montoro MD, et al: Successful outcome of pregnancy in women with hypothyroidism. *Ann Intern Med* 1984; 94:31.

Morris RS, Sauer MV: Oocyte donation in 1990s and beyond. *Assist Reprod Rev* 1993; 3: 211-17.

Mortimer D: Objective analysis of sperm motility and kinematics. In Kell BA, Webster BW, editors: *Handbook of the laboratory: Diagnosis and treatment of infertility.* Boca Raton, 1989, CRC Press.

Mosher W: Fertility and family planning in the United States: Insights from the National Survey of Family Growth. *Fam Plann Perspect* 1988; 20:207.

Mosher WD: Infertility trends among U.S. couples: 1965-1976. *Fam Plann Perspect* 1982; 14:22.

Mosher WD: Reproductive impairments in the United States: 1965-1982. *Demography* 1985; 22:415.

Mosher WD, Pratt WF: Fecundity and infertility in the United States: 1965-1988, DHHS Pub No (PHS)91-1250, Advance Data No 192, Hyattsville, Md: National Center for Health Statistics, 1990.

Mosher WD, Pratt WF: Fecundity and infertility in the United States: Incidence and trends. *Fertil Steril* 1991; 56:192-193.

Mueller BA, Daling JR, Moore DE, et al: Appendectomy and the risk of tubal infertility. *N Engl J Med* 1986; 315:1506-508.

Nakamura K, et al: Menotropin stimulation after prolonged gonadotropin releasing hormone agonist pretreatment for in vitro fertilization in patients with endometriosis. *J Assist Reprod Genet* 1992; 9:113-117.

Nan PM, Cohlen BJ, te Velde ER, et al: Intrauterine insemination or timed intercourse after ovarian stimulation for male subfertility? A controlled study. *Hum Reprod*, 1994; 9:2022-2026.

Neufeld M, MacLaren NK, Blizzard RM: Two types of autoimmune Addison's disease associated with different polyglandular autoimmune (PGA) syndromes. *Medicine* 1981; 60:355.

New MI, et al: Genotyping steroid 21-hydroxylase deficiency: Hormonal reference data. *J Clin Endocrinol Metab* 1983; 57:320.

Newill RG, Katz M: The basal body temperature chart in artificial insemination by donor pregnancy cycles. *Fertil Steril* 1982; 38:431.

Nikolaeva MA, et al: Detection of antisperm antibodies on the surface of living spermatozoa using flow cytometry: Preliminary study. *Fertil Steril* 1993; 59:639.

Novy MJ, et al: Diagnosis of cornual obstruction by transcervical fallopian tube cannulation. *Fertil Steril* 1988; 50:434-440.

Noyes RW, Hertig A, Rock J: Dating the endometrial biopsy. *Fertil Steril* 1950; 1:3.

Nulsen JC, Walsh S, Dumez S, Metzger DA: A randomized and longitudinal study of human menopausal gonadotropin with intrauterine insemination in the treatment of infertility. *Obstet Gynecol* 1993; 82:780-785.

Ogata R, Nakamura G, Uchiumi Y, et al: Therapeutic efficacy of hysterosalpingography (HSG) in infertility: A prospective, randomized, clinical study. *Jpn J Fertil Steril*, 1993; 38:91-94.

O'Herlihy C, Pepperell RJ, Robinson HP: Ultrasound timing of human chorionic gonadotropin administration in clomiphene-stimulated cycles. *Obstet Gynecol* 1982; 59: 40-46.

Olive DL, Lee KL: Analysis of sequential treatment protocols for endometriosis-associated infertility. *Am J Obstet Gynecol* 1986; 154:613-619.

Oliveness F, Kerbrat V, Rufat P, et al: Follow-up of a cohort of 422 children ages 6 to 13 years conceived by in vitro fertilization. *Fertil Steril* 1997; 284-289.

Opsahl MS, Miller B, Klein TA: The predictive value of hysterosalpingography for tubal and peritoneal infertility factors. *Fertil Steril* 1993; 60:444.

Out HJ, Mannarets BM, Driessen SG, Coelingh Bennink HJ: A prospective, randomized, assessor-blind, multicentre study comparing recombinant and urinary follicle-stimulating hormone (Puregon versus Metrodin) in in vitro fertilization. *Hum Reprod* 1995b; 10: 2534-2540.

Out HJ, Mannaerts BM, Driessen SG, Coelingh Bennik HJ: Recombinant follicle stimulating hormone (rFSH; Puregon) in assisted reproduction: More oocytes, more pregnancies: Results from five comparative studies. *Hum Reprod Update* 1996a; 2:162-171.

Padilla SL, Garcia JE: Effect of maternal age and number of in vitro fertilization procedures on pregnancy outcome. *Fertil Steril* 1989; 52: 270-273.

Pal L, Shifren JL, Issacson KB, et al: Impact of varying stages of endometriosis on the outcome of in vitro fertilization—embryo transfer. *J Assist Reprod Genet* 1998; 15:27-31.

Palmer A: Ethiodol hysterosalpingography for the treatment of infertility. *Fertil Steril* 1960; 11:311.

Pellicer I, et al: Exploring the mechanisms of endometriosis-related infertility and analysis of embryo development and implantation and assisted reproduction. *Hum Reprod* 1997; 2: 91-97.

Peterson CM, Hatasaka HH, Jones KP, et al: Ovulation induction with gonadotropins and intrauterine insemination compared with in vitro fertilization and no therapy: A prospective, nonrandomized, cohort study and meta-analysis. *Fertil Steril* 1994; 62:535-544.

Phipps WR, et al: The association between smoking and female infertility as influenced by cause of the infertility. *Fertil Steril* 1987; 48:337.

Phipps WR, Benson CB, McShane PM: Severe thigh myositis following intramuscular progesterone injections in an in vitro fertilization patient. *Fertil Steril* 1988; 49:536-537.

Phung TT, Byrd JR, McDonough PG: Etiologies and subsequent reproductive performance of 100 couples with recurrent abortion. *Fertil Steril* 1979; 132:389.

Pitaway DE, et al: Prevention of acute pelvic inflammatory disease after hysterosalpingography: Efficacy of doxycycline prophylaxis. *Am J Obstet Gynecol* 1983; 47:623.

Platia MP, Krudy AG: Transvaginal fluoroscopic recanalization of a proximally occluded oviduct. *Fertil Steril* 1985; 44:704-706.

Politch JA, et al: Comparison of methods to enumerate white blood cells in semen. *Fertil Steril* 1993; 60:372.

Preutthipan S, Amos N, Curtis P, Shaw RW: A prospective randomized cross over comparison of zygote intrafallopian tube transfer and in vitro fertilization embryo transfer in unexplained infertility. *J Med Assoc Thai*, 1994; 77:599-604.

Radestad A, Bui TH, Nygren KG: Multifetal pregnancy reduction in Sweden: Utilization rate and pregnancy outcome. *Acta Obstet Gynecol Scand* 1994; 73:403-406.

Radwamsla E, Hammond J, Smith P: Single midluteal progesterone assay in the management of ovulatory infertility. *J Reprod Med* 1981; 26:85.

Ransom MX, Blotner MB, Bohrer M, et al: Does increasing frequency of intrauterine insemination improve pregnancy rates significantly during superovulation cycles? *Fertil Steril* 1994; 61:303-307.

Rasmussen F, Lindequist S, Larsen C, Justesen P: Therapeutic effect of hysterosalpingography: Oil- versus water-soluble contrast media: A randomized prospective study. *Radiology* 1991; 179:75-78.

Rice JB, London S, Olive DL: Re-evaluation of hysterosalpingography in infertility investigation. *Obstet Gynecol* 1996; 67:718.

Risquez F, Confino E: Transcervical tubal cannulation, past, present, and future. *Fertil Steril* 1993; 60:211-226.

Ritchie WG: Ultrasound in the evaluation of normal and induced ovulation. *Fertil Steril* 1985; 43:167.

Rizk B, Smitz J: Ovarian hyperstimulation syndrome after superovulation using GnRH-a for IVF and related procedures. *Hum Reprod* 1992; 7:320-327.

Robinson A, Lubs HA, Nielson J, Sorensen K: Summary of clinical findings: Profiles of children with 47,XXY, 47,XXX, and 47,XYY karyotypes. *Birth Defects* 1979; 15:261-266.

Rock J, Menkin MF: In vitro fertilization and cleavage of human ovarian eggs. *Science* 1944; 100:105.

Rock JA, et al: Tubal anastomosis: Pregnancy success following reversal of Fallope ring or monopolar cautery sterilization. *Fertil Steril* 1987; 48:13-17.

Rogers BJ, et al: Analysis of human spermatozoal fertilizing ability using zona-free ova. *Fertil Steril* 1979; 32:664.

Roseboom TJ, Vermeiden JP, Schoute E, et al: The probability of pregnancy after embryo transfer is affected by the age of the patient, cause of infertility, number of embryos transferred and the average morphology score, as revealed by multiple logistic regression analysis. *Hum Reprod* 1995; 10:3035-3041.

Rosenfeld DL, Seidman SM, Bronson RA, et al: Unsuspected chronic pelvic inflammatory disease in the infertile female. *Fertil Steril* 1983; 39:44.

Rosenfeld DL: Abdominal myomectomy for otherwise unexplained infertility. *Fertil Steril* 1986; 46:328-330.

Rossing MA, Daling JR, Weiss NS, et al: Ovarian tumors in a cohort of infertile women. *N Engl J Med* 1994; 331:771-776.

Ruder H, et al: Effects of induced hyperthyroidism on steroid metabolism in man. *J Clin Endocrinol Metab* 1971; 33:382.

Rumke P, et al: Prognosis of fertility of men with sperm agglutinins in the serum. *Fertil Steril* 1974; 25:393.

Sagle M, Hamilton-Fairley D, Kiddy D, Franks S: A comparative, randomized study of low-dose human menopausal gonadotropin and follicle-stimulating hormone in women with polycystic ovarian syndrome. *Fertil Steril*, 1991; 55:56-60.

Santoro N, et al: Intravenous administration of pulsatile gonadotropin-releasing hormone in hypothalanic amenorrhea: Effects of dosage. *J Clin Endocrinol Metab* 1986; 62:109.

Sapienza F, Verheyen G, Tournaye H, et al: An auto-controlled study in in vitro fertilization reveals the benefit of Percoll centrifugation to swim up in the preparation of poor quality semen. *Hum Reprod* 1993; 8:1856-1862.

SART Registry: Assisted reproductive technology in the United States and Canada: 1995 results generated from the American Society for Reproductive Medicine/Society for Assisted Reproductive Technology Registry. *Fertil Steril* 1998; 69:389-398.

Sauer MV, et al: Effect of abstinence on sperm motility in normal men. *Am J Obstet Gynecol* 1988; 158:604-607.

Schenken RS, Asch RH: Surgical induction of endometriosis in the rabbit: Effect on fertility and concentration of peritoneal fluid prostaglandins. *Fertil Steril* 1980; 34:581-587.

Schenken RS, Asch RH, Williams RF: Etiology of infertility in monkeys with endometriosis: Luteinized unruptured follicles, luteal phase defects, pelvic adhesions and spontaneous abortions. *Fertil Steril* 1984; 41:122-127.

Schenken RS, Malinak LR: Reoperation after initial treatment of endometriosis with conservative surgery. *Am J Obstet Gynecol* 1978; 131:416.

Schenker JG, Margalioth EJ: Intrauterine adhesions: An updated appraisal. *Fertil Steril* 1982; 37:593.

Schenker JG, Weinstein D: Ovarian hyperstimulation syndrome: A current survey. *Fertil Steril* 1978; 30:255-259.

Schlaff WD, Hassiakos DK, Damewood MD, Rock JA: Neosalpingostomy for distal tubal obstruction: Prognostic factors and impact of surgical technique. *Fertil Steril*, 1990; 54: 984-989.

Schmidt CL, de Ziegler D, Gagliardi CL, et al: Transfer of cryopreserved-thawed embryos: The natural cycle versus controlled preparation of the endometrium with gonadotropin-releasing hormone agonist and exogenous estradiol and progesterone (GEEP). *Fertil Steril* 1989; 52:609-616.

Schoot DC, Coelingh Bennick HJ, Mannaerts BM, et al: Human recombinant follicle-stimulating hormone induces growth of preovulatory follicles without concomitant increase in androgen and estrogen biosynthesis in a woman with isolated gonadotropin definency. *J Clin Endocrinol Metab* 1992; 74:1471-1473.

Schopohl J, Mehltretter G, von Zumbusch R, et al: Comparison of gonadotropin releasing hormone and gonadotropin therapy in male patients with idiopathic hypothalamic hypogonadism. *Fertil Steril* 1991; 56:1143-1170.

Schwartz D, Mayaux MJ: Female fecundity as a function of age: Results of artificial mammalian in 2193 nulliparous women with azoospermic husbands. Federation CECOS. *N Engl J Med* 1982; 306:404.

Scott JZ, et al: The cervical factor in infertility: Diagnosis and treatment. *Fertil Steril* 1977; 28:1289.

Scott RT, et al: Evaluation of the impact of intraobserver variability on endometrial dating and the diagnosis of luteal phase defects. *Fertil Steril* 1993; 60:652.

Scott RT, Hofmann GE: Prognostic assessment of ovarian reserve. *Fertil Steril* 1995; 63:1-11.

Scott RT, Leonardi MR, Hofmann GE, et al: A prospective evaluation of clomiphene citrate challenge test screening in the general infertility population. *Obstet Gynecol* 1993; 82: 539-545.

Scott RT, Navot D: Enhancement of ovarian responsiveness with microdoses of gonadotropin releasing hormone agonist during ovulation induction for in vitro fertilization. *Fertil Steril* 1994; 61:880-885.

Scott RT, Toner JP, Muasher SH, et al: Follicle stimulating hormone levels on cycle day 3 are predictive of in vitro fertilization outcome. *Fertil Steril* 1989; 51:651-654.

Seibel MM, Berger MJ, Weinstein FG: The effectiveness of Danazol on subsequent fertility in minimal endometriosis. *Fertil Steril* 1982; 38:534-539.

Seracchiolo R, Porcu E, Ciotti P, et al: Gamete intrafallopian transfer: prospective randomized comparison between hysteroscopic and laparoscopic transfer techniques *Fertil Steril* 1995; 64:355-359.

Serhal PF, Katz M, Little V, Woronowski H: Unexplained infertility: The value of Pergonal superovulation combined with intrauterine insemination. *Fertil Steril* 1988; 49:602-608.

Shangold M, Berkley A, Gray J: Both midluteal serum progesterone levels and late luteal endometrial histology should be assessed in all infertile women. *Fertil Steril* 1983; 40:627.

Shapiro BS, Diamond MP, DeCherney AH: Salpingoscopy: An adjunctive technique for evaluation of the fallopian tube. *Fertil Steril* 1988; 49:1076.

Sharara FI, Beaste SN, Leonardi MR, et al: Cigarette smoking accelerates the development of diminished ovarian reserve as evidenced by the clomiphene citrate challenge test. *Fertil Steril* 1994; 62:257-262.

Sharlip ID: What is the best pregnancy rate that may be expected from vasectomy reversal. *J Urol* 1993; 149:1469-1471.

Shaw JM, et al: An association between chromosomal abnormalities in rapidly frozen 2-cell mouse embryos and the ice-forming properties of the cryoprotective solution. *J Reprod Fertil* 1991; 91:9.

Sher G, Knutzen VK, Stratton CJ, et al: In vitro sperm capacitation and transcervical intrauterine insemination for the treatment of refractory infertility. *Fertil Steril* 1984; 41:260-264.

Sherins RJ, Thorsell LP, Dorfmann A, et al: Intracytoplasmic sperm injection facilitates fertilization even in the most severe forms of male infertility: Pregnancy outcome correlates with maternal age and number of eggs available. *Fertil Steril* 1995; 64:369-375.

Shoupe D, et al: Correlation of endometrial maturation with four methods of estimating day of ovulation. *Obstet Gynecol* 1989; 73:88.

Shulman S, et al: Immunologic consequences of vasectomy. *Contraception* 1972; 5:269.

Siegler AM: *Hysterosalpingography*, New York, 1974, Medcon Press.

Silber SH, Cohen R: Microsurgical reversal of female sterilization: The role of tubal length. *Fertil Steril* 1980; 33:598-601.

Silber SJ, Nagy Z, Liu J, et al: The use of epididymal and testicular spermatozoa for intracytoplasmic sperm injection: The genetic implications for male infertility. *Hum Reprod*, 1995; 10:2031-2043.

Silverberg KM, Johnson JV, Olive DL, et al: A prospective, randomized trial comparing two different intrauterine insemination regimens in controlled ovarian hyperstimulation cycles. *Fertil Steril* 1992; 57:357-361.

Singhal V, Li TC, Cooke ID: An analysis of factors influencing the outcome of 232 consecutive tubal microsurgery cases. *Br J Obstet Gynecol* 1991; 98:628-636.

Small DRJ, et al: The interpretation of semen analysis among infertile couples. *Can Med Assoc J* 1987; 136:829.

Smith KD, Rodriguez-Rigau EJ, Steinberger E: Relation between indices of semen analysis and pregnancy rate in infertile couples. *Fertil Steril* 1977; 28:1314.

Smith Levitan M, Kowalik A, Birnholz J, et al: Selective reduction of multifetal pregnancies to twins improves outcome over non-reduced triplet gestations. *Am J Obstet Gynecol* 1996; 175:878-883.

Smitz J, et al: A prospective randomized comparison of intramuscular or intravaginal natural progesterone as a luteal phase and early pregnancy supplement. *Hum Reprod* 1992; 7:168-175.

Sokol RZ, Steiner BS, Bustillo M, et al: A controlled comparison of the efficacy of clomiphene citrate in male infertility. *Fertil Steril* 1988; 49:865-870.

Soliman S, Daya S, Collins J, Hughes EG: The role of luteal phase support in infertility treatment: A meta analysis of randomized trials. *Fertil Steril* 1994; 61:1068-1076.

Soules MR, Spadoni LR: Oil vs. aqueous media for hysterosalpingography: A continuing debate based on many opinions and few facts. *Fertil Steril*, 1982; 38:1.

Soules MR, et al: The corpus luteum: Determinants of progesterone secretion in the normal menstrual cycle. *Obstet Gynecol* 1988; 71: 659.

Southern AL, et al: The conversion of androgens to estrogens in hyperthyroidism. *J Clin Endocrinol Metab* 1974; 38:207.

Staessen C, Janssenswillen C, Van Den Abbeel E, et al: Avoidance of triplet pregnancies by elective transfer of two good quality embryos. *Hum Reprod*, 1993; 8:1650-1653.

Steer CV, Mills CL, Tamn SL, et al: The cumulative embryo score: A predictive embryo scoring technique to select the optimal number of embryos to transfer in an in vitro fertilization and embryo transfer programme. *Hum Reprod* 1992; 7:117-119.

Steptoe PC, Edwards RG: Birth after reimplantation of a human embryo. *Lancet* 1978; 2:366.

Stern J, Peters AJ, Coulam CB: Color Doppler ultrasonography assessment of tubal patency: A comparison study with traditional techniques. *Fertil Steril* 1992; 58:897.

Stern JE, et al: Antisperm antibodies in women: Variability in antibody levels in serum, mucus, and peritoneal fluid. *Fertil Steril* 1992b; 58:950.

Stillman RJ, Hershlag A: Pathology of infertility and adverse pregnancy outcome after in utero exposure to diethylstilbestrol. In Gondos B, Riddick DA, editors: *Pathology of infertility*, New York, 1987, Theime-Stratton.

Stone SC: Peritoneal recovery of sperm in patients with infertility associated with inadequate cervical mucus. *Fertil Steril* 1983; 40:802.

Stumpf PG, March CM: Febrile morbidity following hysterosalpingography: Identification of risk factors and recommendations for prophylaxis. *Fertil Steril* 1980; 33:487.

Surrey E, Meldrum DR: Pregnancy rates after hysterosalpingography with oil and water-soluble contrast media. *Obstet Gynecol* 1987; 69:830.

Svalander PC, Lundin K, Holmes PV: Endotoxin concentration in Percoll density-gradient media used to prepare spermatozoa for human IVF treatment. *Hum Reprod* 1995; 10 (suppl 2):130 (abstract 277).

Svendsen TO, Jones D, Butler L, Muasher SJ: The incidence of multiple gestations after in vitro fertilization is dependent on the number of embryos transferred and maternal age. *Fertil Steril* 1996; 65:561-565.

Swyer GI, Radwanska E, McGarrigle HH: Plasma estradiol and progesterone estimation for the monitoring of induction of ovulation with clomiphene and chorionic gonadotropin. *Br J Obstet Gynecol* 1975; 82:794-799.

Talbot P, Chacon RS: A triple stain technique for evaluating normal acrosome reaction of human sperm. *J Exp Zool* 1981; 215:201.

Tamara L, Callahan BS, Hall JE, et al: The economic impact of multiple-gestation pregnancies and the contribution of assisted-reproduction techniques to their incidence. *N Engl J Med* 1994; 331:244-249.

Tarin JJ: Subzonal insemination, partial zona dissection or intracytoplasmic sperm injection. *Hum Reprod* 1995; 10:165-170.

Taylor PJ: Correlations in infertility, symptomatology, hysterosalpingography, laparoscopy, and hysteroscopy. *J Reprod Med* 1977; 8:339.

Taymor ML, Overstreet JW: Some thoughts on the postcoital test. *Fertil Steril* 1988; 50:702.

Tejada RI, et al: A test for the practical evaluation of male infertility by acridine orange (AO) fluorescence. *Fertil Steril* 1984; 42:87.

Telimaa S: Danazol and medroxyprogesterone acetate in efficacious in the treatment of infertility in endometriosis. *Fertil Steril* 1988; 50:872-878.

Templeton A, Morris J: Reducing the risk of multiple births by transfer of two embryos after in vitro fertilization. *N Engl J Med* 1998; 39:573-577.

Templeton AA, Penny GC: The incidence, characteristics, and prognosis of patients whose infertility is unexplained. *Fertil Steril* 1982; 37:175.

Terquem A, Dadoune JP: Aniline blue staining of human spermatozoa chromatic: Evaluation of nuclear maturation. In Andre J, editor: *The sperm cell*, London, 1983, Martinus Nijhoff.

Tietze C: Reproductive span and rate of reproduction among Hutterite women. *Fertil Steril* 1957; 8:89.

Tomlinson MJ, et al: Round cells and sperm fertilizing capacity: The presence of immature germ cells but not seminal leukocytes are as-sociated with reduced success of in vitro fertilization. *Fertil Steril* 1992; 58:1257.

Toner JP, Philput CB, Jones GS, Muasher SJ: Basal follicle-stimulating hormone level is a better predictor of in vitro fertilization performance than age. *Fertil Steril* 1991; 55:784-791.

Tournaye H, Devroey P, Camus M, et al: Zygote intrafallopian transfer in in vitro fertilization and embryo transfer for the treatment of male-factor infertility: A prospective randomized trial. *Fertil Steril* 1992; 58:344-350.

Treadway EC, et al: Significance of timing of postcoital evaluation of cervical mucus. *Am J Obstet Gynecol* 1975; 121:387.

Tufekci EC, et al: Evaluation of tubal patency by transvaginal sonosalpingography. *Fertil Steril* 1992; 57:336.

Turksoy RN, Biller BJ, Farber M, et al: Ovulatory response to clomiphene citrate during bromocriptine failed ovulation in amenorrhea-galactorrhea and hyperprolactinemia. *Fertil Steril* 1982; 37:441-444.

Uehling DT: Secretory IgA in seminal fluid. *Fertil Steril* 1971; 22:769.

Valle RF: Hysteroscopy and the evaluation of female infertility. *Am J Obstet Gynecol* 1980; 137:425.

Valle RF, Sciarra JJ: Intrauterine adhesions: Hysteroscopic diagnosis, classification, treatment and reproductive outcome. *Am J Obstet Gynecol* 1988; 158:1459-1470.

Van der Elst J, Camus M, Van den Abbeel E, et al: Prospective randomized study on the cryopreservation of human embryos with dimethylsulfoxide of 1,2-propanediol protocols. *Fertil Steril* 1995; 63:92-100.

Van der Merwe JP, Kruger TF, Windt ML, et al: Treatment of male sperm autoimmunity by using the gamete intrafallopian transfer procedure with washed sperm. *Fertil Steril* 1990; 53:682.

Van der Ven HH, et al: Correlation between human sperm swelling in hypoosmotic medium (hypoosmotic swelling test) and in vitro fertilization. *J Androl* 1986; 7:140.

Van der Ven HH, et al: Leucospermia and the fertilizing capacity of spermatozoa. *Eur J Obstet Gynecol Reprod Biol* 1987; 4:49.

Van der Zwalmen P, Bertin-Segal G, Geerts L, et al: Sperm morphology and IVF pregnancy rate: Comparison between Percoll gradient centrifugation and swim up procedures. *Hum Reprod* 1991; 6:581-588.

Van Steirteghem A, Nagy P, Joris H, et al: Results of intracytoplasmic sperm injection with ejaculated, fresh and frozen-thawed epididymal and testicular spermatozoa. *Hum Reprod* 1998; 13:134-142.

Van Uen JFHM, Acosta AA, Swanson RG, et al: Male factor evaluation in in vitro fertilization. *Fertil Steril* 1985; 44:375-383.

Van Voorhis BJ, Syrop CH, Vincent RD, et al: Tubal versus uterine transfer of cryopreserved embryos: A prospective randomized trial. *Fertil Steril* 1995; 63:578-585.

Vauthier-Brouzes D, Lefebvre G, Lesourd S, et al: How many embryos should be transferred in in vitro fertilization? A prospective randomized study. *Fertil Steril* 1994; 62:339-342.

Veeck LL, Mundson CH, Brothman LJ, et al: Significantly enhanced pregnancy rates per cycle through cryopreservation and thaw of pronuclear stage oocytes. *Fertil Steril* 1993; 59:1202-1207.

Venn A, Watson L, Lumley J, et al: Breast and ovarian cancer incidence after infertility and in vitro fertilization. *Lancet* 1995; 346:995.

Verheyen G, DeCroo I, Tournaye H, et al: Comparison of four mechanical methods to retrieve spermatozoa from testicular tissue. *Hum Reprod* 1995; 10:2965-2969.

Vermesh M, et al: Monitoring techniques to predict and detect ovulation. *Fertil Steril* 1987; 47:259.

Vernon MW, Wilson EA: Studies on the surgical induction of endometriosis in the rat. *Fertil Steril* 1985; 44:684-689.

Von Campenhout J, Semard R, Liduc B: The antiestrogenic effect of clomiphene in the human being. *Fertil Steril* 1968; 19:700.

Waldstreicher J, Santoro NF, Hall JE, et al: Hyperfunction of the hypothalmic-pituitary axis in women with polycystic ovarian disease: Indirect evidence for partial gonadotrophic desensitization. *J Clin Endocrinol Metab* 1988; 66:165.

Webster J, Piscitelli G, Polli A, et al: A comparison of cabergoline and bromocriptine in the treatment of hyperprolactinemic amenorrhea. *N Engl J Med* 1994; 331:904-909.

Weir W, Cicchinelli AL: Prognosis for the infertile couple. *Fertil Steril* 1964; 15:625.

Wentz AC: Endometrial biopsy in the evaluation of infertility. *Fertil Steril* 1980; 33:121.

Westrom L: Effect of acute pelvic inflammatory disease on fertility. *Am J Obstet Gynecol* 1983; 146:153.

Westrom L: Incidence prevalence and trends of acute pelvic inflammatory disease and its consequences in industrialized countries. *Am J Obstet Gynecol* 1980; 138:880-892.

Wheeler JM, Malinak LR: Postoperative Danazol therapy in infertility patients with severe endometriosis. *Fertil Steril* 1981; 36:460.

Wheeless CR, Katayama KP: Laparoscopy and tubal sterilization. In Mattingly RF, Thompson JD, editors: *Operative gynecology*, ed 6, Philadelphia, 1985, JB Lippincott.

White PC, New MI, Dupont B: Congenital adrenal hyperplasia. *N Engl J Med* 1987; 316:1519.

Whittemore AS, Harris P, Itnyre J: The collaborative ovarian cancer group: Collaborative analysis of twelve U.S. case control stuides, II: Invasive epithelial cancer in white women. *Am J Epidemiol* 1992; 136:1184-1189.

WHO Scientific Group Report: Consultation on the diagnosis and treatment of endocrine forms of female infertility. *Tech Rep* Series No. 514, 1976.

Wickings EJ, et al: Heterologous ovum penetration test and seminal parameters in fertile and infertile men. *J Androl* 1983; 4:261.

Wilcox A, Weinberg C, Baird D: Timing of sexual intercourse in relation to ovulation, effects on the probability of conception, survival of the pregnancy, and sex of the baby. *N Engl J Med* 1995; 333:1517-1521.

Wilcox AJ, Weinburg CR, O'Connor J, et al: Incidence of early loss of pregnancy. *N Engl J Med* 1988; 319:189-194.

Wilcox LS, Kiely JL, Melvin CL, Martin MC: Assisted reproductive technologies: Estimates of their contribution to multiple births and newborn hospital days in the United States. *Fertil Steril* 1996; 65:361-366.

Wilcox LS, Mosher WD: Use of infertility services in the United States. *Obstet Gynecol* 1993; 82:122.

Witkins SS, Toth A: Relationship between genital tract infections, sperm antibodies in seminal fluid, and infertility. *Fertil Steril* 1983; 40:805.

Wittmaack FM, Kreger DO, Blasco L, et al: Effect of follicular size on oocyte retrieval, fertilization, cleavage and embryo quality in in vitro fertilization cycles: A 6-year data collection. *Fertil Steril* 1994; 62:1205-1210.

Wolf D, et al: Acrosomal status evaluation in normal ejaculated sperm with monoclonal antibodies. *Biol Reprod* 1985; 32:1157.

Wolf H, Anderson DJ: Immunohistologic characterization and quantitation of leukocyte subpopulations in human semen. *Fertil Steril* 1988; 49:497.

Woodward PJ, Wagner BJ, Farley TE: MR imaging in the evaluation of female infertility. *Radiographics* 1993; 13:293-310.

World Health Organization: A double blind trial of clomiphene citrate for the treatment of idiopathic male infertility. *Int J Androl* 1992(a); 15:299-307.

World Health Organization: The influence of varicocele on parameters of fertility in a large group of men presenting to infertility clinics. *Fertil Steril* 1992(b); 57:1289-1293.

Wright CS, Steel SJ, Jacobs HS: Value of bromocriptine in unexplained primary infertility: A double-blind controlled trial. *Br Med J* 1979; 21:1037-1039.

Wu CH, Winkel CA: The effect of therapy initiation day on clomiphene citrate therapy. *Fertil Steril* 1989; 52:564-568.

Yamamoto M, Hibi H, Hirata Y, et al: Effect of varicocelectomy on sperm parameters and pregnancy rate in patients with subclinical varicocele: A randomized prospective controlled study. *J Urol* 1996; 155:1636-1638.

Yanushpolsky E, et al: Effects of endometriomas on oocytes quality, embryo quality and pregnancy rates in in vitro fertilization cycles: A prospective, case controlled study. *J Assist Reprod Genet* 1998; 15:193-197.

Yen SSC: Chronic anovulation caused by peripheral endocrine disorders. In Yen SSC, Jaffe RB, editors: *Reproductive endocrinology*, Philadelphia, 1986, WB Saunders.

Yen, SSC, Vela P, Rankin J: Inappropriate secretion of follicle-stimulating hormone and luteinizing hormone in polycystic ovarian disease. *J Clin Endocrinol Metab* 1970; 30:435.

Young PE, et al: Reconstructive surgery for infertility at the Boston Hospital for Women. *Am J Obstet Gynecol* 1970; 108:1092.

Yovich JL, et al: Pregnancies following pronuclear stage tubal transfer. *Fertil Steril* 1987; 48:851.

Zielmaker GH, Alberda AT, van Gent I, et al: Two pregnancies following transfer of intact frozen thawed embryos. *Fertil Steril* 1984; 42:293-296.

Zinaman MJ, Clegg ED, Brown CC, et al: Estimates of human fertility and pregnancy loss. *Fertil Steril* 1996; 65:503-509.

15

Polycystic Ovary Syndrome and Hyperandrogenism

ANN E. TAYLOR

ANDREA E. DUNAIF

KEY ISSUES

1. Most women with hyperandrogenism have either polycystic ovarian syndrome (PCOS), defined as hyperandrogenism and chronic anovulation when other disorders are excluded, or idiopathic hirsutism, defined as hyperandrogenism and regular ovulatory menstrual cycles.
2. Significant morbid conditions are associated with PCOS, including endometrial hyperplasia, insulin resistance, diabetes mellitus type 2, and probably increased risk for cardiovascular disease.
3. Diagnostic evaluation should be focused on excluding ovarian and adrenal androgen-secreting tumors and screening for associated health risks including glucose intolerance and dyslipidemia.
4. Treatments that improve insulin sensitivity and result in lower serum insulin levels are potentially new therapies for hyperandrogenism.

The most common causes of hyperandrogenism are disorders of unknown cause: polycystic ovary syndrome and idiopathic hirsutism. These disorders affect approximately 5% of premenopausal women (Knochenhauer et al, 1998). In this chapter, we discuss the differential diagnosis of hyperandrogenism, the clinical correlates of the hyperandrogenic state, a diagnostic approach to masculinized women, and therapeutic options.

PATHOPHYSIOLOGY OF HYPERANDROGENISM

Masculinization is defined as clinical evidence of excess androgen action in women; it includes acne and alopecia in addition to hirsutism (Fig. 15-1). True virilization is defined as temporal balding, deepening of the voice, increased muscle bulk, and clitoromegaly, and is the clinical consequence of severe hyperandrogenism. Masculinization results from the effects of either increased androgen production or enhanced androgen use by target tissues. The spectrum of hyperandrogenic conditions ranges from a subtle increase in terminal body hair to true virilization. Because of genetic differences in target tissue number and sensitivity to androgens, there may be no clinical sequelae of hyperandrogenism.

Androgens are steroid hormones synthesized and secreted directly by the adrenal glands and gonads (Longcope, 1986). Potent androgens are also converted from precursors in peripheral tissues, including skin and fat cells. Androgens are defined specifically by their ability in bioassay systems to induce growth and secretion by the prostate and seminal vesicles and to bind tightly to prostatic cytosolic androgen receptors. Like insulin and growth hormone, androgens are anabolic because they cause nitrogen retention.

In humans, testosterone is the biologically important extracellular androgen. It is metabolized into biologically active products and excretory products. The biologically active metabolites include the even more potent androgen, dihydrotestosterone (DHT), formed intracellularly through the 5α-reduction of testosterone, and the estrogen, estradiol (E2), formed through the aromatization of testosterone.

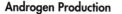

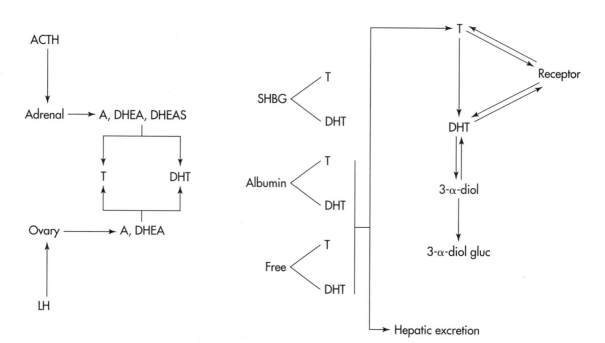

Fig. 15-1. Schema of androgen action. The ovaries and the adrenals secrete the androgen prehormones androstenedione (A) and dehydroepiandrosterone (DHEA) under the control of luteinizing hormone (LH) and adrenocorticotropic hormone (ACTH), respectively. DHEA sulfate (DHEAS) is secreted almost exclusively by the adrenals. Testosterone (T) is secreted by the ovaries and the adrenals and is produced by the peripheral conversion of A and DHEA. Under normal circumstances, dihydrotestosterone (DHT) is formed entirely from the peripheral conversion of A and T. T and DHT circulate tightly bound to the high-affinity binding proteins and sex hormone–binding globulin (SHBG) and are loosely associated with albumin. Free T and that nonspecifically bound to albumin are biologically available to enter target tissues. In most androgen target tissues, T is converted to its more potent metabolite, DHT, by the 5α-reductase enzyme system. Both T and DHT bind to the androgen receptor, initiating androgen action. DHT is metabolized in the periphery to 3α-androstanediol, which is then converted to 3α-androstanediol glucuronide and excreted. (Used with permission of A. Dunaif.)

Other androgens, such as androstenedione, dehydroepiandrosterone (DHEA), and DHEA sulfate (DHEAS), are androgenic by their conversion to testosterone or DHT and, thus, are androgenic prehormones. Androgen production results from glandular secretion and peripheral conversion of these prehormones (mostly androstenedione and DHEA). In normal women, approximately 50% of circulating testosterone is secreted equally by the ovary and the adrenal gland (Longcope, 1986). Androstenedione is also equally secreted by them (Longcope, 1986). In contrast, 50% of DHEA is secreted by the adrenal gland, 20% is secreted by the ovary, and 30% is derived from the peripheral conversion of DHEAS, which is almost completely produced by the adrenal gland (Abraham, 1976). Under normal circumstances, serum DHT is formed entirely from the peripheral conversion of androstenedione (85%) and testosterone (15%) (Ito and Horton, 1971). Thus, androgen production can be increased in abnormal states by the increased glandular secretion of the potent androgen testosterone or by the increased glandular secretion of androgen prehormones such as androstenedione, DHEA, and DHEAS.

In the ovary androgens are precursors of estrogen production, and their production is under the control of luteinizing hormone (LH). Thus, feedback control of ovarian androgens is mediated by the effects of androgen metabolites (*i.e.,* estrogens) on the hypothalamus and the pituitary. In the adrenal cortex, androgen production is under the control of adrenocorticotropic hormone (ACTH). The only known feedback control of adrenal androgen secretion is mediated by cortisol feedback on the hypotholamic-pituitary-adrenal axis.

Biologic availability of androgens is related to the concentration of the high-affinity, androgen-binding protein produced by the liver known as sex hormone–binding globulin (SHBG). Only free androgens and those nonspecifically bound to circulating albumin are able to enter tissues and produce biologic effects (Pardridge, 1981). SHBG has the greatest affinity for DHT, then for testosterone, and then for

E2. There is minimal, if any, binding of androstenedione or DHEA to SHBG. Certain synthetic androgens and progestins (*e.g.,* levonorgestrel, which is contained in several oral contraceptive pills) have high affinities for SHBG and may displace endogenous steroids. Hepatic synthesis of SHBG is decreased by androgens and insulin and increased by estrogens and thyroid hormones. Consequently, testosterone and DHT availability can be enhanced by decreasing SHBG levels or by administering compounds that compete for SHBG binding sites.

The major component of the metabolic clearance rate (MCR) of androgens reflects hepatic metabolism and the renal excretion of metabolites. A smaller component of the MCR results from androgens that leave the circulation to act on target tissues. This extrasplanchnic metabolism is also known as peripheral utilization. Androgen utilization by peripheral tissues is the final determinant of target-tissue androgen action. The pilosebaceous unit consists of a pilary component and a sebaceous component and can differentiate into a terminal hair follicle or a sebaceous follicle. In the pilosebaceous unit, the chief enzyme regulating androgen utilization is 5α-reductase (Kutten et al, 1977; Lobo et al, 1983). In the pilosebaceous unit, the major 5α-reduced androgen DHT is more potent than testosterone. In ovarian granulosa cells, adipose tissue, muscle, and hypothalamus, the aromatase enzyme system converts testosterone to E2 and androstenedione to estrone (E1).

Dihydrotestosterone binds to specific cytosolic androgen receptors that are then translocated to the nucleus. The interaction of DHT with the nuclear androgen receptor (a member of the c-erbA oncogenic hormone receptor superfamily) initiates androgen-specific molecular and cellular responses. Testosterone may also bind directly to the androgen receptor in certain target tissues, such as skeletal muscle, without requiring 5α-reductase conversion to DHT. Individual variation in the masculinizing effects of androgens cannot be explained on the basis of androgen receptor levels. Although the androgen receptor is required for masculinization and its genetic absence results in a female phenotype in genetic males (testicular feminization syndrome), no differences in androgen receptor levels have been detected between hirsute women and normal women or normal men (Mowszowicz et al, 1983). Recent data suggest that in men the functional activity of the androgen receptor can be modulated by the number of polyglutamine tri-nucleotide repeats in the first exon. Hence, longer repeats are associated with decreased sperm counts (Tut et al, 1997), and shorter repeats are associated with increased risk for androgen-dependent prostate cancer (Irvine, 1994). Whether this androgen receptor variability modulates androgen action at the low androgen levels seen in women remains to be determined. Thus, the clinical diversity of response to androgens in women could result from variability in androgen production, androgen bioavailability, peripheral androgen utilization, or, potentially, androgen receptor sensitivity.

> ### BOX 15-1
> ### SIGNS AND SYMPTOMS OF HYPERANDROGENISM
>
> **Nonvirilizing**
>
> Hirsutism
> Oily skin and seborrhea
> Cystic acne
> Diffuse alopecia
> Menstrual irregularities
> Infertility
>
> **Virilizing**
>
> Temporal balding
> Clitoromegaly
> Deepening of the voice
> Skeletal muscle hypertrophy and male body habitus
> Mammary atrophy
> Increased libido

Clinical Features of Hyperandrogenism

Most women with clinical evidence of hyperandrogenism have increased ovarian or adrenal androgen production (Bardin and Lipsett, 1967). In most hyperandrogenic women, SHBG levels are typically low, and free testosterone levels are elevated even when total testosterone levels are normal. Occasional women with normal circulating androgen levels may have isolated increased peripheral compartment (skin and hair follicle) androgen production from increased 5α-reductase activity (Horton et al, 1982) (Box 15-1).

Hirsutism

The most commonly appreciated expression of hyperandrogenism is excess terminal hair in women. Hirsutism is defined as the transformation of vellus (fine, soft, unpigmented) to terminal (coarse, pigmented, longer) hair in androgen-dependent hair areas (*e.g.,* upper lip, chin, chest, back, pubis, thighs). Although the hormonal environment influences the conversion of vellus hairs to terminal hairs, the total number of hair follicles is genetically determined and is not changed by the hormonal environment. Racial and ethnic (but not sex) differences exist in total follicle number; for example, white persons have more follicles than Asians, and persons of Mediterranean descent have more follicles than those of northern European descent. The total hair follicle number influences the severity of the expression of hirsutism in hyperandrogenic women. For example, one fourth to one third of women of British and non-Scandinavian European origin may normally have terminal hair on the upper lip, periareolar area, or linea alba, whereas such hair must be considered abnormal in Asian and Scandinavian women

Idiopathic hirsutism
Polycystic ovarian syndrome
Congenital adrenal hyperplasia (classical and
  nonclassical)
Androgen-secreting neoplasms
Factitious/iatrogenic
Hypertrichosis
Other medical conditions: Hypothyroidism, juvenile hypothyroidism, acute intermittent porphyria, malnutrition, anorexia nervosa, dermatomyositis, epidermolysis bullosa, Cornelia de Lange syndrome, postencephalitis period, onset of multiple sclerosis, nevoid hypertrichosis, and severe insulin resistance.
Medications: Minoxidil, phenytoin, corticosteroids, penicillamine, diazoxide, streptomycin, hexachlorobenzene, psoralens, and cyclosporine

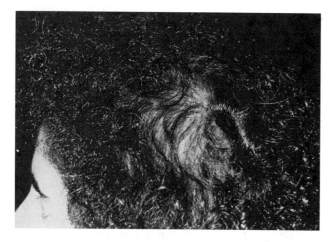

Fig. 15-2. Diffuse androgenic alopecia in a woman with mildly elevated testosterone levels secondary to polycystic ovarian syndrome. She had no signs of true virilization. (Used with permission of A. Dunaif.)

(Ferriman and Gallway, 1961; Carmina et al, 1992). Unlike those areas, the upper abdomen, sternum, back, and shoulders are distinctly unusual sites for terminal hair in women and should be cause for further evaluation, even in women from genetic backgrounds with more baseline hair follicles. Finally, hirsutism must be differentiated from hypertrichosis, which is a generalized increase in vellus (lanugo in the neonate) but not terminal hair. Hypertrichosis may be associated with certain drugs, metabolic disorders, or malignancy (Box 15-2).

Alopecia

Androgen stimulation of the pilosebaceous unit in most parts of the body produces increased hair diameter, pigmen-

tation, rate of growth, and sebaceous gland secretion. Conversely, androgen stimulation of androgen-sensitive hair follicles on the scalp decreases the diameter and rate of hair growth, especially in the temporal area (male pattern baldness). Diffuse hair thinning can also be a sign of mild hyperandrogenism in women (Futterweit et al, 1988) (Fig. 15-2).

Acne

Increased production of sebum leads to acne in susceptible persons; if it is chronic, it can produce scarring. Occasionally, acne is the only sign of severe hyperandrogenism. Lucky et al (1983) found that women with acne alone had elevated free testosterone levels similar to those of women with hirsutism with or without acne.

Menstrual Irregularity and Infertility

Hyperandrogenism is often associated with chronic anovulation that results in menstrual irregularity (Hull, 1987). The anovulatory state can be associated with chronic, unopposed estrogen stimulation of the endometrium, resulting in endometrial hyperplasia, erratic heavy menstrual bleeding, and even endometrial carcinoma (Aiman et al, 1986). In addition, the reduced frequency of ovulation is associated with decreased opportunities for conception. Hyperandrogenism probably has an impact on fertility in addition to anovulation. Many studies suggest a decreased conception rate in spite of induced ovulation, and some suggest an increased risk for spontaneous miscarriage in hyperandrogenic women (Balen et al, 1993; Franks, 1995). The mechanisms for this androgen action remain to be determined.

Virilization

In more severe forms of androgen excess, other masculinizing signs develop. These are referred to as true virilization, and they include increased muscle bulk, clitoromegaly [clitoral length greater than 1 cm or diameter greater than 0.5 cm (Tagatz et al, 1979)], temporal balding, and voice deepening. Clitoromegaly and voice changes are irreversible, even if androgen levels can be reduced to normal. Profound androgen excess may also inhibit breast growth and produce an android distribution of body fat.

Behavior

Behavior may be affected by hyperandrogenism. The major source of data on this question derives from adult women with classic virilizing congenital adrenal hyperplasia, most of whom underwent attempts at surgical correction of clitoromegaly with variable success rates. Hochberg et al (1987) noted various psychological changes in genotypic females with virilizing congenital adrenal hyperplasia. These included altered personality, preadolescent tomboyishness, and injured body image, despite an eventual adjustment to feminine gender identity. Increased sex drive (coital and masturbation frequency), increased satisfaction threshold, and versatility in heterosexual relationships were also described in women with "late-treated" adrenogenital syndrome (Ehrhardt et al, 1968). Whether the poor success rate of their genital correction surgery, resulting in difficult or impossible heterosexual intercourse, confounds these findings is unknown. In the common hyperandrogenic disorders in which androgen levels are only modestly elevated (*e.g.,* testosterone levels ~100 ng/dL), behavioral changes have not been well studied. However, quality of life is compromised in women with PCOS, particularly because of obesity (Cronin et al, 1997).

Differential Diagnosis and Pathophysiology

A woman's concern about androgenic symptoms such as hirsutism or hair loss may differ depending on her ethnic background and her interpretation of normal, which may be influenced by popular images of hairless female beauty. The physician must consider normal racial and ethnic variations in terminal hair distribution and possible causes for hypertrichosis.

Idiopathic Hirsutism

Idiopathic hirsutism (IH) is defined by the maintenance of normal ovulation, despite increased androgen effects on the skin (Lobo, 1986). Regular ovulatory menstrual cycles are reassuring, but never absolute, evidence that serious abnormal causes of hirsutism can be excluded. Women with IH have 5α-reductase activity that is greater than that of normal women but similar to that of normal men (Thomas and Oake, 1974; Kutten et al, 1977) (Fig. 15-3). Although more than 90% of hirsute women have biochemical evidence of hyperandrogenemia (Wild et al, 1983), women with IH tend to have lower androgen production rates (Bardin and Lipsett, 1967). This may explain the absence of ovulatory disturbances in such women. Furthermore, PCOS usually does not develop in women with IH (Dunaif, unpublished observations). Although ultrasonography reveals polycystic ovaries in many women with IH (Adams, 1986), the diagnosis of PCOS cannot be made without some form of anovulation (see later). Recent studies by Legro et al (1998a) have found that hyperandrogenemia with regular menses is an additional familial phenotype in PCOS kindreds. Thus, it may be part of the genetic spectrum of PCOS.

Polycystic Ovary Syndrome and Ovarian Hyperthecosis

These conditions represent a morphologic spectrum of the same process. In 1935, Stein and Leventhal described a syndrome consisting of bilaterally enlarged sclerocystic and polyfollicular ovaries, menstrual dysfunction, and hirsutism (Stein and Leventhal, 1935). Geist and Gaines (1942) noted the association of clinical virilization with islands of luteinized theca cells in the ovarian stroma; this finding subsequently became known as ovarian stromal hyperthecosis.

There is general agreement in the literature that the diagnosis of PCOS requires the presence of hyperandrogenism (elevated serum androgen levels or definitive clinical evi-

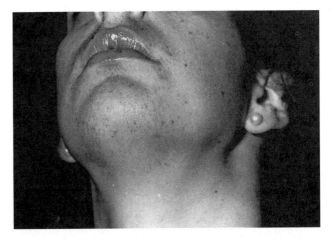

Fig. 15-3. Moderate terminal hair growth on the chin and upper lip of a woman with idiopathic hirsutism. (Used with permission of A. Dunaif.)

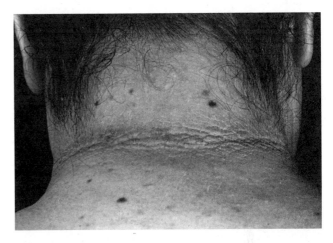

Fig. 15-4. Acanthosis nigricans on the neck of a woman with polycystic ovarian syndrome. (Used with permission of A. Dunaif.)

dence of excess androgen effect) and chronic anovulation (fewer than six to nine menses per year) (Zawadski and Dunaif, 1992). It is now recognized that PCOS represents the most common cause of masculinization in women with a prevalence of approximately 5% of premenopausal women (Knochenhauer et al, 1998).

Women with PCOS are chronically anovulatory, but spontaneous ovulation and conception may occasionally occur. Usually, menstrual irregularities persist from the time of menarche so that a regular pattern of menses is never established. Less often, girls can have primary amenorrhea. Hyperandrogenism may be subtle, and cystic acne may be the only sign. Hyperandrogenism may take several years to produce hirsutism in PCOS or hirtutism may be absent, depending on the 5α-reductase activity in the skin (McKenna et al, 1983). Acanthosis nigricans is evident on clinical examination of the skin in approximately 50% of obese women with PCOS (Dunaif et al, 1987; Stuart et al, 1986; Dunaif et al, 1991) (Fig. 15-4). Acromegaloid features, such

---

BOX 15-3
CLINICAL FEATURES IN WOMEN WITH POLYCYSTIC OVARIAN SYNDROME

Frequent

Hirsutism
Infertility
Oligomenorrhea
Obesity

Common

Amenorrhea
Seborrhea
Acne
Acanthosis nigricans
Alopecia
Impaired glucose tolerance

Rare

True virilization
Acral hypertrophy
Endometrial carcinoma
Hypertension
Non-androgen-secreting ovarian tumors (*e.g.,* dermoid cysts)

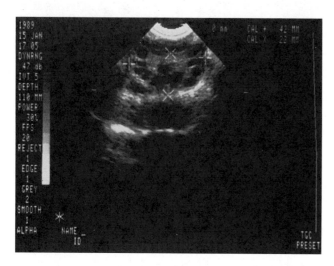

Fig. 15-5. Polycystic ovaries detected by vaginal ultrasonography in a woman with polycystic ovarian syndrome. The ovary is enlarged to 42 mm × 22 mm, and it has eight or more subcapsular follicular cysts 6 to 10 mm in diameter and an increased amount of stromata (Adams criteria). The cysts in this woman completely encircle the ovary, giving it a "pearl necklace" appearance. (Used with permission of A. Dunaif.)

as acral hypertrophy, are found occasionally in women with PCOS. True virilization is uncommon in PCOS and suggests the presence of an adrenal or ovarian tumor. Clinical findings in women with PCOS are summarized in Box 15-3.

In PCOS, classic ovarian morphology includes a thickened cortex, multiple subcapsular follicular cysts, hyperpla-

sia and luteinization of the theca interna, stromal hyperplasia, and multiple immature follicles suggestive of arrested folliculogenesis (Hughesdon, 1982). Ovary size ranges from normal to substantially enlarged. On ultrasonography, these histologic findings appear as a peripheral array of at least eight small follicles (6 to 10 mm in diameter), and there is an increased amount of dense stroma (Adams criteria) (Adams et al, 1986) (Fig. 15-5). Although most women with PCOS have the typical polycystic ovarian morphology, this ovarian morphology is not specific to PCOS. Enlarged polycystic ovaries are seen in women with adult-onset 21-hydroxylase deficiency (Hague et al, 1990) and 20% to 25% of normal controls (Polson et al, 1988). The lack of specificity of ovarian morphologic changes for which this disorder was named emphasizes the importance of defining the biochemical features of PCOS and of excluding other diseases before diagnosis.

The primary androgen-secreting cells of the ovary are thecal and stromal cells, which respond to stimulation by LH (Erickson et al, 1985). Follicles contain granulosa cells that, under normal circumstances, aromatize locally produced androgens to estrogens (primarily E2). The capacity of granulosa cells to aromatize androgens is a function of their maturity, and this is under direct follicle-stimulating hormone (FSH) control (Erickson et al, 1985).

There is considerable overlap in the reported clinical and biochemical features of hyperthecosis and PCOS (Geist and Gaines, 1942; Dunaif et al, 1985). Hyperthecosis has been defined as luteinized cells that are clustered or diffusely scattered away from the follicles in the stroma and that encroach on the hilar region. However, when ovarian sections are examined carefully by histologic analysis, islands of luteinized theca cells (stromal hyperthecosis) can be detected in most ovaries of women with PCOS (Hughesdon, 1982). More extensive stromal hyperthecosis often correlates with more severe androgen excess, producing true virilization. However, stromal hyperthecosis also can be associated with estrogen production alone and may be a cause of postmenopausal vaginal bleeding (Nagamani et al, 1988). Stromal hyperthecosis is more extensive in women with PCOS if there is substantial insulin resistance, and it has been suggested that insulin directly stimulates theca cell growth (Dunaif et al, 1985; Nagamani et al, 1988). Indeed, the extent of theca cell hyperplasia has been shown to be positively related to plasma insulin levels (Nagamani et al, 1988).

Biochemical Features. Characteristic biochemical abnormalities of PCOS include elevated serum androgen levels, decreased SHBG levels, disordered gonadotropin release with increased LH relative to FSH secretion, and acyclic (tonic) estrogen levels in the midfollicular range of the normal menstrual cycle associated with chronic anovulation. Hyperinsulinemia secondary to insulin resistance appears to be a unique feature of PCOS and not of hyperandrogenic states in general (Dunaif et al, 1987). Biochemical abnormalities may wax and wane, and attempts to categorize this disorder by biochemical profiles are problematic.

Elevated Androgens. Plasma levels of testosterone, biologically available testosterone (non–SHBG-bound and free), androstenedione, DHEAS, DHEA, and DHT can be elevated. Typically, testosterone, non–SHBG-bound testosterone, and androstenedione levels are mildly to moderately elevated compared with nonhirsute regularly ovulating women. If serum testosterone levels are *consistently* greater than 150 to 200 ng/dL when measured in an extraction and chromatography assay system or if DHEAS levels are greater than 700 µg/dL (Meldrum and Abraham, 1979; Moltz et al, 1984; Friedman et al, 1985; Derksen et al, 1994), an androgen-secreting neoplasm must be excluded. Peripheral androgen elevations fluctuate with pulsatile adrenal secretion and ovarian menstrual cyclicity so that a single determination may miss androgen excess. Occasionally repeated sampling or pooling of samples may be necessary to detect androgen excess.

By combining the results of a number of studies, it can be seen that there is increased ovarian androgen production in most women with PCOS. Under normal circumstances, more than 90% of serum DHEAS is secreted by the adrenals (Longcope, 1986); thus, its elevation in women with PCOS indicates that there is an adrenal contribution to androgen excess. However, because the adrenals also contribute substantially to circulating testosterone and androstenedione levels, both by direct secretion and by peripheral conversion of prohormones, adrenal hyperandrogenism may occur in the absence of elevated DHEAS levels. Many women with PCOS have an adrenal component to their androgen excess (Ehrmann et al, 1995).

Sex Hormone–Binding Globulin. Serum levels of SHBG are modestly decreased in nonobese women with PCOS and substantially decreased in obese women with PCOS. This is secondary, in part, to the direct action of androgens to decrease hepatic production of SHBG (Andersen, 1974; Winneker et al, 1989). Obesity is also associated with low SHBG levels, which may be attributed to an independent effect of insulin to decrease hepatic SHBG synthesis directly (Plymate et al, 1988; Nestler et al, 1991).

Estrogens. Serum levels of total estrogens are elevated above the range seen in normally menstruating women. Estradiol levels are similar to those seen in the midfollicular phase of the normal menstrual cycle, whereas E1 levels are typically elevated compared with those in normal women (Rebar et al, 1976; Baird et al, 1977). Therefore, on clinical examination, women with PCOS are well estrogenized (*e.g.,* they have moist vaginal mucosa with rugae, and they experience vaginal bleeding after progestin challenge). Because SHBG levels are low, non–SHBG-bound, biologically available E2 levels are increased compared with those in normally ovulating women in the midfollicular phase of the menstrual cycle (Lobo et al, 1981). This may be important in the pathogenesis of the gonadotropin secretory abnormalities of PCOS (Lobo et al, 1981).

Estrogen secretion in PCOS is derived from the ovary and the extragonadal aromatization of androgens (particularly androstenedione to E1). Estrogen production in PCOS is constant and is not cyclic as it is in the normal menstrual cycle. This results in a chronic, unopposed (*i.e.,* no progesterone) effect on the endometrium that can result in endometrial hyperplasia, dysfunctional uterine bleeding, and endometrial neoplasia if left untreated (Jackson and Docherty, 1957).

Gonadotropins. Serum LH levels are increased in most women with PCOS as a function of increased amplitude and increased frequency of pulsatile LH secretion (Waldstreicher et al, 1985; Taylor et al, 1997). Serum FSH levels and pulse frequency are generally in the normal midfollicular range, or they may be slightly low. An increased frequency of LH pulses indicates an increased frequency of hypothalamic gonadotropin-releasing hormone (GnRH) secretion, and, therefore, a hypothalamic site of the abnormality. The increased amplitude of LH pulses may have several causes. First, women with PCOS secrete more LH in response to the same dosage of GnRH (Rebar et al, 1976) or GnRH agonists (Barnes et al, 1989), indicating increased pituitary sensitivity. Second, an increased GnRH pulse frequency has been shown to increase the LH-FSH ratio experimentally, indicating a direct effect of frequency (Spratt et al, 1987). Third, there does not appear to be an increase in the amount of GnRH secreted per pulse because LH is similarly suppressed by small dosages of a GnRH-antagonist in women with PCOS and in normal controls (Hayes et al, 1998). Finally, there does not appear to be an excess secretion of inhibin from PCOS ovaries (Lambert-Messelian et al, 1994).

Insulin Resistance. Insulin resistance is a unique feature of PCOS and not of hyperandrogenic states in general (Dunaif et al, 1987; Dunaif et al, 1989; Robinson et al, 1993). Approximately 40% of women with PCOS have impaired glucose tolerance (31%) or frank diabetes mellitus (7.5%) (Legro et al, 1999). Although obesity and age increase this risk, glucose intolerance, including type 2 diabetes, can be seen in adolescent and nonobese PCOS women (Legro et al, 1999). PCOS is an important risk factor for the development of type 2 diabetes mellitus in women. It is estimated that approximately 10% of diabetes in premenopausal women is PCOS related (Dunaif, 1997).

Pathophysiology of Polycystic Ovary Syndrome. There are four distinct loci of disturbed endocrine functioning in women with PCOS: ovaries, adrenal gland, hypothalamic-pituitary axis, and peripheral insulin-responsive tissues.

Ovarian Function. Theca cells isolated from polycystic ovaries secrete markedly increased amounts of androstenedione and 17-OH progesterone basally and in response to LH (Gilling-Smith et al, 1994). Despite extensive investigation, however, no consistent specific enzymatic defect in steroidogenesis has been found in the majority of ovaries of women with PCOS. A number of steroidogenic pathways are upregulated, consistent with a diffuse hyperresponsiveness rather than a specific enzyme defect (Ehrmann et al, 1995). Many women with PCOS have exaggerated ovarian

17-OH progesterone secretion, suggesting dysregulation of the cytochrome enzyme P450c17 that controls 17 hydroxylation of pregnenolone and progesterone and 17,20 lyase activity to convert 17-OH pregnenolone to DHEA (Ehrmann et al, 1995). This is the rate-limiting enzyme for androgen biosynthesis. No mutations have been found in this enzyme in women with PCOS (Franks et al, 1997; Legro et al, 1998b).

Granulosa cells from polycystic ovaries secrete smaller amounts of estrogen than granulosa cells from normal ovaries. However, the addition of FSH to PCOS granulosa cells results in normal estrogen secretion (Erickson et al, 1985; Mason et al, 1994). This suggests that ovarian responsiveness is normal and that the decreased granulosa cell estrogen production characteristic of PCOS is a functional abnormality secondary to inadequate FSH stimulation.

Adrenal Function. The adrenal glands can contribute to hyperandrogenism in PCOS as indicated by selective venous catheterization studies, elevations of serum DHEAS levels, and studies in which ovarian or adrenal steroid production has been suppressed. Indeed, the nonclassical, late-onset form of adrenal 21-hydroxylase deficiency has clinical, biochemical, and ovarian morphological features indistinguishable from PCOS (Lobo and Goebelsmann, 1980). In the absence of these definable adrenal enzyme defects, women with PCOS often have increased responses to exogenous ACTH of DHEA, 17-OH progesterone, 17-hydroxypregnenolone, and androstenedione (Luckey et al, 1986; Ehrmann et al, 1995). However, these responses do not conform to a pattern for a single adrenal enzyme defect and suggest, instead, generalized adrenal hyperresponsiveness. It is possible that this represents a primary abnormality. Alternatively, insulin has been shown to increase adrenal responsiveness to ACTH (Moghetti et al, 1996).

Function of the Hypothalamic-Pituitary Axis. Several hypotheses have been proposed to explain the neuroendocrine defect of PCOS, including a primary hypothalamic defect, abnormal sex steroid feedback, and abnormal sensitivity to feedback. Spontaneous ovulation (Blankstein et al, 1987; Taylor et al, 1997) or progestin exposure (Christman et al, 1991; Pastor et al, 1998; Daniels and Berga, 1997) can reduce exaggerated LH secretion in women with PCOS but may not normalize it, suggesting that an underlying hypothalamic defect persists regardless of normal feedback. The antiestrogen clomiphene citrate induces a similar rise, and exogenous estrogen produces a similar fall of LH and FSH release in PCOS and in normal ovulatory women in the mid-follicular phase of the menstrual cycle, suggesting that estrogen-negative feedback is intact (Rebar et al, 1976). However, estrogen administration provokes a rise (positive feedback) in LH and FSH levels in women with PCOS 24 hours earlier than it does in normal women in the midfollicular phase. In women with PCOS, there is also increased LH release during GnRH administration than there is in normal women in the midfollicular phase (Rebar et al, 1976). These findings suggest that women with PCOS are "estrogen primed" because both early positive feedback and increased pituitary sensitivity to GnRH can be produced in normal women by exogenous estrogen administration.

Elevated LH and LH-FSH ratios have been described in women with hyperandrogenism of other causes, such as androgen-secreting ovarian neoplasms (Dunaif et al, 1984b) or nonclassical congenital adrenal hyperplasia (Lobo and Goebelsmann, 1980). Androgens are able to distort gonadotropin release by their aromatization to estrogens (Dunaif, 1986). Although androgen levels in the normal male range suppress gonadotropin release in normal women (Serafini et al, 1986), androgen levels in the PCOS range do not directly alter gonadotropin release in women with PCOS or in normal women (Dunaif, 1986). Conversely, the administration of an aromatase inhibitor to women with PCOS results in increases in gonadotropin release characteristic of an antiestrogenic effect (Dunaif, et al, 1984a). However, E1 administration does not alter LH release in women with PCOS (Chang et al, 1982). This suggests that E2 is the major gonadal steroid contributing to the distortion of gonadotropin release in PCOS.

There is growing evidence that gonadotropin secretion in PCOS is also modulated by some factor related to body weight (Taylor et al, 1997; Arroyo et al, 1997). Obese patients tend to have lower mean LH levels, LH-FSH ratios, and LH pulse amplitudes, but they maintain rapid LH pulse frequencies. The inverse correlation of LH secretion with body mass index is similar with percentage body fat and fasting serum leptin levels and is slightly less with fasting insulin levels.

Biochemical-Pathology Correlation. The ovarian pathology findings are consistent with the abnormal hormonal milieu. It is believed that the hyperplastic thecal and stromal tissues are secondary to chronic stimulation by excess LH. It has been suggested by Givens et al (1975) that the gonadotropin-responsive tumors that occasionally coexist with PCOS may be the end result of this stimulation, as are the androgen-secreting luteomas that may occur during pregnancy (see later). Hyperinsulinemia is associated with stromal hyperthecosis in PCOS (Dunaif et al, 1985). Exogenous androgen administration may also result in polycystic ovarian changes (Futterweit and Deligdisch, 1985).

Hypotheses for the Cause of Polycystic Ovary Syndrome. It has been demonstrated that disordered gonadotropin secretion is usually necessary to perpetuate hyperandrogenism in PCOS (Chang et al, 1983) and that either ovarian or adrenal androgen excess can cause gonadotropin release identical to that of PCOS (Lobo and Goebelsmann, 1980; Dunaif et al, 1984b). Thus, a primary central abnormality leading to disrupted gonadotropin secretion or a primary ovarian or adrenal defect leading to hyperandrogenism could be postulated to cause PCOS as follows. First, it has been suggested that a vicious circle is initiated by adrenal androgen excess because of exaggerated adrenarche (Yen, 1980). This causes distorted gonadotropin release with increased LH relative to FSH secretion, resulting in arrested folliculogenesis and LH-dependent ovarian androgen production. Excess androgens are then aromatized peripherally into estrogens. Abnormal gonadal steroid production in turn perpetuates the disordered gonadotropin release. However, gonadotropin secretory abnormalities and hyperandrogenism resume promptly in women with PCOS after medical oophorectomy with long-acting GnRH analogues (Chang et al, 1983). This suggests that there is a primary persistent abnormality in the control of GnRH release or in steroidogenesis in PCOS.

Second, it has been suggested that there is a primary central nervous system alteration that results in PCOS. Indeed, adolescent girls with PCOS have disordered diurnal secretory patterns of LH, suggesting that a neuroendocrine abnormality may be involved (Zumoff et al, 1983). A number of potential neuroendocrine changes have been suggested in PCOS, including decreases in central dopaminergic tone, but these may be secondary to tonic estrogen feedback rather than primary lesions.

Third, there has been renewed interest in a primary ovarian or adrenal enzymatic defect leading to impaired folliculogenesis or increased androgen production. Primary ovarian defects that have been reported in PCOS include abnormal 11β-hydroxylase, 3β-hydroxysteroid dehydrogenase, 17-ketosteroid reductase, 17β-hydroxysteroid dehydrogenase, and 17α-hydroxylase/17-20 lyase activities (Ehrmann et al, 1995). To date, however, there is no strong evidence for primary genetic defects in these ovarian steroidogenic enzymes in PCOS because ovaries appear to function normally in response to FSH (Erickson et al, 1985; Franks, 1995).

Fourth, there has been growing speculation that insulin or insulin-like growth factors (IGFs) play a major role in the pathogenesis of PCOS. Acute infusion of supraphysiologic amounts of insulin can directly alter gonadal steroid secretion in women with PCOS (Dunaif and Graf, 1989). Moreover, lowering insulin levels by weight loss (Kiddy et al, 1992) or the use of pharmacologic agents (Nestler et al, 1989; Dunaif et al, 1996; Nestler et al, 1998) results in decreased circulating androgen levels and the resumption of ovulation.

In summary, PCOS is characterized by masculinization and is differentiated from IH by the presence of oligo-ovulation or anovulation. Only by excluding other causes (Zawodski and Dunaif, 1992) can a diagnosis of PCOS be confirmed. Ultrasonographic documentation of polycystic ovaries supports the diagnosis, but it is not definitive for the disorder.

Metabolic Consequences of Polycystic Ovary Syndrome. The association of PCOS with obesity (Evans et al, 1983), insulin resistance, and glucose intolerance raises the concern that affected women are at increased risk for coronary artery disease and other atherosclerotic conditions. Several large epidemiologic studies have linked hyperinsulinemia with an increased risk for cardiovascular events. However, none of these studies included women, and no long-term prospective studies of cardiovascular risk in women with PCOS have been conducted to address the issue.

Because it takes a long time to complete prospective cardiac event outcome studies, alternative approaches to assess cardiac risk in patients with PCOS have been conducted, including assessment of current cardiovascular risk factors such as hypertension and hyperlipidemia and retrospective studies of all women with symptoms of cardiovascular disease. Some, but not all, studies of fasting lipid levels in women with PCOS, defined by variable criteria, suggest that high-density lipoprotein levels may be reduced and triglyceride levels increased in hyperandrogenic women (Wild, 1995; Talbott et al, 1995). Some of the variability may be explained by the small numbers of patients in some studies and by the lack of weight- and age-matched controls in other studies. Our own data (Graf et al, 1990) suggest that most of the differences in lipid levels between women with PCOS and control subjects can be explained by the differences in body mass index. It remains unclear whether PCOS bestows an increased risk over what would be expected for the degree of insulin resistance and increased prevalence of impaired glucose tolerance and type 2 diabetes. Indeed, 15% of older women with a history consistent with PCOS have diabetes mellitus (Dahlgren et al, 1992b).

Hypertension has also been associated with hyperinsulinemia. However, blood pressure is clearly not increased in young patients with PCOS compared to weight- and body fat–matched controls, even though the patients with PCOS in one study were clearly insulin resistant and hyperinsulinemic (Zimmerman et al, 1992). These results raise the possibility that insulin resistance in women with PCOS, or insulin resistance in women in general, plays a different role in cardiovascular risk than it does in men. However, older women with a history of wedge resection for PCOS may have a prevalence for hypertension that is as high as 39% (Dahlgren et al, 1992b).

More recent studies have addressed other surrogate risk factors for cardiovascular disease, including the production of plasminogen activator-I (PAI-1), which is enhanced by hyperinsulinemia and is associated with a decreased fibrinolytic response to thrombosis. PAI-1 concentration and activity are elevated in women with PCOS (Andersen et al, 1995). Ehrmann et al (1997b) demonstrated reductions in PAI-1 when insulin levels were reduced by troglitazone in patients with PCOS.

To date, two retrospective studies have been reported of women undergoing cardiac catheterization for the evaluation of chest pain. Both are weakened by their small sample size, mixture of premenopausal and postmenopausal subjects, and retrospective assessment of previous hirsutism and menstrual dysfunction. However, both suggest that women who had documented coronary artery disease at the time of catheterization were more likely to have a history consistent with hyperandrogenism. In the first study, Wild et al (1990) reported that there was a significant increase in hirsutism in women with catheterization evidence of coronary artery disease. In the second study, Birdsall et al (1997) found an increase in documented coronary artery disease in women with polycystic ovarian morphology.

Thus, women with PCOS clearly have a proclivity for insulin resistance that may contribute to other risk factors for coronary artery disease and to more coronary atherosclerosis. However, data confirming this hypothesis are unavailable. Current recommendations, given these data, are to consider all cardiovascular risk factors in women with PCOS and to screen vigilantly and treat for obesity, hypertension, hyperlipidemia, and type 2 diabetes mellitus.

Androgen-Secreting Ovarian Tumors

A few ovarian tumors (less than 1%) are capable of producing masculinization by the direct secretion of androgens. These tumors are classified as sex-cord stromal tumors, steroid or lipoid cell tumors, gonadoblastomas, and tumors with functioning stroma. The category of sex-cord stromal tumors contains derivatives of the sex cords (granulosa or Sertoli cells) or stroma singly or in any combination and in various degrees of differentiation. *Lipoid cell tumor* refers to the morphologic features of the steroid-producing cells that make them up, such as luteinized thecoma, Leydig, and adrenal-cortical–like cells. They can be divided into three categories according their cells of origin, known or unknown. Gonadoblastomas are complex tumors composed of sex-cord, stromal, and germ-cell elements. They almost invariably arise in association with gonadal dysgenesis when a Y chromosome–containing cell line is present and produces masculinization from the excessive production of androgens by the Leydig cell elements.

Other Ovarian Tumor Hyperandrogenic Conditions. Several tumors stimulate surrounding stroma into steroid-secreting tissue by human chorionic gonadotropin (hCG)-independent mechanisms. Despite a report of virilizing serous cystadenoma and Brenner tumor without histologic evidence of stromal hyperplasia or luteinization, it is debatable whether these types of ovarian cancer have the necessary steroidogenic enzymes for androgen secretion. Rather, it is generally accepted that neighboring stromata is mechanically stimulated to secrete androgens, as with an expanding follicle, or is trophically stimulated by paracrine or endocrine factors.

Pregnancy. During pregnancy, certain benign ovarian lesions, most commonly luteomas and hyperreactio luteinalis, are capable of androgen hypersecretion (Shortle et al, 1987). These lesions are derived from luteinized stromal cells, present before pregnancy, that respond unusually to placental gonadotropin secretion. Maternal virilization occurs in 10% to 50% of luteomas and in 25% of hyperreactio luteinalis. Fetal masculinization is rare, however, because of the large placental capacity to aromatize androgens into estrogens.

Postmenopause

Postmenopausal women may show masculinization that results from the lowered free estrogen to free androgen ratio caused by declining estrogen secretion in the aged ovary. Androgen secretion may continue at a disproportionately high rate because of stromal stimulation by elevated postmenopausal gonadotropins. Many elderly women experience increased growth of terminal hair on the upper lip and chin, whereas pubic, axillary, and scalp hair are partially lost.

Adrenal Masculinizing Conditions

The principal disorders of the adrenal gland that can cause masculinization in women are congenital adrenal hyperplasia (CAH), Cushing syndrome with significant hyperandrogenism, and testosterone-producing or androgen precursor–producing adrenal tumors. Usually, adrenal hyperandrogenemia is suspected when elevated serum DHEAS levels are found. An isolated elevation in serum testosterone level, however, does not exclude an adrenal source. CAH and adrenal virilizing tumors must be differentiated from premature adrenarche in girls in whom the normal rise in adrenal androgen secretion occurs before 7 years of age. In premature adrenarche, there may be mild acceleration in height and bone age accompanied by precocious pubic hair development, but there is no virilization as there is with CAH and adrenal tumors.

Nonclassical Congenital Adrenal Hyperplasia. Hyperandrogenism resulting from inherited defects in adrenal steroid biosynthesis (predominantly 21-hydroxylase deficiency) can present during adolescence or adulthood (late-onset, attenuated, or nonclassical CAH [NCCAH]) (Fig. 15-6). In these disorders, an enzymatic defect integral to the formation of cortisol causes a slight compensatory increase in pituitary ACTH production and an increased conversion of cortisol precursors to androgens. Women with late-onset CAH may have a history of prepubertal hirsutism but rarely prepubertal virilization.

The most common form of CAH is nonclassical 21-hydroxylase deficiency, which is caused by mutations in the P450c21 gene on chromosome 6 and is inherited as an autosomal recessive trait (New and Speiser, 1986). The nonclassical form of 21-hydroxylase deficiency is not detected until puberty and is not associated with salt wasting, severe virilization, or adrenal insufficiency. This disorder is easily diagnosed by 17-hydroxyprogesterone responses after ACTH administration (see Fig. 15-6). Unstimulated early morning 17-hydroxyprogesterone levels may also be used for diagnosis (Azziz and Zacur, 1989). The incidence of NCCAH among hirsute women ranges from 1% to 5% depending on the ethnic background, with an overall frequency of 0.3% in the general white population and approximately 3% in Jews of European origin (New and Speiser, 1986).

The clinical picture for late-onset 3β-hydroxysteroid dehydrogenase deficiency is indistinguishable from that for PCOS—peripubertal hirsutism and menstrual irregularity (Pang et al, 1985; Zerah et al, 1994). Biochemically, baseline $\Delta5$ steroids (DHEAS and DHEA) are more elevated than $\Delta4$ steroids (androstenedione and testosterone), and the ACTH-stimulated 17α-hydroxypregnenolone-17α-hydroxyprogesterone ratio is elevated to a greater degree than the DHEA-androstenedione ratio. Although this steroid

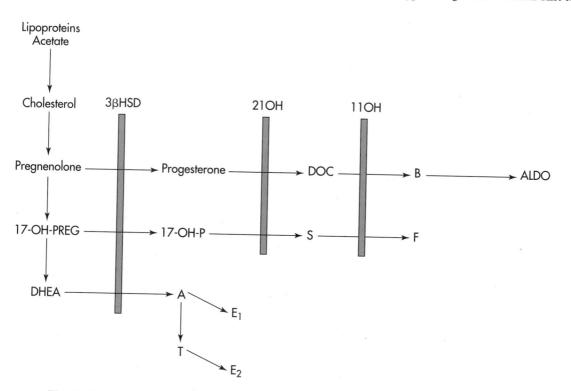

Fig. 15-6. Adrenal steroid biosynthetic pathways and sites of enzyme deficiencies producing the congenital adrenal hyperplasias. Deficiencies of 21-hydroxylase (21OH) can become manifest at birth, in adolescence, or in adulthood. The nonclassical forms of 21-OH deficiency that develop in adolescence or adulthood must be excluded in the evaluation of hyperandrogenism. A, androstenedione; ALDO, aldosterone; B, corticosterone; DHEA, dehydroepiandrosterone; DOC, 11-deoxycorticosterone; E_1, estrone; E_2, estradiol; F, cortisol; 17-OH-P, 17-hydroxyprogesterone; 17-OH-PREG, 17-hydroxypregnenelone; S, 11-deoxycortisol; T, testosterone.

pattern has been reported in as many as 15% of hirsute women based on ACTH stimulation testing (Pang et al, 1985), 3β-hydroxysteroid dehydrogenase gene cloning has demonstrated that mutations in this gene are exceedingly rare (Zerah et al, 1994). Thus, most elevations of Δ5 steroids appear to be caused by functional androgen production defects rather than by enzyme gene mutations. A late-onset form of 11β-hydroxylase deficiency has been reported, though a consistent biochemical response has not been observed. Not all patients have increased 11-deoxycortisol-cortisol ratios.

Cushing Syndrome. Cushing syndrome is caused by the excess, poorly modulated secretion of cortisol due to an adrenal cortisol-producing tumor, an ACTH-secreting pituitary tumor (Cushing disease), an ectopic tumor producing ACTH, or a tumor producing corticotropin-releasing hormone. The effects of chronic hypercortisolism include central obesity, hypokalemic alkalosis, hypertension, impaired glucose tolerance, muscle wasting, thinning of the stratum corneum of the skin, and osteoporosis. In addition, many tumors also secrete androgen, which can produce hirsutism, acne, seborrhea, and true virilization. Some nonandrogen-sensitive hair growth (facial lanugo hair) may occur because of the effect of excess glucocorticoids. It is

estimated that approximately 75% of women with Cushing disease have hirsutism. Hypercortisolism and hyperandrogenism may impact the hypothalamic-pituitary-gonadal axis, producing ovulatory disturbances and menstrual irregularity. When significant virilization occurs in Cushing syndrome, the cause is almost always adrenal carcinoma. Adrenal carcinoma are often palpable because the tissue is steroidogenically inefficient and does not produce sufficient hormones for clinical symptoms until there is considerable tumor mass.

Because the androgens DHEA and androstenedione are derived from 17-hydroxypregnenolone by the action of the P450c17 and 3βHSD genes, any stimulation of low-density-lipoprotein cholesterol uptake and cholesterol side-chain cleavage by ACTH produces a state of cortisol and androgen hypersecretion (Ehrmann et al, 1995). Tumors, on the other hand, are independent of ACTH stimulation and can have varying complements of steroid biosynthetic enzymes. Usually the benign adrenal adenoma that produces hypercortisolism is well differentiated and does not secrete increased androgens. Thus, DHEAS levels are typically suppressed if there are adrenocortical adenomas because of the suppression of ACTH by the elevated plasma cortisol levels. DHEAS levels may be useful in differentiating adrenocortical adenomas from other causes of Cushing syndrome (Yamaji and Ibayashi, 1969). Adrenal carcinomas often produce excess androgens and estrogens, in addition to excess cortisol, but may not be associated with elevated DHEAS levels. Because androstenedione and DHEA are really androgen prehormones, masculinizing and possible virilizing signs of Cushing syndrome result from peripheral conversion to testosterone. Occasionally, a pure testosterone-producing tumor occurs without hypercortisolism or elevated DHEAS levels (see later).

Other Androgen-Secreting Adrenal Tumors. Androgen-secreting adrenal tumors with normal serum cortisol levels can be associated with hypertension mediated by excessive 11-deoxycorticosterone secretion. Pure testosterone-secreting tumors are rare. Approximately 20 cases have been described, usually in postmenopausal women (Gabrilove et al, 1981). Differentiating adrenal testosterone-secreting tumors from ovarian testosterone-secreting tumors is challenging. Such neoplasms may contain LH receptors; hence, hCG may stimulate testosterone secretion in both.

Because of the variable biochemical and clinical picture, 45% of 22 patients with testosterone-secreting adrenal tumors reported between 1975 and 1987 underwent ovarian exploration before the correct diagnosis was made (Mattox and Phelan, 1987). This difficulty underscores the need for initial high-resolution computed tomography (CT) or magnetic resonance imaging (MRI) to exclude an adrenal neoplasm whenever tumoral hyperandrogenemia is suspected because of an elevated serum testosterone level. Usually, pure testosterone-secreting adrenal tumors are benign, whereas adrenal masculinizing tumors whose major androgenic steroid secretory product is DHEA often are malignant.

Hyperprolactinemia

Prolactin excess has been associated with hyperandrogenism (often hirsutism) in a variety of circumstances. Prolactin may augment adrenal androgen secretion by the inhibition of 3β-hydroxysteroid dehydrogenase activity or, less often, through selective action on the sulfation of DHEA in adrenal or extra-adrenal sites (Carter et al, 1977). However, prolactin inhibits FSH-induced ovarian aromatase, leading to intraovarian hyperandrogenemia. In hyperprolactinemic women (prolactin range, 36 to 991 ng/mL) studied by Glickman et al (1982), 40% had androgenic abnormalities of which the most common was elevated free testosterone levels. The next in frequency was depressed SHBG levels and then elevated DHEAS levels.

Modestly increased prolactin levels have been reported in as many as 40% of women with PCOS in the absence of pituitary neoplasms. However, most investigators find substantially fewer women with hyperprolactinemia and, in fact, exclude patients with elevated prolactin levels from the diagnosis of PCOS. It has been suggested that hyperprolactinemia in PCOS is related to decreased central dopaminergic tone (Paradisi et al, 1988), which, in turn, may reflect the tonic estrogenic state.

Hypothyroidism

There are many effects of thyroid disease on adrenocortical and reproductive function. Hypothyroidism is associated with an increased metabolic production rate of testosterone, diversion of testosterone metabolism from androsterone to etiocholanolone, and reduced binding activity and hepatic production of SHBG (Gordon et al, 1969). Hypothyroidism also decreases libido and causes anovulation, infertility, alopecia, and excessive and irregular menstrual bleeding. Despite derangements in androgen metabolism in women with hypothyroidism, masculinization is not significant. Conversely, masculinization may be present in juvenile hypothyroidism. A predominant feature is reversible generalized muscular hypertrophy. Furthermore, juvenile hypothyroidism is sometimes associated with precocious puberty.

Disorders of Sexual Differentiation

Hyperandrogenic symptoms, either prepubertal or postpubertal, may occur in various types of gonadal dysgenesis, among them classic Turner syndrome (streak gonads and a Turner phenotype); pure gonadal dysgenesis (aplastic or absent gonads without the recognizable Turner syndrome phenotype); true hermaphroditism (ovarian and testicular tissue); and hermaphroditism with atypical or mixed gonadal dysgenesis (streak gonad and testis). Thus, it is mandatory to exclude a Y-cell line containing gonadoblastoma in any patient with gonadal dysgenesis who has hyperandrogenism. This can be accomplished only by laparotomy and by removal of the streak gonad because the Y-cell line may occur only there and may not be detectable by peripheral lymphocyte or skin fibroblast chromosomal analysis.

Anorexia Nervosa and Starvation

In general, weight loss is not associated with hyperandrogenism. In anorexia nervosa, however, there is an increase in lanugo hair and amenorrhea and a reduction in breast size.

Insulin Resistance

Hyperandrogenism with true virilization occurs in a number of the rare syndromes of extreme insulin resistance, such as type A insulin resistance, leprechaunism, and partial or complete lipoatrophy syndrome (Barbieri et al, 1986; Dunaif, 1997). In these conditions, insulin levels are strikingly elevated and may increase ovarian androgen production directly or by binding to the IGF-1 receptor. Moderate insulin resistance is also a feature of PCOS and can occur in association with androgen-secreting neoplasms. Thus, the presence of insulin resistance does not aid in the differential diagnosis of hyperandrogenism.

Obesity

Obesity may be both a manifestation of the hyperandrogenic state and a contributor to it. Increased adiposity has been associated with decreased hepatic SHBG synthesis and increased androgen bioavailability (Anderson, 1974). In addition, adipose cell aromatase converts androgens to estrogens, and chronically high levels of estrogen promote adipocyte replication in vitro. This supports the clinical observations of increased menstrual irregularities and of hirsutism in obese women that may be corrected with weight reduction (Rogers and Mitchell, 1952; Glass et al, 1978). However, not every obese woman has hyperandrogenism or ovulatory disturbances (Dunaif et al, 1988). Weight reduction is an effective therapeutic modality for PCOS, but it is not possible to predict which obese women will experience improved menstrual function with weight reduction (Kiddy et al, 1992).

Iatrogenic or Factitious Masculinization

Treatment with various drugs may produce masculinizing features (Box 15-4). Unfortunately, most virilizing side effects are irreversible, even when steroid use is discontinued. In addition to the increasing use of illicit anabolic steroids among women to enhance athletic performance, androgens may be legitimately prescribed for the treatment of menopausal signs and symptoms, breast cancer, aplastic anemia, endometriosis, cystic mastitis, and angioneurotic edema (Wilson, 1988). Hirsutism and acne are side effects of the common progestational oral contraceptive agents that contain levonorgestrel and norgestrel (*e.g.,* Triphasil and Lo-Ovral, respectively). Hirsutism, acne, and alopecia occasionally result from synthetic oral, intravenous, or inhaled glucocorticoids. Fetal virilization can develop if pregnant women ingest progestational or androgenic steroids.

DIAGNOSTIC STRATEGY
Whom to Evaluate

Any woman with hyperandrogenic symptoms should undergo initial evaluation for potentially abnormal causes of increased androgen production (see Box 15-2). In addition, hyperandrogenism should be considered in women with irregular menses, amenorrhea, or infertility. The basic evaluation includes a complete history and physical examination to rule out a serious underlying cause (Fig. 15-7).

Medical History

Important features of the history include age, rapidity of onset of masculinizing symptoms, presence of menstrual dysfunction, and family history including ethnic origin. Hirsutism that is insidious and coincides with puberty suggests a nontumoral cause (*e.g.,* PCOS or NCCAH), whereas rapidly progressive hirsutism with onset after puberty and significant virilizing symptoms, such as increased muscularity and voice deepening, suggests neoplasia. True virilization indicates a severe hyperandrogenic state, whereas the preservation of menstrual cyclicity suggests a more attenuated state. It is also important to determine age at menarche, menstrual and growth histories, fertility (spontaneous or in-

---

> **BOX 15-4**
> **DRUGS WHOSE USE IS ASSOCIATED WITH IATROGENIC MASCULINIZATION**
>
> Synthetic glucocorticoids
> Adrenocorticotropic hormone
> Metyrapone
> Anabolic steroids
> Levonorgestrel-containing oral contraceptive pills
> Maternal use of synthetic progestational agents (fetal virilization)

duced), and libido. If these are normal and hirsutism is present, then IH is likely. If the patient is pregnant, a pregnancy luteoma should be suspected. Any history of endocrinopathy or metabolic disease is particularly important. Drug use, especially oral contraceptive pills and anabolic steroids, should be recorded. Surreptitious anabolic steroid use should be suspected in body builders and competitive athletes.

Physical Examination

Hypertension, bruising, mood changes, and proximal muscle weakness should increase the index of suspicion for Cushing syndrome. Voice pitch should be noted also because a deep voice is suggestive of more severe hyperandrogenism. A masculine, feminine, Cushingoid, or Turner body habitus should be recorded. For example, if a patient has Turner syndrome, hirsutism suggests the presence of a Y-cell line gonadoblastoma. Breasts should be examined for atrophy or galactorrhea. The pelvis and abdomen should be palpated for ovarian or adrenal masses. Skin should be examined for dryness (hypothyroidism), hirsutism, striae, acne or seborrhea/oiliness, alopecia, acanthosis nigricans (Fig. 15-4), or hyperpigmentation (excessive ACTH secretion). Acanthosis nigricans is a cutaneous marker for insulin resistance (Dunaif et al, 1990). Acral hypertrophy can be found in the type A syndrome of insulin resistance, acromegaly, and, occasionally, in PCOS.

External genitalia must be examined carefully for clitoral size, labial development, distribution of pubic hair, and genitourinary malformation. Bimanual examination of the uterus and adnexa is particularly important to find pelvic neoplasms and to disclose genital developmental abnormalities in patients with primary amenorrhea.

Various indices may be used to quantify hirsutism. According to the Ferriman and Gallwey (1961) scoring system, five gradings based on hair density and area are assigned for 11 anatomic regions, and a score is computed from the sum of the gradings. This semiquantitative method is suitable for the initial evaluation, but it is insensitive to changes after treatment because of the limits of visual inspection. It does not assign adequate weight to facial hirsutism because the scores reflect hair growth over the upper lip and chin but not

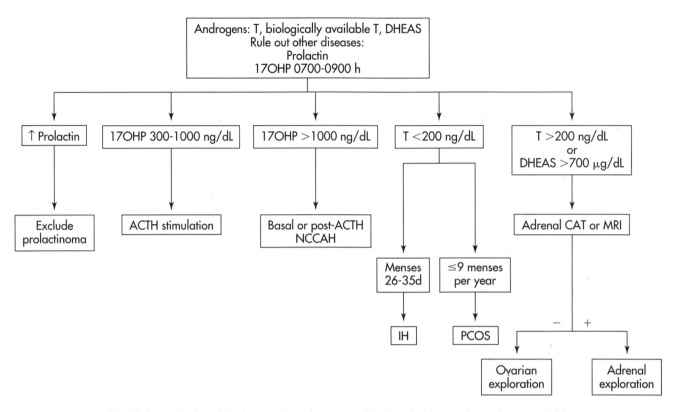

Fig. 15-7. Evaluation of the hyperandrogenic woman. Consider Cushing syndrome in women with recent-onset truncal obesity, easy bruising, and purple striae. T, testosterone; 17OHP, 17 hydroxy-progesterone; DHEAS, dehydroepiandrosterone sulfate; NCCAH, nonclassical 21-hydroxylase deficiency (see Fig. 15-6); IH, idiopathic hirsutism; PCOS, polycystic ovarian syndrome.

BOX 15-5
DIAGNOSTIC EVALUATION OF MASCULINIZED WOMEN

Total testosterone level
Biologically available testosterone level
DHEAS level
7 to 9 AM 17-OH progesterone level
Prolactin level
± FSH level
DHEAS, dehydroepiandrosterone sulfate; 17-OH, 17-hy-droxyprogesterone; FSH, follicle stimulating hormone.

---

on sideburns and cheeks. Finally, the Ferriman-Gallwey score does not account for hair removal. Precise quantitation of hirsutism is generally necessary only in a research study.

Initial Laboratory Studies

The recommended diagnostic evaluation is summarized in Box 15-5. In more than 80% of women with suspected hyperandrogenism, levels of the total or free testosterone or DHEAS are evaluated on a single random determination (Wild et al, 1983). Obtaining other androgen levels, such as androstenedione or 3-α-androstanediol glucuronide, does

not improve diagnostic accuracy. If hyperandrogenism is suspected, measuring circulating androgen levels is important to confirm the diagnosis and to rule out an androgen-secreting tumor. If the serum testosterone level is greater than 150 to 200 ng/dL or the DHEAS level is greater than 700 μg/dL, additional studies must be performed (Friedman et al, 1985) (see below). If a patient has symptoms of Cushing syndrome, a 24-hour urine sample should be collected for urine-free cortisol testing. In addition, other conditions that could cause these clinical symptoms should be ruled out. Specifically, prolactin levels should be measured in all women, and FSH should be measured if menopause is a possibility.

Because of the high frequency of insulin resistance and glucose intolerance, an assessment of glucose tolerance should be considered in all women with PCOS (Legro et al, 1999). A diagnosis of NCCAH does not change clinical management, except for women attempting to conceive (see later). Usually, documenting abnormal adrenal enzyme function with an ACTH stimulation test is unnecessary, and measuring the early morning 17-OH progesterone level can be used to screen for NCCAH (Azziz and Zacur, 1989). A formal ACTH stimulation test should be performed if the morning 17-OH progesterone level is greater than 300 ng/dL. In women of eastern European Jewish origin, however, routine ACTH testing may be appropriate. Ovulatory status may be assessed reliably by measuring the luteal-phase progesterone level on day 21 or 22 of the menstrual cycle. Although an elevated LH-FSH ratio supports a diagnosis of PCOS, single gonadotropin determinations are confounded by pulsatile fluctuations and are generally unnecessary.

Additional Diagnostic Studies

If the initial evaluation demonstrates that a patient's serum testosterone level is greater than 150 ng/dL or the DHEAS level is greater than 700 μg/dL, additional studies are required to rule out an ovarian or adrenal tumor (Friedman et al, 1985).

Dynamic Hormonal Testing

Dynamic hormonal testing is not useful in distinguishing adrenal from ovarian hyperandrogenism because of the considerable overlap in responses. Oral contraceptive pills suppress ovarian and adrenal androgen production and may also suppress androgen-secreting neoplasms (Givens et al, 1975; Wild et al, 1982). Long-acting GnRH agonists (GnRHa) such as Lupron and Synarel selectively suppress ovarian androgen production in the absence of a tumor (Chang et al, 1983). However, androgen-secreting neoplasms have been documented to suppress their steroid production with GnRHa administration (Parr et al, 1988). Ovarian stimulation testing with hCG is nonspecific because similar degrees of stimulation of androgen production can be seen with tumorous and nontumorous causes of ovarian hyperandrogenism. In addition, adrenal virilizing tumors occasionally stimulate their androgen production with hCG (Givens et al, 1974; Gabrilove et al, 1981), whereas ovarian androgen-secreting tumors can respond to changes in ACTH (Tucci et al, 1973). If a patient plans ovulation induction therapy or pregnancy with a partner who also may be carrying CAH genes (e.g., an eastern European Jew), ACTH stimulation testing is necessary if her ethnic background, family history, or unstimulated 17-OH progesterone level raises the probability of a diagnosis of NCCAH. However, the ACTH stimulation test does not distinguish nontumoral from tumoral adrenal entities, nor does it distinguish ovarian hyperandrogenemia from adrenal hyperandrogenemia. The test requires the administration of 250 μg cosyntropin (Cortrosyn) intravenously or intramuscularly, with blood collected for cortisol (to document the receipt of ACTH) and 17-OH progesterone (to assess adrenal 21-hydroxylase function) at 0 and 60 minutes (see Fig. 15-6). A stimulated 17-OH progesterone level greater than 1000 ng/dL is consistent with a P450c21 gene defect (New and Speiser, 1986).

Imaging Studies

Ultrasonography is an inconsistent diagnostic tool for the evaluation of hyperandrogenism. Transabdominal ovarian ultrasonography is relatively insensitive for assessing ovarian morphology, particularly in obese women. Conversely, vaginal ultrasonography is very sensitive for detecting polycystic ovaries (Fig. 15-5). Thus, an experienced sonographer can reliably identify polycystic ovaries using this technique (Adams et al, 1986). However, as discussed in the section on ovarian morphology in PCOS, this finding is not diagnostic of the *syndrome*, it can occur secondary to other causes of hyperandrogenism or chronic anovulation, and it is seen in as many as 20% of normal women (Polson et al, 1988). Finally, ovarian ultrasongraphy cannot exclude the presence of small androgen-secreting neoplasms, which may not even enlarge the ovary containing them.

Most adrenal androgen-secreting neoplasms can be detected by adrenal computerized tomography with contrast (Gabrilove et al, 1981). Computerized tomographic imaging does not accurately image the ovaries. Adrenal CT or MRI must be performed before laparotomy to exclude adrenal lesions in all patients thought to have androgen-secreting neoplasms even when there is isolated testosterone elevation. Magnetic resonance imaging and newer-generation CT are equally effective in disclosing adrenal masses as small as 0.5 cm. Adrenal adenomas are rounded and well circumscribed, whereas adrenal carcinomas usually have irregular borders.

Magnetic resonance imaging is a relatively new technique, and experience with it is limited. Its sensitivity for detecting adrenal masses is similar to that of CT, and it may provide information regarding the tissue type of a mass. It also provides better resolution of pelvic tissues than does CT. Small ovarian cysts and tumoral lesions may be demonstrated using MRI, though the exact usefulness of this technique in excluding ovarian androgen-secreting neoplasms remains to be determined. In fact, instances have been reported in which MRI failed to identify tumors found at surgery. Ovarian scintigraphic localization of tumors has been reported (Mountz et al, 1988), but this procedure requires further validation and is not widely available.

Invasive Procedures

A controversial issue in the evaluation of the masculinized woman is the role of adrenal and ovarian venous sampling. This method is only considered when results from imaging procedures have been equivocal, there is a high suspicion of an adrenal or ovarian tumor, and there is local expertise in its performance. Venous catheterization can localize an androgen-producing tumor by venography and can also delineate effluent or peripheral circulation differences in androgens (Moltz et al, 1984; Wajchenberg et al, 1986). There are several disadvantages to this technique. First, it can cause complications such as bleeding, thrombosis, venous rupture, and renal exposure to contrast dye. Second, technical difficulties can develop in catheterization and sampling of the small vessels because even in expert hands, all four ovarian and adrenal veins can be sampled in only 45% of patients (Sorenson et al, 1986). Third, episodic androgen secretion often causes spurious results. Thus, we recommend that laparotomy and ovarian exploration be performed in any woman thought to have an androgen-secreting neoplasm if adrenal imaging studies exclude an adrenal mass.

Table 15-1   Therapy for Hyperandrogenism

Mechanism of Action	Comments
Ovarian Suppression	
Combination oral contraceptives (OC)	Avoid levonorgestrel-containing agents
GnRHa	Expensive, must combine with estrogen/progestin
Adrenal Suppression	
Glucocorticoids	Antiandrogens more effective for clinical symptoms; reserve for infertility therapy
Androgen Receptor Antagonists	
Spironolactone	Recommended alone or in combination with OC
Cyproterone acetate	Not available in United States
Flutamide	Expensive, potentially hepatotoxic, not recommended
5 α-Reductase Inhibitors	
Finasteride	Expensive, not recommended in fertile women
Androgen Biosynthesis Inhibitors	
Ketaconazole	Expensive, potentially hepatotoxic, not recommended
Insulin-Lowering Agents	
(Efficacy for hyperandrogenic symptoms remains unproven)	
Metformin	Gastrointestinal side effects
Troglitazone	Expensive, potentially hepatotoxic
Other	
Bromocriptine	Not effective
Cimetidine	Not effective

THERAPEUTIC OPTIONS
Goals of Therapy

Except in the rare occurrence of an androgen-secreting tumor, therapy for hyperandrogenic women is directed at the patient's primary symptoms and personal goals (Table 15-1). An elevated serum androgen level is not required to initiate treatment because hyperandrogenic symptoms demonstrate that there is increased androgen use by the target tissue.

In all obese women, weight reduction can substantially improve hyperandrogenism and anovulation (Kiddy et al, 1992). Medical therapy may consist of suppressing LH or ACTH release to reduce glandular secretion interfering with androgen synthesis, increasing SHBG to decreases andro-

gen bioavailability, or decreasing tissue androgen use by inhibiting 5α-reductase activity or blocking androgen action with wider spectrum androgen receptor antagonists. In addition, many cosmetic therapies are available for the symptoms of hirsutism, acne, and alopecia. Nonpharmacologic techniques are particularly useful in conjunction with pharmacologic therapy.

It is essential to ensure that the patient has realistic expectations about the time course and the results of therapy. Once a hair follicle has been transformed by androgen exposure to produce a terminal hair, biochemical control of hyperandrogenism will not result in restoration of vellus hair growth. However, biochemical control will result in a slowing of the rate of hair growth and a decrease in hair diameter and color. Clinical effects on hair growth are not evident until 3 to 6 months of therapy, and maximal effects are not seen for up to 1 year. In most women it takes approximately 1 year for the effects of therapy for alopecia to result in clinically evident changes because of the cyclic nature of scalp hair growth. Conversely, improvements in acne and seborrhea can be seen within 1 to 2 months on therapy. Eradication of terminal hairs requires electrolysis or repeated laser treatments. Because these modalities are expensive, we recommend that the patient wait until biochemical control has been achieved (3 to 6 months) before adding these therapies.

Nonpharmacologic

Techniques used to manage hirsutism include depilation with shaving, tweezers, waxes, or creams; electrocoagulation with diathermy; electrolysis with direct current; repeated bleaching; and laser therapy. Male pattern baldness may be managed surgically with full-thickness, hair-bearing punch autografts obtained from resistant occipital follicles.

In addition, because obesity can unmask or aggravate hyperandrogenic syndromes and insulin resistance associated with PCOS is often observed and has significant health consequences, weight loss should be strongly encouraged from the outset in all overweight patients. Weight loss results in decreased androgen production and insulin levels and in increased SHBG levels, occasionally leading to the complete resolution of symptoms and the resumption of ovulatory menses. As little as a 7% reduction in body weight can lead to a significant decrease in androgen levels and to the resumption of ovulatory menses in obese women with PCOS (Kiddy et al, 1992).

Endometrial Protection

Women with chronic anovulation and continued estrogen production, such as women with PCOS, are at risk for endometrial neoplasia because of the unopposed estrogen effect (Jackson and Docherty, 1957). Thus, regular endometrial shedding must be induced in amenorrheic, hyperandrogenic women with intermittent oral progestin administration (*e.g.,* 5 mg medroxyprogesterone acetate orally for 14 days every 1 to 2 months). The exact frequency of withdrawal bleeding to prevent endometrial hyperplasia has not been established

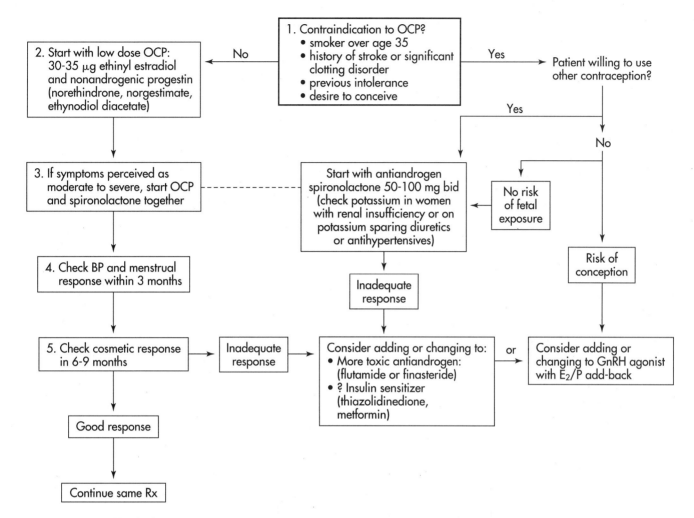

Fig. 15-8. Treatment of hirsutism. OCP, oral contraceptive pills; BP, blood pressure; GnRH, gonadotropin-releasing hormone; E_2, estradiol; bid, twice a day.

in patients with PCOS. Intermittent progesterone withdrawal must be given, in addition to agents for controlling hyperandrogenism, if the latter do not restore regular menses.

Oral Contraceptive Pills

Estrogen and progestin are more effective in combination than either agent is alone in suppressing LH-dependent hyperandrogenemia. Although at least 50 μg ethinyl estradiol (EE) or the equivalent is required to suppress LH, lower estrogen levels (approximately 35 μg EE) can increase serum SHBG and decrease ACTH-dependent adrenal DHEAS production (Wild et al, 1983). Thus, low-dose oral contraceptive pills (30 to 35 μg EE) are usually effective in controlling hirsutism and acne (see Fig. 15-8). Contraceptive pills also induce cyclic uterine withdrawal bleeding and provide contraception.

In women in whom estrogens are contraindicated (see later), high-dose medroxyprogesterone has been used alone with some efficacy. Progesterone inhibits 5α-reductase

activity, which decreases target-tissue androgen use. All progestins have some degree of androgenic action. Levonorgestrel has a relative androgenic activity of 9.4 (methyltestosterone, 100) and has a higher affinity for SHBG than do endogenous steroids. Thus, levonorgestrel increases biologically available potent androgens by competing for binding sites on SHBG and should be avoided in women with PCOS. Oral contraceptive pills containing progestins with acceptable progestational activity and weaker androgenic activity, such as ethynodiol diacetate (androgen activity, 0.63), norethindrone (androgen activity, 1.60), or the newer progestin norgestimate are recommended. We avoid contraceptive pills containing desogestrel because of a potential increased risk for thromboembolism.

The major risks inherent in the use of oral contraceptive pills are related primarily to their estrogen content. Risks include thromboembolic phenomena, gallbladder disease, and exacerbation of hypertension and migraine headaches. They may cause benign hepatic tumors, but this is rare. Less serious but troublesome side effects include nausea and breast tenderness, which typically resolve after the first few months of therapy, and depression and fluid retention, which may persist. Phlebitis, hypertension, and cholelithiasis are relative contraindications to oral contraceptive use. Cigarette smoking significantly increases the risk for thromboembolic phenomena during oral contraceptive use and should be discouraged vigorously. Oral contraceptive agents have been shown to worsen insulin resistance in hyperandrogenic women (Korytkowski et al, 1995; Nader et al, 1997).

In nonsmoking patients with clinically mild to moderate hyperandrogenism who are 35 years of age or younger and who do not have contraindications, oral contraceptive pills with 35 μg EE may be used as first-line therapy. Antiandrogen therapy is usually needed if hirsutism is moderate to severe or if alopecia has developed. Only approximately one third of patients respond to the point that mechanical depilation is not needed. Patients must be informed that a full clinical response may require 6 to 12 months. It is possible to maintain a cosmetic response with oral contraceptives alone after the initial therapy in combination with antiandrogens, usually spironolactone.

Glucocorticoids

Glucocorticoids are used primarily to suppress ACTH-dependent adrenal androgen secretion. They are most commonly indicated for the treatment of CAH. However, recent studies demonstrate that women with NCCAH do just as well or better with antiandrogen therapy (with or without oral contraceptives) as with glucocorticoids, probably because of the difficulty of providing sufficient medication to reduce androgen production without excess glucocorticoid effects. Thus, glucocorticoids are no longer recommended as first-line therapy for NCCAH (Spritzer et al, 1990). Some studies suggest that glucocorticoids significantly improve the ovulatory response of women with NCCAH, and short-term use can be considered in women with infertility. Fertility rates may also be improved by glucocorticoid therapy in conjunction with ovulation induction in hyperandrogenic women who do not have CAH. This may be related to decreasing putative direct negative androgen effects on the uterus, follicle, or hypothalamic-pituitary axis.

The risks and side effects of glucocorticoids range from relative hypoadrenalism with attenuated adrenal stress response (even with dosages in the range of 0.5 mg a day) to iatrogenic Cushing syndrome (with dosages in the range of 0.75 mg a day). The former may be monitored and prevented by titrating the dosage to a cortisol level of more than 2 g/dL between 8 and 9 AM. However, adrenal androgen secretion is more sensitive than cortisol secretion to low-dose glucocorticoid suppression (Rittmaster et al, 1985).

Glucocorticoid replacement, usually with 0.25 to 0.5 mg oral dexamethasone at bedtime, is the specific therapy for women with NCCAH. Clinical improvement may be expected to occur any time between 3 and 12 months after the institution of therapy. Because the clinical response corre-

lates with biochemical control of hyperandrogenemia, if androgen levels do not decrease, this treatment should be discontinued. Dexamethasone is the glucocorticoid of choice because it is virtually devoid of mineralocorticoid activity and can be given in a single bedtime dose. However, as discussed earlier, we only recommend the use of glucocorticoids for the treatment of infertility in hyperandrogenic women.

Antiandrogens

Antiandrogens act primarily by interfering with target tissue binding of androgens to their intracellular receptor. They may be used alone or in combination with oral contraceptive pills for masculinizing signs that are not responsive to a single agent. Antiandrogens can improve insulin sensitivitiy slightly in women with PCOS (Moghetti et al, 1996b).

Spironolactone

The diuretic agent spironolactone is not approved by the Food and Drug Administration (FDA) for use in hirsutism. Nevertheless, it has potent antiandrogen action in high dosages (75 to 200 mg a day) by interfering with androgen synthesis by inhibiting 17α-hydroxylase/17, 20-lyase activity (P450c17) and by competitively inhibiting intracellular testosterone and DHT receptor binding. Moreover, spironolactone may inhibit 5α-reductase activity. When spironolactone is given in high dosages (more than 75 mg daily), there is significant displacement of testosterone from SHBG; however, its overall effect is antiandrogenic. Comparative studies have shown spironolactone to have similar efficacy (alone or in combination with oral contraceptive pills) to cyproterone acetate (O'Brien et al, 1991; Erenus et al, 1996), flutamide (Erenus et al, 1994), and finasteride (Erenus et al, 1997).

Spironolactone has been used for many years and has an excellent safety profile (Cumming et al, 1982). Side effects include dysfunctional bleeding (56%) but not electrolyte disturbances. When the former occurs, the dosage should be decreased and contraceptive pills added, or the drug stopped altogether. Headache (18%), nausea (25%), and lassitude (15%) may occur, but they usually resolve after 1 to 2 months and can be lessened with the concomitant use of oral contraceptive pills (Helfer et al, 1988). The long-term safety of spironolactone is unclear in light of a reported association with breast carcinogenesis in rodents. Spironolactone should not be given during pregnancy because of the potential to interfere with the normal masculinization of a male fetus. Its teratogenic potential is particularly important because spironolactone can lead to a resumption of ovulation in women with PCOS (Evron et al, 1981). However, there is a case report of the delivery of normal male infants in a woman who was administered high-dose spironolactone during pregnancy for Bartter syndrome (Groves and Corenblum, 1995).

A starting dosage of 50 to 100 mg twice a day is recommended (Crosby and Rittmaster, 1991). If side effects do not develop, a maximal dosage of 100 mg twice daily can be used to control hyperandrogenism. If dysfunctional uterine bleeding occurs, the daily dosage should be decreased by 25 mg. A clinical response may be expected to occur approximately 3 to 6 months after therapy is started. Women with IH and PCOS often respond well to this therapy. Because of the risk for teratogenic effects and dysfunctional bleeding, spironolactone is often prescribed in combination with an oral contraceptive pill. Because the two therapies work by different mechanisms, together they are more effective at resolving symptoms than if either therapy is used alone. Generic spironolactone is available and is a cost-effective therapy for hyperandrogenism. In the United States, it is the first-line therapy for moderate to severe hyperandrogenism.

Cyproterone Acetate

The antiandrogen cyproterone acetate is highly effective in the treatment of acne and hirsutism. It also competitively inhibits intracellular androgen receptor function, but it has only 18.6% of the activity of spironolactone. The decrease in LH-dependent androgen synthesis is attributed to the progestational activity of cyproterone and the EE that is administered with it to provide contraception and further suppress LH. This drug is not available in the United States, despite its apparent safe use in Europe. Because it is a progestin, large doses can suppress the hypothalamic-pituitary-adrenal axis. In approximately 10% of patients, the drug is discontinued because it causes fatigue, weight gain, and loss of libido. A clinical response in hirsutism may be expected to occur in 50% to 90% of patients roughly 2 to 3 months after cyproterone acetate is started. The relapse rate 6 months after withdrawal of the drug ranges from 40% to 80%. Acne and seborrhea improve in approximately 60% of patients. It is also teratogenic because of its antiandrogenic actions, and it is always administered in combination with EE in premenopausal women.

Flutamide

Flutamide is a pure antiandrogen that is used primarily in the medical management of prostate cancer. Preliminary clinical trials in hirsutism using 100 mg a day have been promising. Dosages of 250 mg a day have resulted in decreased hirsutism and the resumption of ovulatory menses in adolescents with PCOS (DeLeo et al, 1998). Side effects include liver toxicity, and case reports of hepatic failure leading to transplantion or death have been reported in men and in at least one woman administered flutamide for hirsutism (Wysowski et al, 1993). Flutamide is not FDA approved for the treatment of hirsutism. Given this safety profile, flutamide should be considered only for women in whom all other therapies have failed.

Other Agents
5α-Reductase Inhibitors

Without binding to the androgen receptor, 5α-reductase inhibitors block the conversion of testosterone to DHT. How-ever, there are at least two different isoforms of the 5α-reductase enzyme that are differentially distributed in androgen-sensitive tissues. For example, finasteride was developed for the treatment of prostate hypertrophy, and it was not thought to affect skin 5α-reductase significantly. Surprisingly, recent studies demonstrated that finasteride has an efficacy similar to that of 100 mg/day spironolactone for the treatment of hirsutism (Wong et al, 1995; Erenus et al, 1997). These agents are also teratogenic because they cross the placenta and inhibit fetal 5α-reductase activity, resulting in ambiguous genitalia in a male fetus. These agents are not FDA approved for the treatment of hirsutism.

Ketoconazole

Technically, the antifungal agent ketoconazole is not an antiandrogen because it blocks the synthesis of androgens through the suppression of P450-dependent adrenal and gonadal enzymes such as P450c17. This results in a reduction in serum testosterone levels, whereas 17-hydroxyprogesterone levels increase. Ketoconazole is not FDA approved for the treatment of hirsutism. However, in a study of nine hirsute women treated with 400 to 1200 mg/day, clinical improvement was apparent at 6 months (Martikainen et al, 1988). Because serum DHEAS and cortisol levels did not change, the primary effect was on ovarian androgen synthesis. Low-dose therapy (400 mg a day) is recommended after a 1-month induction period on 1200 mg a day. Untoward effects include nausea, pruritus, and hepatocellular dysfunction. Periodic liver function testing should be performed and the drug discontinued if liver enzyme increases are detected. This drug is not used as the initial choice in the management of women with masculinization, but it may be considered in resistant patients in whom all other measures have failed.

Long-Acting Gonadotropin-Releasing Hormone Analogues

Long-acting GnRHa decrease LH secretion (and, therefore, LH-dependent androgen secretion) by producing gonadotropin desensitization. GnRHa may be used in women in whom primary therapy with oral contraceptive pills or antiandrogens fails. When nafarelin acetate was administered to six hirsute women as a nasal spray at a dosage of 500 μg twice daily, biochemical control occurred in four of the women within 1 to 3 months (Andreyko et al, 1986). This drug also may be useful for women with IH because it decreases androgen delivery to target tissue. Indeed, it was as effective as high-dose cyproterone acetate in one study (Carmina and Lobo, 1997). An important side effect of these agents is osteoporosis because estrogen levels are lower, as are androgen levels. The major limitation is that GnRHa treatment is expensive; it can cost up to $400 per month. The FDA has not approved GnRHa for the treatment of hyperandrogenism. Osteoporosis may be minimized by supplementation with a low-dose estrogen preparation and periodic progesterone withdrawal (Rittmaster, 1995).

Cimetidine

Cimetidine is a weak androgen receptor antagonist (Eil and Edelson, 1984). A controlled clinical study has not found cimetidine to be effective in the treatment of hyperandrogenism (Lissack et al, 1989).

Insulin-Lowering Agents

Troglitazone and metformin lower biologically available testosterone levels by approximately 25% in women with PCOS (Velazquez et al, 1994; Dunaif et al, 1996; Nestler and Jacubowicz, 1996; Ehrmann et al, 1997b). This testosterone lowering correlates with the reduction in insulin levels (Dunaif, 1996) and is not seen without them (Ehrmann, 1997a). It is predicted that this improvement in hyperandrogenemia will be associated with an improvement in hirsutism, but this remains to be documented in more prolonged trials. Resumption of ovulation has been reported in women receiving these agents alone (Dunaif, 1996; Nestler et al, 1998) or in combination with clomiphene citrate (Nestler et al, 1998). Metformin is not consistently effective at lowering insulin levels in PCOS (Crave et al, 1995; Ehrmann et al, 1997a). Only two studies have been conducted on troglitazone in PCOS (Dunaif et al, 1996; Ehrmann et al, 1997b), and to date there have been no comparative studies of efficacy. Metformin can cause lactic acidosis in persons with compromised renal function, and it commonly causes gastrointestinal side effects such as nausea and diarrhea, but these usually do not lead to discontinuation of the drug among patients with PCOS. Troglitazone is well tolerated, but it has been associated with several cases of fatal hepatic necrosis. It is unknown whether this hepatic failure can be predicted by surveillance of liver function tests. Neither of these agents is FDA approved for use in hyperandrogenism.

Ovarian Surgery

Ovarian wedge resection results in transient decreases in androgen levels (Katz et al, 1978). Thus, this procedure is used only as a last resort in infertile women and not for control of hyperandrogenism. Oophorectomy may be considered to manage women with tumors or for those in whom pharmacologic therapy has failed or is contraindicated.

Bromocriptine

Placebo-controlled trials have shown that bromocriptine is no more effective than placebo in controlling hyperandrogenism (Buvat et al, 1986).

Thyroid Hormone Therapy

Thyroid hormones should be given only to women with documented hypothyroidism. The attendant risk for complication limits the use of empiric thyroid hormone therapy designed to promote weight loss or to increase SHBG.

SUMMARY

Hyperandrogenic disorders are common problems in women and are usually secondary to PCOS or IH. These conditions are straightforward to diagnose, and rare serious disorders can be easily excluded. Most of the clinical symptoms can be controlled with therapy. It is important to recognize that women with PCOS are at increased risk for glucose intolerance and cardiovascular disease.

REFERENCES

Abraham GE: Ovarian and adrenal contribution to peripheral androgens during the menstrual cycle. *J Clin Endocrinol Metab* 1976; 39:340-346.

Adams J, Polson DW, Franks S: Prevalence of polycystic ovaries in women with anovulation and idiopathic hirsutism. *BMJ* 1986; 293: 355-359.

Aiman J, Fomey JP, Parker CR: Secretion of androgens and estrogens by normal and neoplastic ovaries in postmenopausal women. *Obstet Gynecol* 1986; 68:1-5.

Andersen P, Seljeflot I, Abdelnoor M, et al: Increased insulin sensitivity and fibrinolytic capacity after dietary intervention in obese women with polycystic ovary syndrome. *Metabolism* 1995; 44:611-616.

Anderson DC: Sex hormone-binding globulin. *Clin Endocrinol (Oxf)* 1974; 3:69-96.

Andreyko JL, Monroe SE, Jaffe RB: Treatment of hirsutism with a gonadotropin-releasing hormone agonist (Nafarelin). *J Clin Endocrinol Metab* 1986; 63:854-859.

Arroyo A, Laughlin GA, Morales AJ, Yen SSC: Inappropriate gonadotropin secretion in polycystic ovary syndrome: Influence of adiposity. *J Clin Endocrinol Metab* 1997; 82: 3728-3733.

Azziz R, Zacur HA: 21-Hydroxylase deficiency in female hyperandrogenism: Screening and diagnosis. *J Clin Endocrinol Metab* 1989; 69:577-584.

Baird DT, Corker CS, Davidson DW, et al: Pituitary-ovarian relationships in polycystic ovary syndrome. *J Clin Endocrinol Metab* 1977; 45:798-809.

Balen A, Tan S, MacDougall J, Jacobs H: Miscarriage rates following in-vitro fertilization are increased in women with polycystic ovaries and reduced by pituitary desensitization with buserelin. *Hum Reprod* 1993; 8: 959-964.

Barbieri RL, Makris A, Randall RW, et al: Insulin stimulates androgen accumulation in incubations of ovarian stroma obtained from women with hyperandrogenism. *J Clin Endocrinol Metab* 1986; 62:904-910.

Bardin CW, Lipsett M: Testosterone and androstenedione production rates in normal women and in idiopathic hirsutism and polycystic ovary syndrome. *J Clin Invest* 1967; 46:891-902.

Barnes RB, Rosenfield RL, Burstein S, Ehrmann DA: Pituitary-ovarian responses to Nafarelin testing in the polycystic ovary syndrome. *N Engl J Med* 1989; 320:559-565.

Birdsall MA, Farquhar CM, White HD: Association between polycystic ovaries and extent of coronary artery disease in women having cardiac catheterization. *Ann Intern Med* 1997; 126:32-35.

Blankstein J, Rabinovici J, Goldenberg M, et al: Changing pituitary reactivity to follicle-stimulating hormone and luteinizing hormone-releasing hormone after induced ovulatory cycles and after anovulation in patients with polycystic ovarian disease. *J Clin Endocrinol Metab* 1987; 65:1164-1167.

Buvat J, Buvat-Herbaut M, Marrolin G, et al: A double-blind controlled study of the hormonal and clinical effects of bromocriptine in the polycystic ovary syndrome. *J Clin Endocrinol Metab* 1986; 63:119-124.

Carmina E, Koyama T, Chang L, et al: Does ethnicity influence the prevalence of adrenal hyperandrogenism and insulin resistance in polycystic ovary syndrome? *Am J Obstet Gynecol* 1992; 167: 1807-1812.

Carmina E, Lobo RA: Gonadotrophin-releasing hormone agonist therapy for hirsutism is as effective as high dose cyproterone acetate but results in a longer remission. *Hum Reprod* 1997; 12:663-666.

Carter JN, Tyson JE, Wayne GL, et al: Adrenocortical function in hyperprolactinemic women. *J Clin Endocrinol Metab* 1977; 45: 973-980.

Chang RJ, Lauger LR, Meldrum DR, et al: Steroid secretion in polycystic ovarian disease after ovarian suppression by a long-acting gonadotropin releasing hormone agonist. *J Clin Endocrinol Metab* 1983; 56:897-903.

Chang RJ, Mandel FP, Lu JKH, et al: Enhanced disparity of gonadotropin secretion by estrone in women with polycystic ovarian disease. *J Clin Endocrinol Metab* 1982; 54:490-494.

Christman GM, Randolph JF, Kelch RP, et al: Reduction of gonadotropin-releasing hormone pulse frequency is associated with subsequent selective follicle-stimulating hormone secretion in women with polycystic ovarian disease. *J Clin Endocrinol Metab* 1991; 72:1278-1285.

Crave J, Fimbel S, Lejeune H, et al: Effects of diet and metformin administration on sex hormone-binding globulin, androgens, and insulin in hirsute and obese women. *J Clin Endocrinol Metab* 1995; 80:2057-2062.

Cronin L, Guyatt G, Griffith L, et al: Development of a health-related quality of life questionnaire for patients with polycystic ovary syndrome. *J Clin Endocrinol Metab* 1998; 83:1976-1987.

Crosby PDA, Rittmaster RS: Predictors of clinical response in hirsute women treated with spironolactone. *Fertil Steril* 1991; 55:1076-1081.

Cumming DC, Yang JC, Rebar RW, et al: Treatment of hirsutism with spironolactone. *JAMA* 1982; 247:1295-1298.

Dahlgren E, Janson PO, Johansson S, et al: Polycystic ovary syndrome and risk for myocardial infarction. *Acta Obstet Gynecol Scand* 1992a; 71:599-603.

Dahlgren E, Johansson S, Lindstedt G, et al: Women with polycystic ovary syndrome wedge resected in 1956 to 1965: A long-term follow-up focusing on natural history and circulating hormones. *Fertil Steril* 1992b; 57:505-513.

Daniels TL, Berga SL: Resistance of gonadotropin releasing hormone drive to sex steroid-induced suppression in hyperandrogenic anovulation. *J Clin Endocrinol Metab* 1997; 82: 4179-4183.

DeLeo V, Lanzetta D, D'Antona D, et al: Hormonal effects of flutamide in young women with polycystic ovary syndrome. *J Clin Endocrinol Metab* 1998; 83:99-102.

Derksen J, Nagesser SK, Meinders AE, et al: Identification of virilizing adrenal tumors in hirsute women. *N Engl J Med* 1994; 331: 968-973.

Dunaif A: Do androgens directly regulate gonadotropin secretion in the polycystic ovary syndrome? *J Clin Endocrinol Metab* 1986; 63:215-221.

Dunaif A: Insulin resistance and the polycystic ovary syndrome: Mechanisms and implications for pathogenesis. *Endocr Rev* 1997; 18:774-800.

Dunaif A, Graf M: Insulin administration alters gonadal steroid metabolism independent of changes in gonadotropin secretion in insulin-resistant women with the polycystic ovary syndrome. *J Clin Invest* 1989b; 83:23-29.

Dunaif A, Graf M, Mandeli J, et al: Characterization of groups of hyperandrogenic women with acanthosis nigricans, impaired glucose tolerance, and/or hyperinsulinemia. *J Clin Endocrinol Metab* 1987; 65:499-507.

Dunaif A, Green G, Futterweit W, et al: Suppression of hyperandrogenism does not improve peripheral or hepatic insulin resistance in the polycystic ovary syndrome. *J Clin Endocrinol Metab* 1990; 70:699-704.

Dunaif A, Green G, Phelps RG, et al: Acanthosis nigricans, insulin action, and hyperinsulinemia: Clinical, histological, and biochemical findings. *J Clin Endocrinol Metab* 1991; 73:590-595.

Dunaif A, Hoffman AR, Scully RE, et al: Clinical, biochemical, and ovarian morphologic features in women with acanthosis nigricans and masculinization. *Obstet Gynecol* 1985; 66:545-552.

Dunaif A, Longcope C, Canick J, et al: The effects of the aromatase inhibitor Δl-testolactone on gonadotropin release and steroid metabolism in polycystic ovarian disease. *J Clin Endocrinol Metab* 1984a; 60:773-780.

Dunaif A, Mandeli J, Fluhr H, et al: The impact of obesity and chronic hyperinsulinemia on gonadotropin release and gonadal steroid secretion in the polycystic ovary syndrome. *J Clin Endocrinol Metab* 1988; 66:131-139.

Dunaif A, Scott D, Finegood D, et al: The insulin sensitizing agent troglitazone: A novel therapy for the polycystic ovary syndrome. *J Clin Endocrinol Metab* 1996; 81:3299-3306.

Dunaif A, Scully RE, Andersen RN, et al: The effects of continuous androgen secretion on the hypothalamic-pituitary axis in women: Evidence from a luteinized thecoma of the ovary. *J Clin Endocrinol Metab* 1984b; 59:389-393.

Dunaif A, Segal KR, Futterweit W, et al: Profound peripheral insulin resistance, independent of obesity, in polycystic ovary syndrome. *Diabetes* 1989a; 38:1165-1174.

Ehrhardt AA, Evers K, Money J: Influence of androgen and some aspects of sexually dimorphic behavior in women with the late-treated adrenogenital syndrome. *Johns Hopkins Med J* 1968; 123:115-122.

Ehrmann DA, Barnes RB, Rosenfield RL: Polycystic ovary syndrome as a form of functional ovarian hyperandrogenism due to dysregulation of androgen secretion. *Endocr Rev* 1995; 16:322-353.

Ehrmann DA, Cavaghan MK, Imperial J, et al: Effects of metformin on insulin secretion, insulin action, and ovarian steroidogenesis in women with polycystic ovary syndrome. *J Clin Endocrinol Metab* 1997a; 82:524-530.

Ehrmann DA, Schneider DJ, Sobel BE, et al: Troglitazone improves defects in insulin action, insulin secretion, ovarian steroidogenesis, and fibrinolysis in women with polycystic ovary syndrome. *J Clin Endocrinol Metab* 1997b; 82:2108-2116.

Eil C, Edelson SK: The use of human skin fibroblasts to obtain potency estimates of drug binding to androgen receptors. *J Clin Endocrinol Metab* 1984; 59:51-55.

Erenus M, Gurbuz O, Durmosoglu F, et al: Comparison of the efficacy of spironolactone versus flutamide in the treatment of hirsutism. *Fertil Steril* 1994; 61:613-616.

Erenus M, Yücelten D, Durmosoglu F, et al: Comparison of finasteride versus spironolactone in the treatment of idiopathic hirsutism. *Fertil Steril* 1997; 68:1000-1003.

Erenus M, Yücelten D, Gurbuz O, et al: Comparison of spironolactone-oral contraceptive versus cyproterone acetate-estrogen regimens in the treatment of hirsutism. *Fertil Steril* 1996; 66:216-219.

Erickson GF, Magoffin DA, Dyer CA, et al: The ovarian androgen producing cells: A review of structure/function relationships. *Endocr Rev* 1985; 6:371-399.

Evans DJ, Hoffman RG, Kalkhoff RK, et al: Relationship of androgenic activity to body fat topography, fat cell morphology, and metabolic aberrations in premenopausal women. *J Clin Endocrinol Metab* 1983; 57:304-310.

Evron S, Shapiro G, Diamant YZ: Induction of ovulation with spironolactone (Aldactone) in anovulatory oligomenorrheic and hyperandrogenic women. *Fertil Steril* 1981; 36:468-471.

Ferriman D, Gallwey JD: Clinical assessment of body hair growth in women. *J Clin Endocrinol Metab* 1961; 21:1440-1447.

Franks S: Polycystic ovary syndrome: A changing perspective. *N Engl J Med* 1995; 333:853-861.

Franks S, Gharani N, Waterworth D, et al: The genetic basis of polycystic ovary syndrome. *Hum Reprod* 1997; 12:2641-2648.

Friedman CI, Schmidt GE, Kim MH, Powell J: Serum testosterone concentrations in the evaluation of androgen-producing tumors. *Am J Obstet Gynecol* 1985; 153:44-49.

Futterweit W, Deligdisch L: Histopathological effects of exogenously administered testosterone in 19 female to male transsexuals. *J Clin Endocrinol Metab* 1985; 62:16-21.

Futterweit W, Dunaif A, Yeh H-C, et al: The prevalence of hyperandrogenism in 109 consecutive female patients with diffuse alopecia. *J Am Acad Dermatol* 1988; 19:831-836.

Gabrilove JL, Seman AT, Sabet R, et al: Virilizing adrenal adenoma with studies on the steroid content of the adrenal venous effluent and a review of the literature. *Endocr Rev* 1981; 2:462-470.

Geist SH, Gaines JA: Diffuse luteinization of the ovaries associated with the masculinization syndrome. *Am J Obstet Gynecol* 1942; 43:975-983.

Gilling-Smith C, Willis DS, Beard RW, et al: Hypersecretion of androstenedione by isolated thecal cells from polycystic ovaries. *J Clin Endocrinol Metab* 1994; 79:1158-1165.

Givens JR, Andersen RN, Wiser WL, et al: A gonadotropin-responsive adrenocortical adenoma. *J Clin Endocrinol Metab* 1974; 38: 126-133.

Givens JR, Andersen RN, Wiser WL, et al: A testosterone secreting, gonadotropin responsive pure thecoma and polycystic ovarian disease. *J Clin Endocrinol Metab* 1975; 41:845-853.

Glass AR, Dahms WT, Abraham G, et al: Secondary amenorrhea in obesity: Etiologic role of weight-related androgen excess. *Fertil Steril* 1978; 30(2):243-244.

Glickman SP, Rosenfeild RL, Bergenstal RM, et al: Multiple androgenic abnormalities, including elevated free testosterone, in hyperprolactinemic women. *J Clin Endocrinol Metab* 1982; 55:251-257.

Gordon GG, Southern AL, Tochimoto S, et al: Effect of hyperthyroidism and hypothyroidism on on the metabolism of testosterone and androstenedione in man. *J Clin Endocrinol* 1969; 29(2):164-170.

Graf M, Brown V, Richards C, et al: The independent effects of hyperandrogenemia, hyperinsulinemia, and obesity on lipid and lipoprotein profiles in women. *Clin Endocrinol (Oxf)* 1990; 33:119-131.

Groves TD, Corenblum B: Spironolactone therapy during human pregnancy. *Am J Obstet Gynecol* 1995; 172:1655.

Hague WM, Adams J, Rodda C, et al: The prevalence of polycystic ovaries in patients with congenital adrenal hyperplasia and their close relatives. *Clin Endocrinol* 1990; 33: 501-510.

Hammerstein J, Meckies J, Leo-Rossberg I, et al: Use of cyproterone acetate in the treatment of acne, hirsutism and virilism. *J Steroid Biochem* 1975; 6:827-836.

Hayes FJ, Taylor AE, Martin KA, et al: Use of a gonadotropin-releasing hormone antagonist as a physiologic probe in polycystic ovary syndrome: Assessment of neuroendocrine and androgendynamics. *J Clin Endocrinol Metab* 1998; 83: 2342-2349.

Helfer EL, Miller JL, Rose LI: Side-effects of spironolactone therapy in the hirsute woman. *J Clin Endocrinol Metab* 1988; 66:208.

Hochberg Z, Gardos M, Benderly A: Psychosexual outcome of assigned females and males with 46,XX virilizing congenital adrenal hyperplasia. *Eur J Pediatr* 1987; 146:497-499.

Horton R, Hawks D, Lobo R: 3-Alpha, 17-beta-androstanediol glucuronide in plasma—a marker of androgen action in idiopathic hirsutism. *J Clin Invest* 1982; 69:1203-1206.

Hughesdon PE: Morphology and morphogenesis of the Stein-Leventhal ovary and of so-called 'hyperthecosis.' *Obstet Gynecol* 1982; 37: 59-77.

Hull MGR: Epidemiology of infertility and polycystic ovarian disease: Endocrinological and demographic studies. *Gynecol Endocrinol* 1987; 1:235-245.

Irvine RA, Yu MC, Ross RK, Coetzee GA: The CAG and GGC micro-satellites of the androgen receptor gene are in linkage disequilibrium in men with prostate cancer. *Cancer Res* 1994;54:2861-2864.

Ito T, Horton R: The source of plasma dihydrotestosterone in man. *J Clin Invest* 1971; 50:162-1627.

Jackson RL, Docherty MD: The Stein-Leventhal syndrome analysis of 45 cases with special reference to association with endometrial carcinoma. *Am J Obstet Gynecol* 1957; 73:161-173.

Katz M, Carr PJ, Cohen BM, et al: Hormonal effects of wedge resection of polycystic ovaries. *Obstet Gynecol* 1978; 51:437-444.

Kiddy DS, Hamilton-Fairley D, Bush A, et al: Improvement in endocrine and ovarian function during dietary treatment of obese women with polycystic ovary syndrome. *Clin Endocrinol (Oxf)* 1992; 36:105-111.

Knochenhauer ES, Key TJ, Kahsar-Miller M, et al: Prevalence of the polycystic ovary syndrome in unselected black and white women of the southeastern United States: A prospective study. *J Clin Endocrinol Metab* 1998; 83:3078-3082.

Korytkowski MT, Mokan M, Horwitz MJ, et al: Metabolic effects of oral contraceptives in women with polycystic ovary syndrome. *J Clin Endocrinol Metab* 1995; 80:3327-3334.

Kuttenn F, Mowszowicz I, Schaison G, et al: Androgen production and skin metabolism in hirsutism. *J Endocrinol* 1977; 75:83-91.

Lambert-Messerlian GM, Hall JE, Sluss PE, et al: Relatively low levels of dimeric inhibin circulate in men and women with polycystic ovary syndrome using a specific two-site enzyme-linked immunosorbent assay. *J Clin Endocrinol Metab* 1994; 79:45-50.

Legro RS, Driscoll D, Strauss JF, et al: Evidence for a genetic basis for hyperandrogenemia in polycystic ovary syndrome. *Proc Natl Acad Sci USA* 1998a; 95:14956-14960.

Legro RS, Kunselman AR, Dodson WC, et al: Prevalence and predictors of risk for type 2 diabetes mellitus and impaired glucose tolerance in polycystic ovary syndrome: A prospective, controlled study in 254 affected women. *J Clin Endocrinol Metab* 1999;84:165-169.

Legro RS, Spielman R, Urbanek M, et al: Phenotype and genotype in polycystic ovary syndrome. *Recent Prog Horm Res* 1998b; 53:217-256.

Lissak A, Sorokin Y, Calderon I, et al: Treatment of hirsutism with cimetidine: A prospective randomized controlled trial. *Fertil Steril* 1989; 51:247-250.

Lobo R: 'Idiopathic hirsutism'—fact or fiction? *Semin Reprod Endocrinol* 1986; 4:179-187.

Lobo RA, Goebelsmann U: Adult manifestation of congenital adrenal hyperplasia due to incomplete 21-hydroxylase deficiency mimicking polycystic ovarian disease. *Am J Obstet Gynecol* 1980; 138:720-726.

Lobo RA, Goebelsmann U, Horton R: Evidence for the importance of peripheral tissue events in the development of hirsutism in polycystic ovary syndrome. *J Clin Endocrinol Metab* 1983; 57:393-397.

Lobo RA, Grange C, Goebelsmann U, et al: Elevations in unbound serum estradiol as a possible mechanism for inappropriate gonadotropin secretion in women with PCOS. *J Clin Endocrinol Metab* 1981; 52:156-158.

Longcope C: Adrenal and gonadal androgen secretion in normal females. *J Clin Endocrinol Metab* 1986; 15:213-228.

Lucky AW, McGuire J, Rosenfield RL, et al: Plasma androgens in women with acne vulgaris. *J Invest Dermatol* 1983; 81:70-74.

Lucky AW, Rosenfeld RL, McGuire J, et al: Adrenal androgen hyperresponsiveness to adrenocorticotropin in women with acne and/or hirsutism: Adrenal enzyme defects and exaggerated adrenarche. *J Clin Endocrinol Metab* 1986; 62: 840-848.

Martikainen H, Heikkinen J, Ruokonen A, et al: Hormonal and clinical effects of ketoconazole in hirsute women. *J Clin Endocrinol Metab* 1988; 66:987-991.

Mason HD, Willis DS, Beard RW, et al: Estradiol production by granulosa cells of normal polycystic ovaries: Relationship to menstrual cycle history and concentrations of gonadotropins and sex steroids in follicular fluid. *J Clin Endocrinol Metab* 1994; 79:1355-1360.

Mattox JH, Phelan S: The evaluation of adult females with testosterone producing neoplasms of the adrenal cortex. *Surg Gynecol Obstet* 1987; 164:98-101.

McKenna TJ, Moore A, Magee F, et al: Amenorrhea with cryptic hyperandrogenemia. *J Clin Endocrinol Metab* 1983; 56:893-896.

Mechanick J, Dunaif A: Masculinization: A clinical approach to the diagnosis and treatment of hyperandrogenic women. In Mazzaferri E, editor: Advances in endocrinology and metabolism, St. Louis, Mosby Year Book.

Meldrum DR, Abraham GE: Peripheral and ovarian nevous concentrations of various steroid hormones in virilizing ovarian tumors. *Obstet Gynecol* 1979; 53: 36-43.

Moghetti P, Castello R, Negri C, et al: Insulin infusion amplifies 17α-hydroxycorticosteroid intermediate response to adrenocorticotropin in hyperandrogenic women: Apparent relative impairment of 17,20-lyase activity. *J Clin Endocrinol Metab* 1996a; 81:881-886.

Moghetti P, Tosi F, Castello R, et al: The insulin resistance in women with hyperandrogenism is partially reversed by antiandrogen treatment: Evidence that androgens impair insulin action in women. *J Clin Endocrinol Metab* 1996b; 81:952-960.

Moltz L, Schwartz U, Sorensen R, et al: Ovarian and adrenal vein steroids in patients with nonneoplastic hyperandrogenism: Selective catheterization findings. *Fertil Steril* 1984; 42: 69-75.

Mountz JM, Gross MD, Shapiro B, et al: Scintigraphic localization of ovarian dysfunction. *J Nucl Med* 1988; 29: 1644-1650.

Mowszowicz I, Melinatou E, Doukani A, et al: Androgen binding capacity and 5-alpha-reductase activity in pubic skin fibroblasts from hirsute patients. *J Clin Endocrinol Metab* 1983; 56:1209-1213.

Nader S, Riad-Gabriel MG, Saad MF: The effect of a desogestrel-containing oral contraceptive on glucose tolerance and leptin concentrations in hyperandrogenic women. *J Clin Endocrinol Metab* 1997; 82: 3074-3077.

Nagamani M, Hannigan EV, Kinh TV, et al: Hyperinsulinemia and stromal luteinization of the ovaries in postmenopausal women with endometrial cancer. *J Clin Endocrinol Metab* 1988; 67:144-153.

Nestler JE, Barlascini CO, Matt DW, et al: Suppression of serum insulin by diazoxide reduces serum testosterone levels in obese women with polycystic ovary syndrome. *J Clin Endocrinol Metab* 1989; 68:1027-1032.

Nestler JE, Jacubowicz DJ, Evans WS, et al: Effects of metformin on spontaneous and clomiphene-induced ovulation in the polycystic ovary syndrome. *N Engl J Med* 1998; 338: 1876-1880.

Nestler JE, Jacubowicz DJ: Decreases in ovarian cytochrome P450c17 activity and serum free testosterone after reduction of insulin secretion in polycystic ovary syndrome. *N Engl J Med* 1996; 335: 617-623.

Nestler JE, Powers LP, Matt DW, et al: A direct effect of hyperinsulinemia on serum sex hormone-binding globulin levels in obese women with polycystic ovary syndrome. *J Clin Endocrinol Metab* 1991; 72: 83-89.

New MI, Speiser PW: Genetics of adrenal steroid 21-hydroxylase deficiency. *Endocr Rev* 1986; 7:331-349.

O'Brien RC, Cooper ME, Murray RML, et al: Comparison of sequential cyproterone acetate/estrogen versus spironolactone/oral contraceptive in the treatment of hirsutism. *J Clin Endocrinol Metab* 1991; 72:1008-1013.

Pang S, Lerner A, Stoner E, et al: Late-onset adrenal steroid 3-beta-hydroxysteroid dehydrogenase deficiency, I: A cause of hirsutism in pubertal and postpubertal women. *J Clin Endocrinol Metab* 1985; 60(3):428-439.

Paradisi R, Grossi G, Venturoli S, et al: Evidence for a hypothalamic alteration of catecholamine metabolism in polycystic ovarian syndrome. *Clin Endocrinol (Oxf)* 1988; 29:317-326.

Pardridge WM: Transport of protein-bound hormones into tissues in vivo. *Endocr Rev* 1981; 2: 103-123.

Parr JH, Abraham RR, Seed M, et al: The treatment of a hyperandrogenic and virilizing state in an elderly female with a synthetic LHRH agonist. *J Endocrinol Invest* 1988; 11:433-436.

Pastor CL, Griffin-Korf ML, Aloi JA, et al: Polycystic ovary syndrome: Evidence for reduced sensitivity of the gonadotropin-releasing hormone pulse generator to inhibition by estradiol and progesterone. *J Clin Endocrinol Metab* 1998; 83:582-590.

Plymate SR, Matej LA, Jones RE, et al: Inhibition of sex hormone-binding globulin production in the human hepatoma (Hep G2) cell line by insulin and prolactin. *J Clin Endocrinol Metab* 1988; 67:460-464.

Polson DW, Wadsworth J, Adams J, Frank S: Polycystic ovaries: A common finding in normal women. *Lancet* 1988; 1:870-872.

Rebar R, Judd HL, Yen SSC, et al: Characterization of the inappropriate gonadotropin secretion in polycystic ovary syndrome. *J Clin Invest* 1976; 57:1320-1329.

Rittmaster R, Loriaux DL, Culter GB Jr: Sensitivity of cortisol and adrenal androgens to dexamethasone suppression in hirsute women. *J Clin Endocrinol Metab* 1985; 61:462-466.

Rittmaster RS: Gonadotropin-releasing hormone (GnRH) agonists and estrogen/progestin replacement for the treatment of hirsutism: Evaluating the results. *J Clin Endocrinol Metab* 1995; 80:3403-3405.

Robinson S, Kiddy D, Gelding SV, et al: The relationship of insulin insensitivity to menstrual pattern in women with hyperandrogenism and polycystic ovaries. *Clin Endocrinol (Oxf)* 1993; 39:351-355.

Rogers J, Mitchell GW: The relation of obesity to menstrual disturbances. *N Engl J Med* 1952; 247:53-55.

Serafini P, Silva PD, Paulson RJ, et al: Acute modulation of the hypothalamic-pituitary axis by intravenous testosterone in normal women. *Am J Obstet Gynecol* 1986; 155:1288-1292.

Shortle BE, Warren MP, Tsin D: Recurrent androgenicity in pregnancy: A case report and literature review. *Obstet Gynecol* 1987; 70:462-466.

Sorensen R, Moltz L, Schwarz U: Technical difficulties in selective venous blood sampling in the differential diagnosis of female hyperandrogenism. *Cardiovasc Intervent Radiol* 1986; 9:75-82.

Spratt DI, Finkelstein JS, Butler JP, et al: Effects of increasing the frequency of low doses of gonadotropin secretion in GnRH-deficient men. *J Clin Endocrinol Metab* 1987; 64:1179-1186.

Spritzer P, Billaud L, Thalabard JC, et al: Cyproterone acetate versus hydrocortisone treatment in late-onset adrenal hyperplasia. *J Clin Endocrinol Metab* 1990; 70:642-646.

Stein IF, Leventhal ML: Amenorrhea associated with bilateral polycystic ovaries. *Am J Obstet Gynecol* 1935; 29:181-191.

Stuart CA, Peters EJ, Prince MJ, et al: Insulin resistance with acanthosis nigricans: The roles of obesity and androgen excess. *Metabolism* 1986; 35:197-205.

Tagatz GE, Kopher RA, Nagel TC, Okagaki T: The clitoral index: A bioassay of androgenic stimulation. *Obstet Gynecol* 1979; 54:562-564.

Talbott E, Guzick D, Clerici A, et al: Coronary heart disease risk factors in women with polycystic ovary syndrome. *Arterioscler Thromb Vasc Biol* 1995; 15:821-826.

Taylor AE, McCourt B, Martin KA, et al: Determinants of abnormal gonadotropin secretion in clinically defined women with polycystic ovary syndrome. *J Clin Endocrinol Metab* 1997; 82:2248-2256.

Thomas JP, Oake RJ: Androgen metabolism in the skin of hirsute women. *J Clin Endocrinol Metab* 1974; 38:19-22.

Tucci JR, Zah W, Kalderon AK: Endocrine studies in an arrhenoblastoma responsive to dexamethasone, ACTH and human chorionic gonadotropin. *Am J Med* 1973; 55:687-694.

Tut TG, Ghadessy FJ, Trifiro MA, et al: Long polyglutamine tracts in the androgen receptor are associated with reduced trans-activation, impaired sperm production, and male infertility. *J Clin Endocrinol Metab* 1997; 82:3777-3782.

Velazquez EM, Mendoza S, Hamer T, et al: Metformin therapy in polycystic ovary syndrome reduces hyperinsulinemia, insulin resistance, hyperandrogenemia, and systolic blood pressure, while facilitating normal menses and pregnancy. *Metabolism* 1994; 43:647-654.

Wajchenberg BL, Achando SS, Okada H, et al: Determination of the source(s) of androgen overproduction in hirsutism associated with polycystic ovary syndrome by simultaneous adrenal and ovarian venous catheterization: Comparison with the dexamethasone suppression test. *J Clin Endocrinol Metab* 1986; 63:1204-1210.

Waldstreicher J, Santoro N, Hall, JE, et al: Hyperfunction of the hypothalamic-pituitary axis in women with polycystic ovarian disease: Indirect evidence for partial gonadotropin desensitization. *J Clin Endocrinol Metab* 1988; 66:165-172.

Wild RA: Obesity, lipids, cardiovascular risk, and androgen excess. *Am J Med* 1995; 98:27S-32S.

Wild RA, Grubb BG, Hartz A, et al: Clinical signs of androgen excess as risk factors for coronary artery disease. *Fertil Steril* 1990; 54:255-259.

Wild RA, Umstot ES, Anderson RN, et al: Adrenal function in hirsutism, II: Effect of an oral contraceptive. *J Clin Endocrinol Metab* 1982; 54:676-681.

Wild RA, Umstot ES, Anderson RN, et al: Androgen parameters and their correlation with body weight in one hundred thirty-eight women thought to have hyperandrogenism. *Am J Obstet Gynecol* 1983; 146:602-606.

Wilson JD: Androgen abuse by athletes. *Endocr Rev* 1988; 9:181-199.

Winneker RC, Wagner MM, Shaw CJ, et al: Antiandrogens do not reverse androgen-induced inhibition of sex hormone-binding globulin levels in adult female rhesus monkeys. *Endocrinology* 1989; 125:715-720.

Wong IL, Morris RS, Chang L, et al: A prospective randomized trial comparing finasteride to spironolactone in the treatment of hirsute women. *J Clin Endocrinol Metab* 1995; 80(1):223-238.

Wysowski DK, Freiman JP, Tourtelot JB, et al: Fatal and non-fatal heptatoxicity associated with flutamide. *Ann Intern Med* 1993; 118(11)860-864.

Yamaji T, Ibayashi H: Plasma dehydroepiandrosterone sulfate in normal and pathological conditions. *J Clin Endocrinol* 1969; 29:273-278.

Yen SSC: The polycystic ovary syndrome. *Clin Endocrinol (Oxf)* 1980; 12:177-208.

Zerah M, Rheaume E, Mani P, et al: No evidence of mutations in the genes for type I and II 3-hydroxysteroid dehydrogenase (3BSHD) in nonclassical 3BHSD deficiency. *J Clin Endocrinol Metab* 1994; 79:1811-1817.

Zawadski JK, Dunaif A: Diagnostic criteria for polycystic ovary syndrome: Toward a rational approach. In Dunaif A, Givens JR, Haseltine FP, Merriam GR, editors (Hershman SM, series editor): *Polycystic ovary syndrome: Current issues in endocrinology and metabolism,* Boston, 1992, Blackwell Scientific.

Zimmerman S, Phillips RA, Wikenfeld C, et al: Polycystic ovary syndrome: Lack of hypertension despite insulin resistance. *J Clin Endocrinol Metab* 1992; 75:508-513.

Zumoff B, Freeman R, Copey S, et al: A chronobiological abnormality in luteinizing hormone secretion in teenage girls with the polycystic-ovary syndrome. *N Engl J Med* 1983; 309:1206-1209.

16

Recurrent Pregnancy Loss

JOSEPH A. HILL

KEY ISSUES

1. The most common cause of spontaneous abortion, whether as an isolated incident (first or second loss) or as another loss in a woman who has had three or more previous losses, is a structural chromosome abnormality, such as trisomy 16 or monosomy X, in the abortus.

2. The only noncontroversial parental factor for recurrent pregnancy loss is an inborn chromosome abnormality such as a balanced translocation. The prognosis for success for couples with a balanced translocation is between 70% and 90%.

3. Evaluation is targeted to assess possible genetic, anatomic, endocrinologic, infectious, and immunologic abnormalities.

4. Potential immunologic causes of pregnancy loss are the most controversial. A scientifically rational assessment includes a lupus anticoagulant, immunoglobulin G and perhaps immunoglobulin M antibodies to cardiolipin and phosphatidylserine, and possible assessment of interferon-γ production to trophoblast stimulation.

5. The prognosis is good for women with a history of recurrent loss, even without therapy. A caring, empathetic attitude from a dedicated medical support team is important for success.

Human pregnancy is largely an inefficient process. Most concepti fail to attain viability (Wilcox et al, 1988). Spontaneous abortion, defined as a clinically recognized pregnancy loss before 20 weeks of gestation, occurs in 10% to 20% of women known to be pregnant (Alberman, 1988) and is the most common complication of pregnancy. Estimates of loss are difficult to determine because the precise timing of implantation is unknown and because different methodologies and criteria are used to document pregnancy.

Historically, recurrent pregnancy loss has been defined as three or more spontaneous abortions, and it occurs in 0.3% of pregnant women (Edmonds et al, 1982). This definition has been changed to two consecutive losses because recurrence risks and subsequent outcomes are similar for women who have two or three previous losses (Regan, 1991; Hill, 1994). Approximately 1% of pregnant women have had at least two spontaneous abortions (Regan, 1991).

Data derived from epidemiologic studies indicate that the risk for subsequent pregnancy loss is approximately 24% after two clinical pregnancy losses, 30% after three, and 40% after four consecutive spontaneous abortions (Warburton and Fraser, 1961; Poland et al, 1977; Regan et al, 1989).

POSSIBLE ETIOLOGIES

Historically, many possible causes of recurrent pregnancy loss have been proposed (Box 16-1). The only one that is not controversial is parental chromosome abnormality. Recurrent pregnancy loss occurs generally at similar developmental stages in consecutive pregnancies. Chromosome abnormalities can result in pregnancy loss throughout gestation, though most occur within the first 11 weeks of pregnancy. Pregnancy loss resulting from a presumed anatomic abnormality may occur in the first or the second trimester. Hormonal deficiencies or excess may result in pregnancy loss earlier than 10 weeks of gestation, whereas pregnancy loss from autoimmunity generally occurs after 10 weeks of pregnancy. Alloimmune pregnancy loss, possibly caused by T helper 1 (Th1) embryotoxic cytokines, may occur any time until 20 weeks of gestation. Pregnancy loss caused by a presumed infectious agent or an environmental insult may occur during any trimester of pregnancy.

Genetic Factors

Chromosome anomalies have been reported in as many as 60% of all first-trimester abortuses (Boue et al, 1975). In a

---

BOX 16-1
**ETIOLOGIES PRESUMED HISTORICALLY FOR
RECURRENT PREGNANCY LOSS**

Genetic Factors

Chromosomal
Single-gene disorders
X-linked
Multifactorial

Anatomic Factors

Congenital
Acquired

Endocrine Factors

Luteal phase insufficiency
Polycystic ovarian syndrome
Thyroid disorders
Diabetes mellitus
Androgen disorders
Prolactin disorders

Infectious Factors

Bacteria
Viruses
Parasites
Zoonoses
Fungi

Immunologic Factors
Autoimmune

Antiphospholipid antibodies
Other autoantibodies

Alloimmune

Blocking antibody deficiency
T-helper immunity (immunodystrophism)

Miscellaneous Factors

Environmental
Stress
Placental abnormalities
Medical illnesses
Male factors
Asynchronous fertilization
Coitus
Exercise

Having one chromosomally abnormal spontaneous abortion may increase the risk for a subsequent loss caused by a chromosome abnormality (Golbus, 1981).

Trisomy 16 is the single most common trisomy found in spontaneous abortion, and it is incompatible with life. After trisomy 16, in descending order of prevalence, are trisomy 22, 21, 15, 14, 18, and 13 (Warburton et al, 1986). Triploidy (69 chromosomes) is also commonly found. All autosomes have been found in trisomic abortuses except trisomy 1.

Triploidy accounts for almost 17% of chromosomally abnormal abortuses, with most triploid fetuses aborted early in pregnancy. Unlike trisomies, triploidy is not associated with maternal age (Hassold et al, 1993). Tetraploidy (92 chromosomes) occurs less often.

Confined placental mosaicism may result in pregnancy loss (Kalausek et al, 1992). The precise mechanism of pregnancy loss in chromosomally abnormal embryos is unknown, but disordered timing of developmental gene regulation has been speculated (Wudl et al, 1977) as has disordered hormonal regulation (Heup et al, 1979). Inborn chromosome aberrations may be inherited or may arise de novo by spontaneous mutations during embryo development. Maternal age-related problems in oocyte spindle formation and meiotic division leading to chromosomally abnormal gametes are well known (Battaglia et al, 1996).

Inborn chromosome abnormalities occur in only 3% to 6% of couples who experience recurrent pregnancy loss (Khuds, 1974; Tho et al, 1979; Stray-Pedersen et al, 1984; Hill et al, 1992; Stephensen, 1996). Neither family history nor reproductive history is sufficient to rule out a chromosome abnormality in the couple. The most common parental chromosome abnormality contributing to pregnancy loss is a translocation, which is the attachment of one chromosome fragment to the broken end of another. Reciprocal translocation involves two chromosomes in a mutual exchange of broken fragments. Robertsonian translocation involves two acrocentric chromosomes, in which breakage occurs close to the centromere in the short arm of one chromosome and in the long arm of another. One of the resultant chromosomes is smaller than normal and is lost in subsequent mitotic divisions. A person with a balanced reciprocal translocation in which no genetic material has been lost will be normal phenotypically. However, depending on the type of meiotic segregation the involved chromosomes undergo, the resultant zygote may be normal (a balanced translocation carrier, like the affected parent), trisomic for part of a chromosome, or monosomic for part of a chromosome. The last two conditions generally lead to pregnancy loss.

Chromomes 6, 7, 9, 16, and 22 are usually involved in reciprocal translocations, and chromosomes 13, 14, 15, 21, and 22 are usually involved in Robertsonian translocations (Connor et al, 1987). In Robertsonian translocations, 58% involve the long arms of chromosomes 13 and 14 (13q 14q). Robertsonian translocations involving homologous chromosomes always result in aneuploidy (either trisomies or monosomies). This is a rare disorder; it was found in only

recent study performed at the Brigham and Women's Hospital, 545 abortuses were successfully karyotyped; of these, 154 were first losses and 45% were found to have an abnormal karyotype. The incidence of aneuploidy was approximately 60% in abortuses of women who had between two and nine previous losses (Rodriquez-Thompson et al, 1999). Trisomies are the most common abnormality found in abortal tissue, and monosomy X (45X) is the next most common.

BOX 16-2
CLASSIFICATION OF CONGENITAL MÜLLERIAN ANOMALIES

Congenital Lesions

Type I.   Agenesis or hypoplasia
Type II.   Unicornuate
Type III.   Didelphys
Type IV.   Bicornuate
Type V.   Septate
Type VI.   Diethylstilbestrol related

Acquired Lesions

Leiomyoma
Adhesions
Endometriosis/adenomyosis

---

1 of 2500 couples with recurrent abortion evaluated at Brigham and Women's Hospital. If a woman has a translocation other than to homologous chromosomes, the risk is approximately 10% that any given conception will be aneuploid, whereas if a man has the abnormality, the risk is 8% that any given clinical pregnancy will be chromosomally abnormal (Simpson et al, 1970). Uncharacterized sperm-selecting factors have been proposed to account for this phenomenon. Couples in whom both partners are balanced translocation carriers are at increased risk for adverse pregnancy and fetal outcomes, but precise risk estimates are unknown.

Other parental structural chromosome anomalies, including mosaicism, may contribute to recurrent pregnancy loss. Chromosome inversions have been thought to represent normal variants, but associations with aneuploid spontaneous abortion have been made.

Single gene disorders may be recognized through analyses of detailed family histories or through particular patterns of anomalies that comprise a syndrome with a known pattern of inheritance. Rarely, X-linked disorders may result in recurrent abortion of male but not of female conceptions. There is also an increased risk for neural tube defects in women with histories of recurrent pregnancy loss (Adam et al, 1995).

Skewed X-chromosome inactivation in which preferential activation of the paternal X-chromosome has been associated with recurrent pregnancy loss maternally inherited through Xq28 (Pegoraro et al, 1997).

Anatomic Factors

Anatomic distortion of the intrauterine cavity has been reported in 10% to 50% of women experiencing recurrent pregnancy loss (Tho et al, 1979; Stray-Pederson et al, 1984; Hill et al, 1992; Stephensen, 1996). The wide range in prevalence of these disorders is most likely the result of selection bias. The incidence of müllerian anomalies in the general population is estimated to be less than 0.5% (Green and Harris, 1976).

Anatomic abnormalities associated with recurrent pregnancy loss have been classified as either congenital (Buttram and Gibbons, 1979; Buttram, 1983) or acquired lesions (Box 16-2).

Other than diethylstilbestrol (DES) exposure, the causes of congenital müllerian anomalies are unknown. Failure of müllerian duct fusion (types II, III and IV) or incomplete caudal-to-cephalad septum reabsorption (type V) have been associated most commonly with recurrent pregnancy loss (Moneschi et al, 1995). A septum has been reported to be associated with a 60% chance of pregnancy loss (Buttram, 1983). Too little information is available to suggest the need for surgical correction of types II, III, and IV anomalies, which are associated typically with obstetric problems other than recurrent spontaneous abortion (Acien, 1993). Resection of an intrauterine septum and cervical cerclage for women exposed in utero to DES has been advocated by many (reviewed in Patton, 1994) based on retrospective and anecdotal case series.

The obstetric outcome of women with congenital uterine malformations after in vitro fertilization and embryo transfer suggests that there are no significant differences in the clinical pregnancy rates when the various forms of uterine malformations are compared. However, the number of study patients included in this report was too small to allow a definitive conclusion (Marcus et al, 1996). Diethylstilbestrol exposure has been associated with subfertility and pregnancy loss (Kaufman et al, 1980), though no specific changes could be related to specific types of pregnancy outcome (Kaufman et al, 1984). Results from in vitro fertilization clinics suggest that implantation and pregnancy outcome are impaired in DES-exposed women with uterine anomalies (Karande et al, 1990).

Congenital uterine abnormalities have been thought to be more commonly associated with second-trimester loss because of the limitation of space and incompetent cervix (Treffers, 1990). However, first-trimester pregnancy loss may occur in a woman with an intrauterine septum because of the poor blood supply to the septum, which may contribute to disordered implantation and poor placental growth including asynchronous hormonal responsiveness (Keller et al, 1979). Incompetent cervix may result from previous cervical trauma or surgery, including cervical conization. A woman with a history of incompetent cervix does not have a higher incidence of first-trimester pregnancy loss.

Acquired anatomic abnormalities associated historically with recurrent pregnancy loss include intrauterine adhesions, leiomyomas, adenomyosis, and endometriosis (March, 1995; Fitzsimmons et al, 1987; Wheeler et al, 1983). Abnormal placentation caused by blood flow abnormalities that result from intrauterine distortions are speculated to bring on uterine contractions and placental abruption. Uterine proteins have also been proposed to be influenced by anatomic distortions caused by endometrial polyps and submucus myomas (Golan et al, 1994). All these proposed mechanisms remain speculative because definitive data are unavailable. The historical association of endometriosis with recurrent pregnancy loss was most likely the result of selection bias. Data from in vitro fertilization clinics indicate that endometriosis is not associated with a higher chance of pregnancy loss (Garcia et al, 1991).

Endocrine Factors

Luteal phase insufficiency, hyperandrogen disorders including the polycystic ovarian syndrome (PCOS), hyperprolactinemia, thyroid dysfunction, and diabetes mellitus have been associated historically with recurrent pregnancy loss. The prevalence of a suspected endocrine problem contributing to recurrent abortion has varied from 15% to 60%, depending on the series (Regan, 1991; Clifford et al, 1994; Hill et al, 1992; Tho et al, 1979; Stray-Pedersen et al, 1984; Stephensen, 1996). Isolated progesterone receptor defects in the endometrium may be a rare cause of recurrent pregnancy loss (Keller et al, 1979).

Human pregnancy is dependent on progesterone production by the corpus luteum and progesterone action on the endometrium after ovulation through rescue by human chorionic gonadotropin (hCG) secretion after implantation until the placenta can take over progesterone production. This luteoplacental shift begins by 6 weeks of gestation and is fully operational by 9 weeks from the last missed period (Csapo et al, 1972; Csapo et al, 1973). Luteal phase insufficiency is speculated to result from abnormal follicle-stimulating hormone (FSH) secretion in the follicular phase, abnormal gonadotropin releasing hormone (GnRH) pulsation, and luteinizing hormone (LH) secretion, which may occur in PCOS and in other hyperandrogenic disorders (Soules et al, 1989; Baird et al, 1991; Regan et al, 1990; Balen et al, 1993). These result in premature ovulation, toxic effects induced by a hyperandrogen environment, disordered resumption of meiosis, endometrial asychrony, disordered estrogen secretion, disordered prostaglandin synthesis, and disordered intraovarian regulation of growth factors and cytokines (Bonney and Franks, 1990). Oligomenorrhea and delayed ovulation have also been associated with pregnancy loss. Oligomenorrhea incidence was found to be inversely proportional to fetal size exclusively in abortions with normal fetal karyotypes (Hasegawa et al, 1992). The role of hyperprolactinemia in recurrent pregnancy loss is thought to be associated with luteal insufficiency.

Abnormal thyroid function has been implicated in some women with reproductive dysfunction (Gilnoer et al, 1991). Mechanisms responsible for such losses remain speculative. The incidence of antithyroid antibodies has been reported to be higher in women with reproductive losses than in women with successful reproductive histories (Stagnaro-Green et al, 1990; Lejeune et al, 1983). In one study, antithyroid antibodies were associated with clinical pregnancy loss but not with biochemical pregnancy loss (Singh et al, 1995).

Women with antithyroid antibodies are at higher risk for thyroiditis after pregnancy loss that was spontaneous, induced, or caused by ectopic gestation (Marqusee et al, 1997). Women with antithyroid antibodies may also be at increased risk for thyroid dysfunction during early pregnancy, but this has not been firmly established.

The incidence of recurrent pregnancy loss is not different between women with well-controlled diabetes mellitus and women without diabetes (Mills et al, 1988). There is also no conclusive evidence that unsuspected diabetes mellitus is a cause of recurrent pregnancy loss (Kalter, 1987). Women with poorly controlled diabetes, as evidenced by elevated plasma glycosylated hemoglobin, have an increased incidence of fetal loss (Mills et al, 1988). In pregnancies that occur after gestational diabetes has been diagnosed, intrauterine deaths were significantly increased than they were in controls, possibly because of the presence of undiagnosed and untreated gestational diabetes (Aberg et al, 1997).

Infectious Factors

Evidence suggests that infection may cause pregnancy loss, especially preterm labor. Whether infection is a cause of recurrent pregnancy loss remains speculative. A woman's immunologic susceptibility to a potentially infectious organism may be the determining factor in whether pregnancy loss occurs. Other probable factors that may play a role in the risk for spontaneous abortion brought on by infection include primary exposure during early gestation, an organism's capability to cause placental infection, the development of an infectious carrier state, and immunocompromise of the person infected (Summers, 1994).

Bacterial, viral, parasitic, fungal, and zoonotic infections have all been associated with recurrent pregnancy loss. Sporadic, random pregnancy loss may have an infectious etiology in some instances. In fact, approximately half of maternal deaths associated with spontaneous abortion are caused by infection (Berman et al, 1985). However, evidence linking infection and recurrent pregnancy loss in humans remains largely anecdotal. Chorioamnionitis, usually resulting from an ascending infection, is a common cause of second-trimester abortion, though hematogenous spread and other direct mechanisms may also contribute. Infection may contribute indirectly to first- or second-trimester pregnancy loss through the activation of inflammatory cytokines and free oxygen radicals, leading directly to cytotoxicity. Infection may indirectly contribute to pregnancy loss through elevation of core body temperature above 39° C, which can be teratogenic and embryocidal (Smith et al, 1978; Milunsky et al, 1992). Infection may also contribute to pregnancy loss through prostaglandin production that culminates in premature labor and delivery (Minkoff, 1983; Romero et al, 1988; Dudley et al, 1996). Alternatively, metabolic byproducts elaborated by pathogenic organisms may weaken chorioamnionitic membrane integrity and lead to the premature rupture of membranes (McGregor et al, 1991; McGregor et al, 1992).

BOX 16-3
POTENTIAL MECHANISMS PROTECTING THE SEMIALLOGENEIC CONCEPTUS FROM IMMUNOLGIC REJECTION

Immune/inflammatory cells
Cytokines/growth factors/hormones
Absence of major histocompatibility class I and class II
Expression of classical human leukocyte antigens
  (HLA E, F, G)
Expression of complement regulatory proteins
fas ligand/*fas* receptor system
Systemic immunosuppression

Organisms commonly associated with adverse reproductive outcome include *Mycoplasma hominis* (Csapo et al, 1972; Sompolinsky et al, 1975) and *Ureaplasma urealyticum* (Kunsdin et al, 1981). Stray-Pedersen et al (1978) reported significantly higher colonization of the endometrium with T-strain mycoplasma in women with histories of recurrent pregnancy loss than in normal controls, which they interpreted as implicating *Mycoplasma* as a cause of abortion. An alternative explanation may be that women who have had spontaneous abortions are more likely to have been in contact with intrauterine instrumentats that could have transferred this organism from the cervix to the uterus because *Mycoplasma* is often found commensally in the human cervical-vaginal environment (McCormack et al, 1972). Thus, unequivocal data substantiating *Mycoplasma* as a cause of human reproductive failure is lacking.

The role of *Chlamydia trachomatis* in endometritis and salpingitis leading to tubal disease is well substantiated, but its role in recurrent pregnancy loss is not determined (Rae et al, 1994). Chlamydiae isolated from human abortal tissue have been demonstrated to cause spontaneous abortion when given to cattle (Page and Smith, 1974). One way chlamydiae may lead to reproductive difficulty is through inflammatory cytokine secretion (Witkin, 1995; Ault et al, 1996).

Other bacterial organisms have been associated with recurrent pregnancy loss. Bacterial vaginosis is more common in women with histories of second-trimester pregnancy loss than in women with successful pregnancies (Llahi-Camp et al, 1996).

Associations between bacterial vaginosis and adverse pregnancy outcome, including chorioamnionitis and preterm labor, have been made (Gibbs, 1993; Hillier et al, 1995), and the induction of inflammatory cytokines has been correlated with adverse pregnancy outcome associated with bacterial vaginosis (Cauci et al, 1996; Imseis et al, 1997).

Group B streptococci have been associated with preterm birth and low birth weight (Regan et al, 1996). Although this organism has not been associated with early pregnancy loss, the finding that infection with group B streptococci in maternal tissues could result in the liberation of proinflammatory cytokines by cells residing in the decidua (Dudley et al, 1997) suggests that it may.

Herpes simplex virus (HSV) infection has been associated with an increased risk for spontaneous abortion (Gronroos et al, 1983). Recently, HSV has been reported to disrupt human leukocyte antigen (HLA)-G expression on a placental trophoblast, which may be a mechanism for pregnancy loss in susceptible women (Schust et al, 1996). Human papillomavirus (HPV) has also been found to be more prevalent in spontaneously aborted tissue than in tissue from electively terminated pregnancies (Hermonat et al, 1998).

The obligate intracellular parasite *Toxoplasma gondii* can invade the placenta and attack the fetus. Associations between toxoplasmosis and recurrent pregnancy loss have been made on the basis of antibody titers to this organism. However, most suggest that it is not a significant factor for loss (Ramirez et al, 1995).

Immunologic Factors

The conceptus is composed of maternal and paternal antigens and its own unique differentiation antigens that are derived genetically. Therefore, the conceptus is semiallogeneic, and it should be expected to be rejected normally because it contains molecules genetically foreign to the maternal host. Therefore, mechanisms (Box 16-3) may be in place to protect the semiallogeneic conceptus from immunologic attack. Both autoimmune and alloimmune mechanisms have been proposed historically for human pregnancy loss. However, few have fulfilled the criteria for causality.

Autoimmune

Of all the immunologic theories proposed for recurrent pregnancy loss, the only one that has most fulfilled the criteria for causality is that involving antiphospholipid antibodies. Whether antiphospholipid antibodies are causes, coincidences, or consequences of reproductive dysfunction is controversial. Controversy also surrounds speculation about the antiphospholipid antibodies involved, the incidence of their occurrence in women with reproductive failure, and by which mechanisms they adversely affect pregnancy.

Antiphospholipid antibodies that are high-titer immunoglobulin (Ig) G or IgM, but not IgA, directed against negatively charged phospholipids, are potentially abnormal. They are characterized by prolonged phospholipid-dependent coagulation in vitro, thrombosis in vivo, thrombocytopenia, and pregnancy loss, which occurs generally after 10 weeks of gestation (Oshiro et al, 1996). The association of antiphospholipid antibodies with one or more of the clinical features listed in Box 16-4 is termed the antiphospholipid syndrome (Harris, 1986).

The incidence of the antiphospholipid syndrome in women who experience recurrent spontaneous abortion varies, depending on which antibodies are measured and the methods used to define a positive value. Using well-defined clinical and laboratory criteria, the incidence is conservatively estimated at less than 5%, though much higher estimates have been given (reviewed in Petri, 1997).

Numerous hypotheses have been proposed to explain the pathophysiologic mechanisms that may be involved in antiphospholipid antibody-mediated pregnancy loss (reviewed in Petri, 1997). Most of these mechanisms involve increased platelet aggregation, decreased endogenous anticoagulant activity, increased thrombosis, and decreased fibrinolysis, culminating in uteroplacental thrombosis and vasoconstriction that results from immunoglobulin binding to platelet and endothelial membrane phospholipids. This binding may lead to membrane instability and hypercoagulability through the inhibition of protein C activation or endothelial prostacyclin synthetase activity (Lockwood et al, 1986), which may inhibit prekallikrein activity and endothelial plasminogen-activator release (Angeles-Caro et al, 1979). Platelet-activating factor may also be released after anticardiolipin-induced platelet adherence, which could worsen thrombosis (Silver et al, 1995). The observation of increased thromboxane and decreased prostacyclin levels in murine placental studies involving antiphospholipid antibodies (Carreras and Vernylan, 1982) has not been supported by studies in humans (Dudley et al, 1990a). Because cardiolipin and most other phospholipids are not expressed on trophoblast cell surfaces, viable endothelial cells, or nonactivated thrombocytes, it is difficult to imagine how these autoantibodies can be involved in pregnancy loss (Christiansen, 1996). This caveat may be why definitive proof that antiphospholipid antibodies are involved in pregnancy loss remains elusive. Alternatively, antiphospholipid antibodies may be markers for other aberrancies leading to pregnancy loss. An anticoagulant protein termed annexin-V is normally present in synctiotrophoblast, where it is theorized to be involved in maintaining intervillous blood flow, but it is reduced in women with antiphospholipid antibodies and recurrent spontaneous abortion (Rand et al, 1994). In women with the antiphospholipid syndrome, IgG can significantly reduce annexin-V expression on syncytiotrophoblast apical membranes in vitro (Rand et al, 1997). The IgM fraction of antiphosphatidylserine also can remove annexin-V and facilitate the binding of prothrombin from human trophoblast (Vogt et al, 1997). This is of potential importance because first-trimester trophoblast cells are capable of externalizing this phospholipid during differentiation (Katsuragawa et al, 1995).

β2-Glycoprotein-1 is a phospholipid cofactor that may be cell-surface expressed; antibodies to this phospholipid cofactor have been associated with recurrent pregnancy loss (Aoki et al, 1995). However, most studies do not support the concept that β2-glycoprotein 1-dependent anticardiolipin antibodies are of greater significance in pregnancy loss than antibodies to cardiolipin alone (Rai et al, 1995).

Monoclonal antibodies against phosphatidylserine inhibit the intercellular fusion of human trophoblast cell lines and cells in vitro (Adler et al, 1995) and can impair trophoblast hormone production and trophoblast invasion in vitro

---

BOX 16-4
CLINICAL FEATURES OF THE
ANTIPHOSPHOLIPID SYNDROME

Nonpregnancy Related	Pregnancy Related
Thrombosis	Spontaneous abortion
Autoimmune thrombocytopenia	Intrauterine fetal demise
Coomb's positive hemolytic anemia	Intrauterine growth restriction
Livedo reticularis	Premature labor
	Fetal distress
	Pregnancy-induced hypertension

From Branch DW, Scott JM, Kochenow NK et al: Obstetric complications associated with the lupus anticoagulants. *N Engl J Med* 1988; 315:1322-1326.

(Katsuragawa et al, 1997). These data provide experimental evidence of a possible mechanism for antiphosphatidylserine-mediated pregnancy loss.

Autoimmunity other than to phospholipids has been associated with recurrent pregnancy loss because of the finding that higher percentages of women who have had recurrent pregnancy losses have autoantibodies to various cell components and organ tissues than do women without reproductive difficulty (reviewed by Geva et al, 1997). Data such as these have led to speculation that autoimmunity to cellular components and tissues other than phospholipids is a cause of reproductive failure or that reproductive difficulty is the first manifestation of some unspecified autoimmune disorder. An alternative explanation is that these associations are either epiphenomena or artifacts related to previous loss. There are no definitive data to substantiate causality nor has a plausible mechanism been proposed to explain how loss occurs because of these purported autoantibodies.

Alloimmune

Th1 cytokines include interleukin (IL)-2, tumor necrosis factor (TNF), and interferon (IFN)-γ. Th2 cytokines include IL-4, IL-5, IL-6, and IL-10. Activated T cells that express the CD4 phenotype secrete these cytokines. CD56 Natural killer (NK) cells can also produce them (reviewed in Mosmann and Coffman, 1989), as can certain endocrinologically responsive tissues (reviewed in Tabibzadeh, 1991; Hill and Anderson, 1990). A dichotomous Th1 and Th2 response to human trophoblast may explain why disease status generally improves in pregnant women with rheumatoid arthritis (Cecere and Persellin, 1981) and why they have a lower incidence of spontaneous abortion than do pregnant women with systemic lupus erythematosus (SLE). Therapeutically administered antibodies directed against TNF-α can cause clinical improvement in rheumatoid arthritis (Rankin et al, 1995), and the absence of TNF and other Th1 cytokines is not as pronounced in women with successful reproductive histories (Hill et al, 1995a). In contrast, diminished IL-2 production in response to recall antigens correlates with SLE activity (Bermas et al, 1994), which generally worsens during pregnancy and is associated with an increased incidence of pregnancy loss (Petri et al, 1991).

In animal models, downregulation of Th1 cytokines has been demonstrated in successful pregnancy (reviewed in Raghupathy, 1997). In approximately 35% to 50% of women with unexplained recurrent pregnancy loss, immune and inflammatory cell responsiveness to trophoblast is activated as evidenced by the increased proliferation (Yamada et al, 1994) and secretion of embryotoxic factors (Hill et al, 1992) such as IFN-γ (Hill et al, 1995a). IFN-γ and TNF have been reported to be toxic to in vitro embryo development (Hill et al, 1987a) and to trophoblast growth (Berkowitz et al, 1988; Haimovici et al, 1991). It has been suggested that they are involved in human reproductive failure in a condition known as immunodystrophism (Hill, 1991), which involves the dichotomous secretion of Th1 cytokines rather than the potentially preferential Th2 cytokines (Hill et al, 1995a).

It is possible that IFN-γ mediates embryotoxicity by limiting the mobility of specific embryonic proteins within cellular membranes (Polgar et al, 1996). Published studies in humans regarding Th1 and Th2 immunity to trophoblast have relied on systemic evidence. Preliminary evidence from our laboratory investigating the role, if any, these cytokines play in reproduction suggests that there is no difference in Th2 cytokine production within the decidua of women who undergo elective abortion and those who have repetitive spontaneous losses. However, we have observed the upregulation of IL-12 in the decidua of some women with recurrent pregnancy loss. This finding, though preliminary, is potentially significant because IL-12 is the major orchestrator of Th1 immunity. An alternative explanation is that IL-12 may be indicative of an inflammatory reaction in response to pregnancy loss and, thus, may be an effect of abortion rather than a contributor to its cause. Further studies are under way to resolve this issue.

Another alloimmune hypothesis for reproductive failure is the concept that blocking antibodies are necessary for successful pregnancy. This hypothesis, proposed by Rocklin et al (1976), was based on suppositions that maternal, antifetal, cellular immune responses develop in all pregnancies that must be blocked by a factor measurable in serum. This serum factor was presumed to be an antibody, and, in the absence of this maternal blocking factor, fetal loss was speculated to result. These suppositions were never substantiated (Sargent et al, 1994). In fact, Rocklin et al (1982) later disproved their own hypothesis, and it has been shown that these purported blocking factors do not develop in 40% of women with successful, uneventful reproductive histories (Amos and Kostyn, 1980). When blocking factors are produced, it generally only happens after 28 weeks of gestation, and they may disappear between normal pregnancies (Regan

et al, 1981). The most compelling data disproving the blocking antibody hypothesis were that women who were incapable of antibody secretion nevertheless achieve successful pregnancy (Rodger, 1985). Thus, the hypothesis that an immunoglobulin effector (*i.e.,* blocking antibody) was necessary for successful pregnancy was scientifically invalidated. Studies from genetically engineered mice, in which specific components of the immune system or the entire immune system are systematically eliminated, indicate that neither the establishment nor the maintenance of pregnancy is dependent on an intact maternal immune system.

Miscellaneous Factors
Environmental

Excessive exposure to lead, mercury, ethylene oxide, ionizing radiation, and dibromochloropropane has been associated with reproductive difficulty by the Occupational Safety and Health Administration (Paul and Kurtz, 1990) and with spontaneous abortion (Polifka and Friedman, 1991). Other occupational exposures that may affect reproduction include anesthetic gases and organic solvents (Paul and Kurtz, 1990). Exposure to electromagnetic fields, such as may occur to persons who live near high-transmission electric power lines or who have prolonged exposure to video display terminals, has been associated historically with pregnancy loss. Inadequate controls and potential errors of recall and memory biases in these retrospective studies limit the adequate interpretation of these reports. Prospective studies have not demonstrated that exposure to electromagnetic fields is associated with an increased risk for pregnancy loss (Lindbolm et al, 1992).

Working during pregnancy is not associated with an increased risk for adverse perinatal outcome unless prolonged periods of standing and long hours are required. Women in these occupations may be at increased risk for preterm delivery of low-birth-weight infants (Gabbe and Turner, 1997). Working women do not have an increased risk for spontaneous abortion, stillbirth, or intrauterine growth restriction (Klebanoff et al, 1990; Klebanoff et al, 1991).

The association of psychosocial issues with pregnancy outcome is controversial. Interpretation of study results is difficult because of the inherent limitations imposed by their retrospective designs, small sample sizes, imprecise definitions of stress, and outcome variables. The Maternal-Fetal Medicine Units' Network of the National Institutes of Child Health and Human Development has reported that maternal psychological stress is associated with spontaneous preterm birth and with low birth weight even after adjustment for maternal demographic and behavioral characteristics (Copper et al, 1996). However, stress has not been associated definitively with spontaneous abortion.

The pathophysiologic mechanisms that would be responsible for stress-induced pregnancy loss are difficult to ascribe, though direct and indirect mechanisms have been theorized. Stress is associated with catecholamine release that could result in vasoconstriction and lead to a disruption in adequate oxygenation and calories to the developing conceptus (Golard et al, 1993). GnRH pulsatility may also be affected by stress and could interfere with the paracrine regulation of human chorionic gonadotropin (hCG) (Barnea and Kaplan, 1989). However, neither maternal concentrations of corticotropin-releasing hormone nor GnRH has been useful in identifying pregnant women at risk for early pregnancy loss (Sorem et al, 1996).

Stress has been reported to increase pregnancy reabsorption in abortion-prone CBA × DBA/2 mice. This effect, though strain specific, appears to be mediated through the upregulation of TNF-α and the downregulation of TGF-β in the decidua (Arck et al, 1995). TNF-α has been reported to inhibit embryo development (Hill et al, 1987a) and trophoblast proliferation (Berkowitz et al, 1988) and to be a component in Th1-type immunity to trophoblast in women with recurrent spontaneous abortion (Hill et al, 1995a). These data suggest the possibility of a psycho-cytokine mechanism for pregnancy loss. Recurrent pregnancy loss is responsible for significant psychological depression in women and significant emotional distress in couples (Klock, 1997). However, more studies are needed before the conclusion can be made that psychological stress is the cause rather than the effect of reproductive difficulty.

Additional environmental factors implicated in spontaneous abortion are ethanol, caffeine, nicotine, and other metabolic products of cigarette smoking. Consumption of more than two alcoholic drinks per day is associated with twice the risk for spontaneous abortion in nonalcohol-consuming controls (Harlop and Shiono, 1980). Low-level alcohol consumption does not appear to be a significant risk factor for spontaneous fetal loss (Cavallo et al, 1995). The minimum threshold dose for increased risk for spontaneous abortion is 2 oz absolute alcohol per week (Kline, 1980). Smoking also has a dose-response relationship with pregnancy complications, including spontaneous abortion (Ferguson et al, 1979). Women who smoke half a pack of cigarettes per day have a higher risk for chromosomally normal spontaneous abortion than women who do not smoke (Kline et al, 1980). There is also a dose-response effect with caffeine consumption, but only if the dose is higher than 300 mg/day (Dlugosz and Bracket, 1992). Consumption of decaffeinated coffee has been associated with pregnancy loss, presumably because of the chemicals added to remove caffeine. Excessive chlorination of drinking water has also been reported to be associated with early pregnancy loss.

Many caveats must be considered before definitive conclusions can be rendered regarding the association of pregnancy loss and any environmental or stress-associated factor. Among them are gestational age at the time of exposure, amount of agent reaching the conceptus, duration of exposure, impact of other factors or agents to which mother and conceptus are simultaneously exposed, physiological status of mother and conceptus, genetic differences, and interrelationship between frequency of exposure, frequency of effect, and recognizability of adverse outcome (Mattison, 1992).

Placental Anomalies

Placental abnormalities are another potential miscellaneous factor in pregnancy loss. Rare abnormalities traditionally have been thought to be associated with second-trimester losses caused by circumvallate placenta and placenta marginata (Torpin, 1955). Defective hemochorial placentation not necessarily linked to fetal chromosome abnormalities has been noted. It has been suggested that spontaneous abortion and pregnancy complicated by preeclampsia or intrauterine growth restriction may be continuums of disorders with similar placental bed abnormalities related to limited depth of invasion (Kong et al, 1987).

Growth-promoting and growth-limiting factors have been detected in uteroplacental tissue. A delicate cytokine balance may exist and facilitate successful pregnancy through the control of trophoblast invasion. In general, Th2-type cytokines and other growth factors, such as colony stimulating factor-1 (CSF-1) and IL-3, may promote trophoblast invasion, whereas Th1-type cytokines may limit trophoblast invasion. Macrophages have been proposed as the pivotal players in this delicate orchestration (Hunt, 1989), possibly through the secretion of IL-12 and TGF-β and the delicate interplay between IL-10 and IFN-γ. Because placental development is a progressive phenomenon and the placenta is not fully developed until the first trimester is complete (Jaffe et al, 1997), abnormalities in the delicate cytokine-growth factor balance—such as too much IL-12, TGF-β, or IFN-γ—may limit trophoblast invasion. If invasion is compromised, increased flow pressure in maternal spiral arteries may dislocate the thin trophoblastic shell. If detachment is widespread, pregnancy loss occurs. If detachment is only partial, placental function may be compromised, increasing the risk for intrauterine growth restriction and pregnancy-induced hypertension (Jaffe et al, 1997).

Placental apoptosis increases significantly as pregnancy progresses, suggesting that it may play a role in normal placental development and placental aging (Smith et al, 1997). Premature induction of apoptosis could theoretically contribute to trophoblast dysfunction and result in early pregnancy loss (Lea et al, 1997). The proto-oncogene product bcl-2, an inhibitor of apoptosis (Wyllie, 1994), has been found to be lower in placental biopsies from women who have had spontaneous abortions than in samples from women who have had elective abortions (Lea et al, 1997). It is also thought that dysregulation of trophoblast protein production is involved in early pregnancy loss.

Maternal Illness

Chronic maternal illness is associated with recurrent pregnancy loss. Women with collagen vascular diseases such as SLE have a higher risk for pregnancy loss. Spontaneous abortion is also a known consequence of severe cardiac, pulmonary, and renal disease. Vascular compromise and poor oxygenation are thought to be the major reasons for loss. Inflammatory bowel disease in pregnant women is associated with an increased frequency of adverse pregnancy outcomes, primarily preterm birth, neonates small for gestational age, and low birth weight (Karnfeld et al, 1997). Whether these adverse outcomes are the result of disease activity, pharmacotherapy, or nutritional status is unknown.

Other rare disorders associated with recurrent pregnancy loss include high copper levels found in Wilson disease (Schagen van Leeunen et al, 1991) and methionine intolerance related to hyperhomocystinemia, a risk factor for first- and second-trimester pregnancy loss (Wouters et al, 1993).

Hematologic disorders are rare, but their diagnosis may be life saving because they are associated with high maternal mortality rates (Mitus and Shafer, 1990). Hypercoagulability may contribute to loss from concomitant medical conditions, such as the antiphospholipid syndrome, or from inherited abnormalities of coagulation in which there is a genetic predisposition to thrombosis, as there is in patients with the factor V Leiden mutation (Dizon-Townson et al, 1997; Ridker et al, 1998). Other contributing factors are defects in the physiological anticoagulant mechanism, such as in antithrombin III, protein C (Rai et al, 1996), and protein S deficiencies, abnormalities of the fibrinolytic system, and dysfibrinogenesis (Gris et al, 1990). Factor XII (Hageman) deficiency, which enhances thrombosis, has been associated with recurrent spontaneous abortion (Schved et al, 1989). Thrombocytosis and thrombocythemia (platelet counts greater than $1 \times 10^6/mm^3$) are also associated with recurrent pregnancy loss (Lishner et al, 1993).

Male Factors

Paternal factors contributing to recurrent pregnancy loss are largely unknown except for chromosome abnormalities as discussed previously. However, paternal alcoholism has been associated with recurrent pregnancy loss even when correcting for maternal consumption (Halmesmaki et al, 1989). Whether these epidemiologic observations are caused by maternal stress or teratogenic effects on spermatozoa are unknown. Men whose partners experience recurrent spontaneous abortion do not have a higher incidence of morphologically abnormal sperm (Hill et al, 1994a), but it is unclear whether the partners of men with teratospermia have a higher frequency of pregnancy loss. Teratospermia has not been associated with chromosomally abnormal sperm (Rosenbusch et al, 1992). Leukocytospermia is also not associated with recurrent abortion, but a higher incidence of elevated T-lymphocyte concentrations have been reported in semen from men whose partners have evidence of Th1 cellular immunity to sperm (Hill et al, 1994a). The significance of this association has not yet been explored.

Asynchronous Fertilization

In some couples, the timing of intercourse may be critical for the establishment of a successful pregnancy. Preovulatory oocyte aging and postovulatory gamete aging may contribute to spontaneous abortion (Guerrero and Rojas, 1975). Nuclear degeneration and meiotic aberrations have been observed in human oocytes (Racowsky and Kaufman, 1992).

Polyspermic fertilization leading to a triploidic or a tetraploidic conceptus is also more likely to occur in aged oocytes because of a defective corticogranular reaction (Lopata et al, 1980). Aged sperm have also been noted to undergo chromosome breakdown before losing their ability to fertilize (Martin-Deleon and Boice, 1982). An increased risk for spontaneous abortion resulting from chromosome anomalies has been noted in humans when implantation occurs too early or too late during the ovulatory cycle, as assessed by basal body temperature recordings (Boue and Boue, 1973). There is no evidence that seasonal variations in conception influence the incidence of spontaneous abortion (Drugan et al, 1989).

Coitus

Coitus during pregnancy could theoretically lead to uterine contractions because of orgasm and excessive catecholamine release or through prostaglandins in semen (Speroff and Rakwell, 1970; Wagner et al, 1976; Omer, 1986). No data are available from studies of women with histories of recurrent pregnancy loss concerning whether coitus during pregnancy is associated with increased risk for loss. Large-scale studies of women who have not had recurrent pregnancy loss suggest that coitus during pregnancy is not associated with adverse outcome.

Exercise

There is no evidence that mild to moderate exercise during pregnancy by healthy women is associated with an increased risk for adverse pregnancy outcome. Running and high-impact aerobics could affect pregnancy adversely by diverting blood flow from the uterus to the peripheral muscles. The American College of Obstetricians and Gynecologists has published guidelines for women who exercise during pregnancy (1994). Contraindications to exercise include illness and many pregnancy-related disorders, but a history of spontaneous abortion, threatened abortion, or first-trimester vaginal bleeding was not addressed. There have been no studies addressing the safety of exercise in women with a history of recurrent pregnancy loss.

EVALUATION

Controversy exists regarding the best time to initiate the evaluation of the couple experiencing pregnancy loss. Investigation has been recommended after three spontaneous abortions, but the origins of this recommendation were not evidenced based. Many, including this author, have recommended the search for possible causes after two consecutive pregnancy losses. This recommendation was based on epidemiologic data indicating that the chance for a subsequent abortion and the potential for discovering a potential cause were equivalent in women experiencing two and three losses. Recent data derived from cytogenetic studies of abortal tissue from women with and without recurrent spontaneous abortion warrant thought and discussion as to whether these recommendations should be further modified.

Approximately 45% to 60% of first miscarriages show chromosome abnormalities (Boue and Boue, 1975; Golbus, 1981; Rodriguez-Thompson et al, 1999). If the first pregnancy loss was chromosomally abnormal, then the second loss has a 75% chance of being chromosomally abnormal. If the first loss was chromosomally normal, there is a 66% chance exists that the next pregnancy loss will be chromosomally normal (Golbus, 1981). In a series of more than 500 pregnancy losses in which a karyotype was obtained of abortal tissue, approximately 60% were found to be abnormal regardless of whether this was the patient's second or ninth pregnancy loss. These findings were related to maternal age; women older than 35 were more likely to have a pregnancy loss associated with an abnormal karyotype than younger women (Rodriguez-Thompson et al, 1999). Based on these findings, consideration should be given to obtaining the karyotype of all pregnancy losses, especially in women older than 35, and to evaluating couples only if a normal abortal karyotype is revealed. If a chromosome abnormality is found in abortal tissue, the couple should be encouraged to reattempt conception without further investigation. For women who have recurrent aneuploic abortions, consideration should be given to obtaining parental karyotypes. However, the incidence of a Robertsonian translocation of homologous chromosomes, which would preclude a successful pregnancy, is rare.

Older women are known to be at increased risk for pregnancy loss (Hansen, 1986). Hence, it may not be surprising to find a higher prevalence of chromosomally abnormal abortuses. Pregnancy loss in older women probably results from chromosome abnormalities in the oocyte, perhaps because the regulatory mechanisms responsible for meiotic spindle assembly are significantly altered during the later reproductive years. Approximately 74% of oocytes recovered from women older than 40 were found to be chromosomally abnormal compared with only 17% of oocytes from women 20 to 25 years of age (Battaglia et al, 1996).

Preconception Assessment

Medical, surgical, psychological, social, and genetic histories should be obtained for each partner in a couple experiencing recurrent pregnancy loss. Questions should be specific regarding chronic medical illness, galactorrhea, previous pelvic infection, uterine instrumentation, and DES exposure. If induced abortion was performed earlier, it is important to reassure the couple that induced first-trimester abortions do not cause subsequent spontaneous losses (Daling and Emanuel, 1977). Menstrual cycle history may give clues regarding oligoovulation, polycystic ovary syndrome, and asynchronous fertilization caused by the imprecise timing of intercourse relative to ovulation. Family history of recurrent pregnancy losses, stillbirths, and birth defects may be informative. Current medications should be recorded, and information concerning illicit drug use, smoking, alcohol

use, and potential occupational exposure should be ascertained. A descriptive sequence of all previous pregnancies is important. This should include the age of gestation and the fetal size (if known). It may be useful to know when each loss occurred because pregnancy loss within persons tends to cluster around the same time in sequential pregnancies. Gestational age may not be as informative because fetal death often happens several weeks before symptoms of expulsion. The time required for conception to take place should be recorded. In rare cases, difficulty in achieving conception may indicate subclinical (peri-implantation) pregnancy loss. Insight into possible genetic abnormalities may be provided by a history of malformed fetuses, especially if neural tube defects occurred. Knowledge of karyotypes of prior abortuses may be helpful. Information about a normal female karyotype should be interpreted cautiously, especially if fetal tissue was not identified definitively. The policy at Brigham and Women's Hospital, if a fetus has not been identified grossly, is to rinse the tissue in physiologic medium and then to examine it under a dissecting microscope so villi can be separated from decidual tissue and removed for culture. Since the implementation of this policy in 1994, the incidence of normal karyotypes identified as normal female (46,XX) has decreased from 70% to 25%. Using molecular biology techniques to compare a known maternal sample with a suspected fetal sample would distinguish definitively whether a female karyotype is maternal or fetal in origin. These techniques, however, are not performed routinely. Alternatively, ultrasound-guided transcervical chorionic villus sampling (CVS) immediately before uterine evacuation may increase the likelihood that fetal rather than maternal tissue is karyotyped. Review of all histologic assessments made on previous abortuses sometimes provides insight into potential causes (Doss et al, 1995).

Physical Examination

Physical examination should include height, weight, blood pressure, and general assessment for signs of metabolic illness. Body habitus should be defined, and the presence of hirsutism or other signs of hyperandrogenism should be noted. Breasts should be examined for galactorrhea, and pelvic examination should focus on signs of previous cervical trauma or DES exposure. Uterine size and shape should also be noted.

Laboratory Testing

Historically, testing has been conducted to look for genetic, anatomic, endocrinologic, infections, and immunologic abnormalities. At the Brigham and Women's Hospital, the tests considered potentially useful in the evaluation of recurrent pregnancy loss are listed in Box 16-5.

Genetic Assessment

Parental cytogenetic testing is warranted in couples where the woman is less than 35 years of age. Karyotype assessment may be unnecessary if prenatal testing would otherwise be suggested for fetal karyotype assessment (for instance, if the woman is older than 35 years). If a cytogenetic anomaly is detected, referral to a genetic counselor should be arranged.

Anatomic Assessment

Hysterosalpingography was the diagnostic procedure used historically for the evaluation of the intrauterine cavity. Hysteroscopic evaluation of the uterine cavity has largely replaced hysterosalpingography because of its higher specificity and lower false-positive and false-negative rates (Raziel et al, 1994). However, both tecniques are limited because they cannot differentiate between a class IV (bicornuate) uterus and a class V (septate) uterus. Laparoscopy has been used to differentiate between these two abnormalities, but the cost of this procedure and the risks involved limit its appeal. Magnetic resonance imaging may be useful (Fielding, 1996), but the associated costs are also high with this modality. Ultrasound evaluation has been reported to be useful, but not by all (Letterie et al, 1995). Recently, sonohysterography has been shown to be very sensitive and specific for the evaluation of müllerian lesions (Keltz et al, 1997). Sonohysterosalpingography is able to distinguish class IV from class V uterine anomalies and has the advantage of providing information about tubal patency if those who experience recurrent pregnancy loss are subfertile.

If hysterosalpingography or sonohysterosalpingography is recommended, it has been our practice to administer a prophylactic antibiotic such as doxycycline against upper genital tract infection from the cervical vaginal environment, even though no data substantiate the necessity of this approach. At the Center for Reproductive Medicine at the Brigham and Women's Hospital, we administer doxycycline 100 mg twice a day beginning the day before the procedure for six doses. Recommending an antiprostaglandin medication, such as 600 mg to 800 mg ibuprofen, 1 hour before the

procedure to assess the intrauterine cavity minimizes patient discomfort associated with intrauterine instrumentation.

Endocrinologic Assessment

Various modalities have been used to diagnose luteal phase insufficiency, among them menstrual cycle history, basal body temperature determination, reproductive hormone level, ultrasound monitoring, and endometrial biopsy. The criterion for assessing the adequacy of the luteal phase is examining the end-organ effect of progesterone on the endometrium through biopsy because of the characteristic endometrial changes brought about by progesterone during the luteal phase. Endometrial biopsies are uncomfortable and expensive, and they are subject to interobserver and intraobserver variation. In addition, endometrial biopsies that exhibit evidence of inadequate luteal phase (a lag of 3 or more days in endometrial development) has been reported in approximately 30% of presumably fertile women (Davis et al, 1989). Timing of the biopsy has varied between studies. Traditionally, the biopsy was obtained 2 days before the anticipated menses. However, a more precise method may be to perform the biopsy 10 days after the LH surge (Jones, 1976). Others have performed the biopsy during the implantation window, compounding the controversy. A sensitive pregnancy test should be performed before a biopsy specimen is taken (Herbert et al, 1990). The endometrial biopsy should not be performed within two cycles of a pregnancy loss because it will be more likely to be out of phase. As many as 45% of women undergo out-of-phase biopsies during this time (Nakajima et al, 1994). This may be related to temporary refractoriness of the pituitary to GnRH (Keye and Jaffe, 1976), persistent hCG (Steier et al, 1984), or persistent decidua, or it may be stress related (Gardiner et al, 1978). Therefore, couples should be advised to avoid conception for two cycles after a loss because luteal phase insufficiency may be enhanced during this time. This recommendation can be modified if ovulation induction is required for conception. Successful pregnancy can result even when conception takes place within two cycles of a loss and even if the endometrium is presumably out of phase (Wentz et al, 1986).

When integrated peripheral blood progesterone levels were used as the standard for assessing luteal phase adequacy, unacceptably low sensitivity and specificity were found for the basal body temperature graphs, luteal phase lengths, and follicular diameters. The endometrial biopsy was acceptable, but the best test for the prediction of a low integrated progesterone level was a single serum progesterone level from the midluteal phase that was less than 10 ng/mL (31.8 nmol/L). An alternative was the sum of three random serum progesterone measurements that amounted to less than 30 ng/mL (95.4 nmol/L) obtained during the luteal phase (Jordan et al, 1994).

Low peripheral blood levels of progesterone have been correlated with out-of-phase endometrial biopsies (Babalioglu et al, 1996). However, normal biopsies are obtained despite low levels of progesterone in peripheral serum (Li et al, 1991). Progesterone in peripheral blood is pulsatile (Soules et al, 1988), and levels in the peripheral circulation are not indicative of levels within the endometrium (Miles et al, 1994). Considerable overlap exists between normal and abnormal peripheral blood levels in women who have successful pregnancies (Azuma et al, 1993). Therefore, ascertaining progesterone levels in the peripheral circulation is not necessarily helpful in determining luteal phase insufficiency.

If luteal phase insufficiency is suspected, serum prolactin, 17-hydroxyprogesterone, and androgen profiles may be warranted. Another diagnostic possibility that should be considered is PCOS, especially if a woman has oligomenorrhea. Preconception LH determinations and ultrasonographic examination have been suggested to facilitate the diagnosis of PCOS (Sagle et al, 1988). A single determination of LH is problematic because, like progesterone, LH is secreted in a pulsatile fashion. However, an LH value greater than 20 mIU/mL during the early follicular or late luteal phase is clearly elevated. Total secretion of LH in the follicular and especially the luteal phase may be more informative but more difficult to obtain. Ultrasonography may be the most sensitive method for diagnosing PCOS in women with recurrent pregnancy loss (Sagle et al, 1980). However, as many as 22% of women with normal reproductive histories are found to have polycystic ovaries by ultrasonographic criteria (Polson et al, 1980).

A glucose tolerance test is not necessary in the evaluation of women with recurrent pregnancy loss because there is no conclusive evidence that unsuspected diabetes or even overt diabetes adequately controlled is a cause of recurrent pregnancy loss (Kalter, 1987). Serum should be assayed for thyroid-stimulating hormone (TSH) with a sensitive assay. Both hypothyroidism and hyperthyroidism have been associated with a greater incidence of spontaneous abortion than occurred in euthyroid controls. Unlike hypothyroidism, however, mild-to-moderate thyrotoxicity generally does not result in reproductive difficulty in women, but severe thyrotoxicosis is associated with an increased risk for early pregnancy loss (Becks and Burrow, 1995). Elevated thyroid peroxidase (TPO) antibody titers have been reported in approximately 24% to 36% of women with recurrent pregnancy loss and in 17% to less than 10% of women with normal reproductive histories (Stagnaro-Green et al, 1990; Bussen and Steck, 1995). The association of TPO antithyroid antibodies with pregnancy loss is controversial. Whether TPO causes loss or is just a marker for subsequent thyroid dysfunction has not been determined (Mazzaferri, 1997). Our clinical experience suggests that pregnancy outcome is not different between women with and without antithyroid antibodies.

Infection Assessment

Cervical cultures are generally not helpful, but they may be taken into consideration if no other abnormalities are revealed or if there is a history of chorioamnionitis or of pre-mature rupture of the membranes. In such cases, consideration should be given for culturing group B β-hemolytic *Streptococcus*, *Mycoplasma*, *Ureaplasma*, and *Chlamydia*, and for seeking signs of bacterial vaginosis. In the absence of clinical infection, TORCH (toxoplasmosis, rubella, cytomegalovirus, and HSV) titers are neither revelatory nor indicated (Sahwi et al, 1995). Trying to detect antibodies to other infections is also not indicated.

Immunologic Assessment

Testing for lupus anticoagulant using either an activated partial thromboplastin time or the more informative Russell Viper Venom Time test and the IgG and perhaps IgM isotypes of anticardiolipin (aCL) and antiphosphatidyl serine (aPS) antibodies should be part of the clinical evaluation of recurrent pregnancy loss. It is imperative that an aCL or an aPS test be repeated to confirm a positive value within a 6- to 8-week interval because it is not uncommon for a low or even a moderate positive value to revert to normal (Rai et al, 1995). Low positive values are not helpful clinically (Rai et al, 1995; Silver et al, 1997). Transiently positive aCL titers are common and can be induced by viral illness (Vaarala et al, 1986). Neither an aCL nor an aPS test serves as a substitute for a lupus anticoagulant test (Cowchuck and Fort, 1994).

Antiphosphatidyl serine is often found in the serum of women with the antiphospholipid syndrome who are seropositive for aCL (Branch et al, 1997), which may indicate autoantibody cross-reactivity. In addition to assessing the lupus anticoagulant and the IgG and IgM isotypes of aCL, assessing the IgG and IgM isotypes of antiphosphatidyl serine may be clinically useful because antiphosphatidyl serine has been shown to inhibit the syncytial formation of placental trophoblast cell lines (Adler et al, 1995; Katsuragawa et al, 1997) and to correlate closely with the pathogenesis of murine pregnancy loss (Silver et al, 1997).

Other autoantibodies, including other antiphospholipid antibodies (phosphatidic acid, phosphatidyl choline, phosphatidyl ethanolanine, phosphatidyl glycerol, phosphatidyl inositol) of all three isotypes (IgG, IgM, IgA), have been detected in the sera of women with reproductive difficulty (Gleicher et al, 1989; Yetman and Kutteh, 1996; Branch et al, 1997). Testing for these other autoantibodies is not justified clinically. Women with recurrent pregnancy loss are no more likely than fertile controls to have elevated levels of these antiphospholipid antibodies once lupus anticoagulant, the IgG isotype of aCL, and an obvious clinical history of autoimmune disease have been excluded (Branch et al, 1997).

The only well-characterized antiphospholipid antibody assay is that for aCL. Positive results for the standard clinical assay for aCL are derived from a calibration curve established for each assay using standard positive sera. This assay achieves acceptable sensitivity and specificity for predicting subsequent thrombosis, thrombocytopenia, and fetal

---

BOX 16-6
IMMUNOLOGIC TESTS THAT LACK CLINICAL BENEFIT BUT ARE NEVERTHELESS ADVERTISED TO COUPLES WHO HAVE RECURRENT PREGNANCY LOSS

Antinuclear antibodies
Immunoglobulin A isotope of anticardiolipin and antiphosphatidyl serine
Antiphosphatidic acid
Antiphosphatidyl choline
Antiphosphatidyl ethanolamine
Antiphosphatidyl glycerol
Antiphosphatidyl inositol
Antihistones
Anti-DNA (SS-DNA, DS-DNA)
Rheumatoid factor
Complement
Smooth muscle antibodies
Antiovarian and antiendometrial antibodies
Antibodies to gonadotropins and gonadosteroids
Antipaternal cytotoxic antibodies (leukocyte antibody detection assay)
Mixed lymphocyte culture reactivities
Human leukocyte antigen profiles, including HLA-DR, HLA-DP, HLA-DQ
Peripheral blood immunophenotype, including peripheral blood CD56(+) natural killer cells
Natural killer cell activity
Embryotoxicity of peripheral serum
Serum cytokine and adhesion molecule assessment

---

loss (*i.e.,* the antiphospholipid syndrome) only at levels six standard deviations above the mean, which is well above the 99th percentile (Harris, 1996). Assessment of other antiphospholipid antibodies relies on a normalized result. A normalized result depends on the cut-off value between what is considered normal and what is considered abnormal. It is perhaps not surprising that a high prevalence of these and other autoantibodies has been detected because of the lack of standardized assays and a critical assessment of what defines a positive value. An attempt to address the arbitrary method of determining a positive value for these tests has been made by using 2.5 multiples of the median, which would place a positive value at approximately the 95th percentile (Kutteh et al, 1994).

The chance for obtaining a false-positive result increases with the number of antigens and their isotypes tested. If one tests, for example, all seven antiphospholipid antibodies and all three of their respective isotypes, 21 determinations would be assessed. If one uses the 95th percentile to indicate a positive value, the likelihood that an independent test would be positive by chance alone would be $1 - (0.95)^{21}$ or 66%. Caution should be applied to interpreting values from different laboratories because of the lack of standardization and the methodological differences used to assign positive values. Until properly standardized assays are developed and a scientific rationale is established for their use, routine clinical assessment of autoantibodies other than lupus anticoagulant and the IgG and IgM isotypes of aCL and aPS should not be made except under specific study protocols. The costs of these tests should be borne neither by the couple seeking care nor by their third-party payors.

In addition to the autoantibodies mentioned previously, other immunologic tests that have been recommended historically, but that are of no clinical benefit, are listed in Box 16-6. Antinuclear antibody titers should not be obtained because these autoantibodies are heterogenous in the population and occur commonly and nonspecifically. Their presence is often transient, and their association with reproductive difficulty has been disproven (Eroglu et al, 1994). Other autoantibody associations with reproductive failure (reviewed in Geva et al, 1997) have not distinguished between cause and effect. These assays are robust with artifacts, rendering proper interpretation difficult. There are no scientific data, either in vitro or in vivo, indicating a potential mechanism of action for reproductive difficulty caused by these other autoantibodies.

There is also no substantive value in obtaining maternal antipaternal leukocyte antibodies by any method, including the leukocyte antibody detection assay (Stephenson et al, 1995). Antipaternal cytotoxic antibodies are rarely seen in women with successful reproductive histories before 28 weeks of gestation, and they may disappear between normal pregnancies (Regan et al, 1981). They are also absent in approximately 40% of women who have successful pregnancies (Amos and Kostyn, 1980). Therefore, if antipaternal cytotoxic antibodies are not formed in 40% of women who have successful pregnancies, how could their absence be a cause of pregnancy loss?

Similarly, obtaining mixed lymphocyte culture reactivities between maternal responder and paternal stimulator cells is unnecessary in couples with recurrent pregnancy loss because the blocking response of these uncharacterized serum factors was found to be the consequence rather than the cause of pregnancy success (Coulam, 1992).

Parental HLA profiles and their association with recurrent pregnancy loss, if parental HLA sharing occurred, received attention in the past. These retrospective reports were of limited sample size and were poorly controlled. Causal mechanisms for loss in cases of sharing were speculative at best. Sharing of HLA-DQA1 alleles between partners experiencing recurrent abortion has been reported in two studies (Christiansen et al, 1994; Steck et al, 1995). A significant deficit of HLA-DQA1-compatible liveborn offspring was observed in one study (Steck et al, 1995), suggesting that HLA-DQA1-compatible fetuses may be aborted early. In another study, Ober's laboratory was unable to find any association between HLA-DQA1 or HLA-DQB1 haplotypes and recurrent pregnancy loss because the distribution of haplotype frequencies did not differ between control subjects, couples with recurrent abortion, and their abortuses (Ober et al, 1993). Others (Takakuwa et al, 1992; Laitnen et al, 1993; Dizon-Townson et al, 1995; Wegenknecht et al, 1997) have confirmed that couples with reproductive failure do not have an increased frequency of HLADQ allele sharing over controls, indicating that HLADQ genotyping is not helpful in the clinical management of recurrent pregnancy loss.

In murine studies assessing embryotoxicity, human serum has been reported to be useful in predicting pregnancy outcome (Chaves and McIntyre, 1984). Immunologists have known since the 1970s that the use of human serum in assays involving murine embryos is not scientifically valid because of the presence of heterophilic antibodies in 40% of all human sera. Human serum complement is toxic to murine embryos, and appropriate collection is critical. The rubber-top vials used for the collection of human serum by laboratories advertising this test on the Internet are also toxic to murine embryos (Haimovici et al, 1989).

Although serum cannot be used to assess embryotoxicity, supernatants from lymphocytes and macrophages may be used. Peripheral blood mononuclear cell activation by cell-surface-expressed protein(s) from the human trophoblast cell line JEG-3 has been reported to stimulate Th1-type cytokine secretion in some women with recurrent pregnancy loss. Supernatants from these stimulated cultures contain IFN-γ that has been shown to be toxic to murine embryo development (Hill et al, 1992). This assay has been used clinically since 1986 at Brigham and Women's Hospital in more than 3000 women with histories of recurrent pregnancy loss. Modifications of this assay have been made that include a quantitative proliferation assay (Yamada et al, 1994) and an enzyme-linked immunosorbent assay in which INF-γ is measured in trophoblast-activated supernatants after subtracting background levels of IFN-γ from unstimulated samples (Hill et al, 1995a). This assay has been named the embryotoxic factor-lymphocyte (ETF-L) assay (Zonagen, Houston, Tex.). Depending on the individual series, Th1-type cytokines are produced in response to trophoblast stimulation in up to 25% of women with otherwise unexplained recurrent pregnancy loss. IFN-γ may also be produced in response to trophoblast stimulation in women with other presumed causes for loss and in fertile controls, but at significantly lower levels.

POSTCONCEPTION MONITORING

Close monitoring is advised once conception has occurred not only for the psychological well-being of the couple, but also to confirm an intrauterine pregnancy. The incidence of ectopic pregnancy in the 3000 couples evaluated in the Recurrent Pregnancy Loss Clinic at Brigham and Women's Hospital was 2.5%. Complete molar gestations have been observed in 5 of the 3000 women thus far. This is an unusually high occurrence of complete moles; the expected inci-

dence in the general U.S. population is 1 in 2000 pregnancies (Bagshawe, 1969). Therefore, recurrent pregnancy loss may be a risk factor for ectopic pregnancy and complete molar gestation. Concerns that women with recurrent pregnancy loss are also at increased risk for intrauterine growth restriction, premature labor and delivery, low-birth-weight neonate, and pregnancy-induced hypertension are not supported by our experience unless they also had the antiphospholipid syndrome.

The endocrinologic events associated with normal pregnancy and pregnancy ending in loss have been studied thoroughly. Gonadotropins and gonadal steroid levels have been reported to be higher in conception cycles than in cycles that do not result in conception. However, these same hormones have not been found to be significantly different between conception cycles that culminate in pregnancy loss and those that end in success (Stewart et al, 1993). Postconception levels of hCG are generally lower in pregnancies ending in early loss. This suggests that the enhanced gonadosteroid secretion noted in conception cycles may be caused by a gonadotropic stimulus from the preimplantation embryo and that embryos with defective postimplantation hCG secretion may have had this defect before implantation (Stewart et al, 1993).

Immunoreactive inhibin levels are not a prognostic indicator of pregnancy outcome, but subnormal hCG is a useful predictor of early pregnancy loss (France et al, 1996). Precisely when the β-subunit for hCG becomes detectable in maternal serum is unknown, but by the time implantation has occurred, β-hCG is detectable. Levels of β-hCG are expected to double every 48 hours for the first 10 weeks of pregnancy (reviewed in Laird and Whittaker, 1990). It is important to remember that this finding of doubling was based on a parametric curve, and an inadequate doubling time, though ominous, does not replace ultrasound monitoring. No hormonal determination predicts pregnancy outcome better than another after fetal heart activity is detected. Postconception LH levels have been compared to preconception levels, with postconception hypersecretion of LH associated more often with early loss (Regan et al, 1990).

In the normal population, once fetal cardiac activity has been detected by ultrasonography, the chance for subsequent delivery is approximately 95%. In women with a history of two or more pregnancy losses, the chance for viable birth after the detection of fetal cardiac activity by ultrasonography is approximately 77% (Laufer et al, 1994). Neither maternal age nor number of previous losses affected this finding. Embryonic heart rates below 90 beats per minute (bpm) at 6 to 8 weeks of gestation have been associated with subsequent loss. The boundary between slow and normal heart rates has not been established, but the lower limit of normal has been estimated at 100 bpm up to 6 weeks of gestation and 120 bpm at 6 to 7 weeks of gestation. This estimation was based on the findings of one series, in which all fetuses with heart rates below 100 bpm at 7 to 8 weeks of gestation died (Doubilet and Benson, 1995).

Doppler ultrasonography to assess the resistive index of the main uterine artery and the subchorionic vessels between 6 and 13 weeks of gestation does not predict pregnancy outcome because of the large overlap between aborted pregnancies and those that progress to viability. Failure to detect a fetal pole and fetal cardiac activity by 7 weeks of gestation is diagnostic for an aembryonic gestation (Pennell et al, 1991). A gestational sac larger than 15 mm or a crown-rump length that exceeds 5 mm without fetal cardiac activity is also diagnostic for an aembryonic pregnancy (Achiron et al, 1993). Even with well-timed intercourse and good dating, ultrasonographic findings may lag 4 to 9 days behind what the dates and timing would otherwise indicate. Such rare events suggest delayed implantation. Repeating the ultrasound examination in 1 week is necessary to distinguish this from true aembryonic pregnancy.

Thyroid function studies have been reported in pregnancy by some, but not all, investigators to be useful in monitoring pregnancy because of the characteristic thyroid profile that occurs in pregnancy, consisting of elevated serum thyroxin (T_4) and thyroxine-binding globulin with lower triiodothyronine resin uptake. Initially, the TSH level may rise before T_4 rises, but it remains in the normal range.

In women who have TPO antithyroid antibodies, monitoring of TSH during the first 8 weeks of pregnancy may be helpful. One percent of women who are TPO positive may not meet the increased demand and use of the thyroid in early pregnancy. These women are also at increased risk for postpartum, postabortal, or postectopic autoimmune thyroiditis (Marqusee et al, 1997). It is not necessary to repeat TPO testing during pregnancy, nor is it necessary to determine antithyroid antibody status using hemagglutination techniques because these have been reported to change during pregnancy, and they are not helpful for predicting subsequent pregnancy outcome (Amino et al, 1978).

Antiphospholipid antibody assessment during pregnancy has been reported to predict outcome. The incidence of antiphospholipid antibody production reportedly was significantly higher at the time of pregnancy termination in those who miscarried than in those who had viable deliveries (Kwak et al, 1994). The conclusion was that downregulation of antiphospholipid antibody production during early pregnancy is associated with a favorable pregnancy outcome (Kwak et al, 1994). An alternative explanation for their data was that low levels of autoantibodies and phospholipids at the time of miscarriage could represent the effect of fetal demise and not its cause. Unfortunately, the possibility that these data represented a transient epiphenomenon was not addressed because follow-up determinations were not performed in any of these women after loss.

Repeating antiphospholipid antibody tests in early pregnancy generally are not helpful in monitoring the pregnancies of women with the antiphospholipid syndrome or of any pregnant woman in whom they were measured before pregnancy.

Reports that NK cell activity could be used to predict pregnancy outcome (Makida et al, 1991; Aoki et al, 1995) led to the suggestion that assessing CD56 (NK cell phenotype), CD16 (Fc receptor, NK cell activation maker), and other immunophenotypes in peripheral blood could predict pregnancy outcomes in women with recurrent pregnancy loss (Coulam et al, 1995a; Kwak et al, 1995). In both reports, small numbers of women with recurrent pregnancy loss, 24 and 35, respectively, were studied. In a recent study performed at The Brigham and Women's Hospital, peripheral blood was obtained from 87 women with histories of recurrent spontaneous abortion (median, 4; range, 3 to 12 previous losses) for immunophenotyping at 6 to 9 weeks of gestation after fetal cardiac activity was documented by ultrasonography. Of these 87 women, 21 subsequently aborted spontaneously, yet there were no differences in the percentages of CD56+, CD16+, or other NK and T cell regulatory activation markers between women who aborted and those who had viable deliveries. When the 21 samples from women who aborted were analyzed with respect to abortal karyotypes (six aneuploid, eight euploid, and seven undetermined), again no significant differences in immunophenotypes could be discerned. Thus, assessment of immunophenotypes is not useful clinically in predicting pregnancy outcome in women with a history of recurrent spontaneous abortion.

Assessment of Th1, Th2, or adhesion molecules in the peripheral serum of pregnant women with a history of reproductive failure is also not useful in predicting subsequent pregnancy outcome (Schust and Hill, 1996). Reports that TNF-α and other inflammatory cytokines were useful (Shaarway and Najui, 1997) were based on results obtained from samples of women who had a diagnosis of inevitable or missed abortion at the time of sample collection. Finding inflammatory cytokines in the peripheral circulation at the time of an inevitable or a missed abortion should not be surprising because of the inflammatory response to fetal demise. Elevated inflammatory cytokines in the peripheral circulation most likely were the result of loss, not the cause.

Complement activation has been associated with pregnancy loss, and levels have been reported to fall before the loss of fetal viability (Tichenor et al, 1995). The clinical implications of this study remain unclear.

Assessment of Th1 immunity to trophoblast (the ETF-L assay) during pregnancy has been reported to be useful in predicting pregnancy outcome (Ecker et al, 1993). The proliferative response of peripheral blood leukocytes to the recall antigens influenza and tetanus, assessed at 6 weeks of gestation, has also been reported to predict pregnancy outcome; loss of responsiveness has been associated with subsequent pregnancy success (Bermas and Hill, 1997).

The clinical practice within the Center for Reproductive Medicine at Brigham and Women's Hospital monitors women with a history of recurrent pregnancy loss weekly or more frequently, if needed, measuring β-hCG level from the day of the missed period until it is between 1000 and 5000 mIU/mL. At that time, pelvic ultrasonography is recommended to confirm an intrauterine gestation, and blood sampling is discontinued unless the patient is part of a specific research study protocol. Ultrasonographic examination is recommended every 2 weeks in conjunction with a visit by a physician or a nurse, and it is continued every 2 weeks until that time during gestation when the patient has lost her previous pregnancies. This close monitoring is conducted for the psychological advantage it provides. Should fetal cardiac activity become absent, intervention can be recommended so that tissue for karyotype assessment may be obtained. For some couples, this level of monitoring is too stressful, and it must therefore be modified to meet each couple's needs. No other blood determinations are necessary once fetal cardiac activity has been identified ultrasonographically. Postconception serum progesterone levels are not useful clinically in the monitoring of early pregnancy because they are pulsatile and are lower than levels attained at the maternal-fetal interface. Preimplantation hormonal profiles also do not differ between pregnancies that end in early loss and those that proceed to viability (Baird et al, 1991). The only possible exception is that a low peripheral progesterone level may be useful in heightening the index of suspicion for an ectopic gestation. A progesterone level greater than 17.5 ng/mL (55.7 nmol/L) in a woman thought to be at risk for ectopic pregnancy may be followed up reasonably without further intervention (McCord et al, 1996).

Later in pregnancy, in addition to ultrasound monitoring, patient care should include the assessment of maternal serum α-fetoprotein levels. High values may indicate neural tube abnormalities, and low values may indicate fetal chromosome anomalies (Merkatz et al, 1984). An unexplained elevation of α-fetoprotein at 16 to 18 weeks of gestation is a risk factor for second-trimester fetal loss (Maher et al, 1984).

Fetal karyotype should be assessed not only in women older than 35 years of age (Hook et al, 1983), it should be considered for all women who have had recurrent pregnancy loss because they are more likely to have subsequent aneuploid pregnancy than are age-matched controls (Drugan et al, 1990). Therefore, recurrent pregnancy loss is a risk factor for subsequent aneuploidy.

Techniques for obtaining material suitable for fetal karyotype assessment include CVS and amniocentesis. Percutaneous umbilical cord blood sampling may be preferable if fetal hydrops is detected ultrasonographically so that the fetus can be evaluated for anemia (D'Alton et al, 1997). Ultrasonography has been reported to be useful for diagnosing aneuploidy (Benacerraf, 1989), but it does not replace direct karyotype assessment. In most instances, the higher complication rate of CVS compared with amniocentesis may be attributed to operator training and experience in performing this procedure. Both CVS and amniocentesis may be performed during the first trimester of pregnancy. However, the earlier the procedure is performed,

the higher the risk for spontaneous loss, which appears to be a variable of the number of attempts to obtain a sufficient sample (Jauniaux, 1997).

Conventional cytogenetic analysis of amniocytes, whether collected by CVS or amniocentesis, relies on metaphase assessment after 7 to 14 days of cell culture. The implementation of fluorescence in situ hybridization on uncultured amniocytes using chromosome-specific probes tagged with fluorochrome provides an adjunct to full metaphase karyotype assessment because results are available for specific aneuploidies within 48 hours of collection (Klinger et al, 1992).

Assessing the fetal karyotype after pregnancy loss is clinically useful and cost effective (Wolf and Harger, 1995). However, because of the high failure rate of fetal karyotyping after spontaneous expulsion or evacuation, consideration should be given to performing a pre-termination procedure, such as CVS, when fetal demise is confirmed (Kyle et al, 1996). In addition to genetic assessment, phenotypic and histologic analysis may be important for the predictive value they may have for future pregnancies and for providing the couple with an explanation for their loss. Morphologic assessment alone does not obviate the need for karyotyping. Neither decidual nor placental lesions are characteristic of an abnormal karyotype. Histologic assessment of abortus material has been used as evidence for the immunologic etiology for pregnancy loss (reviewed in Benirschke and Kaufmann, 1990), especially in cases of decidual vasculitis and massive chronic intervillositis. However, even definitive proof of the antiphospholipid syndrome, as evidenced by decidual vasculopathy and extensive placental infarction (DeWolf et al, 1982), remains elusive (Out et al, 1991). Cause-and-effect mechanisms cannot always be discerned because abnormal histologic findings may be the result of intrauterine fetal death and not necessarily its cause. More work is needed in well-characterized samples from women with and without recurrent pregnancy loss with known abortal karyotypes.

THERAPY

Despite numerous reports claiming efficacy, there is no definitive proof to support any of the therapies for recurrent pregnancy loss because properly designed studies have yet to be performed and published. Individual or committee "expert" opinions based on inadequately designed studies cannot substitute for data derived from a properly designed clinical trial. There are 12 study design criteria that should be fulfilled in a study of therapeutic efficacy for recurrent pregnancy loss (Box 16-7). Naturally, if one were assessing therapeutic efficacy for one of the presumed causes of recurrent pregnancy loss, exclusion of subjects without this presumed cause would be required. No study published to date has fulfilled these study design criteria. Thus, quality level 1 evidence does not exist for a definitive therapy for recurrent pregnancy loss.

BOX 16-7
CRITERIA FOR ASSESSING THERAPEUTIC EFFICACY FOR RECURRENT PREGNANCY LOSS

Scientifically sound rationale for using a particular therapy
Power calculation to ensure a sufficient number of study subjects using reasonable assumptions, such as 60% success without treatment and 80% success with therapy
Exclusion of study subjects with fewer than three unexplained clinical losses
Exclusion of study subjects with presumed causes for previous losses
Prospective study design
Prestratification of participants by age and number of previous losses because both are independent risk factors for subsequent loss
Effective randomization after prestratification
Placebo controlled
Double blind
No concomitant therapy
Karyotype assessment of subsequent losses
Follow-up observation to ensure safety

Modified from Hill JA: Immunology for recurrent pregnancy loss: 'Standard of care or buyer beware.' *J Soc Gynecol Invest* 1997; 4:267-273.

Chromosomal Factors

For the couple with an inborn chromosome abnormality in one or both partners, genetic counseling is warranted. Success is likely when fertilization is synchronized with conception, except when a Robertsonian translocation involving homologous chromosomes is involved. In such rare cases, either donor oocyte or donor sperm is indicated, depending on which partner has the Robertsonian translocation of homologous chromosomes, because the affected partner will always produce aneuploid gametes.

Anatomic Factors

Studies regarding the therapeutic benefits of surgical correction of müllerian anomalies for recurrent pregnancy loss are controversial largely because of inadequate study design and the problems inherent in retrospective studies. The design of studies indicating that surgery was of benefit (Heinonen, 1997) failed to address the problem of regression to the mean (Forrow et al, 1995). Other studies suggesting no benefit (Colacusci et al, 1996) lacked sufficient power to address this issue definitively. No significant difference in pregnancy rates was reported in one study after in vitro fertilization and embryo transfer in women with congenital uterine malformations. However, only five women with a type V (septate) uterus were included in that study (Marcus et al, 1996). None of the studies assessing pregnancy outcome after surgery corrected for the size of the intrauterine lesion in question. This may be important. A residual sep-

tum smaller than 1 cm after hysteroscopic resection has been reported to have had no influence on reproductive outcome compared with a residual septum larger than 1 cm (Fedele et al, 1996). The use of prophylactic antibiotics and postoperative hormonal therapy has been questioned for women undergoing hysteroscopic resection of intrauterine lesions. Postoperative estrogen supplementation, though controversial, may be of benefit after the resection of intrauterine adhesions, but they are probably unnecessary after metroplasty. When hormonal preparations are used, we use 2.5 mg conjugated estrogen daily for 30 days. During the last 10 days, an oral progestin (10 mg medroxyprogesterone) is added. Conception is attempted after withdrawal bleeding. Generally, concomitant laparoscopy is not performed because related complications, such as uterine perforation, develop in less than 1% of patients. If perforation inadvertently occurs, laparoscopy may be necessary to assess possible intraabdominal injury, and the couple is advised that conception be postponed for at least three cycles to allow healing of a uterine perforation.

Cervical cerclage has been recommended for women with recurrent pregnancy loss even in the absence of a typical history of incompetent cervix (Cromblehome et al, 1983) or in the presence of congenital müllerian anomalies (Abramovici et al, 1983). These retrospective studies failed to address the issue of regression to the mean. Cervical cerclage is not a benign procedure, and it should only be performed in patients with existing cervical incompetence or perhaps in patients with uterine anomalies caused by DES exposure (Barth, 1994).

Endocrine Factors

Luteal phase insufficiency has been treated with progesterone, hCG, ovulation induction, or a combination of all three. The efficacy of progesterone therapy for luteal phase insufficiency has not been substantiated because of the lack of uniform case definitions, the failure to control for regression to the mean, and the lack of randomized controlled trials of sufficient power to substantiate a conclusion (Karamardian and Grimes, 1992). Appropriate dosing and route of administration and when to initiate and discontinue progesterone therapy have not been standardized in studies addressing its use. Progesterone supplementation has been advocated (Soules et al, 1997) for luteal phase defects (3- to 4-day out-of-phase endometrial biopsy). Concerns about possible teratogenicity have limited the use of synthetic progestins. The natural 21-carbon molecule, progesterone, though not teratogenic, may have minor side effects in women who take it. Among the side effects are fatigue, fluid retention, and delayed menses. Progesterone may facilitate the growth of leiomyomata and may cause depression in some patients. The route of administration should be vaginal rather than intramuscular or oral. Higher progesterone levels are achieved locally within the uterus after vaginal administration (Miles et al, 1994) because of the direct transit to the uterus through a "first uterine pass effect" (Fanchin et al,

1997). Ideally, administration should begin before implantation but after ovulation (Jones, 1968).

Luteal function has also been stimulated by serial hCG injections. The efficacy of hCG for pregnancy loss was not substantiated in a placebo-controlled trial except for women with oligomenorrhea (Quenby and Farquharson, 1994).

Ovulation induction has been advocated for women with severe luteal phase insufficiency (endometrial biopsy more than 5 days out of phase) (Soules et al, 1997). Downregulation with GnRH agonists has been reported to reduce the rate of pregnancy loss in women with PCOS (Homburg et al, 1993). However, this finding was not substantiated in a randomized control trial of women who had pituitary suppression of LH followed by low-dose ovulation induction and luteal phase progesterone compared with women who had spontaneous ovulation followed by progesterone supplementation (Clifford, et al, 1996). It has been speculated that ovulation induction increases the chance for pregnancy loss from chromosome abnormalities (Boue and Boue, 1973; Racowsky and Kaufman, 1992).

The clinical practice at Brigham and Women's Hospital is to administer 50 mg progesterone vaginal suppositories twice a day beginning 3 days after the LH surge until 10 weeks of gestation if the endometrial biopsy is 3 to 4 days out of phase. If the endometrial biopsy is out of phase 5 days or more or if a patient has oligo-ovulation or PCOS, pituitary desensitization with GnRH agonist is initiated in the luteal phase of a preceding cycle and is followed by ovulation induction with recombinant FSH. Progesterone vaginal suppositories (50 mg twice a day) are begun 3 days after the ovulating dose of hCG is administered until 10 weeks of gestation. Additional studies are needed to substantiate the effectiveness of luteal phase support with or without ovulation induction for luteal phase insufficiency.

Laparoscopic ovarian diathermy has been reported to reduce the incidence of subsequent pregnancy loss in women with PCOS (Amar et al, 1993). Enthusiasm for this approach should be tempered until well-designed studies are performed.

Hypothyroidism should be treated with carefully titrated thyroid medication so that TSH remains in the euthyroid (normal) range. Hyperprolactinemia should be treated to maintain normal prolactin levels. There is no place in the modern medical management of recurrent pregnancy loss for thyroid supplementation or bromocriptine in the absence of hypothyroidism or hyperprolactinemia, respectively.

INFECTIONS

In patients with either *M. hominus* or *U. urealyticum,* treatment with 100 mg doxycycline twice a day was reported to enhance the viable pregnancy rate in comparison with untreated controls (Quin et al, 1983). Unfortunately, this study was neither randomized, double blind, nor placebo controlled, and it failed to correct for regression to the mean. This and other empiric antibiotic treatments have been given to couples with recurrent pregnancy loss. This practice is not warranted in the absence of identifiable infection. If an infectious organism is documented, appropriate antibiotic therapy should be considered for both partners, and post-treatment cultures should be taken to verify elimination of the infection. Appropriately designed clinical trials are needed to substantiate an infectious cause for recurrent pregnancy loss and to determine whether specific antibiotics are able to ameliorate subsequent pregnancy outcome.

Immunologic Factors
Antiphospholipid Syndrome

Because placental damage from thrombosis is thought to be the result of autoimmunity to phospholipids, therapeutic approaches have included prophylactic anticoagulation with aspirin and heparin (Farquharson et al, 1985; Branch et al, 1992; Kutteh, 1996; Rai et al, 1997). Corticosteroids (prednisone, prednisolone) have also been used (Lubba et al, 1983); Hasegawa et al, 1992; Passaleva et al, 1992; Many et al, 1992; Silver et al, 1993; Harger et al, 1995; Laskin et al, 1997), but the maternal side effects of corticosteroids limit their use. Heparin and aspirin have been reported to be more effective than aspirin and corticosteroids for the antiphospholipid syndrome (Lockshin et al, 1989; Cowchuck et al, 1992). Corticosteroids should never be used concomitantly with heparin because of the risk for osteoporosis with these agents. Low-molecular weight heparin may be better than unfractionated heparin because the risk for osteoporosis appears lower when once-a-day dosing is all that is required and it is no longer necessary to monitor coagulation parameters (Weitz, 1997). Heparin has also been reported to bind aCL in vitro, which may explain the decreased levels of aCL reported in women treated with it (Ermel et al, 1995).

Treatment of the antiphospholipid syndrome is not necessarily benign even with aspirin alone because thrombocytopenia may develop, as may subchorionic hematoma formation, which may lead to placental abruption and fetal death. Because placental abruption may occur in women with the antiphospholipid syndrome who do not undergo treatment, the relative risk caused by therapy is difficult to determine. Because of the inherent side effects of anticoagulation therapy even with aspirin alone, the empiric use of these therapies is not justified for women who do not have the antiphospholipid syndrome. Similarly, treating pregnant women with antiphospholipid antibodies of low titer or women who are otherwise at low risk for pregnancy loss, including those who are infertile or who are undergoing in vitro fertilization, cannot be justified (Cowchuck et al, 1997; Denis et al, 1997; Kutteh et al, 1997). Initiating heparin and aspirin before conception is potentially dangerous because of the risk for hemorrhage at the time of ovulation. Therapeutic recommendations include 81 mg aspirin per day followed by 10,000 to 20,000 U heparin per day administered subcutaneously in divided doses. Low-molecular-weight heparin appears to be an effective alternative for obstetric thromboprophylaxis (Nelson-Piercy et al, 1997). The Recurrent Pregnancy Loss

Table 16-1   Results of Prospective, Randomized, Double-Blind, Placebo-Controlled Trials of Leukocyte Immunization for Recurrent Abortion

	Paternal Cells Live Born/Total (%)	Autologous Cells or Saline Live Born/Total (%)
Mobray JF, et al (1985)	17/22 (73)	10/27 (37)
Ho HN, et al (1991)	31/22 (79)	32/47 (65)
Cauchi MN, et al (1991)	13/21 (62)	19/25 (70)
Gatenby PA, et al (1993)	13/19 (68)	9/19 (47)

Clinic at Brigham and Women's Hospital treats the antiphospholipid syndrome with 81 mg aspirin per day followed by either 2500 or 5000 U low-molecular-weight heparin (Fragmin) per day administered subcutaneously once pregnancy has been confirmed after the first missed period.

Other unsubstantiated approaches used to treat the antiphospholipid syndrome include plasmapheresis (Derksen et al, 1987; Ferro et al, 1989) and intravenous immunoglobulin (Scott et al, 1988; Marzusch et al, 1996). Plasmapheresis is no longer considered seriously because the only reports indicating efficacy were compromised by concomitant corticosteroid therapy (Frampton et al, 1987; Ferro et al, 1989), and plasmapheresis alone was not shown to be efficacious (Derksen et al, 1987). Using intravenous immunoglobulin to treat the antiphosphlipid syndrome was predicated on reports of efficacy in other autoimmune-related conditions.

Unfortunately, none of the studies addressing therapy for the antiphospholipid syndrome followed the clinical design criteria for garnering level 1 evidence as outlined in Box 16-7. These studies, though flawed, suggest that anticoagulant therapy is better than no treatment for the antiphospholipid syndrome (Rai et al, 1995; Lockshin, 1997).

Alloimmune Recurrent Pregnancy Loss

Therapy for alloimmune reproductive failure remains anecdotal because a well-designed clinical trial has not been conducted. There is considerable controversy not only on how to treat but on how to diagnose alloimmune recurrent pregnancy loss.

At Brigham and Women's Hospital, Th1 immunity to trophoblast is treated with immunosuppressive doses of progesterone vaginal suppositories (100 mg twice a day beginning 3 days after ovulation until 20 weeks of gestation). Progesterone has been called "nature's immunosuppressant" because concentrations attained at the maternal-fetal interface (10^{-5} mol/L) can inhibit macrophage phagocytosis, lymphocyte proliferation, NK cell function, and cytotoxic T-cell activity (Siiteri et al, 1977). In women with evidence of Th1 immunity to trophoblast (a positive ETF-L assay), progesterone can inhibit Th1 cytokine release and embryotoxic factor production in vitro. How this information can be incorporated clinically awaits testing in a well-designed clinical trial of women with evidence of Th1 immunity to trophoblast.

Even though the hypothesis that blocking antibodies are necessary for successful pregnancy has been disproven, the alloimmunotherapies originally proposed for this continue to be advertised. These alloimmunotherapies include active immunization with either third-party or paternal allogeneic peripheral blood mononuclear cells (leukocytes) and passive immunization with intravenous immunoglobulin (IVIG).

Third-party leukocyte immunization (Taylor and Faulk, 1981) was based on observations that renal allograft rejection could be delayed by third-party blood transfusions (reviewed in Klein, 1994). Paternal leukocyte immunization (Beer et al, 1985) was based on the hypothesis that maternal blocking antibodies were necessary for successful pregnancy (Rocklin et al, 1976). Many anecdotal case series and inadequately designed trials have been published concerning leukocyte immunization (Table 16-1) (Taylor and Faulk, 1981; Beer et al, 1985; Mowbray et al, 1985; Smith and Cowchuck, 1988; Carp et al, 1990; Cauchi et al, 1991; Ho et al, 1991; Gatenby et al, 1993; Christiansen et al, 1993). Meta-analyses (Fraser et al, 1993; The Recurrent Miscarriage Immunotherapy Trialists Group, 1994) and reviews of these analyses (Jeng et al, 1995; Coulam et al, 1996; Hill, 1996; Scott, 1994; Kutteh et al, 1997) have also been published. The efficacy of leukocyte immunization remains speculative at best, and, according to the most recent review (Kutteh et al, 1997) using the 95% confidence intervals from the largest meta-analysis to date (The Recurrent Miscarriage Immunotherapy Trialists Group, 1994), as few as four to as many as 167 women would have to receive leukocyte immunization to achieve one additional live birth.

Adverse side effects caused by leukocyte immunization, which occur in 1 of 50 treated women (The Recurrent Miscarriage Immunotherapy Trialists Group, 1994), are a matter of concern because they may endanger the lives of the mother and her baby. These adverse effects include transfusion reactions, autoimmunity, erythrocyte and platelet sensitization, difficulty in obtaining donor organs should they be needed, infections, intrauterine growth restriction, graft-versus-host disease, and thrombocytopenia leading to neonatal death (Hill and Andersen, 1986; Katz et al, 1992; Kutteh et al, 1997).

As a result of the adverse publicity leukocyte immunization therapy has received (unsubstantiated efficacy, potential for adverse side effects), immunotherapists have advocated IVIG because it has myriad immunomodulating effects (reviewed in Dwyer, 1992). However, studies on the efficacy of IVIG for recurrent pregnancy loss have reported conflicting findings (Mueller-Eckhart et al, 1989; Coulam et al, 1990; Mueller-Eckhardt et al, 1991; Heine and Muller-Eckhardt, 1994; Christiansen et al, 1995; The German RSA/IVIG

Group, 1994; Coulam et al, 1995b; Carp et al, 1996; Kiprov et al, 1996; Perino et al, 1997). Meta-analyses of these studies indicate that IVIG is not efficacious for treating unexplained recurrent pregnancy loss because the 95% confidence interval crosses 1.0 (Clark and Daya, 1998). All these studies have lacked sufficient power to allow a definitive conclusion. None was prestratified according to maternal age or to number of previous losses before randomization. Many lacked proper randomization or were not placebo controlled. Thus, regression to the mean could not be addressed. Few excluded patients with only one or two previous losses, and few corrected for concomitant therapy. Dosage regimens and time frames for therapy had not been standardized. Odds ratios and 95% confidence intervals of the five trials to date and meta-analyses of them do not suggest efficacy. In the United States the cost of IVIG therapy is between $7,000 and $14,000. Nonetheless, the popularity of this therapy has grown to such an extent that a worldwide shortage exists for this blood product, creating difficulty for patients with immunodeficiency who depend on IVIG for survival. Hypotension, nausea, and headache are common adverse side effects. Potentially life-threatening anaphylaxis may develop in IgA-deficient patients (Thornton and Bellow, 1993). Long-term effects of this therapy for pregnant women are unknown. There remains a remote, but realistic, possibility of piron infection, which causes Creutzfeldt-Jakob disease and mad cow disease, because blood from approximately 150 donors is needed to produce one vial of IVIG.

In the future, rapid advances in molecular immunology and transplantation biology will enable novel immunotherapeutic strategies. These strategies may include antigen-based immunointervention and costimulation or tolerance-induction therapies, such as treatment with immune cells, cytokine-growth factors, anticytokines, soluble cytokine receptors, and receptor antagonists. Characterization of the inciting antigen or antigens will be necessary before these strategies can be realized. The development of animal models is prerequisite before translational testing in women. Additional work will be needed to determine adverse side effects and long-term safety issues before any of these strategies can be implemented in appropriately designed clinical trials.

Other Therapeutic Considerations

In vitro fertilization (IVF) and embryo transfer (ET) after ovulation induction with GnRH agonists and gonadotropins has been reported to be useful in treating women with unexplained recurrent spontaneous abortion (Balasch et al, 1996). However, this small (n = 12) observational study was neither randomized nor properly controlled. This study also failed to correct for regression to the mean. In a larger study, 20 couples with unexplained recurrent spontaneous abortion and secondary infertility were subjected to 42 IVF-ET cycles (Raziel et al, 1997). The subsequent reproductive outcomes of these couples were compared with that of cou-

ples who did not have a history of recurrent pregnancy loss. Ages and indications for IVF other than pregnancy loss were similar between groups, as were pregnancy rates (32% and 29% per cycle, respectively). However, the subsequent miscarriage rate was 50% in women with a history of recurrent pregnancy loss, indicating that IVF-ET is not beneficial for recurrent pregnancy loss (Raziel et al, 1997). These data should not be surprising because there are no morphologic criteria for identifying chromosomally normal oocytes and embryos.

Oocyte donation has been reported to be efficacious in treating recurrent pregnancy loss (Remohi et al, 1996). Eight couples with a history of recurrent pregnancy loss were compared to women having donor oocytes due to a low response to gonadotropin stimulation. Each group underwent 12 oocyte donation cycles. Clinical pregnancy and delivery rates per cycle were 75% and 66%, respectively. The delivery rate per patient was approximately 86%, whereas the miscarriage rate was only 11%. The authors suggested that the oocyte may be the origin of reproductive difficulty in these women and questioned the role of other maternal and paternal factors (Remohi et al, 1996). Oocyte donation may obviate chromosome abnormalities that result from advanced maternal age.

An alternative to oocyte donation for women who have adequate ovarian reserve could be IVF, so that preimplantation genetic diagnosis could be performed before ET. It appears that chromosome abnormalities in the abortus are the most common cause of spontaneous abortion (Boue and Boue, 1975), even in women with recurrent pregnancy loss (Rodriguez-Thompson et al, 1999). This is largely an age-related phenomenon because oocytes, and thus embryos, in older women are more likely to be chromosomally abnormal (Battaglia et al, 1996).

Fluorescence in situ hybridization with fluochrome-labeled, chromosome-specific probes that produce different color signals for as many as five chromosomes tested allows numerical chromosome analysis on blastomere biopsy specimens from preimplantation embryos (Munne et al, 1993). Another technique, called comparative genomic hybridization, may one day enable preimplantation genetic diagnosis of all chromosomes on a single blastomere (Reubinoff and Shusan, 1996). Other genetic approaches may include spectral karyotyping of a cell in metaphase arrest or polar body analysis. Genetic analysis of the first polar body would be expected to reveal aneuploides caused by nondisjunction during the first meiotic division. Errors in the second meiotic division, such as trisomy 18, would be revealed through genetic analysis of the second polar body. Polar body analysis, however, does not allow for the detection of aneuploidies that may be derived paternally or after fertilization (Verlinsky et al, 1996). Preimplantation genetic diagnosis has not been used routinely in the treatment of recurrent pregnancy loss primarily because it may entail problems related to mosaicism and because the approach is experimental and its benefits are undocumented.

There is a significant spontaneous pregnancy success rate in couples with recurrent pregnancy loss. This may be enhanced by synchronizing intercourse with ovulation and by providing formalized supportive care (Stray-Pedersen and Stray-Pedersen, 1984; Liddell et al, 1991). Different centers have different success rates even when they use the same intervention therapy and control for maternal age and number of previous losses (Cauci et al, 1995). The emotional care associated with the administration of a placebo can indirectly facilitate successful pregnancy (Perino et al, 1997). This suggests that providing supportive care during early pregnancy may benefit the clinical outcome.

A physician's caring, empathetic attitude is fundamental to healing. Adoption of this attitude by the entire health care team for couples experiencing recurrent pregnancy loss is important. The health care team may bring catharsis to these couples by acknowledging their pain and suffering. Their empathy may help each couple move beyond the stress they feel within themselves, within their relationships, and with friends and family and enable them to incorporate their losses into their lives rather than their lives into their losses. Couples can be encouraged to participate in support groups and to turn to other self-help measures such as adequate diet, meditation, yoga, or exercise. Referrals to behavioral medicine specialists, psychologists, psychiatrists, and licensed social workers who have an interest in the problems they encounter may also be of benefit. These approaches, along with "alternative healing" practices, warrant study in appropriately designed clinical trials.

PROGNOSIS

For couples with recurrent pregnancy loss, the possibility of achieving a successful pregnancy is high. Success depends on maternal age and number of previous losses. The cause of pregnancy loss and intervention therapy may affect the prognosis. Supportive care without pharmacologic or surgical intervention has been shown to benefit pregnancy outcome (Clifford et al, 1997). The probability for viable birth after ultrasound detection of fetal cardiac activity at 5 to 6 weeks from the last menses is approximately 77% (Laufer et al, 1994).

CONCLUSION

Recurrent pregnancy loss is emotionally frustrating for couples and is often a frustrating challenge for their physicians. This often results in the recommendation of unsubstantiated tests and therapies of dubious efficacy. Understanding the potential mechanisms involved in recurrent pregnancy loss and imparting a caring, empathetic attitude toward couples experiencing loss will ameliorate the emotional distress they face and will facilitate a rational, cost-effective assessment that leads to appropriate consultation and ultimately to effective therapy.

REFERENCES

Aberg A, Rydhstrom H, Dallen B, et al: Impaired glucose tolerance during pregnancy is associated with increased fetal mortality in preceding SIDS. *Acta Obstet Gynecol Scand* 1997; 76:212-217.

Abramovici H, Faktor JH, Pascal B: Congenital uterine malformations as indication for cervical suture (cerclage) in habitual abortion and premature delivery. *Int J Fertil* 1983; 28:161-164.

Achiron R, Goldenberg M, Lipitz S, et al: Transvaginal duplex Doppler ultrasonography in bleeding patients suggested of having residual trophoblastic tissue. *Obstet Gynecol* 1993; 81:507-511.

Acien P: Reproductive performance of women with uterine malformations. *Hum Reprod* 1993; 8:122-126.

Adam Z, Poulin F, Papp Z: Increased risk of neural tube defects after recurrent pregnancy losses. *Am J Med Genet* 1995; 55:512-516.

Adler RR, NG Ak, Rote NS: Monoclonal antiphosphatidylserine antibody inhibits intercellular fusion of the choriocarcinoma cell line JAR. Biol Reprod 1995; 53:905-910.

Ailus K, Tulpella M, Palosuot, et al: Antibodies to beta 2-glycoprotein-I and prothrombin in habitual abortion. *Fertil Steril* 1996; 66:937-941.

Alberman E: The epidemiology of repeated abortion. In Beard RW, Bishop F, editors: *Early pregnancy loss: Mechanisms and treatment*, New York, 1988, Springer Verlag.

Amar NA, Rachelin GC: Laparoscopic ovarian diathermy: An effective treatment for antiestrogen resistant anovulatory infertility in women with the polycystic ovary syndrome. *Br J Obstet Gynecol* 1993; 100:161-164.

Amino N, Kwo R, Tanizawa O, et al: Changes of serum antithyroid antibodies during and after pregnancy in autoimmune thyroid diseases. *Clin Exp Immunol* 1978; 31:30-37.

Amos DB, Kostyn DD: HLA: A central immunologic agency of man. *Adv Hum Genet* 1980; 10:137-141.

Angeles-Caro E, Sultan Y, Clauvel JP: Predisposing factors to thrombosis in systemic lupus erythematosus: Possible relation to endothelial cell damage. *J Lab Clin Med* 1979; 92:313-323.

Aohi K, Kajura S, Metsmob Y, et al: Portconceptual natural killer cell activity as a predictor of miscarriage. *Lancet* 1995; 345:1340-1342.

Aoki K, Dudkiewicz AB, Matsuura E, et al: Clinical significance of β_2-glycoprotein-1 dependent cardiolipin antibodies in the reproductive autoimmune failure syndrome: Correlation with conventional antiphospholipid antibody detection systems. *Am J Obstet Gynecol* 1995; 172:926-931.

Arck PC, Merali FS, Stanisz AM, et al: Stress-induced murine abortion associated with substance P-dependent alteration in cytokines in maternal uterine decidua. *Biol Reprod* 1995; 53:814-819.

Ault KA, Taufik OW, Smith-King MM, et al: Tumor necrosis factor-α response to infection with *Chlamydia trachomatis* in human fallopian tube organ culture. *Am J Obstet Gynecol* 1996; 175:1242-1245.

Azuma K, Calderon I, Besanko M, et al: Is the luteo-placental shift a myth? Analysis of low progesterone levels in successful ART pregnancies. *J Clin Endocrinol Metab* 1993; 77:195-198.

Babalioglu R, Varol FG, Ilhan R, et al: Progesterone profiles in luteal-phase defects associated with recurrent spontaneous abortions. *J Assist Reprod Genet* 1996; 13:306-309.

Baird DD, Weinberg CR, Wilcox AJ, et al: Hormonal profiles of natural conception cycle ending in unrecognized pregnancy loss. *J Clin Endocrinol Metab* 1991; 72:793-800.

Balasch J, Crews M, Fabreques F, et al: Antiphospholipid antibodies and human reproductive failure. *Hum Reprod* 1996; 11:2310-2315.

Balen AH, Tan SL, Jacobs HS: Hypersecretion of luteinizing hormones: A significant case of infertility and miscarriage. *Br J Obstet Gynaecol* 1993; 100:1082-1089.

Barnea ER, Kaplan M: Spontaneous, gonadotropin releasing hormone induced and progesterone inhibited pulsatile trimester placenta in vitro. *J Clin Endocrinol Metab* 1989; 69:215-217.

Barth WH Jr: Cervical incompetence and cerclage: Unresolved controversies. *Clin Obstet Gynecol* 1994; 37:831-841.

Battaglia DE, Goodwin P, Klein NA, et al: Influence of maternal age on meiotic spindle assembly in oocytes from naturally cycling women. *Hum Reprod* 1996; 11:2217-2222.

Becks GP, Burrow GN: Diagnosis and treatment of thyroid disease during pregnancy. In DeGroot LJ, editor: ed 3, Philadelphia, 1995, WB Saunders.

Beer AE, Semprini AE, Zho XY, et al: Pregnancy outcome in human couples with recurrent spontaneous abortions: HLA antigen profiles, HLA antigen sharing, female MLR blocking factors, and paternal leukocyte immunization. *Exp Clin Immunogenet* 1985; 2:137-153.

Benacerraf BR: The use of sonography for the antenatal detection of aneuploidy. *Clin Diag Ultrasound* 1989; 25:21-54.

Benirschke K, Kaufmann P: Abortion, placentas of trisomies and immunological considerations of recurrent reproductive failure. In *Pathology of the human placenta*, K. Benirschke, Ed. New York, 1990, Springer Verlag.

Berkowitz RS, Hill JA, Kurtz CB, et al: Effects of products of activated leukocytes (lymphokines and monokines) on the growth of malignant trophoblast cells in vitro. *Am J Obstet Gynecol* 1988; 158:199-203.

Berman SM, MacKay HT, Grimes DA, et al: Deaths from spontaneous abortion in the United States. *JAMA* 1985;n253:3110-3123.

Bermas BL, Hill JA: Proliferative responses to recall antigens are associated with pregnancy outcome in women with a history of recurrent spontaneous abortion. *J Clin Invest* 1997; 100:1330-1334.

Bermas BL, Petri M, Goldman D, et al: T helper cell dysfunction in systemic lupus erythematosus (SLE): Relation to disease activity. *J Clin Immunol* 1994; 14:169-177.

Bonney RC, Franks S: The endocrinology of implantation and early pregnancy. *Bailliere's Clin Endocrinol Metab* 1990; 4:207-301.

Boue J, Boue A: Increased frequency of chromosomal anomalies in abortions after induced ovulation. *Lancet* 1973; 7804:679-680.

Boue J, Boue A, Laser P: Retrospective and prospective epidemiologic studies of 1,500 karyotyped spontaneous abortions. *Teratology* 1975; 11:11-26.

Branch DW, Silver RM, Blackwell JL, et al: Outcome of treated pregnancies in women with antiphospholipid syndrome: An update of the Utah experience. *Obstet Gynecol* 1992; 80:614-620.

Branch DW, Silver R, Dierangeli S, et al: Antiphospholipid antibodies other than lupus anticoagulant and anticardiolipin antibodies in women with recurrent pregnancy loss, fertile controls, and antiphospholipid syndrome. *Obstet Gynecol* 1997; 89:549-555.

Bussen S, Steck T: Thyroid autoantibodies in euthryoid nonpregnant women with recurrent spontaneous abortus. *Hum Reprod* 1995; 10:2938-2940.

Buttram VC Jr: Mullerian anomalies and their management. *Fertil Steril* 1983; 40:159-163.

Buttram VC Jr, Gibbons WE: Mullerian anomalies: A proposed classification (an analysis of 144 cases). *Fertil Steril* 1979; 32:40-46.

Carp HJ, Ahirm R, Mashiach S, et al: Intravenous immunoglobulin in women with five or more abortions. *Am J Reprod Immunol* 1996; 35:360-362.

Carp HJ, Toder V, Bzait E, et al: Immunization by paternal leukocytes for prevention of primary habitual abortion: Results of a matched control trial. *Gynecol Obstet Invest* 1990; 29:16-21.

Carreras LO, Vernylan JG: Lupus anticoagulant and thrombosis: Possible role of inhibition of prostacyclin formation. *Thromb Haemost* 1982; 48:38-40.

Cauci MN, Coulam CB, Cowchuck S, et al: Predictive factors in recurrent spontaneous aborters—a multicenter study. *Am J Reprod Immunol* 1995; 33:165-170.

Cauci MN, Lim D, Kloss YM, et al: The treatment of recurrent abortion by immunization with paternal cells: Controlled trials. *Am J Reprod Immunol* 1991; 25:16-17.

Cauci S, Scrimin F, Priussi S, et al: Specific immune response against *Gardnerella vaginalis* hemolysin in patients with bacterial vaginosis. *Am J Obstet Gynecol* 1996; 175:1601-1605.

Cavallo F, Russo R, Zotti C, et al: Moderate alcohol consumption and spontaneous abortion. *Alcohol* 1995; 30:195-201.

Cecere FA, Persellin RH: The interaction of pregnancy and the rheumatic diseases. *Clin Rheum Dis* 1981; 7:747-748.

Chavez DJ, McIntyre JA: Sera from women with histories of repeated pregnancy losses cause abnormalities in mouse periimplantation blastocyst. *J Reprod Immunol* 1984; 6:273-281.

Christiansen OB: A fresh look at the causes of treatments of recurrent miscarriage, especially its immunologic aspects. *Hum Reprod* 1996; 2:271-293.

Christiansen OB, Mathiesen O, Husth M, et al: Placebo controlled trials of active immunization with third-party leukocytes in recurrent miscarriage. *Acta Obstet Gynecol Scand* 1993; 72:1-8.

Christiansen OB, Mathiensen O, Husth M, et al: Placebo-controlled trial of treatment of unexplained secondary recurrent spontaneous abortions and recurrent late spontaneous abortions with IVF immunoglobulin. *Hum Reprod* 1995; 10:2690-2695.

Christiansen OB, Rasmussen KL, Jersild C, et al: HLA class II alleles confer susceptibility to recurrent fetal loss in Danish women. *Tissue Antigens* 1994; 44:225-233.

Clark DA, Daya S: Is there hope for IVIG? *Am J Reprod Immunol* 1998; 39:65-68.

Clifford K, Rai R, Regan L: Future pregnancy outcome in unexplained recurrent first trimester miscarriage. *Hum Reprod* 1997; 12:387-389.

Clifford K, Rai R, Watson H, et al: Does suppressing luteinizing hormone secretion reduce the miscarriage rate? Results of a randomized controlled trial. *BMJ* 1996; 312:1508-1511.

Clifford K, Rai R, Watson H, Regan L: An informative protocol for the investigation of recurrent miscarriage: Preliminary experience of 500 consecutive cases. *Hum Reprod* 1994; 9:1328-1332.

Colacusci N, DePlacido G, Mollo A, et al: Reproductive outcome after hysteroscopic metroplasty. *Eur J Obstet Gynecol Reprod Biol* 1996; 66:147-150.

Connor JM, Ferguson-Smith MA: *Essential medical genetics,* Oxford, 1987, Blackwell Scientific.

Copper RL, Goldenberg RL, Das A, et al: The preterm prediction study: Maternal stress is associated with spontaneous preterm birth at less than thirty-five weeks' gestation. *Am J Obstet Gynecol* 1996; 175:1286-1292.

Coulam CB: Immunological tests in the evaluation of reproductive disorders: A critical review. *Am J Obstet Gynecol* 1992; 167:1844-1851.

Coulam CB, Goodman C, Roussev RG, et al: Systemic CD56 and cells can predict pregnancy outcome. *Am J Reprod Immunol* 1995a; 33:40-46.

Coulam CB, Krysa L, Stern JJ, et al: Intravenous immunoglobulin for treatment of recurrent pregnancy loss. *Am J Reprod Immunol* 1995b; 34:333-337.

Coulam CB, Peters AJ, McIntyre JA, et al: The use of intravenous immunoglobulins for the treatment of recurrent spontaneous abortion. *Am J Reprod Immunol* 1990; 22:78-82.

Coulam CB, Stephenson M, Stern JJ, et al: Immunotherapy for recurrent pregnancy loss: Analysis of results from clinical trials. *Am J Reprod Immunol* 1996; 35:352-359.

Cowchuck FS, Fort JG: Can tests for IgA, IgG or IgM antibodies to cardiolipin or phosphatidyl serine substitute for lupus anticoagulant assays in screening for antiphospholipid antibodies? *Autoimmunity* 1994; 17:119-122.

Cowchuck FS, Reece EA, Balandan D, et al: Repeated fetal losses associated with antiphospholipid antibodies: A collaborative randomized trial comparing prednisone with low dose heparin treatment. *Am J Obstet Gynecol* 1992; 166:1318-1323.

Cowchuck S, Reece EA for the Organizing Group of the Antiphospholipid Antibody Treatment Trial: Do low-risk pregnant women with antiphospholipid antibodies need to be treated? *Am J Obstet Gynecol* 1997; 176:1099-1110.

Cromblehome WR, Minkoff HL, Delke I, et al: Cervical cerclage: An aggressive approach to threatened or recurrent pregnancy wastage. *Am J Obstet Gynecol* 1983; 146:168-174.

Csapo AI, Pulkkinen MO, Ruttner B, et al: The significance of the corpus luteum in pregnancy maintenance, I: Preliminary studies. *Am J Obstet Gynecol* 1972; 112:1061-1065.

Csapo AI, Pulkkinen MO, Wiest WG: Effects of lutectomy and progesterone replacement therapy in early pregnancy patients. *Am J Obstet Gynecol* 1973; 15:759-763.

Daling JR, Emanuel I: Induced abortion and subsequent outcome of pregnancy in a series of American women. *N Engl J Med* 1977; 97:1241-1245.

D'Alton ME, Malone FD, Chelmow D et al: Defining the role of fluorescence in situ hybridization on uncultured amniocytes for prenatal diagnosis of aneuploides. *Am J Obstet Gynecol* 1997; 176:769-776.

Davis OK, Berkeley AS, Naus GJ, et al: The incidence of luteal phase defect in normal fertile women, determined by serial endometrial biopsies. *Fertil Steril* 1989; 51:582-586.

Denis AL, Guido M, Adler RD, et al: Antiphospholipid antibodies and pregnancy rates and outcome in in vitro fertilization patients. *Fertil Steril* 1997; 67:1084-1090.

Derksen RHWM, Hasselaar P, Blokzijl L, et al: Lack of efficacy of plasma-exchange in removing antiphospholipid antibodies. *Lancet* 1987; 2:222-223.

DeWolf F, Carreras LO, Moerman P, et al: Decidual vasculopathy and extensive placental infarction in a patient with repeated thromboembolic accidents, recurrent loss and a lupus anticoagulant. *Am J Obstet Gynecol* 1982; 42:829-834.

Dizon-Townson DS, Meline L, Nelson LM, et al: Fetal carriers of the factor V Leiden mutation are prone to miscarriage and placental infarction. *Am J Obstet Gynecol* 1997; 177:402-405.

Dizon-Townson D, Nelson L, Scott Jr, et al: Human leukocyte antigens DQ alpha sharing is not increased in couples with recurrent miscarriage. *Am J Reprod Immunol* 1995; 34:209-212.

Dlugosz L, Brachen MB: Reproductive effects of caffeine: A review and theoretical analysis. *Epidemiol Rev* 1992; 4:83-100.

Doss BJ, Greene MF, Hill JA, et al: Massive chronic intervillositis associated with recurrent abortions. *Hum Pathol* 1995; 26:1245-1251.

Doubilet PM, Benson CB: Embryonic heart rate in the early first trimester: What rate is normal? *J Ultrasound Med* 1995; 14:431-434.

Drugan A, Boltums SF, Johnson MP, et al: Seasonal variation in conception does not appear to influence the rates of prenatal diagnosis of nondisjunction. *Fetal Diagn Ther* 1989; 4:195-199.

Drugan A, Koppitch FC III, Williams JC III, et al: Prenatal genetic diagnosis following recurrent early pregnancy loss. *Obstet Gynecol* 1990; 75:381-384.

Dudley DJ, Collmer D, Mitchell MD, et al: Inflammatory cytokine mRNA in human gestational tissues: Implications for term and preterm labor. *J Soc Gynecol Invest* 1996; 3:328-335.

Dudley DJ, Edwin SS, Van Wagoner J, et al: Regulation of decidual cell chemokine production by group B streptococci and purified bacterial wall components. *Am J Obstet Gynecol* 1997; 177:666-672.

Dudley DJ, Mitchell MD, Branch DW: Pathophysiology of antiphospholipid antibodies: Absence of prostaglandin-mediated effects on cultured endothelium. *Am J Obstet Gynecol* 1990; 162:953-959.

Dwyer JM: Manipulating the immune system with immune globulin. *N Engl J Med* 1992; 326:107-116.

Ecker JL, Laufer MR, Hill JA: Measurement of embryotoxic factors is predictive of pregnancy outcome in women with a history of recurrent spontaneous abortion. *Obstet Gynecol* 1993; 81:84-87.

Edmonds DK, Lindsay KS, Miller JF, et al: Early embryonic mortality in women. *Fertil Steril* 1982; 38:447-453.

Ermel LD, Marshburn PB, Kutteh WH: Interactin of heparin with antiphospholipid antibodies from the sera of women with recurrent pregnancy loss. *Am J Reprod Immunol* 1995; 33:14-20.

Eroglu GE, Scopeliltis E: Antinuclear and antiphospholipid antibodies in healthy women with recurrent spontaneous abortion. *Am J Reprod Immunol* 1994; 31:1-6.

Fanchin R, DeZiegler D, Bergeron C, et al: Transvaginal administration of progesterone. *Obstet Gynecol* 1997; 90:396-401.

Farquharson R, Blown A, Compton A: The lupus anticoagulalant: A plan for pregnancy treatment? *Lancet* 1985; ii:842-843.

Fedele L, Bianchi S, Marchini M, et al: Residual uterine septum of less than 1 cm after hysteroscopic metroplasty does not impair reproductive outcome. *Hum Reprod* 1996; 11:727-729.

Ferguson DM, Horwood LJ, Shannon FT: Smoking during pregnancy. *N Z Med J* 1979; 89:41-43.

Ferro D, Quintervelli C, Russe G, et al: Successful removal of antiphospholipid antibodies using repeated plasma exchanges and prednisone. *Clin Exp Rheumatol* 1989; 2:1023-1027.

Fielding JR: MR imaging of mullerian anomalies: Impact on therapy. *Am J Roentgenol* 1996; 167:1491-1495.

Fitzsimmons J, Stahl R, Gocial B, et al: Spontaneous abortion in women with endometriosis. *Fertil Steril* 1987;47:696-700.

Frampton G, Cameron JS, Thom M, et al: Successful removal of antiphospholipid antibody during pregnancy using plasma exchange and low-dose prednisone. *Lancet* 1987;2:1023-1027.

France JT, Keelan J, Sang L et al: Serum concentrations of human chorionic gonadotropin and immunoreactive inhibin in early pregnancy and recurrent miscarriage: A longitudinal study. *Aust N Z J Obstet Gynaecol* 1996; 36:325-330.

Fraser EJ, Grimes DA, Schultz KF: Immunization as therapy for recurrent spontaneous abortion: A review and meta-analysis. *Obstet Gynecol* 1993; 82:854-859.

Gabbe SG, Turner LP: Reproductive hazards of the American lifestyle: Work during pregnancy. *Am J Obstet Gynecol* 1997; 176:826-832.

Garcia JE, Tran T, Smith RD, et al: Relationship of endometriosis staging and in vitro fertilization outcome. *Hum Reprod* 1991; 6:74-75.

Gardiner A, Clarke C, Coven J, et al: Spontaneous abortion and fetal anomaly in subsequent pregnancy. *BMJ* 1978; 1:1056-1060.

Gatenby PA, Cameron K, Simes RJ, et al: Treatment of recurrent spontaneous abortion by immunization with paternal lymphocytes: Results of a controlled trial. *Am J Reprod Immunol* 1993; 29:88-94.

The German RSA/IVIG Group: Intravenous immunoglobulin in the prevention of recurrent miscarriage. *Br J Obstet Gynaecol* 1994; 101:1072-1077.

Geva E, Amit A, Lerner-Gera L, et al: Autoimmunity and reproduction. *Fertil Steril* 1997; 67:599-611.

Gibbs RS: Chorioamnionitis and bacterial vaginosis. *Am J Obstet Gynecol* 1993; 169:460-462.

Gilnoer D, Sato MF, Bourdeaux P, et al: Pregnancy in patients with mid thyroid abnormalities: Maternal and neonatal repercussion. *J Clin Endocrinol Metab* 1991; 73:421-427.

Gleicher N, El-Roiey A, Confino E, et al: Reproductive failure because of autoantibodies unexplained infertility and pregnancy wastage. *Am J Obstet Gynecol* 1989; 160:1376-1385.

Golan A, Halperin R, Herman A, et al: Human decidua-associated protein 200 levels in uterine fluid at hysteroscopy. *Gynecol Obstet Invest* 1994; 38:217-219.

Golard R, Jozak S, Warren W, et al: Elevated levels of umbilical cord anticotropin releasing hormone in growth retarded fetuses. *J Clin Endocrinol Metab* 1993; 77:1174-1179.

Golbus MJ: Chromosome aberrations and mammalian reproduction. In Mastroianni L, Biggers J, Sadler W, editors, *Fertilization and embryonic development in vitro*, New York, 1981, Plenum Press.

Green LK, Harris RE: Uterine anomalies: Frequency of diagnosis and obstetric complications. *Obstet Gynecol* 1976; 47:427-429.

Gris JC, Schred JF, Neven S, et al: Impaired fibrinolytic capacity and early recurrent spontaneous abortions. *BMJ* 1990; 300:1500-1504.

Gronroos M, Honkonen E, Punnoren R: Cervical and serum IgA and serum IgG antibodies to *Chlamydia trachomatis* and herpes simplex virus in threatened abortion: A prospective study. *Br J Obstet Gynaecol* 1983; 90:167-170.

Guerrero R, Rojas OI: Spontaneous abortion and aging of human ova and spermatozoa. *N Engl J Med* 1975; 293:573-575.

Haimovici F, Hill JA, Anderson DJ: The effects of soluble products of activated lymphocytes and macrophages on blastocyte implantation events in vitro. *Biol Reprod* 1991; 44:69-75.

Haimovici F, Hill JA, Anderson DJ: Variables affecting toxicity of human sera in mouse embryo cultures. *J In Vitro Embryo Transf* 1989; 5:202-206.

Halmesmaki E, Valimak M, Roine R, et al: Maternal and paternal alcohol consumption and miscarriage. *Br J Obstet Gynaecol* 1989; 96:188-191.

Hansen JP: Older maternal age and pregnancy outcome: A review of the literature. *Obstet Gynecol Surv* 1986; 41:726-742.

Harger JH, Laifer SA, Bontempo FA, et al: Low-dose aspirin and prednisone treatment of pregnancy loss caused by lupus anticoagulants. *J Perinatol* 1995; 15:463-466.

Harlop S, Shiono PH: Alcohol, smoking, and incidence of spontaneous abortions in the first and second trimester. *Lancet* 1980; 2:173-176.

Harris EN: Syndrome of the black swan. *Br J Rheumatol* 1986; 26:324-326.

Hasegawa I, Takauwa R, Goto S, et al: Effectiveness of prednisolone/aspirin therapy for recurrent aborters with antiphospholipid antibody. *Hum Reprod* 1992; 7:203-207.

Hassold T, Hunt PA, Sherman S: Trisomy in humans: Incidence, origin and etiology. *Curr Opin Genet Dev* 1993; 3:358-403.

Heup RB, Flint AP, Gadsby JE: Embryonic signals that establish pregnancy. *Br Med Bull* 1979; 35:129-130.

Heine O, Muller-Eckhardt G: Intravenous immune globulin in recurrent abortion. *Clin Exp Immunol* 1994; 97(suppl 1):39-42.

Heinonen PK: Reproductive performance of women with uterine anomalies after abdominal or hysteroscopic metroplasty or no surgical treatment. *J Am Assoc Gynecol Laparosc* 1997; 4:311-317.

Hermonat PL, Kechelaus S, Lowery CL, et al: Trophoblasts are the preferential target for human papilloma virus infection in spontaneously aborted products of conception. *Hum Pathol* 1998; 29:170-174.

Hill JA: Immunologic factors in spontaneous abortion. In Bronson AA, Alexander NJ, Anderson DJ, et al, editors: *Reproductive immunology,* Cambridge, 1996, Blackwell Scientific.

Hill JA: Implications of cytokines in male and female sterility. In Chaouat GA, Mowbrary JF, editors: *Cellular and molecular biology of the maternal-fetal relationship,* INSERM/John Libbey Eruotext, 1991, Paris.

Hill JA: Sporadic and recurrent spontaneous abortion. *Curr Prob Obstet Gynecol Fertil* 1994; 17:114-162.

Hill JA, Anderson DJ: Blood transfusions for recurrent abortion: Is the treatment worse than the disease? *Fertil Steril* 1986; 46:152-153.

Hill JA, Anderson DJ: Evidences for the existence and significance of immune cells and their soluble products in reproductive tissues. *Immunol Allerg Clin N Am* 1990;10:1-12.

Hill JA, Anderson DJ, Abbott A, et al: Seminal white blood cells and recurrent abortion. *Hum Reprod* 1994;9:1180-1183.

Hill JA, Anderson DJ, Polgar K: T helper 1-type cellular immunity to trophoblast in women with recurrent spontaneous abortion. *JAMA* 1995a; 273:1933-1936.

Hill JA, Haimovici F, Anderson DJ: Products of activated lymphocytes and macrophages inhibit mouse embryo development in vitro. *J Immunol* 1987; 132:2250-2254.

Hill JA, Melling GC, Johnson PM: Immunohistochemical studies of human uteroplacental tissues from first trimester spontaneous abortion. *Am J Obstet Gynecol* 1995b; 173:90-96.

Hill JA, Polgar K, Harlow BL, et al: Evidence of embryo and trophoblast-toxic cellular immune response(s) in women with recurrent spontaneous abortion. *Am J Obstet Gynecol* 1992; 166:1044-1052.

Hillier SL, Nugent RP, Eschenbach DA, et al: Association between bacterial vaginosis and preterm delivery of a low-birth-weight infant. *N Engl J Med* 1995; 335:1737-1742.

Ho HN, Gill TJ, Hsieh HJ, et al: Immunotherapy for recurrent spontaneous abortion in a Chinese population. *Am J Reprod Immunol* 1991; 25:10-15.

Homburg R, Levy T, Berkowitz D, et al: Gonadotropin-releasing hormone agonist reduces the miscarriage rate for pregnancies achieved in women with polycystic ovarian syndrome. *Fertil Steril* 1993; 59:527-531.

Hook EB, Cross PK, Schreinemachers DM: Chromosomal abnormality rates of amniocentesis and in live-born infants. *JAMA* 1983; 249:2034-2038.

Hunt JS: Cytokine networks in the uteroplacental unit: Macrophages as pivotal regulatory cells. *J Reprod Immunol* 1989; 16:1-17.

Hunt JS, Hsi BL: Evasive strategies of trophoblast cells: Selective expression of membrane antigens. *Am J Reprod Immunol* 1990; 23:57-63.

Imseis H, Creig PC, Livergood CH, et al: Characterization of the inflammatory cytokines in the vagina during pregnancy and labor and with bacterial vaginosis. *J Soc Gynecol Invest* 1997; 4:90-94.

Jaffe R, Jauniaux E, Hustin J: Maternal circulation in the first-trimester human placenta—myth or reality? *Am J Obstet Gynecol* 1997; 176:695-705.

Jauniaux E: Fetal testing in the first trimester of pregnancy. *The Female Patient* 1997; 22:15-24.

Jeng GT, Scott JR, Burmeister LF: A comparison of meta-analytic results using literature vs. individual patient data. *JAMA* 1995; 274:830-836.

Jones CT: Luteal phase defects. In Behrman SJ, Kistner RW, editors: *Progress in infertility,* Boston, 1968, Little, Brown.

Jones GES: The luteal phase defect. *Fertil Steril* 1976; 27:351

Jordan J, Craig K, Clifton DK, et al: Luteal phase defect: The sensitivity and specificity of diagnostic methods in common clinical use. *Fertil Steril* 1994; 62:54-62.

Kalausek DK, Barrett IJ, Gartner AB: Spontaneous abortion and confirmed chromosomal mosaicism. *Hum Genet* 1992; 88:642-646.

Kalter H: Diabetes and spontaneous abortion: A historical review. *Am J Obstet Gynecol* 1987; 150:1243-1246.

Karamardian LM, Grimes DA: Luteal phase deficiency: Effects of treatment on pregnancy rates. *Am J Obstet Gynecol* 1992; 167:1391-1398.

Karande VC, Lester RG, Muasher SJ, et al: Are implantation and pregnancy outcome impaired in diethylstilbestrol-exposed women after in vitro fertilization and embryo transfer? *Fertil Steril* 1990; 54:287-291.

Karnfeld D, Cnattingins S, Ekbom A: Pregnancy outcomes in women with inflammatory bowel disease: A population-based cohort study. *Am J Obstet Gynecol* 1997; 177;942-946.

Katsuragawa H, Kanzaki H, Inoue T, et al: Monoclonal antibody against phosphatidylserine inhibits in vitro human trophoblast hormone production and invasion. *Biol Reprod* 1997; 56:50-58.

Katsuragawa H, Rote NS, Inoue T, et al: Monoclonal antiphosphatidylserine antibody reactivity against human first-trimester placental trophoblasts. *Am J Obstet Gynecol* 1995; 172:1592-1597.

Katz I, Fisch B, Amlt S, et al: Cutaneous graft-versus-host live reaction after paternal lymphocyte immunization for prevention of recurrent abortion. *Fertil Steril* 1992; 57:927-929.

Kaufman RH, Adam E, Binder GL, et al: Upper genital tract changes and pregnancy outcome in offspring exposed in utero to diethylstilbestrol. *Am J Obstet Gynecol* 1980; 137:299-308.

Kaufman RH, Noller K, Adam E, et al: Upper genital tract abnormalities and pregnancy outcome in diethylstilbestrol-exposed pregnancy. *Am J Obstet Gynecol* 1984; 148:973-984.

Keller DW, Wrest WH, Askin FB, et al: Pseudo-corpus luteum insufficiency: A local defect of progesterone action on endometrial stroma. *Fertil Steril* 1979; 48:127-132.

Keltz MD, Olive DL, Kim AH, et al: Sonohysterography for screening in recurrent pregnancy loss. *Fertil Steril* 1997; 67:670-674.

Keye WR Jr, Jaffe RB: Changing patterns of FSH and LH responses to gonadotropin releasing hormone in the puerperium. *J Clin Endocrinol Metab* 1976; 42:1133-1138.

Khudr G: Cytogenetics of habitual abortion. *Obstet Gynecol Surv* 1974; 29:299-310.

Kiprov DD, Nachtigall RD, Weaver RC, et al: The use of intravenous immunoglobulin in recurrent pregnancy loss associated with combined alloimmune and autoimmune abnormalities. *Am J Reprod Immunol* 1996; 36: 228-234.

Klebanoff MA, Shiono PH, Rhoads GG: Outcomes of pregnancy in a national sample of resident physicians. *N Engl J Med* 1990; 323: 1040-1045.

Klebanoff MA, Shiono PH, Rhoads GG: Spontaneous and induced abortion among resident physicians. *JAMA* 1991; 265:2821-2825.

Klein HG: Immunologic aspects of blood transfusion. *Semin Oncol* 1994; 21:16-20.

Kline J, Stein Z, Susser M, et al: Environmental influences in early reproductive loss in a current New York City study. In Porter Ihm, Hook HB, editors: *Human embryonic and fetal death,* New York, 1980, Academic Press.

Klinger K, Landes G, Shook D, et al: Rapid detection of chromosome aneuploidies in uncultured amniocytes using fluorescence in situ hybridization (FISH). *Am J Hum Genet* 1992; 51:55-65.

Klock SC, Chang G, Hiley A, Hill J: Psychological distress among women with recurrent spontaneous abortion. *Psychosomatius* 1997; 38:503-507.

Kong TY, Liddell, Robertson WB: Defective haemochorial placentation as a cause of miscarriage: A preliminary study. *Br J Obstet Gynaecol* 1987; 94:649-655.

Kutteh WH: Antiphospholipid antibody-associated recurrent pregnancy loss: Treatment with heparin and low-dose aspirin vs. superior to low-dose aspirin alone. *Am J Obstet Gynecol* 1996; 174:1584-1589.

Kutteh WH, Werter R, Kutteh CC: Multiples of the media: An alternative method for reporting antiphospholipid antibodies in women with recurrent pregnancy loss. *Obstet Gynecol* 1994; 84:811-815.

Kutteh WH, Yetman DL, Chantilis SJ, et al: Effect of antiphospholipid antibodies in women undergoing in vitro fertilization: Role of heparin and aspirin. *Hum Reprod* 1997; 12:1171-1175.

Kwak JY, Barini R, Gilman-Sachs A, et al: Down-regulation of maternal antiphospholipid antibodies during early pregnancy and pregnancy outcome. *Am J Obstet Gynecol* 1994; 171:239-246.

Kwak JY, Beaman KP, Gilman-Sachs A, et al: Up-regulated expression of CD56+, CD56+/CD16+ and, DC19+ cells in peripheral blood lymphocytes in pregnant women with recurrent pregnancy loss. *Am J Reprod Immunol* 1995; 34:93-99.

Kyle PM, Sepuleda W, Blunt S, et al: High failure rate of postmortem karyotyping after termination for fetal abnormality. *Obstet Gynecol* 1996; 88:859-862.

Laird T, Whittaker PG: The endocrinology of early pregnancy failure. In Huisjes HJ, Lird T, editors: *Early pregnancy failure.* New York, 1990, Churchill Livingstone.

Laitnen T, Koskimier S, Wastmin P: Foeto-maternal compatibility in HLA-DR, -DQ and -DP loci in Finnish couples suffering from recurrent spontaneous abortions. *Eur J Immunogenet* 1993; 20:249-258.

Laskin CA, Bombardier C, Hannah ME, et al: Prednisone and oral aspirin in women with autoantibodies and unexplained recurrent fetal loss. *N Engl J Med* 1997; 357:148-153.

Laufer M, Ecker JL, Hill JA: Pregnancy outcome following ultrasound demonstrated fetal cardiac activity in women with a history of multiple spontaneous abortions. *J Soc Gynecol Invest* 1994; 1:138-142.

Lea RG, Al-Sharekh N, Tulppala M, et al: The immunolocalization of bcl-2 at the maternal-fetal interface in healthy and failing pregnancies. *Hum Reprod* 1997; 12:153-158.

Lejeune B, Grun JP, DeNager PA, et al: Antithyroid antibodies underlying thyroid abnormalities and miscarriage or pregnancy induced hypertension. *Br J Obstet Gynecol* 1983; 100:669-672.

Letterie GS, Haggerty M, Lindee G: A comparison of pelvic ultrasound and magnetic resonance imaging as diagnostic studies for mullerian tract abnormalities. *Int J Fertil Menopausal Stud* 1995; 40:34-38.

Li TC, Dockery P, Cooke ID: Endometrial development in the luteal phase of women with various types of infertility: Comparison with women of normal fertility. *Hum Reprod* 1991; 6:325-330.

Liddell HS, Pattison NS, Zanderigo A: Recurrent miscarriage-outcome after supportive care in early pregnancy. *Aust N Z J Obstet Gynecol* 1991; 31:320-322.

Lindbohm MJ, Heitanen M, Kyyronen P, et al: Magnetic fields of video display terminals and spontaneous abortion. *Am J Epidemiol* 1992; 136:1041-1051.

Lishner M, Amato D, Frine D: Different outcomes of pregnancy in women with essential thrombocytosis. *J Med Sci* 1993; 29;100-102.

Llahi-Camp JM, Rai R, Ison C, et al: Association of bacterial vaginosis with a history of second trimester miscarriage. *Hum Reprod* 1996; 11:1575-1578.

Lockshin MD: Answers to the antiphospholipid syndrome? *N Eng J Med* 1997; 332:1025-1027.

Lockshin MD, Druzin ML, Qamar T: Prednisone does not prevent recurrent fetal death in women with antiphospholipid antibody. *Am J Obstet Gynecol* 1989; 160:439-443.

Lockwood CJ, Reece EA, Romero R, et al: Antiphospholipid antibody and pregnancy wastage. *Lancet* 1986; 2:742-743.

Lopata A, Sathanathan AH, McBain JC, et al: The ultrastructure of the preovulatory human egg fertilized in vitro. *Fertil Steril* 1980; 33:12-20.

Lubba WF, Butler WS, Palmer SJ, et al: Fetal survival after prednisone suppression of maternal lupus anticoagulant. *Lancet* 1983; 1:1361-1363.

Maher JE, Davis RO, Goldenberg RL, et al: Unexplained elevation in maternal serum alpha-fetoprotein and subsequent fetal loss. *Obstet Gynecol* 1984; 83:138-141.

Makida R, Minami M, Takamizawa M, et al: Natural killer cell activity and immunotherapy for recurrent spontaneous abortion. *Lancet* 1991; 338:579-580.

Many A, Pauzner R, Carp H, et al: Treatment of patients with antiphospholipid antibodies during pregnancy. *Am J Reprod Immunol* 1992; 28:216-218.

March CM: Intrauterine adhesions. *Obstet Gynecol Clin N Am* 1995; 22:491-505.

Marcus S, Al Shawaf T, Brinsden P: The obstetric outcome of in vitro fertilization and embryo transfer in women with congenital uterine malformation. *Am J Obstet Gynecol* 1996; 175:85-89.

Marqusee E, Hill JA, Mandel SJ: Thyroiditis after pregnancy loss. *J Clin Endocrinol Metab* 1997; 82:2455-2457.

Martin PA, Shaver EL: Sperm aging in the utero and chromosomal anomalies in rabbit blastocytes. *Dev Biol* 1972; 28:480-486.

Martin-Deleon PA, Bioce MI: Sperm aging the male and cytogenic anomalies: An animal model. *Hum Genet* 1982; 62:70-77.

Marzusch K, Dietl J, Klein R, et al: Recurrent first trimester spontaneous abortion associated with antiphospholipid antibodies: A pilot study of treatment with intravenous immunoglobulin. *Acta Obstet Gynaecol Scand* 1996; 75:922-926.

Mattison DR: Minimizing toxic hazards to fetal health. *Contemp Obstet Gynecol* 1992; 8;81-100.

Mazzaferri EL: Evaluation and management of common thyroid disorders in women. *Am J Obstet Gynecol* 1997; 176:507-514.

McCord ML, Muram D, Buster JE, et al: Single serum progesterone as a screen for ectopic pregnancy: Exchanging specificity and sensitivity to obtain optimal test performance. *Fertil Steril* 1996; 66:513-516.

McCormack WM, Almeida PC, Bailey PE, et al: Sexual activity and vaginal colonization with genital mycoplasmas. *JAMA* 1972; 221:1375-1379.

McGregor J, French J, Jones W, et al: Association of cervicovaginal infections with increased vaginal fluid phospholipase A_2 activity. *Am J Obstet Gynecol* 1992; 167:1588-1594.

McGregor J, Lowellin D, Franco-Buff A, et al: Phospholipase C activity in microorganisms associated with reproductive tract infection. *Am J Obstet Gynecol* 1991; 164:682-686.

Merkatz IR, Mitowsky HM, Marci JN, et al: An association between low maternal serum alpha-protein and fetal chromosome anormalities. *Am J Obstet Gynecol* 1984; 148:886-894.

Merkel PA, Chang Y, Pierangli SS, et al: The prevalence and clinical association of anticardiolipin antibodies in a large inception cohort of patients with connective tissue disease. *Am J Med* 1996; 101:576-583.

Miles RA, Paulson RJ, Lobo RA, et al: Pharmacokinetics and endometrial tissue levels of progesterone after administration by intramuscular and vaginal routes: A comparative study. *Fertil Steril* 1994; 62:485-490.

Mills JL, Simpson JL, Driscoll SE, et al: Incidence of abortion among normal women and insulin-dependent diabetic women whose pregnancies were identified within 21 days of conception. *N Engl J Med* 1988; 319:1617-1623.

Milunsky A, Ulcickas M, Rothman KJ, et al: Maternal heat exposure and neural tube defects. *JAMA* 1992; 268:882-885.

Minkoff H: Prematurity: Infections as an etiologic factor. *Obstet Gynecol* 1983; 62:137-144.

Mitus AJ, Shafer AI: Thrombocytosis and thrombocythemia. *Hematol Oncol Clin North Am* 1990; 4:157-178.

Moneschi F, Zupi E, Marconi D, et al: Hysteroscopically detected asymptomatic mullerian anomalies: Prevalence and reproductive implications. *J Reprod Med* 1995; 40:684-688.

Mosmann TR, Coffman RI: Th1 and Th2 cells: Different patterns of lymphokine secretion lead to different functional properties. *Annu Rev Immunol* 1989; 7:145-173.

Mowbray JF, Gibbings C, Lidlell H, et al: Controlled trial of treatment of recurrent spontaneous abortion by immunostimulation with paternal cells. *Lancet* 1985; 2:941-943.

Mueller-Eckhart G, Hene O, Nepport J, et al: Preventing recurrent spontaneous abortion by intravenous immunoglobulin. *Vox Sang* 1989; 56:151-154.

Mueller-Eckhart G, Huni O, Poltin B: IVIG to prevent recurrent spontaneous abortions. *Lancet* 1991; 1:424-425.

Munne S, Lee A, Rosenwaks Z, et al: Diagnosis of major chromosome aneuploides in human preimplantation embryos. *Hum Reprod* 1993; 8:2185-2191.

Nakajima ST, Molloy MH, OI KH, et al: Clinical evaluation of luteal function. *Obstet Gynecol* 1994; 84:219-221.

Nelson-Piercy C, Letsky EA, de Swiet M: Low-molecular-weight heparin for obstetric thromboprophylaxis: Experience of sixty-nine pregnancies in sixty-one women at high risk. *Am J Obstet Gynecol* 1997; 176:1062-1068.

Ober C, Steck T, Vander Vank, et al: MHC class II compatibility in aborted fetuses and term infants of couples wth recurrent spontaneous abortion. *J Reprod Immunol* 1993; 25:195-207.

Omer H: Possible psychophysiologic mechanisms in premature labor. *Psychosomatics* 1986; 27:580-584.

Oshiro BT, Silver RM, Scott JR, et al: Antiphospholipid antibodies and fetal death. *Obstet Gynecol* 1996; 87:489-493.

Out HJ, Kooijman CD, Bruinse HW, et al: Histopathological findings in placentae from patients with intrauterine fetal death and antiphospholipid antibodies. *Eur J Obstet Gynecol Reprod Biol* 1991; 41:179-186.

Page LA, Smith PC: Placentitis and abortion in cattle inoculated with chlamydiae isolated from aborted human placental tissue. *Proc Soc Exp Biol Med* 1974; 146:246-250.

Passaleva A, Massai G, E'Elios MM, et al: Prevention of miscarriage in antiphospholipid syndrome. *Autoimmunity* 1992; 14:121-125.

Patton PE: Anatomic uterine defects. *Clin Obstet Gynecol* 1994; 37:705-721.

Paul M, Kurtz S: *Reproductive hazards in the work place.* Worcester, Mass., 1990, University of Massachusetts Medical Center, Occupational and Environmental Reproductive Hazards Center.

Pegoraro E, Whitaker J, Mowery-Rushton P, et al: Familial schemed X inactivation: A molecular trait associated with high spontaneous-abortion rate maps to Xq28. *Am J Hum Genet* 1997; 61:160-170.

Pennell RG, Neederman L, Pajak T, et al: Prospective comparison of vaginal and abdominal sonography in normal early pregnancy. *J Ultrasound Med* 1991; 10:63-67.

Perino A, Vassiliadis A, Vucetich A, et al: Short-term therapy for recurrent abortion using intravenous immunoglobulins: Results of a double-blind placebo-controlled Italian study. *Hum Reprod* 1997; 12:2388-2392.

Petri M: Pathogenesis and treatment of the antiphospholipid antibody syndrome. *Med Clin North Am* 1997; 81;151-177.

Petri M, Howard D, Repke J: Frequency of lupus flare in pregnancy: The Hopkins Lupus Pregnancy Center experience. *Arthritis Rheum* 1991; 34:1538-1545.

Poland BJ, Miller JP, Jones DC, et al: Reproductive counseling in patients who had a spontaneous abortion. *Am J Obstet Gynecol* 1977; 127:685-691.

Polgar K, Yacono PW, Golan DE, Hill JA: Immune interferon inhibits lateral mobility of a membrane protein in murine embryos: A potential mechanism for Th1 mediated reproductive failure. *Am J Obstet Gynecol* 1996; 174:282-287.

Polifka JE, Friedman JM: Environmental toxins and recurrent pregnancy loss. *Int Reprod Med Clin North Am* 1991; 2:175-213.

Polson DW, Wedsworth J, Adams J, et al: Polycystic ovaries: A common finding in normal women. *Lancet* 1980; 2:870-872.

Quenby S, Farquharson RG: Human chorionic gonadotropin supplementation in recurrent pregnancy loss: A controlled trial. *Fertil Steril* 1994; 62:708-710.

Quin PA, et al: Efficacy of antibiotic therapy in preventing spontaneous pregnancy loss among couples colonized with genital *Mycoplasma*. *Am J Obstet Gynecol* 1983; 145:239-241.

Racowsky C, Kaufman ML: Nuclear degeneration and meiotic aberrations observed in human oocytes in vitro: Analysis by light microscopy. *Fertil Steril* 1992; 58:750-755.

Rae R, Smith IW, Liston WA, et al: Chlamydial serologic studies and recurrent spontaneous abortion. *Am J Obstet Gynecol* 1994; 170:782-785.

Raghupathy R: Th1-type immunity is incompatible with successful pregnancy. *Immunol Today* 1997; 18:478-482.

Rai RS, Clifford K, Cohen H, et al: High prospective fetal loss rate in untreated pregnancies of women with recurrent miscarriage and antiphospholipid antibodies. *Hum Reprod* 1995; 10:3301-3304.

Rai R, Cohen HR, Dave M, et al: Randomized controlled trial of aspirin and aspirin plus heparin in pregnant women with recurrent miscarriage associated with phospholipid antibodies (or antiphospholipid antibodies). *BMJ* 1997; 314:253-257.

Rai R, Regan L, Hadley E, et al: Second-trimester pregnancy loss in associated with activated C resistance. *Br J Haematol* 1996; 92:489-490.

Rand JH, Wu XX, Guller S, et al: Antiphospholipid immunoglobulin G antibodies reduce annexin-V levels on syncytiotrophoblast apical membrane and in culture media of placental villi. *Am J Obstet Gynecol* 1997; 177:918-923.

Rand JH, Wu XX, Guller S, et al: Reduction of annexin V (placental anticoagulant protein-I) on placental villi of women with antiphospholipid antibodies and recurrent spontaneous abortion. *Am J Obstet Gynecol* 1994; 171:1566-1572.

Raziel A, Arieli S, Bukovsky I, et al: Investigation of the uterine cavity in recurrent aborters. *Fertil Steril* 1994; 62:1080-1082.

Raziel A, Harmon A, Stressburger D, et al: The outcome of in vitro fertilization in unexplained habitual aborters concurrent with secondary infertility. *Fertil Steril* 1997; 67:88-92.

The Recurrent Miscarriage Immunotherapy Trialists Group: Worldwide Collaborative Observational Study and meta-analysis on allogenic leukocyte immunotherapy for recurrent spontaneous abortion. *Am J Reprod Immunol* 1994; 32:55-72.

Regan L: Recurrent miscarriage. *BMJ* 1991; 302:543-544.

Regan L, Brande PR, Hill DP: A prospective study of the incidence, time of, appearance of, significance of anti-paternal lymphocytotoxic antibodies in human pregnancy. *Hum Reprod* 1981; 6:294-298.

Regan L, Braude PR, Trembath PL: Influence of postreproductive performance on risk of spontaneous abortion. *BMJ* 1989; 299:541-545.

Regan JA, Klebanoff MA, Nugent RP, et al: Colonization with group B streptococci in pregnancy and adverse outcome. *Am J Obstet Gynecol* 1996; 174:1354-1360.

Regan L, Owen EJ, Jacobs HS: Hypersecretion of luteinizing hormone, infertility and miscarriage. *Lancet* 1990; 336:1141-1144.

Remohi J, Gallardo E, Levy M, et al: Oocyte donation in women with recurrent pregnancy loss. *Hum Reprod* 1996; 11:2048-2051.

Reubinoff BE, Shushan A: Preimplantation diagnosis in older patients: To biopsy or not to biopsy? *Hum Reprod* 1996; 11:2071-2078.

Ridker P, Miletich JP, Buring JE, et al: Factor V Leiden and risks of recurrent pregnancy loss. *Ann Int Med* 1998; 128:1000-1003.

Rocklin RE, Kitzmiller JL, Carpenter CB, et al: Maternal-fetal relation: Absence of an immunologic blocking factor from serum of women with chronic abortion. *N Engl J Med* 1976; 295:1209-1212.

Rodger C: Lack of a requirement for a maternal humoral immune response to establish and maintain successful allogeneic pregnancy. *Transplantation* 1985; 40:372-375.

Rodriguez-Thompson D: 1998(in press);

Rosenbusch B, Strehler E, Sterzik D: Cytogenetics of human spermatozoa: Correlation with sperm morphology and age of fertile men. *Fertil Steril* 1992; 58:1071-1072.

Sagle M, Bishop K, Ridley N, et al: Recurrent early miscarriage and polycystic ovaries. *BMJ* 1988; 297:1027-1028.

Sahwi SY, Zaki MS, Haiba NY, et al: Toxoplasmosis as a cause of repeated abortion. *J Obstet Gynaecol* 1995; 21:145-148.

Sargent IL, Wilkins T, Redman CWG: Maternal immune responses to the fetus in early pregnancy and recurrent miscarriage. *Lancet* 1994; 2:1099-1104.

Schagen Van Leeunen JH, Christians GCML, et al: Recurrent abortion and the diagnosis of Wilson disease. *Obstet Gynecol* 1991; 78:547-549.

Schust D, Hill JA: Correlation of serum cytokine and adhesion molecule determinations with pregnancy outcome. *J Soc Gynecol Invest* 1996; 3:259-261.

Schust DJ, Hill AB, Ploegh HL: Herpes simplex blocks intracellular transport of HCA-G in platelet derived human cells. *J Immunol* 1996; 157:3375-3380.

Schved J, Gris JC, Neven S, et al: Factor XII congenital deficiency and early spontaneous abortion. *Fertil Steril* 1989; 52:335-336.

Scott JR: Recurrent miscarriage: Overview and recommendations. *Clin Obstet Gynecol* 1994; 37:768-773.

Scott JR, Branch DW, Kochenour NU, et al: Intravenous globulin treatment of pregnant patients with recurrent pregnancy loss due to antiphospholipid antibodies and Rh immunizations. *Am J Obstet Gynecol* 1988; 159:1055-1056.

Shaarway M, Najui AR: Enhanced expression of cytokines may play a fundamental role in the mechanisms of immunologically mediated recurrent spontaneous abortion. *Acta Obstet Gynecol Scand* 1997; 76:205-211.

Siiteri PK, Febres F, Clemens LE, et al: Progesterone and maintenance of pregnancy: is progesterone nature's immunosuppressant? *Ann NY Acad Sci* 1977; 286:384-397.

Silver RK, MacGregor SW, Sholl JS, et al: A comparative trial of prednisone plus aspirin versus aspirin alone in the treatment of anti-cardiolipin antibody positive obstetric patients. *Am J Obstet Gynecol* 1993; 169:1411-1417.

Silver RK, Mullen BA, Caplan MS, et al: Inducible platelet adherence to human umbilical vein endothelium by anticardiolipin-antibody positive sera. *Am J Obstet Gynecol* 1995; 173:702-707.

Silver RM, Pierangeli SS, Edwsin SS, et al: Pathogenic antibodies in women with obstetric features of antiphospholipid syndrome who have negative test results for lupus anticoagulant and anticardiolipin antibodies. *Am J Obstet Gynecol* 1997; 176:628-633.

Simpson JL, Martin AO: Parental diagnosis of cytogenetic disorders. *Clin Obstet Gynecol* 1970; 19:841-853.

Smith DW, Clarren SK, Harvey MA: Hyperthermia as a possible teratogenic agent. *J Pediatr* 1978; 92:878-880.

Smith JB, Cowchuck FS: Immunological studies in recurrent spontaneous abortion: Effects of immunization of women with paternal mononuclear cells in lymphotoxic and mixed lymphocyte reaction blocking antibodies and correlation with sharing of HLA antigens and pregnancy outcome. *J Reprod Immunol* 1988; 14:99-104.

Smith SC, Baker PN, Symmonds M: Placental apoptosis in normal human pregnancy. *Am J Obstet Gynecol* 1997; 177:57-65.

Sompolinsky D, Soloman F, et al: Infections with mycoplasma and bacteria in induced midtrimester and fetal loss. *Am J Obstet Gynecol* 1975; 121:610-614.

Sorem KA, Smikle CB, Spencer DK, et al: Circulating maternal corticotropin releasing hormone and gonadotropin releasing hormone in normal and abnormal pregnancies. *Am J Obstet Gynecol* 1996; 175:912-916.

Soules MR, Clifton DK, Steiner RA, et al: The corpus luteum: Determinants of progesterone secretion in the normal menstrual cycle. *Obstet Gynecol* 1988; 71:659-662.

Soules MR, McLachlan RI, Ek M, et al: Luteal phase defect: Characteristics of reproductive hormones over the menstrual cycle. *J Clin Endocrinol Metab* 1989; 69:804-812.

Soules MR, Wiebe RH, Alesel S, et al: The diagnosis and therapy of luteal phase deficiency. *Fertil Steril* 1997; 28:1033-1037.

Speroff L, Ramwell PW: Prostaglandins in reproductive physiology. *Am J Obstet Gynecol* 1970; 107:1111-1130.

Stagnaro-Green A, Roman SH, Colin RH, et al: Detection of at risk pregnancy by means of highly sensitive assays for thyroid autoantibodies. JAMA 1990; 264:1421-1425.

Steck T, Van der Ven K, Kwak K, et al: HLA-DQA1 and HLA-DQB1 haplotypes in aborted fetuses and couples with recurrent spontaneous abortion. *J Reprod Immunol* 1995; 29:95-104.

Steier JA, Bergsijo P, Myking OL: Human chorionic gonadotropin in maternal plasma after induced abortion, spontaneous abortion and removed ectopic pregnancy. *Obstet Gynecol* 1984; 64:391-395.

Stephensen MD: Frequency of factors associated with habitual abortion in 197 couples. *Fertil Steril* 1996; 66:24-29.

Stephenson MD, Wu V, MacKinnon M, et al: Standardization of flow cytometric cross match (FCXM) for investigation of unexplained habitual abortion. *Am J Reprod Immunol* 1995; 33:1-9.

Stewart DR, Overstreet JW, Nakajima ST, et al: Enhanced ovarian steroid secretion before implantation in early human pregnancy. *J Clin Endocrinol Metab* 1993; 76:1470-1476.

Stray-Pedersen B, Eng J, Reikram TM: Uterine T-mycoplasma colonization in reproductive failure. *Am J Obstet Gynecol* 1978; 130:307-312.

Stray-Pedersen B, Stray-Pedersen S: Etiologies and subsequent reproductive performance in 195 couples with a prior history of habitual abortion. *Am J Obstet Gynecol* 1984; 148:140-146.

Summers PR: Microbiology relevant to recurrent miscarriage. *Clin Obstet Gynecol* 1994; 37:722-729.

Tabidzadeh S: Human endometrium: An active site of cytokine production and action. *Endocrinol Rev* 1991; 12:272-290.

Takakuwa K, Higashino M, Ueda H, et al: Significant compatibility does not exist at the HLA-DQB gene locus in couples with unexplained recurrent abortion. *Am J Reprod Immunol* 1992; 28:12-16.

Taylor C, Faulk MP: Preventing recurrent abortion with leukocyte transfusions. *Lancet* 1981; 40:372-375.

Tho PT, Byrd JR, McDonough PG: Etiologies and subsequent reproductive performance of 100 couples with a prior history of habitual abortion. *Fertil Steril* 1979; 32:389-395.

Thorton CA, Bellow M: Safety of intravenous immunoglobulin. *Arch Neurol* 1993; 50:135-136.

Tichenor JR, Bledsoe LB, Opsahl MS, et al: Activation of complement in humans with a first-trimester pregnancy loss. *Gynecol Obstet Invest* 1995; 39:79-82.

Torpin R: Placenta circumvallata and placenta marginata. *Obstet Gynecol* 1955; 6:277-284.

Treffers PE: Uterine causes of early pregnancy failure: A critical evaluation. In Huisyis HJ, Lind T, editors: *Early pregnancy failure*, Edinburgh, 1990, Churchill Livingstone.

Vaarala O, Palosuo T, Kleemula M, et al: Anticardiolipin response in acute infections. *Clin Immunol Immunopathol* 1986; 41:8-15.

Verlinsky Y, Cieslak J, Freidine M, et al: Polar body diagnosis of common aneuploides by fluorescent in-situ hybridization. *Assist Reprod Genet* 1996; 12:157-162.

Vogt E, Ng AK, Rote NS: Antiphosphatidylserine antibody removes annexin-V and facilitates the binding of prothrombin at the surface of a choriocarcinoma model of trophoblast differentiation. *Am J Obstet Gynecol* 1997; 177:964-972.

Wagner N, Butler J, Sanders J: Prematurity and orgasmic coitus during pregnancy: Data on a small sample. *Fertil Steril* 1976; 27:911-915.

Warburton D, Fraser FC: On the probability that a woman who has had a spontaneous abortion will abort in subsequent pregnancies. *Br J Obstet Gynecol* 1961; 68:784-787.

Warburton D, Kline J, Stein Z, et al: Cytogenetic abnormalities in spontaneous abortions of recognized conceptions. In Porter IH, Hatcher N, Willey A, editors: *Perinatal genetics*, New York, 1986, Academic Press.

Wegenknecht DR, Green KM, McIntyre JA: Analysis of HLA-DQ alleles in recurrent spontaneous abortion couples. *Am J Reprod Immunol* 1997; 37:1-6.

Weitz JI: Low-molecular-weight heparins. *N Engl J Med* 1997; 337:688-697.

Wentz AC, Herbert CM III, Maxson WS, et al: Cycle of conception endometrial biopsy. *Fertil Steril* 1986; 46:196-199.

Wheeler JM, Johnston BM, Malinak LR: The relationship of endometriosis to spontaneous abortion. *Fertil Steril* 1983; 39:656-660.

Witkin SS: Immune pathogenesis of asymptomatic *Chlamydia trachomatis* infections in the female genital tract. *Infect Dis Obstet Gynecol* 1995; 3:169-174.

Wolf GC, Harger EO III: Indications for examination of spontaneous abortion specimens: A reassessment. *Am J Obstet Gynecol* 1995; 175:1364-1368.

Wouters MGAJ, Broers GHJ, Blom HJ, et al: Hyperhomocystinemia: A risk factor in women with unexplained recurrent early pregnancy loss. *Fertil Steril* 1993; 60:820-825.

Wudl LR, Sherman MI, Hillman N: Nature of lethality of T mutations in embryos. *Nature* 1977; 270:137.

Yamada H, Polgar K, Hill JA: Cell-mediated immunity to trophoblast antigens in women with recurrent spontaneous abortion. *Am J Obstet Gynecol* 1994; 170:1339-1344.

Yen SSC: The polycystic ovary syndrome. *Clin Endocrinol* 1980; 12:177-208.

Ywetman DL, Kutteh WH: Antiphospholipid antibody panels and recurrent pregnancy loss: Prevalence of anticardiolipin antibodies compared with other antiphospholipid antibodies. *Fertil Steril* 1996; 66:540-546.

Zlotogora J: Genetic disorders among Palestinian Arabs, I: Effects of consanguinity. *Am J Med Genet* 1997; 68:472-475.

17

Medical Genetics

LOUISE WILKINS-HAUG

KEY ISSUES

1. Testing for genetic mutations is now possible for a growing number of rare disorders and for many commonly encountered diseases of adult onset in women.
2. Fluorescence in situ hybridization and comparative genome hybridization of interphase cells can provide chromosomal information from a single nondividing cell.
3. Uniparental disomy and imprinting play a major role in the control of fetal growth and development.
4. Chromosomal and single-gene abnormalities, particularly cystic fibrosis, should be considered in the infertility evaluation of the couple with identified oligospermia.
5. Preconception genetic screening for disorders of increased prevalence within various populations requires incorporation of test sensitivity, specificity, and knowledge of the ethnic heritage of the person undergoing screening.

The Human Genome Project will likely reach its goal of complete sequencing of the human genome by the year 2005. Our expanding knowledge of the molecular basis of inheritance and the increasing accessibility of gene testing will present a significant challenge to the clinical practice of gynecology. Since the initiation in the early 1990s of the worldwide scientific endeavor to sequence the human genome, gene mutations responsible for inherited diseases have been uncovered at a rapid rate. This information provides an impetus for increased testing of patients by DNA analysis for carrier detection and prenatal diagnosis. The identified mutations involve not only rare diseases but also more common disorders, in particular those conditions occurring with increased frequency among persons of common heritage. Just as important, changes at the gene level represent risk factors for a multitude of adult-onset disorders before a disease state or illness is manifested.

Although the rate of acquisition of genetic knowledge in the past decade has been rapid, references to "familial" disorders have appeared in philosophical writings for several centuries. Medical writings from the early 1800s include the first references to "family passage" of disease states. A scientific approach to inheritance did not appear until the late 1860s with the work of Gregor Mendel. Concurrently during the 1800s, researchers described cell-to-cell transmission of *chromosomes*, a term coined by Waldeyer in 1888. Chromosomes as the carriers of the genetic material integral to Mendel's laws received attention by three investigators in the 1900s—Correns, Tschermark, and deVries (Vogel and Motulsky, 1986). For most of the twentieth century, genetics focused on the identification of human chromosomes and the delineation of DNA as the functional component of the gene. Until 1956, investigators thought human cells contained 48, not 46, chromosomes. The unraveling of gene defects at the molecular level pursued by the Human Genome Project will provide even greater potential for mutation detection and gene therapy.

This chapter lays out the current understanding of various aspects of inheritance including chromosomal, single-gene mendelian, multifactorial, and nonmendelian theories of mitochondrial inheritance, unstable DNA, uniparental disomy, and imprinting. The role of genetic screening is covered, as are its associated ramifications of patient education, test interpretation, and implications after the carrier-affected state is determined. Of specific interest to gynecologists is the increasing role of genetic screening for inherited disorders and for predisposition to various adult-onset diseases and cancers often encountered in women's health care.

GENERAL PRINCIPLES
Cytogenetic Inheritance

It is estimated that each human cell contains 5 to 6 million genes representing a total of 2 million meters of DNA (Simpson and Golbus, 1992). Because each gene comprises a unique sequence of approximately 1000 nucleotide pairs, the physics of transcription, replication, and storage of the human genome within each cell are complex. At least three types of DNA are recognized: unique DNA possessing only a single copy of the nucleotide sequence coding for a particular protein; highly repetitious DNA responsible for packaging; and moderately repetitive DNA that codes for histones or ribosomes (Thompson et al, 1991). Unique coding sequences (exons) are separated from one another by noncoding sequences called introns. Proteins are thus constructed from a discontinuous sequence of unique DNA interrupted by intron sequences. Packaging of the human genome into discrete units, the chromosomes, facilitates the orderly replication and passage of DNA from one generation to the next. Each chromosome is composed of a continuous double strand of DNA containing 1000 to 2000 genes and the associated proteins, the histones. As shown in Fig. 17-1, chromosomes are best visualized during metaphase, the stage during cell division when the DNA is condensed.

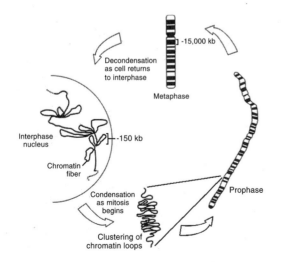

Fig. 17-1. Cycle of condensation and decondensation as a chromosome proceeds through the cell cycle. (From Thompson MW, McInnes RR, Willard HF: *Thompson and Thompson: Genetics in medicine,* ed 5, Philadelphia, 1991, WB Saunders.)

Metaphase spreads can be obtained from any nucleated cell (*e.g.,* peripheral blood lymphocyte, bone marrow, amniotic fluid fibroblast, chorionic villi, skin fibroblast). Because cells spontaneously divide asynchronously and at infrequent intervals, cell division is usually induced by phytohemagglutinin and is halted in metaphase by the use of colcemid, a spindle poison. Cells that are rapidly dividing from bone marrow or chorionic villi do not require the induction of division; thus, the time needed to obtain an analysis is markedly decreased.

Karyotype Analysis

Chromosomes are traditionally displayed as a karyotype, the 23 pairs of chromosomes aligned from largest to smallest (Fig. 17-2). Recognition of a specific chromosome is dependent on its size, shape, and unique banding characteristics. Before banding techniques, chromosomes could be recognized only by their size and shape (Denver nomenclature) and were subdivided into groups (A to G). With subsequent techniques to produce discrete light and dark banding patterns in metaphase chromosomes, each is recognized to have a unique pattern of darkly and lightly stained regions or bands. Giemsa treatment of the chromosomes after trypsin exposure produces G bands. Q banding patterns are similar and are produced by quinacrine mustard, though they require a fluorescence microscope for detection. R bands, produced by denaturation, result in a pattern opposite that of G or Q banding. T and C bands are specific to telomeres (ends of chromosomes) and centromeres, respectively (Fig. 17-3). Stains specific to an individual chromosome, such as DAPI (4'6-diamidino-2-phenylindole-2HCl) and chromosome 15, can further assist in the delineation of a chromosome. Banding patterns are delineated by a standardized nomenclature that allows precise identification of specific regions of a chromosome (Fig. 17-4).

When describing the chromosomal complement of a cell, the following convention is followed:
- number of chromosomes
- sex chromosome pair
- abnormal chromosome

In addition to providing a fingerprint of the individual chromosomes, the banding patterns represent differences in DNA content and probable function. Giemsa (G)- and quinacrine (Q)-positive regions contain moderately or highly repetitive DNA rich in AT sequences. Reverse (R)-positive regions are enriched with guanine and cytosine base pairs and represent unique-sequence DNA (Thompson et al, 1991). Clinical evaluation reveals that alterations in R-positive bands, those regions with unique sequences, carry greater clinical consequences than aberrations in repetitious DNA, the G- and Q-positive bands (Simpson and Golbus, 1992).

Fluorescence in situ hybridization (FISH) offers another means of chromosome identification. Double-stranded DNA, if denatured into single strands, has the innate ability to hybridize preferentially to complementary DNA (Pinkel et al, 1988). DNA can be denatured in situ on a microscope slide without disrupting the chromosomes. Complementary

DNA labeled with a tag and derived from a specific site on a known chromosome is used as the probe during the subsequent hybridization. Hybridization, too, can occur in situ without disrupting the integrity of the microscope preparation (Figs. 17-5, 17-6).

Applications of FISH include the identification of chromosomes in supernumerary markers or in a structural rearrangement previously indiscernible by conventional banding (Schad et al, 1991; Wolff and Schwartz, 1992). Additionally, deletions of chromosomal material below the

resolution of light microscopy can be detected with these sensitive probes (Fig. 17-7). Table 17-1 indicates the range of disorders now recognized as secondary to submicroscopic deletions of specific chromosomal regions. Additional applications of FISH reflect its ability to determine chromosomal number from interphase preparations. Analyses of specific chromosomes reflecting the FISH probes used do not require the time or cell viability needed for conventional karyotype analysis to produce sufficient numbers of metaphase preparations (Guyot et al, 1988), which has led to the use of FISH probes for preliminary amniocyte results in less than 24 hours. This technique, however, is limited by the following constraints: number of chromosomes that can be studied in one cell (commonly 13, 18, 21, X, and Y), specificity of the probe information obtained, and approximately 90% probe sensitivity for these five chromosomes (Lapidot-Lifson, 1996; Ward, 1993; D'Alton, 1997). Furthermore, strict criteria for interpretation eligibility should be followed to prevent obscuring results by maternal cell contamination. Reported sensitivity rates are harder to achieve (Bryndorf, 1997) with adherence to these inclusion criteria.

There have also been advances in the use of FISH for chromosome quantification when cultured tissue cells cannot be obtained (paraffin-embedded sections) and when only small numbers of cells are available (preimplantation biopsy, fetal cells in maternal circulation). Currently under investigation are protocols for multicolor FISH preparations that would allow a greater number of probes to be used in a single cell. A relatively new technique to the field of molecular genetics is the concept of comparative genome hybridization (CGH). As in FISH, interphase cells and the innate abilities of denaturation and hybridization discussed above are used in CGH. In contrast, however, CGH includes

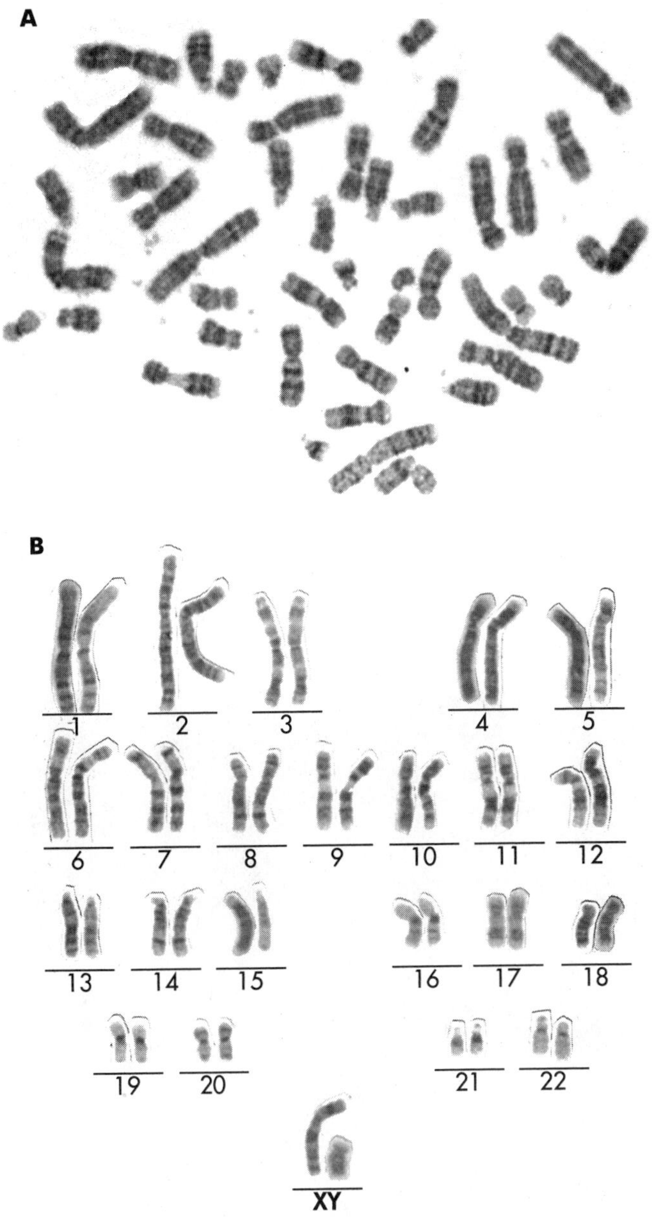

Fig. 17-2. A, Human chromosomes from a peripheral blood lymphocyte culture arrested in metaphase and stained with Giemsa banding technique. **B,** Chromosomes grouped by size and position of centimere and displayed as a karyotype. (Courtesy Morton CC, Cytogenetics, Department of Pathology, Brigham and Women's Hospital, Boston, Mass.)

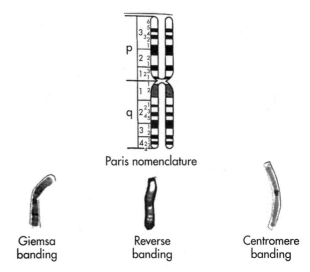

Fig. 17-3. Chromosome 1 displayed with ideogram and various staining technologies. (Courtesy Morton CC, Cytogenetics, Department of Ob-Gyn, Brigham and Women's Hospital, Boston, Mass.)

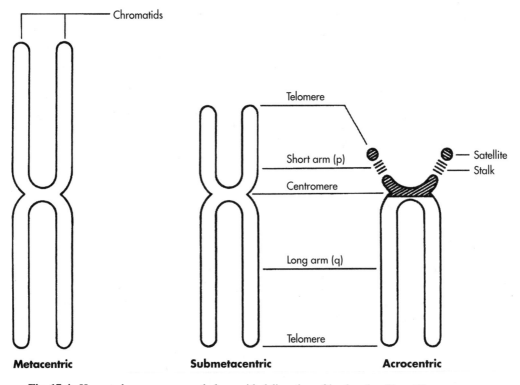

Metacentric   **Submetacentric**   **Acrocentric**

Fig. 17-4. Human chromosome morphology with delineation of landmarks. (From Thompson MW, McInnes RR, Willard MF: *Thompson and Thompson: Genetics in medicine,* ed 5, Philadelphia, 1991, WB Saunders.)

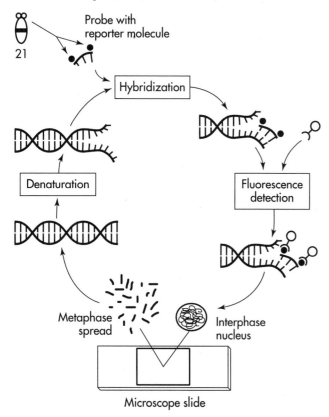

Fig. 17-5. Fluorescence in situ hybridization permits DNA denaturation and hybridization to occur without disruption of the integrity of the microscope preparation.

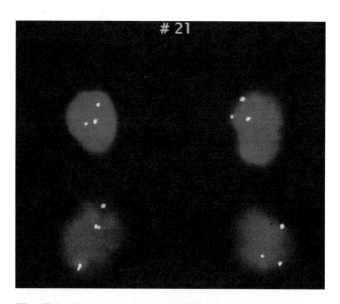

Fig. 17-6. Fluorescence in situ hybridization of interface nucleus spread with a probe derived from an alpha repeat of chromosome 21. (Courtesy Morton CC, Weremowicz S, Departments of Ob-Gyn and Pathology, Brigham and Women's Hospital, Boston, Mass.)

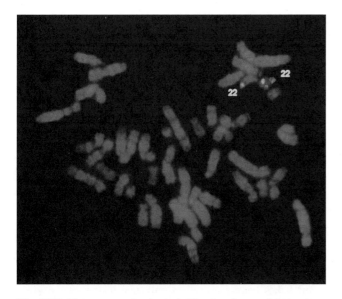

Fig. 17-7. Fluorescence in situ hybridization detects deletion in one of the 22 chromosomes (one fluorescent site) compared to a nondeleted chromosome 22 (two fluorescent sites). (Courtesy Weremowicz S, Cytogenetics, Departments of Ob-Gyn and Pathology, Brigham and Women's Hospital, Boston, Mass.)

Table 17-1   Disorders with Microdeletions Identified

Syndrome	Deletion	Metaphase Detection (%)	FISH (%) Detection
Miller-Dieker (Dobyns, 1993)	17p13.3	56	36
Prader-Willi (Mascari, 1992)	15q11q13	55-70	10
DiGeorge, Velocardiofacial (Driscoll, 1993)	22q11	20-25	60-80

interphase cells from a known normal control, with the sample DNA then acting as a probe. Intrinsic to the technique is the knowledge that if regions of deleted or additional chromosomal material are present, these regions will produce a hybridization pattern and, thus, a fluorescence alteration different from most of the double-stranded genome (Houldsworth, 1994). Progress in this area may advance chromosomal analysis of limited cell numbers; applications are already under way in preimplantation biopsy and fetal cells in maternal circulation.

Abnormalities of Chromosome Inheritance

Meiosis and Mitosis. Delineation of the abnormalities of chromosome inheritance requires an understanding of mitosis and meiosis. Mitosis is the process by which nuclear DNA is copied and passed to a daughter cell. Meiosis allows for two related events—gene recombination on maternally and paternally derived chromosomes and diploid (2N) DNA

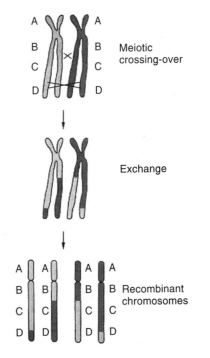

Fig. 17-8. Crossing over between homologous chromosomes during meiosis. (From Thompson MW, McInnes RR, Willard HF: *Thompson and Thompson: Genetics in medicine,* ed 5, Philadelphia, 1991, WB Saunders.)

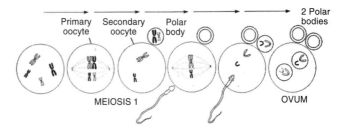

Fig. 17-9. Illustration of human oogenesis and fertilization in relation to meiosis I and II. (From Thompson MW, McInnes RR, Willard HF: *Thompson and Thompson: Genetics in medicine,* ed 5, Philadelphia, 1991, WB Saunders.)

content halving to produce a gamete cell with a haploid complement (N).

During meiosis I (reduction division), each chromosome replicates its DNA and the two sister chromatids are joined at the centromere. A suspended stage of meiosis I (dictyotene) ensues for decades until each ovulatory cycle occurs. As meiosis continues, the homologous pairs align during the diplotene stage, and an exchange of chromatid segments between the homologous chromosomes can take place at crossing-over sites, the chiasmata. For any chromosome pair, crossing over serves to redistribute the genetic material between each member of the chromosome pair (Fig. 17-8). The chromosomes then separate, undergoing disjunction, and each is distributed to one of the two daughter cells. Throughout meiosis I, the centromeres remain intact. Meiosis II is not preceded by DNA synthesis. The chromosomes (now

23 joined sets of sister chromatids per cell) separate at their centromeres, with 23 chromosomes remaining and 23 distributed to the second polar body. Meiosis II is initiated when the sperm nucleus fertilizes and enters the ovum (Fig. 17-9).

Abnormalities of Chromosome Number

Numeric chromosome abnormalities can involve either aneuploidy or polyploidy. *Aneuploidy* refers to the addition or loss of a single chromosome and the resultant alteration in the diploid (2N) complement by one. As shown in Fig. 17-10, an additional chromosome can arise through *nondisjunction*, the failure of chromosomes to segregate to the proper daughter cells during either meiosis I or meiosis II. A chromosome can be lost through *anaphase lag*, the failure of a chromosome to be included during the anaphase stage of meiotic cell division. In humans, cells with 47 chromosomes (2N + 1) are designated as trisomies, and cells with 45 chromosomes (2N − 1) are designated as monosomies. Both Down and Turner syndromes are representative of aneuploidies; the first involves trisomy 21 and the second involves monosomy X. In *polyploidy*, human cells contain one or more copies of each of the 23 chromosomes (2N + N). Partial molar gestations with triploidy (69 chromosomes) in each cell are an example of polyploidy.

Although several theories have been postulated, the mechanisms responsible for either aneuploidy or polyploidy remain unclear. As shown in Table 17-2, the incidence of trisomy 21 and of all other chromosomal trisomies rises with maternal age, but the exact phenomena that increase the rate of nondisjunction in older women is unknown. Postulates include a reduction in crossing over (chiasmata) at meiosis I, an age-related increase in background exposure to environmental agents such as radiation, a factor intrinsic to the aging ovum that involves the integrity of spindle formation, and a genetic predisposition to nondisjunction. Recent studies of DNA polymorphisms have revealed that at least 90% of trisomy 21 originates from a maternal nondisjunction (Sherman et al, 1990), and the have dispelled the earlier theory of decreased recognition and insufficient loss of chromosomally abnormal fetuses in older mothers (Hook et al,

1983). These studies suggest that the aneuploidy-maternal age association is secondary to ovarian nondisjunction during meiosis (Simpson and Golbus, 1992). By contrast, polyploidy, especially triploidy, usually involves an extra set of paternal chromosomes. The most common mechanism for this occurrence is *dispermy*, the fertilization of a normal ovum by two sperm (Kajii and Nikawa, 1977).

The clinical impact of an additional autosomal chromosome is determined by its size and by the specific genes located on that chromosome. In general, full trisomy of only the smaller chromosomes is seen in live-born neonates with Down syndrome (trisomy 21). With an incidence of 1 in 600, this is the most common. Although trisomies of the larger chromosomes (numbers 2 to 12) can be seen in spontaneous abortion, documentation of their existence in live-born neonates is rare. Trisomy of the largest chromosome, number 1, appears to be incompatible with fetal development. It has been reported in only one instance, a six-cell

Table 17-2 Maternal Age and Chromosome Abnormalities in Live Newborns

Maternal Age (Years)	Risk for Down Syndrome	Total Risk for Chromosome Abnormalities
20	1/667	1/526
21	1/667	1/526
22	1/1429	1/500
23	1/1429	1/500
24	1/1250	1/476
25	1/1250	1/476
26	1/1176	1/476
27	1/1111	1/455
28	1/1053	1/435
29	1/1000	1/417
30	1/952	1/417
31	1/909	1/385
32	1/769	1/322
33	1/602	1/286
34	1/485	1/238
35	1/378	1/192
36	1/289	1/156
37	1/224	1/127
38	1/173	1/102
39	1/136	1/83
40	1/106	1/66
41	1/82	1/53
42	1/63	1/42
43	1/49	1/33
44	1/38	1/26
45	1/30	1/21
46	1/23	1/16
47	1/18	1/13
48	1/14	1/10
49	1/11	1/8

From Hook EB: Rates of chromosomal abnormalities at different maternal ages. *Obstet Gynecol* 1981; 58:232. Reprinted with permission from the American College of Obstetricians and Gynecologists (Obstetrics and Gynecology, 1981; 58:232)
*Data not available for 47,XXX at maternal ages 20 to 32.

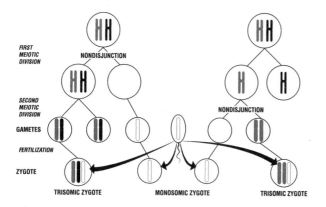

Fig. 17-10. Consequences of nondisjunction occurring in the first or second meiotic division. (From Gelehrter TD, Collins FS: *Principles of medical genetics*, Baltimore, 1990, Williams & Wilkins.)

embryo, and it has never been seen in a spontaneously aborted fetus or a live newborn (Kajii and Nikawa, 1977).

Abnormalities of Chromosome Structure

There can be alterations in chromosome size and shape (Fig. 17-11). Not every structural abnormality is associated with a clinically significant change in physical or mental development (*phenotype*). Particular regions of some chromosomes contain heterochromatic, highly repetitive DNA, and variations in size are common. Known as polymorphisms, these alterations in size and shape of chromosomes 1, 9, and 16 and of the satellite regions of the acrocentric chromosomes can be useful in tracking the segregation of a chromosome (Fig. 17-12).

Similarly, the overall shape of a chromosome can be changed by centromere relocation as the result of an *inversion*. Inversions require two breaks within a chromosome, with a subsequent 180° rotation of the intervening chromosomal segment. Pericentric inversions, which occur on either side of a centromere, alter the shape of the chromosome, whereas paracentric inversions, which do not involve the centromere, alter the banding pattern (see Fig. 17-11). If genetic material is not lost in the process, inversion can occur without phenotypic impact. However, because of meiotic cross-over, inversion carriers are at greater risk for unequal chromosomal distribution and clinical abnormalities in their offspring. This risk is greatest for maternal inversions passed through an affected person. By contrast, inversions passed through clinically unaffected persons may not increase the risk for abnormalities in the neonate. Inversions identified during prenatal testing should be compared to the parental chromosome complements. If these are identical in size and in banding pattern to the parental inversion, the fetus is thought to have a balanced complement. Although the number of cases for study are small, de novo inversions only in the fetus with normal parental karyotypes carry an approximately 10% risk for phenotypic abnormality (Warburton, 1991).

Alterations in chromosome structure involving two chromosomes are referred to as *translocations*. There are two broad categories of translocation: *reciprocal translocation,* in which two chromosomes exchange segments, and *Robertsonian translocation,* in which two chromosomes are joined as one (see Fig. 17-11). If genetic material is not lost during this exchange, the neonate will have a normal phenotype and the genetic complement will be considered balanced. However, exchanged or fused genetic material creates malalignments at meiosis, and the distribution of balanced and unbalanced chromosomal complements to the offspring is possible (Figs. 17-13, 17-14). The risk for conception with an unbalanced segregation is influenced by the type of translocation, the size of the rearrangement, the gender of the parental carrier, and the method of ascertainment (Table 17-3) (Daniel et al, 1989). When a reciprocal translocation is detected de novo in amniotic fluid and given a possible loss of submicroscopic DNA, even apparently balanced rearrangements are associated with a 10% risk for phenotypic abnormality (Warburton, 1991). Maternal carriers of Robertson translocation face a 10% to 25% risk for an imbalance in offspring, depending on the chromosomes involved. In contrast, paternal carriers of Robertsonian translocation have not been clearly shown to be at increased risk for unbalanced segregants (Simpson and Golbus, 1992). Robertsonian translocations involving both members of a chromosome

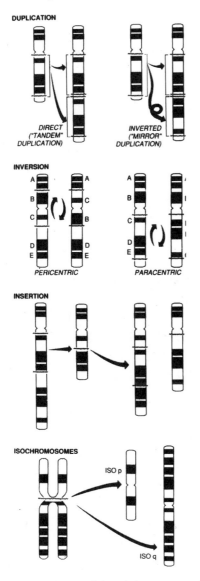

Fig. 17-11. Structural abnormalities of chromosomes depicted by ideograms. (From Gelehrter TD, Collins FS: *Principles of medical genetics,* Baltimore, 1990, Williams & Wilkins.)

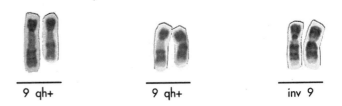

Fig. 17-12. Heterochromatin variants of chromosome 9. (Courtesy CC Morton, Department of Ob-Gyn, Brigham and Women's Hospital, Boston, Mass.)

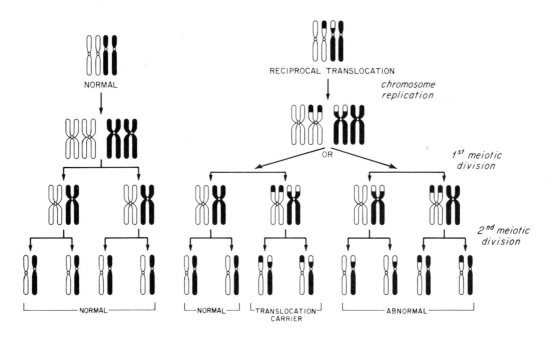

Fig. 17-13. Meiotic division of normal chromosomes and of chromosomes with reciprocal translocation. Shown are two of the four possible abnormal chromosomal complements resulting from random segregation of reciprocally translocated chromosomes.

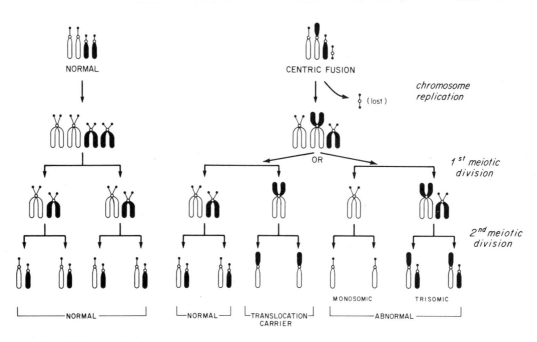

Fig. 17-14. Meiotic division of normal chromosomes and Robertsonian translocation. As in Fig. 17-13, two of the four possible abnormal chromosomal complements are illustrated.

pair (t21q21) carry an essentially 100% recurrence risk for trisomy 21 offspring.

Other structural abnormalities associated with abnormal phenotypes include *deletions,* such as those of the short arm of chromosome 5 that result in cri du chat syndrome. Although some deletions result from an unbalanced segregation from a reciprocal translocation, most chromosomal deletions arise de novo in the affected person. Loss of genetic material from any of the autosomes is characteristi-

cally associated with delays in physical and mental development in the offspring. Agents capable of breaking chromosomes in vitro (clastogens) include radiation, viruses, and some chemicals. However, among live neonates with chromosomal breaks and deletions, an etiologic agent has been difficult to establish.

When centromeres divide horizontally rather than longitudinally, the resultant chromosome contains mirror images of only one arm. Known as *isochromosomes,* these struc-

Table 17-3   Amniocentesis Results for Carriers of Reciprocal Translocation by Parental Origin and Method of Ascertainment

Ascertainment of Rearrangement	Maternal Origin (% Outcomes in Subsequent Pregnancies)			Paternal Origin (% Outcomes in Subsequent Pregnancies)		
	Balanced	*Normal*	*Unbalanced*	*Balanced*	*Normal*	*Unbalanced*
Term, unbalanced infant	41.2	38.9	19.8	40.3	37.5	27.2
Recurrent miscarriages	54.5	40.7	4.8	55.4	43.2	1.4

From Daniel A, Hook EB, Wulf G: Risks of unbalanced progeny at amniocentesis to carriers of chromosome rearrangments: Data from United States and Canadian Laboratories. *Am J Med Genet* 1989; 31:14.

turally abnormal chromosomes contain duplication of one arm and deficiency of the other arm. The most common example of this rearrangement is an isochromosome of the X chromosome (Simpson and Golbus, 1992).

In general, aberrations of autosomes, whether trisomies, deletions, or duplications, are associated with significant disorders in the development of the fetus. To varying degrees, autosomal chromosome abnormalities have in common mental retardation, somatic growth delay, increased structural malformations, and alterations of craniofacial development, leading to various degrees of dysmorphology. Persons with the same chromosomal abnormalities share a remarkable similarity, leading to specific recognizable phenotypes. Descriptions have been made of the various autosomal chromosomal syndromes (Jones, 1988; Yunis, 1977). Abnormalities of the sex chromosomes are discussed in detail in the section on disorders of sexual differentiation.

Mendelian Inheritance

For numerous inherited disorders, the association between the disease state and a specific abnormal protein led to sequencing of the responsible gene and identification of the DNA mutation. Advancements in the understanding of sickle-cell disease are representative of such progress. Eight years after the identification of a hemoglobin abnormality in persons with sickle-cell disease, abnormal electrophoretic migration of sickle hemoglobin was found to reflect an altered hemoglobin configuration. This hemoglobin abnormality resulted from an altered amino acid sequence soon identified to result from a single point mutation in the gene for β-globin (Vogel and Motulsky, 1986). Kan and Dozy (1978) performed prenatal diagnosis of sickle-cell disease by analyzing DNA polymorphisms closely linked to the site of mutation. Specific restriction enzymes that cleave within the sickle-cell gene now provide direct DNA diagnosis of sickle-cell disease (Chang and Yan, 1982).

Diagnostic Technologies

Although the ability to isolate DNA from human cells has existed for several decades, the process of gene identification did not progress substantially until fractionation of a vast quantity of DNA into smaller, more easily analyzed units was developed. Bacterial restriction enzymes (endonu-

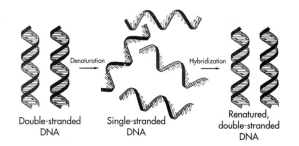

Fig. 17-15. The principle of nucleic acid hybridization. (From Thompson MW, McInnes RR, Willard HF: *Thompson and Thompson: Genetics in medicine,* ed 5, Philadelphia, 1991, WB Saunders.)

cleases), unique in the sequence of bases they recognize and cleave, can with predictable reproducibility separate the human genome into smaller fragments. Using techniques developed by Southern, the resultant segments can be physically separated by electrophoresis migration on agarose gel (Thompson et al, 1991).

Indirect Methodologies. DNA probe technology evolved to identify and retrieve specific sequences of DNA within segments produced by restriction endonucleases. Under appropriate conditions, *DNA probes* (DNA segments, sometimes sequenced, that have known locations on the human genome map) serve as complementary DNA in a denaturation-hybridization sequence (Fig. 17-15). Tagging the probe with a marker allows visual identification by radioactivity or fluorescence (Fig. 17-16) (Simpson and Golbus, 1992).

Restriction fragment length polymorphism (RFLP) is an extension of the concept of DNA fragmentation with endonuclease restriction enzymes and probe identification. In the noncoding regions of DNA, base sequence variation occurs once in every 200 base pairs (Jeffreys, 1979a; Jeffreys, 1979b). When changes in base sequence involve a restriction endonuclease site, thus altering cleaving, the resultant fragments change in size and gel mobility. Useful RFLP is highly variable (polymorphic), lowering the chance that two persons have the same variation at a specific restriction endonuclease site. For genetic diseases in which the DNA sequence has not been determined, RFLP analysis of affected persons and relatives may provide an indirect method of

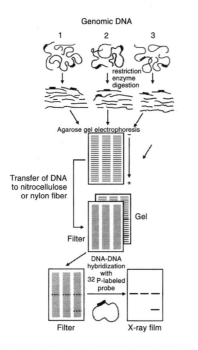

Fig. 17-16. The Southern blotting procedure for analyzing specific DNA sequences in a complex mixture of different sequences such as normal DNA. (From Thompson MW, McInnes RR, Willard HF: *Thompson and Thompson: Genetics in medicine,* ed 5, Philadelphia, 1991, WB Saunders.)

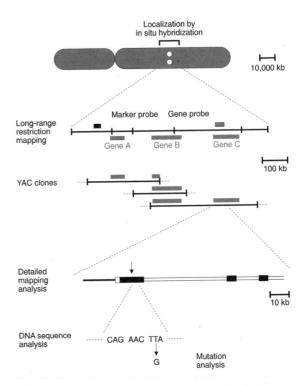

Fig. 17-17. Reversed genetics for cloning analysis of a hypothetical disease gene. (From Thompson MW, McInnes RR, Willard HF: *Thompson and Thompson: Genetics in medicine,* ed 5, Philadelphia, 1991, WB Saunders.)

tracking the abnormal gene through a family. As with genetic linkage, RFLP analysis is confounded by crossing over between the gene in question and the RFLP and the need for multiple family members who can supply that genetic information.

Direct Methodologies. Detection of a genetic disorder by direct analysis of the abnormal gene is the most straightforward approach. The disorders that were first detected by direct DNA analysis were those secondary to a deletion of DNA. Among them are α-thalessemia, Duchenne muscular dystrophy, Becker muscular dystrophy, cystic fibrosis (CF), and growth-hormone deficiency (Milunsky, 1993). Polymerase chain reaction technology has contributed to these advances because it amplifies a predetermined segment of DNA with oligonucleotide primers (short sequences of DNA) that flank the DNA under study (Saiki, 1985). In order to recognize a change in the DNA sequence that does not alter size by deletion or insertion additional steps are required. Provided the DNA mutation has been sequenced, allele-specific oligonucleotide probes can be developed. Once amplified by polymerase chain reaction, the DNA under study can be tested for hybridization pattern by normal and mutant allele-specific oligonucleotide probes to a given gene sequence. In this fashion, direct DNA diagnosis of Tay-Sachs disease (Myerowitz, 1988), α- and β-thalassemia (Kazazian and Boehm, 1988), CF (Kerem et al, 1989), and phenylketonuria is possible (Dilella et al, 1988).

Although direct DNA diagnosis requires knowledge of the mutated sequence, it is sometimes made without knowl-

edge of an associated abnormal protein or of how the disease symptoms are produced. Known as positional cloning (or reverse genetics), initially the abnormal sequence can be localized to a chromosome through somatic cell hybrids—cells that can be created to replicate with individual human chromosomes. In addition, gene mapping to areas of the karyotype can be accomplished with naturally occurring structural chromosome rearrangements and RFLPs. DNA sequences can then be isolated through yeast artificial chromosomes (YAC) (Thompson et al, 1991). This allows the eventual isolation and direct sequencing of the DNA under investigation (Fig. 17-17). Candidate genes for Duchenne muscular dystrophy, CF, and myotonic dystrophy have been sequenced in this fashion.

For many genetic disorders inherited in a mendelian fashion, DNA sequencing has revealed not one but several mutations in a specific gene locus. The molecular genetics of CF emphasize this concept. Sequencing of the DNA responsible for the abnormal protein associated with cystic fibrosis (CFTR) has revealed numerous possible sites of mutation, all of which culminate in CF symptoms. A DNA change at the Δ-508 position, the loss of three bases, is the most common cause of an abnormal CFTR protein in the white population. In persons of northern European heritage, 76% of the CF mutations are Δ-508. The remaining 24% of CF mutations in the white population result from other abnormalities in this gene. Currently, more 400 additional mutations have been identified, each of which is noted in only a minority of patients with CF (Milunsky, 1993). When all probes are analyzed, approximately 90% of CF mutations can be identified. Given the laws of segregation of genes within a population, these estimates are applicable only to the population from which they are derived, generally a northern European white population. Researchers are establishing the frequencies of these mutations in other populations in which CF is less common.

Patterns of Inheritance

A person's chance for inheriting a specific familial condition can be predicted based on Mendel's segregation laws of autosomal recessive, autosomal dominant, sex-linked recessive, or sex-linked dominant inheritance. A gene locus, the DNA sequence responsible for encoding a specific protein, is comprised of two alleles—the DNA sequence on the maternal chromosome and the companion DNA sequence on the paternal chromosome. In general, both alleles must be present for gene function to proceed normally. Production of a disease through the presence of two mutated alleles rather than one mutated allele determines whether the gene has characteristics of recessive or dominant inheritance. The presence of the alleles on sex chromosomes rather than on the autosomes governs some of the intricacies of trait expression based on the sex of the person.

Autosomal Recessive Traits. Often the condition produced by diseases with autosomal recessive inheritance manifests itself during infancy or childhood. Given the early presence of the disease state, the affected person's reproductive fitness and, thus, the capacity to pass mutated alleles to offspring often is limited. Most mutated alleles inherited in an autosomal recessive fashion exist in a population of asymptomatic heterozygotic carriers (Aa). Population studies have shown that everyone carries two to six recessive, deleterious genes in the heterozygotic state (Simpson and Golbus, 1992). Couples in whom both members are heterozygotic for the same abnormal genes have a 25% chance of an affected homozygotic child and a 75% chance of a clinically asymptomatic child. Unless testing proves otherwise, an unaffected sibling of a person with an autosomal recessive disease is thought to have a 66% chance of being a carrier (Fig. 17-18).

In any population, the probability that two random persons carry the same abnormal alleles is governed by two parameters. First, if the persons are related *(consanguineous),* a portion of their DNA is the same, depending on how many generations have intervened between them and their common ancestor. Brothers and sisters share 50% of their gene loci given their common parents, whereas uncles and nieces share 25% of their DNA and first cousins share 12.5%. Second, the gene frequency within a specific population influences the chance that any two persons are heterozygotic for the same recessive allele. For some recessive disorders, the gene may be common in one population, making the carrier frequency relatively high. In another population, the same gene may have a negligible frequency.

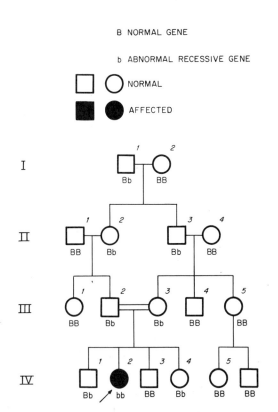

Fig. 17-18. Pedigree illustrating autosomal recessive inheritance.

Autosomal Dominant Traits. A trait or an abnormality produced by only one mutated allele at a gene locus is governed by autosomal dominant inheritance. Because each person with the trait has a normal and an abnormal allele at that locus, the affected person has a 50% chance of segregating the abnormal allele and a 50% chance of segregating the normal allele to offspring. Several characteristics of autosomal disorders can confound the interpretation of a pedigree. Autosomal dominant disorders may not display characteristics of the disease until after a person reaches reproductive age. Additionally, many autosomal disorders have reduced penetrance so that not all persons with the same mutated allele display the same characteristics. A minimally affected parent can have a severely affected child. These attributes of autosomal dominant inheritance can convey the impression that a disorder skips a generation. The intervening person may express minimal symptoms or may die of unrelated causes before symptoms develop. Rarely are dominant pedigrees as clear cut as those depicted in Fig. 17-19.

X-Linked Recessive Traits. X-chromatin inactivation and the Lyon hypothesis govern the intricacies of gene segregation on the sex chromosomes. Women have only one active X chromosome in any cell. Therefore, 46,XX inactivation occurs around the time of implantation, with random variability as to whether the maternally or paternally derived X chromosome is inactivated. All daughter cells, however, maintain the original inactivation. As the last chromosome to replicate in DNA synthesis, the extensive heterochromatin

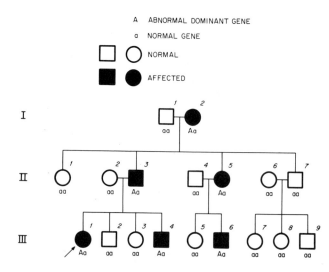

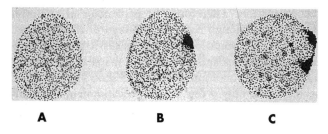

Fig. 17-19. Pedigree illustrating autosomal dominant inheritance.

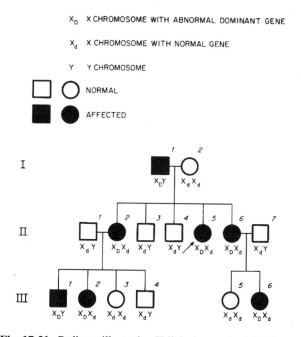

Fig. 17-21. Pedigree illustrating X-linked recessive inheritance.

Fig. 17-20. Sex chromatin (Barr body). **A,** The nucleus of a cell with no sex chromatin (usually a male). **B,** One Barr body (usually a female). **C,** Two Barr bodies (as found in fetuses with three X chromosomes). (From Cavalli-Sforza L, *Elements of human genetics,* Menlo Park, CA, 1977, WA Benjamin.)

of the inactive X chromosome remains visible in the interphase cell as a Barr body (Fig. 17-20). In addition, inactivation of the loci appears to be selective, with most but not all X-chromosome loci involved (Lyon, 1962). Loci for steroid sulfatase and ovarian maintenance determinants on the distal short arm are not inactivated (Simpson and Golbus, 1992). Cell type appears influential. X-inactivation does not occur in fetal germ cells, and there is preferential inactivation of the paternal X chromosome in cytotrophoblast cell lines (Harrison, 1989).

In women who are *heterozygous,* carriers of an X-linked recessive allele, one of two segregations can take place when gametes are formed. Half the gametes can receive the X chromosome with the abnormal allele, and half can receive the X chromosome with the normal allele. The sperm's contribution of either an X (resulting in an XX or female zygote) or a Y (resulting in an XY or male zygote) chromosome will determine whether the abnormal allele results in a carrier or an affected state, respectively. Males with only one X chromosome are considered *hemizygous,* and X-linked disorders will be expressed (Fig. 17-21).

In X-linked recessive disorders, new mutations are fairly common. For an isolated case of an X-linked disorder, the

mutation may have occurred at one of three sites, either on the X chromosome of the affected male offspring or on one of the two maternal X chromosomes. Unless confirmed by diagnostic testing, there is a two-thirds chance that the mother is the carrier of a new mutation X-linked disorder and a one-third chance that the mutation arose in her son. These numbers can be incorporated in a Bayesian calculation when empirically establishing the risk for carrier status in other female relatives. If two males in a family are affected, the intervening females are by definition obligate carriers who have a 50% chance of bearing affected sons and a 50% chance of bearing carrier daughters.

X-Linked Dominant Traits. Rarely have X-liked dominant traits been described. When they appear, females with one abnormal allele also express the disease. In two disorders, Rett syndrome and ornithine transcarbamoylase deficiency, severely affected males generally die shortly after birth (Thompson et al, 1991). Vitamin D-resistant rickets, also inherited as an X-linked dominant trait, though not leading to neonatal demise, displays a more severe course in males than in females (Fig. 17-22).

Multifactorial and Polygenic Inheritance

Many birth defects, though not attributable to a specific mendelian disorder or chromosome abnormality, display marked familial clustering. Exposure to a common environment, especially before birth, is sometimes invoked when several family members have children with the same nonmendelian birth defect, but the genetic constitution of the child also plays a role. Such disorders, referred to as *multifactorial,* include a great number of the isolated structural defects present at birth (Box 17-1).

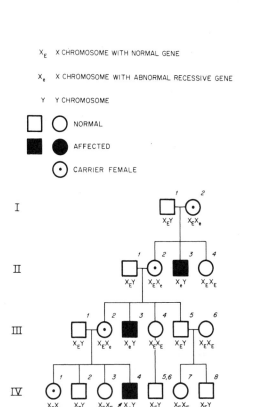

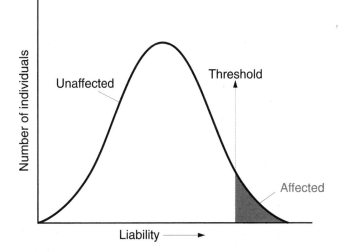

Fig. 17-23. Multifactorial threshold model. Liability to a trait is distributed normally, with a threshold dividing the population into unaffected and affected classes. (From Thompson MW, McInnes RR, Willard HF: *Thompson and Thompson: Genetics in medicine,* ed 5, Philadelphia, 1991, WB Saunders.)

Fig. 17-22. Pedigree illustrating X-linked dominant inheritance.

BOX 17-1
POLYGENIC AND MULTIFACTORIAL TRAITS

Neural tube defects (anencephaly, spina bifida, encephalocele)
Hydrocephaly (except some patients with aqueductal stenosis or Dandy-Walker syndrome)
Cleft lip, with or without cleft palate
Cleft lip (alone)
Cardiac defects (most types)
Diaphragmatic hernia
Omphalocele
Renal agenesis
Ureteral anomalies
Hypospadias (most forms)
Posterior urethral valves
Uterine (müllerian fusion) defects
Hip dislocation
Limb reduction defects (most forms)
Talipes equinovarus (clubfoot)

From Simpson JL, Golbus MS: *Genetics in obstetrics and gynecology,* ed 2, Philadelphia, 1992, WB Saunders.

For multifactorial disorders, twin studies have been useful for examining the role of environmental exposure and genetically determined thresholds (Fig. 17-23). Twins, given their shared prenatal environment, are exposed to the same background of possible deleterious environmental agents. For birth defects in which a genetically determined threshold plays a role, identical (monozygotic) twins would be expected to be similarly affected more often than nonidentical (dizygotic) twins. In general, multifactorial traits, with an approximately 1 in 1000 incidence in live births, have an average recurrence risk of 1% to 5% for both a similarly affected offspring and an affected parent to have an affected offspring. For traits that are more common in one of the sexes, an affected offspring of the less commonly affected sex carries a higher recurrence risk (Simpson and Golbus, 1992).

Polygenic inheritance, distinct from multifactorial, refers to the inheritance of continuously distributed traits controlled by multiple rather than by a single gene locus. Height, weight, blood pressure, age at menarche, and IQ are thought to be governed by polygenic inheritance. Embryonic control of cell growth and differentiation is likely to be polygenic, with alterations in the timing of cell division under genetic control. Familial tendencies for many continuous traits, such as height and weight, may reflect polygenic inheritance. An overlap of polygenic and multifactorial inheritance of noncontinuous traits (such as the birth defects in Box 17-1) may occur if genetically controlled timing of cell differentiation alters a fetus' susceptibility to environmental teratogens, which themselves produce damage only at particular stages (Simpson and Golbus, 1992).

Nonmendelian Inheritance
Mitochondrial

DNA of the mitochondria is circular and predominantly comprised of coding sequences. Thirteen structural genes have been located in the mitochondria. Mitochondria segregate in conjunction with the nucleus of an ovum but not of a sperm. Several diseases, including Leber hereditary optic

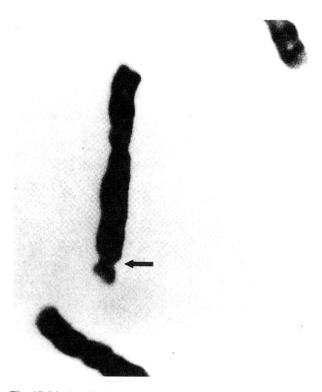

Fig. 17-24. Fragile X site produced under folic acid-deficient media conditions. (From Friedman JM, et al: *Genetics,* Baltimore, 1992, Williams & Wilkins.)

neuropathy, Leigh disease, and myoclonic epilepsy, have been mapped to mitochondrial DNA (Thompson et al, 1991). Inheritance in families is consistent with a cytoplasmic passage from only the mother to her offspring.

Unstable DNA

The transmission of DNA from parent to offspring has traditionally been viewed as a stable process. Alterations in DNA size were considered rare and, if they occurred, were thought to be stable. Several disorders are now recognized to be secondary to the control of gene expression by variable changes in DNA size.

Fragile X Syndrome. Males affected by fragile X syndrome, the most common cause of familial mental retardation, are characterized by large ears and testes, a prominent jaw, and moderate to severe mental retardation (Turner et al, 1986; Webb, 1989). The syndrome is associated with an X chromosome-fragile site (Xq27.3) that can be induced under folate-deficient culture conditions (Fig. 17-24). In affected males and carriers, evidence of the fragile site is variable, and there is a wide range of cells (5% to 60%) that display a break on the long arm of the X chromosome (Sutherland, 1997). Although a locus mapped to the X chromosome is involved, family studies reveal that the abnormal gene is passed through normal transmitting males who are not symptomatic and who do not have cytogenetic evidence of a fragile site. Similarly, in contrast to most X-linked disorders, a large percentage of carrier females can be affected and up

to 35% have mental retardation. Within a family the same X-chromosome mutation in a normal transmitting male, a carrier female, or an affected male producing widely variable phenotypic effects is known as *Sherman's paradox* (Sherman et al, 1985; Sherman et al, 1984).

Initial investigations of the fragile site found the suspect region to be hypermethylated in affected males but not in normal transmitting or unaffected males (Bell et al, 1991; Oberle et al, 1991; Vincent et al, 1991). Sequencing of this region revealed an abundance of cytidine phosphate guanosine (CpG) dinucleotides that, when methylated, halted the expression of adjacent genes (Toniolo et al, 1988). Sequencing within the region of the fragile X identified tandemly arranged arrays of trinucleotides (p[CGG]n) of variable length (Kremer et al, 1991). Direct DNA analysis of families with fragile X found that the largest trinucleotide fragments were associated with the abnormal methylation and full fragile X phenotype. Smaller increases in the fragment length (premutations) were identified in normal transmitting males who had normal methylation patterns and only rare instances of mental retardation. In females, carriers of the premutation had a 3% incidence of mental retardation; those carrying the full mutation had a 50% frequency of mental retardation (Rousseau et al, 1991). Predictions as to the degree of phenotypic expression of the full mutation in females are confounded by X inactivation.

Uniparental Disomy

Uniparental disomy, in which each member of a chromosome pair originates from one parent, was a theory originally proposed by Engel in 1980. Uniparental disomy establishes the potential for single parent contribution of both alleles at a given locus. Because this theory was a radical departure from mendelian biparental inheritance, it received little attention until a decade later when polymorphic DNA probes discerned the parental origin of chromosomes and cases of uniparental inheritance were reported (Engel and DeLozier-Blanchet, 1991). Uniparental origin of a chromosome pair could occur through gamete complementation (fertilization of gametes with complementary loss and gain involving the same chromosome pair) or monosomic duplication or in a conceptus that was initially trisomic. With reference to the latter, postzygotic loss of a chromosome in an originally trisomic conceptus is supported by several reports of uniparental disomy after the documentation of trisomy on chorionic villus sampling (Purvis-Smith et al, 1992; Spence, 1988).

Within a uniparental chromosome pair, each chromosome can be genetically identical (*isodisomy*). This condition results from a nondisjunctional event during a second meiotic division or from a postzygotic nondisjunctional event. Alternatively, each chromosome can be genetically dissimilar (*heterodisomy*) after a first meiotic nondisjunctional event (Spence et al, 1988). Clinical situations that defy mendelian theory and possibly are explained by uniparental disomy include the following:

- Autosomal recessive disorders in the offspring of couples in whom only one parent is a heterozygotic carrier. At least two cases have bee reported of uniparental isodisomy for chromosome 7, which resulted in cystic fibrosis in a child with only one carrier parent (Spence et al, 1988; Voss et al, 1989).
- Transmission of an X-linked disorder from a father to a son as a result of uniparental inheritance of both the X and the Y chromosomes from the father. One case of hemophilia A was reported in a father and a son (Vidaud et al, 1989).
- Expression of X-linked disorders in daughters as a result of inheriting both X chromosomes from a carrier mother.
- Uncovering of imprinted alleles (see below).

Imprinting

At some loci, alterations in gene expression occur not by structural changes in the DNA sequence but as a result of the transient silencing of gene function. When this process occurs during gametogenesis, such modifications are known as imprinting. Imprinted genes produce differences in gene expression determined by parental origin. In mice, at least one quarter of the genome appears to undergo imprinting in which methylation plays a role (Swain et al, 1987; Sapienza, 1989). Imprinted loci appear to undergo selective suppression during oogenesis and spermatogenesis, which can be reversed in somatic cells (Cattanach and Kirk, 1985).

In humans imprinted genes are now recognized by the different phenotypic effects produced, dependent on whether the gene is inherited from the mother or the father. Uniparental disomy, as described in the preceding section, is one mechanism by which imprinted genes may produce abnormal states. The different phenotypes of maternally versus paternally derived uniparental disomy, leading to the Prader-Willi and Angelman syndromes, was one of the first sets of disease states to reflect the uncovering of imprinted genes by uniparental disomy. In Prader-Willi syndrome (PWS), the most common dysmorphic form of obesity, maternal uniparental disomy of the region results in only maternal alleles (and thus no paternal alleles) at the critical site, 15q11q13 (Mascari et al, 1992; Nicholls et al, 1989). Both maternal heterodisomy (two different number 15 homologues from the mother) and maternal isodisomy (identical number 15 homologues from the mother) have been reported, which argues against the supposition that phenotypes result solely from uniparental isodisomy of a recessive gene. More likely, the critical region in PWS is normally imprinted with the inactivation of one set of alleles, resulting in functional hemizygosity. The characteristic PWS phenotype results from the lack of paternal allele at a specific region (15qllql3), either through the presence of a visible or microscopic deletion of the paternal number 15 or through the presence of two copies of the maternal number 15 as a result of uniparental disomy. Similar investigations in Angelman syndrome have also revealed uniparental disomy of chromosome 15 (Malcolm et al, 1991). However, characterized

by dysmorphia, severe mental retardation, paroxysms of laughter, and seizures, Angelman syndrome is phenotypically distinct from PWS (Knoll et al, 1989; Williams et al, 1989). It arises from the lack of maternal genes at a critical region, the one in proximity to that involved in PWS (Malcolm et al, 1991). Paternal uniparental disomy and, thus, functional maternal nullisomy at this region have now been reported in Angelman syndrome (Malcolm et al, 1991; Nicholls et al, 1989). Based on the known location of imprinted genes in the mouse genome and on established homologies between murine and human karyotypes, a role for imprinting has been postulated for several human disease states (Searle et al, 1989). In addition, imprinting may play a fundamental role in human growth potential and survival. In animals, imprinting at certain loci is a critical process for the balanced expression of genes because it affects cell growth and differentiation (Surani, 1991). In at least one overgrowth syndrome, Beckwith-Wiedemann syndrome, which is characterized by gigantism, macroglossia, hemihypertrophy, and visceromegaly, abnormalities of imprinting have been implicated. It has been mapped to 11p15.5, a region that contains insulin-like growth factor 2 (IGF-2), which plays a role in maintaining the proper control of cell growth (Little et al, 1991). IGF-2 is recognized as an imprinted gene with only the paternally derived allele expressed, even though alleles from both parents are present. In three eighths of patients with Beckwith-Wiedemann syndrome, paternal uniparental disomy of region 11p15.5 supports the theory that overexpression of the paternally imprinted IGF-2 is instrumental in the overgrowth noted in this syndrome (Henry et al, 1991).

GENETICS IN GYNECOLOGIC PRACTICE
Disorders of Sexual Differentiation
Embryology

Determination of sexual development is dependent on two factors, the composition of the sex chromosome pair and the proper functioning of autosomal genes controlling sex-differentiating hormones. Sexual differentiation follows an orderly sequence of events. At 6 weeks of development, genital cells migrate from an extraembryonic location to the gonadal ridges and become surrounded by sex cords to form primitive gonads (Thompson et al, 1991). Further differentiation of the bipotential gonad is directed by a testis-determining factor (TDF), most likely a single gene product. Without functional TDF, the gonad differentiates as an ovary. The H-Y antigen on the long arm of the Y chromosome was initially proposed as the TDF. However, current investigation supports the sex-determining region on the short arm of the chromosome as the site for the TDF (Simpson and Golbus, 1992). However, TDF does not operate alone because genes on both the X chromosome and the autosomes are crucial in the differentiation of the testes.

Without TDF the undifferentiated gonad at 6 weeks differentiates into an ovary by 8 weeks (Fig. 17-25). The

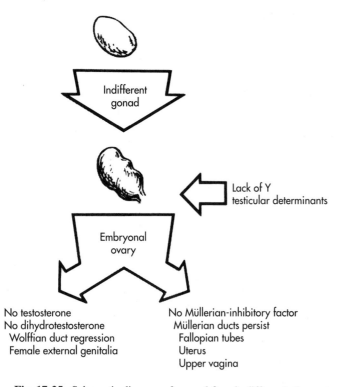

Indifferent gonad

Lack of Y testicular determinants

Embryonal ovary

No testosterone
No dihydrotestosterone
Wolffian duct regression
Female external genitalia

No Müllerian-inhibitory factor
Müllerian ducts persist
Fallopian tubes
Uterus
Upper vagina

Fig. 17-25. Schematic diagram of normal female differentiation. (From Simpson JL, Golbus M: *Genetics in obstetrics and gynecology,* ed 2, Philadelphia, 1992, WB Saunders).

development of the ovary and its germ cells results not from the presence of the two X chromosomes but from the lack of the Y chromosome short arm and TDF. In Turner fetuses with only one X chromosome, ovaries with germ cells develop only to undergo attrition before birth. Thus, although two X chromosomes are not needed to initiate and accomplish ovarian differentiation, they are required for the maintenance of ovarian differentiation. Gene loci for ovarian maintenance are located on both the short and the long arms of the X chromosome and on an autosome (Simpson, 1976). Concomitant with germ cell migration, orderly thickening of the genital ridges occurs and forms the mesonephric (wolffian) and paramesonephric (müllerian) ducts. In the male, the differentiation of seminiferous tubules and Leydig cells is governed by genes separate from those that control gonadal differentiation (Patsavoudi et al, 1985). Progression of the wolffian ducts into the tubular structures of the testes (vas deferens epididymides and seminal vesicles) is initiated by the production of testosterone by the fetal Leydig cells. Leydig cell testosterone production is triggered by placental human chorionic gonadotropin (hCG). Exogenous testosterone at this gestational age results in male tubular differentiation, regardless of the sex chromosome complement. Simultaneous resolution of the müllerian structures (precursors of the uterus and fallopian tubes) is governed by antimüllerian glycoprotein from the Sertoli cells. This glyco-

protein is controlled by a gene located on an autosome (Simpson and Golbus, 1992). Without testosterone and the antimüllerian glycoprotein of the Sertoli cells, and in fact in the complete absence of gonadal development, the fetus develops ductal and genital structures along a female line.

Clinical Disorders of Sexual Differentiation

Disorders of sexual differentiation are numerous, and persons who seek treatment may have normal male, normal female, or ambiguous genitalia. For the practicing gynecologist, disorders of sexual differentiation are generally encountered in women with primary amenorrhea. Evaluations for primary amenorrhea most likely disclose women with gonadal dysgenesis (45,X, 46,XX, or 47,XY), male pseudohermaphroditism, or rare sex chromosome aneuploidies. Less often the gynecologist will have to be familiar with disorders of newborn or childhood genital ambiguity and, in some instances of infertility evaluations, the disorders of sexual differentiation despite male genitalia. The following sections present the mechanisms, clinical characteristics, and variable expressions of these disorders. In-depth reviews can be found in Simpson (Simpson, 1976; Simpson and Golbus, 1992), and the multiple malformation syndromes involving ambiguous genitalia are delineated in Jones (1988).

Gonadal Dysgenesis. Replacement of the gonads by fibrous tissue devoid of germ cells (streak gonads) occurs with 45,X, 46,XX, and 46,XY karyotypes. When identified during evaluation for primary amenorrhea, it is seen that in 40% of patients gonadal dysgenesis results from 45,X, 40% of patients have 46,XX or 46,XY complements, and the remaining 20% have structural rearrangements of the X chromosome (Simpson, 1976). Common to all patients with gonadal dysgenesis, regardless of the karyotype, is the development of female external genitalia, uterus, and fallopian tubes. Because all lack the development of gonadal tissue, elevated levels of gonadotropins are present. Somatic variations in the associated structural abnormalities and phenotypes reflect the differing karyotypes.

The *Turner, 45,X* phenotype, depicted in Fig. 17-26, is characterized by short stature, amenorrhea, and usually normal intelligence. Additional features are presented in Table 17-4. The basis for short stature in the Turner syndrome remains unknown, though loci on a homologous region of the short arms of the X and Y chromosomes may play a role. Because this region does not undergo X inactivation, persons with monosomy X have half the usual number of alleles at this locus (Fisher et al, 1990). Recently, children with monosomy X were treated with human recombinant DNA-derived growth factor to increase their average adult height. However, an underlying abnormality in epiphyseal plates may limit eventual adult height (Simpson and Golbus, 1992). Most persons with monosomy X have normal intelligence, though many score poorly on spatial visual testing. Adult diseases such as hypertension (in one third of adults

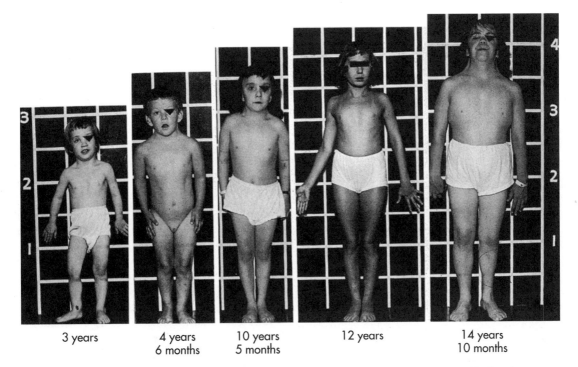

3 years	4 years 6 months	10 years 5 months	12 years	14 years 10 months

Fig. 17-26. Five girls with Turner syndrome. Note the variability of such features as webbed neck and broad chest. (From Jones KL: *Smith's recognizable pattern of malformation*, ed 4, Philadelphia, 1988, WB Saunders.)

with monosomy X) and diabetes should be considered in the long-term health management of these patients.

Generally, ovarian function in Turner syndrome is absent, and there is markedly decreased estrogen and androgen production in the presence of elevated gonadotropins. Without estrogen stimulation at puberty, several somatic features of Turner syndrome are predictable, including decreased quantities of pubic and axillary hair, scant breast tissue, pale areolae, and failure of the müllerian derivatives and external genitalia to differentiate from infantile to adult states (Cornet, 1990; Simpson and Golbus, 1992).

Ovarian function, as reflected by menstruation and breast development in persons with monosomy X, is rarely reported (<5%). In such incidences, undetected mosaic cell lines with normal female complements (46,XX) are proposed but usually not documented. Women with a known combination of 46,XX and 45,X cells (mosaicism) have been shown to have a greater (12%) chance of menstruating, taller adult height, and fewer somatic anomalies (Simpson and Golbus, 1992). Without assisted reproduction in persons with nonmosaic 45,X cells, pregnancy rarely occurs. Whether the incidence of chromosomally abnormal offspring is increased remains unclear because few cases have been studied (Dewhurst, 1978; Simpson and Golbus, 1992). Alternatively, estrogen and cyclic progesterone replacement at puberty can lead to a normal uterine size and to successful pregnancy with donor oocytes (Cornet et al, 1990).

Table 17-4   Turner Phenotype: Major Features and Their Incidence

Feature	Incidence (%)
Small stature, often noted at birth	100
Ovarian dysgenesis with variable degrees of hypoplasia of germinal elements	90+
Transient congenital lymphedema, especially notable over the dorsum of the hands and feet	80+
Shield-like, broad chest with widely spaced, inverted, or hypoplastic nipples	80+
Prominent auricles	80+
Low posterior hairline, giving the appearance of a short neck	80+
Webbing of posterior neck	50
Anomalies of elbow, including cubitus valgus	70
Short metacarpal or metatarsal	50
Narrow, hyperconvex, or deeply set nails	70
Renal anomalies	60+
Cardiac anomalies (coarction of the aorta ination of aorta in 70% of patients)	20+
Perceptual hearing loss	50

From Jones OW, Cahill TC: Basic genetics and patterns of inheritance. In Creasy RK, Resnick R, editors: *Maternal fetal medicine,* Philadelphia, 1994, WB Saunders.

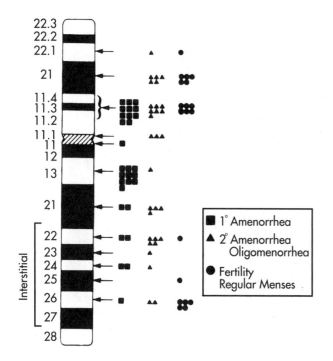

Fig. 17-27. Schematic diagram of X-chromosome showing ovarian function by site of structural abnormality. (From Simpson JL: *Disorders of sexual differentiation: Etiology and delineation,* New York, 1976, Academic Press).

Although a 45,X karyotype results in the full phenotype of Turner syndrome with gonadal dysgenesis and the characteristic constellation of somatic changes (Fig. 17-27), structural abnormalities of the X chromosome can produce some or all of the features of Turner syndrome. Comparison of these structural changes in the X chromosome have enabled delineation of the determinant regions for ovarian maintenance and structural growth (Fig. 17-27) (Wyss et al, 1982). Persons with deletions of the X-chromosome short arm (46,X,del[X]p or 46,X,i[Xq]) generally have a combination of gonadal dysgenesis, short stature, and Turner phenotype. Various deletions of the long arm of the X chromosome suggest an additional site of ovarian function determination. Affected persons have either gonadal dysgenesis or premature ovarian failure, though their adult height is usually normal (Simpson and Golbus, 1992).

Familial gonadal dysgenesis, XX type, develops in karyotypically normal females (46,XX). As in Turner syndrome and other forms of gonadal dysgenesis, affected persons have streak gonads and lack estrogenization of the external female genitalia and the müllerian derivatives. Because it is inherited as an autosomal recessive trait, the first sign is usually primary amenorrhea; normal height and lack of somatic anomalies preclude earlier diagnosis (Purvis-Smith et al, 1992; Simpson, 1976). Autosomal recessive inheritance suggests additional non-X-chromosome gene locations that govern ovarian maintenance. Another component of more complex syndromes may be 46,XX gonadal dysgenesis, such as neurosensory deafness (Perrault syndrome) (Nishi,

1988), with myopathy (Lundgren, 1976), cerebellar ataxia (Skre et al, 1976), and microcephaly-arachnodactyly (Maximilian et al, 1970).

Gonadal dysgenesis with a male karyotype *(Swyer syndrome, 46,XY)* includes features previously described as common to gonadal dysgenesis. Because it is not associated somatic anomalies, when patients seek treatment for primary amenorrhea, the condition is clinically and biochemically indistinguishable from 46,XX gonadal dysgenesis. Loss of testicular tissue before 7 to 8 weeks of gestation appears to be the underlying abnormality. Various modes of inheritance have been proposed, including X-linked recessive and autosomal recessive (Chemke et al, 1970; Espiner et al, 1970; Simpson and Golbus, 1992). The initial differentiation of testicular tissue in the gonad, despite replacement by fibrosis, places these patients at increased risk (20% to 30%) for dysgerminoma or gonadoblastoma. Although an association between the H-Y antigen and the development of neoplasia has been noted (Wachtel, 1983), all patients with 46,XY gonadal dysgenesis should be counseled about gonadectomy, even though retention of the uterus and tubes will allow for future reproductive function by assisted reproductive technologies (Cornet, 1990).

Female Pseudohermaphroditism. Appearing as a discordance between external genitalia and well-differentiated internal gonadal structures, female pseudohermaphrodites have a 46,XX karyotype, masculinized external genitalia, and differentiated ovaries. In general, the karyotype and the internal ductal structures correspond to the gonad: female pseudo-hermaphrodites have ovaries and paramesonephric derivatives (uterus, tubes, upper vagina), regardless of their external genitalia. With some exceptions, female pseudohermaphrodites typically are diagnosed during the newborn or infancy period, when partial virilization of the external genitalia results in ambiguous sexual identification.

Female pseudohermaphroditism can result from exposure to testosterone or its derivatives, either endogenously through a hormonal abnormality or exogenously through maternally ingested hormones. The development of normal ovaries in conjunction with müllerian structures argues against an underlying sex chromosome abnormality. Clinically, the genitalia are characterized by clitoromegaly, displacement of the urethra, and labial fusion. Common hormonal imbalances that produce increased testosterone levels and virilization in affected females are the *adrenogenital syndromes.* Multiple inherited enzyme abnormalities along the pathway of cortisol production from cholesterol can occur. The specific enzyme defect indicates whether other metabolic perturbations are also present (Fig. 17-28). Two deficiencies, one in 21-hydroxylase and one in 11 β-hydroxylase, account for 90% and 5% of congenital adrenal hyperplasia (Levine and Pang, 1993). Although the enzyme deficiencies of the adrenogenital syndrome are inherited in an autosomal recessive fashion with males and females equally affected, only female newborns exhibit evidence of testosterone excess. Production of the adrenal enzymes be-

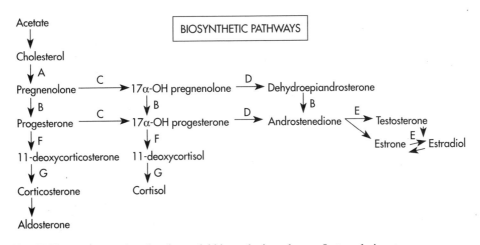

Fig. 17-28. Important adrenal and gonadal biosynthetic pathways. Letters designate enzymes required for the appropriate conversions. A, 20-α-hydroxylase, 22-α-hydroxylase, and 20,22-desmolase. B, 38-β-ol-dehydrogenase. C, 17-α-hydroxylase. D, 17, 20-desmolase. E, 17-keto-steroid reductase. F, 21-hydroxylase. G, 11-hydroxylase. (From Simpson JL: *Disorders of sexual differentiation: Etiology and clinical delineation,* New York, Academic Press, 1976. Reproduced with permission.)

gins by 8 to 9 weeks of gestation so that elevated quantities of testosterone in utero can result in a virilized female newborn with intact müllerian structures and ovaries. Although a few males may be detected at birth to have the increased pigmentation that results from the melanocyte-stimulating properties of adrenocorticotropic hormone, in male newborns without the complications of salt wasting, the diagnosis may otherwise be unsuspected (Simpson and Golbus, 1992).

With a 25% recurrence risk, the prenatal diagnosis of 21-hydroxylase deficiency allows for the detection and the potential treatment of affected females to prevent virilization. Maternal dexamethasone to suppress the fetal pituitary-adrenal axis is needed by 5 weeks' gestation. Either chorionic villus sampling or amniocentesis can then establish the fetal sex and the 21-hydroxylase status by DNA analysis. Affected female fetuses would have to be maintained on maternal dexamethasone therapy (Fig. 17-29). Reported series of such treatment plans have yielded variable results. In approximately two thirds of patients, virilization has been prevented or reduced. However, in one third of patients, virilization was not abated because of differences in dosing regimens, interruptions in medication, delay in treatment, or variability in maternal steroid metabolism (Levine and Pang, 1993). Dexamethasone therapy requires appropriate surveillance for maternal side effects, and the long-term consequences for the fetus remain unexplored.

Exogenous ingestion of masculinizing substances can produce female pseudohermaphroditism. During prenatal development, it has been shown that maternally administered synthetic progestins result in virilization of the female fetus (Grumbach et al, 1959). Testosterone, ethinyl testosterone, norethindrone acetate, and norethindrone, (the latter two are components of several oral contraceptives) may pro-

duce virilization, depending on the dose and the timing of exposure. Rarely associated with virilization are norethynodrel, medroxyprogesterone and 17α-OH-progesterone caproate (Simpson and Golbus, 1992). Maternal tumors rarely virilize a female fetus because women with tumors seldom become pregnant.

Male Pseudohermaphroditism. With a 46,XY karyotype, testes, and female external genitalia, male pseudohermaphrodites also have tubular derivatives corresponding to their internal gonad. In general, their well-differentiated testes are accompanied by mesonephric derivatives (vas deferens epididymides, and seminal vesicles). Rarely is this seen in the newborn with ambiguous genitalia. More often, male pseudohermaphrodites is observed when girls seek treatment for primary amenorrhea; they have normal female or ambiguous genitalia but lack evidence of müllerian structures.

Complete androgen insensitivity (*complete testicular feminization*) is a form of male pseudohermaphroditism. During an evaluation for primary amenorrhea, affected persons can be identified by their lack of müllerian derivatives (absent uterus, tubes, and upper vagina). Their female appearance is characterized by breast development, though the areola is pale, pubic and axillary hair is scant, and the vaginal pouch is shortened. Testes can be documented abdominally in the inguinal canal or in the labia. There is an increased (5%) risk for testicular carcinoma, which typically develops in the second or third decade (Simpson, 1987). Complete testicular feminization syndrome results from end-organ insensitivity to androgens even with normal testosterone levels. In most persons, androgen receptors are absent, but less often a nonfunctional receptor is present. The testosterone receptor gene is located on the X chromosome, and several mutations within this gene are described

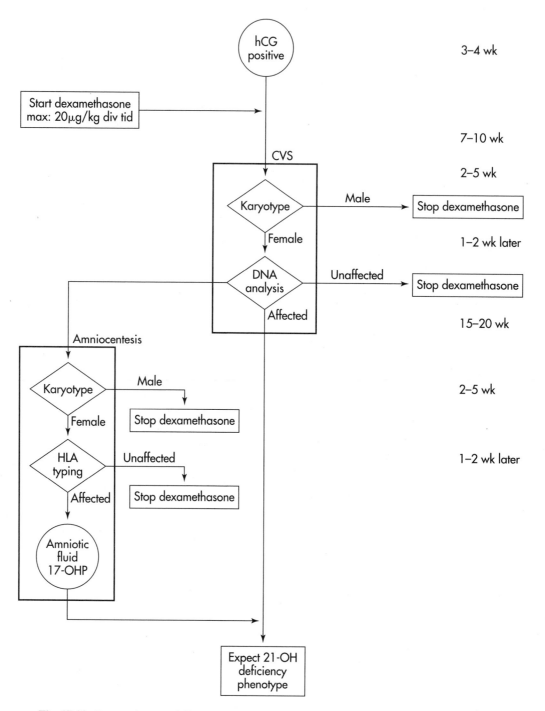

Fig. 17-29. Proposed protocol for management in pregnant women whose fetuses are at risk for congenital adrenal hyperplasia from 21-hydroxylase deficiency. (From Speiser PW, Laforgia N, Kato K, et al: First trimester prenatal treatment and molecular genetic diagnosis of congenital adrenal hyperplasia [21-hydroxylase deficiency]. *J Clin Endocrinol Metab* 1990; 70:838-848.) Copyright © The Endocrine Society.

(Pinsky et al, 1989). Inherited in an X-linked recessive fashion, affected males display complete testicular feminization whereas carrier females generally do not have discernible clinical abnormalities.

Mutations in other regions of the androgen-binding gene can produce partial androgen insensitivity. Also inherited as an X-linked recessive condition, *partial testicular feminiza-*

tion is characterized by initially male or ambiguous genitalia that undergoes feminization and is accompanied by breast development at puberty. As occurs with complete feminization, testes are present though often not descended, müllerian derivatives are absent, and pubertal virilization with development of the secondary sex characteristics fails to occur. Either decreased numbers of androgen receptors or qualitative abnormalities of the receptors have been proposed (Pinsky and Kaufman, 1985).

Less common in an office gynecology practice but encountered in newborns with ambiguous genitalia is male pseudohermaphroditism, caused by *5α-reductase deficiency*. In this condition, although external genitalia may be ambiguous at birth and even a perineal opening resembling a vaginal dimple may exist, müllerian structures are lacking, and at puberty normal virilization occurs. Gynecomastia is absent, in contrast to its presence in other forms of male pseudohermaphroditism. Inherited in an autosomal recessive fashion, male pseudohermaphroditism is caused by a deficiency of 5α-reductase, the enzyme needed for the conversion of testosterone to dihydrotestosterone. Lack of dihydrotestosterone leads to poor virilization of the fetal external genitalia, though testosterone alone is sufficient for the maintenance of the wolffian structures. At puberty the increases in testosterone result in subsequent virilization even in the absence of adequate levels of dihydrotestosterone (Peterson et al, 1977; Simpson and Golbus, 1992).

True Hermaphroditism. The presence of ovarian and testicular tissue and variable external genitalia characterizes true hermaphroditism. Generally, a uterus is present though anomalies of uterine horn development are common. Sufficient normal ovarian tissue may exist to produce estrogen for breast development, menstruation, and ovulation. Conversely, though the testicular tissue produces testosterone and virilization of the external genitalia, it is generally devoid of spermatozoa. Most true hermaphrodites have a normal female karyotype (46,XX); others have various combinations of XY and XX cell lines. Chimerism, the presence of two-cell lines as a result of fusion between two zygotes, has been documented in human twin pairs of opposite sex and may represent one etiology of true hermaphroditism (de la Chapelle, 1988).

Aneuploidies of Sex Chromosomes

Persons with *45,X/46,XY* mosaicism may have Turner phenotypes or ambiguous genitalia or may appear as normally male. In 45,X/46,XY persons with Turner stigmata, given the presence of the 46,XY cell line, the streak gonads are at risk for carcinoma. Neoplasia, which occurrs in 15% to 20% of patients, develops during the first and second decades. Gonadectomy with the retention of müllerian structures to aid in assisted reproduction potential is recommended (Simpson and Golbus, 1992). 45,X/46,XY characteristics may also resemble mixed gonadal dysgenesis and include a streak gonad and dysgenic testes. Especially if it is diagnosed before birth, the most common outcome of 45,X/46,XY is a normal male phenotype. The risk for gonadal carcinoma in these persons is markedly lower; gonadectomy is generally not suggested unless a close clinical evaluation of intrascrotal testes can be performed (Simpson and Golbus, 1992).

Polysomy of the X chromosome *(47,XXX)* happens most often in persons with normal female genitalia. The addi-

tional X chromosome allows proper ovarian maintenance through embryonic and fetal development, though delayed menarche and premature ovarian failure are common. Polysomy of the X chromosome is associated with mental retardation of varying degrees. Persons with polysomy sometimes have IQ levels slightly lower than those of unaffected siblings. With additional X chromosomes (48,XXXX), the prevalence of mental retardation increases; mental delay is always present in persons with 49,XXXXX (Robinson et al, 1979).

Sex chromosome abnormalities with normal or near normal male external genitalia include Klinefelter syndrome (47,XXY). Uncommonly encountered by gynecologists, this condition occurs in 1 in 1000 live male newborns and is identified in 1 in 10 azoospermic males. It is characterized generally by normal male external genitalia in the presence of poorly developed facial hair, female distribution of body fat, and slightly taller than average height (Fig. 17-30). Mental retardation and additional somatic anomalies may develop in some persons. Two thirds of XXY persons are thought to have learning disabilities. Low levels of testosterone are characteristic, and seminiferous tubule degeneration leads to small testes.

Similarly, persons with *47,XYY* also have with normal male external genitalia, taller-than-average height, and azoospermia despite normal testosterone levels. Intelligence may be decreased. The relationship of 47,XYY to mental retardation, mental illness, and antisocial behavior continues to be debated. Although the risk for abnormal behavior is not as high as originally estimated (Jacobs et al, 1965), the rate of incarceration of 47,XYY males continues to be 10 times greater than for 46,XY males (Simpson and Golbus, 1992). However, when 47,XYY males were compared with 46,XY males of comparably reduced intelligence, the percentage of criminal behavior was not found to be different (Witkin et al, 1976).

Reproductive Loss
Spontaneous Miscarriage

Recent studies show that almost one third (31%) of all pregnancies are lost in the first trimester. In a group of women followed up with serial hCG measurements from the time of implantation, a 22% rate of loss before clinical recognition of the pregnancy and a 9% loss rate thereafter was documented (Wilcox et al, 1988). Researchers have long appreciated that chromosome abnormalities have occurred in at least 50% of the latter subgroup of clinically recognized pregnancies lost in the first trimester (Boué et al, 1976). Among losses before the clinical recognition of pregnancy, the frequency of chromosome abnormalities has been more difficult to establish. Karyotype analysis of two- to eight-cell human embryos obtained by in vitro fertilization supports a high rate of chromosome abnormalities in prerecognition losses. Studies have shown that exact numbers remain unclear (Plachot et al, 1987). Autosomal trisomies are the most common cause of karyotypically abnormal

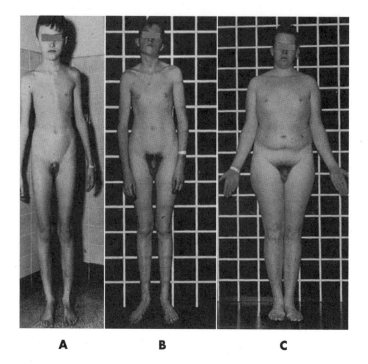

Fig. 17-30. XXY syndrome. **A,** 9-year-old child with XXY syndrome. **B,** 16-year-old with XXY syndrome. **C,** 21-year-old adult with XXY syndrome. (From Jones KL: *Smith's recognizable pattern of malformation,* ed 3, Philadelphia, 1988, WB Saunders.)

Table 17-5   Relative Frequencies of Aberrations in Chromosomally Abnormal Abortuses

Type	Frequency (Approximate) (%)
Aneuploidy	
45,X	20
Autosomal monosomy	<1
Autosomal trisomy	
Total	52
Trisomy 16	16
Trisomy 18	3
Trisomy 21	5
Trisomy 22	5
Other trisomies	23
Triploidy	16
Tetraploidy	6
Structural rearrangements	4

From Thompson MW, McInnes RR, Willard HF. In Thompson and Thompson, editors: Genetics in medicine, ed 5, Philadelphia, 1991, WB Saunders, p. 216. Data chiefly from Boue J, Gropp A: Cytogenetics of pregnancy wastage. *Ann Rev Genet* 1985;14:1-57.

first-trimester miscarriages (50%), with trisomy 16 the most common individual trisomy (Table 17-5). The most common single abnormality is 45,X, and it is identified in 20% of losses (Thompson et al, 1991). Based on the rate of Turner syndrome among live newborns, more than 90% of 45,X concepti are lost through spontaneous abortion. Characteristically, 45,X concepti lost during the first trimester exhibit a

lack of embryonic development with the placenta containing thrombi and hypoplastic villi (Honoré et al, 1976). Later in gestation, a spontaneously aborted fetus with Turner syndrome often is seen to have fetal cystic hygromas and edema. Advanced maternal age is not a feature of Turner syndrome; monosomy X usually results from the loss of the paternal X chromosome (Chandley, 1981).

Pregnancy losses with a triploid complement typically result from dispermy, the fertilization of a normal ovum with two sperm. However, meiotic nondisjunction in either parent may also occur, and cells of the resultant embryo will contain 69 chromosomes. The placenta in triploids with an additional paternal complement is generally hydropic and shows cystic degeneration. Focal hydropic placenta and focal trophoblastic hyperplasia in a fetus constitutes a partial mole, and the current treatment of gestational trophoblastic disease is recommended. In triploidy resulting from an additional maternal complement, severe growth retardation with a small, poorly formed placenta has been seen (McFadden and Kalousek, 1991). These differences between paternally and maternally derived triploids suggest a human example of the imprinting phenomenon observed in mice.

Karyotype analysis of a spontaneous loss often reveals an abnormality. In the rare situations in which an unbalanced structural rearrangement is detected (1.5%), additional evaluation of the couple may reveal that one member is a balanced translocation carrier. For those couples with a karyotypic abnormality, the risk for a subsequent live birth with a karyotype abnormality continues to be debated. Initially, studies of women with a karyotypically abnormal sponta-

Table 17-6   Rate of Chromosome Translocations Among Men with Oligospermia

Author (Year)	(Oligospermia ×10⁶)	N	Autosomal Translocations (%)	Sex Chromosomes (%)	Total Abnormal (%)
Matsuda (1992)	<20	326	11(3.4)	5(1.5)	4.9
Micic (1984)	<20	464	7(1.5)	0	1.5
Bourrouillou (1987)	10-20	406	2(0.5)	0	0.5
Bourrouillou (1987)	<10	594	23(3.9)	11(1.9)	5.8
Abyholm (1981)	<10	180	6(3.3)	5(2.7)	6.1

neous loss followed by a second spontaneous loss were interpreted as showing an 80% likelihood that a second loss would be karyotypically abnormal as well (Hassold, 1980). Reanalysis at the second miscarriage, with adjustment for maternal age, refuted the significance of this earlier finding (Warburton et al, 1987). However, a 1% risk for a live newborn with trisomy 21 after an aneuploid spontaneous loss has been documented in one series (Alberman, 1981). Comparably, after the live birth of a child with trisomy 21, a woman younger than 30 years has a 1% risk for giving birth to a newborn with a nondisjunction event (Stene and Mikkelsen, 1984). Through amniocentesis, parallel evidence from couples with two spontaneous losses and normal parental karyotypes reveals a 1.6% nondisjunction risk versus a 0.3% risk for maternal age-matched controls (Drugan et al, 1990). Underlying mechanisms such as gonadal mosaicism or an inherited tendency to nondisjunction through action on the spindle fibers have been proposed as causes.

Recurrent Spontaneous Abortion

Among couples experiencing repeated spontaneous abortion, balanced translocations are identified in approximately 3% of the women and 2% of the men. This rate is slightly lower if only couples who did not give birth to a live newborn are considered (women 2.4% and men 1.6%). Of note, in one study, if multiple miscarriages occurred in conjunction with a stillbirth or a previous abnormal live newborn, the frequency of translocations increased to 16.7% (Schwartz and Palmer, 1983). A recent review of more than 22,000 couples with two or more spontaneous losses found balanced structural rearrangements in 4.7% (De Braekeleer and Dao, 1990).

Infertility

Oligospermia as the cause of a couple's infertility raises several genetic concerns. As shown in Table 17-6, among men with oligospermia, peripheral blood karyotypes reveal an increased rate of chromosome abnormality (Abyholm, 1981; Bourrouillou et al, 1987; Matsuda et al, 1992; Micic 1984). Abnormal findings are predominantly autosomal reciprocal and Robertsonian translocations, without preference for any specific autosome. The lower the sperm count, the greater the likelihood of a peripheral blood chromosome abnormality. Severe levels of oligospermia (<10 × 10⁶) are associ-

Table 17-7   Rates of Cystic Fibrosis Mutations in Men with Congenital Absence of the Vas Deferens

Author (Year)	N	1 Mutation (%)	2 Mutations (%)	No Mutations (%)
Patrizio (1993)	44	50	9	41
Oates (1994)	49	63	18	18
Mercier (1995)	67	42	24	34
Casals (1995)	30	63	10	27
Chillon (1995)	102	53	19	28

ated with the greatest risk for peripheral blood chromosome translocations (Bourrouillou, 1987). When the partners of these men spontaneously become pregnant, the risk for passing an unbalanced chromosome to the fetus is relatively small (5% to 6%). However, intracytoplasmic sperm injection may circumvent a natural protective mechanism against fertilization by aneuploid sperm, and the true risk for an unbalanced segregation in the intracytoplasmic sperm injection-conceived fetuses may be higher.

Another cause of male infertility is congenital bilateral absence of the vas deferens. Because more than 400 mutations of the CF gene are now recognized, the presence of at least the carrier state, if not the homozygotic affected CF state, is identified in most men with congenital bilateral absence of the vas deferens (Table 17-7). Many investigators think it alone may be one manifestation of the mildest spectrum of CF. Given the carrier frequency of CF in the white population (1 in 29), if a man with congenital bilateral absence of the vas deferens is found to carry one or two mutations of the CF gene, couples may want to pursue DNA testing before proceeding with intracytoplasmic sperm injections. The population-specific limitations of current testing, with the ability to detect most but not all of the mutations of the CF gene, must be considered in calculating a couple's chance of giving birth to a child with CF.

Common Gynecologic Variants and Disorders
Physiological Variants

Polygenic inheritance, in which multiple gene loci function to control a continuous trait, may play a role in the inheritance of the age of menarche. Twin studies have shown identical twins are more similar (concordant) in their menarche age than are nonidentical twins. Elaborate quantitative twin studies have demonstrated that 65% of the variation in timing of menarche is caused by genetic influence (Simpson and Golbus, 1992).

Müllerian Abnormalities

As a result of altered timing of mesonephric duct formation, abnormalities in the development of the müllerian system can occur. Because the defect involves only the fusion of the tubules to form the uterine body, cervix, and upper vagina, normal development is seen in the ovaries and the fallopian tubes, and the external genitalia are feminized. Defects include aplasia, duplication, and incomplete fusion, which can be present as an isolated defect or as a component of several dysmorphology syndromes (Simpson and Golbus, 1992).

True müllerian aplasia *(Rokitansky-Küster-Hauser syndrome)* results in the absence of the upper vagina, cervix, and uterus and the presence of normal ovaries, remnant uterine cords, and feminized external genitalia with a blind vaginal pouch. Renal anomalies such as pelvic kidney and unilateral aplasia develop in 40% of patients, and vertebral anomalies are common. This disorder may be inherited in a polygenic fashion. Theories of autosomal recession and X-linked dominance have been proposed but generally are not accepted for all families (Simpson and Golbus, 1992). True duplication of the müllerian system is rare and involves two separate uteri, each of which possesses two fallopian tubes. More commonly, incomplete fusion of the müllerian system gives rise to two uterine horns, each with only one fallopian tube. In general, if renal anomalies occur, they are seen on the ipsilateral side with the atretic horn. Incomplete fusion anomalies occur in 1 in 1000 female fetuses, and a polygenic inheritance pattern seems likely.

Endometriosis

Although studies of endometriosis have been complicated by biases of ascertainment, difficulty in diagnosis, and population specificities, an inherited tendency to this disease process has been suspected (Gardner et al, 1953). Multifactorial inheritance has been suggested by a 7% recurrence rate among first-degree relatives of affected persons, but incomplete penetrance with a mendelian inheritance pattern has not been excluded (Simpson, 1987). Similarly, concordance in severity among affected persons supports the theory of an inherited disease process (Malinak et al, 1980).

Polycystic Ovarian Syndrome

Although the diagnosis of polycystic ovarian syndrome (PCO) often represents a heterogeneous collection of women, several of the adrenal cortical enzyme abnormalities can resemble a PCO-like clinical picture. Adult-onset 21-hydroxylase deficiency, partial 17α-hydroxylase, and 3β-ol-dehydrogenase may each be accompanied by PCO symptomatology. In essential PCO, a dominant inheritance

pattern, either autosomal or X-linked, has been proposed by some investigators (Simpson and Golbus, 1992). Additional studies with control of population characteristics, diagnostic parameters, and biases will be needed.

Premature Ovarian Failure

Structural abnormalities of the X chromosome and rare cases of XX gonadal dysgenesis can accompany premature ovarian failure. In addition, familial aggregates of premature ovarian failure without chromosome abnormalities exist. Initial studies revealed a greater incidence of POF in women who are carriers of fragile X, though this has not been replicated in all studies (Vianna-Morgante, 1996; Partington, 1996; Kenneson, 1997).

Gynecologic Cancers

The role of inheritance in gynecologic cancer reflects two principles of cancer genetics, Knudson's "two-hit" hypothesis and the identification of cancer genes. During the past 20 years they have been investigated extensively in families with cancer. Although familial aggregates of various cancers, including gynecologic, have been recognized for decades, the contributions of environmental exposure and inherited tendency have yet to be resolved. Most cancers are clonal in origin, arising from a single cell (Fialkow, 1972). With reference to gynecologic neoplasms, both carcinoma of the cervix and leiomyomata have been shown to result from multiple divisions of one cell. Given the premise of single-cell origin of neoplasms, Knudson proposed a two-step process of DNA mutation that leads to uncontrolled cell division (Knudson et al, 1973). In families with aggregates of cancer, the first step most likely is an inherited mutation. In isolated cases of cancer, the first step probably occurs as an acquired mutation from exposure to known oncogens such as radiation, viruses, or chemicals. In each situation, the second step was thought to be an acquired mutation. In familial cancers, though the mutation (Knudson's first step) may be inherited in a mendelian fashion, the development of cancer is dependent on a second mutational event (Fig. 17-31). This theory is also applicable to families whose multiple members have different forms of cancer (Simpson and Golbus, 1992; Thompson et al, 1991).

A second principle integral to the understanding of inherited cancers has been the recent identification of cancer genes, both *oncogenes* and *tumor suppressor genes.* Oncogenes, genomic sequences known to transform normal cells to tumor cells, initially were identified in viruses. Also found in the human genome, oncogenes have close sequence homology to genes that normally control growth and embryonic development. *Protooncogenes* are genomic sequences that become functional oncogenes (c-*onc*) through several mechanisms. Physical relocation of protooncogenes that involve a chromosome translocation may result in the release of surrounding regulatory controls (Guy et al, 1990). Alternatively, incorporation into the human genome of a viral oncogene may trigger protooncogene transformation to a

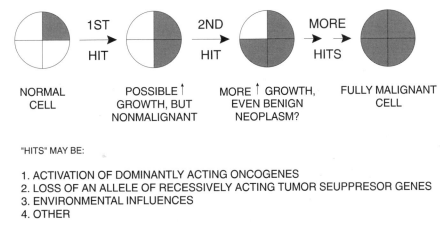

"HITS" MAY BE:

1. ACTIVATION OF DOMINANTLY ACTING ONCOGENES
2. LOSS OF AN ALLELE OF RECESSIVELY ACTING TUMOR SEUPPRESOR GENES
3. ENVIRONMENTAL INFLUENCES
4. OTHER

Fig. 17-31. Diagram of multistep origin of cancer. (From Gelehrter TD, Collins FS: *Principles of medical genetics*, Baltimore, 1990, Williams & Wilkins.)

c-*onc*. Additionally, long terminal repeat sequences have been identified and proposed as triggering factors if they are inserted near a protooncogene (Savard et al, 1987). Oncogenes have been reported in association with embryonal ovarian carcinoma, squamous cervical carcinoma, endometrial adenocarcinoma, ovarian epithelial carcinoma, and choriocarcinoma (Simpson and Golbus, 1992).

Tumor-suppressor genes play a role in cancer through the regulation of genes controlling cell growth. Loss of function of tumor-suppressor genes, which are normally responsible for blocking cell growth, can contribute to malignancy through uninhibited cell growth. The role of tumor-suppressor genes in gynecologic cancer is unknown. Most of the evidence of these genes is found in familial colon cancer, Wilms tumor, and neurofibromatosis (type I) (Thompson et al, 1991).

Ovarian Carcinoma

With regard to specific cancers, the strongest evidence for genetic predisposition to a gynecologic cancer occurs with ovarian epithelial carcinoma. Serous and mucinous forms are the most common, whereas the endometrial form is rarely encountered. However, among families with aggregates of ovarian cancer, serous or undifferentiated types predominate (Simpson and Golbus, 1992). Also supporting the inherited component in familial aggregates are younger age of onset and increased bilaterality of disease (Franceschi et al, 1982).

Chromosome abnormalities that have the potential for translocation of a protooncogene site and thus for activation to an oncogene are commonly seen in transformed ovarian tissue (Wake et al, 1980). A t(6:14)(q21;q24) translocation has been the most commonly reported. Evidence exists as well for alterations of two specific oncogenes, c-*myc* and c-K-*ras*-2 (Filmus and Buick, 1985).

Given the limited means for prospective clinical surveillance, the poor response to therapy, and the significant mortality rates associated with ovarian carcinoma, determination of the risk faced by additional female family members

Table 17-8   Cumulative Age of Risk for Ovarian Cancer in Carriers of BRCA1 and BRCA2 Mutations by Means of Ascertainment

Cumulative Risk	30 Yrs (%)	40 Yrs (%)	60 Yrs (%)	70 Yrs (%)	Lifetime Risk (%)
BRCA1, high risk	0.2	0.6	23	30	63
BRCA1, selected	0	1	13	16	16
BRCA2, high risk	—	—	—	—	10
BRCA2, selected	—	5	8	15	15
Neither, selected	—	—	—	—	1.5

of a person with ovarian carcinoma continues to be pursued. Epidemiologic studies have suggested that 5% to 10% of ovarian cancers have a hereditary basis (Lynch et al, 1987). In rare instances, ovarian cancer is a component of a multiple organ cancer profile such as Peutz-Jeghers syndrome. Affected persons with this dominant inherited disorder have defects of serine-threonine kinase with gastrointestinal polyposis and various forms of cancer including breast, uterus, and ovary. More recently, specific mutations have been found in association with breast and ovarian cancer. These mutations, BRCA1 and BRCA2, were sequenced in 1994 and generally result in truncation of the BRCA1 protein (Albertson, 1994; Jones, 1994). More than 200 mutations have been identified. The functional role of the identified protein is still under investigation. One major hypothesis is that these genes play a role in DNA damage repair and that mutations in this protein alter needed DNA repair mechanisms, setting the stage for unrepaired DNA damaged by extraneous sources. Because these mutations have been identified in families at high risk for breast cancer, the degree of risk conferred by mutations in persons without such family history is still being explored (Table 17-8).

For women with BRCA mutations, consideration is often given to prophylactic oophorectomy once childbearing is completed or at menopause. This approach is based on the rationale that the increased relative risk does not rise until later in life and that the modalities for surveillance of ovarian cancer are limited. Recent decision analysis revealed that if a woman with a BRCA1 or BRCA2 mutation undergoes prophylactic oophorectomy by age 40 (but not after age 60), her life expectancy could be expected to increase by 0.3 to 1.7 years (Schrag, 1997).

For nonepithelial ovarian carcinoma, limited evidence supports an inherited etiology in only benign cystic teratoma and ovarian stroma neoplasias (granulosa cell, Sertoli-Leydig, and fibromas. The bilaterality of benign cystic teratoma (dermoids) suggests an inherited predisposition, and there have been reports of multiple affected family members (Simon et al, 1985). Teratomas originate through parthenogenesis, development from a single germ cell that then undergoes self-replication. Analysis of chromosome markers has shown that dermoids most likely originate from either lack of second polar body formation or reincorporation of the second polar body (Linder et al, 1975).

Gestational Trophoblast Disease

Gestational trophoblast disease (GTD) includes hydatidiform mole, invasive mole, and choriocarcinoma. Whether partial or complete, hydatidiform moles are characterized by avascular hydropic villi and are considered a benign form of GTD. However, 15% of complete moles and 4% of partial moles develop persistent gestational trophoblastic tumor. Partial moles are characteristically triploid (total chromosome count, 69) and almost invariably contain an additional set of haploid chromosomes inherited from the father. Triploid fetuses with the additional complement derived from the mother do not display molar changes but are characterized by severe fetal growth retardation (McFadden and Kalousek, 1991).

In contrast, though complete moles are characteristically diploid, they do not have the normal biparental contribution of chromosomes. The solely paternal origin of the diploid complement in complete moles usually arises from fertilization of an ovum devoid of maternal DNA. Despite the appropriate number of chromosomes, the lack of biparental contribution of the genome, specifically the lack of maternally imprinted chromosomes, leads to the production of hydropic villa and lack of fetal development. These findings are analogous to the classic murine studies in which androgenically produced mice—those created by duplication of the paternal genome without maternal chromosomal contribution—fail to form an organized fetus (Surani et al, 1984).

The recurrence of GTD, whether hydatidiform mole, invasive mole, or choriocarcinoma, appears to be increased over the incidence in the general population. Recurrence of complete moles and partial moles has been reported (Honoré, 1987; Honoré et al, 1988). The risk for recurrence has been estimated at 1.3%, but a possible bias favoring repetitive cases may exist (Sand et al, 1984). Additional studies have shown a recurrence of 28% after two pregnan-

cies complicated by a gestational trophoblast neoplasm (Simpson and Golbus, 1992). More than one family member has been reported with GTD though the significance of these family aggregates has not been studied in a consistent fashion (LeVecchia et al, 1982).

Genetic Screening in Gynecologic Practice
Genetic Diseases of Adult Onset

Assessment of a person's genetic composition to formulate the most appropriate intervention and treatment plan is gaining increased attention. Although many gene mutations produce a specific disease state, most changes in DNA sequences operate at a more subtle level. For many loci, there are now recognized common mutations that may only slightly alter the intrinsic properties of a protein. However, these mutations, in combination with environmental factors or other genetic mutations, culminate in the production of commonly encountered disorders. Genes associated with hypertension, such as Alzheimer disease, thrombosis, and atherosclerosis, have been identified.

Specifically for the gynecologist, one increasingly common situation involves the identification of inherited predispositions to thrombosis. In these patients, oral contraceptives may increase the risk for thrombosis. Until the increased lifetime risk for venous thrombosis with factor V Leiden deficiency was identified, the increased risk for thrombosis through inherited disorders such as protein S, protein C, and antithrombin III was considered rare. However, factor V Leiden mutation leading to activated protein C resistance is present in 4% to 8% of white persons and poses a lifetime risk for thrombosis that is 5 to 7 times greater than in the rest of the population. Among women who have thrombotic events before or after giving birth, the 46.6% rate of factor V Leiden mutation is 4 to 5 times higher than in the rest of the population (Hallack, 1997). However, screening all women for factor V Leiden mutation before prescribing oral contraceptives has not been supported by all centers (Hellegren, 1995; Price, 1997). However, because the prevalence of factor V Leiden deficiency is relatively common, it can be expected that patients have two or more clotting abnormalities. A small portion of the population with factor V Leiden deficiency has concomitant deficiencies of protein S, protein C, and antithrombin III. Combined deficiencies place patients at even greater risk for thrombosis at younger age (Dahlback, 1996). Additionally, patients with homozygotic factor V Leiden deficiency have an eightyfold increased risk for thrombosis (Rosendall, 1995). Taking a family history to identify thrombotic events may help identify patients for whom further testing is needed before oral contraceptives are initiated.

Preconception Counseling

Gynecologists are often provided with an ideal opportunity to undertake preconception counseling with their patients. Although many women seek birth control, this is often a temporary measure because they hope for pregnancy in the

Table 17-9   Disorders of Increased Prevalence Among Persons with Common Heritage

Disorder	Advisory	Population to Screen	Screening Test to Use
Hemoglobinopathies (sickle cell, SC, thalassemias)	ACOG (1996)	• All but those of Northern European ancestry • Universal screening not recommended but at low risk are northern European, Japanese, Inuit (Eskimo), Native American	• MCV (<80) and hemoglobin electrophoresis • Sickle dex inadequate for primary screening
Cystic fibrosis	NIH Consensus Panel (5/97)	• Prenatal population and couples planning pregnancy	• DNA from any source (cheek brushes, peripheral blood, archival cells); >400 mutations identified
	Am College Medical Genetics (11/97)	• Preliminary report: General population screening is premature, but education should be initiated now to assimilate screening into practice over the next 1-3 years	
Tay Sach Disease	ACOG (11/95)	• Serum screening before pregnancy if both partners are of Ashkenazi Jewish, French Canadian, or Cajun descent	• In women who are pregnant or taking oral contraceptives, leukocyte testing must be used
Canava	ACMG (1/98)		DNA analysis

future. Additionally, some women may be attempting to become pregnant or may be undergoing infertility evaluations. All of these situations provide an opportunity to review the patient's and her partner's family, medical, and social histories to determine whether genetic preconception counseling is needed. Whether the gynecologist conducts the counseling or refers the patient to a geneticist or a genetic counselor, identifying the woman at risk is essential. For the specific techniques and risks of prenatal diagnostic testing, the reader is referred to several comprehensive reviews (D'Alton and DeCherney, 1993; Evans et al, 1989; Milunsky, 1993).

Population-Specific Genetic Screening

Closely tied to the scientific initiative to map the entire human genome has been an ongoing effort to ensure balanced integration of genetic testing concepts by patients and providers. A recent task force report from one such group, Ethical, Legal and Social Issues, proposes that written consent be obtained from patients undergoing genetic testing and that testing only be performed by physicians with proven competence in genetics. In addition to becoming familiar with the increasing numbers of disease states for which DNA testing is available, physicians must acquaint themselves and their patients with the concepts of genetic testing. An understanding of the limitations of the test, the influence of heritage on accurate gene determination, the po-

tential insurance and employment implications of the information disclosed, and the impact on family members also at risk should be considered before genetic studies for any disorder are initiated (Elias, 1994).

In populations of various heritages, specific inherited diseases occur with increased frequency (Table 17-9). Determining who should be offered genetic screening and for what disorders remains a complex decision. Influencing the decision are factors such as disease severity, frequency of the carrier state, percentage of carriers detected by available testing, potential for the diagnosis to impact the disease course, and cost of testing. For some disorders, guidelines from various associations, including the American College of Obstetrics and Gynecology and the College of Medical Genetics, are available for the most common disorders. Cystic fibrosis may be of sufficient prevalence to warrant screening in all populations, but constraints concerning lower detection rates in nonwhite populations remain.

Risk for Chromosome Disorders

The association between advanced maternal age and chromosome abnormalities has long been recognized. Although an infant with chromosome abnormalities can be born to a mother of any age, at maternal age 35 years, the risk for trisomy 21 at midtrimester is 1 in 260. This is approximately equal to the 1 in 200 to 400 risk for pregnancy loss after midtrimester amniocentesis. If all chromosome disorders

Table 17-10   Prospective Studies of Maternal Serum Triple Panels for Trisomy 21 (Down Syndrome)

Author (Year)	N	Initial Positive Screen (%)	Positive after Ultrasonography* (%)	Trisomy 21 Detected (%)	PPV (%)
Haddow (1992)	25,207	6.6	3.8	58	2.6
Wald et al (1988)	11,993	4.9	3.3	39	1.7
Phillips et al (1992)	9,993	7.0	3.2	57	1.9

PPV, positive predictive value at amniocentesis.
*Confirmation of gestational age.

are considered, at maternal age 32 years, the risk for a fetus with chromosome abnormalities is 1 in 280. Multiple gestation is not associated with an increased risk for chromosome abnormalities. However, if twins are dizygotic, the risk that either will have trisomy 21 (rarely do both have it) is 1 in 270 at maternal age 32 years (Rodis, 1990).

Sometimes there is an increased risk for chromosome abnormality because of the mother's obstetric history. If a woman has given birth to a live newborn with a nondisjunctional event, or if a parental balanced translocation has been identified, the risk increases for offspring with chromosomal abnormalities. Controversy remains about whether there is an increased risk for aneuploidy in an infant. Factors thought to be associated with such an increased risk are two previous miscarriages (even if both parents have normal karyotypes), previous birth of an infant with triploidy, previous macerated stillbirth without known karyotype, and previous spontaneous abortion of a fetus with chromosome abnormalities. Studies supporting and refuting the increased risk in these situations are discussed elsewhere in this chapter.

For women younger than 35, maternal serum analysis of α-fetoprotein, β-hCG, and estriol provides a screening method for those who may have an infant with trisomy 21. Prospective studies of maternal serum screening have shown that approximately 60% of infants with trisomy 21 have been born to women younger than 35 who have positive results of triple-panel screening (Table 17-10). By comparison, amniocentesis performed in women 35 or older at the time of delivery only detects 20% of infants with Down syndrome. Careful counseling must be part of screening programs for women older than 35 because maternal serum screening does not detect all cases of Down syndrome. It has been estimated that in 20% of women older than 35 who give birth to infants with Down syndrome, results of serum screening are normal (Wald et al, 1992). Other chromosome abnormalities also are associated with an increase in maternal age, and their detection by the serum panel is less well defined. Analysis of fetal chromosomes only by chorionic villus sampling or amniocentesis provides complete detection of chromosome abnormalities if women are 35 years or older at delivery.

Risk for Mendelian Disorders. Gynecologists should be familiar with the more common X-linked recessive disorders, such as Duchenne and Becker muscular dystrophy and the hemophilias. In addition, the complexities of the in-

heritance of fragile X syndrome should be kept in mind when reviewing a patient's family history if members have been diagnosed with mental retardation and, in some cases, developmental delay and autism. Given the rapid advances in genetic testing with DNA analysis, older technologies may have been used if carrier testing was performed in families in the past, and it is recommended that testing be repeated. Additionally, though direct DNA studies are available for some X-linked disorders, tests for a linkage with RFLP may have to be performed. Especially when analyzing multiple family members, it is advantageous to initiate such carrier testing before a pregnancy occurs.

It is rare for an abnormal autosomal recessive gene to segregate to a family, as evidenced by the previous birth of a homozygotic child. The preponderance of children with autosomal recessive disorders are born to couples who are not known to be carriers and to families in whom there is no history of a similarly affected child and no evidence of consanguinity. To this end, screening of persons for autosomal recessive alleles based on the parameters discussed has gained increasing attention.

In many autosomal dominant disorders, disease manifestation often occurs later in life. For this reason, a careful family history is needed to ascertain persons who may be carrying a dominant mutation but are as yet unaffected. These persons may benefit because the disease itself may pose additional risk during pregnancy and because there is a 50% risk for an affected offspring. Family studies with linked markers may be available, or, in an increasing number of cases, direct DNA diagnoses can be offered. Dominant disorders that may be encountered by the gynecologist include Marfan syndrome, myotonic dystrophy, Huntington disease, and adult-onset polycystic kidney disease.

Risk for Multifactorial Diseases

In general, if a couple has one child with a multifactorial birth defect or if the parents themselves are affected, the chance that a subsequent offspring will be similarly affected is approximately 3%. This estimate can be refined for specific conditions based on further knowledge of the defect as in recurrence risks in cardiac anomalies (Table 17-11).

Neural Tube Defects. Although most neural tube defects are presumed to be multifactorial and there is an associated 3% recurrence rate, some are seen in conjunction with a chromosome abnormality or as a component of a genetic

Table 17-11   Recurrence Risks in Cardiac Anomalies

Anomaly	Normal Parents and One Affected Offspring (%)	Affected Parent and No Previously Affected Offspring (%)	
		Mother	Father
Ventricular septal defect	4.4	9.5	2.1
Patent ductus arteriosus	3.4	4.1	2.3
Tetralogy of Fallot	2.7	2.6	1.4
Atrial septal defect	3.2	4.6	1.5
Pulmonic stenosis	2.9	6.5	1.8
Aortic stenosis, valvular	2.2	17.9	2.8
Aortic coarctation	1.8	4.1	1.9
Transposition of the great vessels	1.9		
Atrioventricular canal anomaly (endocardial cushion defect)	2.6		
Tricuspid valve	1.0		
Tricuspid valve, Ebstein anomaly	1.1		
	1.1		
Truncus arteriosus	1.2		
Pulmonary atresia	1.3		
Endocardial fibroelastosis	3.8		

From Nora JJ: Etiologic factors in congenital heart disease. *Pediatr Clin North Am* 1971; 18:1059; Nora JJ, Nora AH: *Genetics and counseling in cardiovascular diseases,* Springfield, 1978, Charles C Thomas (recurrence risk is applied to offspring in this tabulation); Simpson JL, Golbus MS: *Genetics in obstetrics and gynecology,* ed 2, Philadelphia, 1992, WB Saunders.

disorder. Attempts should be made to obtain the karyotype and autopsy results on previously affected infants.

Maternal folic acid supplementation can lower the recurrence risk for neural tube defects in women with a previously affected infant. If supplementation is initiated before conception, the ingestion of 4 mg folic acid per day decreases the chance for recurrence by 72% (MRC Vitamin Study Research Group, 1991). Multivitamins with a lower dose of folic acid (0.36 mg/day) were found to be similarly effective in reducing the risk for neural tube defects in women who did and did not give birth to a previously affected infant (Milunsky et al, 1989). Folic acid supplementation (0.4 to 1 mg per day) for all pregnant women should be considered. Given the early gestational timing of neural tube development, folic acid supplementation must be initiated before conception. With the exception of women with unrecognized B_{12} deficiency, a relatively rare condition among healthy women of reproductive age, 1 to 4 mg folic acid supplementation is not thought to be associated with maternal side effects.

Women at Risk for Teratogen Exposure
Maternal Diseases

Women who are considering becoming pregnant but who have an ongoing medical illness can face an increased risk for giving birth to a child with a congenital anomaly because of the disease process or because of the teratogenic effects of medications needed to treat the disease.

Insulin-dependent diabetes (IDDM) is one disorder in which a teratogenic risk is associated with the disease process itself. Since the mid-1960s, a twofold to threefold increase in congenital malformations has been observed among the children of women with IDDM. Subsequently, several investigators have shown that if IDDM is poorly controlled, reflected by increased hemoglobin A_{1c} levels, children of those patients have the highest rates of malformation (Greene et al, 1989; Ylinen et al, 1984). The mechanism of teratogenicity in poorly controlled IDDM remains unclear. Insulin is not considered teratogenic, and hyperglycemia does not appear to be the sole mechanism. Interactions with other metabolites have been postulated (Sadler, 1980; Sadler et al, 1983). Although there can be a range of anomalies, rates for specific malformations such as caudal regression, situs inversus viscerum, and neural tube defects are increased thirtyfold to 200-fold (Kucera, 1971). Because these anomalies are caused by teratogenic insults within 6 weeks of ovulation, preconception counseling and glycemic control can result in a lower rate of malformation (Gregory and Tattersall, 1992).

If a woman with IDDM is planning pregnancy, patient education or a change in medication can reduce her exposure to medications with proposed or proven teratogenic effects. Phenytoin (hydantoin) is a recognized teratogen associated with a twofold increase in major and minor malformations, specifically developmental delay, skeletal anomalies, cardiac defects, and cleft lip or palate. Other anticonvulsants also have teratogenic effects. Valproic acid has been associated with a characteristic facial dysmorphia, cardiovascular anomalies, and neural tube defects. Carbamazepine recently has been associated with facial dysmorphia and neural tube defects (Jones et al, 1989; Rosa, 1991). A common pathway for the association of birth defects with many of the anticonvulsants may be their involvement in the epoxide pathway. Epoxide itself, rather than the specific anticonvulsant, may be the teratogenic agent. In infants with deficiencies of the epoxide hydrolase enzyme and exposed in utero to anticonvulsants, the highest rate of fetal hydantoin syndrome is noted (Buehler et al, 1990). Changes or discontinuations of anticonvulsants are best attempted before a pregnancy; discontinuation should be considered if it is feasible. If it is not, a change to an agent with a lesser rate of congenital malformations may be possible.

Medications that have teratogenic potential are indicated in Box 17-2. Although patients often reveal during routine history taking that they are taking teratogenic medications for illness, more specific questioning may be necessary for them to disclose that they are taking others such as isotretinoin, an acne medication with known teratogenic potential. Discontinuing or altering the dose of potentially teratogenic medications may be appropriate if a pregnancy is planned. In other patients, specific attention to the continued

BOX 17-2
CHEMICAL TERATOGENS

Definite Relationship to Fetal Abnormalities

Alcohol
Diphenylhydantoin
Folic acid antagonists
Inorganic iodides
Lithium
Organic mercury
Retinoic acid and related compounds
Sex steroids (virilization of female fetuses)
Streptomycin
Tetracyclines
Thalidomide
Thiourea compounds
Trimethadione
Valproic acid
Warfarin

Probable Relationship to Fetal Abnormalities

Alkylating agents
Carbamazepine
Chlorobiphenyls
Aminoglycosides (kanamycin, gentamycin, neomycin)
Methimazole

Possible Relationship to Fetal Abnormalities (Unproven Claims)

Amphetamines
Chlordiazepoxide
Cigarette smoking
Clomiphene
Diazepam
Diphenydramine
Ethionamide
General anesthesia (chronic exposure)
Meprobamate
Metronidazole
Oral hypoglycemic agents
Penicillamine
Phenothiazines
Quinine

No Relationship to Fetal Abnormalities (Proven Safety)

Bendectin
Corticosteroids
General anesthesia (short-term exposure)
Heparin
Isoniazid
Meclizine
Penicillin
Phenobarbital
Sulfonamides
Sex steroids (nongenital anomalies)

From Simpson JL, Globus MS: *Genetics in obstetrics and gynecology*, ed 2, Philadelphia, 1992, WB Saunders.

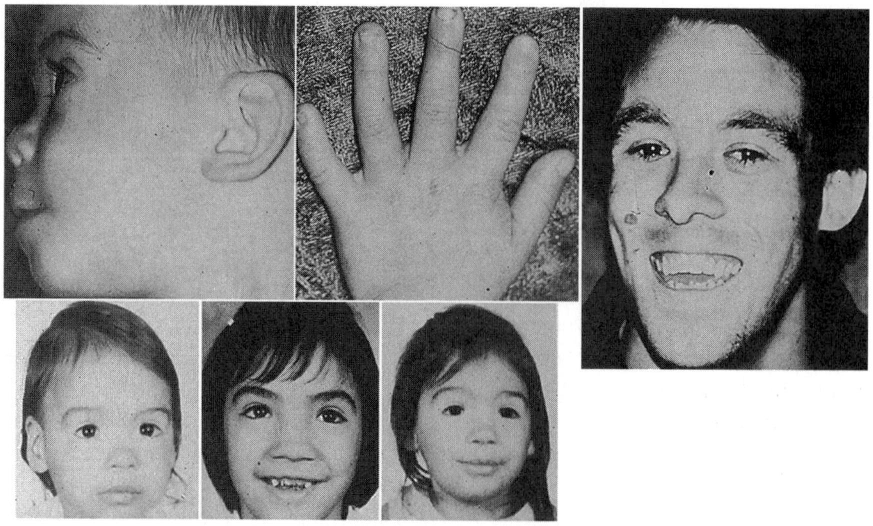

Fig. 17-32. Effects of fetal alcohol syndrome. Changes in the face of the same child from 18 months to 2½ years to 7 years of age. (From Jones KL: *Smith's recognizable pattern of malformation*, ed 4, Philadelphia, 1988, WB Saunders.)

use of a reliable method of birth control is needed for the duration of medication exposure.

Recreational Exposures

Maternal drug abuse also places infants at increased risk for congenital anomalies. Dysmorphology, congenital defects, and growth and developmental delay are known to result when pregnant women use cocaine. One theorized mechanism involves the impact of interrupted vascular supply on embryonic structures, making genitourinary, cardiovascular, and central nervous system anomalies more common (Chasnoff et al, 1985; Little and Snell, 1991). Alcohol is the most common teratogen to which fetuses are exposed by their mothers.

Fetal alcohol syndrome has been estimated at 1 in 3000 live births in the western world (Abel and Sokol, 1991). An estimated 10% to 20% of mental deficiency in the 50 to 80 IQ range has been attributed to fetal alcohol exposure (Olegaard et al, 1979). Fetal alcohol syndrome is characterized by prenatal and postnatal growth deficiency, developmental delay or mental retardation, microcephaly, facial dysmorphia, and minor skeletal malformations (Fig. 17-32) (Jones, 1988). If a pregnant woman consumes two alcoholic drinks a day, lower birth weight is apparent in her newborn. If she consumes four to six alcoholic drinks (5 oz absolute alcohol) a day, other clinical features can be detected. If she consumes eight to 10 alcoholic drinks a day, there is a 30% to 50% chance that her exposed offspring will display some manifestation of FAS, usually mental retardation (Jones, 1988). The prevalence of heavy alcohol consumption in pregnant women is 6% to 11% (Sokol, 1981). At preconception evaluations, identifying women who show evidence of alcohol abuse should be attempted. Most of these women remain undetected, but brief questionnaire screening is possible (Chang, 1997).

REFERENCES

Abel EL, Skol RJ: A revised conservative estimate of the incidence of FAS and its economic impact. *Alcohol Clin Exp Rev* 1991; 15:514-524.

Abyholm T, Stray-Pedersen S: Hypospermiogenesis and chromosomal aberrations: A clinical study of azoospermic and oligospermic men with normal and abnormal karyotype. *Int J Androl* 1981; 4:546-558.

Alberman ED: The abortus as a predictor of future trisomy 21. In De la Cruz F, Gerald P, editors: *Trisomy 21 (Down syndrome)*, Baltimore, 1981, University Park Press.

Alberman ED, et al: Previous reproductive histories in mothers presenting with spontaneous abortions. *Br J Obstet Gynaecol* 1975; 82:366.

Albertsen HM, Smith SA, Mazoyer S, et al: A physical map and candidate genes in the BRCA1 region on chromosome 17q12-21. *Nat Genet* 1994; 7:472-479.

Bell M, et al: Physical mapping across the fragile X: Hypermethylation and clinical expression of the fragile X syndrome. *Cell* 1991; 64:861-866.

Boué J, et al: Phenotypic expression of lethal chromosomal anomalies in human abortuses. *Teratology* 1976; 14:3.

Bourrouillou G, Mansat A, Calvas P, et al: Chromosome anomalies and male infertility: A study of 1,444 subjects. *Bull Assoc Anat* 1987; 71:29-31.

Bové A, Gallino P: A collaborative study of the segregation of inherited chromosome structural rearrangements in 1356 prenatal diagnoses. *Prenat Diagn* 1984; 4:45.

Bryndorf T, Christiensen B, Vad M, et al: Prenatal detection of chromosome aneuploidies by fluorescence in situ hybridization: Experience with 2000 uncultured amniotic fluid samples in a prospective preclinical trial. *Prenat Diagn* 1997; 17:333-341.

Buehler BA, et al: Prenatal prediction of risk of the fetal hydantoin syndrome. *N Engl J Med* 1990; 322:1567.

Carson SA, et al: Heritable aspects of uterine anomalies, II: Genetic analysis of müllerian aplasia. *Fertil Steril* 1983; 40:86.

Caskey CT, et al: The American Society of Human Genetics on cystic fibrosis screening. *Am J Hum Genet* 1990; 46:393.

Cattanach B, Kirk M: Differential activity of maternally and paternally derived chromosome regions in mice. *Nature* 1985; 315:496-498.

Chandley AC: The origin of chromosome aberrations in man and their potential for survival and reproduction in the adult human population. *Ann Genet* 1981; 24:55.

Chang G, Behr H, Goetz MA, et al: Women and alcohol abuse in primary care: Identification and intervention. *Am J Addict* 1997; 6:183-192.

Chang JC, Kin YW: A sensitive new prenatal test for sickle cell anemia. *N Engl J Med* 1982; 307:30.

Chasnoff IJ, et al: Cocaine use in pregnancy. *N Engl J Med* 1985; 313:666.

Chemke J, et al: Familial XY gonadal dysgenesis. *J Med Genet* 1970; 7:105.

Cornet D, et al: Pregnancies following ovum donation in gonadal dysgenesis. *Hum Reprod* 1990; 5:291.

Dahlback B, Hillarp A, Rosen S, Zoller B: Resistance to activate protein C, the FV:Q506 allele and venous thrombosis. *Ann Hematol* 1996; 72:166-176.

D'Alton ME, DeCherney AH: Prenatal diagnosis. *N Engl J Med* 1993; 328:114-120.

D'Alton ME, Malone FD, Chelmow D, et al: Defining the role of fluorescence in situ hybridization on uncultured amniocytes for prenatal diagnosis of aneuploidies. *Am J Obstet Gynecol* 1997; 176:769-776.

Daniel A, Hook EB, Wulf G: Risks of unbalanced progeny at amniocentesis to carriers of chromosome rearrangements: Data from United States and Canadian laboratories. *Am J Med Genet* 1989; 31:14-53.

De Brackeleer M, Dao T-N: Cytogenetic studies in couples experiencing repeated pregnancy losses. *Hum Reprod* 1990; 5:519-528.

de la Chapelle A: The complicated issue of human sex differentiation. *Am J Hum Genet* 1988; 43:1.

Dewhurst J: Fertility in 47,XXX and 45,X patients. *J Med Genet* 1978; 15:132-135.

Dilella AG, Huang WM, Woo SL: Screening for phenylketonuria mutations by DNA amplification with the polymerase chain reaction. *Lancet* 1988; 5:497-499.

Drugan A, et al: Prenatal genetic diagnosis following recurrent early pregnancy loss. *Obstet Gynecol* 1990; 75:381.

Dutrillaux B, Couturier J: Chromosome imbalances in endometrial adenocarcinomas: A possible adaptation to abnormal metabolic pathways. *Ann Genet* 1986; 29:76-81.

Dutrillaux B, Prieur M, Aurias A: Theoretical study of inversions affecting human chromosomes. *Ann Genet* 1986; 29:184-188.

Easton DF, Ford D, Bishop DT: Breast and ovarian cancer incidence in BRCA1-mutation carriers: Breast Cancer Linkage Consortium. *Am J Hum Genet* 1995; 56:265-271.

Elias S, Annas GJ: Generic consent for genetic screening. *N Engl J Med* 1994; 330:1611-1613.

Engel E: A new genetic concept: Uniparental disomy and its potential effect, isodisomy. *Am J Med Genet* 1980; 6:137-43.

Engel E, DeLozier-Blanchet D: Uniparental disomy, isodisomy, and imprinting: Probable effects in man and strategies for their detection. *Am J Med Genet* 1991; 40:432-439.

Espiner EA, et al: Familial syndrome of streak gonads and normal male karyotype in five phenotypic females. *N Engl J Med* 1970; 283:6.

Evans MI, Drugan A, Koppitch EC: Genetic diagnosis in the first trimester: The norm for the 1990s. *Am J Obstet Gynecol* 1989; 160:1332-1336.

Fialkow PJ: Use of genetic markers to study cellular origins and development of tumors in human females. *Cancer Treat Rev* 1972; 15:191-226.

Filmus JE, Buick RN: Stability of C-K-ras amplification during progression in a patient with adenocarcinoma of the ovary. *Cancer Res* 1985; 45:4468-4472.

Fisher EMC, et al: Homologous ribosomal protein genes on the human X and Y chromosomes: Escape from X inactivation and implications for Turner syndrome. *Cell* 1990; 63:1205-1218.

Franceschi S, La Vecchia C, Mangioni C: Familial ovarian cancer: Eight more families. *Gynecol Oncol* 1982; 13:31-36.

Friedman JM, et al: *Genetics.* Baltimore, 1992, Williams & Wilkins.

Gardner GH, Greene RR, Ranney B: The histogenesis of endometriosis. *Obstet Gynecol* 1953; 1:615.

Gartler SM, et al: Evidence of two functional X chromosomes in human oocytes. *Cell Differ* 1972; 1:215.

Gelehrter TD, Collins FS: *Principles of medical genetics.* Baltimore, 1990, Williams & Wilkins.

Greene ME, et al: First-trimester hemoglobin A, and risk for major malformation and spontaneous abortion in diabetic pregnancy. *Teratology* 1989; 39:225-231.

Greene ME, et al: Maternal serum alpha-fetoprotein levels in diabetic pregnancies. *Lancet* 1988; 2:345-346.

Gregory R, Tattersall PB: Are diabetic pre-pregnancy clinics worthwhile? *Lancet* 1992; 340:656-658.

Grumbach MM, Ducharme JR, Moloshok RE: On the fetal masculinizing action of certain oral progestins. *J Clin Endocrinol Metab* 1959; 19:1369.

Guy K, et al: Recurrent mutation of immunoglobulin and c-myc genes and differential expression of cell surface antigens occur in variant cell lines derived from a Burkitt lymphoma. *Int J Cancer* 1990; 45:109-118.

Guyer B, et al: Prenatal diagnosis with biotinylated chromosome specific probes. *Prenat Diagn* 1988; 7:485.

Haddow JE, et al: Prenatal screening for Down's syndrome with use of maternal serum markers. *N Engl J Med* 1992; 327:588.

Hall J: Genomic imprinting and its clinical implications. *N Engl J Med* 1992; 326:827-829.

Hallak M, Senderowicz J, Cassel A, et al: Activated protein C resistance (factor V Leiden) associated with thrombosis in pregnancy. *Am J Obstet Gynecol* 1997; 176:889-893.

Harrison KB: X-chromosome inactivation in the human cytotrophoblast. *Cytogenet Cell Genes* 1989; 52:37-41.

Hassold TJ: A cytogenetic study of repeated abortions. *Am J Hum Genet* 1980; 32:723-730.

Hellegren M, Svensson PJ, Dahlback B: Resistance to activated protein C as a basis for venous thromboembolism associated with pregnancy and oral contraceptives. *Am J Obstet Gynecol* 1995; 173:210-213.

Henry I, et al: Uniparental disomy in a genetic cancer-predisposing syndrome. *Nature* 1991; 351:665-667.

Hertig AT, Rock J: Searching for early human ova. *Gynecol Obstet Invest* 1973; 4:121-139.

Honoré LH: Recurrent partial hydatidiform male: Report of a case. *Am J Obstet Gynecol* 1987; 156:922-924.

Honoré LH, Dill FJ, Poland BJ: Placental morphology in spontaneous human abortuses with normal and abnormal karyotypes. *Teratology* 1976; 14:151-166.

Honoré LH, Lin EC, Morrish DW: Recurrent partial mole. *Am J Obstet Gynecol* 1988; 158:442.

Hook EB, Cross PK, Schreinemachers DM: Chromosome abnormality rates at amniocentesis and in liveborn infants. *JAMA* 1983; 249:2043-2048.

Houldsworth J, Chaganti RS: Comparative genomic hybridization: An overview [comment]. *Am J Pathol* 1994; 145:1253-1260.

Jacobs PA et al: Aggressive behavior, mental subnormality, and XYY male. *Nature* 1965; 208:1351-1352.

Jeffreys AJ: DNA sequence variants in the y, ó, and β globin genes of man. *Cell* 1979a; 18:1.

Jeffreys AJ: DNA sequence variation in the G gamma, A gamma, delta and beta globin genes of man. *Cell* 1979b; 18:131.

Jeffreys AJ, Wilson V, Them SL: Hypervariable minisatellite regions in human DNA. *Nature* 1985; 314:67.

Jones KL: *Smith's recognizable pattern of malformation,* ed 4, Philadelphia, 1988, WB Saunders.

Jones KL, et al: Patterns of malformations in the children of women treated with carbamazepine during pregnancy. *N Engl J Med* 1989; 320:1661.

Jones KA, Black DM, Brown MA, et al: The detailed characterisation of a 400 kb cosmid walk in the BRCA1 region: Identification and localisation of 10 genes including a dual-specificity phosphatase. *Hum Mol Genet* 1994; 3:1927-1934.

Kajii T, Nikawa N: Origin of triploidy and tetraploidy in man: Cases with chromosome markers. *Cytogenet Cell Genet* 1977; 18:109.

Kajii T, et al: Banding analysis of abnormal karyotypes of spontaneous abortions. *Am J Hum Genet* 1973; 25:539.

Kan YW, Dotty AM: Antenatal diagnosis of sickle cell anemia by DNA analysis of amniotic fluid cells. *Lancet* 1978; 2:910.

Kan YW, Dozy AM: Antenatal diagnosis of sickle cell anemia by DNA analysis of amniotic fluid cell. *Am J Hum Genet* 1973; 25:539.

Kazazian HH Jr, Boehm CD: Molecular basis and prenatal diagnosis of beta-thalassemia. *Blood* 1988; 72:1107.

Kenneson A, Cramer DW, Warren ST: Fragile X premutations are not a major cause of early menopause. *Am J Hum Genet* 1997; 61:1362-1369.

Kerem B-S, et al: Identification of the cystic fibrosis gene: Genetic analysis. *Science* 1989; 245:1073.

Knoll J, et al: Angleman and Prader-Willi syndromes share a common chromosome 15 deletion but differ in parental origin of the deletion. *Am J Med Genet* 1989; 32:285-290.

Knudson AG, Strong LC, Anderson DE: Heredity and cancer in man. *Prog Med Genet* 1973; 9:113.

Kremer E, et al: Mapping of DNA instability at the fragile X to a trinucleotide repeat sequence p(CGG)n. *Science* 1991; 252:1711-1714.

Kucera J: Rate and type of congenital anomalies among offspring of diabetic women. *J Reprod Med* 1971; 7:61-70.

Lapidot-Lifson Y, Lebo RV, Flandermeyer RR, et al: Rapid aneuploid diagnosis of high-risk fetuses by fluorescence in situ hybridization. *Am J Obstet Gynecol* 1996; 174:886-890.

LeVeechia C, et al: Gestational trophoblastic neoplasms in monozygous twins. *Obstet Gynecol* 1982; 60:250.

Levine LS, Pang S: Prenatal diagnosis and treatment of congenital adrenal hyperplasia. In Milunsky A, editor: *The fetus,* Baltimore, 1993. John Hopkins University Press.

Linder D, McGaw BR, Hecht F: Parthenogenic origin of benign ovarian teratomas. *N Engl J Med* 1975; 292:63.

Little BB, Snell LM: Cocaine use during pregnancy and congenital anomalies: Further study. *Am J Obstet Gynecol* 1991b:164:350.

Little M, Van Heyningen V, Hastie N: Dads and disomy and disease. *Nature* 1991: 351:609-610.

Matsuda T, Horii Y, Ogura K, et al: Chromosomal survey of 1001 subfertile males: Incidence and clinical features of males with chromosomal anomalies. *Hinyokika Kiyo* 1992; 38:803-809.

Micic M, Micic S, Diklic V: Chromosomal constitution of infertile men. *Clin Genet* 1984; 25:33-36.

Partington MW, Moore DY, Turner GM: Confirmation of early menopause in fragile X carriers. *Am J Med Genet* 1996; 64:370-372.

Phillips OP, et al: Maternal serum screening for fetal Down's syndrome in women less than 35 years of age using alpha-fetoprotein, hCG, and unconjugated estriol: A prospective, 2-year study. *Obstet Gynecol* 1992; 353.

Price DT, Ridker PM: Factor V Leiden mutation and the risks for thromboembolic disease: A clinical perspective. *Ann Int Med* 1997; 127:895-903.

Rosendall FR, Koster T, Vandenbroucke JP, Reitsma PH: High risk of thrombosis in patients homozygous for factor five Leiden (acitate protein C resistance). *Blood* 1995; 85:1504-1508.

Schrag D, Kuntz KM, Garber JE, et al: Decision analysis: Effects of prophylactic mastectomy and oophorectomy on life expectancy among women with BRCA1 or BRCA2 mutations. *N Engl J Med* 1997; 336:1465-1471.

Simpson JL, Elias S: Isolating fetal erythroblasts from maternal blood with identification of fetal trisomy by fluorescent in situ hybridization. *Prenat Diagn* 1992; 12:S34.

Speiser PW, Laforgia N, Kato K, et al: First trimester prenatal treatment and molecular genetic diagnosis of congenital adrenal hyperplasia (21-hydroxylase deficiency). *J Clin Endocrinol Metab* 1990; 70:838-848.

Vianna-Morgante AM, Costa SS, Pares AS, et al: FRAXA premutation associated with premature ovarian failure. *Am J Med Genet* 1996; 64:373-375.

Vogel and Motulskey, 1986.

Wald NJ, et al: Maternal serum screening for Down's syndrome in early pregnancy. *BMJ* 1988; 297:883.

Ward BE, Gersen SL, Carelli MP, et al: Rapid prenatal diagnosis of chromosomal aneuploidies by fluorescence in situ hybridization: Clinical experience with 4,500 specimens. *Am J Hum Genet* 1993; 52:854-865.

18

Gynecologic Infections

RUTH E. TUOMALA

KATHERINE T. CHEN

KEY ISSUES

1. The epidemiology, clinical presentation, and clinical diagnosis of gynecologic infections that are prevalent, have important sequelae, or are considered in the differential diagnosis of more common entities are discussed.
2. Current recommended guidelines for the management and treatment of gynecologic infections are presented.
3. Prevention strategies for gynecologic infections are emphasized.

Gynecologic infections, infectious diseases that affect the female genital tract, are among the most common reasons women seek treatement from health care providers. There are numerous kinds of gynecologic infections, and they fall into two broad categories: those that are sexually transmitted and those that are caused by endogenous flora. In the first part of the chapter, sexually transmitted diseases are discussed. Common sexually transmitted infections in the United States are pelvic inflammatory disease, gonorrhea, chlamydia, herpes, syphilis, genital warts, molluscum, and trichomonas. Diseases more prevalent in developing countries than in the United States are chancroid, lymphogranuloma venereum, and donovanosis. In the second part of the chapter, vaginitis and urinary tract infection are described. Finally, a section on the gynecologic concerns and management of women infected with human immunodeficiency virus (HIV) is presented.

In addition to accurate diagnosis and effective treatment of gynecologic infections, health care providers must em-

phasize preventive medicine and education in the care of their patients. Included in the discussion of each infection is a section on appropriate follow-up for treated patients and on prevention strategies for the prevention of primary and recurrent infections. A general discussion on the prevention of gynecologic infections serves as a focal point with which to begin this chapter.

PREVENTION OF GYNECOLOGIC INFECTIONS

Prevention and control of sexually transmitted diseases (STDs) are based on a few major concepts, as outlined by the Centers for Disease Control and Prevention (CDC): educating patients at risk for STDs on how to decrease their risk; evaluating, treating, and counseling sexual partners of infected patients; and administering vaccines to patients at risk for vaccine-preventable diseases (Centers for Disease Control, 1998).

The most effective way to prevent STDs is to refrain from intercourse with an infected partner. If abstinence is not possible and if there is incomplete knowledge of the infection status of a sexual partner, every effort should be made to decrease infection with the use of barrier methods of contraception. When used consistently and correctly, male condoms are effective in preventing many STDs, including HIV. However, they are not as effective in preventing infections that can be transmitted by skin-to-skin contact. Failures of condoms to prevent the transmission of infection are often the result of improper and inconsistent usage. Condom failures caused by breakage are estimated to be low, in the range of two breaks per hundred condoms used. In limited usage studies, female condoms have also been proven to prevent the transmission of HIV and other sexually transmitted organisms.

Another way to decrease the risk of infection is to refrain from douching. Reports have implicated douching as a risk factor for PID (Wolner-Hanssen et al, 1990, Scholes et al, 1993), chlamydial infection (Scholes et al, 1998), and other STDs (Joesoef et al, 1996).

Notifying and counseling as well as evaluating and treating sexual partners of persons diagnosed with some infections can help prevent reinfection and the further spread of disease. Many public health departments assist patients and health care providers by notifying sexual partners and giving them proper referrals.

Vaccination is one of the most effective yet underused methods of disease prevention. Although vaccination against hepatitis B is available, only 10% of the population at risk has actually received the vaccine despite its greater than 90% effectiveness. A significant number of the 5000 annual deaths caused by hepatitis B infection could be prevented by better use of this vaccine (Fedson, 1994). The CDC advises that all nonimmune persons evaluated for an STD be vaccinated against hepatitis B. The medical community now awaits other vaccines for infectious diseases that can be transmitted through sexual activity.

PELVIC INFLAMMATORY DISEASE

PID affects the upper genital tract and is characterized primarily by infection of the endosalpingeal cells that line the fallopian tubes. Infection may be confined to the tubes (salpingitis) or may involve the ovaries (salpingo-oophoritis). Occasionally, either the endometrium (endometritis) or the ovary (oophoritis) is the sole focus of infection. Infection involves disruption and destruction of the normal architecture on a microscopic or macroscopic level. Even apparently mild disease can lead to functional impairment. Marked inflammation that results in the involvement of contiguous intraperitoneal structures in inflammatory processes and massive suppuration leading to tuboovarian abscess (TOA) formation can totally destroy normal architecture and function.

PID is a disease of sexually active menstruating women. It is rare during pregnancy and in premenarchal, postmenopausal, and celibate women. If it occurs in these other groups of women, it is often secondary and has spread from other foci of intraabdominal sepsis, such as a ruptured appendiceal abscess. The exact incidence of PID in the United States is unknown, although estimates suggest that it accounts for 400,000 outpatient visits per year for a first diagnosis of PID and 5% to 20% of all gynecologic hospital admissions (Rolfs et al, 1992). In 1990, the total direct and indirect costs of diagnosing and treating PID were estimated to be $4.2 billion (Washington and Katz, 1991).

Some risk factors for the occurrence of PID have been delineated and include those related to sexual activity, age,

contraceptive practices, and invasive gynecologic procedures. In addition, recent epidemiologic studies suggest an association between smoking and douching and the occurrence of PID (Marchbanks et al, 1990; Scholes et al, 1992; Scholes et al, 1993).

A history of sexual activity is necessary to consider seriously the diagnosis of PID. The risk is probably largely confined to women who are heterosexually active. Young age at first intercourse, multiple partners, a recent new sexual partner, and frequency of intercourse even within a monogamous relationship all increase risk (Lee et al, 1991). Previous or concomitant documented STD, including previous PID, *Neisseria gonorrhoeae* infection, and *Chlamydia trachomatis* infection (Hillis et al, 1997) increase the risk for PID. Some recent studies strongly suggest that the presence of bacterial vaginosis increases risk for primary and recurrent PID (Larsson et al, 1992; Peipert et al, 1997).

Age is an important risk factor in PID. Peak incidence of PID in the United States is in the 15- to 24-year-old group. After age 25, and particularly after age 30, the incidence of PID markedly declines. It is unclear whether age-related risk is associated with sexual habits, with the development of protective antibodies at the cervical level, or with other factors.

Contraceptive practices influence the risk for PID (Eschenbach et al, 1977; Kelaghan et al, 1981; Rubin et al, 1982), although exact risks are skewed by the fact that the data are based on patients with PID requiring hospitalization. Oral contraceptives and barrier methods decrease the risk for PID compared with no contraceptive method. Although use of oral contraceptives confers a greater risk for *C. trachomatis,* the risk for upper tract infection in women with lower genital tract chlamydial infection is decreased in those who take oral contraceptives (Wolner-Hanssen et al, 1990). In addition, women with PID who use oral contraceptives appear to have milder disease. The use of an intrauterine device (IUD) increases the risk for PID above that of women who use no contraception. This risk is greatest in women who use the Dalkon shield, but risk exists for all types of IUDs and does not differ appreciably among them. The risk for PID is the greatest immediately after IUD insertion. Thereafter, there is a small increase in risk for PID regardless of duration of IUD use, socioeconomic status, and parity. Nulliparous women may be at a greater risk for IUD-associated PID than multiparous women, and they also appear to be at greater risk for tubal factor infertility associated with the IUD. Recent studies suggest that the risk for IUD-associated PID is not as large as previously stated, but instead is largely related to the baseline risks for the acquisition of STDs in individual IUD users (Lee et al, 1988).

All invasive gynecologic procedures are associated with a risk for upper genital tract infection. Such procedures include tubal lavage, hysterosalpingograms, endometrial biopsies, and dilation and curettages (D&Cs) performed either for diagnosis or for therapeutic abortion. Such iatrogenic infections may be associated with endogenous flora or with sexually transmitted organisms. It has been suggested that the presence of *C. trachomatis* in the cervix increases the risk for postabortal PID. It is not clear whether prophylactic antibiotics prevent pelvic infections associated with gynecologic procedures or whether they are even appropriate in these varied settings. In addition, it is uncertain whether the widespread use of antimicrobial prophylaxis for such procedures is cost effective.

Most incidences of PID are thought to be caused by microorganisms that ascend from the lower genital tract through the cervix, along the endometrium to the normally sterile tubes (Eschenbach et al, 1975). Infection also may spread to the tubes and ovaries through the parametrium from cervical vessels and lymphatics. PID is a polymicrobial infection (Eschenbach et al, 1975). Organisms that are sexually transmitted and organisms that are part of the normal endogenous flora of the lower genital tract are participants in PID. Sexually transmitted organisms such as *N. gonorrhoeae* and *C. trachomatis* may be the sole pathogens in PID. Sometimes they occur together, and sometimes they are found along with other nonsexually transmitted organisms. Estimates in the United States are that more than half the cases of PID involve *N. gonorrhoeae* or *C. trachomatis* or both. Which organism is found depends on the prevalence in a particular group. In the inner city or in cases of PID diagnosed in emergency rooms (Soper et al, 1994), it has been suggested that there are higher rates of *N. gonorrhoeae*. In adolescents and college students, *C. trachomatis* may be more prevalent.

Multiple species of aerobic and anaerobic bacteria normally found in the lower genital tracts of asymptomatic women can be found at the site of upper genital tract infection in the presence and the absence of sexually transmitted organisms. PID may be purely aerobic, purely anaerobic, or a mixed aerobic-anaerobic infection. In approximately two thirds of patients, anaerobes are involved. Aerobic endogenous bacteria that are associated with PID include the enterobacteriaceae, particularly *Escherichia coli,* staphylococcal species, and streptococcal species, including the enterococci. Anaerobes that are associated with PID include peptococci, peptostreptococci, anaerobic streptococci, and *prevotella* species formerly known as the *Bacteroides* species (*B. fragilis, B. melaninogenicus,* and *B. bivius*).

Key organisms are probably responsible for the initial invasion of the upper genital tract, and other organisms probably become involved in infection under altered conditions and structure of the upper genital tract (Eschenbach et al, 1977; Gjonnaess et al, 1982). The exact microbial and host factors responsible for tissue invasion and infection are subjects of much ongoing research.

Determining the organisms involved in a particular infection can be ascertained only by direct culture of the infected site. In PID this involves a culture of tubal exudate, tubal biopsy specimen, or cul-de-sac fluid obtained at the time of laparoscopy or laparotomy. Cultures of the lower genital tract do not accurately reflect the organisms present in an upper genital tract infection. Contamination by lower genital tract flora of peritoneal fluid cultures obtained by culdocentesis renders these specimens unacceptable. Although endometrial cultures also suffer from a high degree of lower genital tract contamination, particularly by low-virulence pathogens, endometrial cultures, specifically for *C. trachomatis,* may be helpful. In addition, cervical culture for *N. gonorrhoeae* and cervical assessment for *C. trachomatis* are always appropriate. The presumed microbiology of an individual infection is largely an estimation based on usual organism involvement and, to some extent, on differential clinical presentation.

Diagnosis

The clinical diagnosis of PID is inexact. There are multiple potential symptoms and signs ascribable to PID as predicted by areas of inflammatory involvement. No symptoms or signs are pathognomonic for PID.

Reports in which all clinical diagnoses of PID are confirmed by laparoscopy suggest that in one third of patients, the clinical diagnosis of PID is in error (Jacobson and Westrom, 1969; Sweet et al, 1979). Other conditions that may be diagnosed as PID include appendicitis, ectopic pregnancy, endometriosis, adhesions, and adnexal tumors including ruptured or hemorrhagic functional ovarian cysts. In addition, 10% to 15% of cases of PID are diagnosed initially as other conditions.

For the majority of cases in which PID is erroneously diagnosed, no pelvic pathologic features can be defined by laparoscopy. Without treatment for PID, symptoms in these women resolve and long-term sequelae associated with PID do not ensue. A portion of disease in this group with normal visual findings may be infection confined to the lower genital tract or endometrium, and a portion may involve disease of other organ systems.

The largest such laparoscopy series conducted on an ongoing basis was reported initially by Jacobson and Westrom (1969) in Sweden, and it was updated periodically by Westrom and others (Westrom et al, 1992). When they compared the incidence of various symptoms and signs in women with PID and women with a laparoscopically normal pelvis, few symptoms and signs were seen more often in women with PID (Table 18-1). Although observed in a minority of patients, multiple signs and symptoms in one person indicate the most accurate clinical diagnosis.

Traditional laboratory studies do little to improve the accuracy of a diagnosis of PID. White blood cell (WBC) count is elevated in women with PID and in women without the disease. Often both the erythrocyte sedimentation rate (ESR) and the C-reactive protein (CRP) are elevated in women with PID and may be helpful in judging the response to therapy, but these tests are nonspecific. In virtually all women who have PID, WBCs are present in lower genital tract discharge. If WBCs are not present in this discharge, the diagnosis of PID is unlikely. A recent study found that increased WBCs in vaginal discharge was the most sensitive

Table 18-1   Symptoms and Signs Seen Significantly More Often in Patients with Pelvic Inflammatory Disease Than in Those with Laparoscopically Normal Pelvic Findings

	Pelvic Inflammatory Disease (%)	Visually Normal (%)
Symptoms		
Fever and chills	41.0	20.0
Proctitis	6.9	2.7
Signs		
Adnexal tenderness	92.0	87.0
Palpable mass or swelling	49.4	24.5
Erythrocyte sedimentation rate >15 mm/hr	75.9	52.7
Abnormal discharge	63.2	40.2
Temperature >38° C	32.9	14.1

From Jacobson L, Weström L: Objectivized diagnosis of acute pelvic inflammatory disease: Diagnostic and prognostic value of routine laparoscopy. *Am J Obstet Gynecol* 1969; 105:1088.

BOX 18-1
LAPAROSCOPIC CRITERIA FOR ACUTE PELVIC INFLAMMATORY DISEASE

Minimum criteria
  Erythema of fallopian tubes
  Edema and swelling of fallopian tubes
  Exudate from fimbria or on serosa of fallopian tubes
Scoring
  Mild: minimum criteria, tubes freely movable and patent
  Moderate: minimum criteria more marked, tubes not freely movable, patency uncertain
  Severe: inflammatory mass

From Jacobson L: Differential diagnosis of acute pelvic inflammatory disease. *Am J Obstet Gynecol* 1980; 138:1006-1011.

BOX 18-2
SALPINGITIS: CLINICAL CRITERIA FOR DIAGNOSIS

Abdominal direct tenderness, with or without rebound tenderness	All three necessary for diagnosis
Tenderness with motion of cervix and uterus	
Adnexal tenderness	
	Plus
Gram stain of endocervix: positive for gram-negative, intracellular diplococci	One or more necessary for diagnosis
Temperature (38° C)	
Leukocytosis (>10,000/mm³)	
Purulent material (white blood cells) from peritoneal cavity by culdocentesis or laparoscopy	
Pelvic abscess or inflammatory complex on bimanual examination or by sonography	

From Hager WD, Eschenbach DA, Spence MR, Sweet RL: Criteria for diagnosis and grading of salpingitis. Reprinted with permission from the American College of Obstetricians and Gynecologists (Obstetrics and Gynecology, 1983; 61:114.)

---

laboratory test for PID and that serum WBC was the most specific (Peipert et al, 1996).

Ultrasonography and computed tomography (CT) may aid in detecting the presence and in following up the resolution of TOAs, but they cannot accurately differentiate abscess formation from other causes of pelvic masses.

Diagnostic laparoscopy should be performed when the differential diagnosis of pelvic pain is either PID or a surgical condition and if nonresponse or recurrent clinical disease is not associated with an obvious precipitating cause. The use of laparoscopy in other patients should be individualized, although some investigators suggest that extending the use of laparoscopy to all may prove to be cost effective. Laparoscopic criteria for the diagnosis of PID are listed in Box 18-1.

To establish at least minimal criteria for the diagnosis of PID and to compare better the data between institutions,

Hager et al (1983) proposed baseline criteria for a clinical diagnosis of PID. These criteria are listed in Box 18-2. In addition, classifying disease according to severity either by clinical or laparoscopic criteria may be useful in predicting the duration of therapy and of sequelae based on the prognosis and in developing comparative databases (Soper, 1991). Any grading system should emphasize sensitivity in diagnosing mild disease to minimize adverse outcomes of PID.

In as many as 70% to 85% of selected patients, endometritis is seen in association with salpingitis. In addition, women with signs and symptoms of PID without laparoscopic evidence of the disease may have endometritis (Paavonen et al, 1985; Wolner-Hanssen et al, 1983). Endometritis is assumed to be responsible for symptoms in these patients. The overlap in symptoms between women with laparoscopically documented PID and those with endometritis is such that differential diagnosis by any specific clinical criteria is not possible. Endometritis is strongly associated with the presence of *C. trachomatis* isolated from the cervix, from both the cervix and the endometrium, and from the endometrium alone. To a lesser extent it is associated with *N. gonorrhoeae*. In many women with clinically apparent cervicitis, endometritis is often found on biopsy. Many patients have histopathologic evidence of plasma cell endometritis, although severe endometritis, including even microabscesses, has been described. There is no correlation between the histopathologic severity of endometritis and the degree of tubal damage in cases of coincidental PID. An association between cervicitis, endometritis, and PID and the overlap in symptoms support the ascending theory of infection. An endometrial biopsy diagnostic of endometritis can be helpful in establishing the diagnosis of infection in women with pelvic pain in whom a diagnosis of PID is considered.

Approximately 5% of women with PID have an associated syndrome of perihepatitis called the Fitz-Hugh-Curtis syndrome. This syndrome is an inflammatory, fibrinous perihepatitis associated with right upper quadrant pain, tenderness, and mildly abnormal liver function test results. Eventual scarring results in the classic fibrous "violin string" adhesions between the dome of the liver and the diaphragm. This process is associated with gonococcal and chlamydial PID (Daly et al, 1978; Muller-Schoop et al, 1978). Laparoscopic assessment of women with acute or chronic pelvic pain should include an assessment of the right upper quadrant if a diagnosis of acute or past PID is considered.

The clinical presentation of PID may differ, depending on the primary pathogens involved (Sweet et al, 1986). Gonococcal PID usually becomes acute within 48 hours of the onset of multiple symptoms and signs, including high fever, peritoneal signs, and purulent vaginal discharge. Patients often seek treatment for what appears to be an initial episode of PID. Abscess formation is less common with gonococcal PID, and the therapeutic response is usually prompt. In contrast, chlamydial PID usually involves moderate symptoms and follows a protracted course. Chronic, low-grade pelvic pain, irregular bleeding, subtle signs on physical examination (except for elevated ESR), and severe inflammatory changes identified by laparoscopic examination with a high percentage of tubal scarring all may be features of chlamydial infection. *C. trachomatis* and *N. gonorrhoeae* often are found together in patients with PID, and many of their symptoms overlap. Therefore, the treatment of both organisms is standard rather than the treatment of differential clinical features.

Nongonococcal, nonchlamydial PID is often recurrent and follows a semiacute course. Unlike PID associated with either gonorrhea or chlamydia, in which symptoms usually begin within 7 days of menses, symptoms in other patients with PID often occur more than 14 days after menses. After having symptoms for 5 to 7 days, patients seek medical attention but do not look acutely ill. Fever and peritoneal signs are not prominent, but ESRs often are elevated. Abscess formation is common, and response to therapy often is not dramatic. Anaerobic organisms, particularly bacteroides species, are of concern if a patient has multiple recurrences, is older than 30 years of age, or has abscesses.

The four well-documented, long-term consequences of PID are disease recurrence, pelvic pain, infertility, and ectopic pregnancy. Approximately one fourth of women who have had PID have one or more of these sequelae. Women who have had PID are admitted to hospitals more often for abdominal and pelvic pain, hysterectomy, and ectopic pregnancy than women who have never had PID (Westrom et al,

Table 18-2   Summary of Long-Term Sequelae Seen in 415 Patients with Laparoscopically Documented Pelvic Inflammatory Disease (PID) and in 100 Controls with Laparoscopically Normal Findings on Pelvic Examination

Sequelae	Normal Pelvis	PID
Chronic abdominal pain >6 mo	5.0%	18.1%
Ectopic/intrauterine pregnancy	1/417	1/24
Involuntary infertility related to tubal factor	0%	17.3%

Infertility-Related Episodes of PID		Infertility Related to Severity of PID (first episode only)	
No. of Episodes	% Infertile	Severity of Episodes	% Infertile
1	12.8	Mild	2.6
2	35.5	Moderate	13.1
3+	75.0	Severe	28.6

From Weström L: Effect of acute pelvic inflammatory disease on fertility, *Am J Obstet Gynecol* 1975; 121:707.

1992). As previously mentioned, PID is a recurrent disease despite apparently adequate therapy. Whether aggressive attempts at elucidating and eradicating the microbiologic pathogens and treating sexual partners appreciably decrease the rates of recurrence of upper genital tract infections remains to be seen.

Approximately 20% of all women who have had documented PID have some type of chronic pelvic pain. The pain may be sporadic or cyclic or it may be constant and debilitating, often resulting in hysterectomy (Buchan et al, 1993). PID and its sequelae are responsible for approximately 25% of abdominal hysterectomies performed in the United States each year.

Women who have had PID are at increased risk for infertility because of tubal obstruction. Approximately 20% to 30% of cases of infertility are thought to result from fallopian tube obstruction, usually a consequence of PID. The risk for infertility is related to the number of episodes of infection and to the severity of these episodes (Table 18-2) (Westrom, 1975). Infertility risk is also associated with young age at first intercourse (Safrin et al, 1992), and it is increased in diseases that involve either *C. trachomatis* or TOA (Brunham, 1984; Henry-Suchet and Loffredo, 1980). In women who become pregnant after having had PID, there is an increased incidence of ectopic pregnancy. PID is thought to increase the risk for ectopic pregnancy as much as 10 times; in fact, it is a major factor in the increasing incidence of ectopic pregnancy in the United States. The sequelae of infertility and ectopic pregnancy are increased with a longer duration of symptoms before therapy. At least

---

**BOX 18-3
CENTERS FOR DISEASE CONTROL AND
PREVENTION 1998 RECOMMENDATIONS
FOR THE TREATMENT OF
PELVIC INFLAMMATORY DISEASE**

Inpatient Therapy

A. Uncomplicated acute salpingitis*
Cefotetan 2 g IV q 12 hr

or

Cefoxitin 2 g IV q 6 hr

plus

Doxycycline 100 mg IV or PO q 12 hr
B. Complicated salpingitis (tuboovarian abscess or inflammatory complex)†
Clindamycin 900 mg IV q 8 hr

plus

Gentamicin loading dose of 2 mg/kg IV or IM followed by a maintenance dose of 1.5 mg/kg q 8 hr

Outpatient Therapy

A. Ofloxacin 400 mg PO bid × 14 d

plus

Metronidazole 500 mg PO bid × 14 d
B. Ceftriaxone 250 mg IM × 1 dose

or

Cefoxitin 2 g IM plus probenecid 1 g PO in a single dose

plus

Doxycycline 100 mg PO bid × 14 d

IV, intravenously; *IM*, intramuscularly; *q*, every; *PO*, by mouth; *bid*, twice a day; *qid*, four times a day.
*Parenteral therapy may be discontinued 24 hours after signs of clinical improvement, and oral therapy should continue for a total of 14 days.
†Parenteral therapy should continue for at least 4 days. Subsequent oral therapy of clindamycin 450 mg PO qid or doxycycline 100 mg PO bid should be given for a total of 14 days.

---

one study has suggested that prompt evaluation and treatment of PID associated with chlamydia result in fewer long-term sequelae (Hillis et al, 1993).

Treatment

To date, there are no large-scale comparative trials that support any therapeutic regimen as the most efficacious for the treatment of PID. Essential components of adequate therapy are frequent observation for response, thoughtful use of antibiotics, and notification, screening, and treatment of sexual partners for *N. gonorrhoeae* and *C. trachomatis*.

Suggested antibiotic treatment regimens outlined by the CDC are presented in Box 18-3. Microbiologic rationales for their selection are sound, but these regimens are not con-

sidered to be exclusive. Most authorities support the need for multiple-drug regimens for inpatient or outpatient therapy for PID (Burnakis and Hildebrandt, 1986). Failure rates of 15% to 20% for single-drug therapy are documented and are unacceptably high. The appropriate length of time for adequate antimicrobial therapy, the need for protracted oral therapy in the follow-up of parenteral therapy, and the correlation between resolution of symptoms and length of therapy have not been determined. Antimicrobial regimens that have been studied have clinical cure rates of 75% to 94% and microbiologic cure rates of 71% to 100% (Walker et al, 1993).

Hospitalization for the treatment of PID with parenteral antibiotics and close observation is suggested for all patients with severe disease suggested by nausea and vomiting, high fever, peritoneal signs, or abscess formation. In addition, hospitalization is indicated if the diagnosis is in doubt, if the patient is unable to tolerate oral antibiotics, if close outpatient observation of a monitoring response is difficult, if the initial course of oral therapy has failed, if the patient is immunosuppressed, or if the patient is thought to be pregnant. PID during pregnancy is rare. However, when it occurs it is particularly virulent. It can result in severe morbidity and in high rates of pregnancy loss, and it requires close observation and aggressive antibiotic therapy. Many authorities suggest that all adolescents with PID should be hospitalized because of the concerns regarding compliance with medical care and the grave long-term consequences of lack of compliance (Spence et al, 1990). Some authorities also recommend hospital care for all women with PID who desire future childbearing. Hospitalization for the treatment of PID can provide an opportunity to educate patients about the pathogenesis of PID, thereby reducing risky behaviors and promoting the recognition of early signs and symptoms of acute disease. This is particularly important in the successful long-term treatment of adolescents and in the preservation of fertility.

The best way to treat IUD-associated PID has not been determined. The need to remove an IUD to effect a clinical cure has not been proved, but the resolution of disease may be slower and less complete if an IUD is left in situ. Therefore, it is common practice to remove an IUD when treating PID.

Medical treatment should be instituted for TOA because 75% to 80% of patients with TOA respond to antibiotic therapy (Landers and Sweet, 1985; Reed et al, 1991). Most abscesses smaller than 8 cm respond to acute medical therapy. Ruptured TOAs, TOAs that do not respond to medical therapy within 4 to 5 days, and TOAs that cause chronic pain require surgical extirpation (Thompson et al, 1980). While under observation, 3% of TOAs rupture and require immediate surgical intervention. Rates of "late failures" requiring surgical intervention to cure persistent abscesses or to handle sequelae of persistent pain may be as high as 30%. Because successful pregnancy rates after TOA are only 4% to 15% and because of the potential need for later surgery to deal with persistent symptoms, some authorities advocate more aggressive surgical management of the acute disease. There is no strong evidence that complications from surgery are dependent on the time between the onset of medical therapy and surgical intervention. For these reasons, decisions regarding medical and surgical management of TOA should be individualized.

Total abdominal hysterectomy with bilateral salpingo-oophorectomy as the sole surgical therapy for TOA is now outmoded. Although necessary or desired in some patients, greater conservation is appropriate for most patients. In particular, unilateral adnexectomy with continued medical management is an accepted surgical treatment of unilateral TOA. Some advocate simple drainage of abscess collections with aggressive medical therapy as the best way to maximize ovarian conservation for future reproduction. Laparoscopic and pelviscopic drainage of abscess collections and of pyosalpinxes is increasingly used. Ultrasound-guided transvaginal aspiration of abscesses may also be effective (Aboulghar et al, 1995). After cure of acute PID complicated by TOA, there is justification for fertility surgery and for treatment with procedures aimed at optimizing either natural or in vitro fertilization techniques.

Follow-up and Prevention

All patients with PID who are administered parenteral or oral therapy should have a follow-up examination 48 to 72 hours after therapy begins. If patients do not show substantial improvement in symptoms and signs, they may require additional evaluation.

Notification, evaluation, and treatment of symptomatic and asymptomatic sexual partners is an integral part of PID therapy (Kamwendo et al, 1993) to prevent reinfection. Assessment of male partners should take into account the reservoir of asymptomatic males who harbor gonorrhea and chlamydia, regardless of the organisms isolated from their female partners with PID (Gilstrap et al, 1977). At a minimum, all sexual partners should be assessed for the presence of these organisms. Some authorities advocate presumptive therapy for all sexual partners of women with newly diagnosed PID.

It must be remembered that PID is intimately associated with other STDs. To achieve a decrease in the incidence of PID, successful strategies to decrease the incidence of *N. gonorrhoeae* and *C. trachomatis* are needed. Screening and treating asymptomatic women at risk for *C. trachomatis* infection has been shown to decrease the incidence of PID (Scholes et al, 1996). Women diagnosed with PID should be evaluated for other types of STD. Serosurveys of patients hospitalized with PID suggest HIV positivity rates of 6% to 20.9% (Hoegsberg et al, 1990; Safrin et al, 1990).

RARE ETIOLOGIC AGENTS FOR PELVIC INFLAMMATORY DISEASE

Two rare causes of PID are recognized. They are discussed in turn.

Actinomycosis

Infection by *Actinomyces israelii* is an uncommon cause of disease of the upper genital tract. *Actinomyces* is a gram-positive, nonacid-fast anaerobic bacterium that has a characteristic radially branching filamentous formation. It is typically found in the gastrointestinal tract, including the oral cavity and bowel. Actinomycosis is a sporadic infection of soft tissues and is characterized by an invasion of areas of trauma with chronic, suppurative infection. This infection results in tissue destruction, fibrosis, and the formation of draining sinuses. Active actinomycotic infection usually is polymicrobial; other anaerobic organisms often are involved. Actinomycosis is a rare cause of indolent pelvic infection secondary to the seeding of the upper genital tract from other intraabdominal sources or the hematogenous dissemination of *Actinomyces*. In addition, ascending pelvic actinomycotic infection has been described in patients with IUDs (Berkman et al, 1982; Schiffer et al, 1975; Valicenti et al, 1982).

Colonization of the lower genital tract by *Actinomyces* occurs most often in IUD users or in the presence of other foreign bodies, and it increases with the duration of IUD use. Upper genital tract infection develops in a small percentage of women with actinomycosis in whom colonization occurs. Irregular vaginal bleeding and mild, chronic pelvic discomfort may precede this manifestation. By the time a patient seeks treatment, the pelvic organs may be massively indurated and fibrotic, and there may be a near total destruction of anatomy and adherence to surrounding structures. Because *Actinomyces* tends to invade across tissue planes and boundaries, patients with actinomycotic pelvic infection and ureteric obstruction, rectosigmoid stricture, or retroperitoneal mass have been reported (Ha et al, 1993; Hoffman et al, 1991; Patsner and Giovine 1993; Turnbull and Cohen, 1991). Because medical therapy has only a limited chance of restoring structure and function, surgery is often performed to remove affected organs.

A suggestive Gram stain can lead to the diagnosis of actinomycosis. Histologic sections of actinomycotic infections show central necrosis containing "sulfur granules," which represent microcolonies of actinomyces. With the appropriate anaerobic media and techniques, diagnosis can be confirmed by a culture.

Colonization may be suspected after positive Papanicolaou smear or immunofluorescent slide screening, but treatment with antibiotics has not been shown to eliminate *Actinomyces* effectively from the lower genital tract. Recommendations are to remove IUDs if colonization is suspected and to repeat Papanicolaou smears in 6 weeks to verify the clearance of colonization and to allow subsequent IUD reinsertion (Fiorino, 1996).

When actinomycotic pelvic infection is diagnosed, treatment with antibiotics may be tried first to eliminate the need for surgery, which has been described as difficult, or at least to allow an easier, more conservative surgical procedure later. Actinomycosis is sensitive to penicillin, tetracycline, erythromycin, and clindamycin. High-dose parenteral antibiotics, typically penicillin, are used to treat infection. The exact length of required therapy has not been established, but the slow growth of these organisms and the extensive involvement of infection usually necessitate at least 6 weeks of therapy. Initial parenteral therapy is often completed orally with doxycycline. Treatment of actinomycotic pelvic infection should cover other organisms, particularly anaerobic organisms, typically found in patients with upper genital tract infection. Aggressive medical therapy has resulted in the resolution of obstruction and the shrinkage of large masses that can cure or facilitate later surgical intervention, which often is required for cure.

Genital Tract Tuberculosis

In developed countries, tuberculosis is a rare cause of upper genital tract infection. Today the disease most often develops in older women who were exposed to tuberculosis before the advent of effective chemoprophylaxis and in younger women who emigrate from countries in which tuberculosis is endemic. Approximately one third of the world's population is infected with *Mycobacterium tuberculosis*, and the World Health Organization estimated that in 1996 there were 8 million new cases.

Genital tract tuberculosis is usually secondary to hematogenous spread from pulmonary or from other nongenital tract foci. It rarely spreads to the genital tract from other intraperitoneal foci or from male sexual partners with tuberculous epididymitis. The most common sites of tuberculous involvement in the female genital tract are the fallopian tubes and the endometrium (Agarwal and Gupta, 1993), although the cervix and ovary also can be affected. The vagina and vulva are rarely involved.

Genital tract tuberculosis is an extremely indolent infection. Disease may not become manifest for more than 10 years after the initial seeding of the genital tract. Presenting symptoms may be unusual vaginal bleeding patterns, including altered menses, amenorrhea, and postmenopausal bleeding. Approximately 25% to 35% of women with pelvic tuberculosis have vague, chronic lower abdominal or pelvic pain. The chief symptom of young women with genital tract tuberculosis is infertility (Agarwal and Gupta, 1993; Oosthuizen et al, 1990). Occasionally, women with the disease have tuberculous peritonitis and ascites, although these more commonly are secondary to direct hematogenous seeding of the peritoneum.

The diagnosis of genital tract tuberculosis may be suspected from medical history, travel history, and a chest roentgenogram that shows evidence of healed pulmonary tuberculosis. However, a significant number of patients with pelvic tuberculosis may have no history of tuberculosis infection and may have normal findings on a chest roentgenogram (Saracoglu et al, 1992). Except in debilitated, systemically ill patients, a skin test with a purified protein derivative of tuberculin yields positive findings. A hysterosalpingogram may show characteristic changes suggestive of tuberculous infection, which includes bead-

ing, sacculation, sinus formation, and rigid pipe stem patterning.

Diagnosis can be confirmed by a histologic examination that reveals typical granulomas or by an acid-fast stain or a culture of surgical specimen or endometrial biopsy tissue. Acid-fast stain is less sensitive than culture and histology. Endometrial biopsy specimens and menstrual blood collected in a vaginal or a cervical cup may be submitted for culture. Menstrual fluid is reported to be culture positive more often than biopsy specimens (Oosthuizen et al, 1990).

Treatment of genital tract tuberculosis is primarily medical, and it includes the administration of two or three antituberculosis drugs for 18 to 24 months. Surgery is indicated if the symptoms or the physical examination suggest persistent or increased disease despite adequate therapy or if culture or biopsy results suggest resistant organisms. Surgical therapy often consists of total abdominal hysterectomy and bilateral salpingo-oophorectomy. Early aggressive medical therapy, however, may warrant infertility-related procedures.

GONORRHEA

Gonorrhea is one of the most prevalent STDs in the United States. More than 1 to 1.5 million cases are reported each year. From 1986 to 1989, the incidence of gonorrhea decreased 22% (Gershman and Rolfs, 1991). This reduction continued through 1992, except for adolescents, whose rate increased or remained stable depending on the year and the community. Between 1981 and 1991, 24% to 30% of gonorrhea incidence in the United States occurred in adolescents (Webster et al, 1993). In 1995, gonorrhea remained the most common disease reported among persons 15 to 24 years of age (*MMWR*, 1996). In addition to its association with younger age, gonorrhea is more common in urban population, lower socioeconomic groups, women with multiple sexual partners, women who experienced first intercourse at a young age, and women who have a sexual partner with a urethral discharge or diagnosed gonorrhea.

The causative organism of gonorrhea is *N. gonorrhoeae*, a gram-negative aerobic diplococcus that grows best in carbon dioxide and is sensitive to drying and to extremes in temperature. The organism commonly infects columnar and transitional cells.

Usually gonorrhea is transmitted through sexual activity. An infected male partner transmits infection through vaginal intercourse with approximately 50% efficiency. The incubation period is approximately 3 to 5 days in patients in whom symptoms are recognizable. In women, *N. gonorrhoeae* is harbored chiefly in the endocervix. It is also found in the urethra, rectum, and oropharynx, and occasionally it is found in one of these locations in the absence of cervical gonorrhea. Infection of multiple sites occurs in more than 20% of patients.

Gonorrhea may appear without symptoms or it may appear as a localized infection of the lower genital tract, an invasive infection of the upper genital tract, or a disseminated disease with systemic manifestations.

Manifestations of gonorrhea in most women are subtle, and it occurs more often without symptoms in women than in men. STD clinics report that the prevalence of gonorrhea is higher in those attending as contacts than in those attending with symptoms (Pabst et al, 1992). Endocervical gonorrhea is associated with a purulent cervical discharge, which may or may not be observed as abnormal. Occasionally irregular vaginal bleeding is noted. Urethral gonorrhea or involvement of Skene's glands may be associated with symptoms of lower urinary tract infection, such as dysuria and frequency of urination. Rectal gononorrhea often causes no symptoms. *N. gonorrhoeae* in the oropharynx may cause acute pharyngitis but usually is asymptomatic. Because colonization with *N. gonorrhoeae* produces either no symptoms or vague ones in 80% of patients (Zimmerman et al, 1990), women do not seek medical attention and form a major reservoir of disease transmission. Interpretation of symptoms and diagnosis of gonorrhea may be further complicated by coinfection by other STDs, particularly *C. trachomatis* and *Trichomonas vaginalis.*

Lower genital tract gonorrhea can lead to infection of the Bartholin glands and to the formation of Bartholin abscesses. Bartholin abscesses associated with gonorrhea usually are unilateral, acutely suppurative, and painful. They may spontaneously drain or require incision and drainage, and sometimes they resolve spontaneously.

Acute salpingitis develops in 10% to 20% of women with endocervical gonorrhea. *N. gonorrhoeae* can invade and infect the upper genital tract as a solitary pathogen or as a part of a polymicrobial infection. Some strains of *N. gonorrhoeae* are more pathogenic for the upper genital tract than others. A lipopolysaccharide endotoxin is responsible for local cytotoxicity and inflammation and for fever and systemic toxicity. Furthermore, outer membrane pili proteins and IgA protease facilitate the attachment of the gonococcus to host cells. Certain risk factors in the host that predispose to salpingitis have been previously outlined. The exact microbial and host factors that lead to invasion and to infection of the upper genital tract by *N. gonorrhoeae* are incompletely understood. In the United States, estimates of the incidence of gonococcal salpingitis range from 25% to 80% of all patients with salpingitis.

Although as many as 40% of rectal cultures obtained from women with gonorrhea are positive, some are positive because of perineal contamination and do not reflect true rectal colonization. Rectal colonization may produce symptoms of discharge, bleeding, pain, tenesmus, constipation, and signs such as exudate or mucosal bleeding. However, rectal gonorrhea is usually asymptomatic. Rectal gonorrhea is more likely to be ineffectively treated by tetracycline therapy. In addition, because 30% of treatment failures in women are discovered only by posttreatment rectal culture, some authorities suggest that posttreatment cultures always include a rectal culture.

Pharyngeal carriage of *N. gonorrhoeae* is often asymptomatic. Occasionally it is associated with acute exudative pharyngitis. Pharyngeal gonorrhea is thought to be almost exclusively a result of fellatio with an infected male partner. Largely asymptomatic, pharyngeal gonorrhea is not thought to be contagious or to be a major reservoir of disease transmission. There is evidence that without treatment, spontaneous remission occurs in a 10- to 12-week period. However, there may be a greater tendency for pharyngeal gonorrhea to disseminate because the number of patients with disseminated gonococcal infection (DGI) associated with pharyngeal gonorrhea appears to be disproportionately high. Pharyngeal gonorrhea is more resistant to therapy with standard antimicrobial regimens.

The incidence of DGI in all patients with gonorrhea is approximately 5%. Exact risk factors are unknown, although pregnancy may predispose to DGI. Some series have shown that 28% to 42% of patients with DGI have been pregnant women (Holmes et al, 1971).

DGI usually appears in one of two distinct forms. It may be a systemic illness associated with chills, fever, malaise, asymmetric polyarthralgias, and painful skin lesions. The fingers, toes, hands, wrists, knees, and ankles are often involved in what appears to be tenosynovitis and occasionally frank suppurative arthritis. A skin lesion classically appears as a slightly raised erythematous base with a necrotic center, but it may be petechial, papular, pustular, hemorrhagic, and sometimes bullous. These lesions are lightly scattered about the body, usually number less than 20, and often appear on the extremities. On average 10% to 30%, but as many as 50%, of acutely symptomatic patients with DGI may have positive blood cultures.

The second common clinical syndrome of DGI is septic, monoarticular arthritis. *N. gonorrhoeae* may be the most common cause of septic arthritis in patients younger than 30. Knees are most often involved, although elbows, ankles, and wrists also may be involved. Joint effusion is exudative and often purulent, and the gonococcus is identified by a Gram stain or by a routine culture in approximately 50% of patients. Culture positivity is proportional to the WBC count in the joint fluid. Blood cultures are not positive.

Patients with DGI often lack the typical local symptoms of gonorrhea. If DGI is suspected, all common sites for gonococcal colonization should be cultured. The need to hospitalize everyone with DGI is unclear; however, close observation for the first 48 hours of treatment to judge early therapeutic response and to rule out serious complications is prudent. Disseminated *N. gonorrhoeae* may cause endocarditis, myocarditis, pericarditis, hepatitis, or meningitis.

Diagnosis

The diagnosis of gonorrhea is most accurately made after culture of the organism on selective media such as modified Thayer-Martin agar. This is a chocolate-based agar modified by the addition of antibiotics to inhibit the growth of organisms from sites commonly contaminated by polymicrobial

---

BOX 18-4
CENTERS FOR DISEASE CONTROL AND PREVENTION 1998 RECOMMENDATIONS FOR THE TREATMENT OF GONORRHEA

Uncomplicated urethral, cervical, or rectal infection*
    Cefixime 400 mg PO × 1 dose
        or
    Ceftriaxone 125 mg IM × 1 dose
        or
    Ciprofloxacin 500 mg PO × 1 dose†
        or
    Ofloxacin 400 mg PO × 1 dose†
Pharyngitis*
    Ceftriaxone 125 mg IM × 1 dose
        or
    Ciprofloxacin 500 mg PO × 1 dose†
        or
    Ofloxacin 400 mg PO × 1 dose†
Disseminated gonococcal infection‡
    Ceftriaxone 1 g IM or IV qid
        or
    Cefotaxime 1 g IV q 8 hr§
        or
    Ciprofloxacin 500 mg IV q 12 hr†§
        or
    Ofloxacin 500 mg IV q 12 hr†§
        or
    Spectinomycin 2 g IM q 12 hr§

PO, By mouth; *IM*, intramuscularly; *IV*, intravenously; *q*, every; *qid*, four times a day; *bid*, twice a day; *tid*, three times a day.
*All single-dose regimens for gonorrhea should be followed with azithromycin 1 g PO × 1 dose or doxycycline 100 mg PO bid × 7 days to provide coverage for possible concomitant infection with *Chlamydia*. In pregnant women, erythromycin base 500 mg PO qid × 7 days or amoxacillin 500 mg PO tid × 7 days should be used.
†Quinolones are contraindicated for pregnant and lactating women and for children and adolescents younger than 18 years.
‡Parenteral therapy should continue until the patient has been afebrile and asymptomatic for 24 to 48 hours. Subsequent oral therapy of cefixime 400 mg PO bid, ciprofloxacin 500 mg PO bid, or ofloxacin 400 mg PO bid should be given to complete a total of 1 week of therapy.
§Alternative regimens.

---

growth, such as the cervix or the rectum. The specimen should be plated directly on warmed media and incubated in carbon dioxide without delay to minimize false negative results from improper handling. Growth markedly decreases after 3 hours if the specimen is improperly handled.

Obtaining specimens from multiple sites increases the yield of cultures for suspected gonorrhea. The endocervix is the site that most often produces positive cultures in women, and it should always be sampled. Cultures from the urethra, rectum, and pharynx may be positive despite negative cervical cultures and should be performed when indicated by the history or a strong clinical suspicion of gonococcal disease and in all patients with recurrent disease.

A Gram stain may help in making a tentative diagnosis of gonorrhea in patients who are symptomatic or who are known to have been in contact with gonorrhea. A Gram stain is considered to be positive if intracellular gram-negative diplococci are seen in at least three polymorphonuclear leukocytes per high-power field. Sensitivity and specificity vary by site of isolation. Up to two thirds of women with endocervical gonorrhea have suggestive Gram stains, but specificity in asymptomatic women is as low as 40% to 70%.

Rapid diagnosis by fluorescent monoclonal antibody slides or enzyme assays is of limited value in asymptomatic patients and those at low risk. Chemiluminescent DNA probe assays are reported to be highly specific, to have high positive predictive value, and to have a sensitivity of 90% (Granato and Franz, 1990; Panke et al, 1991). DNA probes may be used for the diagnosis of rectal and pharyngeal gonorrhea, and they have the additional advantage of concomitant assessment for chlamydia (Lewis et al, 1993).

Treatment

Treatment of gonorrhea in the United States has been modified by the emergence of resistant strains of *N. gonorrhoeae* and the need to provide concomitant treatment for *C. trachomatis* when gonorrhea is treated.

Most *N. gonorrhoeae* organisms found in the United States are sensitive to high-dose penicillin. However, a penicillin resistance at rates greater than 3% in most communities has changed the recommendations for therapy (Centers for Disease Control, 1987; Committee on Public Health, 1989). First recognized in 1976, a plasmid-mediated β-lactamase or penicillinase is responsible for most gonococcal resistance. Initially confined to defined urban areas, particularly those in California, New York, and Florida, most cases of penicillinase-producing *N. gonorrhoeae* (PPNG) in other geographic areas were related to travel to the high-risk areas. More than 75% of reported cases of PPNG are associated with endemic contact. Other forms of resistant *N. gonorrhoeae* exist. A chromosomally mediated resistant *N. gonorrhoeae* strain that is resistant to penicillin, tetracycline, and other antibiotics is recognized but is not yet widespread. In addition, plasmid-mediated tetracycline-resistant *N. gonorrhoeae* has recently been reported. Of concern are the recent reports of decreased susceptibility of *N. gonorrhoeae* to fluoroquinolones (Gordon et al, 1996; Fox et al, 1997).

In women, *C. trachomatis* is isolated from 30% to 50% of those from whom gonococcus is isolated. Studies of single-drug therapy for gonorrhea show that the rates of posttreatment isolation of *C. trachomatis* and the occurrence of PID are high if a penicillin, a penicillin derivative, or a cephalosporin is used but low if a tetracycline is used. However, as many as 10% of patients with gonorrhea are not cured if tetracycline is the sole treatment. Therefore, multiple-drug therapies for the treatment of gonorrhea that take into account chlamydia are now standard (Stamm et al, 1984). Current CDC guidelines for treatment of gonorrhea are outlined in Box 18-4.

Follow-up and Prevention

All nonpregnant patients treated with recommended regimens for gonorrhea do not have to return for a test of cure unless symptoms persist. Usually infections identified after treatment with one of the recommended regimens reflect reinfection rather than treatment failure. The prevalence of asymptomatic gonorrhea in male partners may be as high as 20% to 30%. Thus, patients should be instructed to notify sexual partners for evaluation and treatment and to abstain from intercourse until both have completed therapy.

It is advocated that all populations in which the prevalence of culture positivity is more than 1% to 1.5% be screened (Phillips et al, 1989). Screening in high-prevalence populations is justified as cost-effective in decreasing adverse disease outcomes. Targeted screening programs based on risk factors among sexually active women are also proposed (Phillips et al, 1988).

CHLAMYDIA

With an estimated 4 million cases reported each year, chlamydia is now thought to be the most prevalent STD in the United States. The overall prevalence of chlamydia in the female genital tract varies by practice site; it ranges from 2% to 35% in prenatal clinics and 5% to 23% in family planning clinics. In addition, prevalence increases in those presenting with symptoms. Chlamydia is most prevalent in those younger than 25 years of age, and it recurs more often in this age group (Hillis et al, 1993). It is also prevalent in nulliparous and unmarried women, in users of nonbarrier contraceptive methods, and in those with recent multiple or new sexual partners. Unlike gonorrhea, it occurs in a more geographically diverse population (Zimmerman et al, 1990). Chlamydia is often associated with gonorrhea; approximately 30% to 50% of the time, it is cultured from the genital tract after successful therapy for gonorrhea, and the gonococcus is found in 10% to 50% of women with chlamydia. Chlamydia is a major pathogen in postgonococcal and nongonococcal urethritis in the male, and female partners of these males are at high risk for chlamydial colonization and disease.

C. trachomatis is an obligate intracellular bacterial parasite of columnar and transitional epithelial cells. Its role as a pathogen for the genital tract was first recognized as the causative agent of lymphogranuloma venereum (LGV). Non-LGV serotypes of *C. trachomatis* are now associated with asymptomatic carriage in a variety of infections of the female genital tract.

As many as 80% of women colonized with *C. trachomatis* are asymptomatic or have mild, unrecognized symptoms. This is one of the problems in controlling chlamydial infection and its sequelae (Cates and Wasserheit, 1991). Most chlamydial infections in women are identified through screening or contact tracing, neither of which is universal or routine.

C. trachomatis has been associated with cervicitis, which may or may not cause symptoms (Brunham et al, 1988).

C. trachomatis in the cervix is associated with a cervicitis characterized by a hypertrophic-appearing, friable central eversion or ectopy with mucopus. Endocervical mucus that appears yellow against a cotton-tipped applicator (abnormal Q-tip test result) and microscopic examination that reveals the presence of WBCs signify mucopurulence. If both are present, *C. trachomatis* is found 85% of the time. Cervical erythema and friability also are independently correlated with *C. trachomatis.* If signs of cervicitis are seen in a woman with symptoms of PID, chlamydial infection should be suspected.

The female urethral syndrome of dysuria, pyuria greater than 10 WBCs per high-power field, and negative bacterial culture are associated with *C. trachomatis* in as many as 50% of patients. *C. trachomatis* is also implicated as a cause of bartholinitis and late postpartum endometritis. It can be transmitted to neonates at birth through an infected birth canal, and in neonates it is associated with a distinctive conjunctivitis and pneumonitis.

C. trachomatis is associated with as many as 30% to 50% of patients with PID (Märdh et al, 1977), particularly in adolescents. The exact contribution of *C. trachomatis* to morbidity and the long-term sequelae associated with PID are unclear. If PID is treated with antibiotics, which are ineffective against *C. trachomatis,* acute symptoms subside but recurrence is common. Some cases of chlamydial PID are clinically subtle yet are associated with unexpectedly severe disease when patients are examined laparoscopically. The subtle nature of the symptoms possibly contributes to a delay in treatment, which in turn contributes to the high rate of the sequela of infertility seen in some series.

C. trachomatis is found by biopsy or by culture in the endometrium of women with intermenstrual spotting or symptoms of PID with or without laparoscopic confirmation of upper genital tract infection (Krettek et al, 1993; Wolner-Hanssen et al, 1990). Occasionally it is seen in asymptomatic women who have documented clinical disease (Jones et al, 1986).

Silent chlamydial infection is implicated in tubal factor infertility and ectopic pregnancy. Greater presence and higher levels of antichlamydial antibody titer have been linked to both conditions in a population of women, the majority of whom have no known history of PID. In addition, these women are more likely to have visible tubal damage than those without antibody titer (Henry-Suchet and Loffredo, 1980; Phillips et al, 1992; Sheffield et al, 1993; Walters et al, 1988).

One study suggests that an autoimmune response to human heat-shock protein can develop after infection with *C. trachomatis,* probably as a result of cross-reactivity to an epitope of chlamydial heat shock protein with human heat-shock protein (Domeika et al, 1998).

Diagnosis

The presence of *C. trachomatis* is determined most accurately by demonstrating the intracellular organism in cell culture, but this test is complex and costly. Currently, direct

---

BOX 18-5
CENTERS FOR DISEASE CONTROL AND PREVENTION 1998 RECOMMENDATIONS FOR TREATMENT OF CHLAMYDIA

Nonpregnant Women
    Azithromycin 1 g PO × 1 dose
        or
    Doxycycline 100 mg PO BID × 7 d
        or
    Erythromycin base 500 mg PO QID 7 d*
        or
    Erythromycin ethylsuccinate 800 mg PO QID × 7 d*
        or
    Ofloxacin 300 mg PO BID × 7 d*
Pregnant Women
    Erythromycin base 500 mg PO QID × 7 d
        or
    Amoxicillin 500 mg PO TID × 7 d

*Alternative regimens.

---

fluorescent antibody slide staining, enzyme-linked immunosorbent assay techniques, and DNA probe systems are used for rapid chlamydial antigen detection. These tests are more widely available and are less expensive than previous culture techniques. However, sensitivity and specificity are lower when they are used in populations with low prevalence, and they are best ascertained by experienced laboratory personnel with demonstrated ongoing quality control (Lin et al, 1992). The use of rapid tests for the assessment of cure may result in false positive results if they are repeated too soon after successful therapy. False negative results may occur if inappropriate or incomplete therapy temporarily halts organism replication. Polymerase chain reaction has been used to detect *C. trachomatis* in endocervical samples, and it appears more sensitive and more rapid than cell culture for groups at high risk (Witkin et al, 1993; Quinn et al, 1996). Ligase chain reaction in urine samples has also been studied (Lee et al, 1995). It remains to be seen whether these techniques are cost effective.

Treatment

The drugs of choice for treating chlamydia are azithromycin and doxycycline. Both are equally efficacious, yet the effectiveness of doxycycline is diminished if patients are not compliant with the regimen of twice-daily dosing for 7 days. A major advantage of azithromycin, a long-acting macrolide, is its single-dose therapy, but its cost may limit its widespread use. However, a cost-effectiveness analysis found azithromycin to be less expensive than doxycyline because of fewer sequelae associated with untreated chlamydial infections (Magid et al, 1996). Thus, for the noncompliant patient, azithromycin may be more appropriate because

it can provide single-dose, direct, observed therapy. Current CDC recommendations for the treatment of chlamydia are listed in Box 18-5. Treatment to eliminate chlamydia should be based on laboratory documentation. However, when facilities are unavailable or when testing is impractical, presumptive therapy may be instituted for suspected disease in a population at high risk.

Follow-up and Prevention

Patients who are not pregnant do not need a test of cure if they are treated with azithromycin or doxycycline unless symptoms persist or reinfection is likely. Patients should be instructed to refer their partners for evaluation and treatment and to abstain from intercourse until both have completed therapy.

In recognition of the rapidly increasing prevalence of *C. trachomatis* and of the potential reproductive tract sequelae caused by chlamydial infection, strategies to monitor prevalence, control spread, and educate the public have been proposed. These strategies include screening of all groups at risk for chlamydial disease (Kent et al, 1988; Weinstock et al, 1992; Scholes et al, 1996). Additional strategies include the evaluation of all those with referable symptoms, signs, or exposures and the potential empiric treatment of all women and girls at high risk for the disease (Finelli et al, 1996). Suggested risk factors for screening include young age, single state, new sexual partner or mutliple partners in the preceding 3 months, no barrier contraception, cervical friability or ectopy, and purulent vaginal discharge. Suggested clinical criteria for presumptive treatment include diagnosis of cervicitis, PID, or gonococcal infection, having a partner with urethritis, and low likelihood of compliance (Centers for Disease Control, 1993). In the short term, these strategies are more expensive, but long-term benefits should result from averting the high costs associated with the sequelae of untreated chlamydial infections.

GENITAL HERPES

Genital herpes is a sexually transmitted infection of increasing concern for all sexually active women. An estimated 270,000 to 600,000 new cases are reported each year, with the peak incidence occurring in women in their 20s. As many as 46% of women attending an STD clinic and 9% of college students are reported to have antibody evidence of genital herpes. One national survey suggests that in the United States, 21.9% of persons older than 12 years of age have antibody evidence of herpes, an increase of 30% since the late 1970s (Fleming et al, 1997). Of interest, less than 10% of those who were seropositive reported a history of genital herpes. The exact prevalence of genital herpes infection is unknown because not all those with active infection seek medical care and because there is a relatively high proportion of asymptomatic disease. However, some authorities consider the incidence of herpes to be steadily increasing and genital herpes to be one of the most common STDs in the United States today.

Symptomatic genital herpes is the most common cause of painful lesions of the lower genital tract of women in the United States. Herpes infection of the lower genital tract has been associated with cervical cancer, although a causative role remains unproven. In addition, contact with genital herpes during passage through the birth canal has been associated with systemic neonatal infection, which carries major risks of serious morbidity and a high mortality rate.

Genital herpes is caused by the herpes simplex virus (HSV), a member of the DNA-containing Herpesviridae family. There are two major types of HSV, type I (HSV-1) and type 2 (HSV-2). They are closely related and are homologous for approximately 50% of antigens. Although HSV-2 causes the majority of genital herpes lesions and HSV-1 primarily causes orolabial lesions, a significant overlap clearly exists. Approximately 85% to 90% of genital herpes infections are caused by HSV-2, whereas the remainder are caused by HSV-1. This proportion varies. As many as 50% of genital lesions were caused by HSV-1 according to an English survey (Barton et al, 1982).

Genital herpes is a recurrent infection. Periods of active infection are separated by periods of latency during which the inactive virus resides in the dorsal root sacral ganglia. Under the stimulus of various endogenous and exogenous factors, the virus travels down the sensory nerve root to the lower genital area, where it replicates. Outward manifestations of the disease become apparent, and HSV can be identified by culture.

Lesions of genital herpes are typically painful and begin as fluid-filled vesicles or papules, which progress to well-circumscribed, occasionally coalescent, shallow-based ulcers. These ulcers heal by the reepithelialization of mucous membranes or by the crusting over of epidermal surfaces. The virus is shed from active lesions until healing begins, and it can be transmitted during the time of shedding. The clinical manifestation and the duration of active infection vary widely and depend on the virus type, location of presentation, preexistence of antibodies, and presentation as initial or recurrent disease.

Genital herpes infection develops 1 to 45 days (mean, 5.8 days) after exposure to the virus. Manifestations of the initial HSV infection are more severe and last longer than those of the recurrent disease. First episodes are more severe in women than in men. Multiple, painful, usually bilateral lesions occur on the external genitalia. Symptoms tend to peak within 8 to 10 days and gradually decrease in the next week. Crops of new lesions form over a mean of 10 days. Ulcers last 4 to 15 days, and the mean time from the onset of the lesions to total healing is 20 to 21 days. The virus is shed from lesions until the time of crusting over, and the average duration of shedding is 11 days. Usually local lesions are accompanied by bilateral tender lymphadenopathy of the inguinal region and sometimes of the femoral and iliac regions. Adenopathy of the deep inguinal nodes can be

responsible for severe lower pelvic pain. Adenopathy appears after the onset of lesions and often takes longer to resolve, sometimes lasting beyond the period of the lesions themselves.

In most patients local involvement includes urethritis; 82% of urethral cultures are positive. Urination may be problematic either because of periurethral and vulvar edema or because of intense dysuria resulting from urethral herpetic involvement.

In more than 80% of patients, the initial genital herpes infection involves the cervix. Cervical involvement may be clinically apparent because of friability of the cervix, ulcerative and occasionally necrotic lesions of the cervix, and a marked increase in cervical discharge. The exocervix and endocervix also may be involved. In some patients, involvement of the cervix may not be clinically apparent although the virus can be cultured.

Other genital tract sites may be involved. Vaginal lesions develop in 4% of patients. Although HSV has been cultured from the fallopian tube, how often the upper genital tract is involved in the first occurrence of genital herpes is unclear. At present, this is not thought to be a major clinical problem.

Complications of initial HSV infection develop in women more often than in men. These complications may result from local spread or from more distant effects of the virus.

Coincident with the first appearance of symptomatic genital herpes infection in a patient, symptomatic pharyngitis is reported in approximately 10% of patients (Corey, 1988). HSV can be isolated from the pharynx of patients with symptomatic pharyngitis and from those without pharyngeal symptoms. Pharyngitis and pharyngeal viral shedding occur with genital infection with both HSV-1 and HSV-2.

In approximately one fourth of patients, the secondary spread of local lesions to other body sites occurs after the onset of lesions and before they have become encrusted. Extragenital involvement often occurs in sites below the waist, such as the buttocks and the upper legs. However, involvement of the fingers and eyes also has been reported. The secondary spread is thought to happen primarily because of autoinoculation and usually occurs in the second week of disease.

Early in the course of illness, systemic symptoms are apparent in one half to two thirds of patients with genital herpes infection. Fever, malaise, headache, and myalgias are common. Other systemic complications include hepatitis, aseptic meningitis, and autonomic nervous system dysfunction.

Hepatitis appears as typical hepatocellular necrosis after the onset of local genital lesions, usually within the first week of illness. Hepatitis is often accompanied by other systemic symptoms.

Aseptic meningitis is seen more often with HSV-2 than with HSV-1 infections. It develops early in as many as 36% of patients with genital herpes infections. Headache, stiff neck, and photophobia, with or without fever, are typical symptoms. Aseptic meningitis is accompanied by cerebrospinal fluid pleocytosis consisting largely of lymphocytes. Meningitis is self-limited, requires only supportive care, and resolves without permanent neurologic sequelae. Encephalitis is rarely a complication of genital herpes infection.

Sacral autonomic nervous system dysfunction is an uncommon complication of initial genital herpes infection. Typical symptoms include decreased sensation along the sacral nerve route distribution, inability to void as a result of bladder dysfunction (Caplan et al, 1977), and constipation because of bowel dysfunction. Nerve dysfunction is confirmed through electromyography and may last 6 to 8 weeks. Occasionally, sensory involvement may take the form of hyperesthesia in a radicular pattern. Self-limited transverse myelitis with paralysis may also occur.

Recurrent genital herpes infection typically is less severe, is of shorter duration, and involves systemic manifestations less often than the initial disease. One to 2 days to a few hours before the onset of recurrent lesions, prodromal symptoms may occur (Guinan et al, 1981). Symptoms are typically described as a tingling sensation, an itching, or a hyperesthesia of the genital area where lesions later occur. The prodrome may also include sacral dermatomal neuralgia with pain radiating to the buttocks and hips. Recurrent genital lesions are fewer, smaller, and more often unilateral than lesions of the first infection. Recurrent genital herpes lesions may not look like typical ulcers. Instead they may look like fissures or excoriations. Recurrences usually are painful, tend to appear in the same location, and have the same appearance in each episode. Symptoms of recurrent lesions last 4 to 8 days, and there are fewer crops of new lesions. The mean time until recurrent lesions disappear is 9 to 10 days, and viral shedding averages 5 days.

Both urethritis and cervicitis are seen less often with recurrent genital infection than with the first infection. Cervicitis is typically manifest solely as virus positivity. Shedding of the virus from the cervix during recurrent disease occurs in 10% to 15% of patients (Corey, 1988). Tender local adenopathy may occur but is usually less severe and of shorter duration. Systemic manifestations are uncommon, and extragenital involvement is seen in less than 5% of patients.

Frequency of recurrent disease and length of time between recurrences of active infection are highly variable. The average number of recurrences in women who have symptomatic recurrent genital herpes is 5 to 8 per year. Some evidence suggests that the mean time to recurrence is greater from the initial episode to the first recurrence than between subsequent recurrences. Recurrence may be precipitated by an obvious endogenous stimulus, such as cyclic hormonal variation, or by exposure to HSV through sexual contact with an infected partner. Whether contact with exogenous virus precipitates recurrent infection or whether this is actually reinfection with a different viral strain is unclear. Although the general impression is that the frequency of recurrent disease decreases as time from initial infection increases, recurrent disease may be independent of time for at least the first 3 to 4 years.

Approximately 25% of first-time genital herpes infections develop in women who have preexisting antibodies to HSV. Nonprimary first episodes tend to be less severe and to have fewer systemic manifestations than true primary episodes in an antibody-negative patient and may actually represent recurrent infection in a patient with previous asymptomatic HSV-2 infection. In other patients, the presence of antibodies to HSV-1 of oral-labial origin may ameliorate the clinical expression of genital infection. Both primary and nonprimary forms of the disease may be asymptomatic the first time it develops in a patient.

Although the initial presentation of genital herpes infection caused by HSV-1 cannot be distinguished from that caused by HSV-2, HSV-1 is less likely to result in recurrent genital infection (Corey, 1988). Recurrences of infection caused by HSV-1 are less common and less severe. This difference probably is related to virus type and not to antibody response.

In the absence of symptoms and lesions, genital herpes infection is defined by culture-positive viral shedding. The prevalence of asymptomatic shedding is unknown. Such shedding occurs from the cervix and from the vulva, probably with approximately equal frequency. Shedding frequency may peak during the first 3 months after a primary lesion. Thereafter, shedding appears to be sporadic and of brief duration. In one culture survey of women with known genital herpes, daily cultures were positive for HSV on only 1% of days (Brock et al, 1990). Risk factors for asymptomatic shedding are incompletely described, but it is known to be more prevalent with HSV-2 than HSV-1 infection and in women with frequent recurrences, and it is not related to the menstrual cycle.

Virus type and asymptomatic shedding are factors in the transmission of genital herpes. When one partner has genital herpes and the other does not, the overall risk of transmission in monogamous relationships is approximately 10% per year, and it is probably highest when the man is the infected partner (Bryson et al, 1993). The risk of seroconversion appears to be higher in partners with no history of genital herpes and no preexisting antibodies. Transmission is seen less often when infected partners have fewer symptoms. Most transmission occurs during periods of asymptomatic shedding, during the prodromal period, or at the onset of lesion development (Mertz et al, 1988b; Mertz et al, 1992).

Diagnosis

The characteristic clinical presentation and the appearance of lesions often lead to the diagnosis of genital herpes. Virus isolation by tissue culture is the most accurate diagnostic test to confirm the clinical impression. The virus may be isolated from either the vesicle fluid or the base of a wet ulcer. If vesicles are present, they should be unroofed and the fluid should be cultured directly. A single virus culture grown from an appropriate lesion identifies live virus in 85% to 90% of patients. Virus grown in culture can be typed.

The Tzanck smear is less sensitive, but it is helpful when viral cultures are not available. The Tzanck smear relies on cytologic methods to identify changes in cells typically produced by the HSV. Scrapings of viral lesions are gathered and placed on a slide and stained with either Wright's or Giemsa stain. Test results are positive if multinucleated giant cells, atypical keratinocytes, and "ground-glass" cytoplasm are identified. This occurs in up to 50% of patients.

Antibody testing is generally of no value in diagnosing genital herpes infections. Forty percent to 60% of adults have antibodies to HSV-1, and 15% to 35% have antibodies to HSV-2. These represent past exposure that may have resulted in clinically apparent infection or asymptomatic infection. Although it is possible to distinguish HSV-2 antibodies from HSV-1 antibodies, antibody response to type-common antigens leads to a large crossover in identification and to difficulty in detecting new antibody formation in a person with a previous type-common antibody response. Substantial numbers of false-positive and false-negative herpes antibody results and inaccurate viral typing are produced because of the cross-reactivity of common antigens (Ashley et al, 1991). The existence of antibodies to HSV at the onset of an initial genital herpes infection may preclude the identification of this episode as a primary infection in a previously antibody-negative host or a recurrent infection in a previously asymptomatic host. In addition, the presence of HSV antibodies at the onset of a herpes genital lesion may identify past exposure to this virus but may not identify the cause of active lesions. Occasionally, if there is no antibody to HSV at the onset of a suspected primary genital herpes infection, and if antibodies develop during the course of illness, antibody testing can be of some value. Because of the variety of disease expression and because of the inherent inaccuracies in diagnosis by antibody assessment, the timing and the sources of specific infection may be difficult, if not impossible, to determine.

Treatment

There is no therapy that effectively prevents the establishment of latency of genital herpes or that eradicates infection. Acyclovir has been the most widely used antiviral agent that effectively alters the course of genital herpes infection. If given early during the onset of the first episode, acyclovir decreases the duration of symptoms, lesions, viral shedding, and new vesicle formation, but it does not change the course of subsequent recurrences. Limitations of acyclovir include the development of resistant isolates and relatively poor oral bioavailability, necessitating multiple daily doses. Recently, famciclovir and valacyclovir have been introduced to address those issues.

Famciclovir is the well-absorbed form of penciclovir, and valacyclovir is a prodrug of acyclovir. Both have greater absorption and bioavailability than acyclovir, leading to a more convenient dosing schedule, and both are at least as efficacious as acyclovir in the treatment of genital herpes (Cirelli et al, 1996; Beutner, 1995). For the noncompliant patient

and for the patient with acyclovir-resistant isolates, famciclovir or valacyclovir may be the drug of choice.

The CDC-recommended regimens for first-clinical-episode genital herpes include a 7- to 10-day course of acyclovir 400 mg orally three times a day, acyclovir 200 mg orally five times a day, famciclovir 250 mg orally three times a day, or valacyclovir 1 g orally twice a day.

Oral acyclovir, famciclovir, and valacyclovir can be taken either on an acute episodic basis to ameliorate the effects of recurrent disease or on a daily basis to suppress recurrent disease. Episodic therapy for any of the antiviral medications, taken at the earliest sign of recurrence, decreases the duration of lesions, symptoms, and viral shedding and inhibits the formation of new lesions. It does not alter the time period between recurrences (Mertz et al, 1988a; Mertz et al, 1997; Tyring et al, 1998).

Women who take daily suppression therapy have fewer, milder, and shorter recurrences. Many have no recurrences, although asymptomatic shedding can occur even in the absence of recognizable recurrences. It has been suggested that asymptomatic shedding is suppressed with antiviral therapy (Wald et al, 1996), but additional research must be done. There is no evidence that suppression therapy influences the long-term natural history of a recurrent disease, and recurrences occur at the previous level of frequency when suppression is discontinued. The length of time a patient can safely remain on suppression therapy is unknown, but efficacy continues and no cumulative toxicity is apparent with as much as 5 years of acyclovir use (Goldberg et al, 1993). The possibility that resistant viruses will emerge remains a concern. Suppression therapy is suggested for those with more than six recurrences a year, for those with complications associated with recurrent disease, and for those who are immunosuppressed. HIV-infected patients often require high dosages of acyclovir for the suppression of recurrent disease. Suppression therapy should be discontinued periodically to assess the frequency of recurrences and the need for further therapy.

It is recommended that patients with severe disease or with complications requiring hospital stays be administered parenteral therapy with acyclovir 5 to 10 mg/kg intravenously three times daily for 5 to 7 days or until there is clinical improvement. If given at the onset of the first episode, intravenous acyclovir decreases the duration of symptoms, lesions, viral shedding, systemic manifestations, and episodes of new vesicle formation.

The mainstay of therapy for genital herpes infections remains the treatment of local lesions and supportive care through any systemic illness. Local measures such as sitz baths, warm compresses, and analgesics for local relief should be taken to decrease superinfections and to increase comfort. The use of an indwelling bladder catheter may be necessary in severe cases of herpes urethritis. Hospitalization for observation and supportive care during episodes of aseptic meningitis may be necessary. Finally, because the psychological issues associated with genital herpes often are more debilitating than its physical manifestations, appropriate counseling must be provided to meet the emotional and informational needs of patients in whom genital herpes infection is diagnosed (Carney et al, 1994; Kinghorn, 1993).

Follow-up and Prevention

An important part of caring for patients with genital herpes is informing them of the natural history of the disease and of preventive techniques to reduce transmission. They should be informed about the potential for recurrent episodes and asymptomatic viral shedding and the effectiveness of episodic or suppressive antiviral therapy. The risk for neonatal herpes transmission should be explained so patients will understand the importance of telling their obstetricians of their history of herpes infection. They should be encouraged to inform their sexual partners and to abstain from sexual activity when lesions or prodromal symptoms are present. Condoms should be used at all times to decrease the risk of transmission to an uninfected sexual partner, but it cannot guarantee protection against the spread of disease during intercourse because of the varied locations of infection.

SYPHILIS

Syphilis remains a significant cause of morbidity in many developing countries and in some areas of North America and Europe. In the United States, approximately 20,000 to 30,000 new cases of syphilis are reported each year, predominantly in the 15- to 40-year-old group. From 1985 to 1991, reported cases of syphilis and congenital syphilis steadily increased. From 1986 to 1989 the incidence of primary and secondary syphilis increased 59%, but it decreased for the first time in 1991 (Gershman and Rolfs, 1991; Webster and Rolfs, 1993). Most of the increase in syphilis in the late 1980s was seen in urban areas, in women, and in minority populations. From 1981 to 1991, 10% to 12% of reported cases occurred in adolescents (Webster et al, 1993). The increase in syphilis has been strongly associated with illicit drug use and HIV disease, the latter particularly in women and adolescents (Quinn et al, 1990).

Syphilis occurs when the causative organism, the spirochete *Treponema pallidum,* is inoculated into mucous membranes. This occurs most often during sexual activity.

Syphilis exists in well-described stages defined by clinical presentation and by time course. The incubation period from the time of contact to the onset of lesions of primary syphilis ranges from 9 to 90 days, with an average time of 3 weeks. The lesions of primary syphilis are chancres: solitary, painless ulcerations that form at the site of inoculation. A chancre begins as a firm papule and breaks down to become a well-demarcated hard ulcer with a raised, rolled border and a finely granular, erythematous base. The average size of a chancre is 0.5 to 2 cm. Often they occur on the labia, the posterior fourchette, the cervix, or the vagina, although pharyngeal and anal chancres also appear. Bilateral,

firm, nontender regional adenopathy is common. Because chancres are not painful, they often remain unnoticed and undetected. Spirochetes are found at the base of the ulcer, and chancres are infectious. If untreated, chancres heal spontaneously in 2 to 6 weeks.

Nine to 90 days after chancre formation, or an average of 6 to 12 weeks after exposure, hematogenous dissemination of spirochetes occurs, and the onset of symptoms of secondary syphilis begins. The chancre of primary syphilis still may be present. Secondary syphilis has mucocutaneous and systemic manifestations with multiorgan involvement. The most common manifestations of secondary syphilis are rash, lymphadenopathy, and mucous patches of the mouth or of the genital area. Various types of generalized skin lesions may occur. Usually only one type exists at a time, although lesions may evolve. Macular, maculopapular, or primarily papular generalized skin eruptions are typical. Facial sparing and involvement of the palms and soles are classic. Pustular and discoid lesions, as well as alopecia and mucous membrane patches, are well-described variants of the mucocutaneous lesions of secondary syphilis. Another classic lesion of secondary syphilis is the condyloma latum, which is a confluence of raised moist, flat hypertrophic, exuberant granulomatous papular lesions that occur primarily in intertriginous or moist areas. These lesions are infectious. Generalized, usually nontender, lymphadenopathy commonly develops with the skin lesions of secondary syphilis. Influenza-type symptoms, such as fever, malaise, headache, sore throat, arthralgias, leukocytosis, anemia, and occasional splenomegaly, typify the systemic manifestations of secondary syphilis. Manifestations of involvement of other organ systems, such as hepatitis and meningitis, also occur.

After resolution of the signs of secondary syphilis, the infection enters a latent period. Formerly, latent syphilis of up to 4 years' duration was classified as early latent syphilis, and syphilis of more than 4 years' duration was classified as late latent syphilis. Today all types of syphilis of less than 1 year's duration are classified as early syphilis, and little distinction is made for latent syphilis of more than 1 year's duration. Symptoms of secondary syphilis can recur during early syphilis. Otherwise, latent syphilis is asymptomatic and is not infectious. Manifestations of late syphilis are thought to be largely a result of endothelial damage and of ongoing chronic inflammation. Five to 20 years or more after the initial disease occurrence, the consequences of late syphilis develop into single-system or multisystem involvement. Benign, mucocutaneous late disease is accompanied by painless, indolent, destructive lesions. The classic skin lesion of late syphilis is the solitary gumma: a progressive, granulomatous, necrotic ulcer. Lesions also may be nodular and multiple. Gummas and destructive lesions of late syphilis may involve visceral organs, long bones, and joints.

Cardiovascular syphilis and neurosyphilis are two other distinct forms of late syphilis. Cardiovascular syphilis prominently involves the aorta, resulting in aortic insufficiency and in thoracic aortic aneurysms. Neurosyphilis may be asymptomatic, may resemble acute meningitis, or may be responsible for the gradual deterioration of intellectual and motor capacity. Neurosyphilis is probably prevented by the synergy between penicillin therapy for early syphilis and the immune system. Neurosyphilis is of particular concern in the patient with HIV (Holton et al, 1992). Even without symptoms, as many as 50% of patients with syphilis and HIV are estimated to have neurosyphilis. One series showed that 30% of HIV-infected patients with positive serologic test results for syphilis have abnormal cerebral spinal fluid examination results.

Syphilis can be transmitted to the fetus at any stage of pregnancy, resulting in deformities, acute neonatal illnesses, and late manifestations of the disease. Congenital syphilis is prevented or ameliorated by treatment of the mother during pregnancy. For this reason, premarital and prenatal screening for syphilis are mandatory. Because of the increase in congenital syphilis during the late 1980s and the early 1990s, universal prenatal screening multiple times during gestation is recommended.

Diagnosis

A dark-field examination should be performed on secretions from a cleaned lesion. If spirochetes are demonstrated, a diagnosis of syphilis may be made. Positive results of dark-field examination are reported in 78% of chancres of primary syphilis (Anderson et al, 1989). False negative results of dark-field examination can occur, particularly when topical or systemic antimicrobial therapy suppresses the numbers of spirochetes.

The diagnosis of syphilis most often is made by serologic methods. Serologic tests for syphilis are of two types, nontreponemal and treponemal. The nontreponemal tests most widely available are the Venereal Disease Research Laboratory (VDRL) slide tests and the rapid plasma reagin circle card test (RPRCT). These tests detect the presence of cardiolipin, a nonspecific antigen produced during syphilitic infection. These tests are quantitative, and decreasing serial titers may be used to judge therapeutic responses. An abnormal nontreponemal test result is suggestive of, but not specific for, a diagnosis of syphilis. Positive nontreponemal test results for syphilis are associated with various conditions and disorders, including collagen-vascular diseases, lymphomas, drug abuse, and sarcoidosis, and with acute infections such as mononucleosis, *Mycoplasma* infections, HIV infection, and other febrile illnesses.

Testing for the presence of specific antitreponemal antibodies aids in the definitive diagnosis of syphilis. The fluorescent treponemal antibody absorption test (FTA ABS) and the microhemagglutination–*T. pallidum* test (MHA TPS) are the treponemal tests most widely used. They confirm a diagnosis of syphilis with a low false positive rate of 1% to 2%. Once positive results are obtained in a patient, the results of that specific antitreponemal antibody test will always be positive in that patient despite successful therapy.

A serologic test for syphilis predicts the disease in approximately 75% of patients by the fourth week after exposure. By 6 weeks to 3 months, 99% to 100% of serologic test results are abnormal. Although a chancre may be present before seropositivity is revealed, secondary syphilis is usually accompanied by an abnormal serologic test result. If a serologic test result for syphilis remains negative 3 months after suspected exposure, the diagnosis of syphilis is not made. There is no association between the magnitude of the antibody titer and the stage of the disease. In the late stages of syphilis, nontreponemal test results for syphilis may be negative in as many as 30% of patients. However, the treponemal test result is positive in virtually 100% of patients.

When results of a serologic test for syphilis are positive, the stage of disease is determined using historic guidelines. If the patient is asymptomatic and serologic test results determined within the preceding year are negative, or if symptoms of primary or secondary syphilis were present within the preceding year, early syphilis is diagnosed. If normal serologic testing within the preceding year was not documented and if no symptoms of primary or secondary syphilis are documented, syphilis of more than 1 year's duration is presumed. If latent syphilis of prolonged duration is suspected, a lumbar puncture will rule out neurosyphilis. However, the decision to perform this procedure must be individualized (Rudolph, 1976). If no neurologic or psychiatric abnormalities exist and if treatment is with penicillin, a lumbar puncture may be unnecessary because standard penicillin therapy for syphilis of more than 1 year's duration cures most cases of asymptomatic neurosyphilis. However, all patients who have HIV or who are immunosuppressed and have newly diagnosed syphilis should undergo lumbar puncture.

Treatment

Treatment of syphilis will abort acute disease and prevent progression of the disease, but it will not alter the permanent changes produced by tissue destruction. Recommended therapy for all stages of syphilis is parenteral penicillin G. Penicillin-allergic patients who are not pregnant or infected with HIV or who have neurosyphilis are treated with doxycycline or tetracycline. The length of therapy is determined by disease stage. Primary, secondary, and early latent syphilis are treated with benzathine penicillin 2.4 million U intramuscularly in a single dose or with a 2-week course of doxycycline 100 mg orally twice a day or with tetracycline 500 mg orally four times a day. Syphilis of more than 1 year's duration is treated with the penicillin regimen just described once per week for 3 successive weeks or with a 4-week course of doxycycline or tetracycline. Patients with neurosyphilis are given aqueous crystalline penicillin G, 3 to 4 million U intravenously every 4 hours for 10 to 14 days. Penicillin-allergic patients who are pregnant or who have HIV or neurosyphilis may need to be hospitalized for desensitization and treatment with parenteral penicillin for optimal therapy.

The Jarisch-Herxheimer reaction is a well-described phenomenon occurring in some patients treated for primary or secondary syphilis. Approximately 12 hours after therapy, skin lesions become more prominent, and pronounced systemic symptoms of fever, rigors, headache, myalgias, and arthralgias occur. Presumably either the release of treponemal toxins or the formation of circulating antigen-antibody complexes causes the reaction. Symptoms are self-limited and do not recur, and no specific therapy is indicated.

Follow-up and Prevention

After successful therapy, nontreponemal serologic test results revert to normal in a large percentage of patients, depending on the duration of disease (Brown et al, 1985; Fiumara, 1977a; Fiumara, 1980; Romanowski et al, 1991). Within 1 year, 100% of patients with primary syphilis are seronegative. Within 2 years, virtually all patients with secondary syphilis have normal nontreponemal serologic test results. Within 5 years, approximately 45% of patients with latent syphilis are seronegative. Patients should be reexamined clinically and serologically to assess treatment response at 6 months and 12 months or more often if indicated. In patients who have persistent signs and symptoms and a sustained fourfold increase in nontreponemal test titers, previous treatment probably failed or perhaps they were reinfected. Those treated for primary and secondary syphilis and who have nontreponemal test titers that do not decline fourfold within 6 months are at risk for treatment failure. These patients should be reevaluated for HIV infection and retreated for syphillis. Partners of patients diagnosed with syphilis at any stage should be notified and evaluated clinically and serologically.

Syphilis is usually diagnosed through screening and contact tracing. Therefore, it has been suggested that, in addition to premarital and prenatal screening, it would be cost-effective to screen for syphilis in patients in whom other STDs are diagnosed and in areas or populations in which syphilis is diagnosed with unusual frequency (Hibbs et al, 1993).

CHANCROID

Chancroid, characterized by painful genital ulcers, suppurative inguinal lymphadenopathy, and a lack of systemic signs and symptoms, is a sexually transmitted disease caused by the bacteria *Haemophilus ducreyi*. Chancroid is endemic in tropical and subtropical developing countries. The occurrence of chancroid is associated with illicit drug use, prostitution, lack of cleanliness in uncircumcised male partners, syphilis, and HIV infection. In Africa, chancroid is a major risk factor for the heterosexual acquisition of HIV infection. Since 1981, many outbreaks of chancroid in the United States have been documented, usually in urban areas, and have been associated with contact with an infected prostitute (Schulte et al, 1992). Unlike the situation in developing countries, the control and eradication of outbreaks in the United States have been largely successful.

After an incubation period averaging 3 to 7 days, the genital lesions of chancroid appear as small papules or vesicles that become pustular. These lesions rupture and form ulcers within 1 to 3 days of onset. These ulcers are soft, not indurate, and they have irregular, ragged borders with undermined edges. A rim of erythema may surround the ulcer. The base of the ulcer is granulomatous and friable, and it is often covered with gray, adherent, sometimes necrotic, sometimes serosanguineous exudate. Ulcers are painful and tender and may occur individually or in numbers. Contiguous spread results from autoinoculation. Ulcers vary from a few millimeters to 20 millimeters. Most often the labia, the posterior fourchette, and the perianal region are involved, but the cervix, vagina, clitoris, and urethra may be involved. In asymptomatic women, the organism can be present in cervical secretions.

Regional lymph nodes are involved in more than 50% of patients. Bilateral involvement of inguinal nodes is common; however, if genital lesions are unilateral, lymph node involvement is also unilateral. The lymph nodes are superficially tender, increase in size, and may become matted, suppurate, and fluctuant. Overlying skin becomes thinned and necrotic, leading to spontaneous rupture and drainage. If lymph nodes are indurated and fluctuant, they can be aspirated, and a large, chronic, draining sinus may be prevented.

Diagnosis

Using laboratory test results to arrive at a diagnosis of chancroid entails an approximately 80% rate of accuracy (Dangor et al, 1990; Faro, 1989). The diagnosis of chancroid is made either by scraping material from the edges of an ulcer or by collecting material from a suppurating lymph node and culturing it on specific media (Joseph and Rosen, 1994). A Gram stain of this material reveals predominantly gram-negative coccobacillary forms often arranged in a chaining "school of fish" pattern. *H. ducreyi* may be one of many bacterial species present in chancroid lesions; the diagnosis in these patients may be more difficult to document. Experience is being garnered with immunofluorescent staining of lesion material and immunobinding serologic testing. When culture media are not available, the diagnosis of chancroid is often made by the clinical presentation and by the exclusion of other causes of genital ulceration such as genital herpes, LGV, and syphilis (Morse, 1989).

Treatment

If left untreated, ulcers may persist, grow, and form more extensive, erosive lesions. Occasionally, local lesions may run a self-limited course. Treatment used to consist of the administration of sulfa or tetracycline. Tetracycline resistance, however, is widespread, and there are increasing reports of sulfa resistance. Resistance to other antimicrobials is highly variable geographically. Current CDC-recommended therapeutic options include azithromycin 1 g orally in a single dose, ceftriaxone 250 mg intramuscularly in a single dose, ciprofloxacin 500 mg orally twice a day for 3 days, or erythromycin base 500 mg orally four times a day for 7 days. With its oral route and single-dose regimen, azithromycin has major prescribing advantages over the other options.

Follow-up and Prevention

Patients should be reexamined 3 to 7 days after start of therapy. Successful therapy is heralded by subjective improvement in pain and tenderness within 2 to 3 days and objective improvement within 7 days. The organism is rapidly eliminated from lesions and nodes, but complete healing depends on the size of ulcer. Large ulcers require more than 2 weeks to heal. Fluctuance of lymph nodes can occur despite effective therapy; either needle aspiration or incision and drainage with packing can be used for treatment of this complication (Ernst et al, 1995). Sexual partners should be treated even if they do not have symptoms or visible lesions. Patients and their sexual partners should be advised to refrain from intercourse during the treatment period.

LYMPHOGRANULOMA VENEREUM

Lymphogranuloma venereum (LGV), whose major clinical manifestations result from the infection of regional lymph nodes that drain sites of transient local genital infection, is a sexually transmitted disease caused by *C. trachomatis,* specifically immunotypes L1, L2, and L3. Rare in North America and other industrialized countries, LGV is commonly found in tropical and semitropical areas, particularly in developing countries. Because of the increase in immigration from Southeast Asia and South America, the incidence of LGV in the United States is increasing.

The transient mucosal or cutaneous lesion of LGV occurs at the site of inoculation 4 to 21 days after exposure. In women, the lesions are usually isolate, although multiple lesions may develop. Lesions form predominantly on the posterior vulva, the urethral meatus, and the medial labia; sometimes the vagina and the cervix are involved. Lesions are small (less than 6 mm in diameter), vesicular, papular, or pustular. They progress to small, shallow ulcers with irregular borders and erythematous bases. Ulcers usually are not painful and often are not noticed by women. After a short time, local lesions heal spontaneously, and after variable periods of latency, symptoms of local lymphadenitis become manifest.

Symptoms of adenitis vary according to the lymph chains involved and the chronicity of infection. The initial course of lymph node involvement is a 1- to 4-week period during which multiple nodes become inflamed and suppurate, become fixated to overlying skin, and spontaneously rupture and drain. Chronic inflammation of involved lymphatics may lead to obstruction with retrograde edema and occasional ulceration. Involved tissue is often totally replaced by fibrosis and constriction with scarring. Repeated episodes of spontaneous rupture and drainage may lead to chronically draining sinuses, fistula formation, and scarring.

Initial LGV lesions of the anterior vulva and lower portion of the vagina drain into femoral and inguinal lymphatics, resulting in the inguinal syndrome. Multiple nodes of inguinal and femoral regions become firm, adhere to each other, and eventfully form buboes that are fluctuant, painful, and fixed to the skin. If inguinal and femoral areas are involved, buboes are separated by the inguinal ligament forming the pathognomonic groove sign. Involvement most often is unilateral. Chronic inflammation of inguinal lymph nodes can lead to fibrous constriction of the inguinal area, which is often accompanied by draining sinuses. Hypertrophy and edema of vulvar lymphatic tissues can be marked. This is called esthiomene, and when it occurs it is analogous to elephantiasis in men. Overlying vulvar skin may ulcerate. Chronic inflammation in the vaginal and periureteral areas can lead to stricture and fistula formation.

In women the perirectal and pelvic lymph nodes are involved, leading to genitorectal manifestations of LGV. Patients have proctocolitis with bloody diarrhea and perianal discharge or retroperitoneal lymphadenopathy demonstrated by noninvasive imaging techniques. Fibrosis of edematous mucosa eventually leads to stricture formation, and rectovaginal fistulas are common. Unlike chancroid, systemic symptoms may be present when patients seek treatment for LGV. Approximately 50% of patients have fever, malaise, headache, and anorexia at the time of initial lymphadenitis.

Diagnosis

Usually the diagnosis of LGV is based on the results of antibody testing. Complement fixation titers to *C. trachomatis* greater than or equal to 1:128 suggest LGV. Antibody testing by microimmunofluorescence may show an increase in specific IgG titers or the presence of specific IgM antibody. Chlamydial organisms occasionally may be isolated from the exudate of fluctuant or draining buboes, or characteristic chlamydial inclusion bodies can be demonstrated by direct fluorescent antibody staining techniques. Histologic examination of involved nodes may show suggestive palisading aggregates of mononuclear cells surrounding the granulomas or the microabscesses, but they may be fairly nonspecific so biopsy is not the primary mode of diagnosis.

Treatment

Treatment cures infection and prevents the sequelae of nodal involvement. Usual therapy for LGV is with doxycycline 100 mg orally twice a day for at least 3 weeks until the remission of systemic symptoms and local disease. Alternative therapies include erythromycin base 500 mg orally four times a day for 3 weeks, which is also recommended for pregnant women. Aspiration or incision and drainage of fluctuant nodes through normal skin can prevent spontaneous rupture and chronic sinus formation.

Follow-up and Prevention

Patients should be followed up clinically until all signs and symptoms have resolved. Sexual partners of patients diagnosed with LGV should be examined and tested for urethral chlamydial infection, and they should be treated if they had sexual contact with the patient within 30 days of the onset of the patient's symptoms.

DONOVANOSIS

Donovanosis, formerly called granuloma inguinale, is a sexually transmitted diease associated with the encapsulated gram-negative bacillus *Calymmatobacterium granulomatis* and characterized by slowly progressive, hypertrophic ulceration with tissue destruction of the lower genital tract. It is rare in Europe and North America and is most common in tropical and subtropical countries. It tends to occur in small endemic foci and has been associated with a history of syphilis.

The incubation period of donovanosis averages 2 to 4 months, but it may be as long as 6 months. The initial genital tract lesion is a painless, indurated, reddish brown papule that, over a course of days or weeks, erodes and ulcerates. Ulcerations have well-defined borders and clean bases with exuberant, velvety granulation tissue. Most lesions develop on the vulva, are fairly superficial, and spread by contact, autoinoculation, and lymphatic extension. They are not tender unless superinfected. Involved tissue undergoes repeated granulomatous proliferation, ulceration, and scarring; eventually, extensive tissue destruction takes place. Although donovanosis often results in genital ulcers, bleeding from the anogenital tract can occur in as many as 20% of patients (Bassa et al, 1993; Hoosen et al, 1992). Extension to the inguinal area is associated with subcutaneous induration, swelling, and eventual breakdown with pseudobubo formation. Lymph nodes may be slightly enlarged and occasionally tender, but they do not suppurate. Systemic signs are rare, and when they do occur, they are related to extensive disease with secondary infection.

Diagnosis

The diagnosis of donovanosis is established by demonstrating the presence of Donovan bodies in tissue preparations stained with Wright's stain or Giemsa stain. Donovan bodies are mononuclear cells containing large numbers of encapsulated bacilli. Organisms appear in clusters of blue or black, and the entire Donovan body resembles a safety pin. Scrapings of lesions, crush preparations of tissue, or biopsy samples taken from the edge of an ulcer reveal these characteristic formations.

Treatment

Left untreated, lesions of donovanosis appear to undergo periods of spontaneous resolution or healing with subsequent relapses of active disease. Active lesions resolve with antibiotic therapy and relapse less often. Occasionally, prolonged courses of antibiotics are required to heal ulcers and to prevent recurrent disease. One double-strength tablet of trimethoprim-sulfamethoxazole twice a day and 100 mg doxycycline twice a day for at least 3 weeks are the therapies of choice, though ciprofloxacin or erythromycin base are also effective.

Follow-up and Prevention

Patients should be followed up clinically until all signs and symptoms have resolved. Sexual partners of patients who have donovanosis should be examined and treated if they had sexual contact during the 60 days before the onset of patient's symptoms or if they, too, have symptoms and signs of the disease.

GENITAL WARTS

Genital warts, caused by the human papillomavirus (HPV), are among the most common viral STDs in the United States. It is estimated that there are 750,000 new cases every year (CDC, 1994). Approximately, 5% to 20% of people in the 15- to 49-year age group are infected with HPV. Only a small percentage of infected people have clinically evident lesions (Koutsky et al, 1988). Consistently, the highest rates of genital HPV infection have been found in sexually active women younger than 25. In a study of college women who were HPV negative, the cumulative 4-year incidence of HPV infection was 43% (Ho et al, 1998). The major risk factors for acquiring genital HPV infection involve sexual behavior. The more sexual partners a patient has had or the more partners the patient's partner has had, the higher the risk for HPV infection (Kataja et al, 1993; Burk et al, 1996). Another risk factor is immunosuppression. Patients with immune deficiencies have higher rates of HPV than those who are immunocompetent (Lowy et al, 1994).

Once they are sexually transmitted, genital warts have an incubation period ranging from 3 weeks to 8 months (average, approximately 3 months). The transmission rate for genital warts is 25% to 60%, and infectivity may be influenced by the number of lesions and by the ages of the lesions. Genital warts of longer duration tend to be less infectious.

Typical genital warts are exophytic growths that appear as papillary, pink to white, frondlike lesions. These lesions are superficial, and they may be solitary, they may grow in clusters, or they may coalesce into large masses that resemble cauliflowers. Some gross warts appear as discrete, flat-topped, hyperkeratotic papules. The lesions usually are not painful, but they may be pruritic. When exceptionally large, the warts may become necrotic and secondarily infected, leading to superficial bleeding, a discharge, and a fetid odor.

Any part of the vulva, particularly the posterior fourchette, may become infected by HPV and show manifestations of genital warts. The mons, the perineum, and the perianal areas may be involved, as may the vagina, the cervix, and the anal canal. If warts appear near orifices, internal involvement is apparent in 50% to 70% of patients. For this reason, all patients with vulvar warts should undergo speculum examination, and all patients with perianal warts should undergo rectal examination or perhaps anoscopy. Visible warts that develop in the vagina and on the cervix usually appear as flat or papular lesions. Most cervical warts are flat and are visible only by acetic acid staining or by colposcopy.

Genital wart growth is stimulated by heat and moisture and probably by the number, types, and ages of lesions. Autoinoculation may be responsible for contiguous spread. In addition, some genital warts may grow remarkably during pregnancy, only to recede after delivery. Whether this is related to hormonal factors or to changes in local cellular immunity is unclear. The growth of warts tends to slow with time, and as many as one third undergo spontaneous remission within 6 to 12 months. Cellular immune mechanisms are thought to control HPV in part. Diabetic patients, immunosuppressed patients, and those with systemic illness affecting their cellular immunity often experience massive growths of warts that are difficult to control.

HPV has been associated with dysplasia and with cancer of the lower genital tract, particularly of the vulva and the cervix. Among other evidence, there is a statistical association between cervical warts and cervical dysplasia, and HPV DNA is detected in several types of genital malignancy (Reid et al, 1987). Of the more than 80 different types of HPV, some more than others are associated with malignancy. For example, HPV types 6 and 11 are seen in most patients with typical genital warts or in association with mild dysplasia. HPV types 16 and 18 are disproportionately associated with severe dysplasia and cancer of the cervix and the vulva. It is thought that HPV types 16 and 18 encode for two transforming gene products, the E6 protein, which causes rapid degradation of the p53 tumor suppressor protein, and the E7 protein, which binds the retinoblastoma susceptibility gene product (Hartwell et al, 1992). These changes may play a role in the pathogenesis of lower genital tract cancer.

Diagnosis

The diagnosis of genital warts is suggested by a typical gross appearance and by the exclusion of other processes by biopsy. Because most people who have HPV infection do not have clinically evident lesions, the prevalence of HPV genital disease is underestimated (Beutner et al, 1991). To aid with the detection of subclinical HPV infection, colposcopy, cytologic assessment from biopsies and cervical Papanicolaou smears, and HPV DNA tests can document the presence of a virus. Colposcopy can localize vaginal and cervical lesions by the demonstration of acetowhite areas, but this technique is not specific. Histologic features of genital warts include papillomatosis, acanthosis, and parakeratosis with vacuolization of epithelial cells. Papanicolaou smears, by revealing characteristic koilocytotic changes, may suggest the presence of HPV in as many as 1% to 2% of childbearing women. To characterize histologically equivocal lesions, specific HPV detection by DNA probes, in situ hybridization and PCR techniques can help. Typing HPV by DNA probe or by in situ hybridization techniques is in the investigational stage. At present, HPV typing is not clinically helpful in guiding either prognosis or therapy.

Treatment

Genital warts are generally treated with either local cytotoxic agents or ablative therapy. Local application of 10% to 25% podophyllin in benzoin, an antimitotic agent that incorporates into the wart, causes sloughing of the tissue within 3 to 4 days. This treatment is slightly less effective for hyperkeratotic warts and may have to be repeated at weekly intervals for the resolution of larger warts. Repeated patient application of 0.5% podophyllotoxin solution, one of the active components of podophyllin, has been reported to be safe and efficacious (Bonnez et al, 1994). The patient applies the solution twice daily for three consecutive days and repeats the cycle weekly for a maximum of 4 weeks. Trichloroacetic acid and bichloroacetic acid, caustic agents that destory warts by the chemical coagulation of proteins, are of particular value as a treatment for flat warts and for warts on mucosal surfaces. Repeated application every 1 to 2 weeks may be necessary.

Cryocautery, laser therapy, and electrocautery have been used successfully as ablative therapy (Stone et al, 1990; Yliskoski et al, 1989). During cryocautery, the lesions should be frozen to the base. Blistering and resolution of the lesions may take place with initial freezing or may require repeated freezing. Laser therapy and electrocautery attempt to remove lesions completely at the initial therapy. Fewer warts recur after laser therapy if a margin of normal-appearing tissue is also treated (Townsend et al, 1993). All ablative therapies are associated with recurrences of warts to some degree, probably because of latent HPV infection in surrounding tissues. Recurrences are more common in immunosuppressed patients. In addition, recurrences in immunosuppressed patients or in women older than 40 may be associated with malignancy, including squamous disease of the lower genital tract and lymphoproliferative disorders (Marshburn and Trofatter, 1988). Occasionally, large warts require surgical removal. Electrocautery and surgical removal can involve significant blood loss, especially during pregnancy.

Given the high rate of recurrence after common therapies that rely on the physical destruction of HPV lesions, two new methods with direct antiviral activity against HPV—interferon and imiquimod—have been introduced. Interferon is an antiviral, immunomodulatory agent. Studies of interferon suggest that most warts regress with either systemic, topical, or intralesional therapy. However, warts often recur after interferon therapy. Increasing experience suggests that interferon may be useful as adjunct therapy, in addition to ablative therapy, for the treatment of extensive lesions (Week et al, 1988). Adverse systemic side effects and high cost may limit the frequency of interferon administration.

Imiquimod is a potent inducer of interferon-α and other cytokines and is thought to act as an immune-response enhancer. Imiquimod is marketed as a topical 5% cream that patients can apply themselves. The preparation is directly applied to the lesions at bedtime on three alternating days per week for as long as 16 weeks, until the lesions are gone. A double-blind randomized study found topical 5% imiquimod safe and efficacious in clearing lesions. In addition, the recurrence rate at 3 months was low (Edwards et al, 1998). Systemic adverse side effects are unusual because less than 1% of the imiquimod is absorbed.

Follow-up and Prevention

Patients with a history of genital warts should be counseled regarding the need for regular cytologic screening for cervical cancer. Those with persistent or atypical genital warts should be followed up for dysplasia or malignancy, and biopsy specimens of those lesions should be taken. Any associated vaginal infections should be treated concomitantly. Patients should be counseled on ways to decrease local moisture to limit the growth of the lesions that are present. After the initial disappearance or removal of lesions, follow-up of patients and prompt treatment for new or recurrent lesions are necessary. Partner notification is not imperative because treating partners has no effect on the treatment course in women (Krebs and Helmkamp, 1991).

MOLLUSCUM CONTAGIOSUM

Molluscum contagiosum is a benign viral skin infection caused by a DNA-containing pox virus. This infection is spread by intimate, skin-to-skin contact, by autoinoculation, and occasionally by fomites. Perigenital molluscum contagiosum is sexually transmitted, and at least 10% of women with molluscum receive a concomitant diagnosis of another STD (Radcliffe et al, 1991).

Characteristic molluscum lesions are small (2 to 5 mm), flesh-colored or slightly erythematous firm papules. They have umbilicated centers and are found on the epidermal surfaces of the extremities, trunk, or genital areas, including the lower abdomen, pubic area, and inner thighs. Lesions appear 2 to 7 weeks after contact and are usually multiple and asymptomatic. Lesions may occur in crops, and they often spontaneously resolve. The typical course of the disease is 6 to 9 months.

Diagnosis

A diagnosis of molluscum contagiosum is usually made by its clinical appearance. Lesions project into the dermis but do not cross the basement membrane. They can be removed intact, and when crushed onto a slide, Wright's or Giemsa stain reveals molluscum bodies in infected cells. These are ovoid accumulations of replicating virus within the cytoplasm.

Treatment

Most molluscum contagiosum infections resolve if left untreated. However, to contain the spread of lesions or for cosmetic purposes, treatment may be indicated (Billstein and Mattaliatio, 1990). Lesions can be extracted by curette or by incision. Cryotherapy with liquid nitrogen is effective, comfortable, and widely used. The use of laser has also been described.

Widespread distribution of molluscum-like lesions, giant lesions, and occurrence in atypical locations, such as the face, have been associated with the kind of severe cellular immunosuppression seen with HIV infection. A biopsy of such lesions is recommended before treatment to rule out fungal skin infection, in particular *Cryptococcus neoformans* (Peterson and Gerstoft, 1992; Schwartz and Myzkowski, 1992).

VAGINITIS

Vaginitis, characterized by abnormal discharge, vulvovaginal discomfort, or both, is the most common gynecologic problem for which women seek treatment. Vaginitis accounts for more than 10 million office visits each year (Sobel, 1985). Many microorganisms, including those associated with vaginitis, can be cultured from the vagina of asymptomatic women. Unless symptoms are present, the diagnosis of vaginitis should not be made. In addition, because symptoms of vaginitis are nonspecific, the presumptive diagnosis and treatment of vaginitis may not be reliable without laboratory confirmation.

An average of four to seven organisms can be found on routine culturing of the vagina (Bartlett et al, 1977; Galask, 1988; Galask et al, 1976; Larsen and Galask, 1980; Linder et al, 1978). Aerobic and anaerobic bacteria are present. Potential pathogens of the upper genital tract such as gram-negative enteric rods, staphylococcus species, streptococci (including enterococci), anaerobic gram-positive cocci, and bacteroides species are considered normal flora of the vagina. In addition, nonpathogens such as lactobacilli and diphtheroids also are often found. The normal pH of the vagina is 3.5 to 4.5 (Hunter and Long, 1958). The pH of the vagina is influenced by the organic acid byproducts of metabolism, produced by the predominant species in the vaginal flora. Vaginal pH and vaginal flora must be considered when vaginitis is diagnosed. It is increasingly apparent that lactobacilli are regarded as an important microbial defense. Hydrogen peroxide (H_2O_2)-producing species appear to be associated with vaginal health, whereas H_2O_2-negative species are associated with infection and with the organisms present in vaginitis (Hillier et al, 1992). Antibiotics, hormonal changes, douching, vaginal medication, disease states, immunosuppression, and sexual activity may have an influence on vaginal microflora (Galask, 1988; Märdh, 1991; Mead, 1978; Meisels, 1969). Cervical mucus and the presence of normal vaginal discharge must be taken into

Table 18-3 Diagnosis of Vaginitis

	Typical Symptoms	Clinical Findings	Discharge	Wet pH	Preparation	Other
Candidiasis	Itching, irritation, dyspareunia	Erythema, edema	White and clumpy, occasionally watery and clumpy, may be none	<4.5	Potassium hydroxide reveals hyphae, buds	Culture may be of value
Trichomoniasis	Discharge, pain, occasionally itching	Strawberry cervix or vagina	Copious, pooling, frothy gray-white to yellow-green	>5.5	Saline reveals motile *Trichomonas*	>10 WBCs/high-power field
Bacterial vaginosis	Discharge, odor	No mucosal changes	Sticky, homogenous	>4.7	Saline reveals clue cells	Positive whiff test; lack of WCBs and lactobacilli

consideration when interpreting symptoms of vaginitis. Three types of infectious vaginitis are recognized (Table 18-3). These are discussed in turn.

Candidiasis

Candidiasis is the second most common type of vaginal infection. Its usual cause is *Candida albicans,* an organism that can be found in the lower genital tracts of 30% to 80% of women with minimal or no symptoms. A small number of fungal vaginal infections are caused by *Candida glabrata* or by other candidal species.

The hallmark of candidiasis is itching, irritation, or both. Itching may be severe in either the vaginal or the vulvar area, and irritation may be associated with dysuria and dyspareunia. Discharge is commonly described as cottage cheesy or thick, white, and clumpy, although it is not always present with symptomatic candidiasis. Occasionally, it is thin and watery.

Symptoms of candidiasis often begin just before the menses. In addition, numerous precipitating factors have been delineated for symptomatic candidiasis. In those who have *Candida* species in the vagina, some of the precipitating factors for symptomatic candidiasis are those that foster the overgrowth of *Candida.* This overgrowth may result from a suppression of normal bacterial flora, a depression of local cellular immunity, alterations in the metabolic and nutritional milieu of the vagina, and unknown mechanisms. Precipitating factors for symptomatic candidiasis include immunosuppressive or steroid therapy, diabetes mellitus, pregnancy, hormone replacement therapy, oral contraceptive agents, and systemic antibiotics.

Candidiasis often appears as vulvitis or vulvovaginitis. Examination reveals well-demarcated erythema of the vulva with satellite lesions surrounding the major rim of erythema. The vulva can be notably edematous. The vagina also may be edematous and erythematous, with erythema extending onto the squamous exocervix. Excoriations and fissures of

the vulva, and occasionally of the vagina, are not unusual. Even if the patient has noticed no discharge, an adherent clumpy white discharge may be found in the upper portion of the vagina.

When candidiasis is suspected by the clinical presentation, the diagnosis must be confirmed by the finding of normal vaginal pH and positive results on 10% potassium hydroxide (KOH) microscopy. When 1 drop of the discharge is mixed with 1 drop of 10% KOH, covered with a coverslip, and examined under the microscope, normal cellular elements are lysed, and the branching hyphae and buds of the *Candida* are visible. In as many as 25% to 30% of patients with symptomatic candidiasis, the KOH wet preparation is falsely negative. Thus, when a patient has the clinical presentation of candidiasis and a normal vaginal pH but negative microscopy for yeast, diagnostic accuracy can be improved by culture using specific media such as Nickerson's media and Sabouraud's agar.

Various products are available to treat candidiasis. Nystatin vaginal tablets administered for 14 days are one of the oldest and cheapest treatments for uncomplicated candidiasis. More effective initial treatments include local azole antifungal preparations and oral azole agents. The choice of therapy should be based on physician recommendation and patient preference.

Imidazole (miconazole, clotrimazole, butoconazole) and triazole (terconazole) tablets, suppositories, and creams are widely used. Most imidazole preparations are now available over the counter without a prescription. Treatment courses range from 1 to 7 days, with shorter dosing regimens prescribed for doses of increasing concentration. All regimens are approximately equally efficacious with cure rates in excess of 80% (Reef et al, 1993). Shorter-course therapy with higher-dose medication decreases symptoms more rapidly but may be associated with an increased rate of local hypersensitivity reactions. Many experts recommend 7 days of therapy for pregnant patients.

The oral azole antifungal agent fluconazole has been found as efficacious as vaginal preparations in the treatment of vulvovaginal candidiasis (Sobel et al, 1995). Fluconazole is given as a single dose, and it includes uncommon, mild side effects of gastrointestinal intolerance, headache, and rash. It is preferred over oral ketoconazole for initial treatment because ketoconazole is administered over 5 days and has the potential for a serious, yet reversible, side effect of severe hepatotoxicity. The ease of administration of oral fluconazole compared with topical therapies must be contrasted with the desire of some persons to avoid systemic medications. Oral azoles are contraindicated in pregnancy.

Chronic symptoms or recurrent episodes of candidiasis, defined as four or more episodes of symptomatic candidiasis per year, develop in some women. The pathogenesis of recurrent vulvovaginal candidiasis (RVVC) is understood for few patients, such as those with uncontrolled diabetes or cellular immunosuppression. Other theories about its cause include recolonization from the gastrointestinal tract, reinfection from a sexual partner, and transient suppression of local cell-mediated immunity in some patients, with enhanced local allergic responses to *Candida* and other locally applied substances (Fidel et al, 1993; Fong et al, 1992; Witkin, 1987a; Witkin, 1987b; Witkin, 1991; Witkin et al, 1988). Recurrences may also result from infection with non-albicans *Candida* species such as *C. glabrata.* These infections tend to require a longer duration of therapy with available azole agents (Spinillo et al, 1993). It remains to be seen whether drug-resistant *Candida* plays a role in RVVC. Only one case of *C. albicans* resistant to azoles has been reported to date (Sobel and Vazquez, 1996). Cultures for the confirmation of *Candida* and the identification of species are recommended for patients with RVVC.

A number of approaches to RVVC exist (Sobel, 1997). Longer courses (10 to 14 days) of initial therapy, followed by maintenance suppression therapy for 6 months, are advised. The CDC recommends a maintenace regimen of 100 mg ketoconazole per day. Other drugs such as fluconazole, itraconazole, and clotrimazole are under investigation for this use. Interest has also developed in the use of boric acid (600 to 650 mg in a gel capsule used daily for 2 to 6 weeks) to treat RVVC, especially those cases caused by nonalbicans *Candida* species.

Although general dietary changes are not helpful, the daily ingestion of yogurt containing *Lactobacillus acidophilus* has been reported to decrease *Candida* colonization and symptomatic infections (Hilton et al, 1992). Initial results indicate acceptable cure rates. However, a recent prospective study failed to show a correlation between H_2O_2-producing lacotbacilli and *Candida* infections (Hawes et al, 1996). Additional controlled studies are needed before there can be widespread recommendation. Gentian violet-impregnated tampons are messy, and occasionally they irritate, but they are useful in some patients. Applying gentian violet directly to the vaginal vault each week until symp-

toms resolve is inconvenient, but it may be helpful in patients with RVVC.

Once a diagnosis of candidiasis has been made and treatment is started, patients should be instructed to return for follow-up visits only if symptoms persist or recur. Treatment of all sexual partners does not improve the initial response to therapy or decrease the frequency of recurrence. However, treatment of symptomatic partners may be beneficial.

Trichomoniasis

Trichomoniasis, an STD caused by the flagellated parasite *T. vaginalis,* is the third most common cause of vaginitis. It affects 180 million women worldwide and 2 to 3 million American women annually (Lossick, 1990). It is often isolated along with other sexually transmitted organisms, in particular *N. gonorrhoeae.* Risk factors associated with sexual activity, such as multiple or new partners, increase the chances of contracting trichomonas (Barbone et al, 1990).

The incubation period for trichomoniasis is approximately 20 days. Symptoms often peak just after the menses. Classic symptoms of trichomoniasis include a copious, frothy discharge and local pain and irritation. Patients may have dysuria, dyspareunia, and dull lower abdominal pain. Occasionally, itching is the predominant local symptom.

The cervix and the upper portion of the vagina infected by trichomonas may exhibit raised, punctate erythema. This strawberry appearance is pathognomonic for trichomoniasis, but it is found in a minority of patients. Usually, examination of the vulva and vagina reveals a copious, frothy discharge that is white to greenish yellow. The pH of the discharge is greater than 6.0. A wet preparation made by mixing 1 drop of the discharge with 1 drop of normal saline reveals motile trichomonads in most patients with symptomatic trichomoniasis. These parasites are slightly larger than WBCs, are ovoid, and have central, undulating membranes and terminal flagella. In addition, more than 10 WBCs/per high-power field are found on the wet preparations of most patients. Diagnostic accuracy can be improved by culture in specific media, such as Diamond medium or Tichosel broth (Fouts and Kraus, 1980; Krieger et al, 1988). Papanicolau smears occasionally reveal trichomonads but have a false positive rate of 30% to 40% in diagnosing trichomoniasis (Weinberger and Harger, 1993). Confirmatory tests are recommended before initiating treatment for positive Papanicolau smears.

In the United States, the most effective therapy for trichomoniasis is oral metronidazole. The recommended regimen is a single high-dose therapy with 2 g of metronidazole, which effectively eradicates *T. vaginalis* in 90% of patients. Particularly when this therapy is taken with other medications, severe nausea and vomiting occasionally preclude effective use. An alternative regimen of lower-dose longer-term therapy with 500 mg twice daily for 7 days may be used. If the patient cannot tolerate metronidazole, intravaginal clotrimazole or boric acid may provide relief from symptoms and may be curative. Trichomonas infections that are relatively resistant to metronidazole have been described. High-dose therapy repeated for 3 to 5 days, concomitant oral and vaginal therapy, and intravenous metronidazole all have cured resistant trichomoniasis (Muller et al, 1988).

Patients should be instructed to return if symptoms persist after treatment. All sexual partners must be treated even if they are asymptomatic because many women are reinfected by untreated partners. Couples should refrain from intercourse until both have finished treament and are asymptomatic.

Trichomoniasis has been implicated as a risk factor in cuff cellulitis after hysterectomy, cuff abscess, and adverse outcomes of pregnancy, particulary premature rupture of membranes and preterm delivery. Some authorities have proposed routine screening for and therapy of trichomonas before gynecologic surgery and during prenatal care.

Bacterial Vaginosis

Bacterial vaginosis (BV), formerly called *Gardnerella*-associated vaginitis or nonspecific vaginitis, is characterized by excessive discharge and odor. It is the most common cause of vaginitis in women of childbearing age. Despite the fact that BV is seen predominantly in sexually active premenopausal women, it does not appear to be closely associated with sexual activity and it is not considered an STD.

Although for many years the exact microbiologic cause of this infection was unknown, it is now regarded as a result of the synergism among various bacteria, including *Gardnerella vaginalis,* anaerobic gram-negative rods, *Peptostreptococcus* species, *Mycoplasma hominis, Ureaplasma urealyticum,* and *Mobiluncus* species (Hill, 1993). *G. vaginalis* is found as part of the vaginal flora in approximately one third of sexually active women. Without a critical concentration of other vaginal bacteria, particularly anaerobes, this organism is not thought to be responsible for symptoms (Spiegel et al, 1980). The effect bacterial synergy has in causing symptoms is shown using gas-liquid chromatography on specimens from patients with symptomatic disease. Organic acid metabolites of anaerobes predominate in these specimens, and the resolution of symptoms correlates with the appearance of metabolites produced by *Lactobacillus* and streptococcal species. The replacement of lactobacilli by *G. vaginalis,* anaerobes, *Mobiluncus,* and genital mycoplasms is a characteristic feature of bacterial vaginosis (Spiegel, 1991).

Patients with BV may have a variety of symptoms or none at all. As many as 50% may be asymptomatic, whereas 50% to 70% complain of an unpleasant, fishy, or musty vaginal odor. They also report increased vaginal discharge. The onset of odor and discharge associated with BV is evenly distributed throughout the menstrual cycle, and local discomfort is rarely a problem.

The diagnosis of BV is made with a high degree of certainty on examination of the patient and of the discharge.

The discharge of BV is typically homogeneous, grayish white to yellowish white, and partially adherent to the vulva and vaginal walls. Underlying edema or erythema of the vulva or vagina is atypical. The pH of this vaginal discharge is greater than 4.7. When 1 drop of KOH is added to 1 drop of discharge, an intense amine odor produces a positive whiff test result. Typically, on normal saline wet preparation, this discharge has a paucity of WBCs and a predominance of clue cells produced by the adherence of *G. vaginalis* to epithelial cells. By wet preparation, clue cells are best identified by a stippled birefringence that so densely covers the epithelial cell that the normal borders and nuclei are obscured. By Gram stain, clue cells can be identified as epithelial cells almost totally covered by small gram-negative rods. A paucity of other organisms can be seen in the background. Notably there is an absence of lactobacilli. BV can be diagnosed clinically by the presence of three of these four traits: homogeneous discharge, pH >4.7, positive whiff test, and clue cells (Thomason et al, 1990). The single most reliable sign is the presence of clue cells. Laboratory tests that detect the presence of the microbial byproducts unique to BV, such as volatile amines by gas-liquid chromatography, proline aminopeptidase by colorimetric assay, and sialidases, are used on a research basis but are not yet clinically applicable (Thomason et al, 1989). Various scoring systems that assess the presence and concentration of lactobacilli, clue cells, and gram-negative or gram-variable rods or curved organisms consistent with anaerobic *Bacteroides* and *Mobiluncus* species have been proposed (Eschenbach et al, 1988; Hillier, 1993; Nugent et al, 1991). Gram stain assessment is valuable when immediate microscopy is unavailable and for greater reproducibility as a research tool. Culture on a specific medium is rarely useful. BV-associated organisms may be part of the normal vaginal flora, although concentrations are typically higher when BV is present.

The most effective treatment for BV is metronidazole (Pheifer et al, 1978). Metronidazole is thought to cure this infection because of its effect on the vaginal anaerobes. Increasing experience suggests that vaginal therapy with metronidazole gel or clindamycin cream is also effective (Sweet, 1993). CDC-recommended regimens for the treatment of BV include metronidazole orally 500 mg twice a day for 7 days, metronidazole gel 0.75% twice a day for 5 days, and clindamycin cream 2% at bedtime for 7 days. Other treatments include metronidazole 2 g orally in one dose or clindamycin 300 mg orally twice a day for 7 days. In as many as 15% of patients, symptoms recur within 1 month of treatment. The risk factors in recurrence are incompletely understood, but BV may develop more often in users of diaphragms or vaginal contraceptive sponges.

BV has been associated with more invasive infections, including urinary tract infections in diaphragm users, PID, and posthysterectomy infection (Hooten et al, 1989; Soper et al, 1994; Peipert et al, 1997; Soper et al, 1990). It also has been associated with the complications of pregnancy, including preterm labor, preterm birth, intraamniotic infection, and postpartum endometritis (Gravett et al, 1986; Hillier et al, 1995; Hillier et al, 1988; Watts et al, 1990). Results of several investigations indicate that in pregnant women who are at high risk for preterm delivery and who have had a diagnosis of BV, treatment may reduce the risk for prematurity (Hauth et al, 1995; Morales et al, 1994). Thus, screening for and treatment of BV in asymptomatic pregnant women at high risk may be reasonable. The CDC-recommended regimen for the treatment of BV in pregnancy is metronidazole 250 mg orally three times a day for 7 days.

In patients who are not pregnant, follow-up is unnecessary if symptoms resolve after treatment. Because BV is not an STD and the treatment of partners does not reduce recurrence rates in women, their sexual partners do not have to be treated (Vejtorp et al, 1988).

Other Causes of Vaginitis Symptoms

Excessive vaginal discharge may be a manifestation of cervicitis. Organisms associated with cervicitis include *T. vaginalis, N. gonorrhoeae, C. trachomatis,* and herpes simplex virus. If any of these conditions is diagnosed, it should be treated appropriately. In addition, excessive vaginal discharge may be associated with cervical ectopy or eversion, without an apparent infectious cause.

Discharge and odor are associated with the presence of foreign bodies in the vaginal vault. Although this is mainly a concern in pediatric populations, forgotten tampons may also be a source of discharge. In addition to vulvar dystrophies, dysplasias, and vulvar vestibulitis syndrome, vulvar discomfort may be a result of hypersensitivity reactions. These should be considered in women who have undergone numerous courses of topical antiinfection therapy.

URINARY TRACT INFECTION

One in five women will have a urinary tract infection (UTI) at some time in her life, up to 25% of women every year have symptoms of acute dysuria, and more than 7 million office visits to physicians each year are for the evaluation of UTI or related symptoms. Although UTI is not a gynecologic infection, symptoms associated with UTI occur with various gynecologic disorders, so women often visit a gynecologist for the diagnosis of UTI.

The preponderance of symptomatic UTIs, commonly cystitis, develop in the lower urinary tract. UTIs may also appear to be asymptomatic bacteriuria or acute pyelonephritis. In addition, symptoms suggestive of lower UTIs may actually be the result of STDs, various noninfectious urethral syndromes, and vaginitis.

More than 90% of UTIs in women are caused by two organisms, *E. coli* and *Staphylococcus saprophyticus* (Hovelius and Märdh, 1984), with at least 80% caused by *E. coli.*

Women with lower tract UTIs have acute symptoms of dysuria, frequency, and urgency. They also experience gross hematuria, suprapubic pain, and flank or back discomfort.

Pyuria and bacteriuria are present in symptomatic lower tract UTIs.

Approximately 20% of women with UTIs have recurrences of symptoms within variable periods of time. Recurrences are often reinfections, as demonstrated by negative culture findings between episodes and by the isolation of organisms according to biotypes and sensitivity patterns during episodes. These reinfections rarely indicate serious morbidity or renal involvement. Recurrences develop in characteristic clusters of symptomatic UTIs, often during 6- to 12-month time periods. Less often, recurrent symptoms result from the persistence of the same organism. In particular, close intervals of 10 to 14 days between symptomatic episodes may indicate upper tract infection. Persistence of a single organism raises the concern of congenital or acquired structural or functional abnormalities of the urinary tract.

UTIs are dependent on host factors and on the properties of infecting organisms. Bacterial adherence to uroepithelial cells precedes infection. Flora, particularly coliforms, from the gastrointestinal tract colonize the vaginal introital and periurethral-meatal area and ascend into the bladder, causing symptomatic and asymptomatic bacteriuria. Various bacterial adhesions, surface receptor sites, and attachment properties of bacteria have been identified (Märdh and Westrom, 1976; Reid and Sobel, 1987). Women susceptible to UTIs demonstrate an increase in the incidence and density of colonization and more sites for bacterial attachment on uroepithelial surfaces than women without UTIs. The efficiency of bacterial adherence is probably influenced by genetic, hormonal, and other factors. Natural defenses against the bacterial adherence to and the ascent into the urinary tract may be genetically determined. These defenses include various substances produced by the urinary tract, local immunoglobulins, competitive bacterial flora, and normal voiding patterns.

Among sexually active women, most lower UTIs are associated with sexual intercourse (Fihn, 1988; Hooten et al, 1996). Most susceptible women become symptomatic within a short period of time after intercourse. Intercourse is thought to introduce colonizing bacteria into the bladder, and it is shown to increase transiently the numbers of bacteria in the urine up to tenfold.

An independent risk factor for UTI is diaphragm use (Fihn et al, 1985; Strom, 1987). Compared with nonusers, diaphragm users have 2 to 2.5 times the risk for UTI and increased vaginal colonization with coliforms. Other risk factors for UTI include a history of UTI and the failure to void after intercourse. Factors not associated with UTI include perineal hygiene, direction of wiping, and use of tampons and oral contraceptives.

Two percent to 10% of women have asymptomatic bacteriuria, as defined by the presence of 100,000 or more of a single pathogen found on two or more midstream, clean, voided specimens. Asymptomatic bacteriuria may be transient or intermittent, and whether its natural, long-term course is influenced by treatment is unclear. In nonpregnant, nonimmunocompromised women with morphologically normal urinary tracts, asymptomatic bacteriuria does not appear to be associated with UTI or with long-term morbidity and does not require eradication. Among patients with conditions that predispose them to upper UTI, such as pregnancy, attempts at eradication are warranted.

Studies suggest that infection or colonization of the upper urinary tract develops in some women with lower UTI. How often acute pyelonephritis develops if UTI is left untreated is unclear. However, most women with lower UTI appear not to be predisposed to acute pyelonephritis. The occurrence of pyelonephritis is influenced by pathogenic properties of bacteria and by factors in the host that affect bacterial adherence and ascent. Abnormalities of the urinary tract (*e.g.,* such as reflux, obstruction, or stones), abnormalities in host defenses (*e.g.,* diabetes and immunosuppression), and the introduction of virulent bacteria during catheterization or during other instrumentation, are associated with pyelonephritis. Pyelonephritis causes dysuria, frequency, and urgency in 50% of patients. In addition, fever, chills, malaise, and flank or back (costovertebral angle) pain and tenderness are hallmarks. Pyelonephritis causes more morbidity than lower UTI; it increases the risk for bacteremia and long-term sequelae and the need for longer treatment.

Women with dysuria, frequency, and urgency may not have bacterial infection of the lower urinary tract (Komaroff, 1984; Stamm et al, 1980). Urethritis caused by STDs such as *C. trachomatis, N. gonorrhoeae, T. vaginalis,* and HSV can cause identical symptoms. Epidemiologic risk factors, sexual history or history of disease in sexual partners, and associated symptomatology may suggest these diagnoses. Symptoms of urethritis typically occur less acutely, and urinalysis reveals pyuria but rarely hematuria. Urethritis is suspected in symptomatic women who have pyuria with negative urine cultures. In particular, *C. trachomatis* is responsible for symptoms in one third of women with dysuria, pyuria, and negative urine cultures.

Vaginitis also may cause dysuria and urgency. Although vaginitis classically causes external dysuria and UTI causes internal dysuria, this distinction is unreliable. If a urinalysis is properly obtained and if bacteriuria and pyuria are not demonstrable, other symptoms and signs of vaginitis should become apparent by direct history and examination.

Diagnosis

The diagnosis of UTI is made by urinalysis and urine culture. Most women with symptomatic UTI who later are documented to have bacteriuria have pyuria with more than 8 to 10 WBCs per milliliter in unspun urine or 2 to 5 WBCs per high-power field in spun urine sediment. Some authorities suggest that the presence of pyuria be used as a screen to determine which urine specimens should be cultured and which women should be treated presumptively for a UTI. A midstream, clean, voided urine sample, cultured using quantitative techniques, is appropriate for the evaluation of

asymptomatic bacteriuria, pyelonephritis, and most cases of lower UTI. The previously held belief that "significant bacteriuria" necessary for a diagnosis of UTI consists of 100,000 or more organisms per milliliter is clearly erroneous when referring to lower UTI. Although 50% of women with lower UTI have 100,000 or more organisms cultured from urine, approximately one third of women with symptoms of acute dysuria, frequency, and urgency have between 100 and 100,000 organisms by properly obtained culture and warrant a diagnosis of UTI (Stamm, 1989b; Stamm et al, 1982). Studies of bladder urine specimens obtained by suprapubic aspiration or by transurethral catheterization demonstrate that smaller numbers of organisms in symptomatic women are associated with reproducible bladder bacteriuria and pyuria and a predictable response to UTI therapy. The concept of significant bacteriuria or a single-organism colony count of 100,000 or more organisms per milliliter is appropriate only when applied to asymptomatic bacteriuria (Kass and Finland, 1956) or acute pyelonephritis. Thus, urine cultures that reveal 100,000 or more colonies per milliliter of a single pathogen support the diagnosis of UTI in asymptomatic women; cultures that reveal 100 or more colonies per milliliter of a single pathogen support the diagnosis of UTI in symptomatic women. The contamination of urine specimens with multiple organisms may confuse the interpretation of culture results. Clarification by culture of suprapubic aspiration or catheterization specimens may occasionally be of value. Microbiology laboratory technicians should be instructed to identify all bacterial species in urine cultures obtained from symptomatic women and to quantify and identify all *E. coli* and staphylococcal species in cultures obtained from symptomatic women.

Whether recurrences of infection are episodes of reinfection or of persistent infection should be determined. Persistence of infection despite adequate antibiotic therapy or multiple episodes of reinfection, variably defined as more than three to six episodes in 1 year, warrants urologic referral and evaluation for urinary tract abnormality. In addition, episodes of pyelonephritis in nonpregnant women or infections with unusual organisms, such as *Proteus* and other urea splitters associated with stone formation, are indications for urologic consultation.

Most symptomatic lower UTIs are not associated with urinary tract abnormalities. Women with recurrent UTI can predict with 90% accuracy the presence of infection by typical symptoms. If the urinary tract is shown to be normal and if results of previous cultures and patterns of previous infection are known, the initiation of therapy without confirmatory laboratory diagnosis is suggested as a cost-effective and appropriate alternative to repeated laboratory assessments. The proper diagnosis of lower UTI must take into account alternative diagnoses for the symptoms of dysuria, frequency, and urgency. In addition to urinalysis and to urine culture, pelvic examination, wet preparations, and cultures of the organisms that cause STD may be warranted (Table 18-4).

Table 18-4 Differential Diagnosis of Symptoms of Dysuria, Frequency, and Urgency

	Onset	Urinalysis	Urine Culture	Causative Organisms
Lower UTI	Acute	Pyuria, hematuria	≥100 organisms/mL	*E. coli, S. saprophyticus*
Pyelonephritis	Subacute (up to 10 days)	Pyuria, hematuria, casts	≥100,000 organisms/mL	*E. coli*, other gram-negative enterics, enterococci
Urethritis	Acute or subacute	Pyuria	— —	*C. trachomatis, T. vaginalis, N. gonorrhoeae, H. simplex*
Vaginitis	Acute or subacute	—	—	*T. vaginalis, C. albicans*
Other lower urinary tract syndromes	Subacute	— —	— —	—

Treatment

Single-dose antimicrobial therapy or standard dosage schedules of antibiotics for periods of 3, 5, 7, or 10 days all are appropriate therapy for lower UTI. Without antibiotic therapy, symptoms of lower UTI resolve spontaneously in as many as 70% of women. However, treatment eliminates symptoms more quickly. It also may clear an unrecognized upper UTI, and it may decrease the recurrence of symptomatic infection.

Approximately 80% of lower UTI is cured with single-dose therapy (Souney and Polk, 1982). Appropriate single-dose agents include trimethoprim-sulfamethoxazole and fluoroquinolones. Ampicillin, amoxacillin, and cephalosporins are not effective single-agent choices because they are rapidly excreted in the urine. Single-dose therapy is not appropriate for children, pregnant women, or women with underlying medical problems. Symptoms often persist for 2 to 3 days after successful single-dose therapy. This persistence of symptoms does not indicate that therapy has failed.

Standard antibiotic dosage regimens for 3 to 5 days cure 80% to 90% of lower UTI and result in fewer early recurrences than single-dose therapy. Whether 7- to 14-day courses of antibiotics provide additional benefit is unclear. Appropriate choices for standard dosage regimens include nitrofurantoin, trimethoprim-sulfamethoxazole, other sulphas, trimethoprim, penicillins, ampicillin or ampicillin combinations, and cephalosporins. The use of more expensive fluoroquinolones should probably be reserved for recurrent infections, treatment failures, and infections with resistant gram-negative organisms. Pyelonephritis should be treated with standard antibiotic dosage regimens for at least 10 days. Occasionally, patients are admitted for intravenous therapy because of the degree of illness or fever. Intravenous therapy should continue at least until patients are afebrile for 24 hours, and a 10-day course of therapy with oral antibiotics should be completed.

Follow-up and Prevention

Patients with a treated lower UTI who are not pregnant, not immunosuppressed, and without a urinary tract abnormality do not require a follow-up visit or a urine culture unless symptoms persist or recur. Patients with acute pyelonephritis should have a follow-up appointment and a test of cure.

The frequency of recurrent symptomatic lower UTI resulting from reinfection is decreased by low-dose antibiotics given prophylactically either as a single night-time dose or as a single dose after intercourse (Stapleton et al, 1990). Nitrofurantoin and trimethoprim-sulfamethoxazole demonstrate prophylactic benefit. Therapy should be instituted only after the infection has been cured, and it should be empirically continued for 6-month periods. Alternatively, self-medication with short-course therapy at the earliest signs of reinfection may be more cost effective and more acceptable to patients than prophylaxis.

Interest in the ability of cranberry juice to prevent recurrent UTI arose when studies in the 1980s showed that cranberry juice contains substances that inhibit bacterial adherence (Sobota, 1984; Zafriri et al, 1989). A recent randomized, double-blinded controlled trial showed that elderly women who drank cranberry juice every day had less pyuria and bacteriuria and less need for antibiotics (Avorn et al, 1994). Although corroborative studies are needed, women with recurrent UTI may elect to try this nonmedication remedy for the prevention of recurrent disease.

HUMAN IMMUNODEFICIENCY VIRUS INFECTION, INCLUDING ACQUIRED IMMUNODEFICIENCY SYNDROME

Acquired immunodeficiency syndrome (AIDS) is the most advanced stage in a continuum of clinical syndromes caused by the human immunodeficiency virus (HIV-1). These syndromes are characterized by the direct effect of this virus on organ systems and the sequelae of profound alterations in normal immune mechanisms that eventually lead to death.

AIDS was first described in populations of the United States in 1981 even though this disease had existed and was described in other parts of the world, most notably Africa and the Caribbean, before this time. Infection with HIV is now a major worldwide epidemic. Unique medical, societal, economic, legal, and other dilemmas are posed by this virus. Its long latency is part of the reason its pathophysiology and natural history are incompletely understood. Although major advances in the length of symptom-free survival have been made, its cure remains elusive.

In the United States the epidemic largely began within the male homosexual and bisexual communities; the recognition of a large reservoir of disease in the population of intravenous drug users soon followed. By 1988, reported cases of AIDS in women and children accounted for approximately 7% of the total. However, since that time AIDS has increased most rapidly in women. HIV infection in women is a disease of minorities, the disadvantaged, and the young: 70% of AIDS cases are reported in black and Hispanic women, and 80% are reported in women of childbearing age. Transmission occurs in association with intravenous drug use and with heterosexual activity. In asymptomatic women, the transmission of HIV infection is thought to result primarily from heterosexual activity. Heterosexual transmission is often associated with small numbers of sexual partners.

It is known that HIV is transmitted by either of the three following major routes: direct blood contact, sexual transmission, and perinatal transmission from an infected woman to her fetus or newborn through in utero exposure or at the time of parturition. Transmission through infected breast milk also has been documented. Transmission through casual household contact does not occur.

Intravenous drug use with shared needles is the major means by which blood contact leads to HIV infection in the United States. In areas of the country in which HIV disease is particularly prevalent among IV drug users, notably New York City and New Jersey, 50% to 60% of IV drug users are estimated to be infected with HIV. Although medical transfusion of infected blood products accounts for a small proportion of AIDS cases that have been reported, up-to-date screening of blood products since 1985 has continually and markedly reduced this mode of HIV transmission.

Semen and cervical and vaginal secretions can contain the virus (Wofsy et al, 1986); the transmission of HIV during sexual activity has clearly been documented. Both male-to-female and female-to-male transmission can occur. Male-to-female transmission, however, is more efficient. Anal intercourse may be associated with the greatest risk for transmission, but vaginal intercourse can also lead to infection. An exact risk for transmission associated with oral intercourse is unknown.

Epidemiologic risks associated with the heterosexual transmission of HIV include young age, unmarried state, nonintravenous cocaine use, heavy smoking, multiple sexual partners, and unprotected intercourse, specifically the lack of condom use (Hunter et al, 1994) In addition, sex with male partners who themselves have multiple sexual partners or who have not been circumcised, bisexuality, and history of intravenous drug use increases transmission risk (Wood et al, 1993). Increased risk for the sexual transmission of HIV

has been associated with STD history or current disease, particularly any STD associated with the disruption of mucosal integrity or with cervicitis. This list includes syphilis, chancroid, genital herpes, HPV, and, to a lesser extent, *T. vaginalis, N. gonorrheoae,* and *C. trachomatis* (European Working Group on HIV, 1993; Laga et al, 1993).

Other factors influencing the transmission of HIV are poorly understood. Frequency of exposure to the virus, underlying conditions in the exposed person, and the amount and efficiency of the infecting virus all are factors. Progressive immune suppression probably is associated with greater viral shedding and, thus, with greater efficiency of transmission. However, all HIV-infected persons are considered to be potentially infectious through sexual activity.

HIV is a retrovirus with a unique reverse transcriptase that allows its RNA to encode DNA within the infected cell. The virus then becomes irreversibly incorporated within the host DNA. This intertwining of viral and host genetic structures leads to major alterations in function and to the eventual destruction of host cells. It also provides a mechanism for the further infection of target cells within the body. HIV target cell membranes contain a surface molecule, the CD4 receptor. A CD4 envelope protein on the surface of the virus binds to the CD4 receptor. The main target cells within the body for this virus are T_4-helpers, or CD4+ lymphocytes. Gradual alterations in the function and the eventual depletion of this subpopulation of lymphocytes are associated with profound effects on cellular immunity characteristic of HIV infection and with associated life-threatening diseases characteristic of AIDS. Infection of macrophages and other monocytes also occurs and is central to HIV's pathogenicity. HIV has been demonstrated in lymph nodes, bone marrow, spleen, gastrointestinal tissue, lung, brain, retinal tissue, and the placenta.

There is a spectrum of HIV disease whose categorization is still evolving. Primary infection is characterized by high-grade viremia. An average of 14 weeks after the initial infection, many people experience symptoms of primary infection, a self-limited, febrile, nonspecific illness that resembles mononucleosis. After this, HIV infection remains asymptomatic for variable durations despite continual active viral replication. During this time, the virus is sequestered in a variety of organ systems and the amount of measurable, free virus in the bloodstream may decrease. Alterations in the amount of free virus in the periphery and in the number and function of immunocompetent cells gradually occur despite a continuing lack of symptoms. Eventually illnesses associated with defects in cellular immunity or with HIV infection of target organs occur. At any time during the asymptomatic stage or during the early manifestations of illness, abnormal laboratory values associated with immune dysfunction, such as lymphocytopenia with CD4+ cell depletion, thrombocytopenia, and neutropenia, may evolve. Generalized lymphadenopathy, isolated or in conjunction with diffuse, constitutional symptoms, can occur at variable points in the course of the disease.

The last stage of HIV infection is AIDS. A person is said to have AIDS when the absolute CD4+ cell count is less than 200 or when one of a list of illnesses associated with immunosuppression is diagnosed despite the lack of an underlying reason for the immunosuppression, such as age, malignancy, or immunosuppressive medication. These illnesses include key infections such as *Pneumocystis carinii* pneumonia, disseminated viral infections, unusual protozoal and helminthic infections, and atypical mycobacterial infections. They also include atypical malignancies such as Kaposi's sarcoma, non-Hodgkin's lymphoma, primary brain lymphoma, and a number of other clinical findings or diseases indicative of a defect in cell-mediated immunity. In 1987 dementia and a wasting syndrome of inexorable weight loss, persistent, intractable diarrhea, and fever were added to this list. In 1993, invasive cervical cancer became an AIDS-defining condition, and persistent vulvovaginal candidiasis, moderate or severe cervical intraepithelial neoplasia, and PID were added to the list of HIV-related conditions.

Large-scale epidemiologic studies in men suggested that the time from initial infection to a diagnosis of AIDS is 8 to 10 years. Symptom-free survival and the latent period before the manifestation of symptomatic disease and AIDS have been extended because of highly active antiretroviral therapy that makes use of combinations of potent antiretroviral agents in HIV-infected persons judged to be appropriate candidates because of their levels of CD4+ cell counts and free virus as measured by polymerase chain reaction (U.S. Public Health Service, 1997a; U.S. Public Health Service, 1997b). It is assumed that all infected persons will eventually acquire AIDS and die of it despite maximal efforts to control associated conditions without the continual development of new antiretroviral agents. Attempts at immunomodulation and at disease eradication through the aggressive use of combination antiretroviral therapy during primary and early HIV infection are the focus of intensive research. The interaction between disease progression and factors such as age, gender, lifestyle, other infections, and other illnesses is incompletely understood.

Gynecologic care of HIV-infected women is a major part of the health-care management for the HIV population, though gynecologic needs may be ignored. In one study of women whose median CD4+ cell count was 54 and who were admitted to the hospital for AIDS-related concerns, most had not received gynecologic care for 14 to 24 months, even though 44% of these women were sexually active and 66% had gynecologic problems (Frankel et al, 1996). Appropriate gynecologic care necessitates knowledge of the expected frequency of common gynecologic conditions in HIV-infected women and the presentations of gynecologic conditions that may be modified by HIV infection. In addition, discussions of sexuality, contraceptive choices, and decisions regarding reproduction are all part of the comprehensive care.

HIV-infected women are more likely to have a history of gynecologic infections including STDs, PID, and candidia-

sis and physical examination results that reveal genital tract inflammation (Mayer, 1995). Common gynecologic complaints include lower genital tract lesions and symptoms such as discharge, itching, and vulvovaginal pain (Frankel et al, 1996; Cu-Uvin et al, 1996; Greenblatt et al, 1996). In addition to STDs and other genital tract infections, squamous cell abnormalities of the lower genital tract are seen with increasing frequency in women with HIV, and they pose particular concerns for its management. Finally, HIV-infected women themselves are concerned about the effects of HIV infection on menstrual abnormalities. Each of these gynecologic concerns will be considered.

Syphilis, HSV, and genital tract warts, along with other manifestations of HPV, are seen often in HIV-infected women (Hitti et al, 1997; Lindsay et al, 1993; Chirgwin et al, 1995; Fennema et al, 1995; Cronje et al, 1994). In addition to serologic testing for syphilis, assessments for *C. trachomatis, N. gonorrhoeae*, trichomonas, and bacterial vaginosis should be considered in any woman with lower genital tract symptoms or for screening in the case of a new sexual partner or a newly diagnosed pregnancy. All four infections are seen more often, or at least as often, in HIV-infected women as in other women attending gynecologic and obstetric clinics (Deschamps et al, 1993; Laga et al, 1993; Lindsay et al, 1993).

Positive serologic test results for syphilis indicate a risk factor for HIV infection in women, and all women with syphilis should be screened for HIV. There is an increase in biologically false-positive serologic test results for syphilis with HIV infection that is not entirely explained by coexistent intravenous drug abuse (Augenbraun et al, 1994). True positive results, confirmed by a treponemal specific test, must be evaluated in light of the results of any previous syphilis testing. Treatment of active syphilis in a patient with HIV infection must take into account the probable duration of syphilis and the increased rate of neurosyphilis seen in association with HIV infection. Diagnostic testing may have to include lumbar puncture. If neurosyphilis is considered a possibility either because of the duration of syphilis, the stage of HIV infection, or the results of lumbar puncture, intravenous penicillin, rather than intramuscular benzathine penicillin, in doses and of duration appropriate to the treatment of neurosyphilis is administered.

HIV-infected women are more often HSV seropositive than are HIV-negative women (Fennema et al, 1995; Hitti et al, 1997). Primary and recurrent HSV infections are more common, and HSV is the leading diagnosis of genital tract ulcers in HIV-infected women. The clinical course and the response to therapy of HSV infections is influenced by HIV infection. Initial nonprimary and recurrent episodes of genital herpes can result in atypical, large, painful lesions that last for prolonged periods of time. Asymptomatic shedding and recurrent HSV lesons are common; frequency increases with declines in the CD4+ cell count (Augenbraun et al, 1995; LaGuardia et al, 1995). Women with previous asymptomatic HSV disease may experience their first clinical manifestation of disease as the CD4+ count declines. Any ulcer of the lower genital tract, even in women without a history of herpes or of current sexual exposure, should be cultured for herpes. If positive, treatment with high-dose acyclovir is indicated.

Genital ulcer disease has been reported in 14% to 28% of HIV-infected women (Frankel et al, 1996; LaGuardia et al, 1995). Although a number of incidences are related to HSV infection, some patients have unusual manifestations of undefinable cause. Painful genital ulcers in association with low CD4 counts have been reported even without any other mucous membrane lesions. These ulcers have been reported to respond to systemic steroids and to changes in antiretroviral management (Schuman et al, 1996).

The exact association between HIV infection and *N. gonorrhoeae* or *C. trachomatis* is unclear. Increased incidences of these infections in HIV-infected women and increases in the heterosexual transmission of HIV in their presence have been inconsistently observed. In addition, it is unclear whether HIV-infected women have higher rates of gonococcal and chlamydial infections than HIV-negative women treated in similar clinics. *T. vaginalis* is seen more often than either *N. gonorrhoeae* or *C. trachomatis*, and past and current trichomonas infections appear to be seen more often in HIV-infected women (Laga et al, 1993; Cronje et al, 1994; Greenblatt et al, 1996). All three infections can be associated with cervicitis, and the presence of cervicitis has been associated with heterosexual HIV transmission. There is no evidence that treatment of any of these infections is less effective because of HIV infection. Therefore, it seems reasonable to screen sexually active HIV-infected women for *N. gonorrhoeae* and *C. trachomatis*, to diagnose gonorrheal, chlamydial, and trichomonas infection aggressively in symptomatic women, and to treat any documented or presumed cases of infection according to standard protocols.

Bacterial vaginosis is the most prevalent lower genital tract infection in HIV-infected women, yet its presence is not specifically associated with HIV. It has been associated with genital tract inflammation, other STDs, candidiasis, increased numbers of sexual partners, and unprotected sexual intercourse in HIV-infected women, and it has been associated inconsistently with heterosexual transmission (Warren et al, 1996; Greenblatt et al, 1996). A diagnosis of BV should be considered in women with discharge or signs of genital tract inflammation, and effective therapy should be provided.

In studies from the United States, PID resulting in hospital admission is associated with HIV-seroprevalence rates of 6% to 16% (Hoegsberg et al, 1990; Safrin et al, 1990). Whether PID is more prevalent in HIV-infected women is unclear. HIV-infected women in whom PID develops may have a slightly different presentation of disease than women who are HIV negative (Moorman et al, 1993; Irwin et al, 1993; Clarke et al, 1993). Increased rates of concomitant sexually transmitted diseases have been reported as increased rates of histopathologic endometritis and positive endometrial cultures. These women are more likely to have cervicitis, pelvic masses, and high erythrocyte sedimentation rates, and they are more likely to be admitted to the hospital for treatment. There are no apparent differences in the microbiology of the infection, however, and there is no evidence of a need for different antibiotic management or a difference in response to standard therapy.

Lower genital tract colonization with *Candida* is common in HIV-infected women. Most studies suggest that HIV-infected women have some increased risk for symptomatic vulvovaginal candidiasis. In particular, women with low CD4+ cell counts have higher rates of symptomatic disease and more frequent recurrences (Duerr et al, 1997; Spinillo et al, 1994). Occasionally, this condition is the one that prompts women with symptomatic HIV-associated disease to seek treatment (Iman et al, 1990). Despite the concern for infection caused by unusual or resistant organisms, there is no evidence to date of significant numbers of infections with nonalbicans species or of *Candida* that is resistant to commonly used medications. Therapy with weekly fluconazole prevents recurrent, symptomatic candidiasis (Schuman et al, 1997). If there is not concomitant thrush or more invasive fungal disease, many women with recurrent candidiasis are managed successfully with intermittent or chronic use of vaginal antifungals.

Women with HIV infection have high rates of HPV infection, despite the lack of evidence that HIV-infected women are at increased risk to acquire HPV infection (Chirgwin et al, 1995). The prevalence of HPV has been demonstrated to range from 21% to 67% in various populations of HIV-infected women (Frankel et al, 1996; Heard et al, 1997; Branca et al, 1995; Garzetti et al, 1995). The frequency of HPV types, such as HPV-16 and HPV-18, that increase the risk for lower genital tract squamous cell neoplasia is increased in HIV-infected women coinfected with HPV (Miotti et al, 1996; Cohn et al, 1995), and this is a major factor in the increased occurrence and atypical presentations of squamous intraepithelial lesions of the lower genital tract in women. Women with HIV infection have increased manifestations of HPV infection, even with CD4+ cell counts of >500 (Fennema et al, 1995; Chirgwin et al, 1995). Cinically apparent genital warts increase in frequency with worsening immunosuppression (Chirgwin et al, 1995), as do HPV-related squamous cell changes. Genital warts have been observed to be increased 11.6 to 15.9 times in HIV-infected women (Chirgwin et al, 1995; Fennema et al, 1995), and these lesions tend to spread and grow rapidly. There is little evidence to support any different response to therapy. However, it has been noted that the resolution of warts with interferon therapy may be less complete in HIV infection, especially in patients with low CD4+ cell counts (Semprini et al, 1994).

Women with HIV infection are at increased risk for squamous cell abnormalities of the lower genital tract, particularly lesions associated with HPV infection (Vermund et al, 1991; Johnson et al, 1992; Fruchter et al, 1994; Klein et al, 1994; Miotti et al, 1996; Wright et al, 1994; Klevens et al, 1996; Fruchter et al, 1996). Prevalence rates of 18% to 45% of cervical have been reported, with the highest rates seen in women with CD4+ cell counts under 200. Although most cervical abnormalities are either ASCUS or low-grade squamous intraepithelial lesions, multifocal, rapidly progressive, high-grade, and recurrent disease after standard therapy have all been reported, typically in women with the lowest CD4+ cell counts (Maiman et al, 1993). Papanicalaou smears appear to have the same sensitivity in HIV-infected women they have in noninfected women, but they may be more specific because concomitant histopathologic findings indicative of true cervical disease may be more common (Anderson et al, 1996; Fink et al, 1994). Because of the possibility of rapidly progressive and recurrent disease and because it is difficult to predict when these events will occur, it is suggested that patients have frequent Papanicolaou smears taken if they have any abnormalities and that these be followed up by colposcopy and biopsy. Invasive cervical cancer has been reported to occur with increased frequency in association with HIV infection, and it is now an indicator disease for a diagnosis of AIDS. Degree of immunosuppression, however, does not clearly predict risk for invasive cervical cancer, and women with cervical cancer rather than other opportunistic infections or malignancies have higher median CD4+ cell counts (Klevens et al, 1996).

Squamous cell abnormalities develop in the vulva and the anal area. In particular, recurrent and persistent vulvar intraepithelial neoplasia is seen more often in women with HIV infection than without it (Korn et al, 1996). Vulvar intraepithelial neoplasia is seen in association with cervical lesions and by itself, and vulvar lesions may appear as invasive cancer.

Although menstrual abnormalities, including amenorrhea, oligomenorrhea, and intermenstrual and postcoital bleeding are common in HIV-infected women, there is no convincing evidence that these disorders are more common than they are in uninfected women. Baseline and cyclic gonadotropin and progesterone levels are the same in HIV-positive and HIV-negative women (Shelton et al, 1996).

Amenorrhea does not begin to be manifest until women have very low CD4 + cell counts (less than 50) and associated other diseases or wasting (Cohen et al, 1996).

There is some evidence that after the diagnosis of HIV infection, women are less sexually active and have lower pregnancy rates (DeVincenzi et al, 1997; Dahl et al, 1997; Thackway et al, 1997). However, many HIV-infected women remain sexually active, and issues of sexuality, contraception, and HIV transmission must be discussed with them as with all women. Studies that have examined contraception patterns have noted that HIV-positive women are more likely to use condoms than are HIV-negative women. Use rates for condoms remain in the 50% range, and condoms are less likely to be used if other forms of birth control are used, such as tubal ligation and oral contraception. Counseling patients and sexual partners about methods for avoiding the transmission of HIV and other sexually transmitted diseases is important no matter what decisions are made about contraception. One study suggested that 69% of sexual partners were either HIV negative or of unknown status (Dahl et al, 1997).

Counseling women with HIV infection about their reproductive choices involves complex issues, including planning the "best" time for pregnancy according to maternal health and balancing the possible benefits with unknown risks in choosing the appropriate therapy to maximize maternal health and to minimize fetal risk during pregnancy. The risk for the transmission of HIV infection from a pregnant woman to her infant can be minimized through appropriate management. Similarly, though there was a time when the concern for rapidly progressive disease in women and the acceleration of HIV disease by pregnancy were primary factors in the decision not to bear children, it appears that the rate of the clinical progression of disease in women is similar to that in men when both receive comparable medical treatment (Cozzi et al, 1994; Turner et al, 1994; Bastian et al, 1993) and that the influence of pregnancy on the ultimate course of HIV infection is minimal for most women (Stephenson and Griffioen, 1996) Women with HIV infection who once consciously decided to avoid bearing children are now reconsidering options.

REFERENCES

Aboulghar MA, Mansour RT, Serour GI: Ultrasonographically guided transvaginal aspiration of tuboovarian abscesses and pyosalpinges: An optional treatment for acute pelvic inflammatory disease. *Am J Obstet Gynecol* 1995; 172:1501-1503.

Agarwal J, Gupta JK: Female genital tuberculosis: A retrospective clinicopathologic study of 501 cases. *Indian J Pathol Microbiol* 1993; 36:389-397.

Anderson J, et al: Primary and secondary syphilis: 20 years' experience, III: Diagnosis, treatment, and follow-up. *Genitourin Med* 1989; 65:239-243.

Anderson J, et al: Results of routine colposcopic examinations (colpo) in women enrolled in the HIV epidemiology research study (HERS). *Int Conf AIDS* 1996; 11:309.

Ashley R, et al: Inability of enzyme immunoassays to discriminate between infection with herpes simplex virus types 1 and 2. *Ann Intern Med* 1991; 115:520-526.

Augenbraun M, Feldman J, Chirgwin K, et al: Increased genital shedding of herpes simplex virus type 2 in HIV-seropositive women. *Ann Intern Med* 1995; 123:845-847.

Augenbraun MH, DeHovitz JA, Feldman J, et al: Biological false-positive syphilis test results

for women infected with human immunodeficiency virus. *Clin Infect Dis* 1994; 19:1040-1044.

Avorn J, et al: Reduction of bacteriuria and pyuria after ingestion of cranberry juice. *JAMA* 1994; 271:751-754.

Backman LJ Harvey SM: Factors affecting the consistent use of barrier methods of contraception. *Obstet Gynecol* 1996; 88(suppl 3):65S-71S.

Barbone F, et al: A follow-up study of methods of contraception, sexual activity, and rates of trichomoniasis, candidiasis, and bacterial vaginosis. *Am J Obstet Gynecol* 1990; 163:510-514.

Bartlett JG, et al: Quantitative bacteriology of the vaginal flora. *J Infect Dis* 1977; 136:271-277.

Bassa AG, Hjojen AA, Moodley J, et al: Granuloma inguinale (donovanosis) in women: An analysis of 61 cases from Durban, South Africa. *Sex Transm Dis* 1993; 20:164-167.

Bastian L, et al: Differences between men and women with HIV-related *Pneumocystis carinii* pneumonia: Experience from 3,070 cases in New York City in 1987. *J Acquir Immune Defic Syndr Hum Retrovir* 1993; 6:617-623.

Berkman R, et al: The relationship of genital tract actinomycetes slid the development of pelvic inflammatory disease. *Am J Obstet Gynecol* 1982; 143:585-589.

Beutner KR: Valacyclovir: A review of its antiviral activity, pharmacokinetic properties, and clinical efficacy. *Antiviral Res* 1995; 28:281-290.

Beutner KR, Becker TM, Stone KM: Epidemiology of human papillomavirus infections. *Dermatol Clin* 1991; 9:211-218.

Billstein SA, Mattaliatio VJ Jr: The nuisance sexually transmitted diseases: Molluscum contagiosum, scabies, and crab lice. *Med Clin North Am* 1990; 74:1487-1505.

Bonnez W, et al: Efficacy and safety of 0.5% podofilox solution in the treatment and suppression of anogenital warts. *Am J Med* 1994; 96:420-425.

Branca M, et al: Cervical intraepithelial neoplasia and human papillomavirus related lesions of the genital tract in HIV positive and negative women. *Eur J Gynaecol Oncol* 1995; 16:410-417.

Brock BV, et al: Frequency of asymptomatic shedding of herpes simplex virus in women with genital herpes. *JAMA* 1990; 263:418-420.

Brown ST, Zaidi A, Larsen SA: Serologic response to syphilis treatment: A new analysis of old data. *JAMA* 1985; 253:1296-1299.

Brunham RB et al: Mucopurulent cervicitis: The ignored counterpart of urethritis in the male. *N Engl J Med* 1984; 311:1-6.

Brunham RC, et al: Etiology and outcome of acute pelvic inflammatory disease. *J Infect Dis* 1988; 158:510-517.

Bryson Y, et al: Risk of acquisition of genital herpes simplex virus type 2 in sex partners of persons with genital herpes: A prospective couple study. *J Infect Dis* 1993; 167:942-946.

Buchan H, et al: Morbidity following pelvic inflammatory disease. *Br J Obstet Gynaecol* 1993; 100:558-562.

Burk RD, et al: Sexual behavior and partner characteristics are the predominant risk factors for genital human papillomavirus infection in young women. *J Infect Dis* 1996; 174:679-689.

Burnakis TG, Hildebrandt NB: Pelvic inflammatory disease: A review with emphasis on antimicrobial therapy. *Rev Infect Dis* 1986; 8:86-116.

Caplan LR, Kleeman FJ, Berg S: Urinary retention probably secondary to herpes generates. *N Engl J Med* 1977; 297:920-921.

Carney O, et al: A prospective study of the psychological impact on patients with a first episode of genital herpes. *Genitourin Med* 1994; 70:40-45.

Cates W Jr, Wasserheit JN: Genital chlamydial infections: Epidemiology and reproductive sequelae. *Am J Obstet Gynecol* 1991; 164:1771-1781.

Centers for Disease Control: Antibiotic-resistant strains of *Neisseria gonorrhoeae*: Policy guidelines for detection, management, and control. *MMWR Morb Mortal Wkly Rep* 1987; 36(suppl 5):1S-I8S.

Centers for Disease Control 1993: Sexually transmitted disease guidelines. *MMWR Morb Mortal Wkly Rep* 1993; 42:1-102.

Centers for Disease Control and Prevention, Division of JTD/HIV Prevention: Annual Report: Atlanta Ga., Department of Health and Human Services, 1994.

Centers for Disease Control: 1998 guidelines for treatment of sexually transmitted diseases. *MMWR Morb Mortal Wkly Rep* 1998; 47:1-116.

Chirgwin KD, et al: Incidence of venereal warts in human immunodeficiency virus-infected and uninfected women. *J Infect Dis* 1995; 172:235-238.

Cirelli R, et al: Famciclovir: Review of clinical efficacy and safety. *Antiviral Res* 1996; 29:141-151.

Clarke L, et al: Prevalence of selected organisms in HIV+ and HIV− women with pelvic inflammatory disease (PID). 1st National Conference on Human Retroviruses and Related Infections. Dec 12-16, 1993; 98.

Cohen MH, et al: Menstrual abnormalities in women with HIV infection. *Int Conf AIDS* 1996; 11:28.

Cohn J, et al: Screening for cervical neoplasia with Pap smear and HPV DNA assay in HIV infected women. 2nd National Conference on Human Retroviruses and Related Infections. Jan 2, 1995; 152.

Committee on Public Health: Statement on treatment of gonorrhea-penicillin is passé: The New York Academy of Medicine. *Bull N Y Acad Med* 1989; 65:243-246.

Corey L: First-episode, recurrent, and asymptomatic herpes simplex infections. *J Am Acad Dermatol* 1988; 18:169-172.

Cozzi Lepri A, et al: HIV disease progression in 854 women and men infected through injecting drug use and heterosexual sex and followed for up to nine years from seroconversion: Italian Seroconversion Study. *BMJ* 1994; 309:1537-1542.

Cronje HS, et al: Prevalence of vaginitis, syphilis and HIV infection in women in the Orange Free State. *S Afr Med J* 1994; 84:602-605.

Cu-Uvin, S et al: Human immunodeficiency virus infection and acquired immunodeficiency syndrome among North American women. *Am J Med* 1996; 101:316-322.

Dahl K, et al: Sexual behavior and condom use among HIV+ women. 4th Conf Retro and Opportun Infect (1997 Jan 22-26);125:496.

Daly JW, King R, Monif GRG: Progressive necrotizing wound infection in post-medicated patients. *Obstet Gynecol* 1978; 52(suppl):5-8.

Dangor Y, et al: Accuracy of clinical diagnosis of genital ulcer disease. *Sex Transm Dis* 1990; 17:184-189.

Deschamps MM, et al: A prospective study of HIV-seropositive asymptomatic women of childbearing age in a developing country.

J Acquir Immune Defic Syndr Hum Retrovir 1993; 6:446-451.

DeVincenzi I, et al: Pregnancy and contraception in a French cohort of HIV-infected women: SEROCO Study Group. *AIDS* 1997; 11:333-338.

Domeika M, Domeika K, Paavonen J, et al: Humoral immune response to unserved epitopes of *Chlamydia trachomatis* and human 60-KDa heat-shock protein in women with PID. *J Infect Dis* 1998; 177:714-719.

Duerr A, et al: Immune compromise and prevalence of *Candida vulvovaginitis* in human immunodeficiency virus-infected women. *Obstet Gynecol* 1997; 90:252-256.

Edwards L, et al: Self-administered topical 5% imiquimod cream for external genital warts. *Arch Dermatol* 1998; 134:25-30.

Ernst AA, Marvez-Valls E, Martin DH: Incision and drainage versus aspiration of fluctuant buboes in the emergency department during an epidemic of chancroid. *Sex Transm Dis* 1995; 22:217-220.

Eschenbach DA, et al: Diagnosis and clinical manifestations of bacterial vaginosis. *Am J Obstet Gynecol* 1988; 158:819-828.

Eschenbach DA, et al: Polymicrobial etiology of acute pelvic inflammatory disease. *N Engl J Med* 1975; 293:166-171.

Eschenbach DA, Harnisch JP, Holmes KK: Pathogenesis of acute pelvic inflammatory disease: Role of contraceptive and other risk factors. *Am J Obstet Gynecol* 1977; 128:838-850.

European Working Group on HIV Infection in Female Prostitutes: HIV infection in European female sex workers: Epidemiological link with use of petroleum-based lubricants. *AIDS* 1993; 7:401-408.

Faro S: Lymphogranuloma venereum, chancroid and granuloma inguinale. *Obstet Gynecol Clin North Am* 1989; 16:517-530.

Fedson DS: Adult immunization: Summary of the National Vaccine Advisory Committee Report. *JAMA* 1994; 272:1133-1137.

Fennema JS, et al: HIV, sexually transmitted diseases and gynecologic disorders in women: Increased risk of genital herpes and warts among HIV-infected prostitutes in Amsterdam. *AIDS* 1995; 9:1071-1078.

Fidel PL Jr, et al: Systemic cell-mediated immune reactivity in women with recurrent vulvovaginal candidiasis. *J Infect Dis* 1993; 168:1458-1465.

Fihn SD: Behavioral aspects of urinary tract infection. *Urology* 1988; 32(suppl 3):168.

Fihn SD, et al: Association between diaphragm use and urinary tract infection. *JAMA* 1985; 254:240-245.

Finelli L, et al: Selective screening versus presumptive treatment criteria for identification of women with chlamydial infection in public clinics: New Jersey. *Am J Obstet Gynecol* 1996; 174:1527-1533.

Fink JM, et al: The adequacy of cytology and colposcopy in diagnosing cervical neoplasia in HIV-seropositive women *Gynecol Oncol* 1994; 55:133-137.

Fiorino AS: Intrauterine contraceptive device-associated actinomycotic abscess and *Actinomyces* detection on cervical smear. *Obstet Gynecol* 1996; 87:142-149.

Fiumara NJ: Reinfection primary, secondary, and latent syphilis: The serologic response after treatment. *Sex Transm Dis* 1980; 7:111-115.

Fiumara NJ: Treatment of seropositive primary syphilis: An evaluation of 196 patients. *Sex Transm Dis* 1977; 4:92-95.

Fleming DT, et al: Herpes simplex virus type 2 in the United States, 1976-1994. *N Engl J Med* 1997; 337:1105-1111.

Fong IW, McCleary P, Read S: Cellular immunity of patients with recurrent or refractory vulvovaginal moniliasis. *Am J Obstet Gynecol* 1992; 166:887-890.

Fouts AC, Kraus SJ: *Trichomonas vaginalis:* Reevaluation of its clinical presentation and laboratory diagnosis. *J Infect Dis* 1980; 141:137-143.

Fox KK, et al: Antimicrobial resistance in *Neisseria gonorrhoeae* in the United States, 1988-1994: The emergence of decreased susceptibility to the fluoroquinolones. *J Infect Dis* 1997; 175:1396-1403.

Frankel RE, Selwyn PA, Mezger J, Andrews S: High prevalence of gynecologic disease among hospitalized women with HIV disease. Comorbid gynecologic disease in hospitalized HIV-infected women. 3rd Conf Retro and Opportun Infect, Jan 1, 1996. *Clin Infect Dis* 1997; 25:706-712.

Fruchter RG, et al: Characteristics of cervical intraepithelial neoplasia in women infected with the human immunodeficiency virus. *Am J Obstet Gynecol* 1994; 171:531-537.

Fruchter RG, et al: Multiple recurrences of cervical intraepithelial neoplasia in women with the human immunodeficiency virus. Obstet Gynecol 1996; 87:338-344.

Galask RP: Vaginal colonization by bacteria and yeast. *Am J Obstet Gynecol* 1988; 158:993-995.

Galask RP, Larsen B, Ohm MJ: Vaginal flora and its role in disease entities. *Clin Obstet Gynecol* 1976; 19:61-81.

Garzetti GG, et al: Cervical dysplasia in HIV-seropositive women: Role of human papillomavirus infection and immune status. *Gynecol Obstet Invest* 1995; 40:52-56.

Gershman KA, Rolfs RT: Diverging gonorrhea and syphilis trends in the 1980s: Are they real? *Am J Public Health* 1991; 81:1263-1267.

Gilstrap LC, et al: Gonorrhea screening in male consons of women with pelvic infection. *JAMA* 1977; 238:965-966.

Gjonnaess H, et al: Pelvic inflammatory disease: Etiologic studies with emphasis on chlamydial infection. *Obstet Gynecol* 1982; 59:550-555.

Goldberg LH, et al: Long-tem suppression of recurrent genital herpes with acyclovir: A 5-year benchmark. *Arch Dermatol* 1993; 129:582-587.

Gordon SM, et al: The emergence of *Neisseria gonorrhoeae* with decreased suscepibility to ciprofloxacin in Cleveland, Ohio: Epidemiology and risk factors. *Arch Int Med* 1996; 125:465-470.

Granato PA, Franz MR: Use of the gen-probe page system for the detection of *Neisseria gonorheae* in urogenital samples. *Diagn Microbiol Infect Dis* 1990; 13:217-221.

Gravett MG, et al: Preterm labor associated with subclinical amniotic infection and with bacterial vaginosis. *Obstet Gynecol* 1986; 67:220-237.

Greenblatt RM, et al: Lower genital tract infections among HIV-infected women and high risk seronegatives: The women's interagency HIV study (WIHS). *Int Conf AIDS* 1996; 11:126.

Guinan ME, et al: The course of untreated recurrent genital herpes simplex infection in 27 women. *N Engl J Med* 1981; 304:759-763.

Ha HK, et al: Abdominal actinomycosis: CT findings in 10 patients. *Am J Roentgenol* 1993; 161:791-794.

Hager WD, Eschenbach DA, Spence MR, Sweet RL: Criteria for diagnosis and grading of salpingitis. *Obstet Gynecol* 1983; 61:114.

Hartwell L: Defects in a cell cycle checkpoint may be responsible for the genomic instability of cancer cells. *Cell* 1992; 71:543-546.

Hauth JC, Goldenberg RL, Andrews WW: Reduced incidence of preterm delivery with metronidazole and erythromycin in women with bacterial vaginosis. *N Engl J Med* 1995; 333:1732-1736.

Hawes SE, et al: Hydrogen peroxide-producing lactobacilli and acquisition of vaginal infections. *J Infect Dis* 1996; 174:1058-1063.

Heard I, et al: High rate of persistence of HPV infection in HIV-seropositive women. *4th Conf Retro and Opportun Infect*, Jan 22-26, 1997. 1997; 125:332.

Henry-Suchet J, Loffredo V: Chlamydial and *Mycoplasma* genital infection in salpingitis and tubal sterility. *Lancet* 1980; 1:539-543.

Hibbs JR, et al: Emergency department-based surveillance for syphilis during an outbreak in Philadelphia. *Ann Emerg Med* 1993; 22:1286-1290.

Hill GB: The microbiology of bacterial vaginosis. *Am J Obstet Gynecol* 1993; 169:450-454.

Hillier SL, et al: Association between bacterial vaginosis and preterm delivery of low-birth-weight infants. *N Engl J Med* 1995; 333:1737-1742.

Hillier SL, et al: A case-control study of chorioamniotic infection and chorioamnionitis in prematurity. *N Engl J Med* 1988; 319:972-978.

Hillier SL, et al: The relationship of hydrogen peroxide-producing lactobacilli to bacterial vaginosis and genital microflora in pregnant women. *Obstet Gynecol* 1992; 79:369-373.

Hillis SD, et al: Delayed care of pelvic inflammatory disease as a risk factor for impaired fertility. *Am J Obstet* 1993; 168:1503-1509.

Hilton E, et al: Ingestion of yogurt containing *Lactobacillus acidophilus* as prophylaxis for candidal vaginitis. *Ann Intern Med* 1992; 116:353-357.

Hitti J, et al: Herpes simplex virus seropositivity and reactivation at delivery among pregnant women infected with human immunodeficiency virus-1. *Am J Obstet Gynecol* 1997; 177:450-454.

Ho GYF, et al: Natural history of cervicovaginal papillomavirus infection in young women. *N Engl J Med* 1998; 335:468-474.

Hoegsberg B, et al: Sexually transmitted diseases and human immunodeficiency virus infection among women with pelvic inflammatory disease. *Am J Obstet Gynecol* 1990; 163:1135-1139.

Hoffman MS, et al: Advanced actinomycotic pelvic inflammatory disease simulating gynecologic malignancy: A report of two cases. *J Reprod Med* 1991; 36:543-545.

Holmes KK, Counts GW, Beaty HN: Disseminated gonococcal infection. *Ann Intern Med* 1971; 4:979-993.

Holton PD, et al: Prevalence of neurosyphilis in human immunodeficiency virus-infected patients with latent syphilis. *Am J Med* 1992; 93:9-12.

Hook EW III, Holmes KK: Gonococcal infections. *Ann Intern Med* 1985; 102:229-243.

Hoosen AA, Bassa A, Moodley J: Granuloma inguinale (donovanosis): An analysis of 64 cases from Durban, South Africa. *Int Conf AIDS* 1992; 8:91.

Hooten TM, et al: Association between bacterial vaginosis and acute cystitis in women using diaphragms. *Arch Int Med* 1989; 149:1932-1936.

Hooten TM, et al: A prospective study of risk factors for symptomatic urinary tract infection in young women. *N Engl J Med* 1996; 335:468-474.

Hovelius B, Märdh, PA: *Staphylococcus saprophyticus* as a common cause of urinary tract infections. *Rev Infect Dis* 1984; 6:328-337.

Hunter DJ, et al: Sexual behavior, sexually transmitted diseases, male circumcision and risk of HIV infection among women in Nairobi, Kenya. *AIDS* 1994; 8:93-99.

Hunter CA, Long KR: Vaginal and cervical pH in normal women and in patients with vaginitis. *Am J Obstet Gynecol* 1958; 75:872-874.

Iman N, et al: Hierarchical pattern of mucosal candida infections in HIV-seropositive women. *Am J Med* 1990; 89:142-146.

Irwin K, et al: Comparison of clinical presentation and course of PID in HIV+ and HIV− women: Updated results from an ongoing multicenter study. *1st Natl Conf Hum Retroviruses Relat Infect,* Dec 12-16, 1993. 1993; 98.

Jacobson L, Westrom L: Objectivized diagnosis of acute pelvic inflammatory diseases: Diagnostic and prognostic value of routine laparoscopy. *Am J Obstet Gynaecol* 1969; 105:1098-1098.

Joesoef MR, Sumampuuw H, Linnan M, et al: Douching and STDs in pregnant women in Sura Baya, Indonesia. *Am J Obstet Gynecol* 1996; 174:115-119.

Johnson JC, et al: High frequency of talent and clinical human papillomavirus cervical infections in immunocompromised human immunodeficiency virus-infected women. *Obstet Gynecol* 1992; 79:321-327.

Jones RH, et al: Recovery of *Chlamydia trachomatis* from the endometrium of women at risk of chlamydial infection. *Am J Obstet Gynecol* 1986; 155:36.

Joseph AK, Rosen T: Laboratory techniques used in the diagnosis of chancroid granuloma inguinale, and lymphogranuloma venereum. *Dermatol Clin* 1994; 12:1-8.

Kamwendo F, et al: Gonorrhea, genital chlamydial infection, and pollspecific urethritis in male partners or women hospitalized and treated for acute pelvic inflammatory disease. *Sex Transm Dis* 1993; 20:143-146.

Kass EH, Finland M: Asymptomatic infections of the urinary tract. *Trans Assoc Am Physicians* 1956; 69:56-64.

Kataja V, Syrjanen S, Yliskoski M, et al: Risk factors associated with cervical human papillomavirus infections: A case-control study. *Am J Epidemiol* 1993; 138:735-745.

Kelaghan J, et al: Barrier-method contraceptives and pelvic inflammatory disease. *JAMA* 1981; 248:184-187.

Kent GP, et al: Screening for *Chlamydia trachomatis* infection in a sexually transmitted disease clinic: Comparison of diagnostic tests with clinical and historical risk factors. *Sex Transm Dis* 1988; 15:51-57.

Kinghorn GR: Genital herpes: Natural history and treatment of acute episodes. *J Med Virol* 1993; 1:33-38.

Klein RS, et al: Risk factors for squamous intraepithelial lesions on Pap smear in women at risk for human immunodeficiency virus infection. *J Infect Dis* 1994; 170:1404-1409.

Klevens RM, et al: Characteristics of women with AIDS and invasive cervical cancer. *Obstet Gynecol* 1996; 88:269-273.

Komaroff AL: Acute dysuria in women. *N Engl J Med* 1984; 310:368-375.

Korn AP, Abercrombie PD, Foster A: Vulvar intraepithelial neoplasia in women infected with human immunodeficiency virus-1. *Gynecol Oncol* 1996; 61:384-386.

Koutsky LA, Galloway DA, Holmes KK: Epidemiology of genital human papillomavirus infection. *Epidemiol Rev* 1988; 10:122-163.

Krebs HB, Helmkamp BF: Treatment failure of genital condylomata acuminata in women: Role of the male sexual partner. *Am J Obstet Gynecol* 1991; 165:337-339.

Krettek JE, et al: *Chlamydia trachomatis* in patients who used oral contraceptives and had intermenstrual spotting. *Obstet Gynecol* 1993; 81:728-731.

Krieger JN, et al: Diagnosis of trichomoniasis: Comparison of conventional wet-mount examination with cytologic studies, cultures, and monoclonal antibody staining of direct specimens. *JAMA* 1988; 259:1223-1227.

Laga M, et al: Non-ulcerative sexually transmitted diseases as risk factors for HIV-1 transmission in women: Results from a cohort study. *AIDS* 1993; 7:395-402.

LaGuardia KD, et al: Genital ulcer disease in women infected with human immunodeficiency virus. *Am J Obstet Gynecol* 1995; 172:(1):553-562.

Landers DV, Sweet RL: Current trends in the diagnosis and treatment of tuboovarian abscess. *Am J Obstet Gynecol* 1985; 151:1098-1110.

Larsen B, Galask RP: Vaginal microbial flora: Practical and theoretic relevance. *Obstet Gynecol* 1980; 55(suppl):100S-113S.

Larsson PG, et al: Incidence of pelvic inflammatory disease after first trimester legal abortion in women with bacterial vaginosis after treatment with metronidazole: A double-blind, randomized study. *Am Obstet Gynecol* 1992; 166:100-103.

Lee HH, Chernesy MA, Schacter J: Diagnosis of *Chlamydia trachomatis* genitourinary infection in women by ligase chain reaction assay of urine. *Lancet* 1995; 345:213-216.

Lee NC, Rubin GL, Borucki R: The intrauterine device and pelvic inflammatory disease revisited: New results from the Women's Health Study. *Obstet Gynecol* 1988; 72:1-6.

Lee NC, Rubin GE, Grimes DA: Measures of sexual behavior and the risk of pelvic inflammatory disease. *Obstet Gynecol* 1991; 77:425-430.

Lewis JS, et al: Direct DNA probe assay for *Neisseria gonorrhoeae* in pharyngeal and rectal specimens. *J Clin Microbiol* 1993; 31: 2783-2785.

Lin JS, et al: Underdiagnosis of *Chlamydia trachomatis* infection: Diagnostic limitations in patients with low-level infection. *Sex Transm Dis* 1992; 19:259-265.

Linder JGEM, et al: Quantitative studies of the vaginal flora of healthy women and of obstetric and gynaecological patients. *J Med Microbiol* 1978; 11:233-241.

Lindsay MK, et al: The risk of sexually transmitted diseases in human immunodeficiency virus-infected parturients. *Am J Obstet Gynecol* 1993; 169:1031-1035.

Lossick JG: Epidemiology of urogenital trichomoniasis. In Honigsberg BM, editor, *Trichomonads parasitic in humans*, New York, Springer-Verlag, 1990.

Lowy DR, Kirnbauer R, Schiller JT: Genital human papillomavirus infection. *Proc Natl Acad Sci USA* 1994; 91(7)2436-2440.

Magid D, Douglas JM, Schwartz JS: Doxycycline compared with azithromycin for treating women with genital *Chlamydia trachomatis* infections: An incremental cost-effectiveness analysis. *Ann Intern Med* 1996; 124:389-399.

Maiman M, et al: Human immunodeficiency virus infection and invasive cervical carcinoma. *Cancer* 1993; 71:402-406.

Marchbanks PA, Lee NC, Peterson HB: Cigarette smoking as a risk factor for pelvic inflammatory disease., *Am J Obstet Gynecol* 1990; 162:639-644.

Märdh P-A: The vaginal ecosystem. *Am J Obstet Gynecol* 1991; 165:1163-1168.

Märdh P-A, et al: *Chlamydia trachomatis* infection in patients with acute salpingitis. *N Engl J Med* 1977; 296:1377-1379.

Märdh P-A, Westrom L: Adherence of bacteria to vaginal epithelial cells. *Infect Immunol* 1976; 13:661-666.

Marshburn PB, Trofatter KF Jr: Recurrent condyloma acuminatum in women over age 40: Association with immunosuppression and malignant disease. *Am J Obstet Gynecol* 1988; 159:429-433.

Mayer KH: Genital tract inflammation (GTI) in HIV infected women. 2nd *Natl Conf Hum Retroviruses Relat Infect,* Jan 2, 1995, 1995; 153.

Mead PB: Cervical-vaginal flora of women with invasive cervical cancer. *Obstet Gynecol* 1978; 52:601-604.

Meisels A: Dysplasia and carcinoma of the uterine cervix, IV: A correlated cytologic and histologic study with special emphasis on vaginal microbiology. *Acta Cytol* 1969; 13:224-234.

Mertz GJ, et al: Oral famciclovir for suppression of recurrent genital herpes simplex virus infection in women: A multicenter, double-blind, placebo-controlled trial: Collaborative Famciclovir Genital Herpes Research Group. *Arch Intern Med* 1997; 157:343-349.

Mertz GJ, et al: Prolonged continuous versus intermittent oral acyclovir treatment in normal adults with frequently recurring genital herpes simplex virus infection. *Am J Med* 1988a; 85:14-19.

Mertz GJ, et al: Risk factors for the sexual transmission of genital herpes. *Ann Intern Med* 1992; 166:197-202.

Mertz GJ, et al: Transmission of genital herpes in couples with one symptomatic and one asymptomatic partner: A prospective study. *J Infect Dis* 1988b; 157:1169-1177.

Miotti PB, et al: Cervical abnormalities, human papillomavirus, and human immunodeficiency virus infections in women in Malawi. *J Infect Dis* 1996; 173:714-717.

Moorman AC, et al; The microbiologic etiology of pelvic inflammatory disease (PID) in HIV + and HIV − women: Updated results from an ongoing multicenter study. *1st Natl Conf Hum Retroviruses Relat Infect* Dec 12-16, 1993, 1993; 99.

Morales WS, Schorr S, Albritton J: Effect of metronidazole in patients with preterm birth preceding pregnancy and bacterial vaginosis. *Am J Obstet Gynecol* 1994; 171:345-349.

Morse SA: Chancroid and *Haemophilus ducreyi. Clin Microbiol Rev* 1989; 2:137-157.

Muller M, Lossick JG, Gorrell TE: In vitro susceptibility of *Trichomonas vaginalis* to metronidazole and treatment outcome in vaginal trichomoniasis. *Sex Transm Dis* 1988; 15: 17-24.

Muller-Schoop JW, et al: *Chlamydia trachomatis* as possible cause of peritonitis and perihepatitis in young women. *Br Med J (Clin Res)* 1978; 1:1022-1024.

Nugent RP, Krohn MA, Hillier SL: Reliability of diagnosing bacterial vaginosis is improved by a standardized method of gram stain interpretation. *J Clin Microbiol* 1991; 29:297-301.

Oosthuizen AP, Wessels PH, Hefer JN: Tuberculosis of the female genital tract in patients attending an infertility clinic. *S Afr Med J* 1990; 77:562-564.

Paavonen J, et al: Prevalence and manifestations of endometritis among women with cervicitis. *Am J Obstet Gynecol* 1985; 152:280-286.

Pabst KM, et al: Disease prevalence among women attending a sexually transmitted disease clinic varies with reason for visit. *Sex Transm Dis* 1992; 19:88-91.

Panke ES, et al: Comparison of gen-probe DNA probe test and culture for the detection of *Neisseria gonorrhoeae* in endocervical specimens. *J Clin Microbiol* 1991; 29:883-888.

Patsner B, Giovine AP: Pelvic actinomycosis presenting as a primary retroperitoneal mass: A case report. *J Reprod Med* 1993; 38:159-162.

Peipert JF, et al: Bacterial vaginosis as a risk factor for upper genital tract infection. *Am J Obstet Gynecol* 1997; 177:1184-1187.

Peipert JF, et al: Laboratory evaluation of acute upper genital tract infection. *Obstet Gynecol* 1996; 87:730-735.

Peterson CS, Gerstoft J: Molluscum contagiosum in HIV-infected patients. *Dermatology* 1992; 184:19-21.

Pheifer TA, et al: Nonspecific to vaginitis: Role of *Haemophilus vaginalis* and treatment with metronidazole. *N Engl J Med* 1978; 298:1429-1434.

Phillips RS, et al: *Chlamydia trachomatis* cervical infection in women seeking routine gynecologic care: Criteria for selective testing. *Am J Med* 1989; 86:515-520.

Phillips RS, et al: The effect of cigarette smoking, *Chlamydia trachomatis* infection, and vaginal douching on ectopic pregnancy. *Obstet Gynecol* 1992; 79:85-90.

Phillips RS, et al: Gonorrhea in women seen for routine gynecologic care: Criteria for testing. *Am J Med* 1988; 85:177-182.

Quinn TC, et al: The association of syphilis with risk of human immunodeficiency virus infection in patients attending sexually transmitted disease clinics. *Arch Intern Med* 1990; 150:1297-1302.

Quinn TC, et al: Epidemiologic and microbiologic correlates of *Chlamydia trachomatis* infection in sexual partnerships. *JAMA* 1996; 276:1737-42.

Radcliffe KW, Daniels D, Evans BA: Molluscum contagiosum: A neglected sentinel infection. *Int J STD AIDS* 1991; 2:416-418.

Reed SD, Landers DV, Sweet RL: Antibiotic treatment of tuboovarian abscess: Comparison of broadspectrum-lactam agents versus clindamycin-containing regimens. *Am J Obstet Gynecol* 1991; 164:1556-1561.

Reef SE, Levine WC, McNeil MM: Treatment options for vulvovaginal candidiasis. *Clin Infect Dis* 1993; 20:S80-S90.

Reid G, Sobel JD: Bacterial adherence in the pathogenesis of urinary tract infection: A review. *Rev Infect Dis* 1987; 9:470-487.

Reid R, et al: Sexually transmitted papillomaviral infections, I: The anatomic distribution and pathologic grade of neoplastic lesions as secreted with different viral types. *Am J Obstet Gynecol* 1987; 156:212-222.

Rolfs RT, Galaid EI, Zaidi AA: Pelvic inflammatory disease trends in hospitalizations and office visits, 1979 through 1988. *Am J Obstet Gynecol* 1992; 166:983-990.

Romanowski B, et al: Serologic response to treatment of infectious syphilis. *Ann Intern Med* 1991; 114:1005-1009.

Rubin GL, Ory HW, Layde PM: Oral contraceptives and pelvic inflammatory disease. *Am J Obstet Gynecol* 1982; 114:630-635.

Rudolph AH: Examination of the cerebrospinal fluid in syphilis. *Cutis* 1976; 17:749-752.

Safrin S, et al: Long-term sequelae of acute pelvic inflammatory disease: A retrospective cohort study. *Am J Obstet Gynecol* 1992; 166:1300-1305.

Safrin S, et al: Seroprevalence and epidemiologic correlates of human immunodeficiency virus infection in women with acute pelvic inflammatory disease. *Obstet Gynecol* 1990; 75:666-670.

Saracoglu OF, Mungan T, Tanzer F: Pelvic tuberculosis. *Int J Gynaecol Obstet* 1992; 37:115-120.

Schiffer MA, et al: Actinomycosis infections associated with intrauterine contraceptive devices. *Obstet Gynecol* 1975; 45:67-71.

Scholes D, Dailing JR, Stergachis AS: Current cigarette smoking and risk of acute pelvic inflammatory disease. *Am J Public Health* 1992; 82:1352-1355.

Scholes D, et al: Prevention of pelvic inflammatory disease by screening for cervical chlamydial infection. *N Engl J Med* 1996; 334:1362-1366.

Scholes D, et al: Vaginal douching as a risk factor for acute pelvic inflammatory disease. *Obstet Gynecol* 1993; 81:601-606.

Scholes D, Stergachis A, Ichikawa L, et al: Vaginal douching as a risk factor for *Chlamydia trachomatis* infection. *Obstet Gynecol* 1998; 91:993-997.

Schulte JM, Martich FA, Schmid GP: Chancroid in the United States, 1981-1990: Evidence for underreporting of cases. *MMWR CDC Surveill Summ* 1992; 41:57-61.

Schuman P, Christianson C, Sobel JD: Apthous vaginal ulceration in two women with acquired immunodeficiency syndrome. *Am J Obstet Gynecol* 1996; 174:1660-1663.

Schuman P, et al: Weekly fluconazole for the prevention of mucosal candidiasis in women with HIV infection: A randomized, double-blind, placebo-controlled trial: Terry Beirn Community Programs for Clinical Research on AIDS. *Ann Intern Med* 1997; 126:689-696.

Schwartz JJ, Myskowski PL: Molluscum contagiosum in patients with human immunodeficiency virus infection: A review of 27 patients. *J Am Acad Dermatol* 1992; 27:583-588.

Semprini AE, et al: Treatment with interferon for genital HPV in HIV-positive and HIV-negative women. *Eur J Obstet Gynecol Reprod Biol* 1994; 53:135-137.

Sheffield PA, et al: The association between *Chlamydia trachomatis* serology and pelvic damage in women with tubal ectopic gestations. *Fertil Steril* 1993; 60:970-975.

Shelton M, et al: Menstrual cycle hormone patterns in HIV-infected women. *3rd Conf Retro and Opportun Infect,* Jan 1, 1996, 1996; 134.

Sobel JD: Candidal vulvovaginitis. *Clin Obstet Gynecol* 1993; 36:153-165.

Sobel JD: Epidemiology and pathogenesis of recurrent vulvovaginal candidiasis. *Am J Obstet Gynecol* 1985; 152:924-935.

Sobel JD: Vaginitis. *N Engl J Med* 1997; 337:1896-1903.

Sobel JD, et al: Single oral dose fluconazole compared with conventional clotrimazole topical therapy of *Candida* vaginitis. *Am J Obstet Gynecol* 1995; 172:1263-1268.

Sobel JD, Vazquez JA: Symptomatic vulvovaginitis due to fluconazole resistant *Candida albicans* in a female who was not infected with human immunodeficiency virus. *Clin Infect Dis* 1996; 22:726-727.

Sobota AE: Inhibition of bacterial adherence by cranberry juice: Potential use for treatment of urinary tract infections. *J Urol* 1984; 131:1013-1016.

Soper DE: Diagnosis and laparoscopic grading of acute salpingitis. *Am J Obstet Gynecol* 1991; 164:1370-1376.

Soper DE, Bump RC, Hurt WG: Bacterial vaginosis and trichomoniasis vaginitis and risk factor for cuff cellulitis after abdominal hysterectomy. *Am J Obstet Gynecol* 1990; 163:1016-1021.

Soper DE, et al: Observation concerning the microbial etiology of acute salpingitis. *Am J Obstet Gynecol* 1994; 170:1008-1014; discussion 1014-1017.

Souney P, Polk BE: Single-dose antimicrobial therapy for urinary tract infections in women. *Rev Infect Dis* 1982; 4:29-34.

Spence MR, Adler J, McLellan R: Pelvic inflammatory disease in the adolescent. *J Adolesc Health Care* 1990; 11:304-309.

Spiegel CA: Bacterial vaginosis. *Clin Microbiol Rev* 1991; 4:485-502.

Spiegel CA, et al: Anaerobic bacteria in nonspecific vaginitis. *N Engl J Med* 1980; 303:601-607.

Spinillo A, et al: Clinical and microbiological characteristics of symptomatic vulvovaginal candidiasis in HIV-seropositive women. *Genitourin Med* 1994; 70:268-272.

Spinillo A, et al: Epidemiologic characteristics of women with idiopathic recurrent vulvovaginal candidiasis. *Obstet Gynecol* 1993; 81:721-727.

Stamm WE: Protocol for diagnosis of urinary tract infection reconsidering the criterion for significant bacteriuria. *Urology* 1989; 32(suppl 2):6-12.

Stamm WE, et al: Causes of the acute urethral syndrome in women. *N Engl J Med* 1980; 303:409-415.

Stamm WE, et al: Diagnosis of coliform infection in acutely dysuric women. *N Engl J Med* 1982; 307:463-468.

Stamm WE, et al: Effect of treatment regimens for *Neisseria gonorrhoeae* on simultaneous infection with *Chlamydia trachomatis. N Engl J Med* 1984; 310:545-549.

Stapleton A, et al: Postcoital antimicrobial prophylaxis for recurrent urinary tract infection. *JAMA* 1990; 264:703-706.

Stephenson JM, Griffioen A: The effect of HIV diagnosis on reproductive experience: Study Group for the Medical Research Council Collaborative Study of Women with HIV. *AIDS* 1996; 10:1683-1687.

Stone KM, et al: Treatment of external genital warts: A randomised clinical trial competing podophyllin, cryotherapy, and electrodesiccation. *Genitourin Med* 1990; 66:16-19.

Strom BL: Sexual activity, contraceptive use, and other risk factors for symptomatic and asymptomatic bacteriuria. *Ann Intern Med* 1987; 107:816-823.

Sweet RL: New approaches for the treatment of bacterial vaginosis. *Am J Obstet Gynecol* 1993; 169:479-482.

Sweet RL, et al: The occurrence of chlamydial and gonococcal salpingitis, during the menstrual cycle. *JAMA* 1986; 255:2062-2064.

Sweet RL, et al: Use of laparoscopy to determine the microbiologic etiology of acute salpingitis. *Am J Obstet Gynecol* 1979; 134:68-78.

Thackway SV, et al: Fertility and reproductive choice in women with HIV-1 infection. *AIDS* 1997; 11:663-667.

Thomason JL, Gelbart SM, Broekhuizen FF: Advances in the understanding of bacterial vaginosis. *J Reprod Med* 1989; 34:581-586.

Thomason JL, et al: Statistical evaluation of diagnostic criteria for bacterial vaginosis. *Am J Obstet Gynecol* 1990; 162:155-160.

Thompson SE, et al: The microbiology and therapy of acute pelvic inflammatory disease in hospitalized patients. *Am J Obstet Gynecol* 1980; 36:179-186.

Townsend DE, Smith LH, Kinney WK: Condylomata acuminata: Roles of different techniques of laser vaporization. *J Reprod Med* 1993; 38:362-364.

Turner BJ, et al: Health care delivery, zidovudine use, and survival of women and men with AIDS. *J Acquir Immune Defic Syndr Hum Retrovir* 1994; 7:1250-1262.

Tyring SK, et al: A randomized placebo-controlled comparison of oral valacyclovir and acyclovir in immunocompetent patients with recurrent genital herpes infections: The Valacyclovir International Study Group. *Arch Dermatol* 1998; 134:185-191.

Vejtorp M, Bollerup AC, Vejtorp L: Bacterial vaginosis: A double-blinded randomized trial of the effect of treatment of sexual partners. *Br J Obstet Gynaecol* 1988; 95:920-926.

Vermund SH, et al: High risk of human papillomavirus infection and cervical squamous intraepithelial lesions among women with symptomatic human immunodeficiency virus infection. *Am J Obstet Gynecol* 1991; 165: 393-400.

Wald A, et al: Supression of subclinical shedding of herpes simplex virus type 2 with acyclovir. *Ann Int Med* 1996; 124:8-15.

Walker CK, et al: Pelvic inflammatory disease: Metaanalysis of antimicrobial regimen efficacy. *J Infect Dis* 1993; 168:969-978.

Walters MD, et al: Antibodies to *Chlamydia trachomatis* and risk for tubal pregnancy. *Am J Obstet Gynecol* 1988; 159:942-946.

Warren D, et al: High prevalence of abnormal vaginal flora and bacterial vaginosis in women with or at risk for HIV infection. *Int Conf AIDS* 1996; 11:219.

Washington AE, Katz P: Cost of and payment source for pelvic inflammatory disease: Trends and projections, 1983 through 2000. *JAMA* 1991; 266:2565-2569.

Watts DH, et al: Bacterial vaginosis as a risk factor for post-cesarean endometritis. *Obstet Gynecol* 1990; 75:52-58.

Webster LA, Berman SM, Greenspan JR: Surveillance for gonorrhea and primary and secondary syphilis among adolescents: United States, 1981-1991. *MMWR CDC Surveill Summ* 1993; 42:1-11.

Webster LA, Rolfs RT: Surveillance for primary and secondary syphilis United States, 1991. *MMWR CDC Surveill Summ* 1993; 42:13-19.

Week PK, Buddin DA, Whisnant JK: Interferons in the treatment of genital human papillomavirus infections. *Am J Med* 1988; 85:159-164.

Weinberger MN, Harger JH: Accuracy of the Papanicolaou smear in the diagnosis of asymptomatic infection with *Trichomonas vaginalis*. *Obstet Gynecol* 1993; 82:425-429.

Weinstock HS, et al: *Chlamydia trachomatis* infection in women: A need for universal screening in high prevalence populations? *Am J Epidemiol* 1992; 135:41-47.

Westrom L: Effect of acute pelvic inflammatory disease on fertility. *Am J Obstet Gynecol* 1975; 121:707-713.

Westrom L, et al: Pelvic inflammatory disease and fertility: A cohort study of 1844 women with laparoscopically verified disease and 657 control women with normal laparoscopic results. *Sex Transm Dis* 1992; 19:185-192.

Witkin SS: Immunologic factors influencing susceptibility to recurrent candidal vaginitis. *Clin Obstet Gynecol* 1991; 34:662-668.

Witkin SS: Immunology of recurrent vaginitis. *Am J Reprod Immunol Microbiol* 1987a; 15:34-37.

Witkin SS: Transient, local immunosuppression in recurrent vaginitis. *Immunol Today* 1987b; 8:360.

Witkin SS, et al: Detection of *Chlamydia trachomatis* by the polymerase chain reaction in the cervices of women with acute salpingitis. *Am J Obstet Gynecol* 1993; 168:1438-1442.

Witkin SS, Jeremias J, Ledger WJ: A localized vaginal allergic response in women with recurrent vaginitis. *J Allergy Clin Inmunol* 1988; 81:412-416.

Wofsy GB, et al: Isolation of AIDS-associated retrovirus from genital secretions of women with antibodies to the virus. *Lancet* 1986; 1:527-529.

Wolner-Hanssen P, et al: Association between vaginal douching and acute pelvic inflammatory disease. *JAMA* 1990; 263:1936-1941.

Wolner-Hanssen P, et al: Decreased risk of symptomatic chlamydia pelvic inflammatory disease associated with oral contraceptive use. *JAMA* 1990; 263:54-59.

Wolner-Hanssen P, et al: Laparoscopy in women with chlamydial infection and pelvic pain: A comparison of patients with and withut salpingitis. *Obstet Gynecol* 1983; 61:299-303.

Wood RW, et al: HIV transmission: Women's risk from bisexual men. *Am J Public Health* 1993; 83:1757-1759.

Wright TC Jr, et al: Cervical intraepithelial neoplasia in women infected with human immunodeficiency virus: Prevalence, risk factors, and validity of Papanicolaou smears: New York Cervical Disease Study. *Obstet Gynecol* 1994; 84:591-597.

Yliskoski M, et al: Cryotherapy and CO2-laser vaporization in the treatment of cervical and vaginal human papillomavirus (HPV) infections. *Acta Obstet Gynecol Scand* 1989; 68:619-625.

Zafriri D, et al: Inhibitory activity of cranberry juice on adherence of type I and type P fimbriated *E. coli* to eukaryotic cells. *Antimicrob Agents Chemother* 1989; 33:92-98.

Zimmerman HL, et al: Epidemiologic differences between chlamydia and gonorrhea. *Am J Public Health* 1990; 80:1338-1342.

19

Endometriosis

MARK D. HORNSTEIN
ROBERT L. BARBIERI

KEY ISSUES

1. Treatment of pelvic pain in patients with endometriosis is complex and often requires a multidisciplinary approach. Combinations of nonnarcotic analgesics with hormonal treatments such as danazol, the gonadotropin-releasing hormone (GnRH) agonists, and progestins have been successful. Long-term treatment with GnRH-agonists is possible using hormonal "add-back" therapy.
2. The pregnancy rates in endometriosis-associated infertility are improved by operative laparoscopic treatment. Hormonal treatment of endometriosis should be reserved for patients not attempting conception.
3. Empiric therapies for infertile patients with endometriosis are often successful. These include ovulation induction with clomiphene citrate and intrauterine inseminations (IUI), gonadotropins and IUI, and in vitro fertilization.

Although endometriosis was described in detail more than 100 years ago, it continues to be one of the unsolved enigmatic diseases affecting women. The first known report was written by Rokitansky (Rokitansky, 1860). After this, only a few scattered reports appeared until almost 1900, when Cullen (1896) published extensive descriptions of his findings. Yet 40 years later, Cattell and Swinton were able to document fewer than 20 reports of endometriosis in the world literature (Cattell and Swinton, 1936). In 1921, Sampson published the first of his series of reports and recorded for posterity his theory of retrograde menstruation as the causative factor in the disease (Sampson, 1921). His articles awakened wide interest, even controversy, and today his theory kindles as much heated debate among physicians as it did after the publication of his first reports.

Endometriosis may be defined as the presence of functioning endometrial tissue outside the uterus. It is usually confined to the pelvis in the region of the ovaries, uterosacral ligaments, cul-de-sac, and uterovesical peritoneum. The development and extension of endometrial tissue into the myometrium is termed adenomyosis. This disease entity is probably unrelated histogenetically and is characterized by a different clinical situation. It should be iterated that the term endometriosis implies proliferating growth and function (usually bleeding) in an extrauterine site. An endometrioma may be defined as an area of endometriosis, usually in the ovary, that has enlarged sufficiently to be classified as a tumor. When an endometrioma is filled with old blood, resembling tar or chocolate syrup, it is commonly known as a chocolate cyst.

ETIOLOGY

The two most popular theories of histogenesis are the retrograde menstruation theory and the coelomic metaplasia theory. The retrograde menstruation theory states that viable fragments of endometrium are carried to intraperitoneal sites by retrograde menstruation through the oviducts or by transport through the lymphatics or vascular channels. Most endometrial implants are thought to arise from the regurgitation of small fragments of endometrium through the fallopian tubes. In support of the transport theory are the following:

During menstruation, retrograde regurgitation of desquamated endometrium has been observed at laparoscopy and laparotomy.

Some desquamated menstrual endometrium is viable and can seed and grow in intraperitoneal locations.

Endometrial tissue can be found in pelvic lymphatic channels.

The transport theory also provides a possible explanation for the presence of endometriosis in old laparotomy or laparoscopy sites and in such distant sites as the lung, pleura, arm, thigh, and pelvic lymph nodes.

The coelomic metaplasia theory states that the ovarian epithelium and pelvic peritoneal mesothelium are capable of differentiating into müllerian elements (*e.g.*, endometrium). Stimuli that cause the transformation of these epithelial elements into endometrium are poorly described. Inflammatory processes, however, such as the irritation of the pelvic peritoneum by regurgitated menstrual blood or by acute infection may be important stimuli for metaplasia.

Most authorities favor the retrograde transport theory over the coelomic metaplasia theory as the most likely explanation for the original source of endometrial implants. However, a number of findings have yet to be explained by supporters of the retrograde transport theory, the most important of which is that endometriosis does not develop in all women with retrograde menstruation. This occurs because of a dose-response effect; endometriosis develops only in those women whose retrograde menstruation involves large amounts of endometrium. Epidemiologic evidence that supports this concept is presented later. Recently, Nisolle and Donnez (1997) have suggested different causes of endometriosis, depending on its location within the pelvis. Using morphologic data, they hypothesize that peritoneal endometriosis is best explained by the transport theory, whereas ovarian endometriosis and nodules on the rectovaginal septum result from metaplasia of ovarian epithelium and müllerian remnants.

Another possibility is that immunologic surveillance varies among women. Small implants of endometrium that are regurgitated into the peritoneal cavity are not eradicated in women with local deficiencies in certain immune functions. One candidate for an immune mediator in endometriosis is the macrophage. Macrophages are present in high concentrations in peritoneal fluid. There they serve as phagocytic cells and scavengers. In addition, they produce locally active products, such as interleukins, cytokines, and prostaglandins, that may serve as local mediators of inflammation. Numerous investigators note an increased concentration of macrophages, particularly well-differentiated activated macrophages, in the peritoneal fluid of women who have endometriosis. This suggests a possible immune mechanism in the etiology of endometriosis (Halme et al, 1983).

Regardless of the presumed cause of endometriotic tissue, it appears likely that endometriomas are monoclonal in origin (Jimbo et al, 1997). Using the human androgen receptor gene as a marker, these investigators showed that all epithelial cell samples from endometriomas, and even cells from multiple distant sites within the same endometrioma, displayed identical patterns for the marker gene. These observations suggest that endometriomas arise from a single cell or from an identical cluster of cells.

A key concept in understanding the cause of endometriosis is that hormonal factors are of central importance in the pathogenesis of this disease. The importance of hormonal factors is highlighted by the following clinical observations: Endometriosis is uncommon before the menarche and rarely occurs after menopause.

Ovarian ablation usually results in complete and prompt regression of ectopically located endometrial glands and stroma (though scar tissue may persist).

Endometriosis is rarely observed in amenorrheic women but is common in women who have uninterrupted cyclic menstruation for more than 5 years.

Endometriosis improves or stabilizes during episodes of physiologically induced (pregnancy) or artificially induced (hormonal) amenorrhea.

Frequent pregnancy, if initiated early in reproductive life, appears to prevent the development of endometriosis.

Little experimental evidence is available concerning the hormonal requirements of endometrial implants, but it is known that normal endometrium and the endometrial implants contain estrogen, androgen, and progesterone receptors. It is likely that the endometrial implants retain patterns of hormonal responsiveness similar to those of normal endometrial cells. The following observations are true in the normal endometrium (Table 19-1):

In physiologic doses estrogen stimulates endometrial hyperplasia in a dose-dependent fashion if unopposed by progesterone.

Androgens produce atrophy of the endometrium.

Physiologic doses of progesterone support endometrial growth and secretory changes.

Pharmacologic doses of progestational agents produce a decidual reaction when there is adequate estrogen, and they produce atrophy in a hypoestrogenic environment.

To test the hypothesis that endometrial implants retain hormonal responses similar to those of normal endometrium, DiZerega et al (1980) studied the effects of estrogen, progesterone, and placebo on the growth of peritoneal endometrial implants in castrated monkeys. Estrogen alone was able to support the growth of the endometrial tissue in the peritoneal cavity. In a hypoestrogenic, hypoprogestational environment, the endometrial tissue atrophied. Progesterone alone was also able to support the growth of the endometrial tissue. These hormonal responses of endometrial tissue form the physiologic underpinning for effective hormonal therapy.

Table 19-1 Effects of Estrogens, Androgens, and Progestins on Endometrial Tissue

	Physiologic Doses	Pharmacologic Doses
Estrogens	Growth	Hyperplasia
Androgens	—	Atrophy
Progestins	Secretory changes	Decidual reaction

The pelvic peritoneum and the ovary are the most common anatomic sites of endometriosis. Both the peritoneal fluid and the ovaries contain high concentrations of estradiol. In a woman with normal ovulatory cycles, the circulating estradiol concentration usually does not exceed 400 pg/ml. However, the concentration of estradiol in cul-de-sac fluid is in the range of 1000 pg/ml, and the concentration of estradiol in ovarian follicular fluid can be 1000-fold higher (1,000,000 pg/ml). The high local concentration of estradiol in peritoneal fluid and in the ovary probably plays an important role in supporting the growth of endometrial implants.

EPIDEMIOLOGY

The epidemiology of endometriosis is poorly defined, and the incidence and risk factors for endometriosis are the subjects of much controversy. The main problem hindering a clear exploration of the epidemiology of endometriosis is that this disease can only be definitively diagnosed by a surgical procedure (laparoscopy or laparotomy). Ethical considerations preclude random laparoscopy of large groups of women. Until a highly reliable noninvasive method of diagnosing endometriosis is discovered, investigation of the epidemiology of endometriosis will be hampered by methodologic problems.

Endometriosis can develop in girls and women between the ages of 10 and 60 years. The average age at first diagnosis is 27 years. Most women with endometriosis have had symptoms of the disease for 2 to 5 years before diagnosis.

Endometriosis is an exceedingly common gynecologic problem, but precise incidence and prevalence figures are unavailable. A study of discharge records from acute care, nonfederal hospitals in 1980 revealed that approximately 8% of all women with gynecologic admissions had endometriosis as a discharge diagnosis (Cramer, 1987). Of all women admitted to the hospital, 0.6% had a discharge diagnosis of endometriosis. Of all girls and women between the ages of 15 and 44 years, 0.9% carried this discharge diagnosis. These and similar data suggest that in the general population of reproductive-age girls and women, the prevalence of endometriosis is at least 1%. In certain populations at high risk, the prevalence of endometriosis is much higher. For example, in female partners of infertile couples, the prevalence of endometriosis is estimated to be as high as 30% to 50%.

Genetic factors may play a role in endometriosis. Familial clustering of endometriosis is a common clinical observation. In families with endometriosis, the disease is often confined to the maternal line and is seven times more common in first-degree relatives than in the general population. In future studies, the evaluation of DNA polymorphism may identify specific genes involved in the development of endometriosis. In an intriguing study, Cramer et al (1996) observed that women with endometriosis were twice as likely as controls to carry a specific mutation in the galactose-1-phosphate uridyl transferase (GALT) gene. Mutations in this enzyme, involved in galactose metabolism, have also been implicated in patients with müllerian anomalies, suggesting a familial association in endometriosis and a possible mechanism for its development in some women.

Menstrual factors appear to play an important role in the development of endometriosis. Women with the disease more often report menstrual cycles of less than 27 days with more than 8 days of menstrual flow (Table 19-2) (Cramer et al, 1986). Women with müllerian anomalies, in whom normal menstrual egress is blocked by cervical stenosis or vaginal septa, often have endometriosis. Of special interest, women with double uteri and only one blocked uterine outflow tract often have endometriosis on the pelvic structures contralateral to the blocked outflow tract but not on the contralateral pelvic structures. Other evidence in support of the retrograde menstruation theory comes from a mathematical model of factors that control the directionality of menstrual flow. At small cervical os diameters, a greater flow was seen through the fallopian tubes. This suggests that women with reduced cervical os diameters may be at greatest risk for the development of endometriosis (Barbieri et al, 1992). These findings support the concept that increasing amounts of retrograde menstruation increase the risk for endometriosis.

Other epidemiologic studies suggest that multiple pregnancies and the prolonged use of low-dose oral contraceptives may decrease the risk for endometriosis. Both exposures probably decrease the cumulative lifetime amount of retrograde menstruation. Of special interest are recent studies that suggest that conditioning exercise may be associated with a decreased risk for endometriosis. For example, Cramer et al observed that women who exercise regularly, started exercising before age 15, and exercise more than 7 hours a week are at a low risk for endometriosis (Cramer

Table 19-2 Menstrual Characteristics in Relation to Relative Risk for Endometriosis

Menstrual Characteristics	Relative Risk for Endometriosis
Cycle (days)	
≤27	2.1
28-34	1.0
≥35	0.6
Duration of flow	
≤7	1.0
≥8	2.4
Menstrual pain	
None	1.0
Mild	1.7
Moderate	3.4
Severe	6.7

From Cramer DW: Epidemiology of endometriosis. In Wilson EA, editor: *Endometriosis,* New York, 1987, Alan R. Liss.

et al, 1986). These findings have important public health implications.

PATHOLOGY

Endometriosis refers to ectopic endometrium. Its abnormal features, largely those of endometrium, consist of endometrial epithelium and stroma.

The four basic structures seen microscopically in endometriosis are endometrial epithelium, glands or glandlike structures, stroma, and hemorrhage (Fig. 19-1). Continuing function in areas of endometriosis tends to destroy its microscopic characteristics. If totally excised and properly oriented for the pathologist, early lesions, particularly those in the cul-de-sac, usually demonstrate classic histology. However, the large endometrial cysts of the ovary, which are obvious to the gynecologist during surgery, may show only hemosiderin-laden macrophages with varying amounts of fibrous connective tissue and inflammatory cells. It is important to remember that the endometrial stroma, not the glands or the epithelium, is responsible for bleeding in endometriosis. Based on the stroma alone, an experienced gynecologic pathologist can usually make the diagnosis of endometriosis without difficulty. A decidual reaction or a typical "naked nuclei" cellular pattern surrounded by a delicate reticulum or by spiral arterioles with adjacent predecidua, with or without old or recent hemorrhage, is sufficient to permit the diagnosis to be made without examination of the glands.

The most common site of endometriosis is the ovary; in approximately 50% of patients, both ovaries are involved. Other areas and organs affected (in order of incidence) are posterior cul-de-sac, anterior uterovesicle peritoneum, posterior broad ligament, uterosacral ligaments, fallopian tube, uterus, rectovaginal septum, sigmoid colon, cervix, vulva, vagina, umbilicus, small intestine, laparotomy or episiotomy scars, ureter and bladder mucosa, arm, leg, pleura, and lung (Fig. 19-2).

Endometriosis has many visual manifestations. The classic visual appearance of endometriosis is the powder-burn lesion, a small, punctate, brown or purple discoloration of the peritoneum or ovarian surface. Attention in recent years has focused on the diagnosis of atypical endometriosis. Atypical lesions may be red, white, or even glandular (Jansen and Russell, 1986). Histologic confirmation of endometriosis with atypical lesions has been reported in more than 75% of biopsies of red and white areas, with less common confirmation of biopsies of adhesions (Martin et al, 1989). Endometrial lesions may be invisible to the human eye. Published reports describe the occurrence of microscopic endometrial foci on the pelvic peritoneum that cannot be detected visually by the surgeon.

In recent years there has been an increased appreciation of deep endometriosis. These lesions may be nodular, and they extend beneath the peritoneal surface. They consist primarily of fibromuscular tissue and include extensions of endometrial glandular and stromal tissue. Typically such lesions develop in the rectovaginal septum and the uterosacral ligaments. Because of their deeply invasive nature, they may contribute to considerable pelvic pain and may be difficult to treat (Brosens, 1994).

Benign endometrial cysts of the ovary vary from microscopic sizes to masses 8 to 10 cm in diameter. They may be multiple in the early stages of the disease but subsequently coalesce into a single large cyst. During the early stage of development, endometrial cysts are usually mobile and have smooth surfaces. As they grow and surface bleeding occurs,

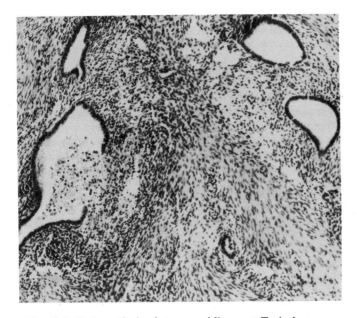

Fig. 19-1. Endometriosis of uterosacral ligament. Typical endometrial glands and stroma are evident in the fibrous connective tissue of the ligament.

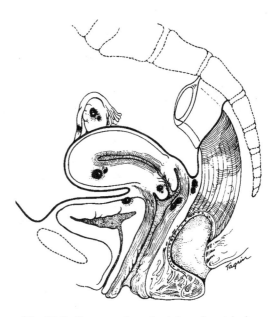

Fig. 19-2. Common sites of pelvic endometriosis.

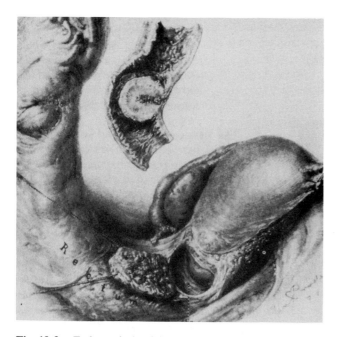

Fig. 19-3. Endometriosis of the sigmoid extending deeply into the bowel lumen. Extensive cul-de-sac endometriosis is shown invading the vagina and rectum. (From Cullen TS: The distribution of adenomyosis containing uterine mucosa. *Arch Surg* 1920; 215.)

the cyst may densely adhere to the surrounding structures, including the serosa of the sigmoid colon. The lateral aspect of the ovary is often involved and may adhere to the ileum or the lateral pelvic peritoneum. Often, the ovary has multiple areas that resemble powder burns because of changes in blood pigment. Minute red or blue cystic areas (raspberry or blueberry spots) with adjacent puckering may be identified on ovarian surfaces but are noted more often on the uterosacral ligaments or the pelvic peritoneum. The lining of the endometrial cyst varies from red to dark brown, depending on the extent and duration of bleeding. The cyst wall may be thin and smooth or thick and velvety, depending on the preponderance of fibrous tissue or functioning endometrium within it. If discrete papillary or polypoid lesions are found within the cyst cavity, the possibility of malignancy should be considered. Cyst contents are usually thick and resemble chocolate syrup or tar—hence, the commonly used descriptive term chocolate cyst. A hemorrhagic corpus luteum may have an identical gross appearance; therefore, unless confirmed by pathologic findings, chocolate cysts should not be thought of as caused by endometriosis. Even in true endometriomas, the histologic picture may be confusing; endometrial glands and stroma may become compressed by the pressure of the trapped blood, and the pathologist may be unable to make a specific diagnosis. If the endometriosis is not completely burned out, close examination of the wall usually reveals numerous hemosiderin-laden macrophages, lymphocytes, and patches of condensed endometrial stroma without glands.

The uterosacral ligaments or the rectovaginal peritoneum may be involved separately, or there may be a fused mass incorporating both structures (Fig. 19-3). The discovery of bluish-red or brown nodules with surrounding areas of puckering on the uterosacral ligaments, adjacent cul-de-sac, peritoneum, or serosa of the sigmoid is a characteristic finding. If these reach adequate size, they may be palpated easily on rectovaginal examination.

Occasionally, the lower genital tract is the site of endometriosis; lesions of the cervix, vagina, and vulva have been reported. Usually the patient has a history of antecedent trauma such as cervical cauterization or conization, vulvar surgery, or episiotomy. Surface endometriosis of this variety is almost certainly derived from the implantation of viable endometrium and generally responds actively to estrogen and progesterone. Such lesions may bleed in synchrony with the menses. When endometriosis involves the portio vaginalis of the cervix, the gross examination is usually pathognomonic; blue-black, elevated nodules, either discrete or confluent, are evident on speculum examination.

Small bowel involvement is rare (approximately 0.1% to 0.2%) but may lead to an erroneous diagnosis before surgery. Scar tissue often twists or coils around the lesion and results in symptoms of nausea, diarrhea, and crampy midabdominal or periumbilical pain. When lesions invade the bowel mucosa, patients may have rectal bleeding. Cyclic monthly hematochezia associated with the menses is highly suggestive of intestinal endometriosis. Colonoscopy combined with biopsy specimens is usually diagnostic. On gross examination, the mucosal surface is usually smooth, and there is subjacent fibrosis and scarring. In extensive pelvic endometriosis, several loops of ileum may be involved by contiguity so that resection of the areas is necessary. Similarly, the serosa of the appendix is often involved.

Urinary tract endometriosis is uncommon but probably occurs more often than is reported in the literature. The involvement of the serosal surface of the bladder is often seen, but it is usually asymptomatic. By the time the muscularis or mucosa is involved, the patient has usually noted cyclic hematuria and pain. Cystoscopy may show typical bluish "mulberry" lesions, and endoscopic biopsy usually confirms the diagnosis. Ureteral involvement has been reported and probably explains some cases of idiopathic, unilateral hydronephrosis (Fig. 19-4). Cyclic flank pain, fever, and pyuria may occur as a result of intermittent ureteral obstruction. The excretory urogram may show early ureteral dilation if it is obtained at the optimum time in the cycle. Several cases of biopsy-proven pleural and pulmonary endometriosis, in which a hematogenous or lymphatic mode of dissemination must be postulated, are now on record.

In summary, the abnormal process of endometriosis, though microscopically benign, produces havoc in the pelvis as important structures become involved. It is unique in that it spreads like cancer and produces fibrosis and scarring. The end result may be ovarian destruction, oviduct defor-

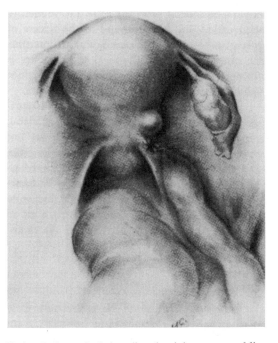

Fig. 19-4. Endometriosis invading the right uterosacral ligament, with fibrosis producing marked hydroureter. (Courtesy Dr. Thomas Leavitt.)

mity, bladder dysfunction, large bowel obstruction, and ureteral constriction.

Only limited data are available on the natural course of endometriosis. Thomas and Cooke (1987) reported that in 8 of 17 patients treated with a placebo, progression of the disease was revealed by second-look laparoscopy after a 6-month interval. In three patients, new adhesions developed during the observation period. The magnitude of the disease progression, however, was small. A retrospective review of seven patients who underwent repeated laparoscopic examinations of varying intervals without any treatment estimated that the disease progressed at a rate of 0.3 points per month using the revised American Fertility Society's staging system (American Fertility Society, 1985). Overall, in 5 of 7 women the disease progressed during the period under observation (Hoshiai et al, 1993).

Malignancy in endometriosis is rare. Criteria for the diagnosis of carcinoma arising from endometriosis were outlined by Sampson (1925), namely that the ovary must be the site of benign endometriosis, that there must be a genuine adenocarcinoma, and that a transition from benign to malignant areas must be demonstrated. Of interest is the observation that many cases of clear cell carcinoma of the ovary are associated with endometriosis (Scully et al, 1966).

Pathologists have noted that approximately 4% of all endometrial lesions demonstrate features of epithelial atypia, including cellular crowding, pseudostratification, hyperchromatic nuclei, and pleomorphism (Czernobilsky and Morris, 1979). Women with endometrial lesions demon-

strating epithelial atypia may be at high risk for epithelial malignancies of the pelvis, such as clear cell or endometrioid carcinoma (LaGranade and Silverberg, 1988). Long-term follow-up of 10 women with endometriosis and epithelial atypia showed that two of the women subsequently had clear cell carcinoma and one woman subsequently had endometrioid carcinoma. Jiang et al (1996) recently investigated the clonal status of endometrial implants. They examined DNA from 40 patients with endometriosis for clonal status and allelic losses of tumor suppressor loci, and they found that most endometriotic cysts and normal endometrial glands were monoclonal, suggesting that both develop from a single progenitor cell. They also found loss of heterozygosity in 28% of patients, suggesting that tumor suppressor gene inactivation may play a role in a subset of patients with endometriosis.

CLINICAL FEATURES
Symptoms

Characteristic symptoms associated with endometriosis are progressive, acquired, severe pain associated with or occurring just before menstruation; dyspareunia; painful defecation; premenstrual staining and hypermenorrhea; suprapubic pain, dysuria, and hematuria; and infertility (Table 19-3). Some patients do not have "acquired" dysmenorrhea but state that they have always had painful periods. Most, however, have had a recent increase in the severity of their pain. In many patients, the pain cannot be classified as dysmenorrhea because it is actually premenstrual. The pain, which is usually bilateral, varies from mild to severe discomfort in the lower abdomen and is often associated with rectal pressure. Many affected women complain of lower back and leg pain. A constant soreness in the lower abdomen or pelvis throughout the cycle, which is aggravated just before the menses or during coitus, may be the only complaint. The cause of pain with endometriosis is unknown, but it is probably related to miniature menstruation and bleeding and to the release of prostaglandins. That the pain is caused by intermittent stimulation and withdrawal of hormones is substantiated by clinical improvement in most patients if amenorrhea is induced.

Pain is not always associated with endometriosis even when the disease is extensive. Bilateral large ovarian endometriomas are often asymptomatic unless rupture occurs. On the other hand, incapacitating pelvic discomfort may be associated with minimal amounts of active endometriosis. Often the surgeon can find only a few implants or red lesions to account for the multiplicity of symptoms.

Signs

Endometriosis cannot be definitively diagnosed by physical examination; however, many women with endometriosis have physical findings that suggest the presence of the disease (Box 19-1). Women with endometriosis may have

Table 19-3 Management Strategies in the Treatment of Endometriosis Based on the Presenting Symptom

	Pelvic Pain*		
Stages	Family Completed	Family Not Completed	Infertility
I and II	Hormonal therapy	Hormonal therapy	Expectant management, ovulation induction, or laparoscopic surgery
III and IV	Hormonal therapy, surgery, or both	Hormonal therapy, surgery, or both (TAH-BSO considered)	Conservative surgery with preoperative or postoperative (or both) ovulation induction; IVF

*Fertility not an immediate issue.

BOX 19-1
SYMPTOMS AND SIGNS OF ENDOMETRIOSIS

Symptoms
Dyspareunia
Infertility
Painful defecation
Premenstrual staining and hypermenorrhea
Progressive dysmenorrhea
Suprapubic pain, dysuria, and hematuria

Signs
Cul-de-sac induration
Fixed ovarian masses
Uterosacral ligament nodularity

---

tender uterosacral ligaments that are thickened (banjo strings) and nodular. Rectovaginal examination may demonstrate a thickened rectovaginal septum and an indurated cul-de-sac. Deep lesions may be more easily appreciated during menses. In women with endometriomas, fixed adnexal masses may be noted. In addition, some women with endometriosis may also have a laterally displaced cervix, perhaps because of the foreshortening of the uterosacral ligaments (Propst et al, 1998).

DIAGNOSIS AND STAGING

Although the diagnosis of endometriosis may be suggested by medical history and physical examination, it can be made definitively only by laparoscopy or laparotomy. In patients with mild to moderate endometriosis, laparoscopy reveals the classic powder-burn lesions. These consist of small (less than 5 mm) purple, blue, or red spots that are visible on the pelvic peritoneum. Scarring and adhesions are commonly seen in patients with moderate to severe endometriosis. Evaluation of ovarian masses by laparoscopy is difficult, and the definitive diagnosis of ovarian endometriomas should be confirmed by pathologic evaluation. Aspiration of ovarian masses at the time of laparoscopy may increase the number

of endometriomas accurately diagnosed during this procedure. A biopsy specimen of small endometrial lesions taken through the laparoscope can help to confirm the diagnosis. It should be remembered that some endometrial implants may contain only stroma with hemorrhage, thus making the diagnosis difficult for the pathologist.

Intensive efforts are under way to develop noninvasive methods of diagnosing endometriosis. In women with endometriomas, ultrasonography can help confirm the mass and can provide a noninvasive method of observing its size. Pelvic ultrasonography, however, is of little value in screening for endometriosis because ultrasonography cannot detect peritoneal implants or adhesions. Transvaginal ultrasonography has shown promise in distinguishing endometriomas from other adnexal masses. A recent report demonstrated that this technique correctly identified endometriomas with a sensitivity of 84% and a specificity of 90% in women with ovarian masses (LaGranade and Silverberg, 1988). Studies also suggest that magnetic resonance imaging (MRI) may be the noninvasive procedure with the highest sensitivity and specificity for diagnosing endometriosis (Nishimura et al, 1987). Many endometrial implants have unique and intense relaxation signals that identify them. Fat-saturation techniques appear to improve the distinction between blood and fat within ovarian masses. This may aid in the detection and characterization of endometriosis by MRI (Sugimura et al, 1993). More research is needed to clarify the role of MRI in the diagnosis of endometriosis. The high cost of MRI studies may preclude the widespread clinical application of this technique.

Recently, the potential clinical usefulness of the measurement of serum CA-125 for the diagnosis of endometriosis was described. In the late 1970s, Bast and Knapp produced a panel of monoclonal antibodies to membrane antigens of human ovarian epithelial cancer. Evaluation of hundreds of antibody clones revealed one that was of particular interest. This monoclonal antibody was designated OC-125 (Bast et al, 1981). In adult human tissue, CA-125 was detected in the endocervix, endometrium, fallopian tube, peritoneum, pleura, and pericardium. In human fetal tissue, CA-125 was detected in the müllerian epithelium, amnion, umbilical epithelium, peritoneum, pleura, and pericardium. Normal adult and fetal ovaries were negative for CA-125. Most human epithelial ovarian cancers were positive for CA-125. Endometriomas were also noted to stain with the antibody OC-125 (Fig. 19-5).

Bast et al (1983) hypothesized that CA-125 may be present in the peripheral circulation because of the shedding of CA-125 from membrane surfaces. To test this hypothesis, they developed a sensitive immunoradiometric assay to detect CA-125 in the blood. Evaluation of the blood test for CA-125 revealed that more than 80% of patients with ovarian cancer had elevated blood levels of CA-125 and less than 1% of apparently healthy controls had elevated blood levels of CA-125 (Bast et al, 1983). Modest elevations in blood CA-125 levels were occasionally noted in four clinical situations other than ovarian carcinoma: during the first trimester of pregnancy, in acute pelvic inflammatory disease, after gynecologic surgery, and sometimes in endometriosis.

To investigate further the relationship between elevated blood CA-125 levels and endometriosis, Barbieri et al (1986) prospectively measured serum CA-125 before surgery in 147 consecutive patients undergoing diagnostic laparoscopy or laparotomy. They noted that patients with advanced (stages III and IV) endometriosis had elevated blood CA-125 levels compared with women in whom laparoscopy revealed normal diagnoses. Patients with stage II endometriosis also had serum CA-125 levels higher than those in controls, but there was a considerable overlap in the CA-125 levels between these two groups. For the diagnosis of stages III and IV endometriosis, serum CA-125 measurements had a sensitivity of 0.54, a specificity of 0.96, a positive predictive value of 0.58, and a negative predictive value of 0.96 in a population with a 9% prevalence of stage III and IV endometriosis (Barbieri et al, 1986). Menstrual-related cyclicity of serum CA-125 levels has also been observed in patients with endometriosis. CA-125 levels tend to be higher during menses and lower in the follicular and luteal phases of the menstrual cycle. However, the use of CA-125 values obtained during menses does not improve the diagnostic acuity of the test for endometriosis (Hornstein et al, 1992).

Serum CA-125 measurements may also be valuable in monitoring disease activity. Investigators have observed that after effective surgical or medical therapy for endometriosis, serum CA-125 levels decrease. Recurrence of disease is often associated with an increase in the serum CA-125 level (Barbieri et al, 1986).

Most patients with endometriosis have stage I or stage II disease. The major problem with the clinical application of serum CA-125 measurements for the diagnosis of endometriosis is that serum CA-125 has a low sensitivity (0.17) for the diagnosis of stage I and stage II disease. It is, therefore, not useful as a screening test for endometriosis. It may be possible to develop a more sensitive and specific blood test for endometriosis. If endometrial lesions contain membrane antigens that are specific to the disease, it may be possible to develop antibodies to these antigens. Indeed, radiolabeled monoclonal antibodies to CA-125 have been

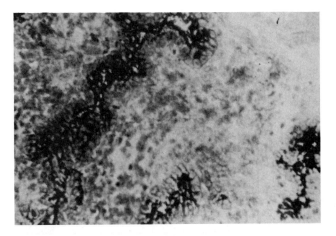

Fig. 19-5. Cryostat section of ovarian endometrioma stained with OC-125 antibody and the avidin-biotin immunoperoxidase technique and counterstained with hematoxylin. Normal ovarian tissue in the upper right portion of the figure does not stain with OC-125 antibody. The endometrioma tissue stains with the OC-125 antibody. (From Barbieri RL, et al: Elevated concentrations of CA-125 in patients with advanced endometriosis. *Fertil Steril* 1986; 45:630.)

used with immunoscintigraphy. Although severe endometriosis has been detected by this technique, it remains investigational (Kennedy et al, 1988). If these antigens appear often in the circulation of patients with endometriosis but not in patients without endometriosis, a useful blood test for endometriosis could be developed. A reliable blood test for endometriosis would represent a significant advance in gynecology.

A critical concept is that endometriosis is a heterogeneous disease that ranges in severity from minimal to severe. Therefore, surgical pathologic staging is of utmost importance for planning therapy, determining prognosis, communicating with other physicians, and standardizing research reporting. In the 1970s both Acosta and Kistner proposed descriptive clinical staging systems. These systems have generally been replaced by the revised American Society for Reproductive Medicine (ASRM) staging system (Fig. 19-6) (American Society for Reproductive Medicine, 1997), most recently updated in 1996.

In the ASRM system, points are assigned for the severity of endometriosis based on the size and depth of the implant and for the severity of adhesions. Points are summed, and patients are assigned to one of four stages: stage I—minimal disease, 1 to 5 points; stage II—mild disease, 6 to 15 points; stage III—moderate disease, 16 to 40 points; and stage IV—severe disease, more than 40 points. Although the new classification scheme does not alter the staging of the disease, it does allow for the inclusion of atypical lesions in the point system. The ASRM system standardizes the reporting of endometriosis and allows quantification of endometriosis staging in clinical research. Recently, however, the reproducibility of the system has been examined. Although observers generally agreed on the assessment of peritoneal endometriosis and pelvic adhesions, quantifying the degree of

Patient's name _____ Date _____

Stage I (Minimal) - 1-5
Stage II (Mild) - 6-15
Stage III (Moderate) - 16-40
Stage IV (Severe) - >40
Total _____

Laparoscopy _____ Laparotomy _____ Photography _____
Recommended treatment _____
_____
Prognosis _____

PERITONEUM	ENDOMETRIOSIS		<1 cm	1-3 cm	>3 cm
	Superficial		1	2	4
	Deep		2	4	6
OVARY	R	Superficial	1	2	4
		Deep	4	16	20
	L	Superficial	1	2	4
		Deep	4	16	20
	POSTERIOR CULDESAC OBLITERATION		Partial		Complete
			4		40
	ADHESIONS		<1/3 Enclosure	1/3-2/3 Enclosure	>2/3 Enclosure
OVARY	R	Filmy	1	2	4
		Dense	4	8	16
	L	Filmy	1	2	4
		Dense	4	8	16
TUBE	R	Filmy	1	2	4
		Dense	4*	8*	16
	L	Filmy	1	2	4
		Dense	4*	8*	16

*If the fimbriated end of the fallopian tube is completely enclosed, change the point assignment to 16.

Additional endometriosis: _____
_____
_____
_____

Associated pathology: _____
_____
_____
_____

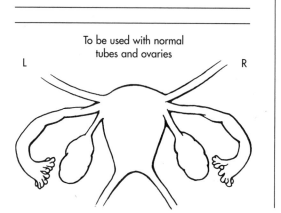

To be used with normal
tubes and ovaries

L   R

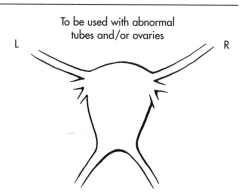

To be used with abnormal
tubes and/or ovaries

L   R

Fig. 19-6. Revised American Society for Reproductive Medicine classification of endometriosis. (Courtesy American Society for Reproductive Medicine.)

ovarian endometriosis proved less consistent in the earlier version of the classification (Hornstein et al, 1993).

CLINICAL PRESENTATION

Most patients with endometriosis have pelvic pain, infertility, or a pelvic mass. Therapeutic considerations differ for each presentation (Table 19-3).

Pelvic Pain

Pelvic pain is one of the most common symptoms of women with endometriosis. Women with pelvic pain unrelieved by antiprostaglandins (*e.g.,* ibuprofen) or that causes significant disability (*e.g.,* absenteeism from work or school) should consider undergoing a laparoscopy. The American Fertility Society has developed a form for use in recording the type, site, and volume of lesions seen at surgery. This instrument

EXAMPLES & GUIDELINES

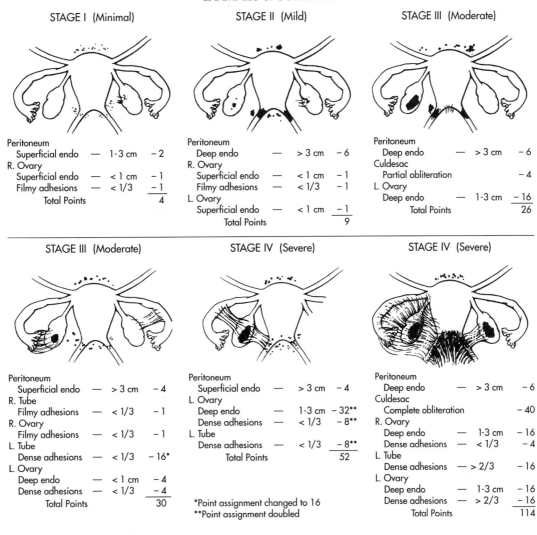

Fig. 19-6, cont'd. For legend, see opposite page.

allows the clinician to compare the clinical location and severity of pain with the anatomic findings at surgery (American Society for Reproductive Medicine, 1996). If endometriosis is diagnosed, it should be treated to the extent possible during laparoscopy. Interestingly, the extent of pain does not correlate with the extent of disease. Patients with stage I or stage II disease often have more pain than those with advanced disease (Fedele et al, 1990; Fukaya et al, 1993). There may be more pain associated with active lesions in mild disease than with adhesions in severe endometriosis. The latter may represent burned-out endometriosis that may, in the absence of fresh active lesions, result in less pain for the patient. In young women with endometriosis and severe pelvic pain, long-term hormonal therapy may be required. Surgery to remove endometrial implants and scar tissue may provide temporary relief from pain. However, as is the case after hormonal treatment, endometriosis and its ensuing pain usually recur. In general, women with severe endometriosis and unrelenting pain who

are older than 40 and who have completed their families are probably best treated by definitive surgery (*e.g.*, hysterectomy and bilateral oophorectomy).

Infertility

Any discussion of infertility in the patient with endometriosis is complicated by the observation that endometriosis does not usually present an absolute barrier to conception. Nonetheless, clinical evidence suggests that endometriosis can cause subfertility and infertility. In normal couples, monthly fecundability—the monthly chance to achieve pregnancy—is approximately 0.15 to 0.20 (Schwarz and Mayaux, 1982). In most studies of women with endometriosis and infertility who did not undergo treatment, however, the monthly fecundability diminishes to 0.02 to 0.1 (Pittaway et al, 1989). This suggests an association between endometriosis and infertility. The mechanisms responsible for this association include mechanical factors and a host of other poorly defined processes. For example, it is clear that if both ovaries are completely covered by adhesions, the egg and the sperm will be unable to interact. This results in infertility. Less clearly defined is the possibility that an ovarian endometrioma disrupts egg maturation by intraovarian mechanisms.

Despite the large body of clinical data associating high-stage endometriosis with infertility, convincing data that associate minimal and mild endometriosis with infertility are less prevalent. In an exhaustive review of infertility diagnoses and treatments, Hull (1992) concluded that even patients with so-called minor endometriosis had lower conception rates than the normal population. Patients with more severe disease who did not undergo treatment fared predictably worse. Additional evidence of subfertility in patients with minimal endometriosis came from a study of patients undergoing artificial insemination by donor. Women with minimal endometriosis had a monthly fecundity less than one third (0.036) that of normal controls (0.12) (Jansen, 1986). Similar results were reported in women who had stage I or stage II disease and underwent donor insemination. Patients with endometriosis had a monthly fecundity of 0.06 compared with a monthly fecundity of 0.14 in controls (Toma et al, 1992).

In patients in whom obvious mechanical factors for infertility are absent, the cause of endometriosis-related subfertility is unclear. Although several hypotheses have been advanced to explain the origins of infertility in these women, none has conclusively accounted for their subfertility.

Some investigators propose that ovulation disorders contribute to infertility in patients with endometriosis. Some women with endometriosis may be oligoovulatory, but most women with endometriosis have regular ovulatory cycles. In fact, the incessant endometrial reflux associated with regular menses may play a role in the implantation of ectopic endometrium.

A subtle ovulation abnormality, the luteal-phase defect, may be associated with endometriosis. However, in 100 consecutive patients with endometriosis from whom endometrial biopsy specimens were taken during the late luteal phase of the cycle, none had an out-of-phase endometrium. This suggests that luteal-phase deficiency is not especially common in women who have endometriosis (Barbieri et al, 1982).

Increasingly, the peritoneal environment of women with endometriosis is being evaluated. Pelvic endometriosis is often associated with diffuse pelvic inflammation, an increase in peritoneal fluid volume, and the number of activated peritoneal macrophages. These activated peritoneal macrophages are capable of phagocytosis of sperm, impaired sperm motility and transport, impaired oocyte capture, and secretion of esterases, peroxidases, proteolytic enzymes, cytokines, and lymphokines. Such secretions may create an environment hostile to egg and sperm function and interaction, impaired fertilization, and, ultimately, diminished embryo survival (Haney, 1988).

In addition, the concentration of lymphocytes and lymphocyte subpopulations is elevated in patients with stage I and stage II endometriosis (Hill et al, 1988). Numerous investigators have tried to correlate higher levels of peritoneal leukocyte products with endometriosis. Studies attempting to correlate peritoneal prostaglandin concentrations with endometriosis have produced contradictory results. It is hoped that further investigation will clarify the roles of the immune system and its products in the cause of endometriosis-associated subfertility.

Sporadic reports have suggested that endometriosis may be associated with an increased incidence of spontaneous abortion and luteal-phase defect. Recent studies suggest that the association between endometriosis and an increased risk for spontaneous abortion is spurious and probably resulted from selection bias (Hornstein, 1991; Pittaway, 1988).

Pelvic Mass

During physical examination, it is disclosed that some patients with endometriosis have a palpable pelvic mass, no pelvic pain, or a history of infertility. Some women with an asymptomatic pelvic mass are found at surgery to have an endometrioma and extensive endometriosis. The management of the patient with pelvic pain, however, should be directed at verifying that malignancy is not present. If present, it must be properly treated. The evaluation and treatment of such patients is covered elsewhere in this text.

TREATMENT

Patients with endometriosis typically have pelvic pain, infertility, or a pelvic mass. Therapeutic interventions should be designed to resolve the patient's specific problem.

Pelvic Pain

Therapy for endometriosis-associated pelvic pain has been shown to be efficacious and will be discussed under four headings: prophylaxis, observation and analgesia, hormonal therapy, and surgical treatment. An algorithm for the treatment of pelvic pain is presented in Fig. 19-7.

Prophylaxis

Manipulations that produce amenorrhea or cause endometrial atrophy are likely to decrease the risk for endometriosis. Early and frequent pregnancies may decrease the incidence of endometriosis, but this therapeutic strategy is incompatible with the life plans of most women. Exercise-induced amenorrhea may prove to be an effective prophylactic modality, but it also may be difficult for many women to achieve (Cramer et al, 1986).

There is suggestive evidence that women who have been taking oral contraceptives for prolonged periods of time, especially those with a potent progestin and a minimal amount of estrogen, may have a diminished risk for endometriosis. This is based on the observation that these agents produce endometrial atrophy and lessen menstrual flow, thus preventing tubal reflux of menstrual debris into the peritoneal cavity.

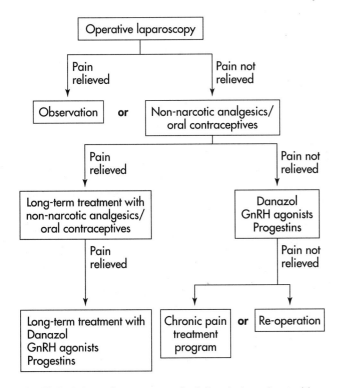

Fig. 19-7. Schema for treatment of pelvic pain in patients with endometriosis who do not desire fertility.

Observation and Analgesia

For some women with endometriosis, expectant management is a viable therapeutic option. For instance, some women with pelvic pain and minimal endometriosis may prefer therapy with analgesics over hormonal therapy with danazol, GnRH agonists, or high-dose progestins. For some young women with infertility and minimal or mild endometriosis, the best way to improve their fecundability may be to diagnose and treat any other confounding infertility factors rather than to treat the endometriosis medically.

Nonsteroidal antiinflammatory drugs (NSAIDs) should be considered the first-line therapy for pain relief in women with endometriosis. The antiprostaglandin effects of this class of analgesics often provides excellent relief of dysmenorrhea, and their antiinflammatory activity is helpful in reducing pelvic pain. Ibuprofen in dosages up to 2400 mg per day or naproxen sodium in dosages up to 1100 mg per day are excellent choices for most patients. These agents are usually well tolerated, but they should be used with caution for any patient who has a history of peptic ulcer disease or uncontrolled hypertensive renal disease or who is on anticoagulation therapy. These medications tend to work best when prescribed on a scheduled rather than an as-needed basis if pain may be expected, such as during menses.

A second-line agent to be considered is tramadol. It binds to the opiate receptor but is itself nonopiate. Therefore, it is thought to entail less potential for abuse than narcotics. Usual dosages are 100 to 200 mg per day. Tramadol should be prescribed with caution to patients taking monoamine ox-

idase inhibitors, patients prone to seizures, or patients taking medications that may lower the seizure threshold.

Patients unresponsive to NSAIDs or tramadol may require oral narcotics. These agents are highly addictive and should be prescribed with caution. Combinations of acetaminophen with codeine hydrocodone and oxycodone usually provide excellent pain relief for patients with acute pain.

Finally, patients with chronic pelvic pain caused by endometriosis often benefit from a multidisciplinary team approach. Numerous pain treatment centers offer multiple therapies for the patient with chronic pain. An important part of the approach to the patient involves psychological assessment and counseling to understand and treat the pain better.

Hormonal Therapy

During the past 40 years, the medical management of endometriosis has become significantly more sophisticated. In the early 1950s, the high-dose estrogen regimen of Karnaky was the only available hormonal treatment for endometriosis. In the 1960s and 1970s, Kistner's "pseudopregnancy" and "progestin-only" regimens dominated the medical management of endometriosis (Kistner, 1960). During the 1980s, danazol became the primary hormonal agent used in the treatment of endometriosis. In the 1990s, the GnRH agonists have become the most commonly used drugs for the treatment of endometriosis. These advances have significantly expanded the hormonal armamentarium of the gynecologist treating endometriosis. Proper use of these agents requires a thorough understanding of the hormonal responses of endometrial tissue and an appreciation of the pharmacologic properties of the available agents.

The central dogma that guides the hormonal therapy of endometriosis is the belief that steroid hormones are the major regulators of the growth and function of endometrial tissue. Most endometrial implants contain estrogen, progesterone, and androgen receptors. In general, estrogen stimulates the growth of these implants, and androgens induce their atrophy. The role of progesterone in the regulation of endometrial tissue is controversial. Progesterone alone may actually support the growth of endometrial tissue. However, the synthetic 19-norprogestogens, which are derivatives of testosterone and have androgenic properties, appear to inhibit the growth of endometrial tissue.

The polarity of response of endometrial tissue to androgens and estrogens is the basis of all current hormonal therapies of endometriosis. Three observations complicate this simplistic conceptualization. First, a small percentage of endometrial implants (approximately 5%) do not contain significant concentrations of either estrogen or progesterone receptors. These lesions may be relatively resistant to hormonal therapy. Second, microheterogeneity within endometrial lesions may make the steroid receptor-positive cell populations more susceptible to hormonal manipulations than the steroid receptor-negative cell populations. Third, some endometrial lesions that contain progesterone

Table 19-4   Hormone Strategies for Endometriosis Treatment

Hormone Strategy	Examples	Estradiol Concentration (pg/ml)	Unwanted Effects
Low estrogen, low androgen	Gonadotropin-releasing hormone agonists	20	Vasomotor symptoms, bone loss
	Bilateral oophorectomy	20	Irreversible sterility, vasomotor symptoms, bone loss, lipid changes
Low estrogen, high androgen	Danazol	40	Weight gain, acne, oily skin, hirsutism, voice changes

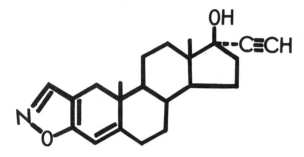

Fig. 19-8. Structure of danazol.

receptors do not demonstrate typical functional or structural responses to progesterone stimulation. This observation suggests that in some endometrial implants, the intranuclear steroid receptors are uncoupled from their site of action (DNA).

The polarity of response of endometrial tissue to androgens and estrogens is the basis for the two hormonal strategies most often used to treat endometriosis. One basic strategy is to create an acyclic, low-estrogen hormonal environment. Low estrogen levels cause atrophy of the endometrial tissues. The acyclic environment helps minimize the chance of miniature "menstruation" in the endometrial implants and prevents the reseeding of implants from the retrograde transport of normal endometrium during menstruation. An acyclic, low-estrogen environment is best produced by bilateral oophorectomy or by the use of GnRH agonists. The second basic strategy is to produce a hormonal environment high in androgens. Danazol therapy is the best example of this strategy. High-androgen environments directly produce atrophy of endometrial implants. High-androgen strategies also result in low, acyclic estrogen levels by interfering with ovarian follicular development. Table 19-4 summarizes these different strategies.

Danazol. Danazol is an isoxazole derivative of the synthetic steroid 17-ethinyl-testosterone (Fig. 19-8). The pharmacology of danazol is exceedingly complex and is best discussed in terms of the molecular pharmacology of the drug (Barbieri and Ryan, 1981). Current laboratory findings suggest that danazol interacts with only two major classes of proteins, steroid hormone receptors and enzymes of steroidogenesis. The entire pharmacologic profile of danazol

(and its metabolites) can be explained by danazol's interaction with these two classes of proteins.

Danazol and steroid-binding proteins. Systematic screening of the interaction of danazol with steroid-binding proteins found that danazol binds to intracellular androgen, progesterone, and glucocorticoid receptors (Barbieri and Ryan, 1979). Numerous investigators have confirmed these original findings.

The interaction of a steroid with an intracellular steroid receptor system can result in three possible outcomes: the steroid can produce the biologic effects characteristic of that intracellular receptor system (agonist); the steroid can block the biologic effects typically seen after stimulation of the receptor system (antagonist); and the steroid can produce a mixed pattern of agonistic and antagonistic effects. As previously noted, androgens induce atrophy in endometrial implants. The androgenic effect of danazol is one of the main pharmacologic means by which this drug produces atrophy in endometrial tissue.

Danazol has been reported to bind to intranuclear estrogen receptors. However, the affinity of the danazol-estrogen receptor interaction is so weak that this interaction is not thought to have clinical significance. Danazol interacts with glucocorticoid receptors; preliminary evidence suggests that it is a weak glucocorticoid agonist. Danazol also binds to intranuclear progesterone receptors, but its effects in bioassays for progesterone are exceedingly complex. In some bioassays, danazol induces secretory changes in the endometrium, which suggests that danazol is a progesterone agonist. In other systems, danazol is able to block the effect of progesterone, which means it behaves as an antiprogesterone. Given these diverse bioassay findings, it may be best to classify danazol as a mixed agonist-antagonist with respect to the progesterone receptor system.

In addition to binding to intracellular steroid receptors, danazol interacts with circulating steroid hormone-binding globulins. Danazol can displace testosterone from sex hormone-binding globulin (SHBG) and cortisol from corticosteroid-binding globulin. Of these two interactions, the danazol-induced increase in the percentage of bioavailable testosterone is clinically the more important. In normal women, 40% of testosterone is bioavailable (non-SHBG bound). In women taking danazol, 80% or more of the circulating testosterone is bioavailable (Nilsson et al, 1982). Therefore, part of the androgenic properties of danazol in the human may result from the dramatic increase in bioavailable androgens caused by danazol. In addition, the observation that danazol can bind to circulating steroid-binding proteins significantly complicates the interpretation of serum total steroid concentrations in patients receiving this drug.

In summary, danazol is an androgen, a glucocorticoid agonist, and a mixed agonist-antagonist with respect to the progesterone receptor system. Part of danazol's androgenic behavior results from its ability to displace testosterone from SHBG, which results in an increase in bioavailable testosterone. Danazol's poor ability to bind to estrogen receptors suggests that it has no significant effect on this receptor system. Steroid receptors regulate cell function in a large number of diverse tissues. The effects of danazol on cell function in a variety of steroid receptor-containing tissues will be reviewed briefly.

By acting as an androgen agonist, danazol decreases luteinizing hormone (LH) and follicle-stimulating hormone (FSH) secretions in castrated animals. One of danazol's main metabolites, ethinyl-testosterone, also suppresses LH and FSH secretions in castrated animals by acting as a progesterone agonist (Desaulles and Krahenbuhl, 1964). Although danazol suppresses LH and FSH levels in castrated animals, the effects of danazol on LH and FSH levels in animals with intact gonads are complex. The weight of evidence suggests that in women with ovaries, danazol administration does not produce a significant decrease in basal serum LH or FSH levels. This can be explained by the fact that danazol exerts a mild suppressive effect on pituitary secretion of LH and FSH, but simultaneously it causes a decrease in circulating, estradiol levels (by direct actions on the ovary). This, in turn, stimulates a rise in LH and FSH levels. The overall effect is that danazol does not produce any significant change in basal serum LH or FSH levels in premenopausal women receiving this drug; however, the mid-cycle surges of LH and FSH are blocked in patients taking danazol.

Danazol's androgenic properties directly suppress the growth of endometriosis and endometrial tissues. Danazol's lack of estrogenic effect facilitates the androgen-mediated inhibition of growth.

Its androgenic properties probably contribute to the decreased high-density lipoprotein (HDL) cholesterol levels observed in women receiving danazol. The atherogenic risk caused by the decrease in HDL cholesterol levels must be fully quantified, but patients with low HDL cholesterol levels may be at increased risk for atherosclerosis. Danazol's androgenic and mixed progestational effects probably contribute to the mild increase in insulin resistance observed in women receiving it.

Danazol and enzymes of steroidogenesis. In 1977 it was first reported that danazol inhibits multiple enzymes of steroidogenesis (Barbieri et al, 1977a, 1977b). Con-

centrations of danazol similar to those in the circulatory systems of women taking 800 mg/day (2 μmol/L) of the drug inhibit multiple enzymes involved in ovarian, testicular, and adrenal steroidogenesis. These enzymes include 3β-hydroxysteroid dehydrogenase isomerase; the 17-hydroxylase, 17-20-lyase complex; 17β-hydroxysteroid dehydrogenase; 11β-hydroxylase; and 21-hydroxylase (Barbieri et al, 1980; Barbieri and Ryan, 1981). Steingold et al (1986) followed up these in vitro experiments by demonstrating that danazol inhibits steroidogenesis in vivo.

An acyclic, high-androgen, low-estrogen environment is extremely hostile to the growth of endometrial tissue. Danazol produces a high-androgen environment because it is inherently androgenic, and it produces high levels of bioavailable testosterone by displacing testosterone from SHBG. A high-androgen environment directly inhibits the growth of endometrial tissue. Danazol produces a low-estrogen environment by inhibiting follicular growth, thereby decreasing LH and FSH secretion, and by inhibiting follicular estrogen secretion through direct action on follicular steroidogenesis. In addition, the acyclic endocrine environment produced by danazol minimizes the chance of menstruation, which prevents the reseeding of the peritoneum with new implants of the retrograde transported endometrium. The acyclic endocrine environment may also decrease pelvic pain by inhibiting bleeding in the endometriotic implants.

Guidelines concerning the use of danazol continue to evolve. The following discussion highlights the areas of consensus and the breadth of disagreement concerning the use of danazol.

Initiation of therapy. Danazol should be initiated after the completion of a normal menstrual cycle. It is important that danazol not be administered to a pregnant woman. Female pseudohermaphroditism is common in daughters of mothers treated with danazol during the first or second trimester (Duck and Katayama, 1981). Danazol is an effective contraceptive agent (less than a 1% incidence of ovulation) at dosages of 400 to 800 mg/day. However, patients with poor medication compliance can become pregnant on these doses of danazol because they are taking the drug in an intermittent fashion. At dosages less than 400 mg/day, the incidence of ovulation is substantial; thus, barrier contraception must be used. In addition, women taking more than 400 mg/day danazol should use a barrier contraception if their medication compliance is poor.

Dosage. Danazol in dosages of 200 mg/day or more produces pain relief in most patients with endometriosis. However, dosages of at least 400 mg are required to induce amenorrhea reliably (Biberoglu and Behrman, 1981). Given these considerations and a desire to minimize costs, most patients are started on 200 mg danazol two to three times a day. For patients with severe endometriosis, consideration can be given to using danazol at a dosage of 200 mg four times daily. Cessation of menses and serum estradiol levels are good clinical and laboratory monitors of danazol therapy. Many experienced clinicians believe that the maximal therapeutic effect of danazol occurs if menses are completely suppressed. The greater the degree of estrogen suppression, the greater the likelihood that amenorrhea will occur. The interval between drug administration appears to play an important role in determining the degree of estrogen suppression. For example, in one study the mean serum estradiol concentration was 40% lower in patients receiving 200 mg danazol every 6 hours than in patients receiving 400 mg danazol every 12 hours (Dickey et al, 1984).

Duration of therapy. Initial trials investigating the efficacy of danazol evaluated a 6-month therapy regimen. This therapy interval need not be followed rigidly. Individualization of care is important when danazol is used to treat endometriosis. For example, in the patient with advanced endometriosis who is scheduled for repeat surgery, an 8- to 12-week preoperative course of danazol may be appropriate. For the patient with painful endometriosis who does not desire pregnancy and who is adamantly opposed to surgery, a 52- to 78-week course of danazol is reasonable if side effects and laboratory parameters are carefully monitored.

Side effects. More than 75% of patients receiving danazol have one or more side effects (Barbieri et al, 1982). Major side effects seen with danazol therapy (in decreasing order of frequency) are weight gain, edema, decreased breast size, acne, oily skin, hirsutism, deepening of the voice, headache, hot flashes, changes in libido, and muscle cramps. Significant weight gain (2 to 10 kg) is not uncommon. All these side effects are reversible with the exception of voice changes. The time course for the resolution of androgenic symptoms may be long; 6 months or more is usual.

Contraindications. In nonpregnant, nonbreast-feeding patients with documented endometriosis, relatively few absolute contraindications to danazol therapy exist. Danazol is metabolized largely by hepatic mechanisms, and it has been reported to produce mild changes in liver function test results (elevated serum transaminase levels) in some patients. Therefore, danazol is contraindicated for patients with hepatic dysfunction. Because danazol can induce marked fluid retention, any patient with severe hypertension, congestive heart failure, or borderline renal function may experience deterioration in her medical condition after the initiation of therapy.

Timing of attempts at conception after completion of therapy. Dmowski and Cohen (1978) reported a high number of second- and third-trimester intrauterine fetal deaths in patients who conceived within the first three cycles after the discontinuation of danazol therapy. They suggested that this degree of fetal wastage may be secondary to implantation in an atrophic endometrium; after a course of danazol, one full menstrual cycle with normal flow and duration should be observed before any attempt is made to conceive. In contrast to these observations, Daniell and Christianson (1981) observed no increase in fetal wastage in patients who conceived within 3 months of completing a course of danazol. Barbieri et al (1982) confirmed that danazol therapy was not associated with increased fetal wastage. Additional information is needed to resolve these discrepancies.

Danazol and surgery for the treatment of the infertility of endometriosis. In infertile patients with advanced stages of endometriosis, surgery is usually necessary to repair anatomic abnormalities and to remove endometriotic implants. Few experimental data concerning the value of danazol in the preoperative or postoperative management of endometriosis are available. Some experienced clinicians suggest that danazol has little value in the preoperative management of endometriosis. Others think danazol may improve the prognosis for infertile women with endometriosis by decreasing the number and size of endometrial areas, thereby minimizing the extent of surgery. In addition, the preoperative use of danazol eliminates the chance of traumatizing a corpus luteum. Use of danazol in the postoperative management of the infertile patient with endometriosis is also controversial. Most conceptions that take place after surgery occur within the first 12 months of surgery. By treating patients with danazol for prolonged periods after surgery, the time interval with the highest fertility potential may be passed over. Therefore, danazol may be used in patients before surgery, but short courses of postoperative danazol therapy should be reserved for women with residual disease who are not attempting conception.

Use in the treatment of endometriosis in patients not desiring fertility. For the patient who is older than 40 years, has symptomatic endometriosis, and has completed her family, definitive therapy consisting of total abdominal hysterectomy and bilateral salpingo-oophorectomy (TAH-BSO) is usually recommended. However, some patients may want to postpone or avoid major surgery. For these patients, a trial of danazol may be reasonable. For the young, symptomatic patient with endometriosis who intends to delay pregnancy, danazol therapy is highly effective in relieving symptoms and physical findings.

Treatment of endometriomas. There has been no systematic study assessing the effect of danazol on endometriomas. Clinical experience suggests that danazol can often reduce the size of small endometriomas, but it is unusual for danazol to cause complete regression of an endometrioma. In general, danazol is more effective in causing peritoneal endometrial implants of small diameter to regress than in ablating cysts. Large ovarian masses generally require surgical exploration.

Use in metastatic endometriosis. For most patients with endometriosis that involves organs outside the pelvis, TAH-BSO is necessary. Some patients refuse surgery, and others are extremely poor candidates. In these patients, danazol therapy may be used as a last resort. Danazol has been successful in the treatment of pulmonary endometriosis, bowel obstruction, and ureteral obstruction caused by endometriosis. However, once hormone therapy is discontinued, the disease often recurs.

Recurrence rates after therapy for endometriosis. A major problem in the treatment of endometriosis is that the disease tends to recur unless definitive surgical therapy is performed. After a course of danazol therapy, the recurrence of symptoms and physical findings is at least 20% per year and is generally higher in patients with endometriomas (Barbieri et al, 1982). A second course of danazol therapy is often successful in inducing a remission of disease symptoms and physical findings.

Danazol versus pseudopregnancy. Few data that directly compare the efficacy of danazol versus a pseudopregnancy regimen in the treatment of endometriosis are available. The results of one small, prospective, randomized trial of danazol versus a combination of mestranol and norethynodrel were reported by Noble and Letchworth (1979). Eighty-six percent of the patients treated with danazol reported improvement in their symptoms. Only 30% of the pseudopregnancy group reported symptomatic improvement, and improvement in objective findings was demonstrated in 84% of patients treated with danazol compared with only 18% of patients on the pseudopregnancy regimen. Side effects were a major problem for patients on both therapeutic regimens. Only 4% of the danazol group, but 41% of the pseudopregnancy group, discontinued therapy because of side effects.

Gonadotropin-Releasing Hormone Agonist Therapy. GnRH is a hypothalamic decapeptide that stimulates pituitary LH and FSH secretion. In primates, pulses of GnRH in the range of one pulse per hour are associated with a normal pattern of LH and FSH secretion, normal follicular and corpus luteum development, and cyclic menses. Administration of GnRH at a high pulse rate (more than five pulses per hour) or in a continuous fashion produces an initial agonist response with an increase in LH and FSH secretion. This is followed by a drastic decrease in LH and FSH secretion with the cessation of ovarian follicular activity, hypoestrogenism, and amenorrhea. This may be the result of the downregulation or the desensitization of pituitary GnRH receptors by a continuous infusion of GnRH (Knobil, 1980).

The natural decapeptide GnRH has a short half-life because of its degradation by tissue and circulating peptidases. Therefore, it is difficult to produce a constant circulating concentration using native GnRH. By the chemical alteration of amino acid 6 of GnRH, analogues can be synthesized that have two useful properties, high affinity for the pituitary GnRH receptor and a long half-life because of the resistance to cleavage by endopeptidases. Initially, many investigators thought these synthetic derivatives of GnRH would be superagonists and potent fertility-enhancing agents—hence, the term GnRH agonists. Unexpectedly, GnRH agonists proved to be potent inhibitors of gonadal function. Their administration to men or women causes a transient 1- to 2-week increase in the production of LH and FSH by the pituitary gland and then a dramatic and sustained decrease in pituitary production of bioactive LH and FSH. The ability of the GnRH agonists to downregulate pituitary secretion of gonadotropins has not been fully explained. Numerous GnRH agonists, including nafarelin, leuprolide, buserelin, goserelin, histrelin, and triptorelin, are available or are under evaluation in clinical trials (Table 19-5). No GnRH agonist is effective when given orally. These agents, however, can be administered by monthly intramus-

Table 19-5   Structures of Gonadotropin-Releasing Hormone Agonists with Documented Efficacy in the Treatment of Endometriosis

	p Glu-His-Trp-Spr-Tyr-Gly-Leu-Arg-Pro-Gly-NH2	
Native GnRH	6	10
Leuprolide	D-Leu	−NHEt
Buserelin	D-Ser(t-Bu)	−AzA-Gly
Nafarelin	D-NAL(2)	

Table 19-6   Doses of Gonadotropin-Releasing Hormone Agonists Used in the Treatment of Endometriosis

Leuprolide acetate	0.5-1.0 mg subcutaneously daily
Leuprolide acetate- Depo formulation	3.75-7.5 mg intramuscularly monthly
Nafarelin	0.4-0.8 mg intranasally daily

cular depot injections or implants, or by daily subcutaneous injections or nasal sprays (Table 19-6).

Treatment with GnRH agonists results in the reversible suppression of gonadal steroid production in men and women. Consequently, many diseases that are modulated by the gonadal steroids testosterone and estradiol can be successfully treated with GnRH agonists.

For example, GnRH agonists have been reported to be successful in the treatment of leiomyomata uteri, polycystic ovarian syndrome, precocious puberty, and premenstrual syndrome and as adjuvants for the induction of ovulation in women and in the treatment of prostatic cancer in men. The first report of the use of a GnRH agonist in the treatment of endometriosis came from Meldrum et al (1982). Although used for only a 1-month trial, the study demonstrated the efficacy of this class of compounds as therapy for endometriosis.

Henzl et al (1988) reported on the comparative efficacies of danazol and the GnRH agonist nafarelin in the treatment of endometriosis. The study was large, randomized, and double blind, and it included an objective assessment of the response to therapy by a comparison of laparoscopic examinations performed before and after treatment. The investigators tested two dosages of nasal nafarelin (400 and 800 μg/day) and one dosage of oral danazol (800 mg/day). Drug therapy was continued for 6 months. More than 80% of the patients treated with either nafarelin or danazol had symptomatic and objective improvement in their condition. Nafarelin and danazol were found to be quantitatively similar in efficacy (Fig. 19-9), but the side effects of the two drugs differed substantially. Women who received danazol reported weight gain, edema, and myalgia. They had increased circulating levels of serum aspartate aminotransferase and alanine aminotransferase and decreased levels of

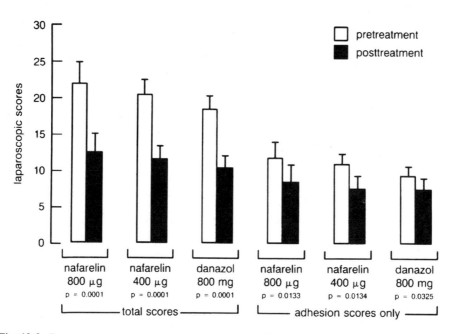

Fig. 19-9. Pretreatment and posttreatment American Fertility Society endometriosis scores in women receiving 6 months of nasal nafarelin or oral danazol therapy. (From Henzl M, et al: Administration of nasal nafarelin as compared with oral danazol for endometriosis: A multicenter double-blind comparative clinical trial. *N Engl J Med* 1988; 318:485.)

HDL cholesterol. In contrast, the principal side effects reported by women who received nafarelin were hot flashes, decreased libido, and vaginal dryness.

Similar prospective, randomized, comparative trials of other GnRH agonists and danazol report efficacy and side effects comparable to those of Henzl et al (1988). Matta and Shaw (1986) used buserelin, Wheeler et al (1992) used leuprolide depot, the Nafarelin European Endometriosis Trial group (1992) studied nafarelin, and Rock et al (1993) investigated goserelin. In all cases, the GnRH agonists proved efficacious and safe.

The major safety concern raised with this class of drugs relates to their hypoestrogenic effects. The initial experience with the GnRH agonists demonstrated that patients using the agonists experience a variety of hypoestrogenic symptoms, including hot flashes and vaginal dryness. In addition, urinary calcium studies suggested an increase in calcium excretion similar to that seen in menopausal women. There is thus a concern that patients taking GnRH agonists are at risk for losing trabecular bone (Steingold et al, 1987). The spongy trabecular portion of bone that is found in the spine and hip is more sensitive to the loss of estrogen than the cortical bone found in the shaft of the long bones. Numerous investigators have examined the extent of bone loss during short courses of GnRH agonist therapy. Although the sites measured, the method of measurement, and the drug used have differed, most studies demonstrate an approximate 2% to 7% loss in bone density during 6 months of GnRH agonist treatment, with substantial recovery in a 6-month, follow-up interval (Fogelman, 1992).

Because of the concern about hypoestrogenic effects, most notably on bone, there has been a recent trend to combine hormonal "add-back" therapy with the use of GnRH analogues. One strategy has been to combine progestins with GnRH agonists. The combination of medroxyprogesterone acetate with GnRH agonist treatment diminished hot flashes and protected bone but failed to improve endometrial symptoms (Cedars et al, 1990). The use of a different progestin, norethindrone, produced symptomatic relief but failed to protect bone density (Surrey and Judd, 1990). In another study, the same progestin (norethindrone) used in a higher dosage of 5 to 10 mg/day yielded symptomatic relief of endometriosis, with laparoscopically proven efficacy, and had a protective effect on bone (Surrey and Judd, 1992). However, this high dose of norethindrone led to adverse effects on serum lipids and cholesterol subfractions.

An alternative approach has been to use the antiresorptive properties of an organic bisphosphonate in combination with a progestin. Such a combination allows a reduction in the dose of the progestin while sparing bone density and reducing the adverse effects of the progestin on lipids. In a prospective, randomized study, a 2.5 mg daily dosage of norethindrone and the bisphosphonate sodium etidronate reduced pelvic pain and vasomotor symptoms while it protected against bone loss (Surrey et al, 1995). Lipid profiles were less adversely affected than with high-dose progestin therapy. The long-term safety of bisphosphonates in women who want to postpone childbearing has not been established.

Another strategy in reducing the hypoestrogenic effects of GnRH analogues has been to add back small doses of es-

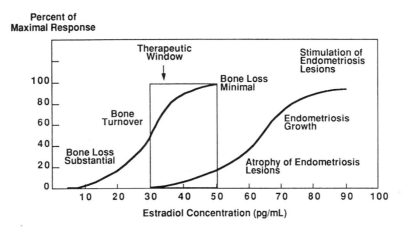

Fig. 19-10. Estradiol therapeutic window. The concentration of estradiol required to cause growth of endometriosis lesions may be greater than the concentration required to stabilize bone mineral density. (From Barbieri RL: Hormone treatment of endometriosis: the estrogen threshold hypothesis. *Am J Obstet Gynecol* 1992; 166:742.)

trogens, in addition to progestins, to alleviate the adverse effects of severe hypoestrogenemia while preserving the beneficial effects of GnRH agonist therapy. This treatment regimen is predicated on the hypothesis that estrogen-dependent tissues vary in their responsiveness to estrogen. An estrogen threshold may exist for each estrogen-dependent disease; clinical improvement in the underlying disease may occur with only minimal adverse effects of hypoestrogenism (Barbieri, 1992) (Fig. 19-10). Thus, an estradiol therapeutic window may exist in which maximal benefit can occur with minimal hypoestrogenic sequelae. Several recent studies have suggested that such an estrogen-progestin add-back is efficacious and safe. Howell et al (1993) showed that patients who had endometriosis and were treated for 6 months with goserelin combined with transdermal estradiol and medroxyprogesterone acetate experienced less bone loss than women treated with goserelin alone (Howell et al, 1993). A multicenter Finnish study used norethisterone and 17-β-estradiol in combination with the GnRH-agonist, goserelin acetate (Kiiholma et al, 1995). This combination produced improved American Fertility Society endometriosis scores on repeat laparoscopy and reduced pelvic pain scores. A reduction in vasomotor symptoms in the add-back group was also seen compared with the GnRH-agonist alone group. Unfortunately, this study did not assess bone mineral density.

A recently published multicenter, randomized, double-blind study compared three hormonal add-back regimens to a GnRH-agonist without add-back in a 1-year trial (Hornstein et al, 1998). Each group received leuprolide acetate depot monthly. The first group received placebos for estrogen and progestin; the second group received norethindrone acetate 5 mg daily and placebo for estrogen; the third group received norethindrone acetate 5 mg daily and conjugated equine estrogens 0.625 mg; and the fourth group received norethindrone acetate 5 mg and conjugated equine estrogen 1.25 mg daily. Patients in all three add-back groups

had reductions in their endometriosis pain scores comparable to those of the group treated with the GnRH-agonist alone. However, more patients in the high-estrogen add-back group left the study prematurely because of a lack of improvement in symptoms. Hot flashes were suppressed in all the add-back groups. Of significance was the fact that none of the add-back groups lost bone mineral density through the 1-year course of the study, whereas mean bone density decreased more than 6% in the GnRH-agonist only group. This study demonstrated the efficacy and safety of low-dose progestin and low-dose estrogen-progestin add-back therapy.

The large numbers of recent publications on the use of the GnRH agonists for endometriosis serve to emphasize that the use of these agents continues to evolve. Nonetheless, it is now possible to present some guidelines for the use of these compounds with the caveat that many disagreements among experts still exist. The format below is similar to that used in the discussion of danazol and may allow the reader to contrast the clinical use of these two pharmacologic approaches.

Initiation of therapy. It is possible to initiate GnRH analogues at two points during the menstrual cycle. Patients may begin taking the agonists during a normal menses or in the midluteal phase of the cycle. Because these agents produce temporary elevations in gonadotropin levels and because it generally takes 8 to 15 days for full pituitary down-regulation to occur, it is best not to have the agonist effect coincide with the ovulatory midcycle gonadotropin surge. This is best accomplished with an early follicular or midluteal start. Depot preparation should be given at the time of menses. Although malformations associated with GnRH agonist use have not been reported, the safety of its use in early pregnancy has not been established. Thus, it is prudent to avoid inadvertent use in early gestation.

Dosage. The recommended dosages of the GnRH agonists available in the United States appear in Table 19-6.

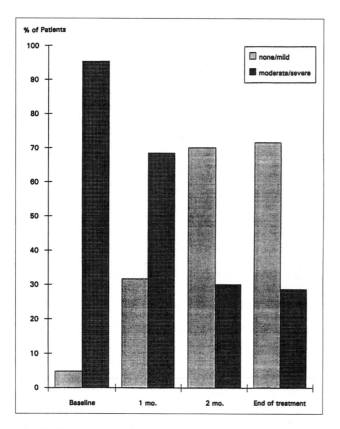

Fig. 19-11. Severity of endometriosis symptoms during retreatment with nafarelin. The total severity score is the sum of the scores for each of five signs or symptoms: dysmenorrhea, dyspareunia, pelvic pain, pelvic tenderness, and pelvic induration. Each of the five was scored as follows: 0, absent; 1, mild; 2, moderate; 3, severe. The total severity score was interpreted as follows: 0, no symptoms; 1 or 2, mild; 3 to 5, moderate; 6 to 10, severe; 11 to 15, very severe. (From Hornstein, et al: Retreatment with nafarelin for recurrent endometriosis symptoms: Efficacy, safety and bone mineral density. *Fertil Steril* 1997; 67:1016.)

These doses have been shown to produce estradiol levels in the range of 15 to 30 pg/ml and to produce amenorrhea in most patients.

Duration of therapy. The Food and Drug Administration has approved nafarelin, leuprolide depot, and goserelin for a 6-month course of therapy for endometriosis. This regimen was based on early studies that used this duration of treatment and took into account the concerns regarding the long-term loss of bone. Under some circumstances, shorter courses of therapy may be desirable to reduce the side effects of the GnRH agonists. A prospective, randomized, double-blind trial demonstrated that 3-month courses of a GnRH-agonist are equally as efficacious as a six-month course (Hornstein et al, 1995) and that the duration of pain relief is not diminished with the shorter course. Furthermore, the shorter treatment resulted in less bone loss (Orwell et al, 1994). For patients with no or minimal loss in bone density or with bone density above the fracture threshold after 6 months of therapy, additional treatment may be considered with the

patient's consent, followed by careful monitoring of bone density every 6 months. Alternatively, appropriate hormonal add-back regimens may be considered. Repeated cycles of GnRH agonist are possible, with the confirmation of healthy bone density before therapy is reinitiated (Henzl, 1992). Two recent studies have demonstrated the efficacy and safety of GnRH-agonist retreatment. In a 3-month retreatment, 95% of patients reported moderate or severe pain at the beginning of the retreatment, but only 29% reported moderate or severe pain at the conclusion of the 3-month trial (Hornstein et al, 1997a) (Fig. 19-11). There was no significant bone loss in the retreated patients. These findings have subsequently been confirmed (Adamson et al, 1997).

Side effects. The profound hypoestrogenia seen with these agents leads to predictable side effects of hot flashes (90%), vaginal dryness, and decreased libido. In addition, more than 20% of patients taking GnRH agonists experience headaches (Henzl and Kwei, 1990). Women with a history of migraines seem to be predisposed to a worsening of their headaches. Androgenic side effects such as acne, oily skin, and hirsutism are predictably rare in women treated with GnRH agonists.

Contraindications. As mentioned previously, GnRH agonists are contraindicated in pregnancy. In addition, women who are breast-feeding or who have undiagnosed vaginal bleeding should not take these agents. Hypersensitivity reactions to GnRH agonists have been reported.

Timing of attempts at conception after therapy cessation. Menses generally resume approximately 6 weeks after the completion of a course of GnRH analogues. Increased fetal wastage has not been reported with these medications as it has with danazol.

Use of GnRH agonists with surgery in the treatment of endometriosis. There are no large-scale clinical findings to evaluate the efficacy of GnRH analogues, before or after surgery, in patients who have endometriosis. Because the optimal time to attempt conception is during the first 12 months after surgery and because menses do not immediately return after GnRH agonist therapy, it seems prudent to refrain from the postoperative use of these drugs in infertile patients. However, postoperative use of the analogues is efficacious for patients in whom pelvic pain returns rapidly after surgery. A randomized, placebo-controlled study has examined the use of a GnRH-agonist after laparoscopic surgery for endometriosis (Hornstein et al, 1997b) (Fig. 19-12). The median length of time patients required alternative medical or surgical treatment for pain was 11.7 months in the placebo-treated patients versus more than 24 months in patients treated postoperatively for 6 months.

Treatment of endometriomas. Medical therapy is unlikely to produce the complete regression of large endometrial cysts. Patients with such ovarian masses should have surgical exploration. This is usually possible by laparoscopy. One study, however, demonstrated a reduction in the size of ovarian cysts, presumed to be endometriomas, in patients treated with buserelin (Donnez et al, 1989). In general, the cysts were small (3 to 4 cm), and only a small (1 to 2 cm) diminution in their size was reported.

Use in metastatic endometriosis. Endometriosis outside the pelvis generally requires TAH-BSO; however, the use of GnRH agonists for extrapelvic endometriosis has been suggested (Markham, 1991). An interesting case of catamenial pneumothorax, recurrent pneumothorax associated with menstruation, that was treated by leuprolide depot has recently been reported (Dotson et al, 1993). Episodes of pneumothorax ceased during the year the patient was treated with GnRH agonists, but it recurred when her therapy was changed to daily norethindrone.

Recurrence rates after medical therapy. It is difficult to appreciate fully the recurrence rate after medical therapy for endometriosis. Pelvic pain resulting from other causes may lead to overestimates of recurrence rates, whereas the recurrence of disease not leading to symptoms may underestimate the reactivation of disease. Waller and Shaw (1993) have reviewed the research related to patients with laparoscopically proven endometriosis who were treated with GnRH agonists between 1985 and 1987; recurrence rates up to 7 years from the initial treatment were reported. They found that the cumulative recurrence rate for the fifth year of treatment was 53%. Patients with minimal disease and severe disease had recurrence rates of 37% and 74%, respectively. This long-term study suggests that the recurrence of endometriosis after medical therapy is common and more likely in patients with more severe disease.

GnRH agonists versus pseudopregnancy. Although the relief of pain with pseudopregnancy (oral contraceptive [OC] use) does occur, severe cases of endometriosis are better treated with danazol or a GnRH agonist. OCs, especially used in an acyclic manner, benefit many women with mild degrees of endometriosis. A single study directly comparing OCs and GnRH agonists for the treatment of endometriosis has been published. Vercellini et al (1993) prospectively compared goserelin and a low-dose OC that contained 0.02 mg ethinyl estradiol and 0.15 mg desogestrel. Significant pain reduction occurred in both groups, but women with deep dyspareunia reported better relief with goserelin than with OCs. The reduction in nonmenstrual pain and the return of symptoms was similar in both groups. Both drugs were well tolerated, and only one patient (in the OC group) withdrew because of side effects. This study again demonstrated the efficacy of OCs in the treatment of endometriosis, but it also demonstrated that in more severe cases the GnRH agonists may provide greater symptomatic relief.

Pseudopregnancy Regimens. In response to chronic, acyclic stimulation by estrogen and progesterone, the endometrium becomes inactive and demonstrates decidualization. Figs. 19-11 and 19-12 illustrate this phenomenon. This observation is the basis for the use of acyclic, combined estrogen-progestogen agents in the treatment of endometriosis (Kistner, 1958; Kistner, 1960). There is no evidence that a particular preparation of an estrogen-progestogen pill is uniquely effective in the treatment of endometriosis. Any

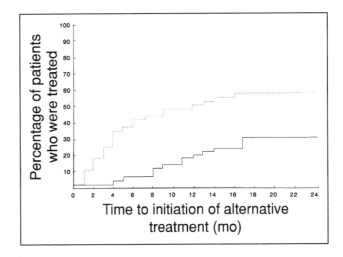

Fig. 19-12. Time to initiation of alternative treatment for patients who were treated with nafarelin (———) or placebo (··········). (From Hornstein, et al: Use of nafarelin versus placebo after reductive laparoscopic surgery for endometriosis. *Fertil Steril* 1997; 68:862.)

combined estrogen-progestogen preparation may be used; however, an OC that includes an androgenic progestin has theoretical appeal. A standard regimen would use 0.03 mg ethinyl estradiol with 0.3 mg norgestrel (Lo/Ovral) daily. Hormones are given every day for 3 to 4 months. The medication is discontinued for 1 week, and light menstrual bleeding may occur at this time. The medication is then reinstituted for another course. If clinically significant breakthrough bleeding occurs, the hormone dosage can be increased to 0.05 mg ethinyl estradiol with 0.5 mg norgestrel (Ovral) daily. Such an acyclic use of oral contraceptives has two advantages. First, it reduces the number of menstrual cycles, thus reducing the frequency of painful periods. Second, the reduction in the number of menstrual cycles may reduce reseeding of the pelvis with endometrium.

A pseudopregnancy regimen is especially useful in the management of dysmenorrhea caused by endometriosis in the young patient. For example, a 17-year-old girl with mild endometriosis and incapacitating dysmenorrhea can be put on a pseudopregnancy regimen as previously described. For the adolescent patient, a pseudopregnancy regimen is less expensive and often better tolerated than danazol or a GnRH agonist.

Progestin-only Regimens. Numerous progestins (e.g., medroxyprogesterone acetate, norethindrone acetate, norgestrel acetate, and lynestrenol) are used as single agents for the treatment of endometriosis (Semm and Mettler, 1980). In general, these agents produce a hypoestrogenic-acyclic hormonal environment by suppressing ovarian follicular activity through the inhibition of LH and FSH secretion. In addition, these agents may have direct effects on endometrial tissue via estrogen, androgen, and progesterone receptors. As noted earlier, many synthetic progestins are weak androgen agonists.

A major problem with the use of progestins as single agents is that large doses must be given to produce an acyclic hypoestrogenic environment. These high doses are often associated with side effects such as bloating, weight gain, and irregular uterine bleeding. Aggravation of depression can be pronounced in some patients. Parenteral administration of large doses of medroxyprogesterone acetate in depot form can be effective in the treatment of endometriosis (a dosage range of 150 mg every 3 months to 150 mg every month). However, this drug is not recommended as a first-line agent in women who have not completed their families because it can produce prolonged amenorrhea after therapy is terminated, and the long-term safety of the agent is still controversial. Oral administration of 30 to 50 mg medroxyprogesterone acetate daily can be effective in the treatment of endometriosis (Luciano et al, 1988). In general, a course of progestins is less expensive than similar treatment with danazol and the GnRH agonists.

Surgical Treatment

In contemplating the surgical treatment of endometriosis, one should always bear in mind that functioning ovarian tissue is necessary for the continued activity of the disease. Therefore, the successful treatment of endometriosis depends on acknowledging when it is reasonably safe and desirable to maintain ovarian function and when it is necessary to eliminate it. It is obvious that ovarian function should be conserved when endometriosis is treated early and there are minimally symptomatic lesions and that it should be eliminated when the pelvic organs are hopelessly invaded by endometriosis or when fertility is no longer a concern. Unfortunately, from the standpoint of definite surgical indications, most cases fall between the two extremes and may present problems in surgical judgment seldom encountered in any other pelvic disease. As knowledge of the life history of endometriosis increases, there is a tendency to become more conservative, particularly in the treatment of early and borderline cases. In general, it is thought that one should err on the side of the conservation of ovarian function. This belief is based on the fact that endometriosis usually progresses slowly over a period of years, rarely becomes malignant, and regresses at menopause. Surgical options include laparoscopic surgery, conservative surgery by laparotomy, and extirpative surgery.

Laparoscopic Surgery. The diagnosis of endometriosis requires laparoscopy or laparotomy. At the time of a diagnostic laparoscopy, an attempt should be made to excise all endometrial implants and adhesions. Laparoscopy for advanced endometriosis requires several hours of surgery, expert technical skills on the part of the surgeon, and specialized equipment. Minimal and mild endometriosis can often be surgically treated at the time of laparoscopy without significantly prolonging operative time and with a minimum of special skills and equipment. Laparoscopic treatment of endometriosis uses a two- or three-puncture technique. Two lower abdominal incisions are often necessary to grasp specific pelvic organs and to allow the use of unipolar or bipolar electrocautery or laser for the lysis of adhesions and the ablation of implants. There are no studies that directly compare the efficacy of electrocautery and laser in the treatment of endometriosis-associated infertility.

Conservative Surgery. If the childbearing function is to be preserved, surgical procedures should be as conservative as possible. The approach can usually be through a suprapubic transverse incision. A thorough exploration of the pelvic and abdominal organs should be routinely performed, and a decision should be reached about the performance of either conservative or definitive surgery. Good surgical technique is important. Gentle handling of tissues and meticulous hemostasis are important to minimize the subsequent formation of adhesions. A full description of surgical techniques may be found in most gynecologic surgery textbooks.

Extirpative Surgery. The treatment of choice for most women with advanced endometriosis who have completed their families is TAH-BSO. From a pathophysiologic viewpoint, it is the bilateral oophorectomy and the concomitant hypoestrogenism that provide relief from the disease process. Many authorities recommend TAH or TAH-unilateral salpingo-oophorectomy (USO) for the treatment of endometriosis. These authorities argue that leaving one or both ovaries in situ will prevent the sequelae of early surgical menopause. Although this is true, approximately 50% of women treated with TAH alone require reoperation because of persistent endometriosis (Montgomery and Studd, 1987). In a recently reported study, 63% of women who had ovarian preservation at the time of hysterectomy for endometriosis had recurrent symptoms, and nearly half of those women required repeat surgery (Namnoum et al, 1993). A 50% failure rate makes this an unattractive treatment option for advanced endometriosis; however, in cases of mild to moderate endometriosis, TAH-USO may be a reasonable treatment choice.

When definitive surgery for advanced endometriosis is performed, it is important to remove all functioning ovarian tissue. Many women who have advanced endometriosis and who allegedly had TAH-BSO have persistent symptoms of disease activity. Uniformly, these women have serum estradiol and FSH concentrations in the premenopausal range. These laboratory studies demonstrate the presence of residual ovarian activity.

From the standpoint of surgery, early or moderately advanced endometriosis offers no unusual difficulties, but extensive endometriosis may present many technical problems. Endometriosis, in contrast to pelvic inflammatory disease, produces an extremely dense type of pelvic adhesion with an almost complete absence of planes of cleavage. Therefore, much of the dissection must be performed with sharp instruments, and the danger of damage to adherent structures is thereby increased. This hazard may be diminished by the use of preoperative danazol or GnRH agonists.

Hysterectomy and BSO can usually be performed on patients with large ovarian endometrial cysts and extensive

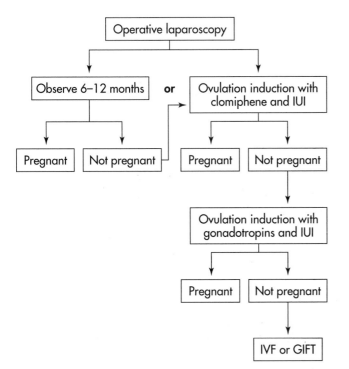

Fig. 19-13. Schema for the treatment of infertility in stage I and stage II endometriosis.

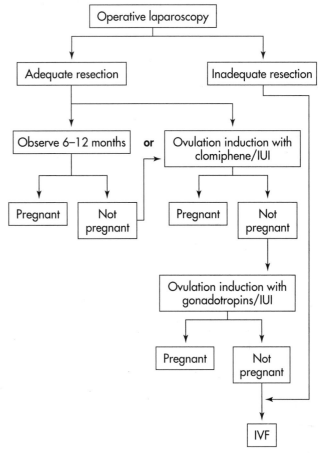

Fig. 19-14. Schema for the treatment of infertility in stage III and stage IV endometriosis.

pelvic adhesions and even on those with marked invasion of the rectovaginal septum. This may be facilitated by incising the posterior peritoneum above the insertion of the utero-sacral ligaments. The endopelvic fascia and rectosigmoid may then be reflected, minimizing the danger of fistula formation. At times it may be necessary to leave a considerable portion of the implants attached to the bowel or other pelvic structures. The fact that these remnants will regress along with other müllerian tissue in the pelvis after removal of the ovaries is of great importance in the treatment of this disease. A few patients in whom this atrophy did not occur have been reported; however, it is possible that ovarian tissue was incompletely removed in some of these patients. Low-dose pelvic external radiation may be useful in irradiating ovarian function in such instances.

As emphasized, hypoestrogenism "cures" most cases of endometriosis. Paradoxically, most women who have undergone TAH-BSO for advanced endometriosis can use low-dose estrogen replacement therapy without reactivating endometriosis. To reduce hot flashes and to try to reduce residual disease, a course of medroxyprogesterone acetate, 20 mg per day for 3 months, may prove beneficial. At that time, 0.625 mg of conjugated equine estrogen (CEE) daily or its equivalent is prescribed. With this regimen, less than 10% of patients should have a reactivation of disease. If the disease does recur, hormone replacement therapy can be discontinued. Some authorities think that residual endometriotic implants can undergo malignant transformation when stimulated by continuous unopposed estrogen replacement. These authorities recommend adding a cyclic progestin to

the CEE. No well-controlled scientific data to evaluate this practice are available.

Infertility

In reviewing treatment options for patients with endometriosis and infertility, it is useful to distinguish between patients with minimal and mild disease (ASRM stages I and II) and those with moderate and severe endometriosis (ASRM stages III and IV). In patients with mild disease, the absence of severe anatomic distortion and the less certain nature of the causal relationship between endometriosis and infertility may allow a more empiric management course. In patients who have more severe disease with extensive adhesions, endometriomas, and a clearer cause of infertility, a primary surgical approach appears prudent. Often this may be followed directly by IVF. Algorithms for the treatment of infertility in stages I and II and stages III and IV endometriosis are presented in Figs. 19-13 and 19-14.

The first step in treatment is the visual confirmation of endometriosis. Laparoscopy is usually the first-choice method of surgery. There has been a long-standing controversy about whether the surgical treatment of endometriosis contributes to improved pregnancy rates in low-stage disease.

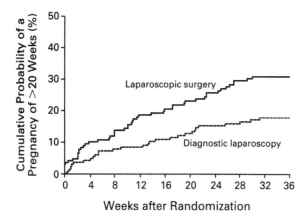

Fig. 19-15. Cumulative probability of a pregnancy carried beyond 20 weeks in the 36 weeks after laparoscopy in women with endometriosis, according to study group. Six women assigned to the laparoscopic surgery group and one woman assigned to the diagnostic laparoscopy group became pregnant during the cycle in which laparoscopy was performed. In these women, the actual interval between laparoscopy and the date of last menstrual period ranged from 0 to 14 days. (From Marcoux S, Maheux R, Berube S, et al: Laparoscopic surgery in infertile women with minimal or mild endometriosis. *N Engl J Med* 1997; 337:221.)

Older studies analyzing fertility in women treated laparoscopically for endometriosis-associated infertility were hampered by the use of crude pregnancy rates rather than fecundability, variable classification systems, lack of randomized studies, and, most significantly, lack of proper controls. A recent study by the Canadian Collaborative Group on Endometriosis, however, seems to have settled the issue. Marcoux et al (1997) analyzed the pregnancy outcomes in 341 patients with endometriosis randomized to undergo laparoscopic surgery to resect or ablate lesions and adhesions or diagnostic laparoscopy for stage I or stage II endometriosis (Fig. 19-15). The pregnancy rate was significantly higher in the surgical group (31%) than in the nontreated group (18%) at the 36-week follow-up point (see Fig. 19-11); this improvement in fecundity suggests that infertile patients with endometriosis undergoing laparoscopy should undergo surgical correction of their disease. Thus, an initial operative approach seems prudent in these patients. If conception does not occur in a reasonable amount of time, perhaps 6 to 12 months, completion of the infertility work-up followed by one of the empiric therapies appears warranted. In older women of reproductive age, it is reasonable to begin infertility investigation and treatment more rapidly.

An alternative to surgery is medical management of endometriosis-associated infertility. However, there are no controlled clinical studies demonstrating that the medical treatment of mild or moderate endometriosis improves fertility. According to the few randomized prospective studies that have been completed, hormonal treatment using danazol, medroxyprogesterone acetate, or GnRH agonists for women with minimal or mild endometriosis does not improve fecundability in comparison with women with en-

dometriosis who were not treated (Dodson et al, 1993; Hull, 1987; Seibel et al, 1982). Adamson et al (1993) have shown that expectant management and surgery result in higher pregnancy rates than ovarian suppression in patients with low-stage endometriosis (Adamson et al, 1993). In addition, a meta-analysis confirmed the finding that medical treatment does not improve pregnancy outcomes (Adamson and Pasta, 1994).

A better alternative to medical treatment in women with stage I or stage II endometriosis is ovulation induction, coupled with intrauterine inseminations (IUI). This approach does not directly treat endometriosis, but it may overcome the minor abnormalities associated with follicular development or ovulation in these women. It may allow a concentrated fraction of motile sperm to have better access to the upper female reproductive tract. One randomized, controlled study noted improved pregnancy rates in patients with endometriosis who were treated with clomiphene citrate and IUI (Deaton et al, 1990).

Recently, several investigators have advocated combining superovulation and human menopausal gonadotropin (hMG) or FSH with IUI in the treatment of minimal or mild endometriosis. This achieves cycle fecundity rates of 0.12 to 0.40 (Chaffkin et al, 1991; Dodson et al, 1987; Hurst et al, 1993; Hurst and Wallach, 1990). The benefit of superovulation in this setting has been confirmed by Fedele et al (1992), who conducted a randomized, prospective trial in which patients with stage I or stage II endometriosis were randomized to receive superovulation with hMG or expectant management for three cycles. Treated patients had significantly higher monthly fecundability (0.15) than controls (0.05). In a randomized, prospective trial, Tummon et al (1997) compared superovulation with FSH and IUI and no treatment for patients with low-stage endometriosis. Patients were either treated or observed for one to four cycles. Pregnancy occurred in 11% of treated cycles versus 2% of control cycles, and the cumulative pregnancy rate was 30% for patients who underwent FSH-IUI and 10% for the patients who were merely observed (Fig. 19-16). Finally, Kemmann et al (1993) found higher fecundity rates in women with stage I or stage II endometriosis who underwent ovulation induction after laparoscopic surgery. Treatment with hMG yielded a fecundity rate of 0.114 compared with 0.066 in clomiphene cycles and 0.028 in untreated cycles. Their highest pregnancy rates occurred among patients treated by IVF. One group of investigators did not find a significantly improved pregnancy rate in patients with minimal endometriosis who were treated with one of several ovulation-induction agents in comparison with untreated controls (Serta et al, 1992).

For patients with minimal or mild endometriosis who do not conceive with combined gonadotropins and IUI therapy, the assisted reproductive technologies of IVF or gamete intrafallopian transfer are the next step. Pregnancy rates for patients with endometriosis who undergo IVF are similar to those with other infertility diagnoses. In fact, the French national IVF registry (FIVNAT, 1993) and the U.S. IVF registry (Medical Research International and Society for Assisted Reproductive Technology, 1991) have reported identical success rates for patients with endometriosis and tubal factor infertility. Most IVF centers use one of the GnRH agonists in either a long protocol in which the GnRH-agonist is used for 10 to 14 days before gonadotropin stimulation or a short protocol using the GnRH agonist for 1 to 3 days before stimulation. Recently, several investigators have proposed that longer treatment with a GnRH-agonist for patients with endometriosis before they undergo IVF may improve pregnancy rates by improving oocyte quality or by enhancing endometrial receptivity. Dicker et al (1992) reported a significantly higher pregnancy rate in women treated with a GnRH agonist for 6 months than in patients not followed up with a GnRH agonist. Nakemura et al (1992) reported a 67% pregnancy rate in patients treated at least 60 days versus 27% in patients treated with a standard GnRH agonist protocol. Slightly higher pregnancy rates were also reported by others (Chedid et al, 1995; Marcus and Edwards, 1994) using an ultra-long GnRH agonist protocol. The results of these small studies suggest a possible benefit with the use of longer courses of GnRH agonist downregulation before IVF. However, a large-scale, prospective, randomized trial is needed to settle the issue.

As a result of the often severe anatomic distortions seen with advanced endometriosis, the primary therapy for patients with stage III (moderate) or stage IV (severe) disease should be surgery. As equipment and surgical techniques become more sophisticated and gynecologists gain increased laparoscopic skills, an initial operative laparoscopic approach is usually warranted. The same principles of good surgical technique apply whether the resection of endometriosis is by laparoscopy or laparotomy. After surgery, concerted attempts at conception should be made. In general, postoperative medical therapy for couples attempting pregnancy should be discouraged because most conceptions that take place after surgical correction for endometriosis occur in the first postoperative year (Barbieri et al, 1982). If conception fails to occur in 6 to 12 months, empiric therapy using superovulation may be considered.

Approximately 40% of women with advanced endometriosis and infertility are unable to conceive, even after surgical and medical therapy. For these women, IVF with embryo transfer is a viable treatment option. In fact, the greater efficacy of IVF for patients with endometriosis is in those who also have bilateral tubal disease (Soliman et al, 1993). In the early days of IVF, several centers reported lower pregnancy rates among patients with severe endometriosis (Oehninger et al, 1988; Matson and Yovitch, 1986). These studies, however, did not include GnRH agonists, and laparoscopy rather than ultrasonography was used for egg retrieval. The latter point is crucial because in patients with advanced endometriosis, laparoscopic access to the ovaries may be difficult, and the number and quality of oocytes obtained may be reduced. More recent studies using

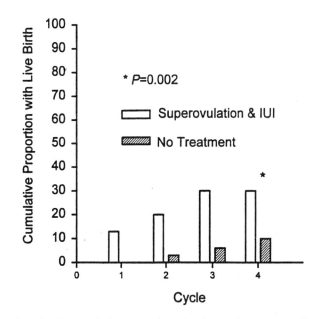

Fig. 19-16. Cumulative proportion of patients whose pregnancies culminated in live birth. (From Tummon IS, Asher LJ, Martin JSB, et al: Randomized controlled trial of superovulation and insemination for infertility associated with minimal or mild endometriosis. *Fertil Steril* 1997; 68:10.)

GnRH agonists and ultrasound-guided retrieval revealed similar pregnancy rates in patients with stages I and II and stages III and IV disease (Geber et al, 1995; Olivennes et al, 1995; Pal et al, 1998). The rate of live births among women with endometriosis is in the range of 20% per oocyte retrieval. One exception to this observation is that women with advanced endometriosis who have undergone multiple ovarian cystectomies for endometriomas often respond poorly to ovarian hyperstimulation and produce less than the expected number of mature ovarian follicles. In turn, the poor response to ovulation induction decreases the clinical pregnancy rate for this group of women. The mechanism or mechanisms responsible for this are unclear. However, multiple ovarian cystectomies for endometriomas may be associated with the resection of a significant proportion of the total oocyte population (Hornstein et al, 1989).

Pelvic Mass

For most women with a persistent adnexal mass, surgical removal is the treatment of choice. Surgical removal of adnexal masses is simultaneously diagnostic and therapeutic. Surgical removal of an endometrioma should be followed by the development of a long-term treatment plan because there is usually a recurrence within several years. Sequential resection of multiple recurrent endometriomas may result in premature menopause. For young patients, long-term hormonal therapy may be necessary to prevent the recurrence of endometriomas and repeat surgery. In many instances, this can be accomplished after the resection of an endometrioma by instituting a long-term acyclic course of combined estrogen-progestogen oral contraceptives.

REFERENCES

Adamson GD, Heinrichs WL, Henzl MR, et al: Therapeutic efficacy and bone mineral density response during and following a three month retreatment of endometriosis with nafarelin (Synarel). *Am J Obstet Gynecol* 1997; 177: 1413-1418.

Adamson GD, Hurd SJ, Pasta DJ, et al: Laparoscopic endometriosis treatment: Is it better? *Fertil Steril* 1993; 59:35-44.

Adamson GD, Pasta DJ: Surgical treatment of endometriosis-associated infertility: Meta-analysis compared with survival analysis. *Am J Obstet Gynecol* 1994; 171:1488-1505.

American Fertility Society: Management of endometriosis in the presence of pelvic pain. *Fertil Steril* 1993; 60:952-955.

American Fertility Society: Revised American Fertility Society classification of endometriosis. *Fertil Steril* 1985; 43:351-352.

American Society for Reproductive Medicine: Revised American Society for Reproductive Medicine classification of endometriosis: 1996. *Fertil Steril* 1997; 67:817-821.

Barbieri RL: CA-125 in patients with endometriosis. *Fertil Steril* 1986; 45:767-769.

Barbieri RL: Hormone treatment of endometriosis: The estrogen threshold hypothesis. *Am J Obstet Gynecol* 1992; 166:740-745.

Barbieri RL, Callery M, Perez SE: Directionality of menstrual flow: Cervical os diameter as a determinant of retrograde menstruation. *Fertil Steril* 1992; 57:727-730.

Barbieri RL, Canick, Makris A, et al: Danazol inhibits steroidogenesis. *Fertil Steril* 1977a; 28:809-813.

Barbieri RL, Canick JA, Ryan KJ: Danazol inhibits steroidogenesis in the rat testis in vitro. *Endocrinology* 1977b; 101:1676-1682

Barbieri RL, Evans S, Kismer RW: Danazol in the treatment of endometriosis: Analysis of 100 cases with a 4-year follow-up. *Fertil Steril* 1982; 37:737-746.

Barbieri RL, Lee H, Ryan KJ: Danazol-binding to rat androgen, glucocorticoid progesterone, and estrogen receptors: Correlation with biological activity. *Fertil Steril* 1979; 31:182-186.

Barbieri RL, Niloff JM, Bast RC Jr, et al: Elevated serum concentrations of CA-125 in patients with advanced endometriosis. *Fertil Steril* 1986; 45:630-634.

Barbieri RL, Osathanondh R, Canick JA, et al: Danazol inhibits human adrenal 21- and 11-hydroxylation. *Steroids* 1980; 35:251-263.

Barbieri RL, Osathanondh R, Ryan KJ: Danazol inhibition of steroidogenesis in the human corpus luteum. *Obstet Gynecol* 1981; 57:722-724.

Barbieri RL, Ryan KJ: Danazol: Endocrine pharmacology and therapeutic applications. *Am J Obstet Gynecol* 1981; 141:453-463.

Bast RC Jr, Feeney M, Lazarus H, et al; Reactivity of a monoclonal antibody with human ovarian carcinoma. *J Clin Invest* 1981; 68: 1331-1337.

Bast RC Jr, Klug TL, St. John E, et al: A radioimmunoassay using a monoclonal antibody to monitor the course of epithelial ovarian cancer. *N Engl J Med* 1983; 309:883-887.

Biberoglu KO, Behrman SJ: Dosage aspects of danazol therapy in endometriosis: Short-term and long-tem effectiveness. *Am J Obstet Gynecol* 1981; 139:645-654.

Brosens IA: New principles in the management of endometriosis. *Acta Obstet Gynecol Scand* 1994; 159(suppl):18-21.

Cattell RB, Swinton NW: Endometriosis with particular reference to conservative treatment. *N Engl J Med* 1936; 241:341.

Cedars M, Lu JK, Meldrum DR, et al: Treatment of endometriosis with a long-acting gonadotropin releasing hormone agonist plus medroxyprogesterone acetate. *Obstet Gynecol* 1990; 75:641-645.

Chaffkin LM, Nulsen JC, Luciano AA, et al: A comparative analysis of the cycle fecundity rates associated with combined human menopausal gonadotropin (hMG) and intrauterine insemination (IUI) versus either hMG or ICI alone. *Fertil Steril* 1991; 55:252-257.

Chalas E, Chumas J, Barbieri R, et al: Nucleolar organizer regions in endometriosis, atypical endometriosis, and clear cell and endometrioid carcinomas. *Gynecol Oncol* 1991; 40:260-263.

Chedid S, Comus M, Suritz J, et al: Comparison among different ovulation stimulation regimens for assisted procreation procedures in patients with endometriosis. *Hum Reprod* 1995; 10:2406-2411.

Cramer DW: Epidemiology of endometriosis. In Wilson EA, editor: *Endometriosis,* New York, 1987, Alan R. Liss.

Cramer DW, Wilson E, Stillman RJ, et al: The relation of endometriosis to menstrual characteristics, smoking, and exercise. *JAMA* 1986; 225:1904-1908.

Cramer DW, Hornstein MD, Ng WG, et al: Endometriosis associated with the N314D mutation of galactose-1-phosphate uridyl transferase (GALT). *Mol Hum Reprod* 1996; 2:149-152.

Cullen TS: Adenomyoma of the round ligament. *Bull Johns Hopkins* 1896; 7:112.

Czernobilsky B, Morris WJ: A histologic study of ovarian endometriosis with emphasis on hyperplastic and atypical changes. *Obstet Gynecol* 1979; 53:318-323.

Daniell JF, Christianson G: Combined laparoscopic surgery and danazol therapy for pelvic endometriosis. *Fertil Steril* 1981; 35:521-525.

Deaton JL, Gibson M, Blackmer KM, et al: A randomized, controlled trial of clomiphene citrate and intrauterine insemination in couples with unexplained infertility or surgically corrected endometriosis. *Fertil Steril I* 1990; 54:1083-1088.

Desaulles PA, Krahenbuhl C: Comparison of the antifertility and sex hormone activities of sex hormones and derivatives. *Acta Endocrinol* 1964; 47:444-456.

Dicker D, Goldman JA, Levy T et al: The impact of long-term gonadotropin-releasing hormone analogue treatment on preclinical abortions in patients with severe endometriosis undergoing in vitro fertilization-embryo transfer. *Fertil Steril* 1992; 57:597-600.

Dickey RP, Taylor SN, Curole DN: Serum estradiol and danazol, I: Endometriosis responses, side effects, administration interval, concurrent spironolactone, and dexamethasone. *Fertil Steril* 1984; 42:709-716.

DiZerega CS, Barber DL, Hodgen GD: Endometriosis: Role of ovarian steroids in initiation, maintenance, and suppression. *Fertil Steril* 1980; 33:649-653.

Dmowski WP, Cohen MR: Antigonadotropin (danazol) in the treatment of endometriosis. *Am J Obstet Gynecol* 1978; 130:41-48.

Dodson WC, Whitesides DB, Hughes CL Jr, et al: Superovulation with intrauterine insemination in the treatment of infertility: A possible alternative to gamete intrafallopian transfer and in vitro fertilization. *Fertil Steril* 1987; 48:441-445.

Donnez J, Nisolle-Pochet M, Clerckx-Braun F, et al: Administration of nasal buserelin as compared with subcutaneous buserelin implant forendometriosis. *Fertil Steril* 1989; 52:27-30.

Dotson RL, Petersen M, Doucette RC: Medical therapy for recurring catamenial pneumothorax following pleurodesis. *Obstet Gynecol* 1993; 82:656-658.

Duck SC, Katayama KP: Danazol may cause pseudohemaphroditism. *Fertil Steril* 1981; 35:230.

Fedele L, Bianchi S, Marchini M, et al: Superovulation with human menopausal gonadotropins in the treatment of infertility associated with minimal or mild endometriosis: A controlled randomized study. *Fertil Steril* 1992a; 58:28-31.

Fedele L, Parazzini F, Bianchi S, et al: Stage and localization of pelvic endometriosis and pain. *Fertil Steril* 1990; 53:155-158.

Fedele L, Parazzini F, Radici E, et al: Buserelin acetate versus expectant management in the treatment of infertility associated with minimal or mild endometriosis: A randomized clinical trial. *Am J Obstet Gynecol* 1992b; 166:1345-1350.

Fedele L, Vercellini P, Arcaini L, et al: CA-125 in serum, peritoneal fluid, active lesions, and endometrium of patients with endometriosis. *Am J Obstet Gynecol* 1988; 158:166-170.

FIVNAT (French In Vitro National): French national IVF registry: Analysis of 1986 to 1990 data. *Fertil Steril* 1993; 59:587-595.

Fogelman I: Gonadotropin-releasing hormone agonists and the skeleton. *Fertil Steril* 1992; 57:715-724.

Fukaya T, Hoshiai H, Yajima A: Is pelvic endometriosis always associated with chronic pain: A retrospective study of 618 cases diagnosed by laparoscopy. *Am J Obstet Gynecol* 1993; 169:719-722.

Geber S, Paraschos T, Atkinson G, et al: Results of IVF in patients with endometriosis: The severity of the disease does not affect outcome, or the incidence of miscarriage. *Hum Reprod* 1995; 10:1507-1511.

Halme J, Backer S, Hammond MG, et al: Increased activation of pelvic macrophages in infertile women with mild endometriosis. *Am J Obstet Gynecol* 1983; 145:333-337.

Haney AF: Pelvic endometriosis etiology and pathology. *Semin Reprod Endocrinol* 1988; 6:287.

Henzl MR: Gonadotropin-releasing hormone analogs: Update on new findings. *Am J Obstet Gynecol* 1992; 166:757-761.

Henzl MR, Corson SL, Moghissi K, et al: Administration of nasal nafarelin as compared with oral danazol for endometriosis: A multi-center double-blind comparative clinical trial. *N Engl J Med* 1988; 318:485-489.

Henzl MR, Kwei L: Efficacy and safety of nafarelin in the treatment of endometriosis. *Am J Obstet Gynecol* 1990; 162:570-574.

Hill JA, Faris HM, Schiff I, et al: Characterization of leukocyte subpopulations in the peritoneal fluid of women with endometriosis. *Fertil Steril* 1988; 50:216-222.

Hornstein MD: Endometriosis and spontaneous abortion. In Friedman AJ, editor: *Recurrent pregnancy loss, infertility, and reproductive medicine clinics of North America,* Philadelphia, 1991, WB Saunders.

Hornstein MD, Barbieri RL, McShane PM: The effects of previous ovarian surgery on the follicular response to ovulation induction in an in vitro fertilization program. *J Reprod Med* 1989; 34:277-281.

Hornstein MD, Gleason RE, Oray J, et al: The reproducibility of the revised American Fertility Society Classification of Endometriosis. *Fertil Steril* 1993; 59:1015-1021.

Hornstein MD, Hemmings R, Yuzpe AA, et al: Use of nafarelin versus placebo after reductive laparoscopic surgery for endometriosis. *Fertil Steril* 1997; 68:860-864

Hornstein MD, Surrey ES, Weisberg GW, et al: Leuprolide acetate depot and hormonal add-back in endometriosis: A 12-month study. *Obstet Gynecol* 1998; 91:16-24.

Hornstein MD, Thomas PP, Gleason RE, et al: Menstrual cyclicity of CA-125 in patients with endometriosis. *Fertil Steril* 1992; 58:279-283.

Hornstein MD, Yuzpe AA, Burry KA, et al: Prospective randomized double-blind trial of 3 versus 6 months of nafarelin therapy for endometriosis associated pelvic pain. *Fertil Steril* 1995; 63:955-962.

Hornstein MD, Yuzpe AA, Burry K, et al: Retreatment with nafarelin for recurrent endometriosis symptoms: Efficacy, safety and bone mineral density. *Fertil Steril* 1997; 67:1013-1018.

Hoshiai H, et al: Laparoscopic evaluation of the onset and progression of endometriosis. *Am J Obstet Gynecol* 1993; 169:714-719.

Howell R, et al: A randomized controlled trial of goserelin (Zoladex) with add-back hormone replacement therapy (HRT) for endometriosis effect on bone density. Presented at the 49th Annual American Fertility Society Meeting, Montreal, October 11-14, 1993.

Hull ME, Moghissi KS, Magyar DF, et al: Comparison of different treatment modalities of endometriosis in infertile women. *Fertil Steril* 1987; 47:40-44.

Hull MGR: Infertility treatment: relative effectiveness of conventional and assisted conception methods (Review). *Hum Reprod* 1992; 7:785-796.

Hurst BF, Bollmann A, Ciangiola C: Treatment of infertility patients with hMG-IUI in a private practice. *Int J Fertil* 1993; 38:28.

Hurst BF, Wallach EE: Superovulation with intrauterine insemination: Empiric therapy for infertile couples. *Postgrad Obstet Gynecol* 1990; 22:1.

Jansen RPS: Minimal endometriosis and reduced fecundability: Prospective evidence from an artificial insemination by donor program. *Fertil Steril* 1986; 46:141-143.

Jansen RPS, Russell P: Nonpigmented endometriosis: Clinical, laparoscopic, and pathologic definition. *Am J Obstet Gynecol* 1986; 155:1154-1159.

Jiang X, Hitchcock A, Bryan EJ, et al: Microsatellite analysis of endometriosis reveals loss of heterozygosity of candidate ovarian tumor suppressor gene loci. *Cancer Res* 1996; 56:3534-3539.

Jimbo J, Hitami Y, Yoshikawa H, et al: Evidence for monoclonal expansion of epithelial cells in ovarian endometrial cysts. *Am J Pathol* 1997; 150:1173-1178.

Kemmann E, Chazi D, Corsan G, et al: Does ovulation stimulation improve fertility in women with minimal/mild endometriosis after laser laparoscopy? *Int J Fertil Menopausal Stud* 1993; 38:16.

Kennedy SH, Soper MD, Mojiminiya OA, et al: Immunoscintigraphy of ovarian endometriosis: A preliminary study. *Br J Obstet Gynaecol* 1988; 95:693-697.

Kiilhoma P, Tuimala R, Kiuinen S, et al: Comparison of the gonadotropin-releasing hormone agonist goserelin acetate alone versus goserelin combined with estrogen-progesterone add-back therapy in the treatment of endometriosis. *Fertil Steril* 1995; 64:903-908.

Kistner RW: The use of newer progestins in the treatment of endometriosis. *Am J Obstet Gynecol* 1958; 75:264.

Kistner RW: The use of steroidal substances in endometriosis. *Clin Pharmacol Ther* 1960; 1:525.

Knobil E: The neuroendocrine control of the menstrual cycle. *Recent Prog Horm Res* 1980; 36:53-88.

LaGranade A, Silverberg G: Ovarian tumors associated with atypical endometriosis. *Hum Pathol* 1988; 19:1080-1084.

Luciano AA, Turksay RN, Carico J: Evaluation of oral medroxy-progesterone acetate in the treatment of endometriosis. *Obstet Gynecol* 1988; 72:323-327.

Mais V, Guerriero S, Ajossa S, et al: The efficiency of transvaginal ultrasonography in the diagnosis of endometrioma. *Fertil Steril* 1993; 60:776-780.

Malkasian GD Jr, Podratz KC, Stanhope CR, et al: CA-125 in gynecologic practice. *Am J Obstet Gynecol* 1986; 155:515-518.

Marcoux S, Maheux R, Berube S, et al: Laparoscopic surgery in infertile women with minimal or mild endometriosis: Canadian Collaborative Group on Endometriosis. *N Engl J Med* 1997; 337:217-222.

Marcus SF, Edward GR: High rates of pregnancy after long-term downregulation of women with severe endometriosis. *Am J Obstet Gynecol* 1994; 171:812-817.

Markham SM: Extrapelvic endometriosis. In Thomas EJ, Rock JA, editors: *Modern approaches to endometriosis,* Boston, 1991, Kluwer Academic.

Martin DC, Hubert GD, Vander Zwaag R, et al: Laparoscopic appearances of peritoneal endometriosis. *Fertil Steril* 1989; 51:63-67.

Matson PL, Yovick JL: The treatment of infertility associated with endometriosis by in vitro fertilization. *Fertil Steril* 1986; 46:432-434.

Matta WH, Shaw RW: A comparative study between buserelin and danazol in the treatment of endometriosis. *Br J Clin Pract* 1986; 41(suppl 48):69.

Meldrum DR, Chang RJ, Lu J, et al: "Medical oophorectomy" using a long-acting GnRH agonist: A possible new approach to the treatment of endometriosis. *J Clin Endocrinol Metab* 1982; 54:1081-1083.

Montgomery JC, Studd JWW: Oestradiol and testosterone implants after hysterectomy for endometriosis. *Contrib Gynecol Obstet* 1987; 16:241-246.

The Nafarelin European Endometriosis Trial Group (NEET): Nafarelin for endometriosis: A large-scale, danazol-controlled trial of efficacy and safety, with 1-year follow-up. *Fertil Steril* 1992; 57:514.

Nakamura K, Oosawa M, Kandou I, et al: Menotropin stimulation after prolonged gonadotropin releasing hormone agonist pretreatment for in vitro fertilization in patients with endometriosis. *J Assisted Reprod Genet* 1992; 9:113-117.

Namnoum AB, et al: Incidence of symptom recurrence following hysterectomy for endometriosis. Presented at the 49th Annual American Fertility Society Meeting, Montreal, October 11-14, 1993.

Nilsson B, Sodergard R, Damber MG, et al: Danazol and gestagen displacement of testosterone and influence of sex hormone-binding capacity. *Fertil Steril* 1982; 38:48-53.

Nishimura K, Togashi K, Itoh K, et al: Endometrial cysts of the ovary: MR imaging. *Radiology* 1987; 162:315-318.

Nisolle M, Donnez J: Peritoneal endometriosis, ovarian endometriosis, and adenomyotic nodules of the rectovaginal septum are the different entities. *Fertil Steril* 1997; 68:585-596.

Noble AD, Letchworth AT: Medical treatment of endometriosis: A comparative trial. *Postgrad Med J* 1979; 55(suppl 5):37-39.

Oehninger S, Acosta AA, Kreiner D, et al: In vitro fertilization and embryo transfer (IVF/ET): An established and successful therapy for endometriosis. *J In Vitro Fertil Embryo Transf* 1988; 5:249-255.

Olive DC, Haney AF: Endometriosis associated infertility: A critical review of therapeutic approaches. *Obstet Gynecol* 1986; 41:538-555.

Olivennes F, Feldberg D, Liu HC, et al: Endometriosis: A stage by stage analysis—The role of in vitro fertilization. *Fertil Steril* 1995; 64:392-398.

Orwoll ES, Yuzpe AA, Burry KA, et al: Nafarelin therapy in endometriosis: Long term effects on bone mineral density. *Am J Obstet Gynecol* 1994; 171:1221-1225.

Pal L, Shifren JL, Isaacson KB, et al: Impact of varying stages of endometriosis on the outcome of in vitro fertilization-embryo transfer. *J Assist Reprod Genet* 1998; 15:27-31.

Pittaway DE: Endometriosis and spontaneous abortion. *Semin Reprod Endocrinol* 1988; 6:257.

Pittaway DE, Fayez JA: The use of CA-125 in the diagnosis and management of endometriosis. *Fertil Steril* 1986; 46:790-795.

Propst AM, Storti KA, Barbieri RL: Lateral cervical displacement: An association with endometriosis. *Fertil Steril* 1998; 70:568-570.

Rock JA, Truglia JA, Caplan RJ, et al: Zoladex (goserelin acetate implant) in the treatment of endometriosis: A randomized comparison with danazol. *Obstet Gynecol* 1993; 82:198-205.

Rokitansky C: Uber Uterusdrusen-Neubilding im Uterus und Ovarialsarcomen. *ZKK Gesellch d Arzte zu Wein* 1860; 37:577.

Sampson JA: Endometrial carcinoma of the ovary arising in endometrial tissue in that organ. *Arch Surg* 1925; 10:1.

Sampson JA: Perforating hemorrhagic (chocolate) cysts of the ovary. *Arch Surg* 1921; 3:245.

Schwartz D, Mayaux MJ: Female fecundity as a function of age: Results of artificial insemination in 2193 nulliparous women with ezpospermic husbands. *N Engl J Med* 1982; 306:404-406.

Scully RE, Richardson GS, Barlow JF: The development of malignancy in endometriosis. *Clin Obstet Gynecol* 1966; 9:384-411.

Seibel MM, Berger MJ, Weinstein FG, et al: The effectiveness of danazol on subsequent fertility in minimal endometriosis. *Fertil Steril* 1982; 38:534-537.

Semm K, Mettler L: Technical progress in pelvic surgery via operative laparoscopy. *Am J Obstet Gynecol* 1980; 138:121-127.

Serta RT, Ruto S, Seibel MM: Minimal endometriosis and intrauterine insemination: Does controlled ovarian hyperstimulation improve pregnancy rates? *Obstet Gynecol* 1992; 80:37-40.

Shaw RW: Zoladex Endometriosis Study Team: An open randomized comparative study of the effect of goserelin depot and danazol in the treatment of endometriosis. *Fertil Steril* 1992; 58:265-272.

Soliman S, Daya S, Collins J, et al: A randomized trial of in vitro fenilization versus conventional treatment for infertility. *Fertil Steril* 1993; 59:1239-1244.

Steingold KA, Cedars M, Lu JK, et al: Treatment of endometriosis with a long-acting gonadotropin-releasing hormone agonist. *Obstet Gynecol* 1987; 69:403-411.

Steingold KA, Lu JK, Judd HL, et al: Danazol inhibits steroidogenesis by the human ovary in vivo. *Fertil Steril* 1986; 45:649-654.

Sugimura K, Okijuka H, Imaoka I, et al: Pelvic endometriosis: Detection and diagnosis with chemical shift MR imaging. *Radiology* 1993; 188:435-438.

Surrey ES, Gambone JC, Lu JK, et al: The effects of combining norethindrone with a gonadotropin-releasing hormone agonist in the treatment of symptomatic endometriosis. *Fertil Steril* 1990; 53:620-626.

Surrey ES, Judd HL: Reduction of vasomotor symptoms and bone mineral density loss with combined norethindrone and long-acting gonadotropin-releasing hormone agonist therapy of symptomatic endometriosis a prospective randomized trial. *J Clin Endocrinol Metab* 1992; 75:558-563.

Surrey ES, Voigt B, Fournet N, et al: Prolonged gonadotropin releasing hormone agonist treatment of symptomatic endometriosis: The role of cyclic sodium etidronate and low-dose norethindrone "addback" therapy. *Fertil Steril* 1995; 63:347-355.

Thomas EJ, Cooke ID: Impact of gestrinone on the course of asymptomatic endometriosis. *BMJ* 1987; 294:272-274.

Toma SK, Stovall DW, Hammond MG: The effect of laparoscopic ablation or pregnancy rates in patients with stage I or II endometriosis undergoing donor insemination. *Obstet Gynecol* 1992; 80:253-256.

Tummon IS, Asher LJ, Martin JSB, et al: Randomized controlled trial of superovulation and insemination for infertility associated with minimal or mild endometriosis. *Fertil Steril* 1997; 68:8-12.

Vercellini P, Trespidi L, Colombo A, et al: A gonadotropin-releasing hormone agonist versus a low-dose oral contraceptive for pelvic pain associated with endometriosis. *Fertil Steril* 1993; 60:75-79.

Waller KG, Shaw RW: Gonadotropin-releasing hormone analogs for the treatment of endometriosis: Long-term follow-up. *Fertil Steril* 1993; 59:511-515.

Wheeler JM, Knittle JD, Miller JD: Depot leuprolide versus danazol in treatment of women with symptomatic endometriosis, I: Efficacy results. *Am J Obstet Gynecol* 1992; 167:1367-1371.

20

Psychological Aspects of Women's Reproductive Health

SUSAN CARUSO KLOCK

KEY ISSUES

1. Women are twice as likely as men to suffer from depression.
2. Recent research highlights new and effective treatments for premenstrual dysphoric disorder.
3. Psychological and social factors are paramount in the management of postpartum depression.
4. The relationship between stress and infertility remains unclear. Recent advances in reproductive technology have resulted in an increased need for psychological counseling to aid patients in decision making.
5. Menopause does not cause an increase in depression.

A woman's primary health care provider, whether obstetrician, gynecologist, internist, or family practitioner, is often the first person she consults about medical and psychological problems. Therefore, the primary care provider is in a unique role to identify, assess, treat, or refer, if appropriate, psychological disorders among women. In addition, as Mathis (1967) noted, reproduction-related events are emotionally laden topics:

Sex, reproduction, and the reproductive system are almost synonymous with emotional reactions in our culture. . . . The woman who seeks medical attention for her reproductive system deserves a physician who understands the total significance of femininity as well as they know the anatomy and physiology of the female. The physician who assumes this responsibility automatically becomes involved in emotional processes unequaled in any other branch of medicine.

Unfortunately, many physicians feel ill-prepared to address psychological issues with their patients. In addition, a physician in a busy practice often has little time to spend with his or her patients or to keep up to date on the continually evolving diagnostic and treatment issues in women's health psychology.

The woman's primary care provider should be well versed in psychological issues related to reproduction. Women are becoming more active and more educated consumers of health care, and they expect their health-care providers to attend to the physical and psychological aspects of their health (Boston Women's Health Book Collective, 1992). The woman's role as a patient has shifted from one of a passive recipient of information to that of an active consumer. This has been brought about by social changes that include questioning of the traditional patriarchal medical model, increased awareness of women's health issues, increased dissemination of health information to the public, and increased focus on holistic medicine. All these changes have brought about an increase in specialty clinics for disorders such as premenstrual syndrome and menopausal problems, increased use of nontraditional forms of healing, and multidisciplinary case management.

There has been a long history of interaction between psychiatry and obstetrics and gynecology, though psychiatric consultation is often underused (Cohen, 1988; Stewart and Stotland, 1993). The interaction began as advances in the management of obstetrics were developed. In the late nineteenth century, the advent of forceps for delivery, medication for sepsis, and anesthesia for pain control marked the medicalization of reproduction. During this time, psychiatrists Breuer and Freud considered the role of the female reproductive cycle and sexual functioning as critical parts of theories of personality and development (Cohen, 1988). Case reports by obstetricians and surgeons claimed cures of hysteria and other maladies through hysterectomy. During the 1950s and 1960s, obstetricians began using psychological methods to increase women's preparation and control over childbirth by promoting relaxation and breathing techniques and by providing psychosocial support during labor and delivery. During this time as well psychiatrists and psychologists began investigating disorders such as postpartum depression and premenstrual syndrome. Today there is the subspecialty of women's health psychology, which focuses on psychological issues related to women's health from the prevention and treatment perspectives. The psychology of women includes postfeminist concepts emphasizing women's unique interpersonal social roles. Some women have broken away from traditional roles to enjoy increased career and family choices. This increased freedom and decision making has had positive and negative effects. Although women may enjoy increased autonomy, economic freedom, and self-efficacy, they still experience high rates of depression, spousal abuse, economic discrimination, and poverty. Cultural and racial differences still exert influence over women's opportunities for education, economic advancement, and access to health services. The health care provider must be aware of these differences and must be sensitive to the fact that one woman's experience is not prototypical of all women.

All health care providers should be aware that women, in general, are twice as likely as men to suffer from depression, with lifetime prevalence rates of 21% in women and 13% in men (Kessler et al, 1994). Women are at increased risk for depression because of economic, social, psychological, and biologic factors. Therefore, a biopsychosocial approach should guide clinical thinking about women and depression (McGrath et al, 1990). From a biologic perspective, the hypothalamic-pituitary-gonadal hormone axis and changes in this system that span a woman's reproductive life may provide the neuroendocrinologic backdrop for vulnerability to depression. From a psychological perspective, women have been shown to have personality and cognitive styles that may cause or perpetuate depression. Examples of these are avoidance, passive-dependent behavior patterns and pessimistic, negative-cognitive styles. Often they use emotion-based coping mechanisms that focus more on depressed feelings and not enough on action and on mastering problems. Social and cultural factors also play a role. Physical, sexual, and spousal abuse may be potent precipitants to depression. The responsibilities of marriage and child rearing, combined with the social and economic demands of the workplace, can lead to role strain and conflict that may contribute to depression. Cognizance of these factors can help the health practitioner to realize the multifactorial causes of depression and to be aware of the base rate of depression among women seen in clinical practice.

This chapter provides a specific review of the psychological literature concerning the four reproduction-related affective syndromes that occur during a woman's life. These four topics are premenstrual syndrome, postpartum depression, psychological sequelae of infertility, and menopause. The purpose of this chapter is to provide the physician with a general overview of the research and the clinical findings related to these topics.

PREMENSTRUAL DYSPHORIC DISORDER

Premenstrual syndrome (PMS) was described more than 50 years ago (Frank, 1931). Frank is credited with coining the phrase *premenstrual tension* as he reported "indescribable tension" and increased seizure activity in the late luteal phase among a group of women with seizure disorder. He reported that the tension increased during the late luteal phase and remitted with the onset of menses. Since the publication of Frank's article, there have been thousands of studies investigating various aspects of PMS.

The definition and diagnostic criteria of the disorder have evolved significantly in the past 20 years. The term is used to describe mild, negative changes that are primarily somatic in nature, such as bloating, breast tenderness, and headache that occur during the premenstruum. Premenstrual dysphoric disorder (PDD) is a psychiatric diagnosis used to indicate serious premenstrual distress with associated deterioration in functioning (American Psychiatric Association, 1994). The first point to be determined before making the diagnosis of PDD is differentiating between normal premenstrual somatic, psychological changes and problematic premenstrual symptoms (Brooks-Gunn, 1986). Blechman et al (1988) emphasized the importance of clearly defining terms for diagnostic accuracy and clarity. She defined *premenstrual changes* as any physical or behavioral experience that is discriminably different during the premenstruum than it is at other times in the menstrual cycle. Premenstrual changes can be positive or negative. It is estimated that 75% of women experience some type of premenstrual change (Steiner, 1997). *Premenstrual symptoms* are those changes that are perceived by the woman to be negative or severe or that limit functioning.

More than 100 symptoms have been identified as part of the PMS-PDD profile (Halbriech et al, 1982). Common symptoms include feelings of depression or irritability, decreased concentration, increased food and alcohol consumption, breast pain, edema, headaches, and fatigue. Although some researchers have argued that there are several subtypes of PMS, most patients have a unique combination of symptoms with varying degrees of intensity and duration (Halbriech and Endicott, 1982).

After symptoms have been identified, a diagnosis of PDD can be considered. Before a diagnosis of PDD can be made, the patient has to document daily symptoms for at least two menstrual cycles. Her primary symptom must be mood related, such as irritability, depression, or lability. She also must report 5 of the 11 symptoms characteristic of PDD. The symptoms should have occurred with most menstrual cycles during the past year and must be of sufficient severity to interfere with a woman's functioning in relationships, work, or other areas of her life. A diagnosis of PDD can be made only if four conditions are met: the symptoms are reliably related to the luteal phase of the menstrual cycle, they remit shortly after the onset of menses, they are separate from a preexisting psychiatric disorder, and they significantly impair functioning and involve at least a 30% increase in symptom severity from the follicular to the luteal phases. In 1994 the American Psychiatric Association included research diagnostic criteria for PDD in the appendix of its *Diagnostic and Statistical Manual*, 4th edition (see Box 20-1) (American Psychiatric Association, 1994).

It is estimated that 10% to 30% of women have PMS, though rates vary depending on the stringency of the diagnostic criteria and the accuracy of the assessment (Smith and Schiff, 1989). With its more severe symptom profile, PDD is estimated to affect only 3% to 8% of women in the general population and 24% of women in the psychiatric population (Eckerd et al, 1989; Rivera-Tovar and Frank, 1990; Steiner, 1997). In a recent multicenter study, the prevalence of PDD was estimated among a sample of 670 women seeking evaluation for PMS (Hurt et al, 1992). The typical patient in this study was 34 years old, white, employed, college educated, had two children, and had an 8-year history of premenstrual difficulties. Using three different scoring methods for daily symptoms, the rates of PDD varied from 14% to 38%. Of note, 27% of the sample had a coexisting psychiatric disorder and 50% had a history of other psychiatric disorders. Some investigators have noted the high prevalence of personality and other psychiatric disorders among this group of patients (Eckerd et al, 1989). Therefore, it is important to differentiate PDD from other psychiatric disorders.

Given the confusion surrounding the definitions of PMS and PDD, it is not surprising that the assessments of both have changed significantly in the past three decades. In the 1950s, Dalton (1964) simply asked her patients whether they had symptoms that varied with their cycles to confirm a diagnosis of PMS. Unfortunately, as recent research has demonstrated, retrospective reports of premenstrual symptoms are often inaccurate (Ruble, 1977). Other studies have compared the relationship between prospective and retrospective ratings of symptoms and found that they are not highly correlated (Valda, 1987). Therefore, it is recommended that the assessment of PDD include a complete gynecologic examination to rule out somatic cause(s) for the symptoms, daily rating of symptoms for three consecutive cycles, and a psychological evaluation (Keye, 1987).

An example of a daily symptom rating sheet is given in Fig. 20-1 (Reid, 1987). This form is easy for the patient to use and is readily interpreted by the clinician. Other measures, such as the Premenstrual Assessment Form and the Daily Rating Form, the Moos Menstrual Distress Questionnaire, and visual analogue scales are available (Caspar and Powell, 1986; Halbriech and Endicott, 1982; Moos, 1968). In addition, psychometric tests such as the Minnesota

---

BOX 20-1
DIAGNOSTIC CRITERIA FOR PREMENSTRUAL DYSPHORIC DISORDER

A. In most menstrual cycles during the past year, five (or more) of the following symptoms were present for most of the time during the last week of the luteal phase, began to remit within a few days after the onset of the follicular phase, and were absent in the week after menses, and at least one of the symptoms was either (1), (2), (3), or (4):

  (1) markedly depressed mood, feelings of hopelessness, or self-deprecating thoughts

  (2) marked anxiety, tension, feelings of being "keyed up" or "on edge"

  (3) marked affective lability (*e.g.,* feeling suddenly sad or tearful or increased sensitivity of rejection)

  (4) persistent and marked anger or irritability or increased interpersonal conflicts

  (5) decreased interest in usual activities (*e.g.,* work, school, friends, hobbies)

  (6) subjective sense of difficulty in concentrating

  (7) lethargy, easy fatigability, or marked lack of energy

  (8) marked change in appetite, overeating, or specific food cravings

  (9) hypersomnia or insomnia

  (10) subjective sense of being overwhelmed or out of control

  (11) other physical symptoms, such as breast tenderness or swelling, headaches, joint or muscle pain, a sensation of "bloating," weight gain

Note: In menstruating females, the luteal phase corresponds to the period between ovulation and the onset of menses, and the follicular phase begins with menses. In nonmenstruating females (*e.g.,* those who have undergone hysterectomy), the timing of luteal and follicular phases may require measurements of circulating reproductive hormones.

B. The disturbance markedly interferes with work or school or with the usual social activities and relationships with others (*e.g.,* avoidance of social activities, decreased productivity and efficiency at work or school).

C. The disturbance is not merely an exacerbation of the symptoms of another disorder, such as major depressive disorder, panic disorder, dysthymic disorder, or personality disorder (though it may be superimposed on any of these disorders).

D. Criteria A, B, and C must be confirmed by prospective daily ratings during at least two consecutive symptomatic cycles. (The diagnosis may be made provisionally before this confirmation.)

From American Psychiatric Association: *Diagnostic and statistical manual of mental diseases,* ed. 4, Washington, D.C., 1994, American Psychiatric Association Press.

PRISM
CALENDAR

Name: _____

Baseline weight on day 1: _____ lb or kg (circle one)

		1	2	3	4	5	6	7	8	9	10	11	12	13	14	15	16	17	18	19	20	21	22	23	24	25	26	27	28	29	30	31	32	33	34	35	36	37	38	39	40	41	42	43	44	45	46	47	48	49
BLEEDING Day of Menstrual Cycle Month: Date:																																																			
WEIGHT CHANGE																																																			
SYMPTOMS																																																			
Irritable																																																			
Fatigue																																																			
Inward anger																																																			
Labile mood (crying)																																																			
Depressed																																																			
Restless																																																			
Anxious																																																			
Insomnia																																																			
Lack of control																																																			
Edema or rings tight																																																			
Breast tenderness																																																			
Abdominal bloating																																																			
Bowels: const. (c) loose (l)																																																			
Appetite: up ↑ down ↓																																																			
Sex drive: up ↑ down ↓																																																			
Chills (C)/sweats (S)																																																			
Headaches																																																			
Crave: sweets/salt																																																			
Feel unattractive																																																			
Guilty																																																			
Unreasonable behavior																																																			
Low self-image																																																			
Nausea																																																			
Menstrual cramps																																																			
LIFESTYLE IMPACT																																																			
Aggressive towards others Physically																																																			
Verbally																																																			
Wish to be alone																																																			
Neglect housework																																																			
Time off work																																																			
Disorganized, distractable																																																			
Accident prone/clumsy																																																			
Uneasy about driving																																																			
Suicidal thoughts																																																			
Stayed at home																																																			
Increased use of alcohol																																																			
LIFE EVENTS																																																			
Negative experience																																																			
Positive experience																																																			
Social activities																																																			
Vigorous exercise																																																			
MEDICATIONS																																																			

INSTRUCTIONS FOR COMPLETING THIS CALENDAR

1. On the first day of menstruation prepare the calendar. Considering the first day of bleeding as day 1 of your menstrual cycle enter the corresponding calendar date for each day in the space provided below.
2. Each morning: Take weight after emptying bladder and before breakfast. Record WEIGHT CHANGE from baseline.
3. Each evening: At about the same time complete the column for that day as described below.

> BLEEDING: Indicate if you have had bleeding by shading the box above that days date ■; for spotting use an ⊠.
> SYMPTOMS: If you do not experience any symptoms, leave the corresponding square blank. If present indicate severity:

> MILD: 1 (noticeable but not troublesome)
> MODERATE: 2 (interferes with normal activity)
> SEVERE: 3 (temporarily incapacitating)

LIFESTYLE IMPACT: If the listed phrase applies to you that day enter an ⊠.
LIFE EVENTS: If you experienced one of these events that day enter an ⊠.

> Experiences: For positive (happy) or negative (sad or disappointing) experiences unrelated to your symptoms specify the nature of the events on the reverse side of this form.
> Social activities: Imply events such as special dinner, show, or party, etc. involving family or friends.
> Vigorous exercise: Implies participation in a sporting event or exercise programme lasting more than 30 minutes.

MEDICATION: In the bottom 3 rows list medications if any and indicate days when taken by entering an ⊠.

Fig. 20-1. The Prospective Record of the Impact and Severity of Menstrual Symptomatology (PRISM). (From Reid R: Premenstrual syndrome. *Endocrinol Metab* 1987; 5:1. Reprinted with permission.)

Multiphasic Personality Inventory can be used to determine the presence of a coexisting psychopathologic disorder (Choung, 1988). Despite the widespread recognition of PMS and PDD and their inclusion in the psychiatric nomenclature, the causes of and treatments for the disorders remain unclear. Several thorough reviews of the causes of PMS and PDD are available (Reid, 1981; Rubinow and Schmidt, 1992; Smith and Schiff, 1989; Steiner, 1997). Box 20-2 includes a summary of the most common theories of the cause of PDD.

The three most commonly proposed theories to explain PDD are the ovarian hormone hypothesis, the serotonin hypothesis, and the psychosocial hypothesis. The ovarian hormone hypothesis refers to the belief that PDD is caused by an imbalance in the ratio of estrogen to progesterone, with a relative deficiency in progesterone. This theory was first popularized by Dalton, who believed that PMS resulted from a deficiency of progesterone and who treated her patients with progesterone suppositories (Dalton, 1964). Recent studies investigating the levels of estrogen and progesterone among women with PMS have been inconclusive because of methodological difficulties, including inconsistent diagnostic criteria, lack of matched controls groups, lack of daily ratings of premenstrual symptoms, and inconsistent assessment of the duration and severity of symptoms (Maxson, 1987; Morse, 1991; Rubinow and Schmidt, 1992).

The serotonin theory (Steiner, 1997) hypothesizes that normal ovarian hormone function is the cyclical trigger for PDD-related biochemical events within the central nervous system and other target tissues. Changes in the hypothalamic-pituitary-gonadal axis in altering central neurotransmitters have been studied extensively. Evidence suggests that serotonin may be important in the development of PDD (Rapkin, 1992). Reduced platelet uptake of serotonin has been observed during the week before menstruation in women with premenstrual syndrome (Taylor, 1984), and women with this disorder also have lower levels of platelet serotonin content (Ashby et al, 1988). A blunted serotonin response to fenfluramine challenge among women with PDD has recently been reported (FitzGerald et al, 1997). Taken together, this evidence may provide a common pathway for understanding PDD as a variant of other affective disorders.

A final group of hypotheses regarding the cause of PMS concerns the psychosocial theories (Abraham and Mira, 1989). Early psychoanalytic theorists thought PMS was a conscious manifestation of a woman's unconscious conflicts about femininity and motherhood (Rodin, 1992). Psychoanalytic thinkers proposed that the premenstrual physical changes reminded the woman that she was not pregnant and, therefore, was not fulfilling her traditional feminine role. Although this hypothesis was compelling to many psychoanalytically oriented clinicians, it was impossible to substantiate by scientific methods.

Cognitive and social learning theory models have also been proposed (Blechman, 1988; Reading, 1992). These models suggested that the onset of menses was an aversive

---

BOX 20-2
THEORIES OF THE CAUSE OF PREMENSTRUAL SYNDROME

Excess estrogen
Progesterone deficiency
Fluid retention
Hyperprolactinemia
Vitamin B_6 deficiency
Hypoglycemia
Prostaglandin deficiency
Prostaglandin excess
Endogenous hormone allergy
Endogenous opiates
Psychogenic
Thyroid abnormality
Serotonin deficiency

From Smith S, Schiff I: The premenstrual syndrome: Diagnosis and management. *Fertil Steril* 1989; 52:527.

---

psychological event for the woman susceptible to PMS or PDD. The woman dreaded the onset of menses and began to search for signals that it was about to begin. She then developed an increased psychological arousal and vigilance for cues that menses was about to begin. Over time the cues that menses was about to begin were paired with the aversive event (menses), and normal premenstrual changes became premenstrual symptoms. In addition, it was theorized that these women might have had negative cognitive expectative sets that further reinforced the aversiveness of premenstrual symptoms. The reporting of symptoms was reinforced by reliably predicting the aversive event (menses). It was thought that women then developed maladaptive coping strategies, such as mood changes, social withdrawal, missed work, and increased eating to reduce the immediate stress. The immediate reduction of stress in the short term reinforced these behaviors, and over time they occurred regularly during the premenstruum.

From a sociocultural perspective, some writers have noted that PMS and PDD are manifestations of the negative attitudes and beliefs about menstruation that are pervasive in our culture (Williams, 1983). Others have speculated that PMS and PDD are cultural expressions of women's anger and discontent over traditional female roles in American society (Gottlieb, 1988) and over the constant role strain between being productive workers and fulfilling traditional roles in which child-rearing activities are central (Johnson, 1987). Feminist thinkers argue that PMS and PDD are disorders created by the medical establishment to medicalize a normal biologic process and to make up a psychiatric disorder that helps prevent women from engaging in activities with responsibility and power within society (Faludi, 1991). In addition, the diagnosis of PDD has been cited as discriminatory because only women can be found to have it.

Blechman et al (1988) objected to the creation of a new diagnostic category for a premenstrual disorder. Their objection is based on their premise that many women experience premenstrual symptoms at other times during the menstrual cycle and, therefore, that a diagnosis implying a premenstrual causal factor is inappropriate.

There is a wide range of treatments for PMS and PDD, including lifestyle changes, psychotherapy, and medication (Keye, 1989). Lifestyle changes include dietary modifications such as avoiding simple carbohydrates, eating frequent small meals, and reducing or eliminating salt, caffeine, sugar, and alcohol. They also include decreasing tobacco use, increasing aerobic exercise (20 to 30 minutes three times per week) (Prior et al, 1987; Steege and Blumenthal, 1993), and practicing stress management techniques such as assertiveness training, time management, progressive muscle relaxation, and guided imagery (Goodale et al, 1990).

In terms of medication, several studies have investigated the use of progesterone to treat premenstrual symptoms. Although they reported positive results, these studies are marred by several methodological problems including nonrandom assignment to treatment groups, small sample sizes, and lack of placebo control groups (Greene, 1953; Maddocks et al, 1986; Maxson, 1987; Sampson, 1979). Recently Freeman et al (1990) demonstrated in a double-blinded, placebo-controlled study that progesterone suppositories were an ineffective treatment for PMS. Other hormonal preparations such as the oral contraceptive pill and GnRH agonists have been used to alter ovarian hormone function. Results using oral contraceptives are inconclusive; in some patients improvement has been reported, yet in others symptoms have worsened (Graham and Sherwin, 1992; Paige, 1971). The use of GnRH agonists has been reported to result in a complete relief of symptoms (Hammarback and Backstrom, 1987; Muse et al, 1984), but the long-term use of these agents is of questionable value because of the side effects of maintaining a hypoestrogenic state. Many psychotropic medications such as fluoxetine, nortryptyline, and alprazolam have been used to treat PMS and PDD (Harrison et al, 1990; Menkes et al, 1992; Smith and Schiff, 1989; Wood et al, 1992). These medications are given in a variety of regimes to target specific symptoms. Recently, several investigators have reported effective treatment with the selective serotonin reuptake inhibitors antidepressants (Pearlstein and Stone, 1994; Steiner et al, 1995; Yonkers et al, 1996).

In summary, many women may report premenstrual changes but only 5% to 10% meet the criteria for PDD. Prominent symptoms of PDD are emotional lability, depression or irritability, and numerous physical and behavioral symptoms that occur the week before the beginning of menses and that remit shortly after menses begins. Careful documentation of symptoms is necessary to establish the relationship between symptom onset and remission relative to the menstrual cycle. Symptoms must also be present for two to three consecutive cycles. Although the cause of PDD is unclear, several treatments have been developed. Progester-

one and other hormone preparations have had mixed effectiveness. Lifestyle changes and psychotherapy also have mixed results. Psychoactive medications may be used if lifestyle changes have been ineffective or if symptoms are severe. Careful diagnosis, including the exclusion of a preexisting psychological disorder, is crucial.

POSTPARTUM DEPRESSION

Pregnancy and childbirth are significant developmental milestones for most women. Physical, intrapersonal, and relational adaptations are needed to adjust successfully to pregnancy and delivery. The stresses of a new mother are numerous, including disruption in routine, sleep deprivation, decreased independence, social isolation, and change in status at the workplace. The well-adjusted woman is able to anticipate these changes and to prepare for them accordingly. Some women, though, may experience postpartum depression, a serious psychiatric disorder. Pregnancy, delivery, and postpartum care are medical events controlled or overseen by an obstetrician or other health care provider. Therefore, it is important for medical personnel to be well versed in the course and treatment of postpartum depression.

Postpartum depression should be screened for and treated as early as possible for several reasons. It can cause significant suffering for the woman who experiences it, it has a relatively high prevalence, it can be of long duration, and it can have deleterious consequences for the newborn (Susman, 1996). The adverse impact of postpartum depression on infants has been noted and is receiving increased attention in the literature (Cooper et al, 1988; Murray, 1988; Robson and Kumar, 1980).

Postpartum depression is characterized by depressed affect, loss of interest in activities, change in appetite, fatigue, sleep difficulties, difficulty caring for the baby, guilt, low self-esteem, difficulty concentrating, psychomotor retardation or agitation, and suicidal ideation. It is more serious and persistent than the "maternity blues," a transient emotional reaction that women experience shortly after they give birth that subsides without intervention (Hopkins et al, 1984). Hayworth et al (1980) noted that postpartum depression may begin 2 to 8 weeks after delivery and may persist from 2 weeks to several months. The *Diagnostic and Statistical Manual of Mental Disorders* (DSM)-IV specifies postpartum depression as a variation of major depression (American Psychiatric Association, 1994). Estimates of the prevalence of postpartum depression vary, depending on the method of assessment. Based on self-report data, Dalton reported that 7% of women were depressed in the postpartum period (Dalton, 1971). Cutrona (1983) reported that 3.5% of her sample of pregnant women were depressed during their pregnancy and the postpartum period based on DSM-III depression criteria. O'Hara et al (1984) found a rate of 9% of depression during pregnancy and 12% in the postpartum period using research diagnostic criteria. Using research diagnostic criteria in a prospective study, Gotlib et al (1989) found that 10% of women were depressed during pregnancy and 7% were depressed in the postpartum period. The percentages rose to 22% during pregnancy and 26% during the postpartum period with the Beck Depression Inventory, a self-report measure of depression. In general, the base rate of postpartum depression is approximately 10% (O'Hara, 1993).

Several factors have been investigated as possible causes of postpartum depression. Biologic variables, including hormones and neurotransmitters, have been investigated for their hypothesized relationship to postpartum depression. Dalton (1971) proposed that progesterone played a significant role in the cause of postpartum depression, though she did not report any data supporting her hypothesis. Nott et al (1976) measured levels of luteinizing hormone, follicle-stimulating hormone, estrogen, progesterone, and prolactin in a prospective study and correlated them with symptoms of depression. They found a moderate correlation between irritable mood and estrogen and an inverse correlation between progesterone and depression. Unfortunately, none of their subjects met criteria for clinically significant depression. Gordon et al (1986) found that estriol levels were moderately inversely correlated with crying spells in the postpartum period. In a series of prospective studies, O'Hara et al (1989, 1990, 1991) studied plasma estrogen, progesterone, prolactin, and cortisol. Of these, only estrogen showed a relationship to postpartum depression. Estrogen levels in subjects with postpartum depression were significantly lower than in those who did not experience it.

Others have investigated the relationship between postpartum depression and tryptophan, the precursor to serotonin and the rate-limiting agent in its production (Handley et al, 1977; Handley et al, 1980; Stein et al, 1976). A decrease in serotonin has been associated with symptoms of depression in psychiatric patients (Coppen et al, 1976; Riley and Shaw, 1976). Stein et al (1976) found that women with severe postpartum depression had tryptophan levels similar to those of depressed psychiatric inpatients. Plasma tryptophan levels and depression scores had a correlation coefficient of −0.60, suggesting a moderate relationship. Handley et al (1977) found that tryptophan levels were low before delivery and then rose rapidly on postpartum days 1 and 2. In another study, Handley et al (1980) found that plasma tryptophan levels rose from the second to fifth postpartum days, though none of their patients could be classified as having postpartum depression. The absence of a tryptophan peak after delivery was significantly correlated with the occurrence of maternity blues and subsequent depression in the next 6 months (Handley et al, 1977). Treadway et al (1969) found no significant correlation between plasma catecholamines and postpartum mood.

The relationship between postpartum depression and psychosocial variables has also been studied. Hopkins et al (1984) provided a thorough review of the literature on postpartum depression and predisposing psychosocial variables. They concluded that there are no significant relationships

between postpartum depression and demographic factors such as age or parity. There does appear to be a relationship between postpartum depression and relationship quality. Several studies have found that a poor marital relationship precedes postpartum depression (Kumar and Robson, 1984; O'Hara, 1986; Watson et al, 1984). In addition, lack of support from the male partner has been associated with an increased severity of postpartum depression (O'Hara et al, 1983a; O'Hara, 1986). Cutrona (1983) reported that lack of perceived social support during pregnancy was associated with the degree of postpartum depression.

Another significant predictor of postpartum depression is depression during pregnancy (Cutrona, 1983; O'Hara et al, 1983b; O'Hara et al, 1984). Watson et al (1984) also reported that symptoms of depression during pregnancy predicted a later diagnosis of postpartum depression. Gotlib et al (1991) followed up a group of 360 women during and after pregnancy to determine the predictors of depression. They found that 10% of women met criteria for depression during pregnancy and that 7% were depressed during the puerperium. Only half the cases of postpartum depression were of new onset; the remainder of the women who were depressed during the puerperium were depressed during pregnancy. These investigators also found that different variables predicted depression during pregnancy and during the postpartum period. Factors that predicted depression during pregnancy were young age, limited education, multiparity, and lack of outside employment. These variables were not significant predictors of postpartum depression.

Hopkins et al (1987) investigated the relationship between infant-related stressors and postpartum depression. In a cross-sectional study, they compared life-event stress, neonatal risk status, infant temperament, and social support in groups of depressed and nondepressed women between 6 and 8 weeks postpartum. They found that infant-related stressors such as medical complications and maternal perceptions of infant temperament were significantly related to postpartum depression. Interestingly, in this study, life-event stress and social support were not related to postpartum depression.

Another study looked at predictors of postpartum depression in a sample of 115 primiparous women (Whiffen, 1988). In this study marital adjustment, cognitive attributional style, life stress, maternal expectation and perception of infant behavior, and symptoms of depression were investigated. In this sample, 6% of the women had major depression at 8 weeks postpartum. Many variables were related to postpartum symptoms of depression, but the only variables related to the *diagnosis* of postpartum depression were poor marital adjustment and the presence of symptoms of depression during the pregnancy.

In a prospective study, Gotlib et al (1991) followed up a group of 730 women during pregnancy through 4 weeks postpartum. In this study, 10% of the subjects were diagnosed with depression during pregnancy. An additional 5% of women became depressed during the puerperium. Women who were depressed during the postpartum period reported higher scores for symptoms of depression during pregnancy, higher perceived stress during pregnancy, lower levels of marital satisfaction, and more use of escape as a coping strategy than nondepressed women. During the puerperium, these two groups also differed on current perceived stress and marital satisfaction.

In the only study using a matched control group, O'Hara et al (1990) compared a group of pregnant women with a group of nonpregnant controls to determine whether pregnancy and the postpartum periods were times of increased stress and depression. Women were assessed during the second trimester of pregnancy and again 9 weeks postpartum. Eight percent of the pregnant subjects met criteria for depression during the second trimester; 6% of the controls were depressed during the same time period. Ten percent of the pregnant women were depressed at 9 weeks postpartum compared with 8% of the control subjects. The rates, time of onset, and duration of depression were not significantly different between the two groups. During the postpartum assessment, 26% of the pregnant women had the maternity blues and 8% of the controls had the "blues." The authors concluded that the prevalence of clinical depression may not significantly increase after childbirth but that symptoms of depression or the maternity blues are more likely.

O'Hara et al (1991) proposed a diathesis-stress model of postpartum depression that has also been used to describe the cause of other types of depression. In this model, diatheses (vulnerability factors) such as a familial predisposition for depression, history of depression episodes, or dysfunctional cognitive attributional style may predispose a woman to depression, which then emerge as the woman has to cope with stressors related to pregnancy and motherhood. Common stressors during the pregnancy and postpartum are presented in Table 20-1 (Arrizmendi and Affonso, 1987). The preexisting vulnerability to depression in combination with acute stressors may lead to the development of depression. O'Hara et al (1991) tested this model of postpartum depression in a study of childbearing women with postpartum depression. In the study they assessed demographic, psychiatric, social, and cognitive vulnerability variables. In addition, they measured stress from current life events, peripartum stress, and childcare stress. Hormonal assays were also conducted on prolactin, estradiol, progesterone, and cortisol at 34, 36, and 38 weeks of gestation and several days postpartum. Their results indicated that history of depression, depression during pregnancy, childcare-related stressors, and peripartum stressors accounted for 40% of the variance in the diagnosis of postpartum depression. None of the hormonal variables were significantly different for the depressed versus the nondepressed women.

Powell and Drotar (1992) conducted a final study investigating the impact of psychosocial variables on postpartum depression. In this study women were asked about their mood, stressors, social support, and "daily hassles." Results indicated that prepartum depression, social support, and daily hassles were the strongest predictors of postpartum depression. This provides additional evidence for the diathesis-stress model and suggests that predisposing vulnerability factors and current stressors must be considered when screening women for postpartum depression.

In summary, the base rate for postpartum depression is approximately 10%. It is unclear whether the postpartum period is a time of increased clinical depression among women, though an increase in reporting symptoms of depression is common. For those women who have postpartum depression, the common variables associated with the disorder are history of depression (including depression during pregnancy), poor marital relationship, difficulties with childcare, inadequate social support, and numerous daily stressors. Women with one or some of these factors may need increased attention during pregnancy and the postpartum period. The diagnosis of depression is made when the symptoms of depressed mood, emotional lability, decreased interest in activities, poor concentration, sleep or appetite changes, and difficulty caring for the newborn are present at moderate to severe intensity and are of at least 2 weeks' duration. It is particularly important to determine whether the woman is still able to care for herself and her newborn. The physician can help detect cases of postpartum depression by addressing it at postpartum follow-up appointments. After completion of the physical examination, a few questions, such as "Have you had any problems with depression since the baby has been born?" or "Do you feel that you have adjusted well to becoming a mother?" can open the door to assessing symptoms of depression. In addition, the brief (10-item) Edinburgh postnatal depression scale can be used as a simple screening tool (Box 20-3) (Cox et al, 1987; Cox et al, 1996). Studies have indicated that using a cut-off score of 12 or 13 on this measure is useful in identifying women with postpartum depression (Warner et al, 1996).

Various treatments are available for postpartum depression (Appleby et al, 1997; Elliot, 1989; Wisner et al, 1996). Individual cognitive-behavioral psychotherapy can provide the patient with increased social support, emotional expression, stress management skills, and improved cognitive and behavioral coping strategies that can increase feelings of efficacy and control. Within the context of psychotherapy, antidepressant medications can be used. Sichel (1992) recommended early psychopharmacologic stabilization with tricyclic antidepressants. Medication use is often limited among mothers who breast-feed because of concerns about the effects of psychoactive medications ingested by the newborn through breast milk. Despite a recent review of the available literature suggesting that the use of amitriptyline, nortriptyline, desipramine, clomipramine, dothiepin, and sertraline have not been associated with adverse side effects for nursing infants, the authors continue to recommend that pharmacotherapy be considered on a case-by-case basis after an examination of the relative risks and benefits. Stowe and Nemeroff (1995) summarized dosing and breast-feeding ratings for several

Table 20-1   Postpartum Stressors

Category	Examples of Items Reported	Category	Examples of Items Reported
Physical symptoms	Fatigue	Labor-delivery	Fears
	Nausea-vomiting		Pain-discomfort
	Bodily pain-discomfort		Complications
	Rest-sleep disturbances		Waiting
	Physical restrictions		Cesarean
	Eating disturbances		Outcomes
	Gastrointestinal disturbances	Social stressors	Decrease in social opportunities
	Bowel/bladder		Friends' reactions, advice
Changes in living patterns	Housing (space, rearrange house)		Others (communications of strangers)
	Activities (diet, exercise, smoking)		Single parenting (reactions)
	Time schedules (responsibilities)	Job-career-school	Work (fatigue, limitations, relationships)
	Relocation to new residence		Change in career plans
Body image	Weight gain		School (decisions to finish, quit, examinations)
	Negative feelings (fat, unattractive, distorted size)		Time constraints (impact on relationships)
	Wardrobe not fitting	Mate-spouse issues	Reactions-comments (emotional needs)
	Getting back into shape		Arguments-marital problems
	Physical marks on body		Sex life (attractiveness, discomfort, decreased frequency)
Monetary stressors	Money to buy things		Miscellaneous (husband's responsibility with household, working too much)
	Bills	Parenting concerns	Mothering role and responsibilities
	Concern over insurance coverage		Breast-feeding concerns
	Loss of regular income		Child-care concerns
Family stressors	Parents (reactions, pressures, getting along)		Newborn care
	Support (lack of, far away, too helpful)		Night feedings
	In-laws		Miscellaneous (pediatric care, driving with baby, baby classes)
	General worries	Newborn behaviors	Baby crying
Emotional stressors	Changes (moody, irritable, sensitive, lack of patience)		Identifying infant distress signals
	Fears-worries-concerns (baby, coping, control)		Colicky behaviors
	Anger, frustration-ambivalence		Health (baby okay?)
	Depression, loneliness	Baby welfare	Normality (abnormal baby, birth defects)
	Guilt		Effects on baby (nutrition, diseases)
Pregnancy concerns (PG)	Fear of miscarriage		Anticipation-expectations
	Complications—risks		Sick baby (prematurity, intensive care)
	Preterm labor	Other children	Care-responsibilities
	High blood pressure		Sibling rivalry (children fighting)
	Insufficient weight gain		Reactions to new baby
	Baby's due date		
	Birth control (spacing)		
	Miscellaneous (technology)		

From Arrizmendi T, Affonso D: Stressful events related to pregnancy and postpartum. J Psychosom Res 1987; 31:743.

The Edinburgh Postnatal Depression Scale (EPDS) has been developed to assist primary care health professionals to detect mothers suffering from postnatal depression, a distressing disorder more prolonged than the 'blues' (which occur in the first week after delivery) but less severe than puerperal psychosis.

Previous studies have shown that postnatal depression affects at least 10% of women and that many depressed mothers remain untreated. These mothers may cope with their baby and with household tasks, but their enjoyment of life is seriously affected, and there may be long-term effects on the family.

The EPDS was developed at health centers in Livingston and Edinburgh. It consists of short statements. The mother underlines which of the four possible responses is closest to how she has been feeling during the past week. Most mothers complete the scale without difficulty in less than 5 minutes.

The validation study showed that mothers who scored above a threshold 12/13 were likely to be suffering from a depressive illness of varying severity. Nevertheless the EPDS score should *not* override clinical judgment. A careful clinical assessment should be carried out to confirm the diagnosis. The scale indicates how the mother has felt *during the previous week,* and in doubtful cases it may be usefully repeated after 2 weeks. The scale will not detect mothers with anxiety neuroses, phobias, or personality disorders.

Instructions for Users

1. The mother is asked to underline the response that comes closest to how she has been feeling in the previous 7 days.
2. All 10 items must be completed.
3. Care should be taken to avoid the possibility of the mother discussing her answers with others.
4. The mother should complete the scale herself, unless she has limited English or has difficulty with reading.
5. The EPDS may be used at 6-8 weeks to screen postnatal women. The child health clinic, postnatal check-up or a home visit may provide suitable opportunities for its completion.

Edinburgh Postnatal Depression Scale (EPDS)
J. L. Cox, J. M. Holden, R. Sagovsky
Department of Psychiatry, University of Edinburgh

Name:
Address:
Baby's age:

Because you have recently had a baby, we would like to know how you are feeling. Please UNDERLINE the answer that comes closest to how you have felt IN THE PAST 7 DAYS, not just how you feel today.

Here is an example, already completed.
I have felt happy:
   Yes, all the time
   <u>Yes, most of the time</u>
   No, not very often
   No, not at all
This would mean: "I have felt happy most of the time" during this past week. Please complete the other questions in the same way.

In the past 7 days:
* 1. I have been able to laugh and see the funny side of things
   As much as I always could
   Not quite so much now
   Definitely not so much now
   Not at all
* 2. I have looked forward with enjoyment to things
   As much as I ever did
   Rather less than I used to
   Definitely less than I used to
   Hardly at all
* 3. I have blamed myself unnecessarily when things went wrong
   Yes, most of the time
   Yes, some of the time
   Not very often
   No, never
* 4. I have been anxious or worried for no good reason
   No, not at all
   Hardly ever
   Yes, sometimes
   Yes, very often
* 5. I have felt scared or panicky for no very good reason
   Yes, quite a lot
   Yes, sometimes
   No, not much
   No, not at all
* 6. Things have been getting on top of me
   Yes, most of the time I haven't been able to cope at all
   Yes, sometimes I haven't been coping as well as usual
   No, most of the time I have coped quite well
   No, I have been coping as well as ever
* 7. I have been so unhappy that I have had difficulty sleeping
   Yes, most of the time
   Yes, sometimes
   Not very often
   No, not at all
* 8. I have felt sad or miserable
   Yes, most of the time
   Yes, quite often
   Not very often
   No, not at all
* 9. I have been so unhappy that I have been crying
   Yes, most of the time
   Yes, quite often
   Only occasionally
   No, never
*10. The thought of harming myself has occurred to me
   Yes, quite often
   Sometimes
   Hardly ever
   Never

Response categories are scored 0, 1, 2, and 3 according to increased severity of the symptom.
Items marked with an asterisk are reverse scored (i.e. 3, 2, 1 and 0). The total score is calculated by adding together the scores for each of the 10 items. Users may reproduce the scale without further permission providing they request copyright (which remains with the *British Journal of Psychiatry*) by quoting the names of the authors, the title, and the source of the paper in all reproduced copies.

From Cox JL, Holden JM, Sagovsky R: Detection of postnatal depression: Development of the 10 item Edinburgh Postnatal Depression Scale (EPDS). *Br J Psychiatry* 1987; 150:762.

Table 20-2   Recommended Dosing and Use-in-Pregnancy and Breast-Feeding Ratings for Antidepressant Medications

Generic Name	Daily Dose (mg/day)	Half-Life (hours)*	FDA Risk Category	Effect of Drug on Nursing Infants†
Tricyclic/heterocyclic antidepressants				
Amitriptyline (Elavil, Endep)	150-300	10-22	D	Unknown but of concern
Imipramine (Tofranil)	150-330	11-25	D	Unknown but of concern
Desipramine (Norpramin)	150-300	12-76	C	Unknown but of concern
Nortriptyline (Pamelor, Aventyl)	75-150	15-93	D	NA
Clomipramine (Anafranil)	150-250	19-37	C	Compatible
Doxepin (Sinequan, Adapin)	150-300	11-23	C	Unknown but of concern
Maprotiline (Ludiomil)	140-225	21-66	B	NA
Protriptyline (Vivactil)	15-60	54-198	C	NA
Monoamine oxidase inhibitors				
Phenelzine (Nardil)	45-90	NA‡	C	—
Tranylcypromine (Pamate)	30-60	NA‡	C	—
Selective serotonin reuptake inhibitors				
Fluoxetine (Prozac)	20-60	24-95§	B	Unknown but of concern
Fluvoxamine (Luvox)	50-300	17-22	C	Unknown but of concern
Paroxetine (Paxil)	20-50	24	C	—
Sertraline (Zoloft)	50-200	26§	B	—
Other antidepressants				
Bupropion (Wellbutrin)	150-450	8-24§	B	—
Trazodone (Desyrel)	200-300	4-13	C	Unknown but of concern
Venlafaxine (Effexor)	150-375	5-11	C	—
Nefazodone (Serzone)	300-600	2-4	C	—

From Stowe ZN, Nemeroff CB: Psychopharmocology during pregnancy and lactation. In Schatzberg AF, Nemeroff CB, editors: *Textbook of psychopharmacology,* Washington, D.C., 1995, American Psychiatric Press.

FDA, US Food and Drug Administration; *NA,* not applicable; —, not available.

*Half-life of elimination is listed for parent compound.

†Based on the 1994 American Academy of Pediatrics Committee on Drugs report on the use of medications during breast-feeding.

‡Duration of action is based on irreversible enzyme inhibition; half-life of elimination is not applicable.

§Elimination half-life of active metabolites of fluoxetine (4 to 16 days), sertraline (2 to 4 days), and bupropion (>3 days).

antidepressant medications. Their summary is presented in Table 20-2.

In addition to individual psychotherapy, psychoeducational groups can provide valuable information about parenting and childcare. Support groups can be helpful in letting the patient share her feelings with others and learning that she is not alone in her adjustment to parenthood. Couples counseling can be used when relationship issues play a significant role in the depression. One study demonstrated that women whose husbands take an active role in childcare responsibilities are less prone to postpartum depression (Paykel et al, 1980). Couples therapy can help the couple learn to communicate clearly with one another and to share in household and childcare activities according to a mutually agreeable arrangement. Finally, if outpatient management is not possible because of the severity of the depression (*i.e.,* if a woman is unable to take care of herself or her baby, if she is suicidal or homicidal, or if she has psychotic delusions), hospitalization is indicated.

To summarize, numerous variables have been investigated as predisposing factors for postpartum depression. There is no unequivocal evidence of a hormonal cause for postpartum depression. Depression during pregnancy, history of depression, quality of the marital relationship, perceived social support, and daily stressors do appear to be related to postpartum depression. Early identification of and treatment for postpartum depression are critical for the welfare of the mother and the baby.

INFERTILITY

Fertility is highly valued in most cultures, and the desire for a child is one of the most basic of all human motivations. For women, pregnancy and motherhood are developmental milestones that are highly emphasized by our culture (Strauss et al, 1992; Veevers, 1980). When attempts to have a child fail, the experience can be emotionally devastating (Mahlstedt, 1985; Menning, 1982).

Infertility is defined as 12 months of appropriately timed intercourse that does not result in conception. Approximately 16% of couples in the United States have difficulty conceiving a child (National Center for Health Statistics, 1982). This appears in part to have resulted from the trend among some women to delay childbirth until their middle to late thirties and from the associated decrease in fertility after the age of 35. Although there is the perception that infertility is on the rise, this perceived increase is actually an artifact of the large number of women currently in the childbearing years because of the baby boom of the 1950s and early 1960s. The base rate of infertility among women has remained the same, but the absolute number of women in the reproductive years has increased (Mosher and Pratt, 1990). Approximately 40% of infertile couples have female factor infertility, 40% have male factor infertility, and 20% have a combination or they have infertility of unknown cause. For decades clinicians have thought that infertility, particularly that of unknown cause, could result from psychological distress (Benedek, 1952; Mai et al, 1972; Sandler, 1968). Investigators tried to identify "unconscious" or other psychological variables that caused infertility (Edelmann et al, 1991; Moller and Fallstrom, 1991; Shatford et al, 1988). In the mid-1980s clinicians and researchers began questioning the hypothesis that psychological distress *caused* infertility. Instead they found that psychological distress was a *consequence* of infertility. Mental health clinicians have become increasingly involved in providing care to infertile patients (Greenfeld et al, 1984; Klock and Maier, 1991a).

The emotional impact of infertility has been described by studies conducted through clinical observation and empirical research. Based on her clinical observation of infertile couples, Mahlstedt (1985) described a series of losses (self-esteem, relational, health, and financial) experienced by the infertile couple. First the infertile person experiences a challenge to self-esteem, and then possibly an erosion of self-esteem, because of repeated failed attempts to have a child. It can be significantly worse in persons who have been highly successful in other areas of life and who have not developed the coping skills to deal with failure and loss.

A second loss can be the real or feared loss of important relationships. This includes the marital relationship and relationships with family and friends. The marital relationship can be strained or lost because of fears that the fertile partner will leave the infertile partner. Inability to discuss their feelings about infertility, blaming one another, and sexual difficulties related to infertility treatment can strain the couple's relationship. Several writers have noted that infertile couples have sexual difficulties (Daniluk, 1988; Fagan et al, 1986; Reading, 1993; see Klock [1993] for a review of female sexual dysfunction). Sex may become a reminder of the couple's failure to have a child. In addition to marital difficulties, the infertile couple may feel strain in their relationships with family and friends. For example, an infertile woman may avoid contact with her mother and sister because they are continually asking whether she is pregnant.

The infertile couple may avoid friends who are pregnant because they are reminders that others can get pregnant with ease. The infertile woman's loss of relationships can deprive her of social support that may compound her feelings of isolation and depression.

A third loss related to infertility is the loss of health. A woman may spend a great deal of time in the infertility clinic for tests and treatments. Although she is not "sick," she may begin to identify with that role and begin to feel that her physical health is compromised. In addition, women may report feeling ill because of the side effects of some of the hormonal medications used to enhance fertility.

A fourth loss is the loss of financial security. Infertility treatment, especially in states that do not mandate insurance coverage of infertility treatment, can be extremely expensive (Gennaro et al, 1992). One cycle of in vitro fertilization (IVF) costs approximately $10,000. Accompanying financial problems are concerns about job security. Because the woman is often the primary focus of evaluation or treatment, she often misses considerable amounts of work, which places her job in jeopardy. In addition, she may fear telling her employer the reason for her absences because the employer may assume the treatment will be successful and the woman will be leaving her job. If the employer assumes she will be leaving her job to have a child, the woman may be vulnerable to firing or layoff.

Losses related to infertility and its psychological sequelae can adversely impact the infertile woman. Moller and Fallstrom (1991a) provide a useful schema for understanding the interactive effects of biologic and psychosocial precursors and consequences of infertility. Their model is presented in Fig. 20-2.

Much of the empirical research on the psychological impact of infertility has focused on patients who undergo IVF. Freeman et al (1985) found that approximately half the women in their sample rated infertility as the most stressful experience of their lives. In addition, she found that 18% of men and 16% of women had significant psychological distress that included high levels of depression and somatization. Leiblum et al (1987) found that more women than men reported depression before and after infertility treatment and that 34% of the women in her study rated IVF as being "very stressful." A third study of the psychological impact of IVF was conducted by Baram et al (1988), who surveyed couples after the completion of one cycle of IVF. As an indirect measure of how stressful the procedure was, couples were asked whether they would undergo IVF again. Thirty-eight percent reported that they would not because it was too expensive, the success rate was too low, and they were unwilling to resubmit themselves to the emotional pain of the procedure. In addition, 18% of the couples reported that infertility had a negative impact on their marriages. Sixty-six percent of women reported that they became depressed after the procedure, and 13% reported that they had suicidal ideation after an unsuccessful procedure.

After documenting that infertility and IVF were psychologically stressful, researchers began looking at variables

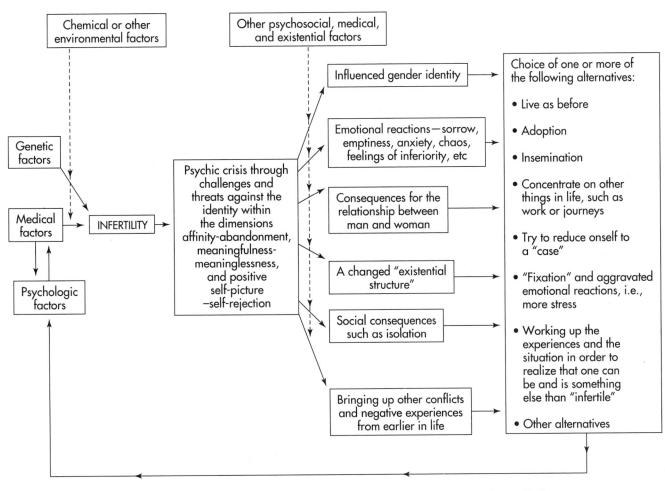

Fig. 20-2. Schema of infertility precursors and consequences. (From Moller A, Fallstrom K: Psychological factors in the etiology of infertility: A longitudinal study. *J Psychosom Obstet Gynecol* 19911 12:13. Reprinted with permission.)

that would predict the development of psychological distress among infertile patients. Newton et al (1990) investigated psychological factors preceding IVF that were related to post-IVF adjustment. They found that 14% of women had clinically significant levels of anxiety, and 24% had clinically significant levels of depression. He found that the development of anxiety and depression after IVF were best predicted by the presence of anxiety and depression before IVF. Men did not report clinically significant anxiety or depression.

Two recent studies have investigated the stressfulness of infertility using a stress and coping model (Lazarus, 1984). Based on this model, a situation is stressful if it is perceived as a threat to the person and if the person does not feel confident about having the coping skills to adapt to it. In this model, infertility is stressful because it threatens the person's highly valued plan to have a child.

The extent to which infertility is stressful is impacted by the coping skills the person uses. This model identifies a priori those persons for whom infertility would be psychologically stressful. In a study by Litt et al (1992), several variables were assessed to determine their contribution to post-IVF distress. Variables that were assessed included demographic and reproductive history, general appraisal (optimism), situational appraisal (chances for success), and coping skills. After an unsuccessful IVF cycle, 20% of women were clinically depressed. Results indicated that general optimism and perceived responsibility for the cause of the infertility protected against post-IVF distress. Feelings of loss of control, perceived contribution to the failure of IVF, and use of escape as a coping strategy were related to increased post-IVF distress. In this study, optimism seemed to protect women from the psychological distress of infertility. Only one coping strategy, escape, was related to post-IVF outcome; women who used escape as a coping strategy experienced greater distress.

In a cross-sectional study of infertile patients, investigators found that for women the most important factors mitigating against psychological distress were perceived personal control, optimism that they would eventually have a child, and intensity of motivation to have a child (Abbey et al, 1992). High levels of perceived personal control and optimism were related to lower levels of distress, and high levels of motivation to have a child were associated with

---

BOX 20-4
GUIDELINES FOR INFERTILITY COUNSELING

The following guidelines for referral indicate which issues are typically the most stressful or are most likely to cause significant emotional distress and disruption during infertility treatment. They are intended to provide the medical professional with a guide to those issues likely to warrant referral to a qualified infertility counselor.

1. Patients entering treatment by assisted reproductive technology: Assisted reproductive technology includes treatment with in vitro fertilization, gamete intrafallopian transfer; other affiliated programs such as treatment with donor gametes (sperm and ovum), surrogacy, and gestational carrier programs; and any other medically assisted means of noncoital reproduction. Considerable research has shown that treatment with assisted reproductive technology is often psychologically and physically demanding. Furthermore, the treatment may be perceived by the couple and their caregivers as a last chance at parenthood and may be considered only after several years of infertility and myriad medical treatments. Not all couples need supportive and educational counseling. Any couple requesting counseling, showing overt distress, or meeting the description in the following guidelines would probably profit from referral to a qualified infertility counselor.
2. Psychiatric illness (past and present)
   A. History of psychiatric illness with clear vulnerability to the current stressor
   B. Current significant psychiatric symptoms or illness
3. History of pregnancy complications or loss
   A. History of traumatic perinatal or fetal loss
   B. History of unresolved bereavement associated with abortion or perinatal death
   C. Current multiple pregnancy in which the patient is considering fetal reduction
   D. Patient undergoing in vitro fertilization or genetic screening
4. Significant physical illness (past and present)
   A. Significant illness making pregnancy dangerous
   B. Request for donor gametes because of significant illness or genetic disorder
5. Sexual abuse (past or present)
   A. History of unresolved rape, incest, or sexual abuse
   B. Current sexual abuse
6. Conflicted gender identity, homosexuality, or bisexuality
   A. Homosexuality or bisexuality interfering with marital stability and infertility treatment
   B. Atypical sexual behavior compromising fertility or infertility treatment
7. Chemical abuse or dependency
   A. Repeated failed attempts at treatment and continued or current abuse
   B. Inability to meet demands of medical treatment owing to abuse or dependence
   C. Even occasional use of drugs that are teratogenic
   D. A pattern of unstable behavior owing to chemical dependency
   E. Drug-seeking behavior
8. Pregnancy after 40 years of age
9. Chaotic social or familial functioning
10. Single lifestyle

From Burns L: An overview of the psychology of infertility. *Infertil Reprod Med Clin North Am* 1993; 4:433.

---

increased distress. In other words, the more important it was to the woman to have a child, the more distress she reported from the infertility experience.

Several published studies have addressed the relationship between psychological stress (high versus low) and outcome (pregnancy versus no pregnancy) (Edelmann et al, 1991; Moller, 1991b; Strauss et al, 1992). It is commonly perceived among patients and clinicians that if a couple will "just relax," they will get pregnant. There is the implicit assumption that psychological stress may prevent a woman from attaining and maintaining a pregnancy. In a nonrandomized, uncontrolled study, Domar et al (1990) reported decreases in anxiety and depression and a subsequent 34% pregnancy rate among a group of infertile women who attended a 10-session relaxation program. Facchinetti et al (1997) reported that women who conceived through IVF had lower cardiovascular vulnerability to psychological stress, as measured by a cognitive stress task on the day of egg retrieval, than women who did not conceive. Finally, Boivin and Takefman (1995) concluded that psychological stress was related to IVF outcome in a group of women who kept daily ratings of stress throughout an IVF cycle.

Although these studies suggest that there may be a relationship between psychological stress and outcome among women who undergo, they are incomplete because they do not assess physiological markers of anxiety. It has been hypothesized that psychological stress alters levels of cortisol, prolactin, and progesterone, which in turn has an adverse affect on pregnancy outcome. Few studies assess the physiological and the psychological aspects of anxiety during IVF and relate them to pregnancy outcome. One study found that levels of anxiety, prolactin, and cortisol increased significantly from baseline to the time of egg retrieval during IVF (Demyttenaere et al, 1991). Harlow et al (1996) also found that levels of state anxiety, prolactin, and cortisol all increased during IVF but that there was no relationship between increased anxiety, hormones, and pregnancy outcome. Additional studies are needed to assess the intricate relationship between psychological anxiety, stress, hormones, and pregnancy outcome during IVF.

Many of the studies of infertility have focused on women because they are the primary recipients of infertility treatment. Male factor infertility is also stressful and has been studied in the context of donor insemination (Berger, 1978; Klock and Maier, 1991b). Studies have indicated that male infertility can have a detrimental effect on a man's self-esteem and sexual functioning (Klock, 1993).

In addition to the stress of routine infertility treatment, third-party reproduction such as donor insemination, donor oocyte, and gestational carrier also entails psychological risks and rewards. As reproductive technologies have expanded, so have the ways in which a couple can have a child (Lantos, 1990). These options have added layers of psychological, social, ethical, and legal entanglements that do not encumber traditional reproduction. Society has not yet caught up with the advances in technology. Therefore, the psychological risk of these treatments is increased as patients are used as test cases to expand the boundaries of parenthood. Additional research and discussion are needed to determine the consequences of these treatments and to develop a language to describe the relationships between parent and child, for now "parent" can mean gamete donor, gestational carrier, or psychosocial parent. Psychologists and psychiatrists can help screen patients, educate and prepare them for treatment, and treat psychological disorders that may develop during the course of treatment.

The physician should remember that infertility is a stressful life event for women and men. Women are more likely than men to report psychological distress in the forms of depression and anxiety. Approximately 20% of women experience reactive clinical depression after a failed IVF attempt. Marital and sexual adjustment can be compromised by infertility. Because infertility is a problem that affects the couple, it is recommended that the couple be seen together for evaluation and treatment and that the emphasis be placed on infertility as the *couple's* problem. Perceived control is protective against psychological distress in infertility treatment. Therefore, providing the patient with opportunities to control treatment-related events may be helpful.

Takefman et al (1990) demonstrated that providing patients with basic information about the procedures is helpful in increasing their knowledge about infertility and decreasing their negative feelings about the experience. Last, it is as important to talk about when to end treatment as it is to talk about the treatment itself (Burns, 1993). The physician can discuss in broad terms the average number of cycles for various types of treatment. In addition, the physician can encourage the couple to discuss between themselves how much time, money, and emotional energy they are willing to devote to infertility treatment. Couples should be encouraged to take breaks from treatment, as time permits, to allow for physical rest and for the renewal of psychological resilience.

In terms of psychological services for infertility patients, a mandatory psychological consultation is recommended for anyone considering third-party reproduction (Burns, 1993; Klock and Maier, 1991a). In addition psychological consultation may be indicated for any patient who has had a difficult reproductive history (numerous pregnancy losses), significant psychiatric problems (substance abuse, sexual assault, or psychiatric illness), or significant marital instability. Box 20-4 provides a useful summary of guidelines for referrals to a mental health professional.

MENOPAUSE

Midlife is a time of significant biologic and psychological change for women (Hutchinson, 1993). Menopause is the time when a woman's menstrual cycle ends because of estrogen deficiency. Estrogen deficiency also produces vaginal atrophy, vasomotor instability (hot flashes), loss of bone mass, and changes in cardiovascular risk (Greendale and Sowers, 1997). Along with these biologic changes, significant psychosocial events occur during midlife, such as changes in her relationships with her children, loss or illness of parents, and marital instability or widowhood. The menopause has been described as a psychologically difficult time during which women are subject to moodiness, irritability, and depression (Strickland, 1988). In the late nineteenth century, psychiatrists Maudsley and Kraeplin described a clinical syndrome of depression or melancholia that occurred during the climacteric (Schmidt and Rubinow, 1989). Kraeplin is credited with coining the phrase involutional melancholia, which was used to refer to patients who had depression during the menopause. These patients were described as having rigid, obsessive personalities and symptoms of agitated depression with hypochondriacal or nihilistic delusions. Involutional melancholia gained validity as a distinct psychiatric entity by its inclusion in the first and second editions of the DSM (American Psychiatric Association, 1994). From the gynecologic perspective, Kupperman et al (1959) included psychiatric symptoms in their description of the menopause, as did other textbooks of gynecology. Although it was clinical lore in gynecology and psychiatry that menopause was a time of increased risk for depression, few empirical studies had investigated the relationship between menopause and depression. In the past two decades, there has been an increase in the study of the biologic and psychological aspects of menopause.

From a psychiatric perspective, investigators tried to determine whether there was a unique menopausal mood disorder. Weissman (1979) studied more than 400 psychiatric outpatients. She divided the sample into two groups, those younger than 45 and those 45 or older, and assessed history and current symptoms of depression. She found that there was no difference in the rates of depression between the two groups. Although she used these findings to question the existence of involutional melancholia, a major flaw in this study is the classification of subjects into premenopausal (younger than age 45) and menopausal (45 or older) categories based on age alone. Therefore, it is unclear whether the two groups were significantly different in terms of menopausal status. Winokur (1973) also studied a group of women admitted to a psychiatric hospital and found that there was no greater risk for an episode of depression during the menopause than at other times during a woman's life.

In a study using nonclinical subjects of all ages, Neugarten and Kraines (1965) found that menopausal women and adolescent girls had the highest scores on a symptom checklist assessing psychological symptoms associated with the menopause. Although menopausal women had high symptom scores, postmenopausal women had low symptom scores indicating that the increase in symptoms at the time of menopause is not long lasting. More recent studies of community samples of middle-aged women have demonstrated that depression is no more likely during menopause than at other times. For a critical review of this literature, see Nicol-Smith (1996). A recent epidemiological study found that the dysphoric mood aspect of menopause is distinct from the vasomotor symptoms related to menopause, suggesting different etiologies for these changes (Porter et al, 1996). These authors also found that 51% of the sample reported experiencing depression in the last 6 months, but only 22% described it as a problem. Depression was more often reported by women who used hormone replacement therapy, had a history of depression, had other medical problems, had self-rated poor health. Women with medically or surgically induced menopause were more likely to report problematic menopausal symptoms.

Recent studies have suggested that women who have used or are using hormone replacement therapy (HRT) report more symptoms of depression (Pearlstein et al, 1997). Because of the cross-sectional nature of these studies, the causal direction of this relationship is unknown. It may be that women who experience depression are more likely to seek help and to use HRT as a way of treating the symptoms, or it may be that HRT causes depression. Longitudinal studies are needed to clarify the relationship between HRT and symptoms of depression. These studies also point out the difficulty of generalizing to all menopausal women based on studies using clinical samples.

If depression is experienced at greater levels or among a specific subgroup of women during menopause, then questions regarding the cause of depression arise. Researchers have hypothesized that depression during the menopause is caused by declining levels of gonadal hormones or is secondary to fatigue and loss of sleep from nocturnal hot flashes (Hutchinson, 1993; Schmidt and Rubinow, 1989). Others think that symptoms of depression during the menopause result from stressful life events and the transitions of aging (Morse and Dennerstein, 1989). To determine whether gonadal hormones play a role in menopausal depression, many studies have investigated the impact of HRT on mood among menopausal women (Coope, 1981; Schneider et al, 1977; Strickland, 1988). Unfortunately these studies were marred by numerous methodologic problems.

Sherwin (1988) and Sherwin and Gelfand (1984) conducted two rigorous studies on the effects of exogenous hormone treatment on menopausal mood symptoms. In the latter, 38 women who underwent total hysterectomy were divided into four groups and were treated with estrogen, androgen, estrogen and androgen, or placebo. Ten women with intact ovaries served as controls. Treatment was administered for 3 months. During the fourth month, all patients received a placebo and then were crossed over to a different treatment. Mood symptoms and plasma levels of estrone, estradiol, and testosterone were assessed four times during the study. Results indicated that estrone and estradiol levels were equivalent across treatment groups and that, as expected, the control group had significantly higher levels of estrogen. They also indicated that the estrogen and androgen and the androgen alone treatment groups had significantly higher levels of testosterone than the other groups. In terms of symptoms of depression, all subjects were within the normal range of mood symptoms, though post hoc tests indicated that the placebo group had significantly higher depression scores than the other groups. The placebo group's higher depression scores correlated with lower levels of estradiol, estrone, and testosterone. The authors concluded that exogenous estrogen may help to maintain higher central levels of serotonin, thereby attenuating depression.

Another study by Sherwin et al (1988) investigated the use of estrogen and androgen, estrogen alone, or no treatment in a group of 44 women who underwent complete hysterectomy. Treatment was provided and hormone levels and psychological symptoms were assessed at monthly intervals. Results indicated that there was a significant correlation between estrogen levels and composure, elation, and clearheadedness for the treatment groups. Women in the treatment groups also reported feeling more elated, energetic, composed, and confident than women in the placebo group.

Investigators studied the effects of estrogen and progesterone on women undergoing natural menopause (Siddle et al, 1990). Each woman received estrogen continuously for the first month. After that, half the subjects received 20 mg dydrogesterone for the first 12 days of the cycle for 3 months and the other half received 10 mg dydrogesterone for the first 12 days of the cycle for 3 months. Results indicated that the two levels of progesterone treatment resulted in no significant differences in psychological symptoms. After collapsing the data across the two progesterone groups, no differences were found in levels of psychological symptoms between the estrogen alone and the estrogen and progesterone groups.

Sherwin (1991) looked at the effects of combined estrogen and progesterone treatment on menopausal symptoms. Women undergoing natural menopause were assigned to four treatment groups of conjugated estrogens and medroxyprogesterone or placebo. Hormonal assays and assessment of psychological symptoms were conducted at regular intervals throughout the study. Women taking estrogen and the higher dose (5 mg) of medroxyprogesterone acetate reported significantly more dysphoria than women taking estrogen alone. The study also found that regardless of treatment group, women experienced greater sexual desire during weeks 1 and 2 of the treatment month than in week 4, when no hormones were taken. Mood scores of women administered low (0.625 mg) and high (1.25 mg) doses of estrogen did not differ significantly. On the other hand, mood scores of women administered low doses of estrogen (0.625 mg) and high doses of progesterone (5 mg) revealed significantly more dysphoria than did mood scores of women administered high doses of estrogen (1.25 mg) alone. The author concluded that progesterone has a mood-dampening effect on menopausal women. She also noted that the changes in mood were not caused by changes in the frequency of hot flashes because all groups reported similar reductions in hot flashes. Other studies investigating the effect of combined estrogen and progesterone treatment of menopausal women indicate that women receiving estrogen and progesterone have more dysphoric moods than women taking estrogen alone (Dennerstein et al, 1979; Holst et al, 1989; Magos et al, 1986).

Pearlstein et al (1997) described a mechanism for action of estrogen and dysphoric mood. They reviewed the literature, primarily from animal models, and suggested that monamine oxidase activity increases and serotonin levels decrease in menopausal women after estrogen administration levels of serotinon increase. Pearlstein et al (1997) concluded that decreased serotonin responsivity after menopause could expose a woman to depression.

In addition to hormonal changes, psychological changes take place during menopause. Dennerstein and Burrows (1978) have noted nervousness, irritability, depression, and decreased social adaptation among menopausal women. Another factor that may influence the occurrence of psychological changes with menopause are the negative expectations about menopause prevalent in our culture. Women may come to dread the changes that they have heard about from other women. This may make them more susceptible to experiencing those changes. Interestingly, cross-cultural studies have shown that women in non-Western cultures do not have significant difficulties during menopause. In fact, in cultures in which women's status rises after menopause, there is no noted psychological change in functioning

(Davis, 1982; Van Keep and Kellerhals, 1974; Wilbush, 1982). The National Institute on Aging is sponsoring the Study of Women's Health across the Nation, which began in 1994. This study addresses numerous aspects in the experience of menopause, including ethnic differences. Preliminary results indicate that black women have more estrogen-related symptoms than other women. Fewer women of Asian descent report significantly debilitating symptoms than white (2% to 3%) or black (12% to 14%) women (DeAngelis, 1997).

Changes in sexual desire and arousal may have an impact on mental health during menopause (Bachman et al, 1985; McCoy and Davidson, 1985; Sarrel, 1982; Sarrel, 1990). Sarrel (1990) noted that approximately 20% of women referred to a general sexual dysfunction clinic had sexual function problems related to menopause. Bachmann et al (1985) found that 20% of women in their study reported decreases in sexual desire. McCoy and Davidson (1985) found that among 16 women experiencing natural menopause, sexual desire and frequency decreased during and after menopause. Overall, five changes have been noted to take place during the menopause: diminished sexual responsiveness, dyspareunia, decreased sexual frequency, decreased sexual desire, and dysfunction among the male partner (Sarrel, 1990). These changes are thought to be influenced by the hormonal, psychological, and social changes that take place during menopause. In terms of physical changes, decreases in genital engorgement, delayed reaction time of the clitoris, and decreased vaginal secretions can be attributed to the lower levels of estrogen and its effect on peripheral blood flow.

The clinical management of menopausal women can focus on physical and psychological difficulties. First, specific symptoms and their severity should be documented. Then an evaluation between the relative risk and the relative benefit of HRT can be considered. If the relative benefit outweighs the relative risk, the initial HRT trial may help alleviate somatic symptoms and improve psychological adjustment. If mood symptoms continue to be problematic after the successful initiation of HRT, psychological consultation may be considered. Contributory psychosocial problems may be assessed. In addition, if indicated, antidepressant therapy may be initiated after HRT has been established.

SUMMARY

The interface among obstetrics, gynecology, and psychiatry presents many challenges to the physician and the mental health professional. This chapter has reviewed the research and clinical literature in four areas relatively common in the obstetrics and gynecology practice or in other primary care practices. Women's health psychology continues to grow as a subspecialty and to increase our knowledge of the health and psychological needs of women (Stewart and Stotland, 1993). Physicians play an important role in identifying and treating psychological disorders that occur across the reproductive life span. Because of their important role in women's health care, physicians should be particularly knowledgeable of and sensitive to the emotional needs of patients. In addition, a good consultative relationship with a psychologist or a psychiatrist is often helpful in providing multidisciplinary treatment of psychological disorders.

It can be difficult to establish a collaborative relationship between the obstetrician-gynecologist and the psychiatrist or psychologist. During the course of a busy day in which a patient is experiencing an acute psychological crisis, it is difficult to establish a relationship with a mental health professional. The pressing concern at that time is patient care. There may not be time for discussions of treatment philosophy, training experience, and role boundaries. Unfortunately, this may prevent an effective collaboration from taking place. Instead of trying to develop a consultative relationship in the midst of a patient crisis, a physician should proactively establish a collaborative relationship with a colleague in psychology or psychiatry. In general, psychologists or psychiatrists with doctorates (Ph.D. or M.D.) have the most extensive background and training. Psychologists specialize in many modalities of psychother-apy, including psychoanalytical, cognitive, behavioral, couples, and group therapy. They also administer psychological tests to assess personality and psychological functioning. A referral to a psychiatrist is necessary if medication is to be part of the psychological treatment. The most important part of the psychiatric consultative relationship is the ability of the psychologist or psychiatrist to work well with the patient and the referring physician. In the context of a collaborative relationship, it is useful to discuss the roles of each provider to clarify the primary relationship of the physician with the patient and the role of the mental health professional as a consultant. The patient may be informed that the providers will be working together and sharing information on an ongoing basis. This helps to reassure the patient that her care is monitored and that her providers are well informed. The development of a collaborative relationship between the primary care provider and the mental health professional can ensure high-quality patient care. In this time of increasing demands on the time and energy of the physician and increased attention on patient satisfaction with medical care, the psychological consultant can be an important adjunct in the health care of women.

REFERENCES

Abbey A, Halman L, Andrews F: Psychosocial, treatment and demographic predictors of the stress associated with infertility. *Fertil Steril* 1992; 57:122-127.

Abraham S, Mira M: Psychosocial forces in premenstrual syndrome. In Demers L, McGuire J, Phillips A, Rubinow D, editors: *Premenstrual, postpartum and menopausal mood disorders,* Baltimore, 1989, Urban & Schwarzenberg, pp. 65-80.

American Psychiatric Association. *Diagnostic and statistical manual of mental diseases,* editions I to IV, Washington, D.C., 1952, 1968, 1987, 1994, American Psychiatric Association Press.

Appleby L, Warner R, Whitton A, et al: A controlled study of fluoxetine and cognitive/behavioral counselling in the treatment of postnatal depression. *BMJ* 1997; 314:932-936.

Arrizmendi T, Affonso D: Stressful events related to pregnancy and postpartum. *J Psychosom Res* 1987; 31:743-750.

Ashby CR, Carr LA, Cook CL, et al: Alteration of platelet serotonergic mechanisms and monoamine oxidase actitivity on premenstrual syndrome. *Biol Psychiatry* 1988; 24:225-228.

Bachmann G, Leiblum S, Sandler B, et al: Correlates of sexual desire in post-menopausal women. *Maturitas* 1985; 7:211-220.

Baram D, Tourelot E, Muechler E, et al: Psychosocial adjustment following unsuccessful in in vitro fertilization. *J Psychosom Obstet Gynecol* 1988; 9:181-190.

Benedek T: Infertility as a psychosomatic defense. *Fertil Steril* 1952; 3:527-541.

Berger D: Psychiatric and psychological aspects of male infertility. *Prog Reprod Biol* 1978; 3:157-162.

Blechman E: Premenstrual syndrome. In Blechman E, Brownell K, editors: *Handbook of behavioral medicine for women,* New York, 1988, Pergamon Press, pp. 80-91.

Boivin J, Takefman J: Stress levels across stages of in vitro fertilization in subsequently pregnant and nonpregnant women. *Fertil Steril* 1995; 64:802-806.

Boston Women's Health Book Collective. *The new our bodies, ourselves,* New York, 1992, Touchstone.

Brooks-Gunn J: Differentiating premenstrual symptoms and syndromes. *Psychosom Med* 1986; 48:385-390.

Burns L: An overview of the psychology of infertility. *Infertil Reprod Med Clin North Am* 1993; 4:433-454.

Casper R, Powell AM: Premenstrual syndrome: Documentation by linear analog scale compared with two descriptive scales. *Am J Obstet Gynecol* 1986; 155:862-867.

Choung C, Colligan R, Coulam C, et al: The MMPI as an aid in evaluating patients with premenstrual syndrome. *Psychosomatics* 1988; 29:197-199.

Cohen R: A brief history of the relationship between obstetrics and the mental health professions. In Cohen R, editor: *Psychiatric consultation in childbirth settings,* New York, 1988, Plenum, pp.13-19.

Coope J: Is oestrogen therapy effective in the treatment of menopausal depression? *J Roy Col Gen Pract* 1981; 31:134-140.

Cooper P, Campbell E, Day A, et al: Nonpsychotic psychiatric disorders after childbirth: A prospective study of prevalence, incidence, course and nature. *Br J Psychiatry* 1988; 152:799-806.

Coppen A, Eccleston E, Peet M: Total and free tryptophan in unipolar illness. *Lancet* 1976; 2:1249-1250.

Cox JL, Chapman G, Murray D, et al: Validation of the Edinburgh postnatal depression scale (EPDS) in non-postnatal women. *J Affect Disord* 1996; 39:185-189.

Cox JL, Holden JM, Sagovsky R: Detection of postnatal depression: Development of the 10 item Edinburgh Postnatal Depression Scale. *Br J Psychiatry* 1987; 150:782-786.

Cutrona C: Causal attributions and perinatal depression. *J Abnormal Psychol* 1983; 92:161-172.

Dalton K: *The premenstrual syndrome.* Springfield, 1964, Charles Thomas.

Dalton K: Prospective study into puerperal depression. *Br J Psychiatry* 1971; 118:689-694.

DeAngelis T: Menopause symptoms vary among ethnic groups. *APA Monitor*, November 16, 1997, p.16.

Daniluk J: Infertility: Intrapersonal and interpersonal impact. *Fertil Steril* 1988; 49:982-990.

Davis D: Women's status and experience of the menopause in a Newfoundland fishing village. *Maturitas* 1982; 4:207-216.

Demyttenaere K, Nijs P, Evers-Kiebooms, et al: Coping, ineffectiveness of coping and the psychoendocrinological stress responses during in vitro fertilization. *J Psychsom Res* 1991; 35:231-243.

Dennerstein L, Burrows G: A review of studies of the psychological symptoms found at menopause. *Maturitas* 1978; 1:55-61.

Dennerstein L, Burrows G, Hyman G, et al: Hormone therapy and affect. *Maturitas* 1979; 1: 247-254.

Domar AD, Seibel MM, Benson H: The mind/body program for infertility: A new behavioral treatment approach for women with infertility. *Fertil Steril* 1990; 53:246-253.

Eckerd M, Hurt S, Severino S: Late luteal phase dysphoric disorder: Relationship to personality disorder. *J Personal Disord* 1989; 3:338-342.

Edelmann R, Connolly K, Cooke I, et al: Psychogenic infertility: Some findings. *J Psychosom Obstet Gynecol* 1991; 12:163-166.

Elliot S: Postnatal depression: Consequences and intervention. In Demers L, McGuire J, Phillips A, Rubinow D, editors: *Premenstrual, postpartum and menopausal mood disorders,* Baltimore, 1989, Urban & Schwarzenberg, pp. 153-162.

Facchineti F, Volpe A, Matteo ML, et al: An increased vulnerability to stress is associated with a poor outcome of in vitro fertilization and embryo transfer treatment. *Fertil Steril* 1997; 67:309-315.

Fagan P, Schmidt C, Rock J, et al: Sexual functioning and psychological evaluation of in vitro fertilization couples. *Fertil Steril* 1986; 46:668-672.

Faludi S: *Backlash: An undeclared war against American women.* New York, 1991, Crown.

FitzGerald M, Malone KM, Li S, et al: Blunted serotonin response to fenfluramine challenge in premenstrual dysphoric disorder. *Am J Psychiatry* 1997; 154:556-558.

Frank R: The hormonal cause of premenstrual tension. *Arch Neurol Psychiatry* 1931; 26: 1053-1057.

Freeman E, Boxer A, Rickels K, et al: Psychological evaluation and support in a program of in vitro fertilization and embryo transfer. *Fertil Steril* 1985; 43:48-53.

Freeman E, Rickels K, Sondheimer S, et al: Ineffectiveness of progesterone suppository treatment for premenstrual syndrome. *JAMA* 1990; 264:349-353.

Gennaro S, Klein A, Miranda L: Health policy dilemmas related to high technology infertility services. *Image: J Nurs Sch* 1992; 24:191-199.

Goodale I, Domar A, Benson H: Alleviation of premenstrual syndrome symptoms with the relaxation response. *Obstet Gynecol* 1990; 75:649-655.

Gordon R, Gordon K, Gordon-Hardy L, et al: Predicting postnatal emotional adjustment with psychosocial and hormonal measures in early pregnancy. *Am J Obstet Gynecol* 1986; 155:80-85.

Gotlib I, Whiffen V, Mount J, et al: Prevalence rates and demographic characteristics associated with depression in pregnancy and the postpartum. *J Consult Clin Psychol* 1989; 57:269-274.

Gotlib I, Whiffen V, Wallace P: Prospective investigation of postpartum depression: Factors involved in onset and recovery. *J Abnorm Psychol* 1991; 100:122-132.

Gottlieb A: American premenstrual syndrome : A mute voice. *Anthropol Today* 1988; 4:10-22.

Graham C, Sherwin B: A prospective treatment study of premenstrual symptoms using a triphasic oral contraceptive. *J Psychosom Res* 1992; 36:257-263.

Greendale G, Sowers M: The menopause transition. *Endocrin Metab Clin North Am* 1997; 26:261-277.

Greene R, Dalton K: Premenstrual syndrome. *BMJ* 1953; 1:1007-1009.

Greenfeld D, Mazure C, Haseltine F, et al: The role of the social worker in the in vitro fertilization program. *Soc Work Health Care* 1984; 10:71-78.

Halbriech U, Endicott J: Classification of premenstrual syndromes. In Friedman R, editor: *Behavior and the menstrual cycle,* New York, 1982, Marcel Dekker, pp. 26-33.

Halbriech U, Endicott J, Schacht S, et al: The diversity of premenstrual changes as reflected in the Premenstrual Assessment Form. *Acta Psychiatr Scand* 1982; 65:46-65.

Hammarback S, Backstrom T: Induced anovulation as treatment of premenstrual tension syndrome: A double-blinded, crossover study of LRH agonist versus placebo. Presented at the Second International Symposium on Premenstrual, Postpartum and Menopausal Mood Disorders, Kiawah Island, S.C., Sept. 9, 1987.

Handley S, Dunn T Waldron G, et al: Mood changes in puerperium and plasma tryptophan and cortisol concentrations. *BMJ* 1977; 2: 18-21.

Handley S, Dunn T, Waldron G, et al: Tryptophan, cortisol, and puerperal mood. *BMJ* 1980; 136:498-500.

Harlow CR, Fahy UM, Talbot WM, et al: Stress and stress related hormones during in vitro fertilization treatment. *Hum Reprod* 1996; 11:274-279.

Harrison W, Endicott J, Nee J: Treatment of premenstrual dysphoria with alprazolam. *Arch Gen Psychiatry* 1990; 47:270-275.

Hayworth J, Little B, Bonham-Carter S, et al: A predictive study of postpartum depression: Some predisposing characteristics. *Br J Med Psychol* 1980; 53:161-167.

Holst J, Backstrom T, Hammarback S, et al: Progestogen addition during oestrogen replacement therapy: Effects on vasomotor symptoms and mood. *Maturitas* 1989; 11: 13-21.

Hopkins J, Campbell S, Marcus M: Role of infant related stressors in postpartum depression. *J Abnorm Psychol* 1987; 96:237-241.

Hopkins J, Marcus M, Campbell S: Postpartum depression: A critical overview. *Psychol Bull* 1984; 95:498-515.

Hurt S, Schnurr P, Severino S, et al: Late luteal phase dysphoric disorder in 670 women evaluated for premenstrual complaints. *Am J Psychiatry* 1992; 149:525-531.

Hutchinson K: Psychological aspects of menopause. *Infertil Reprod Med Clin North Am* 1993; 4:503-516.

Johnson T: Premenstrual syndrome as a Western culture-specific disorder. *Cult Med Psychiatry* 1987; 11:337-341.

Kessler RC, McGonagle KA, Zhao S, et al: Lifetime and 12-month prevalence of DSM-III R psychiatric disorders in the United States. *Arch Gen Psychiatry* 1994; 51:8-12.

Keye W: General evaluation of premenstrual symptoms. *Clin Obstet Gynecol* 1987; 30:396-401.

Keye W: Management of premenstrual syndrome. In Demers L, McGuire J, Phillips A, Rubinow D, editors: *Premenstrual, postpartum and menopausal mood disorders,* Baltimore, 1989, Urban & Schwarzenberg, pp. 81-103.

Klock S: Psychological aspects of donor insemination. *Infertil Reprod Clin North Am* 1993; 4:455-470.

Klock SC: Female sexuality and sexual counseling. *Curr Prob Obstet Gynecol Fertil* 1993; 16:99-139.

Klock S, Maier D: Guidelines for the provision of psychological services for infertility patients at the University of Connecticut Health Center. *Fertil Steril* 1991a; 56:680-685.

Klock S, Maier D: Psychological aspects of donor insemination. *Fertil Steril* 1991b; 56:489-495.

Kumar R, Robson K: A prospective study of emotional disorders in childbearing women. *Br J Pscyhiatry* 1984; 144:35-47.

Kupperman H, Wetchler B, Blatt M: Contemporary therapy of the menopausal syndrome. *JAMA* 1959; 171:1627-1630.

Lantos J: Second generation ethical issues in the new reproductive technologies. In Stotland N, editor: *Psychiatric aspects of reproductive technology,* Washington, D.C., 1990, American Psychiatric Association, pp. 87-96.

Lazarus R, Folkman S: *Stress, appraisal and coping,* New York, 1984, Springer.

Leiblum S, Kemmann E, Lane M: The psychological concomitants of in vitro fertilization. *J Psychosom Obstet Gynecol* 1987; 6:165-178.

Litt M, Tennen H, Affleck G, et al: Coping and cognitive factors in adaptation to in vitro fertilization failure. *J Behav Med* 1992; 15:171-187.

Maddocks S, Hahn P, Moller F, et al: A double blind placebo controlled trial of progesterone suppositories in the treatment of premenstrual syndrome. *Am J Obstet Gynecol* 1986; 154:573-580.

Magos A, Brewster E, Singh R, et al: The effects of norethisterone in postmenopausal women on oestrogen replacement therapy: A model for the premenstrual syndrome. *Br J Obstet Gynecol* 1986; 93:1290-1292.

Mahlstedt P: The psychological component of infertility. *Fertil Steril* 1985; 43:335-346.

Mai F, Munday R, Rump E: Psychosomatic and behavioural mechanisms in psychogenic infertility. *Br J Psychiatry* 1972; 120:199-204.

Mathis J: Psychiatry and the obstetrician-gynecologist. *Med Clin North Am* 1967; 51:1375-1381.

Maxson W: The use of progesterone in the treatment of premenstrual syndrome. *Clin Obstet Gynecol* 1987; 30:465-477.

McCoy N, Davidson J: A longitudinal study of the effects of menopause on sexuality. *Maturitas* 1985; 7:203-210.

McGrath E, Keita GP, Strickland B, et al: *Women and depression: Risk factors and treatment isues.* Washington, D.C., 1990, American Psychological Association.

Menkes D, Taghavi E, Mason P, et al: Fluoxetine treatment of severe premenstrual syndrome. *BMJ* 1992; 305:346-347.

Menning B: Psychosocial impact of infertility. *Nurs Clin North Am* 1982; 17:155-163.

Moller A, Fallstrom K: Psychological consequences of infertility: A longitudinal study. *J Psychosom Obstet Gynecol* 1991a; 12:27.

Moller A, Fallstrom K: Psychological factors in the etiology of infertility: A longitudinal study. *J Psychosom Obstet Gynecol* 1991b; 12:13-21.

Moos R: The development of a menstrual distress questionnaire. *Psychosom Med* 1968; 30:853-861.

Morse C: A critical review of methodological issues and approaches to managing premenstrual syndrome. *J Psychsom Obstet Gynecol* 1991; 12:133-142.

Morse C, Dennerstein L: Psychosocial aspects of the climacteric. In Demers L, McGuire J, Phillips A, Rubinow D, editors: *Premenstrual, postpartum and menopausal mood disorders,* Baltimore, 1989, Urban & Schwarzenberg, pp. 179-191.

Mosher W, Pratt W: Fecundity and infertility in the United States, 1965-1988. *Advance Data* 1990; 192:1-9.

Murray L: Effects of postnatal depression on infant development. In Kumar R, Brockington I, editors: *Motherhood and mental illness,* vol. 2, London, 1988, John Wright.

Muse K, Cetel N, Futterman, L, et al: The premenstrual syndrome: Effects of medical ovariectomy. *N Engl J Med* 1984; 311:345-349.

National Center for Health Statistics: *Reproductive impairments among married couples.* United States Vital and Health Statistics, Public Health Service, Washington D.C., 1982, U.S. Government Printing Office.

Neugarten B, Kraines F: Menopausal symptoms in women of various ages. *Psychosom Med* 1965; 27:266-273.

Newton C, Hearn M, Yuzpe A: Psychological assessment and follow-up after in vitro fertilization: Assessing the impact of failure. *Fertil Steril* 1990; 54:879-886.

Nicol-Smith L: Causality, menopause and depression: A critical review of the literature. *BMJ* 1996; 313:1229-1232.

Nott P, Franklin M Armitage C, et al: Hormonal changes and mood in the puerperium. *Br J Psychiatry* 1976; 128:379-384.

O'Hara M: Postpartum mood disorders: An overview. Presented at the Psychiatric Disorders Associated with Female Reproductive Function Course. Boston, Massachusetts General Hospital/Harvard Medical School, June 12, 1993.

O'Hara M: Psychologic and biologic factors in postpartum depression. In Demers L, McGuire J, Phillips A, Rubinow D, editors, *Premenstrual, postpartum and menopausal mood disorders,* Baltimore, 1989, Urban & Schwarzenberg, pp. 139-152.

O'Hara M: Social support, life events and depression during pregnancy and the puerperium. *Arch Gen Psychiatry* 1986; 43:569-573.

O'Hara M, Neunaber D, Zekoski E: Prospective study of postpartum depression: Prevalence, course and predictive factors. *J Abnormal Psychol* 1984; 93:158-171.

O'Hara M, Rehm L, Campbell S: Postpartum depression: A role for social network and life stress variables. *J Nerv Ment Dis* 1983a; 171:336-341.

O'Hara M, Rehm L, Campbell S: Predicting depressive symptomatology: Cognitive behavioral models and postpartum depression. *J Abnorm Psychol* 1983b; 91:457-461.

O'Hara M, Schlechte J, Lewis D, et al: Controlled prospective study of postpartum mood disorders: Psychological, environmental and hormonal variables. *J Abnorm Psychol* 1991; 100:63-73.

O'Hara M, Zekoski E, Phillips L, et al: Controlled prospective study of postpartum mood disorders: Comparisons of childbearing and nonchildbearing women. *J Abnorm Psychol* 1990; 99:3-15.

Paige K: The effects of oral contraceptives on affective fluctuations associated with the menstrual cycle. *Psychosom Med* 1971; 33:515-518.

Paykel ES, Emms EM, Fletcher J, et al: Life events and social support in puerperal depression. *Br J Psychiatry* 1980; 136:339-346.

Pearlstein T, Rosen K, Stone A: Mood disorders and menopause. *Endocrinol Metab Clin North Am* 1997; 26:279294.

Pearlstein TB, Stone AB: Long term fluoxetine treatment of late luteal phase dysphoric disorder. *J Clin Psychiatry* 1994; 55:332-335.

Porter M, Penney G, Russell D, et al: A population based survey of women's experience of the menopause. *Br J Obstet Gynecol* 1996; 103:1025-1028.

Powell S, Drotar D: Postpartum depressed mood: The impact of daily hassles. *J Psychosom Obstet Gynecol* 1992; 13:255-262.

Prior J, Vigna Y, Sciarretta D, et al: Conditioning exercise decreases premenstrual symptoms: A prospective, controlled 6 month trial. *Fertil Steril* 1987; 47:402-407.

Rapkin A: The role of serotonin in premenstrual syndrome. *Clin Obstet Gynecol* 1992; 35:146-153.

Reading A: Cognitive model of premenstrual syndrome. *Clin Obstet Gynecol* 1992; 35:693-701.

Reading A: Sexual aspects of infertility and its treatment. *Infertil Reprod Med Clin North Am* 1993; 4:559-568.

Reid R: Premenstrual syndrome. *Endocrinol Metab* 1987; 5:1-21.

Reid R, Yen S: Premenstrual syndrome. *Am J Obstet Gynecol* 1981; 139:85-105.

Riley G, Shaw D: Total and nonbound tryptophan in unipolar illnes. *Lancet* 1976; 2:1249-1251.

Rivera-Tovar A, Frank E: Late luteal phase dysphoric disorder in young women. *Am J Psychiatry* 1990; 147:1634-1642.

Robson K, Kumar R: Delayed onset of maternal affection after childbirth. *Br J Psychiatry* 1980; 136:347-354.

Rodin M: The social construction of premenstrual syndrome. *Soc Sci Med* 1992; 35:693-699.

Rubinow DR, Schmidt PJ: Premenstrual syndrome: A review of endocrine studies. *Endocrinologist* 1992; 2:47-54.

Ruble D: Premenstrual symptoms: A reinterpretation. *Science* 1977; 197:291-293.

Sampson G: Premenstrual syndrome: A double-blind controlled trial of progesterone and placebo. *Br J Psychiatry* 1979; 135:209-215.

Sandler S: Emotional stress and infertility. *J Psychosom Res* 1968; 12:51-59.

Sarrel P: Sex problems after menopause: A study of fifty married couples treated in a sex counseling programme. *Maturitas* 1982; 4:231-237.

Sarrel P: Sexuality and menopause. *Obstet Gynecol* 1990; 75(suppl):26-29.

Schmidt P, Rubinow D: Menopausal mood disorders. In Demers L, McGuire J, Phillips A, Rubinow D, editors: *Premenstrual, postpartum and menopausal mood disorders,* Baltimore, 1989, Urban & Schwarzenberg, pp. 193-203.

Schneider M, Brotherton P, Hailes J: The effects of exogenous oestrogens on depression in menopausal women. *Med J Austr* 1977; 2:162-163.

Shatford L, Hearn M, Yuzpe A, et al: Psychological correlates of dysfunctional infertility diagnosis in an in vitro fertilization program. *Am J Obstet Gynecol* 1988; 158:1099-1107.

Sherwin B: Affective changes with estrogen and androgen replacement therapy in surgically menopausal women. *J Affect Dis* 1988; 14:177-187.

Sherwin B: The impact of different doses of estrogen and progestin on mood and sexual behavior in postmenopausal women. *J Clin Endocrinol Metab* 1991; 72:336-343.

Sherwin B, Gelfand M: Sex steroids and affect in the surgical menopause: A double-blind, cross-over study. *Psychoneuroendocrinology* 1984; 10:325-335.

Sichel D: Psychiatric issues of the postpartum period. *Curr Affect Illness* 1992; 11:5-10.

Siddle N, Fraser D, Whitehead M, et al: Endometrial, physical and psychological effects of postmenopausal oestrogen therapy with added dydrogesterone. *Br J Obstet Gynecol* 1990; 97:1101-1107.

Smith S, Schiff I: The premenstrual syndrome—diagnosis and management. *Fertil Steril* 1989; 52: 527-535.

Steege J, Blumenthal J: The effects of aerobic exercise on premenstrual symptoms in middle aged women. *J Psychosom Res* 1993; 37:127-133.

Stein G, Milton F, Bebbington P, et al: Relationship between mood disturbances and free and total plasma tryptophan, cortisol and puerperal mood. *BMJ* 1976; 2:457-464.

Steiner M: Premenstrual syndromes. *Ann Rev Med* 1997; 48:447-455.

Steiner M, Steinberg S, Stewart, et al: Fluoxetine in the treatment of premenstrual dysphoria. *N Engl J Med* 1995; 332:1529-1534.

Stewart D, Stotland N: The interface between psychiatry and obstetrics-gynecology: An introduction. In Stewart D, Stotland N, editors: *Psychological aspects of women's health care.* Washington, D.C., 1993, American Psychiatric Association Press.

Stone A, Pearlstein T, Brown W: Fluoxetine in the treatment of late luteal phase dysphoric disorder. *J Clin Psychiatry* 1991; 52:290-293.

Stowe ZN, Nemeroff CB: Psychopharmocology during pregnancy and lactation. In Schatzberg AF, Nemeroff CB, editors: *Textbook of psychopharmology,* Washington, D.C., 1995, American Psychiatric Press.

Strauss B, Appelt H, Ulrich D: Relationship between psychological characteristics and treatment outcome in female patients from an infertility clinic. *J Psychosom Obstet Gynecol* 1992; 13:121-132.

Strickland B: Menopause. In Blechman E, Brownell K, editors: *Handbook of behavioral medicine for women,* New York, 1988, Pergamon, pp. 41-47.

Susman JL: Postpartum depressive disorder. *J Fam Pract* 1996; 43(suppl): S17-S24.

Takefman J, Brender W, Boivin J, et al: Sexual and emotional adjustment of couples undergoing infertility investigation and the effectiveness of preparatory information. *J Psychosom Obstet Gynecol* 1990; 11:275-290.

Taylor DL, Mathew RH, Ho BT Weinman M: Serotonin levels and platelet uptake during premenstrual tension. *Neuropsychobiology,* 1984; 12:16-18.

Treadway R, Kane F, Jarrehi-Zadeh A, et al: A psychoendocrine study of pregnancy and puerperium. *Am J Psychiatry* 1969; 125:86-91.

Valda J, Youdale M, Freeman R: Premenstrual assessment form typological categories: Classification of self-defined premenstrually symptomatic and asymptomatic women. *J Consult Clin Psychol* 1987; 55:418-422.

Van Keep P, Kellerhals J: The impact of sociocultural factors on symptom formation. *Psychother Psychosom* 1974; 23:251-263.

Veevers J: *Childless by choice.* Toronto, 1980, Butterworth.

Warner R, Appleby L, Whitton A, et al: Demographic and obstetric risk factors for postnatal psychiatric morbidity. *Br J Psychiatry* 1996; 168:607-611.

Watson J, Eliot S, Rugg A, et al: Psychiatric disorders in pregnancy and the first postnatal year. *Br J Psychiatry* 1984; 144:453-462.

Weissman M: The myth of involutional melancholia. *JAMA* 1979; 242:742-744.

Whiffen V: Vulnerability to postpartum depression: A prospective multivariate study. *J Abnormal Psychol* 1988; 97:467-474.

Wilbush J: Climacteric expression and social context. *Maturitas* 1982; 4:195-205.

Williams J: *Psychology of women*, ed. 2, New York, 1983, W.W. Norton, 1983.

Winokur G: Depression in the menopause. *Am J Psychiatry* 1973; 130:92-93.

Wisner KL, Perel JM, Findling RL: Antidepressant treatment during breast-feeding. *Am J Psychiatry* 1996; 153:1132-1137.

Wood S, Mortola J, Chan Y, et al: Treatment of premenstrual syndrome with fluoxetine: A double-blind, placebo-controlled, crossover study. *Obstet Gynecol* 1992; 80:339-344.

Yonkers KA, Halbriech U, Freeman E, et al: Sertaline in the treatment of premenstrual dysphoric disorder. *Psychopharmacol Bull* 1996; 32:41-46.

21

Menopause

BRIAN W. WALSH
ELIZABETH S. GINSBURG

KEY ISSUES

1. Because women are living longer, they are spending an increasing proportion of their lives in the post-menopausal state.
2. The loss of estrogen at the menopause has multiple consequences. A woman's immediate quality of life can be compromised, and her long-term risks for developing osteoporosis and heart disease will increase.
3. Estrogen treatment has multiple benefits but also some risks. Selective estrogen receptor modulators have the potential to provide some of the benefits with fewer risks.
4. For women who are unable or unwilling to take hormonal treatments, nonhormonal options are available.

Menopause is defined as the permanent cessation of menses. This is only one aspect of the climacteric, during which time women undergo endocrine, somatic, and psychological changes that span several years. Because these changes are related both to aging and to estrogen depletion, it is difficult to quantify the respective effects of each. This chapter addresses the consequences of declining estrogen production in postmenopausal women and the risks and benefits of hormonal replacement therapy.

AGING OF THE OVARY

The mean age of women at menopause is 51 years; approximately 4% of women undergo natural menopause before they are 40 years of age (Fig. 21-1) (McKinlay et al, 1972).

Menopause tends to occur earlier in women who smoke. It is slightly delayed in women who have had children or used oral contraceptives because they have had fewer ovulations earlier in life (Cramer et al, 1995). Although life expectancy rose considerably in the twentieth century, the average age at menopause has not changed significantly since antiquity (Amundsen and Piers, 1970). Today women in industrialized countries can expect to spend more than one third of their lives after menopause.

The ovary's aging process appears to begin during fetal development. Although 7 million oogonia are present at 20 weeks' gestation, only 700,000 remain at birth (Schiff and Wilson, 1978). After birth, the number of oocytes continues to decline even before the onset of puberty.

For several years before menopause, estradiol and progesterone production decline despite the occurrence of ovulatory cycles (Sherman et al, 1976). This waning of ovarian follicular activity reduces the negative feedback inhibition of estradiol and inhibin on the hypothalamic-pituitary system, resulting in a gradual rise in follicle-stimulating hormone (FSH). The remaining ovarian follicles are increasingly those less responsive to FSH; menopause occurs when the residual follicles are refractory to elevated concentrations of FSH.

Estrogen production by the postmenopausal ovary is minimal (Fig. 21-2). The major source of postmenopausal estrogens is adrenal androgens, particularly androstenedione, which undergoes aromatization by peripheral tissues to estrone. Typically, 2.8% of androstenedione is converted to estrone, but higher rates are seen in obese women who have more adipose tissue to aromatize androgens (Groden et al, 1973). This explains in part why obese women have fewer menopausal symptoms than thin women (Erlik et al, 1982). The mean postmenopausal concentration of estrone (35 pg/mL) is higher than the mean concentration of estradiol (13 pg/mL) (Vermeulen, 1976). This estradiol is produced by conversion from estrone.

The postmenopausal ovary continues to produce testosterone and androstenedione primarily from stromal and hilar cells (Fig. 21-3). The mean concentration of testosterone in postmenopausal women (approximately 250 pg/mL) is slightly lower than it is in premenopausal women. In contrast, the mean postmenopausal concentration of

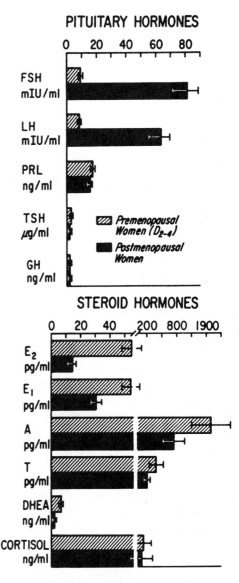

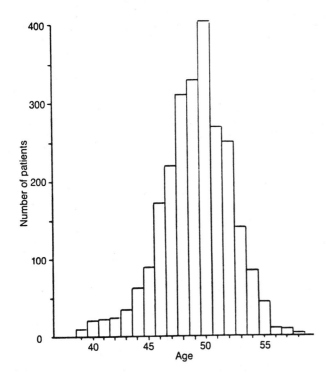

Fig. 21-1. Age of menopause in 2000 women during a natural menopause. (From Gambrell RD Jr: The menopause: Benefits and risks of estrogen-progesterone replacement therapy. *Fertil Steril* 1982; 32:457.) Copyright © 1982, American Medical Association.

Fig. 21-2. Circulating concentrations of pituitary and steroid hormones in premenopausal (menstrual cycle day 2 to 4) and postmenopausal women. (From Yen SSC: The biology of menopause. *J Reprod Med* 1977; 18:28.)

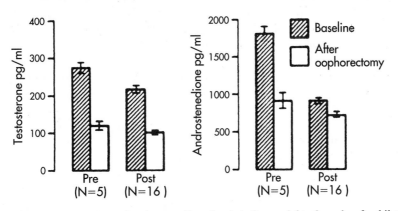

Fig. 21-3. Serum testosterone and androstenedione levels before and 6 to 8 weeks after bilateral oophorectomy. Five premenopausal (Pre) and 16 postmenopausal (Post) women were studied. (From Judd HL, Lucas WE, Yen SSC: Effect of oophorectomy on testosterone and androstenedione levels. *Am J Obstet Gynecol* 1974; 118:793.)

androstenedione (850 pg/mL) is approximately half the concentration in premenopausal women (1500 pg/mL) (Vermeulen, 1976). Because they are no longer opposed by estrogens, these postmenopausal androgens may lead to increased hair growth on the upper lip and the chin.

VASOMOTOR FLUSHES

Vasomotor flushes are one of the most common and troublesome symptoms for women at the climacteric; approximately 80% of women experience hot flashes within 3 months of a natural or a surgical menopause. Of these women, 85% have them for more than 1 year, and 25% to 50% have them for as long as 5 years (Thompson et al, 1973). For most women, the onset of hot flashes occurs before the final menstrual period. Hot flashes lessen in frequency and intensity with advancing age, unlike the other sequelae of menopause that progress with time.

Definitions and Pathophysiology

Hot flashes are the subjective sensation of intense warmth of the upper body that typically last for 4 minutes and that range in duration from 30 seconds to 5 minutes (Chang and Judd, 1979). They often follow a prodrome of palpitations or a sensation of pressure within the head, and they may be accompanied by weakness, faintness, or vertigo. They usually end in sweating and a cold sensation.

The frequency of hot flashes varies from several per year to many per day. They tend to occur at night when they may cause awakening. This was shown by Erlik et al (1981b), who monitored the stages of sleep with a sleep polygraph (electroencephalogram, electromyelogram, and electrooculogram) while simultaneously recording finger temperature and skin resistance as objective indices of vasomotor flushes (Fig. 21-4). Waking episodes were indeed temporally associated with the occurrence of hot flashes. The resultant poor quality of sleep may lead to chronic fatigue, characterized by symptoms such as irritability, poor concentration, and impaired memory.

A *vasomotor flush* is the objective component of this phenomenon and is characterized by a visible ascending flush of the thorax, neck, and face. First peripheral blood flow increases, particularly to the fingers, and skin temperature reaches a maximum 5 minutes later. This increase in blood flow appears to be limited to the cutaneous vasculature and does not involve blood flow to muscle; thus, blood pressure remains stable during a flush. Loss of body heat through the skin causes the core body temperature to fall (Mashchak et al, 1985a). The final event occurs when the plasma luteinizing hormone level rises and reaches its peak 12 minutes after the flush begins.

Etiology

Hot flashes result from the withdrawal of estrogens, not from hypoestrogenism per se. They accompany the menopause, whether it be natural, surgical, or medical (i.e.,

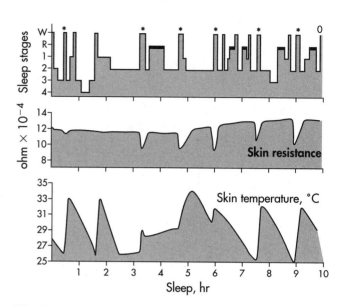

Fig. 21-4. Sleepgram and recordings of skin resistance and temperature in a postmenopausal subject with severe hot flashes. Asterisks denote objectively measured hot flashes. (From Erlik Y, Tatarun IV, Meldrum DR, et al: Association of waking episodes with menopausal hot flushes. *JAMA* 1981b; 245:1741.) Copyright © 1981, American Medical Association.

hypoestrogenism induced by the use of long-acting gonadotropin-releasing hormone agonists or by danazol). Discontinuation of exogenous estrogens may precipitate flashes; for example, women with Turner syndrome, who are hypoestrogenic, do not have hot flashes unless exogenous estrogens have been prescribed and later are withdrawn (Yen, 1977).

Obese women usually are less troubled by hot flashes (Erlik et al, 1982) than thin women because they tend to have higher levels of estrogen. This appears to result because the increased adiposity of obese women allows for greater peripheral conversion of adrenal androgens into estrogens (Grodin et al, 1973) and because their sex hormone-binding globulin levels are typically lower. As a result, a greater proportion of their estrogens are unbound and are free to act on target tissues (Fig. 21-5) (Davidson et al, 1981).

Men also may have hot flashes, but these are a consequence of testosterone withdrawal. They develop in three quarters of men with prostate cancer who are treated by orchiectomy (Charig et al, 1989) or with GnRH agonists (Smith, 1984), which lower serum testosterone to castrate levels. Similarly, 62% of men in whom testicular insufficiency has been developing have flashes, which are considerably alleviated by testosterone replacement (Norcross and Schmidt, 1986). Treatment with estrogens provides relief, but symptoms may return when estrogen treatment is discontinued (Huggins et al, 1941). Androgens do not have to be converted to estrogen to suppress hot flashes because a nonaromatizable androgen, fluoxymesterone, effectively relieves them (Defazio et al, 1984).

Vasomotor flushes are caused by an acute lowering of the set point of the thermoregulatory center located in the hypo-

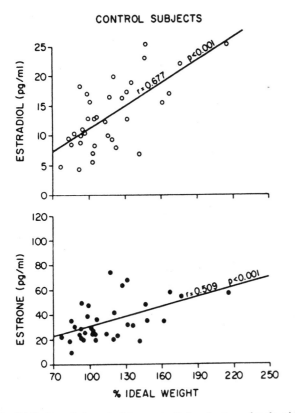

CONTROL SUBJECTS

Fig. 21-5. Correlation of plasma estradiol and estrone levels with percentage of ideal weight in postmenopausal women. (From Judd HL, Davidson BJ, Frumar AM, et al: Serum androgens and estrogens in postmenopausal women. *Am J Obstet Gynecol* 1980; 36:859.)

thalamus, which is precipitated by estrogen withdrawal. The presence of estrogen may stabilize the thermoregulatory center by maintaining hypothalamic opioid activity. Loss of estrogen at menopause may cause a hypothalamic "opioid withdrawal" that leads to thermoregulatory instability. This hypothesis is supported by the observation that estrogen prescribed in physiologic amounts induces hypothalamic opioid activity (D'Amico et al, 1991).

Estrogen's stabilizing effect on the hypothalamic thermoregulatory center can be mediated by neurotransmitters such as norepinephrine. As shown in Fig. 21-6 (Berkow, 1987), the intraneuronal level of norepinephrine is regulated by the balance between the enzymes tyrosine hydroxylase (the rate-limiting step of norepinephrine synthesis from tyrosine) and monoamine oxidase (which irreversibly degrades norepinephrine to inactive metabolites). After synthesis, norepinephrine is stored in prejunctional vesicles; when released into the synaptic cleft, it binds to postjunctional receptors to propagate a response, either excitatory or inhibitory. This action is terminated by the rapid reuptake of norepinephrine into the postjunctional neuron.

In animals, estrogen has multiple effects on norepinephrine neurons. It stimulates tyrosine hydroxylase activity (Beattie et al, 1972), thereby increasing norepinephrine synthesis. In addition, estrogen reduces monoamine oxidase activity (Luine and McEwen, 1977) and so retards norepinephrine degradation. Each of these actions increases the intraneuronal level of norepinephrine. Estrogen also augments norepinephrine release (Paul et al, 1979) and inhibits

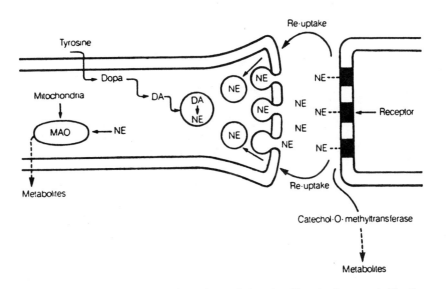

Fig. 21-6. Schematic representations of an adrenergic junction. Tyrosine is converted by the enzyme tyrosine hydroxylase to 3,4-dihydroxyphenylalanine (Dopa), decarboxylated to dopamine (DA), hydroxylated to form norepinephrine (NE), and stored in vesicles. On release, norepinephrine interacts with adrenergic receptors. This action is terminated by reuptake of norepinephrine into the prejunctional neurons. Norepinephrine is degraded into inactive metabolites by monoamine oxidase (MAO) and catechol-O-methyltransferase. (From Berkow R, editor: *The Merck manual of diagnosis and therapy,* Rahway, NJ, 1987, Merck, Sharp & Dohme Research Laboratories, p. 2474.)

norepinephrine reuptake (Nixon et al, 1974), thereby potentiating its effect on postjunctional receptors. Finally, estrogen appears to increase the number of hypothalamic α_2 postsynaptic receptors (Johnson et al, 1985). All these actions of estrogen enhance α_2 adrenergic activity. Estrogen withdrawal appears to cause vasomotor flushes by reducing α_2 adrenergic activity. This explains why α_2 agonists, such as clonidine (Clayden et al, 1974), aldomet (after conversion to its active form, methylnorepinephrine) (Hammond et al, 1984), and lofexidine (Jones et al, 1985) suppress hot flashes and why yohimbine, which inhibits presynaptic α_2 receptors, provokes hot flashes (Freedman and Woodward, 1992). This further explains why estrogen treatment must be given for 2 to 4 weeks before hot flashes are maximally relieved (Haas et al, 1988) because it does not act directly but must alter central norepinephrine metabolism. This alteration of norepinephrine metabolism may persist for a short time after estrogen withdrawal, explaining why relief of hot flashes continues for a few weeks after estrogens are discontinued.

Diagnosis

Patient history and physical examination should be sufficient to make the diagnosis and to exclude other conditions that may resemble hot flashes, such as thyrotoxicosis, carcinoid tumor, pheochromocytoma, anxiety, diabetic insulin reaction, alcohol withdrawal, and diencephalic epilepsy. Any drug or process that releases histamine, vasoactive peptide (substance P), or prostaglandin may induce flushes; these include nitroglycerine, nifedipine, niacin, vancomycin, calcitonin, ethanol, monosodium glutamate, disulfiram, and corticotropin-releasing hormone. Menopause may be con-

firmed, if necessary, by an elevated serum FSH level. However, a low serum estradiol level is not diagnostic because premenopausal women often have low levels during menses.

Treatment
Estrogens

Because hot flashes result from estrogen withdrawal, the obvious choice for therapy is estrogen replacement; this results in greater than 95% efficacy. By relieving hot flashes, particularly those occurring at night, estrogen replacement improves sleep quality. Estrogen treatment has been shown to reduce sleep latency and to increase rapid eye movement sleep (Schiff et al, 1979). In a double-blinded, placebo-controlled study, estrogen use decreased insomnia, irritability, and anxiety, and improved memory (Campbell and Whitehead, 1977). Thus those symptoms that appear to result from chronic sleep disturbance are significantly improved by estrogen replacement.

Treatment with estrogen does not produce immediate relief of hot flashes (Fig. 21-7) (Haas et al, 1988). Hot flash frequency is not reduced until after 2 weeks of treatment and is not maximal until 4 weeks. Treatment for 1 month is necessary before the adequacy of any dose can be evaluated. After 1 month, the dose may be increased (there appears to be a dose-response relationship between the dose of estrogen and the degree to which hot flashes are suppressed). For example, 3-week treatment with transdermal estradiol 0.025 mg reduces the occurrence of flashes by 40%, 0.05 mg reduces them by 53%, 0.10 mg reduces them by 83%, and 0.20 mg reduces them by 91% (Steingold et al, 1985).

Estrogen replacement is not a permanent cure for hot flashes; they return when treatment is discontinued. The pa-

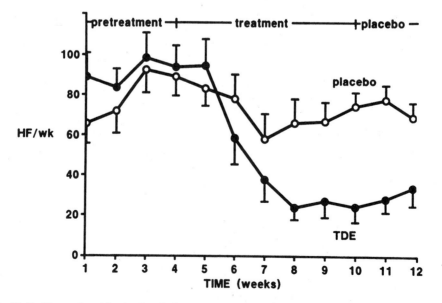

Fig. 21-7. Change in subjective hot flashes (HF) recorded by postmenopausal women treated with transdermal estrogen (TDE) and placebo. (From Haas S, Walsh B, Evans S, et al: The effect of transdermal estradiol on hormone and metabolic dynamics over a 6-week period. Reprinted with permission from the American College of Obstetricians and Gynecologists [Obstetrics and Gynecology, 1988; 71:671].)

tient should be advised of this when terminating estrogen therapy. The return of hot flashes may be minimized by slowly tapering the dose over a period of several weeks.

Progestins

Women with endometrial cancer who were treated with depo-medroxyprogesterone acetate (depo-MPA) were incidentally noted to have relief from their hot flashes. A clinical trial later found that depo-MPA has a dose-dependent effect; 50 mg reduced flashes by 60%, 100 mg by 75%, and 150 mg by 85% (Morrison et al, 1980). The frequency of hot flashes was reduced within 2 weeks of injection, became maximal at 4 weeks, and remained suppressed for the remainder of the 12 weeks of observation. The temporal relationship and the dose-dependency in the relief of hot flashes resembled that seen with transdermal estrogens. Oral MPA, 10 mg daily, has also been found to reduce flush frequency by 87% (Albrecht et al, 1981).

The mechanism of action of progestins is unknown. It has been hypothesized that they, too, may act through central neurotransmitters because they raise the hypothalamic thermoregulatory set point during the luteal phase of ovulation. Progestins are useful for patients for whom estrogen is contraindicated, but they may cause irregular vaginal bleeding, abdominal bloating, constipation, breast tenderness, and mood changes.

α-Adrenergic Agonists

Women treated with antihypertensive medicines were noted to have fewer hot flashes. It is hypothesized that these drugs alter hypothalamic neurotransmitters, thereby "stabilizing" the thermoregulatory center. They may also act directly on the peripheral vasculature to block cutaneous vasodilation. Clonidine, an α-adrenergic agonist, is known to reduce the frequency of hot flashes by 30% to 40% when used at doses of 0.1 mg and 0.2 mg twice daily. At these doses, patients often complain of dizziness and dry mouth (Laufer et al, 1982). For this reason, the initial dose should be 0.05 mg twice daily; it can be increased to 0.1 mg twice daily if hot flashes persist and if there are no side effects. Similarly, another α-adrenergic agonist, lofexidine, was found to reduce hot flashes by as much as 66% (Jones et al, 1985). The initial dose of lofexidine (0.1 mg twice daily) was increased by increments of 0.1 mg (up to a maximum of 0.6 mg) every 2 weeks until flashes ceased or until side effects such as dry mouth, fatigue, and headache were intolerable. Methyldopa (250 mg three times a day) has also been found to reduce hot flashes by 20% (Hammond et al, 1984). Because the use of α-adrenergic agonists is limited by their side effects, patients with hypertension are the best candidates for this nonhormonal treatment.

Veralipride

Veralipride, an antidopaminergic drug, has been found to reduce the frequency of hot flashes significantly in premenopausal women treated with GnRH agonists (Vercellini et al, 1992) and in postmenopausal women (Boukobza, 1986). The usual dose is 100 mg daily. Neither study compared veralipride with placebo.

Bellergal

Bellergal, a preparation of ergotamine tartrate, belladonna alkaloids, and 40 mg phenobarbital, is 50% effective when given as one tablet twice daily (Lebherz and French, 1969). Which of the components is responsible for its effect is unknown. This medicine is rarely used because it has addictive potential and safer alternative treatments are available.

Herbs

Dong quai, derived from the root of *Angelica sinensis,* was evaluated in a randomized, double-blinded, placebo-controlled study of 71 postmenopausal women. It was found to be no better than placebo in relieving menopausal hot flashes or vaginal atrophy, and it did not cause endometrial thickening. In addition, estradiol, estrone, and sex hormone-binding globulin levels were unchanged by dong quai treatment (Hirata et al, 1997). Soy flour, which contains the phytoestrogen daidzin, was compared to wheat flour in a randomized, double-blinded, 12-week study of 58 subjects. Both treatments significantly reduced the frequency of hot flashes—by 40% in the soy group and by 25% in the wheat flour group. The reduction from soy occurred earlier, by 6 weeks (Murkies et al, 1995). Anecdotally, ginseng black cohash and St. John's Wort, available in health food stores, have been touted to relieve hot flashes; however, no scientific data are available. It is tempting for patients to seek alternative therapies, and they often assume that if a product is "natural" or plant derived, it is free of side effects or potential harm. This is potentially dangerous thinking. For example, ginseng may have estrogen-like effects on gene expression in breast cancer cell lines, and it was not found to cause cell proliferation in a breast cancer cell line. However, it did have estradiol-like effects on ps2 gene RNA production (Duda et al, 1996).

Agents such as tricyclic antidepressants and oxazepam have been proposed for the treatment of hot flashes. Because they have not been compared with placebo, their therapeutic efficacy remains unproven. Comparison with placebo is important because many investigators have shown that placebo significantly reduces hot flashes. Nonmedical treatments are under evaluation for the treatment of hot flashes. One of them, paced respiration, has been found useful in relieving flushes (Freedman et al, 1992).

OSTEOPOROSIS
Definition and Etiology

Osteoporosis is a systemic skeletal disease characterized by low bone mass and microarchitectural deterioration of bone tissue, with a consequent increase in bone fragility and susceptibility to fracture. The World Health Organization suggests that osteoporosis be defined as a bone mineral density

2.5 standard deviations or more below the young adult peak mean and that low bone density, or osteopenia, be defined as a bone mineral density between 1 and 2.5 standard deviations below the young adult mean. Osteoporosis develops when the rate of bone resorption exceeds the rate of bone formation. It affects trabecular bone earlier than cortical bone, and its major consequence is increased risk for fracture. The most common sites of fracture are the vertebral bodies, the distal radius, and the femoral neck.

Primary osteoporosis results from estrogen deficiency and constitutes 95% of all cases. Because estrogen receptors are present in bone, estrogen may act on bone directly (Komm et al, 1988). Estrogen may also act by any of three additional mechanisms. First, it may decrease the sensitivity of bone to parathyroid hormone without changing the amount of circulatory parathyroid hormone. Second, it may increase calcitonin levels. This is evident by three findings: high estrogen states, produced by oral contraceptives and pregnancy, are associated with elevated calcitonin levels (Lindsay and Sweeney, 1976a); men, who have greater bone mass than women, have higher calcitonin levels (Hillyard et al, 1978); calcitonin levels decline with age (Deftos et al, 1980) and with menopause and rise with estrogen replacement (Stevenson et al, 1990). Third, estrogen may directly increase intestinal calcium absorption.

Secondary osteoporosis constitutes the minority of cases and may result from any of the following: glucocorticoid (Mateo et al, 1993) or heparin use, renal failure, hyperthyroidism (endogenous or iatrogenic) (Schneider et al, 1994), primary hyperparathyroidism, and hyperadrenalism. It also may occur as a result of dietary calcium deficiency or upper intestinal surgery.

Incidence

At all ages, women have less bone mass than men. Both sexes achieve peak bone mass at age 30 and progressively lose bone mass at a rate of approximately 1% to 2% per year after age 40 (Heanly, 1976). In women this rate increases to 3% to 9% per year for 6 years after menopause (Fig. 21-8) (Horsman et al, 1977).

Anyone with lower peak bone mass is more likely to develop significant osteoporosis. Thus, women are at higher risk than men, white and Asian persons are at higher risk than black persons (Smith et al, 1973), and thin women are at higher risk than obese women (Tremollieres et al, 1993). The greater bone mass of obese women may be a consequence of their increased weight, which mechanically stresses their axial skeleton. It also may be a consequence of their higher levels of endogenous estrogen, which result from increased peripheral aromatization of androstenedione to estrogen (Grodin et al, 1973) and from lower sex hormone-binding globulin levels with the concomitantly greater free estradiol levels (Davidson et al, 1981). Women with prior fractures are twice as likely to have subsequent fractures than women with equivalent bone density (Lauritzen et al, 1993).

Rates of bone loss vary greatly. Women who smoke (Hopper and Seeman, 1994), drink alcohol, are sedentary (Krall and Dawson-Hughes, 1993), or consume two or more cups of coffee per day lose bone mass more quickly (Barrett-Connor et al, 1994). In addition, low calcium consumption and high-protein or high-phosphate diets accelerate bone loss in women (Licata et al, 1981). Family history is also a significant risk factor, perhaps because of the presence of one or both alleles for a "low-activity" vitamin D receptor protein gene. A study of 117 women, most of whom were Anglo-Irish, found that 74% of those women who did not have this allele had bone densities above the fracture threshold, whereas 61 % of women with both of these alleles had bone densities below that threshold (Mundy, 1994). Future studies are needed to demonstrate that this allele is a reliable marker for fracture risk.

Twenty-five percent of women older than 60 show vertebral fractures on x-ray examination, as do 50% of women older than 75 (Alffam, 1964; Iskrant, 1968). Twenty-five percent of women older than 80 have had hip fractures (Gambrell, 1982); the annual incidence is 1.3% after age 65 and 3.3% after age 85 (Lindsay et al, 1984). One of six women dies within 3 months of a hip fracture (Gallagher and Nordin, 1973). The annual health care cost in the United

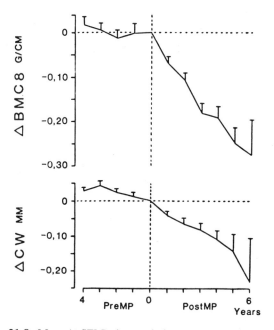

Fig. 21-8. Mean (±SEM) changes in bone mass, measured as bone mineral content (g/cm³) of the proximal (BMC8) forearm and mean conical width (CW) (millimeters) of metacarpals 2, 3, and 4 of both hands. Δ, changes from the last premenopausal (PreMP) yen. Broken horizontal line gives values for the last premenopausal year (0), and the broken vertical line indicates the last premenopausal year. (From Falch JA, Oftebro H, Haug E: Early postmenopausal bone loss not associated with decrease in vitamin D. *J Clin Endocrinol Metab* 1987; 64:836.)

States for these fractures is estimated to be more than 10 billion dollars.

Diagnosis

Once osteoporosis develops, significant reversal may not be possible. Unfortunately, known risk factors for osteoporosis (age, weight, calcium intake, caffeine intake, alcohol and tobacco use, and urinary markers of bone turnover) do not identify 30% of women with low bone mass (Slemenda et al, 1990). Radiologic techniques are used to detect early loss of bone mass before significant osteoporosis develops. Early detection provides the opportunity to initiate treatment before fractures occur. For every standard deviation below mean peak bone density, the risk for fracture is increased twofold. Because osteoporosis affects trabecular bone earlier than cortical bone, those modalities that preferentially measure trabecular bone are the most informative.

Single-photon absorptiometry of the distal radius is inexpensive and easy to perform, and it requires only 5 mrem of radiation. Because the distal radius consists of 75% cortical bone and only 25% trabecular bone, measurement at this site may not detect early bone loss. In skilled hands, it is accurate within 5% and has a precision of 2% to 4% (Dequeker and Johnston, 1981). Dual-photon absorptiometry of the second to fourth vertebral bodies offers an advantage because these sites consist of 60% cortical bone and 40% trabecular bone. It is more expensive, requires 5 to 15 mrem of radiation, is accurate within 5% to 7%, and has a precision of 2% to 5% (Dequeker and Johnston, 1981).

Computerized tomography of the vertebral body measures 5% cortical bone and 95% trabecular bone. Therefore, it may detect changes in as brief an interval as 6 months (Cann et al, 1980). It has the greatest radiation exposure

(200 mrem), is the most expensive modality, and has a precision of 1% to 3%.

The most recent modality to be developed, quantitative digital radiography, has become the technique of choice. It provides high-resolution images with excellent precision (1% to 2%) and low radiation exposure (1 to 3 mrem) (Mazess et al, 1992). It requires less than 8 minutes per study, which is considerably shorter than the 20 to 45 minutes needed for dual-photon absorptiometry.

Ultrasound densitometry is under investigation because it uses no ionizing radiation, is portable, and is low in cost (Schott et al, 1993). Nearly all studies are performed using the os calcis (heel) because it is easily accessible and it consists of trabecular bone. A prospective study of 3100 women, ages 45 to 75, found that the relative risk of spine fractures was 1.9 per 1 standard deviation decrease in density measured by heel ultrasonography (Thompson et al, 1996).

Measurement of a woman's bone density today has limited predictive value for future bone density. To identify women who are "fast bone losers" (*i.e.,* greater than 3.1% loss of forearm bone mineral content per year) a nonradiologic method has been evaluated (Christiansen et al, 1987). A single measurement of a fasting urinary calcium-creatinine ratio greater than 270 mmol/ mol, a fasting urinary hydroxyproline-creatinine ratio greater than 11.2 mol/mol, a serum alkaline phosphatase greater than 120 μg/L, *and* a fat mass index less than 0.222 (calculated from height and weight) correctly identified 79% of the "fast losers" and 78% of the "slow losers." Unfortunately, the predictive value of this approach is only 53%.

Patients who have osteoporosis or osteoporosis-related fractures should undergo careful history and physical examination to exclude an underlying cause. Measurements of serum calcium, phosphate, alkaline phosphatase, creatinine, erythrocyte sedimentation rate, thyroid studies, or serum protein electrophoresis may assist in identifying any underlying disorder, but values will be normal in patients with primary osteoporosis.

Treatment

Because established osteoporosis may not be significantly reversed, medical management should emphasize prophylaxis rather than treatment. Patients should be advised to stop smoking, reduce the intake of dietary phosphates, and exercise regularly to preserve bone mass.

Estrogens

Estrogens have been shown to prevent the loss of bone mass and to reduce the incidence of osteoporotic fractures. They act by decreasing bone resorption (Fig. 21-9) (Christiansen et al, 1981), by increasing intestinal calcium absorption, and by reducing renal calcium excretion (Lobo et al, 1983). Low doses of estrogen appear to be as effective as higher doses; 0.625 mg and 1.25 mg of conjugated equine estrogen (CEE)

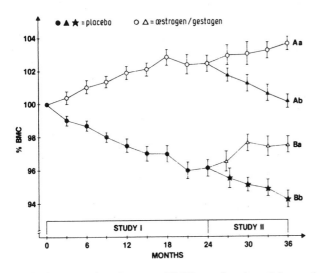

Fig. 21-9. Bone mineral content (BMC) as a function of time and treatment in 94 (study I) and 77 (study II) women soon after menopause. (From Christiansen C, Christiansen MS, Transbol I: Bone mass in postmenopausal women after withdrawal of estrogen-gestagen replacement therapy, *Lancet* 1981; 1:459.)

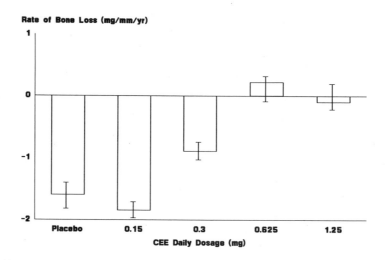

Fig. 21-10. Mean annual change (±SEM) in bone mass in women treated daily with placebo or with 0.15, 0.3, 0.625, or 1.25 mg oral CEE. Bone mineral content measured by single-photon absorptiometry at the midpoint of the third right metacarpal. (From Lindsay R, Hart DM, Clark DM: The minimum effective dose of estrogen for prevention of postmenopausal bone loss. Reprinted with permission from the American College of Obstetricians and Gynecologists [Obstetrics and Gynecology 1984; 63:759].)

are equally effective in preventing bone loss and in reducing the incidence of fractures (Fig. 21-10) (Weiss et al, 1980). An even lower dose of estrogen, 0.3 mg oral esterified estrogen given daily for 2 years, was found to increase bone density of the spine by 1% (Genant et al, 1997). Although ethinyl estradiol and mestranol are also effective (Lindsay et al, 1976b), conjugated estrogens and estradiol are preferred because they have less impact on the liver.

Because bone loss is irreversible, estrogen treatment initiated shortly after menopause will maximize the amount of bone preserved. Treatment should be taken for at least 6 years to reduce substantially the lifetime risk for fracture (Fig. 21-11) (Felson et al, 1993; Weiss et al, 1980). No method identifies all patients in whom osteoporosis will develop; hence, most postmenopausal women are potential candidates for this therapy. A measurement of baseline bone density may help patients for whom the decision to initiate estrogen replacement is difficult. However, normal bone density does not rule out the future development of osteoporosis.

Progestins

Used alone, progestins do not appear to preserve bone mass; 20 mg MPA daily for 2 years, was equivalent to placebo treatments (Gallagher et al, 1991). However, these investigators found that MPA, when combined with estrogen, may act synergistically to conserve bone mass, allowing a lower estrogen dose (*e.g.,* CEE 0.3 mg daily) to be used. A proposed mechanism is that progesterone may block glucocorticoid receptors located on bone (Monolagas et al, 1978), preventing endogenous glucocorticoids from exerting their inhibitory effects on bone metabolism.

Many women cannot or choose not to take hormonal treatment and are at risk for osteoporosis. For those women, multiple alternative therapies have been proposed. The following treatments have been evaluated recently for efficacy in preventing or treating osteoporosis: raloxifene, bisphosphonates, calcitonin, calcium, vitamin D, fluoride, and thiazides.

Raloxifene

See p. 561.

Bisphosphonates

Etidronate, a bisphosphonate, controls Paget disease of the bone because it retards osteoblastic and osteoclastic activity, which are both abnormally high in patients with this condition. However, when etidronate is given in low doses, the antiosteoclastic activity predominates so that bone mass may increase. Etidronate, prescribed four times per year in cycles of 400 mg daily for 2 weeks, increased vertebral bone density by 2% per year for 2 to 3 years. During that time, fracture rates were reduced by 50% to 70% (Storm et al, 1990; Watts et al, 1990). With longer durations of use, etidronate may cause focal osteomalacia from impairment of mineralization. Newer bisphosphonates, such as alendronate (Harris et al, 1993) and risedronate, may be superior to etidronate because they are more potent in suppressing osteoclast activity and they entail less inhibition of bone formation and mineralization. Alendronate, given as 10 mg daily for 3 years, increased the density of the spine by 8.8% and the femoral neck by 5.9% (Liberman et al, 1995). Vertebral fracture rates were reduced by 47%, with similar decreases in hip and wrist fractures (Black et al, 1996). Because alendronate can cause esophagitis (deGroen et al, 1996), the patient should take it with a glass of water and remain upright for 30 minutes after drinking. Bisphosphonates may offer promise as alternatives to estrogen in the prevention of osteoporosis, adjunctive treatments for women who have bone loss while taking estrogen, and treatments for established osteoporosis.

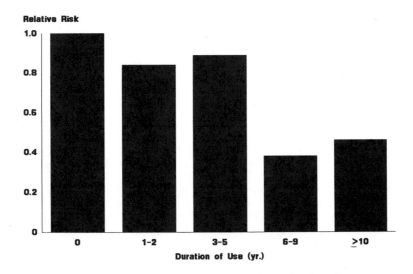

Fig. 21-11. Relative risk for hip or forearm fracture according to duration of postmenopausal estrogen use. (Data from Weiss NS, Ure CL, Bullard JH, et al: Decreased risk of fractures of the hip and lower forearm with postmenopausal use of estrogen. *N Engl J Med* 1980; 303:1195.)

Calcitonin

Calcitonin is a peptide hormone secreted by the C cells of the thyroid gland. Its main physiologic role is to protect against hypercalcemia, primarily by inhibiting bone resorption. It exerts this action by binding to high-affinity receptors on osteoclasts and markedly inhibiting osteoclast activity. Treatment with calcitonin has been found to increase bone mass to a variable extent; the greatest increases are seen in women with the highest rates of bone turnover (Civitelli et al, 1988). It appears to have a direct analgesic effect among patients with acute fractures. The usual dose is 50 to 100 U/day or every other day. Approximately 10% to 20% of patients have headache, nausea, and flushing when given the injectable form. A calcitonin nasal spray has been developed and is more acceptable. When given as 200 IU daily, it appeared to increase spine density by 2% over 2 years. In that study, there was a trend toward fewer vertebral and nonvertebral fractures (Chestnut et al, 1993).

Calcium

The efficacy of calcium in preventing postmenopausal bone loss has been controversial. One well-designed study found that oral calcium supplementation in early postmenopausal women with adequate dietary calcium intakes did not prevent bone loss (Fig. 21-12) (Riis et al, 1987). However, calcium use may prevent bone loss in selected patients as shown in a 2-year clinical trial of 300 healthy postmenopausal women who were given either placebo or 500 mg calcium carbonate or calcium citrate maleate (Dawson-Hughes et al, 1990). Calcium treatment did not prevent bone loss in women who had undergone menopause within the preceding 5 years or in those who consumed more than 400 mg calcium per day. For women who were 6 or more years into menopause and who consumed less than 400 mg calcium, calcium supplementation did prevent bone loss.

Calcium citrate maleate was more effective than calcium carbonate, possibly because of better gastrointestinal absorption. Thus it appears that calcium supplementation may reduce "age-related" bone loss several years after the menopause in women who have low dietary calcium intakes. Although calcium supplementation cannot prevent "estrogen-related" bone loss occurring shortly after the menopause, it may permit the use of a lower dose of estrogen (*e.g.,* 0.3 mg CEE) (Ettinger et al, 1984). Caution should be used with patients who have a history of renal stones.

That calcium may prevent "age-related" bone loss was also suggested in a study of 37 healthy premenopausal women between ages 30 and 42 (Baran et al, 1990). Half of these women were instructed to increase their dietary calcium intake by an average of 610 mg/day; age- and weight-matched controls maintained their usual diets. After 3 years, vertebral bone density was unchanged in the women who raised their calcium intake but was 3% lower in controls. The increase in dietary calcium was accompanied by an increased consumption of calories (28%), fat (38%), and protein (60%). In addition, the group with increased calcium gained 4.2 kg versus 3.4 kg for the control group over the 3 years. Thus, the prevention of age-related bone loss seen in this study may have resulted from increased body fat because of higher caloric consumption. The possibility does exist, however, that increasing dietary calcium peak bone mass in the third decade may reduce the age-related bone loss and perhaps lessen the incidence of osteoporotic fractures later in life.

Vitamin D

The biologically active form of vitamin D is 1, 25-dihydroxycholecalciferol. Its physiologic action is to increase the efficiency of intestinal calcium absorption and to increase osteoblast activity. A clinical trial in 3200 elderly

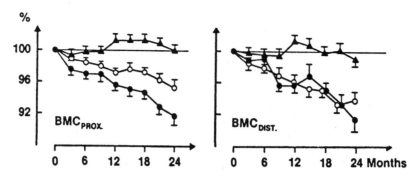

Fig. 21-12. Bone mineral content of the proximal (BMC$_{PROX}$) and distal (BMC$_{DIST}$) radius of post-menopausal women treated with percutaneous estrogens (solid triangle), calcium (open circle), and placebo (solid circle). (Data from Riis B, Thomsen K, Christiansen C: Does calcium supplementation prevent postmenopausal bone loss? *N Engl J Med* 1987; 316:173.)

women evaluated the effect of 18 months of treatment with vitamin D, 20 μg (800 IU)/day. Vitamin D intake significantly decreased the incidence of new hip fractures by 43% and nonvertebral fractures by 32% (Chapuy et al, 1992). Lower doses of vitamin D have been studied in other clinical trials and generally have not been effective. Because higher doses carry a risk for hypercalciuria and even hypercalcemia, this agent should be prescribed with caution.

Fluoride

Fluoride stimulates bone formation and increases cancellous bone mass as much as twofold (Briancon and Meunier, 1981). However, the bone formed is structurally abnormal, weak, and more likely to fracture. This was shown in a study of 200 postmenopausal women with osteoporosis who were randomized to treatment with sodium fluoride 75 mg/day or to placebo (Riggs et al, 1990). Although fluoride treatment increased vertebral bone density by 35%, it did not reduce the incidence of vertebral fractures. Most worrisome was that the incidence of nonvertebral fractures was three-fold higher in the fluoride group. This was attributed to a fluoride-induced loss of cortical bone suggested by a 4% decrease in density of the radial shaft. Fluoride increases cancellous bone at the expense of cortical bone. Not only is the additional cancellous bone structurally weak, which does not prevent vertebral fractures, but the loss of cortical bone increases the risk for fracture of nonvertebral bones. Therefore, fluoride does not appear to be effective in the prevention or treatment of osteoporosis.

Thiazide Diuretics

Thiazide diuretics may prevent osteoporosis because they reduce the urinary excretion of calcium. Two studies suggest that thiazides may prevent osteoporotic fractures. Lacroix et al (1990) prospectively studied 9500 elderly men and women for 4 years and identified 242 with hip fractures. After controlling for the greater body weight and the lower incidence of tobacco use of thiazide users, they found that the relative risk (RR) of hip fracture in thiazide users was significantly reduced to 0.68 and that the 95% confidence interval (CI) was 0.49 to 0.94. Felson et al (1991) analyzed 176 patients with hip fracture and 672 age-matched controls from the Framingham Study Cohort. Recent high-dose thiazide use reduced the risk for hip fracture (RR, 0.31; 95% CI, 0.11 to 0.88), but past use had no effect. Surprisingly, low-dose thiazide use appeared to increase the risk for hip fracture (RR, 2.23; 95% CI, 1.26 to 3.94), which may be a spurious finding. A clinical trial is necessary to define the optimal thiazide dose and the minimum treatment duration that preserves bone mass and to determine how long the benefit persists after treatment is discontinued. Whether thiazides should be used to prevent bone loss must take into account their potentially deleterious effects: increased plasma cholesterol, triglyceride, glucose, and uric acid levels; decreased high-density lipoprotein levels; and potassium depletion, which may predispose to arrhythmia. If the efficacy of thiazide diuretics in preventing fractures is confirmed by clinical trials and this benefit outweighs the risks inherent in thiazide use, then thiazides may be particularly beneficial in the medical treatment of postmenopausal women with hypertension.

GENITAL ATROPHY
Pathogenesis

The tissues of the lower vagina, labia, urethra, and trigone derive from a common embryonic origin, the urogenital sinus, and are all estrogen dependent (Iosef et al, 1981). After the loss of estrogen at menopause, the vaginal walls become pale because of diminished vascularity and thin (typically only three or four cells thick). Vaginal epithelial cells contain less glycogen, which, before menopause, had been metabolized by lactobacilli to create acidic pH, thereby protecting the vagina from bacterial overgrowth. Loss of this protective mechanism leaves the thin, friable tissue vulnerable to infection and ulceration. The vagina also loses its rugae and becomes shorter and inelastic.

Patients may have symptoms secondary to vaginal dryness, such as dyspareunia and vaginismus. These can compromise sexual satisfaction and lead to diminished libido.

They may also have symptoms secondary to vaginal ulceration and infection, such as vaginal discharge, burning, itching, and bleeding.

The urethra and the urinary trigone undergo atrophic changes similar to those of the vagina. Dysuria, urgency, frequency, and suprapubic pain may occur in the absence of infection. Presumably this occurs because the markedly thin urethral mucosa allows urine to come in close contact with sensory nerves. In addition, the menopausal loss of the resistance to urinary flow by thick, well-vascularized urethral mucosa has been hypothesized to contribute to urinary incontinence (Zinner et al, 1980).

Diagnosis

Atrophic vaginitis may be diagnosed by its typical appearance. Atrophy may be confirmed, if necessary, by a vaginal cell maturation index obtained by scraping the lateral vaginal wall at the level of the cervix. Exfoliated cells may be classified by degree of maturation, with a small proportion of superficial cells indicating a high degree of vaginal atrophy. If atypical lesions are present, samples should be taken for biopsy to establish a diagnosis. If a discharge is present, it should be evaluated for pathogens such as *Candida, Neisseria gonorrhoeae, Chlamydia, Trichomonas,* and *Gardnerella.* If *Candida* is found, the patient should be screened for diabetes because the low glycogen content of nonestrogenized vaginal epithelial cells ordinarily will not support its growth. Atrophic urethritis or trigonitis is diagnosed by ruling out the presence of infection. Urethroscopy is usually unnecessary but would reveal a pale, atrophic urethra.

Treatment

Estrogen therapy is effective; the dose required is generally lower than that needed to treat hot flashes or osteoporosis. Treatment for these conditions usually relieves genital atrophy and improves sexual satisfaction (Nathorst-Boos et al, 1993). Estrogen treatment has been found to reduce the incidence of recurrent urinary tract infections (Raz and Stamm, 1993). If atrophy is the only indication for estrogen treatment, daily use for a minimum of 2 to 12 weeks is needed to reverse the atrophic changes. Once atrophy is relieved, therapy may be tapered to two to three times per week. Usual daily oral doses are as follows: CEE, 0.3 mg or 0.625 mg; estrone, 0.3 mg, 0.625 mg, or 1.25 mg; or micronized estradiol, 1 mg or 2 mg (Carr and MacDonald, 1983). Transdermal estradiol, 50 μg twice weekly, is also effective. Estrogens such as CEE 0.3 mg (Fig. 21-13) (Mandel et al, 1983) or micronized β-estradiol 0.2 mg may be administered vaginally (Gordon et al, 1977). Although most of the estrogen acts locally, some of it is rapidly absorbed into the systemic circulation and may stimulate endometrial growth (Schiff et al, 1977). Generally, progestins should be given intermittently with vaginal estrogens for patients with an intact uterus and repeated for as long as the patient has withdrawal bleeding.

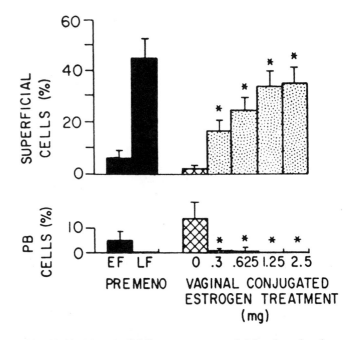

Fig. 21-13. Mean ($\pm$SEM) percentage superficial and parabasal (PB) cells from vaginal exfoliative cytology. Premenopausal controls in the early follicular (EF) and late follicular (LF) phases of their cycles are compared with postmenopausal women before and after vaginal administration of various doses of conjugated estrogen. *Indicates significant difference (<0.05) from the untreated postmenopausal value. (From Mandel FP, et al: Biologic effects of various doses of vaginally administered conjugated equine estrogens in postmenopausal women, *J Clin Endocrinol Metab* 1983; 57:133.)

If estrogens are contraindicated, synthetic mucopolysaccharides or water-soluble lubricants such as Replens (Warner-Lambert: Morris Plains, N.J.) may relieve dyspareunia. In fact, one double-blinded, randomized comparison of Replens and Premarin (Wyeth-Ayerst: Radnor, Pa.) vaginal cream, used three times per week for 3 months, found both agents to have the same effect on vaginal maturation scoring, pH, and moisture (Nachtigall, 1994). Vaginal stenosis may be improved by the use of graduated vaginal dilators.

ATHEROSCLEROSIS

Cardiovascular disease (CVD) is the leading cause of death among women in industrialized countries; more than 50% of postmenopausal women die of CVD. Estrogens have been hypothesized to protect against atherosclerosis because the incidence of CVD is low before menopause. The CVD mortality rate of premenopausal women is approximately one fifth that of men, but in postmenopausal women it rises exponentially to approach that of men (Fig. 21-14) (Lerner and Kannel, 1986). One explanation is that a premenopausal woman's estrogen confers protection lost at menopause. This is supported by the observation that women who undergo premature surgical menopause (bilateral oophorectomy) and

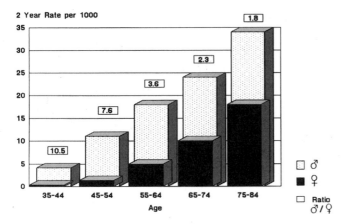

Fig. 21-14. Incidence of myocardial infarctions (MI) by age and sex (female, solid bar; male, stippled bar). Ratio of male-to-female MIs for each age group is noted at top of graph. (From Lerner DJ, Kannel WB: Patterns of coronary disease morbidity and mortality: A 26-year follow-up of the Framingham population. *Am Heart J* 1986; 111:383.)

do not use estrogen replacement have twice as much CVD as do age-matched premenopausal controls. If they use estrogen replacement, however, the incidence of CVD is the same as it is premenopausal women of the same age. Premature natural menopause, in contrast, has not been found to increase CVD risk when controlled for age, smoking, and estrogen use (Colditz et al, 1987).

Epidemiological Studies

Most epidemiological studies have found that there is a lower incidence of CVD in postmenopausal women who use estrogen than in those who do not. The Nurses' Health Study (Stampfer et al, 1991), the largest cohort study (it followed up 121,000 women for as long as 18 years) identified 425 cases of fatal myocardial infarction (MI). The adjusted relative risk for death caused by coronary heart disease was significantly reduced to 0.47 (95% CI, 0.32 to 0.69) for current hormone use but was unchanged at 0.99 (95% CI, 0.75 to 1.30) for past use. The greatest decrease was seen in women who had at least one risk factor for heart disease (current smoking, hypercholesterolemia, hypertension, diabetes, parenteral history of premature MI, obesity). Substantially less benefit was seen in women with no risk factors. Concomitant progestin use did not appear to detract from this benefit.

The benefit of estrogens was also observed in a prospective study of more than 8000 postmenopausal women living in an affluent retirement community in southern California (Henderson et al, 1991). More than 1400 women died during 7 years of observation. All-cause mortality rates were 20% lower for women who at some point took postmenopausal estrogens than for women who did not (RR of death, 0.80; 95% CI, 0.70 to 0.87). The greatest reductions in mortality rates were seen with current use and with long duration of use; current use for more than 15 years was associated with a 40% lower mortality rate. This reduction was not dependent on estrogen dose; high ($\geq$1.25 mg/day) and low

($\leq$0.625 mg/day) doses of oral CEE (the most common estrogen used) were associated with nearly equal reduction. This is an interesting observation because 0.625 mg and 1.25 mg conjugated estrogens produce nearly equal increases in high-density lipoprotein (HDL) levels and nearly equal decreases in low-density lipoprotein (LDL) levels (Walsh et al, 1991). Because few women in this cohort took progestins or parenteral estrogens, their effects cannot be determined from this study. The reduced mortality rate among estrogen users seen in this study reflected fewer deaths from occlusive atherosclerotic vascular disease. Cancer mortality rates, observed for many malignancies including those of the breast, were 20% lower among estrogen users (RR, 0.81). One possible explanation for this finding is that estrogen users may have had greater health awareness or increased medical surveillance and so had less extensive disease at the time of diagnosis. As expected, estrogen users had increased mortality rates from endometrial cancer (RR: 3.0).

This study (Henderson et al, 1991) also found that women who underwent menopause before age 45 showed the greatest benefit from estrogen use. For women whose menopause occurred after age 54, estrogen treatment did not reduce mortality. Estrogen use also appeared to reduce mortality rates for women who smoked, had hypertension, or who had a history of angina or MI so that their risk approached that of healthy women who did not use estrogen (Table 21-1). This is a significant finding; at one time hypertension, tobacco use, and coronary disease were considered to be relative contraindications to estrogen replacement therapy. This was based on the increased incidence of stroke and heart attack in women taking high-dose oral contraceptives and in men taking high-dose conjugated estrogens prescribed for secondary prevention of MI (The Coronary Drug Project, 1973). This does not appear to be a concern with the much lower doses of estrogen prescribed for postmenopausal use.

Findings of epidemiological studies suggest that the postmenopausal women who would benefit most from hormone replacement therapy (HRT) are those who underwent menopause before age 45 or those who have risk factors for CVD. These findings further argue for continuous, long-term treatment because this is associated with additional reductions in mortality. It should be remembered that these studies are epidemiological observations of estrogen users and nonusers and are *not* clinical trials. Although investigators control for many potential confounding factors, the possibility exists that healthier women are more likely to seek and be prescribed estrogens. Proof that estrogen reduces CVD requires a long-term, large-scale, placebo-controlled clinical trial.

Angiographic Studies

Sullivan et al (1990) provided evidence that women with preexisting atherosclerosis may benefit from estrogen replacement. Earlier these investigators reported that women who use estrogen and undergo coronary catheterization are less likely to have coronary occlusion than women who do not use estrogen (RR, 0.44; 95% CI, 0.29 to 0.67) (Sullivan et al, 1988). In their most recent study, they retrospectively analyzed the all-cause mortality rates of women who underwent catheterization in the preceding 10 years. Unfortunately, few of their subjects were estrogen users—defined as estrogen use at the time of catheterization (5% of subjects) or sometime thereafter (another 5% of subjects). The adjusted 10-year survival rate of women with severe coronary stenosis who used estrogens was 97%, compared with only 60% for nonusers. In women with mild to moderate coronary stenosis, the 10-year survival rate was 95% for those who used estrogen and 85% for those who did not. Although these findings suggest that women with coronary atherosclerosis may benefit from estrogen use, it must be recognized that this is a retrospective study with potential bias. The decreased mortality rate seen in estrogen users may have been in part a self-fulfilling prophecy because estrogen nonusers who lived the longest after catheterization had the greatest opportunity to begin estrogen treatment and to be classified as estrogen users.

Clinical Trials

The first clinical trials to reduce CVD by estrogen treatment were performed in men. Early studies enrolling men after MI showed that estrogen treatment reduced serum cholesterol but not the incidence of a second event (Stamler et al, 1980). The Coronary Drug Project (1973), consisting of 1101 survivors of MI, was terminated when excess thrombotic events, particularly pulmonary emboli, were seen in the estrogen-treated group; the incidence of CVD was not reduced. A similar observation was made in men with prostate cancer treated with the estrogen diethylstilbestrol, which increased CVD, possibly by causing excessive fluid accumulation that led to congestive heart failure or by increasing thromboembolism (DeVogt, 1986). This adverse action of estrogen in men may have been the consequence of the highly potent estrogens used and may not reflect the action of estrogen at physiologic levels.

Recently, clinical trials to reduce CVD by hormone treatment have been initiated in women. The HERS trial (Heart and Estrogen/Progestin Replacement Study) enrolled 2763 postmenopausal women with established heart disease who had not undergone hysterectomy (Hulley et al, 1998). Their average age was 67. They were randomly assigned to treatment with either placebo or to 0.625 mg CEE combined with 2.5 mg MPA daily. Mean duration of enrollment was 4.1 years. The primary endpoint was nonfatal or fatal MI, which overall was unchanged by hormone treatment (RR 0.99; 95% CI, 0.80 to 1.22). Adjustment for differences in baseline CVD risk factors reduced the RR to 0.95 (0.76 to 1.17). Hormone treatment lowered LDL by 11% and raised HDL by 10%, as expected. Women who were assigned hormone treatment were less likely to be prescribed hypolipidemic agents; adjustment for this reduced the RR to 0.94 (95% CI, 0.76 to 1.17). Restriction of the analysis to those subjects who took

Table 21-1   Relative Risk for Death from All Causes by Selected Characteristics and History of Use of Estrogen Replacement Therapy

	Estrogen Replacement Therapy Ever Used	
	No	Yes
Elevated blood pressure		
No	1.00*	0.79†
Yes	1.54‡	1.15
Angina/MI history		
No	1.00*	0.81§
Yes	1.62‡	1.02
Smoking		
Never	1.00*	0.74‡
Ever	1.28	1.05
Alcohol		
No	1.00*	0.56‡
Yes	0.61‡	0.39‡
Quetelet's index: wt/ht² × 1000		
35	1.14‡	0.92
≥35	1.00*	0.72†
Exercise, h/d		
<0.5	1.00*	0.73‡
0.05-0.09	0.67‡	0.61‡
≥1.0	0.56‡	0.43‡
Age at last menstrual period		
<45	1.0*	0.71§
45-54	0.81†	0.65‡
≥55	0.75‖	0.75‖

From Henderson BE, Paganini-Hill A, Ross RK: Decreased mortality in users of estrogen replacement therapy. *Arch Intern Med* 1991; 151:75-78.
*Reference group.
†P < 0.01; ‡ P < 0.0001; § P < 0.001; ‖ P < 0.05.

at least 80% of the study drug lowered the RR to 0.87 (0.67 to 1.11). There did appear to be a marked effect of treatment duration: the RR for hormone use was increased at 1.52 for year 1, unchanged at 1.00 for year 2, decreased at 0.87 for year 3, and decreased at 0.67 for years 4 and 5. One possible explanation for this apparent null result is that cardioprotection by HRT is primarily lipid mediated, and this takes time (more than 2 years) to confer benefit. This is consistent with other clinical trials of hypolipidemic drugs, which found that the reduction in CVD requires at least 2 years to become evident. An alternative explanation is that daily MPA may negate the cardioprotective effect of estrogen. Most of the epidemiological data suggesting a cardioprotective effect of hormone use was based on unopposed estrogen use or, more recently, on cyclic progestin use.

Mechanisms of Action of Estrogen

Because men and women have an equal incidence of CVD when matched for lipoprotein concentrations (Gordon et al,

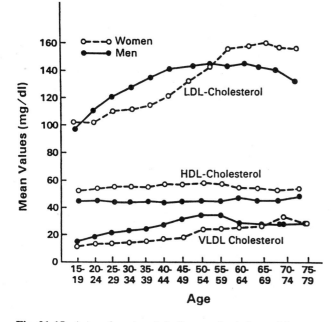

Fig. 21-15. Age and sex trends in lipoprotein cholesterol fractions, Framingham study. (From Kannel WB: Risk factors for coronary disease in women: Perspective from the Framingham study. *Am Heart J* 1987; 114:413.)

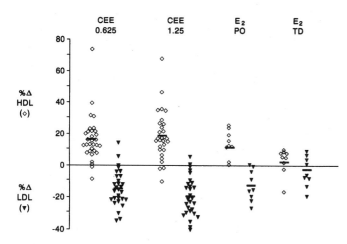

Fig. 21-16. Effect of estrogen treatments on plasma low-density lipoprotein (LDL) and high-density lipoprotein (HDL) cholesterol concentrations. Each point represents the individual percentage change with estrogen compared with placebo. The horizontal bar denotes the mean of the percentage changes. (From Walsh BW, Schiff I, Rosner B, et al: Effects of postmenopausal estrogen replacement on the concentrations and metabolism of plasma lipoproteins. *N Engl J Med* 1991; 325:1196.)

1977), the sex difference in the incidence of CVD may be a consequence of the characteristic sex differences in serum lipoprotein concentrations. Premenopausal women appear to be protected against CVD by their typically lower LDL levels and higher HDL levels than men of the same age (Fig. 21-15). However, coincident with the loss of estrogen at menopause, LDL levels in women rise to exceed those of men (Matthews et al, 1989). Loss of estrogen may cause this increase in LDL because estrogen replacement lowers LDL

levels by 15% to 19% by increasing the clearance of LDL from the circulation (Fig. 21-16) (Walsh et al, 1991). In contrast, HDL levels in women decline by only 5% at menopause (Matthews et al, 1989). Hence, the HDL-raising effect of oral estrogens (typically 16% to 18%) (Walsh et al, 1991) appears to be a pharmacological action of the high portal estrogen concentrations presented to the liver after intestinal absorption. Therefore, if endogenous estrogens protect against CVD, the likely mechanism is an effect on LDL rather than on HDL. In contrast, the lower incidence of CVD among postmenopausal women who use estrogen may result from increases in HDL levels and decreases in LDL levels. Using the regression coefficients determined by clinical trials in which cholesterol levels were improved by drug treatment, the magnitude of the lipid changes induced by oral estrogen treatment would be expected to lower the incidence of CVD by as much as 40%. Reductions of this magnitude have been observed among women who use estrogen (Henderson et al, 1991; Stampfer et al, 1991). In addition, postmenopausal estrogen treatment has been found to reduce plasma levels of lipoprotein (a), a highly atherogenic particle (Sacks et al, 1994).

An alternative explanation has been proposed for the sex difference in the incidence of CVD. A semilogarithmic plot of cardiovascular deaths of women against age shows that the rate of increase in the rate of CVD is constant throughout a woman's lifetime and is not accelerated after menopause. In comparison, there is a decline in the rate of increase of CVD in men after the onset of the male climacteric, when testosterone levels wane (Fig. 21-17) (Heller and Jacobs, 1978). This decline in androgens may be a major factor responsible for the lower female-male CVD ratio seen with increasing age. Androgens are known to affect serum lipoproteins adversely; exogenous use (*e.g.,* testosterone enanthate and methyltestosterone) and endogenous increases in androgens (occurring during puberty) have been found to lower HDL levels (Bagatell et al, 1992; Kirkland et al, 1987).

Estrogens may protect against cardiovascular disease independent of their beneficial actions on lipoprotein levels. In addition, they may retard the oxidation of LDL, thereby decreasing its atherogenicity. This was shown in healthy postmenopausal women who underwent intravenous estradiol infusion; LDL oxidation was significantly delayed (Sack et al, 1994). Estrogens may suppress the uptake of LDL by blood vessel walls, impairing the development of endothelial atheroma (Wagner et al, 1991). There is also evidence that estrogens act directly to promote vasodilation, as demonstrated in estrogen-treated castrated female monkeys (Williams et al, 1992). This may be mediated indirectly by estrogen-induced alterations in prostaglandin metabolism by increasing the levels of prostacyclin (a vasodilator) and decreasing the levels of thromboxane (a vasoconstrictor) (Steinleitner et al, 1989). The vasodilatory effect of estrogen may be more direct because estrogen receptors are present throughout the vascular system (McGill, 1989). The binding

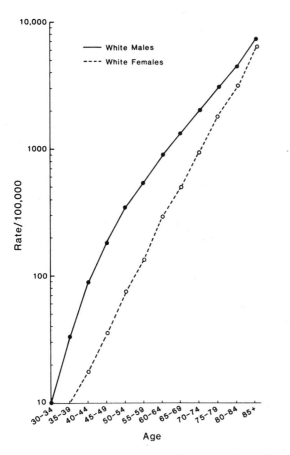

Fig. 21-17. Age-specific mortality rates for ischemic heart disease by sex (white persons only, United States, 1977). (From Ross RK, Paganini-Hill A: Estrogen replacement therapy and coronary heart disease. *Semin Reprod Endocrinol* 1983; 1:19.)

of estrogen to endothelial estrogen receptors could stimulate the release of nitric oxide, a potent endogenous vasodilator. This was suggested by work on female rabbits, in which endogenous estrogens were found to promote an increase in the basal release rates of nitric oxide (Hyashi et al, 1992).

Results of epidemiological studies suggest that estrogen use prevents the development of heart disease. However, the only randomized clinical trial of postmenopausal HRT did not clearly prove this beneficial effect. Instead this trial suggested that the concomitant administration of a progestin may detract from the cardioprotective action of estrogen. There is a concern that progestins, particularly the androgenic 19-nortestosterone derivatives, may do so by lowering HDL levels or by preventing estrogen-induced vasodilatation. It is to be hoped that results from the Women's Health Initiative will clarify the effects of hormone treatment on CVD.

COGNITION

It has been suggested that estrogen replacement may conserve cognitive function after menopause. At present, this is unproven. Case-control studies have been hampered by numerous methodologic problems and have produced mixed results (Brenner et al, 1994; Honjo et al, 1995). Two

community-based prospective studies have shown a protective effect of estrogen replacement on the development of Alzheimer's disease (Honjo et al, 1995; Sherwin, 1996). In the Leisure World cohort study (Henderson VW et al, 1994) estrogen users were found to have a lower incidence of Alzheimer's disease and related dementia (odds ratio [OR], 0.69; 95% CI, 0.46 to 1.03). The lowest incidence of dementia was seen in women taking estrogens for the longest duration (greater than 7 years) and at the highest dose (1.25 mg/day conjugated estrogens) (Paganini-Hill et al, 1994). In the Baltimore Longitudinal Study of Aging (Kawas et al, 1997), the relative risk for Alzheimer's disease in estrogen users compared with nonusers was 0.46 (95% CI, 0.21 to 0.99), but no duration effect was observed. A small study of nine women with Alzheimer's disease found that verbal memory was significantly better in women taking ERT than in women who were not (Henderson et al, 1996). However, one prospective study of 800 normal postmenopausal women in Rancho Bernardo found no association of estrogen therapy with cognitive function (Barrett-Connor and Kritz-Silverstein, 1993). Other studies have found that postmenopausal estrogen therapy may enhance short-term verbal (Jacobs et al, 1998; Kampen and Sherwin, 1994; Phillips and Sherwin, 1992) and visual memory (Resnick et al, 1997) and name and word recall (Robinson et al, 1994). Until results from randomized, controlled clinical trials are known, it is too soon to advocate the use of estrogen for the prevention or treatment of Alzheimer's disease in women. A trial funded by the National Institute on Aging (Alzheimer's Disease Cooperative Study Unit) is in progress to study this.

SKIN EFFECTS

Estrogen replacement may prevent skin wrinkling by retarding the loss of elastic fibers that occurs with aging and menopause. This is suggested by the fact that facial (Henry et al, 1997) and forearm (Pierard et al, 1995) skin elasticity is greater in estrogen users than it is in nonusers. In addition, estrogen users have thicker skin than do nonusers (Callens et al, 1996). Skin collagen content was found to be increased by HRT in a study of 73 women who underwent 312 skin biopsies (Castelo-Branco et al, 1992). This was also observed in a small study of 10 women in whom type III collagen in skin was increased significantly after 6 months of treatment with estradiol and testosterone implants (Savvas et al, 1993). The ability of the most superficial layer of the skin, the stratum corneum, to retain water may be improved by estrogen replacement, facilitating the barrier functions of the skin (Pierard-Franchimont et al, 1995). A recent cross-sectional study evaluated skin wrinkling, senile dry skin, and atrophy in 3875 postmenopausal women observed from 1971 to 1974 (Dunn et al, 1997). After adjustment for age, body mass index, and sun exposure, the OR for dry skin in estrogen users compared with nonusers was 0.76 (95% CI, 0.60 to 0.97), and for skin wrinkling it was 0.68 (95% CI,

0.52 to 0.89). After adjustment for smoking, winkling was still significantly less in white women (OR, 0.59; 95% CI, 0.38 to 0.91). Atrophy was not significantly lower in users than in nonusers. However, there are conflicting data. One study found that the thickness of the papillary dermis of the skin was increased by mestranol and glucocorticoid but was decreased by mestranol alone (Cortes-Gallegos et al, 1996). It should be noted that these studies reflect estrogen use at higher doses unopposed by progestins. Although these studies suggest that estrogen appears to decrease skin aging, proof would require a randomized clinical trial.

ESTROGENS
Pharmacology

Many estrogen preparations are available—conjugated estrogens, synthetic estrogens, and micronized estradiol. All of them may be given orally or parenterally, continuously or cyclically. Because oral estrogens have been prescribed for more than 30 years, most of the demonstrated long-term benefits of estrogens are based on experience with oral use. The daily doses of the most common estrogens taken orally are CEE 0.625 mg, micronized estradiol 1 mg, and piperazine estrone sulfate 1.25 mg. These doses are usually effective in relieving menopausal symptoms such as hot flashes and vaginal atrophy and in preventing osteoporosis. Generally, CEEs are twice as potent per unit weight than pure estrone preparations (Mashchak et al, 1982). As many as half consist of the potent equine estrogens equilin and 17-dihydroequilin sulfates, and the remainder are estrone sulfate. These equine estrogens have a prolonged action caused in part by storage and slow release from adipose tissue. They have been detected in the blood as long as 13 weeks after administration (Whittaker et al, 1980).

Orally administered estradiol is rapidly converted to estrone in the intestinal mucosa. Oral estrogens are then presented to the liver, where 30% of an initial dose is conjugated with glucuronide on the first pass (Siddle and Whitehead, 1983). These conjugates undergo rapid renal and biliary excretion. The biliary conjugates are hydrolyzed by intestinal flora, allowing 80% to be reabsorbed and returned to the liver. They may then be reconjugated and excreted or they may enter the systemic circulation. This enterohepatic circulation contributes to the prolonged effect of orally administered estrogens. Thus, patients with altered gut flora (*e.g.,* from antibiotic therapy) may not sufficiently hydrolyze these conjugates, and reabsorption may be prevented. As a result, these patients may require higher doses to achieve a therapeutic effect. In addition, patients chronically maintained on phenytoin have enhanced glucuronidation and excrete estrogens more rapidly (Englund and Johansson, 1987). They, too, may require higher doses.

Women who smoke may also require higher estrogen doses. Postmenopausal women who smoke and use estrogen have half the serum estrogen levels of women who use estrogen and do not smoke (Jensen et al, 1985). Smoking is thought to stimulate 2-hydroxylation of estradiol, yielding 2-hydroxy estrogens that have minimal estrogenic activity and are rapidly cleared from the circulation (Michnovicz et al, 1986). This explains why smokers have higher incidences of osteoporosis and menopausal symptoms and may require higher estrogen doses.

Women who consume alcohol and use estrogen replacement therapy may have higher circulating levels of estrogens than are desirable. This may explain why it is more likely that breast cancer will develop in women who consume alcohol. When women treated with transdermal estradiol drink alcohol, estradiol levels increase by 40% above levels after the ingestion of calorie-matched placebo drinks (Ginsburg et al, 1995a). This may be explained in part by the finding that the half-life of estradiol is prolonged by 54% (from 4.1 hours to 6.3 hours) in women who consume alcohol (Ginsburg et al, 1995b). In women using oral estradiol replacement, a similar vodka-containing drink increases circulating estradiol levels by 327% (Ginsburg et al, 1996) (Fig. 21-18). Mechanisms responsible for the interactions between alcohol and estrogen are not yet known.

After oral ingestion, the concentration of estrogen in the portal circulation is four to five times higher than it is in the general circulation. Thus, hepatocytes are exposed to higher levels of estrogen after oral estrogen administration than are other cells. Estrogens administered orally will have a more profound effect on hepatic metabolism than those administered parenterally. Although many of these actions—for instance, stimulating the production of renin-substrate and coagulation factors—may be deleterious to the liver, some effects may be beneficial, such as increased HDL production and increased LDL catabolism (Walsh et al, 1991). The effect each of these has on lipoproteins may reduce cardiovascular risk.

Synthetic estrogens are chemical derivatives of estradiol and are the estrogens currently used in oral contraceptives. Ethinyl estradiol (EE) results from the addition of a 17-ethinyl group, which impedes catabolism by the liver, leading to its long half-life of 48 hours. The other commonly used synthetic estrogen, mestranol, must undergo demethylation by the liver to become EE, its active form. Because this demethylation is only 50% complete, mestranol has only half the potency of EE (Schwartz and Hammerstein, 1973). When administered orally, these synthetic estrogens are more than 100 times as potent on a per-weight basis as natural estrogens in stimulating the production of hepatic proteins (Mashchak CA et al, 1982 Because the minimum dose (10 μg) for therapeutic effect (*e.g.,* to reduce urinary calcium excretion) exceeds the lowest dose that markedly elevates hepatic globulins (5 μg), synthetic estrogens are not often used (Mandel et al, 1982b).

Parenteral estrogens may be administered by the vaginal, transdermal, or subcutaneous route. Vaginal estrogens are absorbed into the systemic circulation and achieve one fourth of the circulatory level of an equal dose given orally (Deutsch et al, 1981). However, they exert a potent local ef-

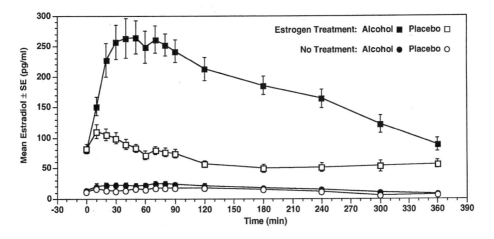

Fig. 21-18. Circulating estradiol levels before and after alcohol and placebo drink ingestion in women who do and do not use estrogen. (From Ginsburg ES, Mello NK, Mendelson JH, et al: Effects of alcohol ingestion on estrogens in postmenopausal women. *JAMA* 1996; 276:1747. Copyright © 1996, American Medical Association.)

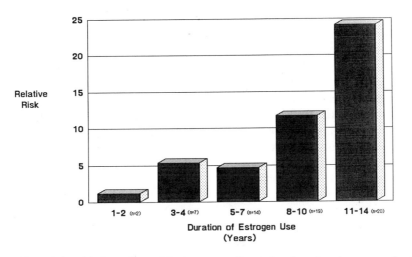

Fig. 21-19. Relative risk for endometrial cancer according to duration of postmenopausal estrogen use. (From Weiss NS, Szekely DR, English DR, et al: Endometrial cancer in relation to patterns of menopausal estrogen use. *JAMA* 1979; 242:261. Copyright © 1996, American Medical Association.)

fect; 0.3 mg CEE given vaginally produces the same degree of epithelial maturation as 1.25 mg given orally (Geola et al, 1980; Mandel et al, 1983). Continuous vaginal use of estrogen leads to increased circulatory levels because of the enhanced transfer across a healthier, more vascularized epithelium (Siddle and Whitehead, 1983).

Twenty-five-milligram subdermal estradiol pellets have been found to be effective, but they have variable life spans of 3 to 6 months and are difficult to remove. Transdermal skin patches applied twice weekly are more convenient. They provide constant serum estrogen levels; the 50 μg/240 patch produces a mean serum estradiol level of 70 pg/mL and an estrone level of 50 pg/mL. These levels are usually effective in relieving hot flashes (Haas et al, 1988) and in preventing bone loss (Stevenson et al, 1981). Whether parenteral estrogens reduce the incidence of CVD has yet to be demonstrated.

Possible Side Effects

Estrogens may cause nausea, mastalgia, headache, and mood changes. More serious risks include the following.

Endometrial Neoplasia

Unopposed estrogen use (*i.e.,* without the addition of a progestin) may induce endometrial hyperplasia and ultimately adenocarcinoma. Retrospective case-control studies have found that unopposed estrogen use increases the risk for endometrial cancer twofold to fourfold, from a baseline incidence of 1/1000 women (ages, 50 to 74 years) per year to 4/1000 women per year. The increase in risk appears to be related to the dose and the duration (minimum, 1 to 2 years) of estrogen use (Fig. 21-19) (Weiss et al, 1979). The relative risk for endometrial cancer is 1.2 with 0.625 mg conjugated estrogens daily, and it is 3.8 with 1.25 mg daily (Rubin, 1990). This elevated risk persists for more than 6 years after therapy is discontinued. Women who use oral contraceptives for more than 12 months and later take unopposed post-menopausal estrogens do not have a greater risk for endometrial cancer than nonusers. The risk for endometrial cancer associated with unopposed estrogen use is low for women using 0.625 mg CEE, particularly if they previously used oral contraceptives (Rubin, 1990).

Most of the carcinomas associated with estrogen use are early stage and low grade and have not deeply invaded the myometrium (Chu et al, 1982). The adjusted 5-year survival rate for women with endometrial cancer who use estrogen is 94% compared with 81% for women with endometrial cancer who do not use estrogen (Elwood and Boyes, 1980). This may be the result of one or more of the following: women prescribed estrogens generally are in better health than nonusers; they are evaluated more frequently, allowing for earlier diagnosis; only well-differentiated endometrial neoplasms retain estrogen receptors by which an exogenous estrogen can provide a stimulus.

Progestins can prevent and reverse endometrial hyperplasia. Studd et al (1980), in observing 855 women with annual endometrial biopsies for as long as 5 years, found an annual 15% incidence of hyperplasia among women taking 1.25 mg unopposed conjugated estrogen. The addition of a progestin for 7 days per month reduced this incidence to 3%. Ten days of progestin treatment per month lowered the incidence to 2%, and 13 days of treatment reduced this to essentially zero (Fig. 21-20). Based on these data, progestins are typically given for 13 days per month. Progestin treatment has also been successful in completely reversing established endometrial hyperplasia in 94% of 258 women with hyperplasia (Gambrell et al, 1980). Women who use estrogens combined with progestins have a significantly lower incidence of endometrial cancer (71 per 100,000) than women who use estrogens alone (434 per 100,000) or women who use no hormones (242 per 100,000) Gambrell, 1982a). Women who use estrogens and progestins are considered not to be at increased risk for endometrial cancer.

Progestins appear to protect the endometrium by reversing the induction of estradiol and progesterone receptors produced by estrogen (Whitehead et al, 1981). Progestins, in addition, increase the activity of estradiol and isocitric dehydrogenases of the endometrium, thereby inactivating estradiol. The magnitude of these effects is more dependent on the duration of progestin therapy than on the dose. The minimum effective doses are 1 mg for norethindrone and 0.15 mg for norgestrel.

Ovarian Neoplasia

Estrogen replacement may increase the risk for endometrioid cancer of the ovary, which comprises 10% to 20% of all ovarian malignancies. This has *not* been conclusively established (Weiss et al, 1982). It is unknown whether progestin use reduces this risk, if it indeed exists.

Breast Neoplasia

Whether postmenopausal estrogen use increases the risk for breast cancer has been actively debated. There has been a suspicion, based on the following theoretical grounds, that estrogen use increases the risk for breast cancer:

Breast cancer can be an estrogen-sensitive tumor.

Estrogens can induce mammary tumors in rodents.

Women with prolonged endogenous estrogen exposure (e.g., early menarche, late menopause, nulliparity) are at increased risk for breast malignancy.

More than 20 studies have been conducted to resolve this controversy. Nearly all found that postmenopausal estrogen replacement does not substantially increase the risk for breast cancer. The largest epidemiological study focused on 1960 patients with breast cancer and 2258 matched controls, identified through a breast-screening program with 280,000 participants (Brinton et al, 1986). The RR of breast cancer

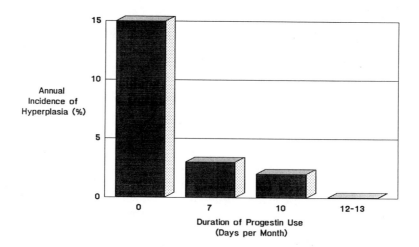

Fig. 21-20. Annual incidence of endometrial hyperplasia according to duration of progestin use per month. (From Studd JWW, Thorn MH, Patterson MEL, et al: The prevention and treatment of endometrial pathology. In Pasetto N, Paoletti R, Ambrus JL, editors: *The menopause and post-menopause,* Lancaster, U.K., 1980, MTP Press, p. 127.)

for all postmenopausal women who used estrogen (1.03) was not increased. However, there was a statistically significant increase in breast cancer risk with increasing duration of estrogen use. For women exposed for 10 to 14 years, the RR was 1.28. For women exposed longer than 20 years, the RR was 1.47. This increase is relatively small; the average is approximately 2% per year of estrogen use. The Nurse's Health Study (Colditz et al, 1990) also found duration of estrogen treatment to increase the risk for breast cancer. Estrogen use for more than 5 years increased the risk for breast cancer; concomitant use of a progestin did not alter this increased risk. For women taking estrogens, self-breast examination and mammography are especially important. Because death rates from CVD are more than four times those of endometrial and breast cancer combined, any adverse carcinogenic effect of estrogen would be far outweighed by its reduction of CVD.

Gallbladder Disease

During the first year of use, estrogen treatment increases the risk for cholelithiasis by 20% (95% CI, 0.7 to 2.1) (Kakar et al, 1988). The relative risk for gallbladder disease with combination estrogen-progestin treatment is 1.38 (95% CI, 1.00 to 1.92) (Hulley et al, 1998). Cholelithiasis probably occurs because estrogens increase the hepatic excretion of LDL cholesterol (Walsh et al, 1991). In addition, estrogens reduce the amount of chenodeoxycholic acid in bile, which keeps cholesterol in aqueous solution (Bennion, 1977).

Thromboembolic Disease

Estrogen replacement increases the activity of the coagulation and fibrinolytic systems (Caine et al, 1992). In a placebo-controlled clinical trial of conjugated estrogen-medroxyprogesterone, the RR of venous thromboembolic disease was increased at 2.89 (95% CI, 1.50 to 5.58) (Hulley et al, 1998).

Hypertension

Estrogen replacement in general may modestly lower blood pressure in many women (Mashchak and Lobo, 1985b), but it may induce or exacerbate hypertension in others (Crane et al, 1971). This idiosyncratic reaction to oral estrogens may be mediated by an increase in the hepatic production of renin substrate or by the production of an aberrant form (Shionoiri et al, 1983). In any case, this elevation in blood pressure is usually reversible with the discontinuation of estrogen.

Glucose Tolerance

Although oral contraceptives are associated with impaired carbohydrate metabolism (Spellacy, 1976), the lower doses used for estrogen replacement have not been linked to impaired glucose tolerance (Spellacy et al, 1978). Diabetes does not appear any more likely to develop in postmenopausal women who use estrogen than in those who do not (Manson et al, 1992). For those postmenopausal women who already have diabetes, there is either no change or improvement of the disease with estrogen use, as evidenced by lower glucose levels or reduced insulin requirements (Cantilo, 1941). This is consistent with the observation that estrogen appears to increase the binding of insulin to its receptor (Bellejo et al, 1983). Moreover, animal models have shown that estrogen improves experimentally induced hyperglycemia (Paik et al, 1982).

Contraindications

Postmenopausal estrogen replacement therapy is absolutely contraindicated if a patient has any of the following conditions:

Known or suspected breast cancer: However, women with breast cancer may be treated with tamoxifen citrate, which has been found to conserve bone mass (Love et al, 1992), induce a beneficial lipoprotein profile (Thangaraju et al, 1994), and reduce the incidence of cardiac morbidity by 31%.

Endometrial carcinoma, if it has spread beyond the uterine corpus. Postmenopausal women who have stage I endometrial cancer and who take estrogen have been found to have higher 5-year survival rates than women who do not (Creasman et al, 1986). Women who have endometrial cancer confined to the uterus at the time of diagnosis and who remain disease free for at least 2 years are highly likely to be cured of their cancer. They may be considered for estrogen treatment if sufficient benefits exist.

Undiagnosed genital bleeding

Active liver disease

Active thromboembolic disease or a history of estrogen-related thromboembolic disease

Postmenopausal estrogen replacement therapy is relatively contraindicated if a patient has any of the following conditions:

Chronic liver dysfunction: Impairment of the liver's ability to metabolize estrogen leads to excessive levels of estrogen. This may be offset by the administration of smaller, less frequent doses.

Poorly controlled hypertension

History of thromboembolic disease: Although the absolute incidence of thrombosis is generally low with postmenopausal estrogen use, it may be significantly higher in a woman whose history indicates she is at increased risk for a thrombotic event. If it is thought that estrogen treatment would confer significant benefits, it may be prescribed transdermally because this route does not stimulate the hepatic production of coagulation factors.

Preexisting uterine leiomyomata or active endometriosis: Estrogen use may prevent the involution of these conditions, which occurs after menopause. Estrogen treatment may be initiated after waiting a short interval (*i.e.,* 3 to 12 months). Patients who have submucous leiomyomata may experience heavy or irregular bleeding with hormone replacement.

Acute intermittent porphyria: Estrogens may precipitate attacks.

PROGESTOGENS

Progestins are used to prevent endometrial stimulation, which may be induced by estrogen treatment. They may also be used to relieve hot flashes in patients who are not candidates for estrogen replacement.

Available Preparations

Progesterone and its derivatives are absorbed through the oral, vaginal, rectal, and intramuscular routes. Although convenient, oral absorption is highly variable; there is as much as a threefold difference among patients (Whitehead et al, 1980), and different clinical effects may be seen in patients given the same oral dose. After absorption, oral progestins are transported to the liver in high concentrations, where they may alter the hepatic metabolism of serum lipoproteins and, in particular, may lower HDL cholesterol levels. Progestins are then rapidly metabolized by the liver to deoxycorticosterone (Ottosson et al, 1984).

Medroxyprogesterone acetate, 5 mg daily for cyclic treatment, is the most commonly used progestin in the United States. It is effective against hyperplasia, and it has modest effects on serum lipids. MPA given intramuscularly as its depot form is well absorbed but has a highly variable duration of effectiveness and often causes irregular vaginal bleeding. The usual dose is 50 to 150 mg intramuscularly every 1 to 3 months (the 50-mg dose is sufficient to relieve hot flashes) (Morrison et al, 1980). Megestrol acetate (40 to 80 mg daily) or micronized progesterone (200 to 300 mg daily) may be substituted for MPA. Micronized progesterone offers promise as an ideal progestin because it is active against hyperplasia without significantly altering serum lipid levels (Writing Group for PEPI, 1995).

The 19-nortestosterone derivatives are the potent progestins used in oral contraceptives. Available in the United States in low doses in the form of progestin-only oral contraceptives, they have partial androgenic properties and lower HDL cholesterol levels. Norethindrone is available as either Micronoror (Ortho Pharmaceutical: Roritan, N.J.) or Nor-QD (Suntex: Humacao, Puerto Rico), each of which contains 0.35 mg norethindrone. Typically, three tablets daily are needed to protect against hyperplasia. Norgestrel is available as Ovrette (Wyeth-Ayerst: Radnor, Pa.), which contains 0.075 mg; two tablets daily are needed for endometrial protection (Whitehead et al, 1981). Three 19-nortestosterone-derived progestins that are less androgenic and are used in Europe will soon become available in the United States: desogestrel, norgestimate, and gestodene.

Adverse Effects

Progestins may produce abdominal bloating, mastalgia, headaches, mood changes, and acne. More important, all progestins, particularly the 19-nortestosterone derivatives (*e.g.*, norgestrel and norethindrone), negatively affect serum lipids by lowering HDL levels. High-density lipoprotein levels are lowered by 9% to 16% with 10 mg MPA daily (Silfverstope et al, 1982; Tikkanen et al, 1981), by 17% to 20%

with 0.5 mg norgestrel daily (Hirvonen et al, 1981; Ottosson et al, 1985), and by 20% to 36% with 10 mg norethindrone daily (Hirvonen et al, 1981; Silfverstope et al, 1982). These doses of norgestrel and norethindrone are higher than necessary because 0.15 mg norgestrel and 1 mg norethindrone are as effective against hyperplasia as the higher doses (Whitehead et al, 1981). It is unknown what effects the lower doses have on lipids.

The net effect of a hormonal regimen on lipids depends on the estrogen and progestin used and on the dose, route, and frequency of administration. In general, progestins may negate in whole or in part the beneficial effect of estrogen on HDL and LDL. This may compromise the possible reduction in CVD observed with estrogen replacement. Because there is no proof that progestins protect against breast cancer, progestins should be used only for the woman with an intact uterus for whom prevention of endometrial cancer is needed.

HORMONE TREATMENT REGIMENS

Before initiating hormonal therapy, the patient should be evaluated by taking a detailed history and conducting a physical examination, including blood pressure, breast and pelvic examination, stool guaiac, and Papanicolaou smear. Mammography should be performed to prevent prescribing estrogens to a patient with preexisting subclinical cancer of the breast; this examination should be repeated annually. Serum cholesterol level should be measured at least once every 5 years as long as it remains below 200 mg/dL; if serum cholesterol exceeds this level or if the HDL cholesterol level is below 35 mg/dL, follow-up should be arranged. An endometrial biopsy specimen should be taken before treatment if there is a history of abnormal vaginal bleeding or if the patient is at increased risk for having unrecognized endometrial hyperplasia. This may be accomplished either by endometrial aspiration, if it is technically feasible, or by fractional dilation and curettage. Before instituting therapy, biopsy specimens should be taken from patients receiving unopposed estrogens for extended periods of time, regardless of bleeding; biopsies should be taken every year because the annual incidence of hyperplasia is 30% (Schiff et al, 1982).

In the United States, the most common HRT schedule for women with intact uteri is cyclic and consists of 0.625 mg CEE daily and 5 mg MPA for the first 13 or 14 calendar days of each month. Most patients on this regimen have withdrawal bleeding on the tenth and twentieth days of the month (Archer et al, 1984). If bleeding occurs at any other time, an endometrial biopsy should be taken. For patients who have previously undergone hysterectomy, no progestin is needed.

Another estrogen may be substituted for CEE, and another progestin may be substituted for MPA. Appropriate doses of other oral estrogens are 0.5 or 1 mg micronized estradiol, 0.3 or 0.625 mg esterified estrogens, or 1.25 mg piperazine estrone sulfate. Parenteral estrogens (*e.g.,* transdermal estradiol) are particularly useful for women in whom the hepatic effects of oral estrogens should be avoided, such as those with a history of hepatic dysfunction, thrombosis, or hypertension. The typical starting dose of transdermal estradiol is 0.05 mg applied twice weekly; this may be increased to 0.10 mg after 1 month, if necessary.

To avert withdrawal bleeding, continuous rather than cyclic hormonal treatment is used. A typical regimen is 0.625 mg CEE daily with 2.5 or 5 mg MPA daily. Irregular vaginal bleeding results in more than half the patients initially, but within 1 year 75% to 85% will be amenorrheic (Archer et al, 1984). Women most likely to become amenorrheic are those who are many years past menopause or who are given the higher progestin dose. Alternatively, norethindrone, 0.35 to 1.05 mg daily, may be substituted for MPA. It is available as Micronor, a progestin-only oral contraceptive. If vaginal bleeding develops after a patient has been amenorrheic on this regimen, an endometrial biopsy should be taken; 2 of 41 women who had irregular bleeding after several years of continuous estrogen and progestin treatment were found to have endometrial adenocarcinoma (Leather et al, 1991).

Transvaginal ultrasound monitoring has been evaluated as a modality to screen postmenopausal women for endometrial disease. This technique uses a high-frequency ultrasound transducer placed in the vagina, where it is in proximity to the uterus and can provide high-resolution imaging. This method is superior to transabdominal imaging because it overcomes the difficulties encountered in imaging women who are obese, have excessive bowel gas, or have inadequate bladder filling as a result of discomfort or incontinence (Mendelson et al, 1988). Ultrasonography accurately measures endometrial thickness within 1 mm of the actual thickness seen on pathologic examination (Nasri and Coast, 1989). Two large series evaluated postmenopausal vaginal bleeding by transvaginal ultrasonography before diagnostic dilatation and curettage in 205 and 215 women, respectively (Grandberg et al, 1991; Klug and Leitner, 1989). In women with endometrial cancer, endometrial thickness was 18 ± 16 mm; in women with endometrial atrophy, it was 3 ± 1 mm. Neither series found endometrial cancer in women whose endometria were thinner than 8 mm. Because 70% of women with postmenopausal vaginal bleeding have endometria thinner than 5 mm, a substantial number of dilatations and curettages can be avoided. A 5-mm threshold in women undergoing HRT was found to have a positive predictive value of 9% for detecting any abnormality, with 90% sensitivity, 48% specificity, and a negative predictive value of 99% (Langer et al, 1997). Whether this modality is cost effective has yet to be demonstrated.

RALOXIFENE

Although postmenopausal estrogen use may protect against osteoporosis and heart disease, it may increase the risks for breast and endometrial cancers. In fact, many women discontinue hormone treatment because of lingering concerns about these long-term hazards or because of unacceptable side effects such as vaginal bleeding and breast tenderness. Because estrogen is not an ideal treatment, drugs have been sought that have an estrogenic effect in some tissues, such as bone and cardiovascular system, but not in others, such as breast and endometrium. Drugs that have these tissue-specific effects have been termed *selective estrogen receptor modulators.* Potentially, the benefits of estrogen can be derived without the accompanying risks. This tissue selectivity is biologically possible because the conformation of a drug-estradiol receptor complex determines the particular DNA response elements to which it can bind. Raloxifene, a benzothiophene that binds to the estrogen receptor (Kauffman et al, 1995) is a selective estrogen receptor modulator. The raloxifene-estrogen receptor complex does not bind to the estrogen-response element. Instead, it binds to a unique area of DNA, the raloxifene response element, to have estrogen-antagonist effects on breast and endometrium and estrogen-agonist effects on bone and cholesterol.

Raloxifene was first studied in humans in a limited fashion in 1982 as a possible treatment for metastatic breast cancer. Large-scale clinical trials were not initiated until 1994, primarily to assess its efficacy in the prevention and treatment of osteoporosis in otherwise healthy postmenopausal women. To date, more than 14,000 women worldwide have been enrolled in raloxifene studies; of these, 8,000 women were assigned treatment with raloxifene. Although most of these studies are ongoing, interim and short-term results have recently been published.

Effects on Bone

Raloxifene preserves bone density in postmenopausal women. Treatment with 60 mg daily for 2 years significantly increases bone density (compared with calcium-supplemented placebo groups) of the lumbar spine by 2.4%, the total hip by 2.4% (Fig. 21-21), the femoral neck by 2.5%, and the total body by 2%. This study also evaluated the 30-mg and 150-mg daily doses of raloxifene and found them to have a similar on the bone density to the 60-mg dose (Delmas et al, 1997). A second study randomly assigned women to treatment with 0.625 mg CEE daily, 60 mg raloxifene daily, or to calcium-supplemented placebo. Compared to the placebo group, treatment with raloxifene 60 mg daily for 2 years was found to increase bone density of the total hip by 1.5%, which is half the 3% increase seen with estrogen (Eli Lilly, 1997, data on file). Based on these data, the Food and Drug Administration granted approval in December 1997 for the use of 60 mg raloxifene daily for the *prevention* of osteoporosis. More recently, raloxifene has been found to reduce the incidence of vertebral fractures by 50% (Ettinger et al, 1998). This was expected because histomorphic evaluation findings of iliac crest bone biopsies obtained from 10 women treated with raloxifene for 6 months were normal, with no evidence of mineralization defects, woven

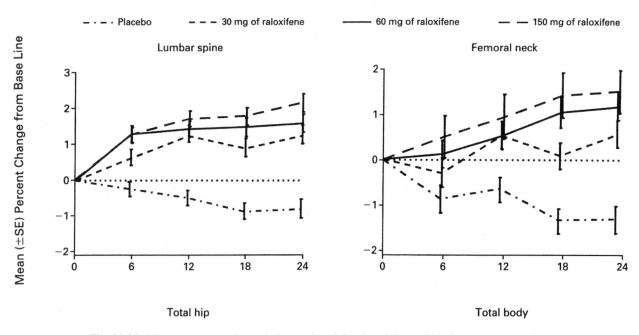

Fig. 21-21. Mean percentage change in bone mineral density of the total hip in postmenopausal women given raloxifene or placebo for 2 years. Bars show the standard errors for the median changes. (Modified from Delmas PD, Bjarnason NH, Mitlak BH, et al: Effects of raloxifene on bone mineral density, serum cholesterol, and uterine endometrium in postmenopausal women. *N Engl J Med* 1997; 337:1644. Copyright © 1997 Massachusetts Medical Society. All rights reserved.)

bone, marrow fibrosis, osteomalacia, or osteocyte damage (Eli Lilly, 1997). The bone formation rate per unit of bone volume and the activation frequency were decreased to a lesser extent with raloxifene than with estrogen treatment (Eli Lilly, 1997).

Effects on Cardiovascular Risk Markers

Raloxifene favorably alters several markers of cardiovascular risk in healthy postmenopausal women by lowering the levels of LDL-cholesterol, fibrinogen, and lipoprotein (a) and by not raising triglyceride levels. However, in contrast to HRT, raloxifene has no effect on HDL-C and PAI-1 levels, and it has a lesser effect on HDL₂-C and lipoprotein (a) levels. This was shown in a clinical trial (Walsh et al, 1998) (Figs. 21-22 and 21-23) of 390 healthy postmenopausal women who received one of four possible treatments for 6 months: raloxifene 60 mg/day, raloxifene 120 mg/day, HRT (CEE 0.625 mg/day and MPA 2.5 mg/day), or placebo. Compared with placebo, both doses of raloxifene significantly lowered LDL-C by 12% (similar to the 14% reduction with HRT) and lipoprotein (a) by 7% (less than the 19% decrease with HRT). The decrease in LDL-cholesterol induced by raloxifene would be expected to reduce the risk for coronary artery disease. Epidemiological studies have found that the levels of LDL-C are related to risk for coronary artery disease among men and women. Moreover, clinical trials that lowered LDL-cholesterol levels in women have been found to reduce the incidence of a second cardiac event. One such trial of a lipid-lowering agent found that a 30% reduction in LDL-cholesterol levels in women was as-

sociated with a 46% reduction in cardiovascular events (Sacks et al, 1996). This suggests that the 12% reduction in LDL levels observed in this study, if sustained over time, may lower the incidence of heart disease by as much as 18%. The 7% reduction in lipoprotein (a) levels may reduce this risk even more.

Raloxifene increased HDL₂-C by 15% to 17%, less than the 33% elevation with HRT. Raloxifene did not significantly change HDL-C, triglycerides, and PAI-1, whereas HRT increased HDL-C by 10%, increased triglycerides by 20%, and decreased PAI-1 by 19%. Raloxifene significantly lowered fibrinogen by 10% to 12%, unlike HRT, which had no effect. This decline in fibrinogen may be cardioprotective. Fibrinogen levels are an independent risk factor for heart disease, with a reduction of 0.5% for every 0.01 g/L decrease in fibrinogen levels (Kannel et al, 1987). The 0.42 g/L reduction in fibrinogen induced by raloxifene could reduce cardiovascular events by 21%. This is speculative. There is no evidence from any clinical trial to show that lowering a woman's fibrinogen level reduces her cardiovascular risk.

The effect of raloxifene on markers of cardiovascular risk resembles the pattern seen with tamoxifen more than it does with HRT (Grey et al, 1995; Mannucci et al, 1996; Shewmon et al, 1994) (Table 21-2). In particular, the raloxifene and tamoxifen effect on HDL-C, HDL₂-C, and apolipoprotein A1 are both distinctly smaller than estrogen's effect. The overall similarity of the effects of raloxifene and tamoxifen is noteworthy because the changes induced by tamoxifen on cardiovascular risk markers could be responsi-

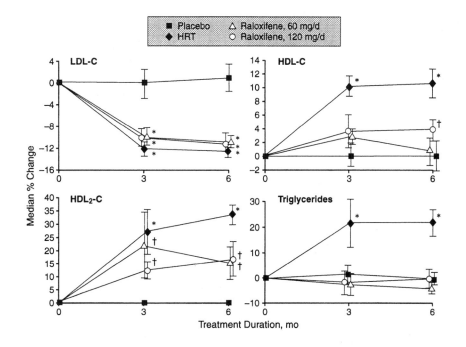

Fig. 21-22. Median percentage changes in LDL-C, HDL-C, HDL$_2$-C, and triglyceride levels in healthy postmenopausal women during 6 months of treatment with raloxifene 60 mg/day, raloxifene 120 mg/day, hormone replacement therapy (conjugated equine estrogen 0.625 mg/day and medroxyprogesterone acetate 2.5 mg/day), or placebo. Bars show the standard errors for the median changes. LDL, low-density lipoprotein; HDL, high-density lipoprotein. (From Walsh BWW, Kuller LH, Wild RA, et al: Effects of raloxifene on serum lipids and coagulation factors in healthy postmenopausal women. *JAMA* 1998; 279:1448. Copyright © 1998, American Medical Association.)

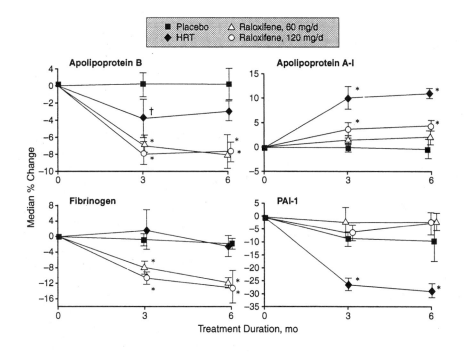

Fig. 21-23. Median percentage changes in apolipoproteins A-I and B, fibrinogen, and plasminogen activator inhibitor (PAI-1) levels in healthy postmenopausal women during 6 months of treatment with raloxifene 60 mg/day, raloxifene 120 mg/day, hormone replacement therapy (conjugated equine estrogen 0.625 mg/day and medroxyprogesterone acetate 2.5 mg/day), or placebo. Bars show the standard errors for the median changes. (From Walsh BWW, Kuller LH, Wild RA, et al: Effects of raloxifene on serum lipids and coagulation factors in healthy postmenopausal women. *JAMA* 1998; 279:1448. Copyright © 1998, American Medical Association.)

Table 21-2   Comparison of the Effects of Raloxifene, Tamoxifen, and Hormone Replacement Therapy on Markers of Cardiovascular Risk in Healthy Postmenopausal Women: Percentage Change Compared with Placebo Treatment

Cardiovascular Risk Marker	Tamoxifen 20 mg/day	Raloxifene 60 mg/day	Hormone Replacement Therapy
LDL-cholesterol	**−16***	−12	**−14**
HDL-cholesterol	+2*	0	+10
HDL$_2$-cholesterol	+2*	+15	+33
Triglycerides	0*	−4	+20
Apolipoprotein A1	+7*	+3	+12
Apolipoprotein B	−7†	**−9**	−3
Lipoprotein (a)	**−32†**	−7	**−19**
Fibrinogen	**−24***	−10	−1
Plasminogen activator inhibitor-1	−15‡	+8	**−19**
Prothrombin fragments 1 and 2	+1‡	+5	+19
Fibrinopeptide A	+11‡	−4	+3

Data on raloxifene and hormone replacement therapy (conjugated equine estrogen 0.625 mg/day and medroxyprogesterone acetate 2.5 mg/day) are from the current study. Data on tamoxifen are from Grey et al (1995),* Mannucci et al (1996),† and Shewmon et al (1994),‡ who reported the effect of 3 to 6 months' treatment. Statistically significant changes are shown in boldface type.
LDL, Low-density lipoprotein; *HDL,* high-density lipoprotein.

ble for its apparent cardioprotective effect. In randomized, controlled clinical trials in postmenopausal women with breast cancer, tamoxifen reduced the incidence of fatal myocardial infarction (OR, 0.37; 95% CI, 0.18 to 0.77) (McDonald and Stewart, 1991) and hospital admissions from cardiac disease (RR, 0.68; 95% CI, 0.48 to 0.97) (Rutqvist and Mattsson, 1993). A third such trial (Constantino et al, 1997) found a trend toward fewer cardiovascular deaths in women administered tamoxifen, but this did not reach statistical significance (RR, 0.85; 95% CI, 0.47 to 1.58). Recently, the Tamoxifen Breast Cancer Prevention Trial (Fisher B, 1998) showed no difference in myocardial infarction rates between the tamoxifen and placebo groups, which could have resulted from the young age and premenopausal status of the participants and the limited duration of treatment. Proof that raloxifene reduces the risk for heart disease would require a clinical trial with a cardiovascular event endpoint. Such a study is under way.

Effects on Venous Thromboembolic Disease

To date, 51 women enrolled in raloxifene trials have experienced episodes of venous thromboembolic disease (VTE). Nineteen had pulmonary emboli, and 32 had deep vein thrombosis (Lilly Research Laboratories, data on file). The relative risk of VTE with raloxifene treatment is 3.4 (95% CI, 1.5 to 8.0), which is similar to that of 2.9 reported for postmenopausal estrogen treatment (Hulley et al, 1998). The greatest risk for VTE appeared during the first 4 months of

treatment. Many incidences occurred in women who had a history of thrombophlebitis. For this reason, a history of VTE is one of the few contraindications to raloxifene treatment (the others are hepatic dysfunction and premenopausal use). Because of this risk, patients should be advised to discontinue raloxifene at least 72 hours before prolonged immobilization (*e.g.,* for elective surgery) and to resume taking it only when fully ambulatory.

Effects on the Uterus

Raloxifene does not appear to stimulate the endometrium. In the course of 2 years, the incidence of vaginal bleeding was 3% with the 60-mg dose and 2.2% with placebo (Delmas et al, 1997). In a 6-month study with an estrogen-progestin treatment arm, the rates of bleeding in women with intact uteri was 6% for 60 mg raloxifene and for placebo. This was considerably lower than the 64% incidence with hormone treatment (Walsh et al, 1998). Thus, episodes of vaginal bleeding that occur during raloxifene treatment warrant clinical evaluation.

Endometrial biopsies from 206 women randomly assigned raloxifene in a 1-year placebo-controlled clinical trial all showed atrophy. In contrast, endometrial hyperplasia developed in 23 of 100 women assigned to unopposed estrogen, and 39 had proliferative changes (Eli Lilly, 1997). Endometrial thickness was also assessed in a 2-year study of 831 women who underwent transvaginal ultrasonography every 6 months. Endometrial thickness was unchanged and indistinguishable between the raloxifene and the placebo-treated groups. (Delmas et al, 1997). There have been 12 new reports of endometrial cancer in women enrolled in raloxifene studies. The relative risk for endometrial cancer for raloxifene users was not increased and remained at 0.84 (95% CI, 0.25 to 2.87) (Lilly Research Laboratories, data on file).

Effects on the Breast

Raloxifene does not cause breast tenderness. The incidence of breast tenderness in 2 years was 3.3% with the 60-mg dose and 2% with placebo (Delmas et al, 1997). In a 6-month study with an estrogen-progestin treatment arm, the rate of breast tenderness was 4% for 60-mg raloxifene and 6% for placebo, much lower than the 38% incidence seen with hormone treatment (Walsh et al, 1998). To date, there have been 45 new reports of breast cancer in women enrolled in raloxifene studies. The relative risk for breast cancer for raloxifene users was significantly lower, at 0.33 (95% CI, 0.19 to 0.52), than the relative risk for the group given placebo. Of those 45 new incidences of breast cancer, 25 women had taken the study drug for more than 18 months. For this subgroup, the relative risk for breast cancer was even lower at 0.23 (95% CI, 0.10 to 0.49). The apparent protective effect of raloxifene appeared to be limited to estrogen receptor-positive tumors. Inclusion and exclusion of the small number of patients with ductal carcinoma in situ did not alter the results (American Society of Clinical Oncology, 1998).

Table 21-3   Tamoxifen Breast Cancer Prevention Trial: Clinical Outcomes

Outcome	Placebo Group	Tamoxifen Group	Relative Risk
Malignancies (total)	256	203	0.79
Breast, invasive	154	85	0.55
Endometrial	14	33	2.36
Other	88	85	0.97
Breast, ductal carcinoma in situ	59	31	0.52
Thromboembolic events			
Pulmonary emboli	6	17	2.8
Deep vein thrombosis	19	30	1.6
Cardiovascular events			
Myocardial infarction	28	27	0.96
Anginal surgery	12	12	1.00
Stroke	24	34	1.41
Fractures (total)	71	47	0.66
Hip	20	9	0.45
Colles'	12	7	0.58
Spine	39	31	0.79

Effect on Central Nervous System

Raloxifene increases the incidence of hot flashes and is not a treatment for women who seek relief from menopausal symptoms. The difference in the incidence of hot flashes between the raloxifene- and placebo-treated groups is 5% to 6% in earlier studies (Delmas et al, 1997; Walsh et al, 1998). The effect of raloxifene on cognitive functioning and on the incidence of Alzheimer's disease is unknown.

TAMOXIFEN
Clinical Studies

In the United States, tamoxifen has been used for the treatment of advanced breast cancer since 1978. It has been found to prolong survival for women with node-positive and node-negative breast cancer and to prevent the occurrence of contralateral breast cancer (Early Breast Cancer Trialist Group, 1992). Initially, there were concerns that tamoxifen, acting as an estrogen-antagonist, could predispose patients to osteoporosis and heart disease. On the contrary, tamoxifen was actually found to increase bone density (Love et al, 1992), lower LDL-cholesterol and fibrinogen levels (Grey et al, 1995), and reduce the incidence of myocardial infarction (McDonald and Stewart, 1991; Rutqvist and Mattsson, 1993). However, tamoxifen was also found to increase the incidence of endometrial cancer (van Leeuwen et al, 1994). Therefore, it appears that for most organs (except, most notably, for the breast), tamoxifen acts like an estrogen.

Because tamoxifen has been found to prevent contralateral breast cancer, it may play a role in the prevention of breast cancer in women at high risk. To answer that question, a multicenter study enrolled 13,000 women in a placebo-controlled clinical trial. Subjects were required to be older than 35 years and to be at increased risk for breast cancer, equal to that of the average 60-year-old woman. Many subjects were premenopausal, and 40% were younger than 49 years. The study was terminated 14 months early because a clear treatment benefit for the reduction of breast cancer was observed. The mean duration of treatment was 4 years. Relative risk for breast cancer with tamoxifen treatment was reduced in all age groups: for women 49 and younger, RR was 0.65 (95% CI, 0.43 to 0.98); for women 50 to 59, RR was 0.52 (95% CI, 0.32 to 0.85); and for women 60 and older, RR was 0.47 (95% CI, 0.29 to 0.77) (Fisher et al, 1998). This reduction was observed for invasive breast cancer and for ductal carcinoma in situ (Table 21-3). Tamoxifen treatment was also found to increase endometrial cancer (RR, 2.4) and to decrease bone fractures (RR, 0.66). There was no difference in myocardial infarction rates between the tamoxifen and the placebo groups; this could be because of the young age and premenopausal status of many of the participants and the limited duration of treatment.

CONCLUSIONS

Estrogen replacement offers significant benefits to many postmenopausal women, especially to those in whom menopause occurred before age 45. The increased risk for endometrial and breast cancer seen with estrogen replacement appears to be small in comparison with its benefits. For women unable or unwilling to take estrogen treatment, the selective estrogen receptor modulators and the bisphosphonates may be useful. Benefits and risks of these treatments should be reviewed with each patient in detail, for ultimately she must decide whether to initiate therapy and to give her informed consent.

REFERENCES

Albrecht BH, Schiff I, Tulchinsky D, Ryan KJ: Objective evidence that placebo and oral medroxyprogesterone acetate therapy diminish menopausal vasomotor flushes. *Am J Obstet Gynecol* 1981; 139:631.

Alffam PH: An epidemiologic study of cervical and interochanteric fractures of the femur in suburban populations. *Acta Orthop Scand* 1964; 65:1.

Jordan VC, Gusman JE, Eckert S, et al: Incident Primary breast cancers are reduced by raloxifent: Integrated data from multicenter, double-blind, randomized trials in Presented at American Society of Clinical Oncology Meeting, Los Angeles, April 1998.

Amundsen DW, Diers CJ: The age of menopause in classical Greece and Rome. *Hum Biol* 1970; 42:79.

Anderson JJ, Ferguson DJP, Raab GM: Cell turnover in the resting human breast: Influence of parity, contraceptive pill, age, and laterality. *Br J Cancer* 1982; 46:376.

Archer DF, Pickar JH, Bottiglioni F: Bleeding patterns in postmenopausal women taking continuous combined or sequential regimens of conjugated estrogens with medroxyprogesterone acetate, *Obstet Gynecol* 1984; 83:686-692.

Bagatell CJ, Knopp RH, Vale WW, et al: Physiologic testosterone levels in normal men suppress high-density lipoprotein cholesterol levels. *Ann Intern Med* 1992; 116:967-973.

Ballejo G, Saleem TH, Khan-Dawood FS, et al: The effect of sex steroids on insulin-binding by target tissues in the rat. *Contraception* 1983; 28:413.

Baran D, Sorenson A, Grimes J, et al: Dietary modification with dairy products for preventing vertebral bone loss in premenopausal women: A 3-year prospective study. *J Clin Endocrinol Metab* 1990; 70:264-270.

Barrett-Connor E, Chang JC, Edelstein SL: Coffee-associated osteoporosis offset by daily milk consumption. *JAMA* 1994; 271:280-283.

Barrett-Connor E, Kritz-Silverstein D: Estrogen replacement therapy and cognitive function in older women. *JAMA* 1993; 269: 2637-2641.

Beattie CW, Rodgers CH, Soyka LF: Influence of ovariectomy and ovarian steroids on hypothalamic tyrosine hydroxylase activity in the rat. *Endocrinology* 1972; 91:276.

Bennion LJ: Changes in bile lipids accompanying oophorectomy in premenopausal women. *N Engl J Med* 1977; 297:709.

Berkow R, editor: *The Merck manual of diagnosis and therapy,* Rahway, N.J., 1987, Merck, Sharp & Dohme Research Laboratories.

Black DM, Cummings SR, Karpf DB, et al: Randomised trial of effect of alendronate on risk of fracture in women with existing vertebral fractures: Fracture Intervention Trial Research Group. *Lancet* 1996; 348:1535-1541.

Boukobza G: Efficacy and tolerance of veralipride in the treatment of flushing in the menopause. *Rev Fr Gynecol Obstet* 1986; 81:413-417.

Brenner DE, Kukull WA, Stergachis A, et al: Postmenopausal estrogen replacement therapy and the risk of Alzheimer's disease: A population-based case-control study. *Am J Epidemiol* 1994; 140:262-267.

Briancon D, Meunier PJ: Treatment of osteoporosis with fluoride, calcium, and vitamin D. *Orthop Clin North Am* 1981; 12:629-648.

Brinton LA, Hoover R, Fraymeni JF: Menopausal oestrogens and breast cancer risk: An expanded case-control study. *Br J Cancer* 1986; 54:825.

Caine YG, Bauer KA, Barzeger S, et al: Coagulation activation following estrogen administration to postmenopausal women. *Thromb Haemost* 1992; 68:392-395.

Callens A, Vaillant L, Lecomte P, et al: Does hormonal skin aging exist? A study of the influence of different hormone therapy regimens on the skin of postmenopausal women using non-invasive measurement techniques. *Dermatology* 1996; 193:289-294.

Campbell S, Whitehead M: Estrogen therapy and the postmenopausal syndrome. *Clin Obstet Gynecol* 1977; 4:31.

Cann CE, Genant HK, Ettinger B: Spinal mineral loss in oophorectomized women: Determination by quantitative computer tomography. *JAMA* 1980; 244:2056.

Cantilo E: Successful responses in diabetes mellitus of the menopause provided by the antagonistic action of sex hormones on pituitary activity. *Endocrinology* 1941; 28:20.

Carr BR, MacDonald PC: Estrogen treatment of postmenopausal women. *Adv Intern Med* 1983; 28:491.

Castelo-Branco C, Duran M, Gonzalez-Merlo J: Skin collagen changes related to age and hormone replacement therapy. *Maturitas* 1992; 15:113-119.

Chang RJ, Judd HL: Elevation of skin temperature of the finger as an objective index of postmenopausal hot flushes: Standardization of the techniques. *Am J Obstet Gynecol* 1979; 135:713.

Chapuy MC, et al: Vitamin D and calcium to prevent hip fractures in elderly women. *N Engl J Med* 1992; 327:1637-1642.

Charig CR, Rundle JS: Flushing: Long-term side effect of orchiectomy in treatment of prostatic carcinoma. *Urology* 1989; 33:175-178.

Christiansen C, Christiansen MS, Transbol I: Bone mass in postmenopausal women after withdrawal of estrogen/gestagen replacement therapy. *Lancet* 1981; 1:459.

Christiansen C, Riis BJ, Rodbro P: Prediction of rapid bone loss in postmenopausal women. *Lancet* 1987; 1:1105.

Chu J, Schweid Al, Weiss NS: Survival among women with endometrial cancer: A comparison of estrogen users and nonusers. *Am J Obstet Gynecol* 1982; 143:569.

Civitelli R, Gonelli S, Zacchei F, et al: Bone turnover in postmenopausal osteoporosis: Effect of calcitonin treatment. *J Clin Invest* 1988; 82:1268.

Clayden JR, Bell JW, Pollard P: Menopausal flushing: Double-blind trial of a nonhormonal medication. *BMJ* 1974; 1:409.

Colditz GA, Hankinson SE, Hunter DJ, et al: The use of estrogens and progestins and the risk of breast cancer in postmenopausal women. *N Engl J Med* 1995; 332:1589-1593.

Colditz GA, Willett WC, Stampfer MJ, et al: Menopause and the risk of coronary heart disease in women. *N Engl J Med* 1987; 316:1105.

Constantino JP, Kuller LH, Ives DG, et al: Coronary heart disease mortality and adjuvant tamoxifen therapy. *J Natl Cancer Inst.* 1997; 89:776-782.

The Coronary Drug Project Research Group: Findings leading to discontinuation of the 2.5 mg/day estrogen group. *JAMA* 1973; 226:652.

Cortes-Gallegos V, Villanueva GL, Sojo-Aranda I, et al: Inverted skin changes induced by estrogen and estrogen/glucocorticoid on aging dermis. *Gynecol Endocrinol* 1996; 10:125-128.

Cramer DW, Xu H, Harlow BL: Does "incessant" ovulation increase risk for early menopause? *Am J Obstet Gynecol* 1995; 172(part 1):568-573.

Crane MG, Harris JJ, Windsor W: Hypertension, oral contraceptive agents, and conjugated estrogens. *Ann Intern Med* 1971; 74:13.

Creasman WT, Henderson D, Hinshaw W, et al: Estrogen replacement therapy in the patient treated for endometrial cancer. *Obstet Gynecol* 1986; 67:326-330.

D'Amico JF, Grendale GA, Lu JK, et al: Induction of hypothalamic opioid activity with transdermal estradiol administration in postmenopausal women. *Fertil Steril* 1991; 55: 754.

Davidson BJ, Gambone JC, Lagasse LD: Free estradiol in postmenopausal women with and without endometrial cancer. *J Clin Endocrinol Metab* 1981; 52:404.

Dawson-Hughes B, Dallal GE, Krall et al: A controlled trial of the effect of calcium supplementation on bone density in postmenopausal women. *N Engl J Med* 1990; 323:878-883.

DeFazio J, Meldrum DR, Winer JH, et al: Direct action of androgen on hot flashes in the human male. *Maturitas* 1984; 6:8.

Deftos LJ, Weisman MH, William GW, et al: Influence of age and sex on plasma calcitonin in human beings. *N Engl J Med* 1980; 302:1351.

deGroen PC, Lubbe DF, Hirsh LJ, et al: Esophagitis associated with the use of alendronate. *N Engl J Med.* 1996; 335:1016-1021.

Delmas PD, Bjarnason NH, Mitlak BH, et al: The effects of raloxifene on bone mineral density, serum cholesterol, and uterine endometrium. *N Engl J Med.* 1997; 337:1641-1647.

Dequeker JV, Johnston CC, editors: *Noninvasive bone measurements,* Oxford, 1991, IRL Press.

Deutsch S, Ossowski B, Benjamin I: Comparison between degree of systemic description of vaginally and orally administered estrogens at different dose levels in postmenopausal women. *Am J Obstet Gynecol* 1981; 139:967.

DeVogt HJ, et al: Cardiovascular side effects of diethylstilbestrol, cyproterone acetate, and medroxyprogesterone acetate used for treatment of prostatic cancer. *J Urol* 1986; 135:303.

Duda RB, Taback B, Kessel B, et al: Ps2 expression induced by American ginseng in MCF-7 breast cancer cells. *Ann Surg Oncol* 1996; 3:515-520.

Dulbecco R, Henahan M, Armstrong B: Cell types and morphogenesis in the mammary gland. *Proc Natl Acad Sci USA* 1982; 79:7346.

Dunn LB, Damesyn M, Moore AA, et al: Does estrogen prevent skin aging? Results from the first National Health and Nutrition Examination Survey (NHANES I). *Arch Dermatol* 1997; 133:339-342.

Early Breast Cancer Trialists' Collaborative Group: Systemic treatment of early breast cancer by hormonal, cytotoxic, or immune therapy: 133 randomized trials involving 31,000 recurrences and 24,000 deaths among 75,000 women. *Lancet* 1992; 339:71-85.

Eli Lilly and Company. Evista (raloxifene hydrochloride) tablets prescribing information, Indianapolis, Ind., Dec. 10, 1997.

Elwood JM, Hayes DA: Clinical and pathologic features and survival of endometrial cancer patients in relation to prior use of estrogens. *Gynecol Oncol* 1980; 10:173.

Englund DE, Johansson EDB: Plasma levels of oestrone, oestradiol, and gonadotropins in postmenopausal women after oral and vaginal administration of conjugated equine estrogens. *Br J Obstet Gynaecol* 1987; 85:957.

Erlik Y, Meldrum DR, Judd HL: Estrogen levels in postmenopausal women with hot flushes. *Obstet Gynecol* 1982; 59:403.

Erlik Y, Meldrum DR, Lagasse LD, et al: Effect of megestrol acetate on flushing and bone metabolism in postmenopausal women. *Maturitas* 1981a; 3:167.

Erlik Y, Tataryn IV, Meldrum DR, et al: Association of waking episodes with menopausal hot flushes. *JAMA* 1981b; 245:1741.

Ettinger B, Black D, Cummings S, et al: Raloxifene reduces the risk of incidental vertebral fractures: 24-month interim analyses [abstract]. *Osteoporosis International* 1998; 8 (suppl. 3):n.p.

Ettinger B, Cann L, Genant K: Menopausal bone loss: Effects of conjugated estrogen and/or high calcium diet. *Maturitas* 1984; 6:108.

Felson DT, Sloutskis D, Anderson JJ, et al: Thiazide diuretics and the risk of hip fractures: Results from the Framingham study. *JAMA* 1991; 165:370-373.

Felson DT, Zhang Y, Hannan MT, et al: The effect of postmenopausal estrogen therapy on bone density in elderly women. *N Engl J Med* 1993; 329:1141-1146.

Fisher B, Costantino JP, Wickerham DL, et al: Tamoxifen for prevention of breast cancer: Report of the National Surgical Adjuvant Breast and Bowel Project P-1 Study. *J Natl Cancer Inst* 1998; 90:1371-1388.

Freedman RR, Woodward S, Sabharwal SC: Alpha 2-adrenergic mechanism in menopausal hot flushes. *Obstet Gynecol* 1992; 76:573.

Freedman RR, Woodward S: Behavioral treatment of menopausal hot flushes: Evaluation by ambulatory monitoring. *Am J Obstet Gynecol* 1992; 167:436-439.

Gallagher JC, Kable WT, Goldgar D: Effect of progestin therapy on cortical and trabecular bone: Comparison with estrogen. *Am J Med* 1991; 90:171-178.

Gambrell RD: Clinical use of progestins in the menopausal patient. *J Reprod Med* 1982a; 27:531.

Gambrell RD, Massen FW, Castaneda TA: The use of the progestin challenge test to reduce the risk of endometrial cancer. *Obstet Gynecol* 1980; 55:732.

Gambrell RD Jr: The menopause: Benefits and risks of estrogen-progesterone replacement therapy. *Fertil Steril* 1982; 32:457.

Genant HK, Lucas J, Weiss S, et al: Low-dose esterified estrogen therapy. *Arch Intern Med* 1997; 157:2609-2615.

Geola FL, et al: Biological effects of various doses of conjugated equine estrogens in postmenopausal women. *J Clin Endocrinol Metab* 1980; 51:620.

Ginsburg ES, Mello NK, Mendelson JH, et al: Effects of alcohol ingestion on estrogens in postmenopausal women. *JAMA* 1996; 276: 1747-1751.

Ginsburg ES, Walsh BW, Gao X, et al: The effects of acute ethanol ingestion on estrogen levels in postmenopausal women using transdermal estradiol. *J Soc Gynecol Invest* 1995a; 2:26-29.

Ginsburg ES, Walsh BW, Gao X, et al: The effects of ethanol on the clearance of estradiol in

postmenopausal women. *Fertil Steril* 1995b; 63:1227-1230.

Gordon T, et al: High density lipoprotein as a protective factor against coronary heart disease. *Am J Med* 1977; 62:707.

Gordon G, Vaughan C: *Clinical management of the osteoporoses,* Acton, Mass., 1976, Publishing Sciences Group.

Grandberg S, et al: Endometrial thickness measured by endovaginal ultrasound for identifying endometrial abnormality. *Am J Obstet Gynecol* 1991; 164(part 1):47-52.

Grey AB, Stapleton JP, Evans MC, Reid IR: The effect of the anti-estrogen tamoxifen on cardiovascular risk factors in normal postmenopausal women. *J Clin Endocrinol Metab* 1995; 80:3191-3195.

Grodin JM, Siiteri PK, MacDonald PC: Source of estrogen production in postmenopausal women. *J Clin Endocrinol Metab* 1973; 36:207.

Grodstein F, Stampfer MJ, Colditz GA, et al: Postmenopausal hormone therapy and mortality. *N Engl J Med* 1997; 336:1769-1775.

Haas S, et al: The effect of transdermal estradiol on hormone and metabolic dynamics over a six-week period. *Obstet Gynecol* 1998; 71: 671.

Hammond MG, Hatley L, Talbert LM: A double-blind study to evaluate the effect of methyldopa on menopausal vasomotor flushes. *J Clin Endocrinol Metab* 1984; 58:1158.

Harris ST, et al: The effect of short-term treatment with alendronate on vertebral density and biochemical markers on bone remodeling in early postmenopausal women. *J Clin Endocrinol Metab* 1993; 76:1399-1406.

Harris ST, et al: Four year study of intermittent cyclic etidronate treatment of postmenopausal osteoporosis: Three years of blinded therapy followed by one year of open therapy. *Am J Med* 1993; 95:557-567.

Heanly RP: Estrogens and postmenopausal osteoporosis. *Clin Obstet Gynecol* 1976; 19:791.

Heller RF, Jacobs HS: Coronary heart disease in relation to age, sex, and the menopause. *BMJ* 1978; 1:472.

Henderson BE, Paganini-Hill A, Ross RK: Decreased mortality in users of estrogen replacement therapy. *Arch Intern Med* 1991; 151: 75-78.

Henderson VW, Paganini-Hill A, Emanuel CK, et al: Estrogen replacement therapy in older women: Comparisons between Alzheimer's disease cases and nondemented control subjects. *Arch Neurol* 1994; 51:896-900.

Henderson VW, Watt L, Buckwalter JG: Cognitive skills associated with estrogen replacement in women with Alzheimer's disease. *Psychoneuroendocrinology* 1996; 21:421-430.

Henry F, Pierard-Franchimont C, Cauwenbergh G, et al: Age related changes in facial skin contours and rheology. *J Am Geriatr Soc* 1997; 45:220-222.

Hillyard CJ, Stevenson JC, MacIntyre I: Relative deficiency of plasma calcitonin in normal women. *Lancet* 1978; 1:961.

Hirata JD, Swiersz LM, Zell B, et al: Does dong quai have estrogenic effects in postmenopausal women? A double-blind, placebo-controlled trial. *Fertil Steril* 1997; 68:981-986.

Hirvonen E, Malkonen M, Manninen V: Effects of different progestins. *N Engl J Med* 1981; 304:560.

Honjo J, Tanaka K, Kashiwagi T, et al: Senile dementia—Alzheimer's type and estrogen. *Horm Metab Res* 1995; 27:204-207.

Hopper JL, Seeman E: The bone density of female twins discordant for tobacco use. *N Engl J Med* 1994; 330:387-392.

Horsman A, Simpson M, Kirby PA: Nonlinear bone loss in oophorectomized women. *Br J Radiol* 1977; 50:504.

Huggins C, Stevens RE, Hodges CU: Studies of prostatic cancer, II: The effects of castration in advanced carcinoma of the prostate. *Arch Surg* 1941; 43:209.

Hulley S, Grady D, Bush T, et al: Randomized trial of estrogen plus progestin for secondary prevention of coronary heart disease in postmenopausal women. *JAMA* 1998; 280:605-613.

Hyashi T, et al: Basal release of nitric oxide from aortic rings is greater in female rabbits than in male rabbits: Implications for atherosclerosis. *Proc Natl Acad Sci USA* 1992; 89:11259-11263.

Iosif CS, et al: Estrogen receptors in the human female lower urinary tract. *Am J Obstet Gynecol* 1981; 141:817.

Iskrant AP: The etiology of fractured hips in females. *Am J Public Health* 1968; 58:485.

Jacobs DM, Tang MX, Stern Y, et al: Cognitive function in nondemented older women who took estrogen after menopause. *Neurology* 1998; 50:368-373.

Jensen J, Christiansen C, Rodbro P: Cigarette smoking, serum estrogens, and bone loss during hormone-replacement therapy early after menopause. *N Engl J Med* 1985; 313:973-975.

Johnson AE, et al: Estradiol modulation of noradrenergic receptors in the guinea pig brain assessed by tritium-sensitive film autoradiography. *Brain Res* 1985; 336:153.

Jones KP, Ravnikar VA, Schiff I: Effect of lofexidine on vasomotor flushes. *Maturitas* 1985; 7:135.

Kakar F, Wass NS, Strite SA: Noncontraceptive estrogen use and risk of gallstone disease in women. *Am J Public Health* 1988; 78:564.

Kampen DL, Sherwin BB: Estrogen use and verbal memory in healthy postmenopausal women. *Obstet Gynecol* 1994; 83:979-983.

Kannel WB, Wolf PA, Castelli WP, d'Augustino RB: Fibrinogen and risk of cardiovascular disease. *JAMA* 1987; 258:1183-1186.

Kauffman RF, Bryant HU: Selective estrogen receptor modulators. *Drug News Perspect* 1995; 8:531-539.

Kawas C, Resnik S, Morrison A, et al: A prospective study of estrogen replacement therapy and the risk of developing Alzheimer's disease: The Baltimore Longitudinal Study of Aging. *Neurology* 1997; 48:1517-1521.

Keene GS, Parker MJ, Pryor GA: Mortality and morbidity after hip fractures. *BMJ* 1993; 307:1248-1250.

Kirkland RT, et al: Decrease in plasma high-density lipoprotein cholesterol levels at puberty in boys with delayed adolescence: Correlation with plasma testosterone levels. *JAMA* 1987; 257:502.

Klug PW, Laurier G: Comparisons of vaginal ultrasound and histologic findings of the endometrium. *Geburtshilfe Frauenheilkd* 1989; 49:797-802.

Komm BS, et al: Estrogen binding, receptor MRNA, and biologic response in osteoblast-like osteosarcoma cells. *Science* 1988; 241:81.

Krall EA, Dawson-Hughes B: Walking, bone mineral density and bone loss. *J Bone Miner Res* 1993; 8(suppl 1):SI50.

Lacroix AZ, et al: Thiazide diuretic agents and the incidence of hip fracture. *N Engl J Med* 1990; 322:286-290.

Langer RD, Pierce JJ, O'Hanlon KA, et al: Transvaginal ultrasonography compared to en-dometrial biopsy for the detection of endome-trial disease. *N Engl J Med* 1997; 337:1792-1798.

Laufer LK, et al: Effect of clonidine on hot flashes in postmenopausal women. *Obstet Gynecol* 1982; 60:483.

Lauritzen JB, et al: Radial and humeral fractures as predictors of subsequent hip, radial or humeral fractures in women and their seasonal variation. *Osteoporosis Int* 1993; 3:133-137.

Leather AT, Savvas M, Studd JW: Endometrial histology and bleeding patterns after 8 years of continuous combined estrogen and progestogen therapy in postmenopausal women. *Obstet Gynecol* 1991; 78:1008-1010.

Lebherz TB, French LT: Nonhormonal treatment of the menopausal syndrome: A double-blind evaluation of an autonomic system stabilizer. *Obstet Gynecol* 1969; 33:795.

Lerner DJ, Kannel WB: Patterns of coronary dis-ease morbidity and mortality: A 26-year fol-low-up of the Framingham population. *Am Heart J* 1986; 111:383.

Liberman UA, Weiss SR, Broll J, et al: Effect of oral alendronate on bone mineral density and the incidence of fractures in postmenopausal osteoporosis. *N Engl J Med* 1995;333:1437-1443.

Licata AA, et al: Acute effects of dietary protein on calcium metabolism in patients with osteo-porosis. *J Gerontol* 1981; 36:14.

Lindsay R, et al: Incidence, cost and risk factors of fracture of the proximal femur in the USA. In Christiansen C, et al, editors: *Osteoporosis,* Denmark, 1984, Aalborg Stoftsbogturkkeri.

Lindsay R, et al: Long-term prevention of post-menopausal osteoporosis by estrogens. *Lancet* 1976b; 1:1038.

Lindsay R, et al: Comparative effects of oestro-gen and a progestagen on bone loss in post-menopausal women. *Clin Sci Mol Med* 1978; 54:193.

Lindsay R, Sweeney A: Urinary cyclic AMP in osteoporosis. *Scott Med J* 1976a; 21:231.

Lobo RA, Brenner PF, Mishell DR: Metabolic parameters and steroid levels in post-menopausal women receiving lower doses of natural estrogen replacement. *Obstet Gynecol* 1983; 62:94.

Love RR, Mazess RB, Barden HS, et al: Effects of tamoxifen on bone mineral density in post-menopausal women with breast cancer. *N Engl J Med* 1992; 326:852-856.

Luine VN, McEwen BS: Effect of estradiol on turnover of type A monamine oxidase in brain. *J Neurochem* 1977; 28:1221.

Mandel FP, et al: Biologic effects of various doses of vaginally administered conjugated equine estrogens in postmenopausal women. *J Clin Endocrinol Metab* 1983; 57:133.

Mandel FP, et al: Biologic effects of various doses of ethinyl estradiol in postmenopausal women. *Obstet Gynecol* 1982; 59:673.

Mannucci PM, Bettega D, Chantarangkul V, et al: Effect of tamoxifen on measurements of hemostasis in healthy postmenopausal women. *Arch Intern Med* 1996; 156:1806-1810.

Manolagas SC, Anderson DG: Detection of high-affinity glucocorticold binding in rat bone. *J Endocrinol* 1978; 76:379.

Manson JE, et al: A prospective study of post-menopausal estrogen therapy and subsequent incidence of non-insulin-dependent diabetes mellitus. *Ann Epidemiol* 1992; 2:665-673.

Mashchak CA, et al: Comparison of pharmaco-dynamic properties of various estrogen formu-lations. *Am J Obstet Gynecol* 1982; 144:511.

Mashchak CA, Lobo RA: Estrogen replacement therapy and hypertension. *J Reprod Med* 1985b; 30(suppl):805.

Mashchak CA, et al: The relation of physiologi-cal changes to subjective symptoms in post-menopausal women with and without hot flushes. *Maturitas* 1985a; 6:301.

Mateo L, et al: Bone mineral density in patients with temporal arteritis and polymyalgia rheumatica. *J Rheumatol* 1993; 20:1369-1373.

Matkovic V, et al: Bone status and fracture rates in two regions of Yugoslavia. *Am J Clin Nutr* 1979; 32:540.

Matthews KA, et al: Menopause and risk factors for coronary heart disease. *N Engl J Med* 1989; 321:641-646.

Mazess RB, et al: Enhanced precision with dual-energy x-ray absorptiometry. *Calcif Tissue lnt* 1992; 51:14-17.

McDonald CC, Stewart HJ, for the Scottish Breast Cancer Committee. Fatal myocardial infarction in the Scottish adjuvant tamoxifen trial. *BMJ* 1991; 303:435-437.

McGill HC: Sex steroid hormone receptors in the cardiovascular system. *Postgrad Med* 1989 (April); :64-68.

McKinlay S, Jeffreys M, Thompson B: An inves-tigation of the age of menopause. *J Biosoc Sci* 1972; 4:161.

Mendelson EB, et al: Endometrial abnormalities: Evaluation with transvaginal sonography. *Am J Roentgenol* 1988; 150:139-142.

Michnovicz JJ, et al: Increased 2-hydroxylation of estradiol as a possible mechanism for the anti-estrogenic effect of cigarette smoking. *N Engl J Med* 1986; 315:1305-1309.

Morrison JC, et al: The use of medroxyproges-terone acetate for the relief of climacteric symptoms. *Am J Obstet Gynecol* 1980; 138:99.

Mundy GR: Osteoporosis: Boning up on genes. *Nature* 1994; 367:216-217.

Murkies AL, Lombard C, Strauss BJ, et al: Di-etary flour supplementation decreases post-menopausal hot flushes: Effect of soy and wheat. *Maturitas* 1995; 21:189-195.

Nachtigall LE: Comparative study: Replens® versus local estrogen in menopausal women. *Fertil Steril* 1994; 61:178-180.

Nasri MN, Coast GJ: Correlation of ultrasound findings and endometrial histopathology in postmenopausal women. *Br J Obstet Gynecol* 1989; 96:1333-1338.

Nathorst-Boos J, et al: Is sexual life influenced by transdermat estrogen therapy: A double blind placebo controlled study in post-menopausal women. *Acta Obstet Gynecol Scand* 1993; 72:656-660.

Nixon RL, Jamowsky DS, David JM: Effects of progesterone, estrogen, and testosterone on the uptake and metabolism of ³H-norepineph-ritic, ³H-dopamine, and ³H-serotonin in rat synaptosomes. *Res Common Chem Pathol Pharmacol* 1974; 7:233.

Norcross WA, Schmidt JD: Hot flashes in men with testicular insufficiency. *West J Med* 1986; 145:515-516.

Ottosson UB, et al: Conversion of oral proges-terone into deoxycorticosterone during post-menopausal replacement therapy. *Acta Obstet Gynecol Scand* 1984; 63:577.

Ottosson UB, Johanson BG, Schoultz B: Sub-fraction of high-density lipoprotein choles-terol: A comparison between progesterone and natural progesterone. *Am J Obstet Gynecol* 1985; 151:746-750.

Overgaard K, Hansen MA, Jensen SB, et al: Ef-fect of calcitonin given intranasally on bone mass and fracture rates in established osteo-porosis: A dose-response study. *BMJ* 1992; 305:556-561.

Paik SG, et al: Induction of insulin-dependent di-abetes by streptozotocin: Inhibition by estro-gens, potentiation by androgens. *Diabetes* 1982; 31:724.

Paul SM, et al: Estrogen-induced efflux of en-dogenous catecholamines from the hypothala-mus in vitro. *Brain Res* 1979; 178:499.

Phillips SM, Sherwin BB: Effects of estrogen on memory function in surgically menopausal women. *Psychoneuroendocrinology* 1992; 17:485-495.

Pierard GE, Letawe C, Dowlati A, et al: Effect of hormone replacement therapy for menopause on the mechanical properties of skin. *J Am Geriatr Soc* 1995; 43:662-665.

Pierard-Franchimont C, Letawe C, Goffin V, et al: Skin water-holding capacity and transder-mal estrogen therapy for menopause: A pilot study. *Maturitas* 1995; 22:151-154.

Raz R, Stamm WE: A controlled trial of intra-vaginal estriol in postmenopausal women with recurrent urinary tract infections. *N Engl J Med* 1993; 329:753-756.

Resnick SM, Metter EJ, Zonderman AB: Estro-gen replacement therapy and longitudinal de-cline in visual memory: A possible protective effect? *Neurology* 1997; 49:1491-1497.

Riggs BL, et al: Effect of fluoride treatment on the fracture rate in postmenopausal women with osteoporosis. *N Engl J Med* 1990; 322:802-809.

Riis B, Thomsen K, Christiansen C: Does calcium supplementation prevent post-menopausal bone loss? *N Engl J Med* 1987; 316:173.

Robinson D, Friedman L, Marcus R, et al: Estro-gen replacement therapy and memory in older women. *J Am Geriatr Soc* 1994; 42:919-922.

Rubin GL: Estrogen replacement therapy and the risk of endometrial cancer: Remaining contro-versies. *Am J Obstet Gynecol* 1990; 162:148-154.

Rutqvist LE, Mattsson A, for the Stockholm Breast Cancer Study Group: Cardiac and thomboembolic morbidity among post-menopausal women with early stage breast cancer in a randomized trial of adjuvant ta-moxifen. *J Natl Cancer Inst* 1993; 85:1398-1406.

Sack MN, Rader DK, Cannon RO: Oestrogen and inhibition of oxidation of low-density lipoproteins in postmenopausal women. *Lancet* 1994; 343:269-270.

Sacks FM, McPherson R, Walsh BW: Effect of postmenopausal estrogen replacement of plasma lipoprotein (a) concentrations. *Arch Intern Med* 1994; 154:1106-1110.

Sacks FM, Pfeffer MA, Moye LA, et al: The effect of pravastatin on coronary events after myocardial infarction in patients with average cholesterol levels: Cholesterol and Recurrent Events Trial investigators. *N Engl J Med* 1996; 335:1001-1009.

Schiff I, et al: Effects of estrogens on sleep and psychological state of hypogonadal women. *JAMA* 1979; 242:2405.

Schiff I, et al: Endometrial hyperplasia in women on cyclic or continuous estrogen regimens. *Fertil Steril* 1982; 37:79.

Schiff I, Tulchinsky D, Ryan KJ: Vaginal absorption of estrone and 17α-estradiol. *Fertil Steril* 1977; 28:1963.

Schiff I, Wilson E: Clinical aspects of aging of the female reproductive system. In Schneider EL, editor: *The aging reproductive system,* New York, 1978, Raven Press.

Schneider DL, Barrett-Connor EL, Morton DJ: Thyroid hormone use and bone mineral density in elderly women. *JAMA* 1994; 271:1245-1249.

Schott AM, Hans D, Sornay-Rendu E, et al: Ultrasound measurements on os calcis: Precision and age-related changes in a normal female population. *Osteoporosis Int* 1993; 3:249-254.

Schwartz U, Hammerstein J: The estrogenic potency of ethinyl estradiol and mestranol—a comparative study. *J Acta Endocrinol* 1973; 72:118.

Sherman BW, West JH, Korenman SG: The menopausal transition: Analysis of LH, FSH, estradiol, and progesterone concentrations during menstrual cycles of older women. *J Clin Endocrinol Metab* 1976; 42:629.

Sherwin BB: Hormones, mood, and cognitive function in postmenopausal women. *Obstet Gynecol* 1996; 87(suppl): 20S-26S.

Shewmon DA, Stock JL, Rosen CJ, et al: Tamoxifen and estrogen lower circulating lipoprotein(a) concentrations in healthy postmenopausal women. *Arterioscler Thromb* 1994; 14:1586-1593.

Shionoiri H, et al: An increase in high-molecular weight renin substrate associated with estrogenic hypertension. *Biochem Med* 1983; 29:14.

Siddle N, Whitehead M: Flexible prescribing of estrogens. *Contemp Ob Gyn* 1983; 22:137.

Silfverstolpe G, et al: Lipid metabolic studies in oophorectomized women: Effect on serum lipids and lipoproteins of three synthetic progestogens. *Maturitus* 1982; 4:103.

Slemenda CW, et al: Predictors of bone mass in perimenopausal women: A prospective study of clinical data using photon absorptiometry. *Ann Intern Med* 1990; 112:96-101.

Smith DM, Nance WE, Kang KW: Genetic factors in determining bone mass. *J Clin Invest* 1973; 52:2800.

Smith JA: Androgen suppression by a gonadotropin releasing hormone analogue in patients with metastatic carcinoma of the prostate. *J Urol* 1984; 131:110.

Spellacy WN: Carbohydrate metabolism in male infertility and female fertility-control patients. *Fertil Steril* 1976; 27:1132.

Spellacy WN, Butri WC, Birk SA: Effect of estrogen treatment for one year on carbohydrate and lipid metabolism in women with normal and abnormal glucose tolerance test results. *Am J Obstet Gynecol* 1978; 131:87.

Stamler J, et al: Effects of long-term estrogen therapy on serum cholesterol-lipid-lipoprotein levels and mortality in middle aged men with previous myocardial infarction. *Circulation* 1980; 22:658.

Steingold KA, et al: Treatment of hot flashes with transdermal estradiol. *J Clin Endocrinol Metab* 1985; 61:627.

Steinleitner A, et al: Decreased in vitro production of 6-keto prostaglandin by uterine arteries from postmenopausal women. *Am J Obstet Gynecol* 1989; 161:1677-1681.

Stevenson JC, et al: Calcitonin and the calcium-regulating hormones in postmenopausal women: Effect of estrogens. *Lancet* 1981; 1:693.

Stevenson JC, et al: Effects of transdermal versus oral hormone replacement therapy on bone density in spine and proximal femur in postmenopausal women. *Lancet* 1990; 336:256-269.

Storm T, et al: Effect of intermittent cyclical etidronate therapy on bone mass and fracture rate in women with postmenopausal osteoporosis. *N Engl J Med* 1990; 322:1265-1271.

Studd JWW, et al: The prevention and treatment of endometrial pathology. In Pasetto N, Paoletti R, Ambrus JL, editors: *The menopause and postmenopause,* Lancaster, U.K., 1980, MTP Press.

Sullivan JM, et al: Estrogen replacement and coronary artery disease. *Arch Intern Med* 1990; 150:2557-2562.

Sullivan JM, et al: Postmenopausal estrogen use and coronary atherosclerosis. *Ann Intern Med* 1988; 108:358-363.

Thangaraju M, et al: Effect of tamoxifen on plasma lipids and lipoproteins in postmenopausal women with breast cancer. *Cancer* 1994; 73:659-663.

Thompson B, Hart SA, Durno D: Menopausal age and symptomatology in general practice. *J Biol Sci* 1973; 5:71-82.

Thompson P, Taylor J, Fisher A: A prospective study of fracture prediction using heel ultrasound in postmenopausal women. *J Bone Miner Res* 1996; 11:1829.

Tikkanen MJ, et al: Different effects of two progestins on HDL. *Atherosclerosis* 1981; 40:365.

Tremollieres FA, Pouilles JM, Ribot C: Vertebral postmenopausal bone loss is reduced in overweight women: A longitudinal study in 155 early postmenopausal women. *J Clin Endocrinol Metab* 1993; 77:683-686.

van Leeuwen FE, Benraadt J, Coebergh JWW, et al: Risk of endometrial cancer after tamoxifen treatment of breast cancer. *Lancet* 1994; 343:448-452.

Vercellini P, et al: Veralipride for hot flushes during gonadotropin-releasing hormone agonist treatment. *Gynecol Obstet Invest* 1992; 34:102-104.

Vermeulen A: The hormonal activity of the postmenopausal ovary. *J Clin Endocrinol Metab* 1976; 42:247.

Wagner JD, et al: Estrogen and progesterone replacement therapy reduces low density lipoprotein accumulation in the coronary arteries of surgically postmenopausal cynomolgus monkeys. *J Clin Invest* 1991; 88:1995-2002.

Walsh BW, Kuller LH, Wild RA, et al: Effects of raloxifene on serum lipids and coagulation factors in healthy postmenopausal women. *JAMA* 1998; 279:1445-1451.

Walsh BW, Schiff I, Rosner B, et al: Effects of postmenopausal estrogen replacement on the concentrations and metabolism of plasma lipoproteins. *N Engl J Med.* 1991; 325:1196-1204.

Watts NB, et al: Intermittent cyclical etidronate treatment of postmenopausal osteoporosis. *N Engl J Med J* 1990; 323:73-79.

Weiss NS, et al: Decreased risk of fractures of the hip and lower forearm with postmenopausal use of estrogen. *N Engl J Med* 1980; 303:1195.

Weiss NS, et al: Endometrial cancer in relation to patterns of menopausal estrogen use, *JAMA* 1979; 242:261.

Weiss NS, et al: Noncontraceptive estrogen use and the occurrence of ovarian cancer. *J Natl Cancer Inst* 1982; 68:95.

The Writing Group for the PEPI Trial. Effects of estrogen and estrogen/progestin regimens on heart disease risk factors in postmenopausal women. *JAMA.* 1995; 273:199-208.

Whitehead MI, et al: Absorption and metabolism of oral progesterone. *BMJ* 1980; 280:825.

Whitehead MI, et al: Effects of estrogens and progestins on the biochemistry and morphology of the postmenopausal endometrium. *N Engl J Med* 1981; 305:1599.

Whittaker PG, Morgan MR, Dean PD: Serum equiline, estrone, and estradiol levels in postmenopausal women receiving conjugated equine estrogens. *Lancet* 1980; 1:14.

Williams JK, et al: Short-term administration of estrogen and vascular responses of atherosclerotic coronary arteries. *J Am Coll Cardiol* 1992; 20:452-457.

Yang NN, Venugopalan M, Hardikar S, Glasebrook A: Identification of an estrogen response element activated by metabolites of 17β-estradiol and raloxifene. *Science* 1996; 273:1222-1225.

Yen SSC: The biology of menopause *J Reprod Med* 1977; 18:28.

Zinner NN, Sterling AM, Ritter RC: Role of urethral softness in urinary incontinence. *Urology* 1980; 16:115.

22

Urogynecology and Pelvic Floor Dysfunction

MARIE-ANDRÉE HARVEY

EBOO VERSI

KEY ISSUES

1. What disruptions in pelvic floor anatomy result in incontinence and prolapse?
2. What new management strategies are employed in the treatment of genuine stress incontinence?
3. What are painful bladder syndromes?
4. New examination and imaging techniques are utilized for management of disorders of pelvic floor support.
5. Can anal incontinence be prevented? New diagnostic approaches are discussed.

Urogynecology has been a rapidly evolving field, and it now encompasses all disorders involving the pelvic floor. In addition to aspects of lower urinary tract function and dysfunction, it includes disorders of pelvic organ support and anal incontinence, primarily as they are related to the trauma of childbirth.

Obviously, there are situations in which the interface between the urogynecologist, the urologist, and the proctologist becomes blurred. In such situations, surgeons from these specialties must work together, and such collaboration is to be encouraged.

EPIDEMIOLOGY
Urinary Incontinence
Prevalence

Most published data on urinary incontinence address prevalence rates in defined groups. Although they are useful, these studies do not yield reliable information on the global problem of female urinary dysfunction. It is generally understood that incontinence is underreported, but inaccuracies can also arise from the data collected through mailed questionnaires in which reliance is placed on the patient's assessment of urine leakage rather than on objective demonstration.

In children between 5 and 14 years of age, 6.9% of boys and 5.1% of girls have regular incontinence, whereas 10.9% of boys and 11.2% of girls have occasional incontinence (Thomas et al, 1980) (Fig. 22-1). From 15 years of age on, the prevalence of urinary incontinence increases with age and is higher in women than it is in men (Brocklehurst et al, 1968). However, stress incontinence is more common than urge incontinence, although the prevalence of the latter does tend to rise in the elderly (Kondo et al, 1992).

Menopause has often been proposed as a cause of incontinence, but there is no good epidemiological evidence to suggest that the menopause per se (i.e., estrogen deficiency) results in incontinence (Versi, 1994). The reason for this association is that the prevalence of stress incontinence reaches a peak in the fifth and sixth decades and is coincident with the menopause. However, rates decline thereafter (Jolleys, 1988), which is contrary to what would be expected if this were an estrogen-deficiency symptom. Analysis of studies in postmenopausal women using hormone replacement therapy for the treatment of genuine stress incontinence does not show a consistent beneficial effect (Cardozo and Versi, 1993). The prevalence of urge incontinence and detrusor instability appears to rise after the menopause, but this may be an age-related rather than a hormone-related phenomenon.

Psychosocial

The psychosocial impact of incontinence is considerable, with 34% of patients complaining that it interferes significantly with household chores and other daily activities (Minaire and Jacquelin, 1992). The psychological reaction to incontinence resembles reactive depression. Psychological symptoms associated with urinary incontinence are

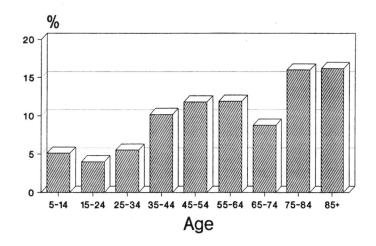

Fig. 22-1. The prevalence of female urinary incontinence at different ages. (Modified from Thomas TM, Plymat KR, Blannin J, et al: Prevalence of urinary incontinence. *BMJ* 1980; 281:1243.)

tension and sleep disorders. This was confirmed in a report showing that incontinence-related psychoneurosis resulted from decreased quality of life rather than from underlying personality traits (Kelleher et al, 1993). With regard to quality of life, middle-aged women experience more deleterious effects than older women, and it is the incontinence itself, not the frequency or the severity, that causes this negative impact.

Costs

It is difficult to estimate the total cost of urinary incontinence because reliable data are lacking. However, in 1995 it is known that $26.3 billion was spent on incontinence in direct costs for the over-65 population in the United States (Wagner and Hu, 1998). In 1983 the cost of palliative care in France was $35 million, and the anticipated growth was 30% per annum (Minaire and Buzelin, 1992). Overall in the western world, significant incontinence probably afflicts between 4% and 8% of the population, yet only 5% of these persons have a precise medical diagnosis (Veilas et al, 1989). Thus the problem of incontinence is widespread and expensive.

Pelvic Floor Prolapse

Although it accounts for more than 400,000 surgical procedures annually in the United States (Mallet and Bump, 1994), the prevalence of genital prolapse has not been the subject of many studies. Only two studies have reported on the prevalence of utero-vaginal prolapse, but none have addressed the general climacteric population. Bump (1993), in a comparison of black and white women, disclosed a 24% and 23% prevalence of severe prolapse, respectively. However, this was a population referred for genito-vaginal prolapse, and it was not representative of the general climacteric population. The National Health Interview Survey Data (Kjerulff et al, 1996) reported a prolapse prevalence rate of 2.1 per 1000 women, and the estimated annual incidence of

the condition was 97,034 women per year. However, this was based on in-home interviews of noninstitutionalized patients. Diagnoses were reported by patients and were not verified by chart review, and the study excluded women who were older than 50 (range, 18 to 50 years); hence, they were not relevant to the majority who experience the problem.

We have studied the prevalence of pelvic organ prolapse in 285 climacteric women without primary urogenital symptoms (data not published). Our study established 51%, 27%, and 20% prevalence rates of anterior wall, posterior wall, and apical prolapse, respectively, almost all of which were minor (not protruding through the hymen). No increase with advancing menopausal age was documented as significant, though a trend was noted for anterior and apical prolapse.

Anal Incontinence

Anal incontinence is the involuntary loss of feces or flatus. If urinary incontinence is just coming out of the closet, anal incontinence remains taboo; therefore epidemiological data are scant. Among women older than 45, 11% are found to be incontinent to flatus and feces, and 2% have weekly episode of fecal incontinence (Denis et al, 1992). Ten percent to 33% of institutionalized elderly women had fecal incontinence.

EMBRYOLOGY OF THE LOWER URINARY TRACT
Kidneys and Ureters

Kidneys and ureters are formed through a three-stage process that recapitulates development of the excretory system in primitive vertebrates. During the third week of embryonic life, the mesoderm forming the nephrogenic cord along the dorsal body wall gives rise to several pairs of tubules, the pronephros. This system is transient and nonfunctioning in the human (Crelin, 1978). Formation and degeneration of the pronephros proceeds in a cranial-to-caudal sequence and is

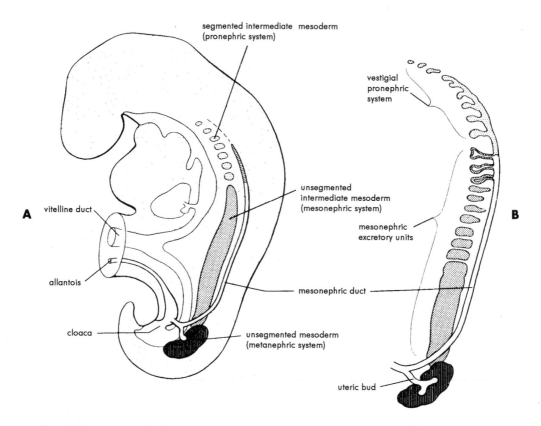

Fig. 22-2. A, Schematic diagram of the intermediate mesoderm shows the relationship among the pronephric, mesonephric, and metanephric systems. In the cervical and upper thoracic regions, the intermediate mesoderm is segmented. In the lower thoracic, lumbar, and sacral regions, it forms a solid, unsegmented mass of tissue, the nephrogenic cord. Note the longitudinal collecting duct, initially formed by the pronephros but later taken over by the mesonephros. **B,** Schematic representation of the excretory tubules of the pronephric and mesonephric systems in a 5-week-old embryo. The ureteric bud penetrates the metanephric tissue. Note the remnant of the pronephric excretory tubules and the longitudinal collecting duct.

complete by the end of the fourth week. The only persistent component of this system is the pronephric duct. Initially, it comprises the union of the pronephric tubules, but, as they degenerate, the duct continues to grow caudally to join the cloaca during the fifth week. Subsequently, it is retained as the mesonephric duct.

The second primitive kidney, the mesonephros, develops within the nephrogenic cord caudal to the pronephros, beginning in the fourth week. The tubules begin as blind vesicles that grow to join the mesonephric duct laterally. Medially each tubule forms a Bowman's capsule and associates with a vascular glomerulus. The mesonephros probably functions to produce urine in the human fetus during the third and fourth months (DeMartino and Zamboni, 1966). In the female, the entire system degenerates, leaving only vestigial remnants. The persistent tubules may be identified in the mesovarium of the adult as the epoöphoron and paroöphoron, whereas the mesonephric duct becomes Gartner's duct within the broad ligament and the lateral paravaginal tissues. In the male, the mesonephros also degenerates, but the duct persists and, under the influence of androgens, develops into the male genital duct system.

The third and permanent kidney, the metanephros, arises from the metanephric mesenchyme, the most caudal portion of the mesodermal nephrogenic cord. Its collecting system, the ureter, develops as an outgrowth of the mesonephric duct. The ureteric bud arises from the caudal end of the mesonephric duct (Fig. 22-2). It grows cranially, pushing into the metanephric mesenchyme and induces this tissue to differentiate into permanent nephrons (Grobstein, 1955). Factors originating in the metanephric mesenchyme then induce a series of dichotomous subdivisions in the cranial portion of the ureter that ultimately form the calyceal collecting system. The distal portion elongates to form the permanent ureter. Apparent ascent and medial rotation of the metanephros to its permanent position occur as a result of rapid growth of the caudal structures of the embryo over the ensuing weeks. The metanephros produces urine by the fourth month of fetal life.

Bladder and Urethra

The bladder and the urethra are primarily derived from endodermal tissue. The expanded distal portion of the hindgut—the cloaca—is divided by the urorectal fold into

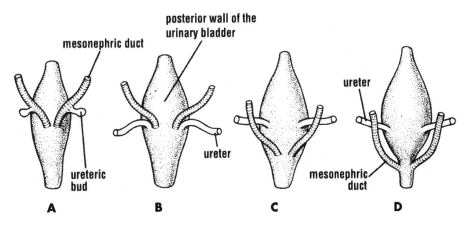

Fig. 22-3. Schematic drawings show the relationship between the ureters and the mesonephric ducts during development. Initially, the ureter is formed by an outgrowth of the mesonephric duct, but with time it obtains a separate entrance into the urinary bladder. (From Sadler TW: *Langman's medical embryology,* ed 5, Baltimore, 1985, Williams & Wilkins.)

the anterior urogenital sinus and the posterior rectum during the fourth week (Vaughn and Middleton, 1975). The urogenital sinus is further divided into the vesicourethral canal that forms the bladder and upper urethra and into the definitive urogenital sinus that forms most of the urethra, the paraurethral glands, and the vestibule. Within the base of the bladder is a specialized structure, the trigone, that derives partly from mesoderm. The urorectal fold becomes the perineal body that separates the vestibule and the rectum (DeLancey, 1989).

The vesicourethral canal receives the allantois cranially. By the fourth month of fetal life, attenuation and elongation of the allantois results in formation of a ligamentous structure called the urachus. It runs from the bladder dome to the umbilicus. The urachus persists in adult life as the median umbilical ligament of the anterior abdominal wall.

Bilaterally the vesicourethral canal receives the orifices of the mesonephric ducts. The metanephric duct (the ureter) arises as an outgrowth of the mesonephric duct just cranial to this junction. However, differential growth of the ducts results in the establishment of an independent orifice between the metanephric duct and the developing bladder (Fig. 22-3). The mesonephric duct orifice becomes displaced distally and opens into the upper urethra. In the female most of the mesonephric duct undergoes degeneration. The terminal portion ultimately becomes incorporated into the bladder wall and gives rise to a part of the trigone and posterior upper urethra (Tanagho and Smith, 1969). Thus this segment of the bladder is of mesodermal origin.

Distally the vesicourethral canal elongates and contributes to the formation of the upper anterior urethra. Most of the urethra, however, derives from the urogenital sinus. Paraurethral glands (Skene's glands) arise as outgrowths of the urethral mucosa and are probably homologues of the male prostate gland (Huffman, 1948). The posterior segment of the urogenital sinus further differentiates into the vestibule and the distal vagina.

HISTOLOGY

The histologic structure of the urinary tract from the renal calyces to the urethra is consistent and varies only by an increase in thickness. It is well suited to the functions of storage and the propulsion of urine. Three component layers are identified-mucosa, muscularis, and adventitia (Hurt, 1988).

The mucosal lining is transitional epithelium, three to five cells thick in the ureters and up to eight cells thick in the bladder. In the contracted state, the epithelium is compact and the cells are round. As the viscus distends to accommodate stored urine, the epithelium becomes thin and the individual cells flatten parallel to the surface. There is no discernible basement membrane. The lamina propria is composed of collagen and elastin fibers. The distal trigone and urethra are lined by nonkeratinizing stratified squamous epithelium. Like vaginal mucosa, they are estrogen sensitive; this is consistent with their common embryologic derivation from the urogenital sinus (Dixon and Gosling, 1990).

The muscularis is composed of an inner longitudinal and an outer circular layer. An additional outer longitudinal layer begins in the distal ureter and continues into the bladder. The layered arrangement is less discrete in the urinary tract than in the gastrointestinal tract. This results in a more interlaced, anastomosing pattern in the bladder. The inner longitudinal layer of each ureter flattens as it enters the bladder to form the sheetlike trigone. This layer continues downward into the proximal urethra.

The muscularis is surrounded by a fibroelastic adventitia. At the bladder dome, this layer provides loose attachments to accommodate the mobility necessary for physiologic filling and emptying. In the periurethral area an extensive vascular plexus courses through the adventitia. When the vessels are engorged, they may contribute to urethral closure pressure by creating forces of extrinsic compression (Rud et al, 1980), thus taking part in urethral coaptation.

The bladder outlet lacks a discrete circumferential sphincter, yet several elements compensate for this function.

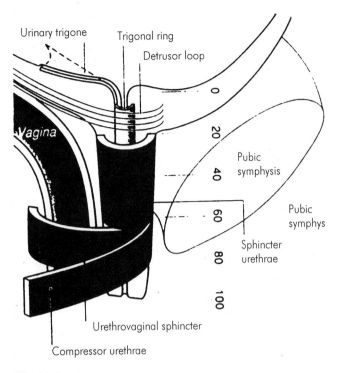

Fig. 22-4. Diagrammatic representation of the components of the internal and the external urethral sphincters. (From DeLancey JOL: Anatomy and physiology of urinary continence. *Clin Obstet Gynecol* 1990; 33:302.)

In the bladder neck, elastin fibers comprise a passive mechanism that maintains closure at rest (Gosling et al, 1977). In the urethra, four components contribute to the sphincter mechanism: the epithelium, connective and vascular tissue, smooth muscle, and striated muscle. The outer circular layer of the detrusor muscle is continuous with the urethra and may contribute to the smooth muscle sphincter. However, this layer is poorly developed in females, and its contribution to urethral closure is doubted because the detrusor and the sphincter muscles function reciprocally (Dixon and Gosling, 1990). It is likely that the smooth muscle around the bladder neck opens this structure during micturition. The urethra also contains the striated urogenital sphincter, comprising approximately 20% to 80% of total urethral length (Fig. 22-4). It is composed primarily of slow-twitch muscle fibers capable of maintaining prolonged basal tone (Gosling et al, 1981). Additional voluntary sphincter function is provided by the decussation of striated muscle fibers of the compressor urethrae and the urethrovaginal sphincter muscle of the urogenital diaphragms. The hormonally sensitive epithelium forms the ultimate watertight closure of the urethral valve, along with the submucosal vascular plexuses, the latter providing an "inflatable cushion" (DeLancey, 1996). The epithelium must be supple and moist to achieve a hermetic seal. Finally, abundant collagen and elastin fibers intrinsic to the urethral wall add a passive mechanism that contributes to closure.

URINARY TRACT ANATOMY
Ureters

The ureters are bilateral tubes that function as conduits to convey urine from the kidneys to the urinary bladder. Each ureter is 30 to 34 cm in length and 6 to 10 mm in diameter and lies retroperitoneal from the renal pelvis to the bladder. Each ureter has an abdominal portion and a pelvic portion. The abdominal portion comprises the superior 15 cm and runs caudally anterior to the psoas muscle, crossing the genitofemoral nerve. The right ureter is crossed over by the duodenum, the right colic and ileocolic vessels, and the terminal ileum. The left ureter is crossed by the left colic vessels and the sigmoid mesentery and vessels.

The pelvic ureter begins near the sacroiliac articulation at the linea terminalis of the iliac bone. As it descends into the true pelvis along the lateral wall, it is crossed over by the ovarian vessels coursing within the infundibulopelvic ligament. It crosses the common iliac artery near its bifurcation to lie medial to the visceral branches of the anterior division of the internal iliac artery. As the ureter continues into the pelvis, it travels along the superior surface of the levator ani muscle in the cardinal ligament, the most inferior portion of the broad ligament. Here it is surrounded by the extensive venous plexus of the uterus and is crossed superiorly by the uterine artery at approximately the level of the internal cervical os, 1 to 1.5 cm lateral to the cervix (DeLancey, 1990). Each ureter then turns medially and anteriorly, coursing closely to the anterior vaginal fornix to enter the base of the bladder. The interstitial portion of the ureter is approximately 1 cm in length and traverses an oblique, anteromedial course to open through a slitlike orifice at the bladder trigone (Woodburne, 1968).

Bladder

The bladder is a highly distensible, hollow organ that changes shape and its superior relations as it fills with urine. The superior segment, or dome, of the bladder consists of the detrusor muscle. Its surface is covered with visceral peritoneum that reflects onto the bladder from the anterior abdominal wall and off the bladder into the vesicouterine pouch. The inferior surfaces are not covered by peritoneum. Anteriorly the bladder is separated from the pubic bone by a potential retroperitoneal space called the space of Retzius. Posteriorly it is related to the anterior surface of the uterine cervix and the anterior fornix of the vagina.

The trigone is a specialized area at the base of the bladder that represents the continuation of the muscular layer of the ureters as they are incorporated into the bladder wall (Woodburne, 1968). It lies over the anterior vaginal wall. A triangular area, it is delineated by the ureteral orifices, the interureteric ridge forming the base, and the internal urethral meatus at the apex (Fig. 22-5). Ureteral orifices are approximately 3 cm apart. Because it forms a relatively fixed, unyielding segment of the bladder, the trigone is important in supporting the outlet during storage of urine and in coordi-

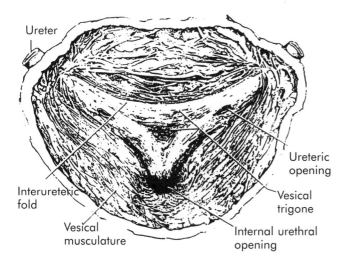

Fig. 22-5. View of the bladder trigone showing ureteral orifices and internal urethral meatus. (From Woodburne RT: Anatomy of the bladder and bladder outlet. *J Urol* 1968; 100:478. ©American Urological Association, Inc.)

nating the funneling effect necessary for efficient emptying of the bladder (Tanagho and Smith, 1969).

Urethra

The female urethra is approximately 4 cm long. It runs from the bladder base to the vestibule and is positioned behind the pubic symphysis anterior to the vagina. The external urethral meatus forms a slitlike orifice in the vestibule approximately 2 cm posterior to the clitoris. Paraurethral Skene's glands are inconstant, but they usually open to the posterior urethra just within the meatus.

Two muscle groups surround the urethra, the internal smooth muscle and the external striated muscle. The internal smooth muscle consists of two layers—the circular muscle, which is poorly differentiated in the female urethra, and the longitudinal muscle, which is well developed and lies inside the circular layer. The longitudinal muscle probably functions to shorten the urethra during micturition, facilitating bladder emptying. Evidence of cholinergic innervation in that area (Ek et al, 1977) supports this hypothesis.

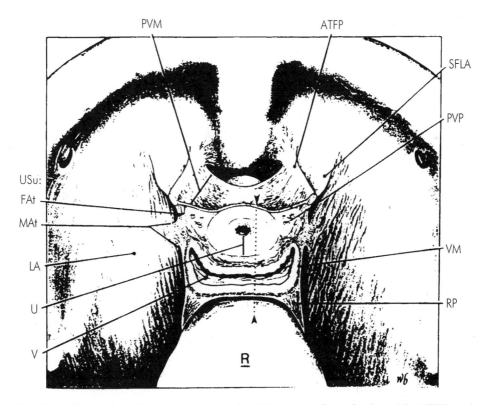

Fig. 22-6. Cross-section of the urethra (U), vagina (V), arcus tendineus fasciae pelvis (ATFP), and superior fascia of levator ani (SFLA) just below the vesical neck (drawn from cadaver dissection). The pubovesical muscles (PVM) lie anterior to the urethra and anterior and superior to the paraurethral vascular plexus (PVP). The urethral supports (USu) (the pubourethral ligaments) attach the vagina and vaginal surface of the urethra to the levator ani muscles (MAt, muscular attachment) and to the superior fascia of the levator ani (FAt, fascial attachment). R, rectum; RP, rectal pillar; VM, vaginal wall muscularis; LA, levator ani. (Dotted line indicates a plane of section not shown in this chapter.) (From DeLancey JOL: Anatomy and physiology of urinary continence. *Clin Obstet Gynecol* 1990; 33:300.)

Parasympathetic stimulation not only results in contraction of the detrusor, it also results in contraction of the longitudinal urethral smooth muscle, which shortens the urethra and which, in turn, results in decreased resistance to flow to facilitate voiding. For its part, the circular smooth muscle contains some adrenergic receptors that may be involved in maintaining basal tone. However, in contrast to its male counterpart, the circular smooth muscle is attenuated and its role in continence is less profound.

Striated urethral muscle is divided in two portions, a proximal sphincter and a distal archlike muscle fibers (DeLancey, 1990). The first part is called the sphincter urethrae, and it extends to the proximal half of the urethral length. Located in the distal third of the urethra, the second part consists of an arch of muscle over the anterior surface of the urethra. Lateral attachment to the vaginal wall (urethro-vaginal sphincter muscle) and to the ischiopubic ramus (compressor urethrae) provides a compressive effect. Muscle fibers are composed of slow-twitch units that provide resting tone and fast-twitch fibers that exert additional occlusion at times of stress (*e.g.,* cough) (Fig. 22-4). Urethral support is dual: the distal third of the urethra is fixed in position, and the proximal two thirds is mobile. The perineal membrane provides support to the distal urethra. Connective tissue attachment arises from the anterior distal urethra and inserts onto the pubic bones. This attachment lies just beneath the compressor urethrae and the urethro-vaginal sphincter. The proximal urethra is supported by a system that includes connective tissue (endopelvic-fascia and arcus tendineus fascia pelvis) and muscles (levator ani). The endopelvic fascia, which bounds the urethra and the vagina, attaches laterally to the arcus tendineus fasciae pelvis, called the paravaginal attachment (Richardson et al, 1981), and to the levator ani. The resting tone of the levator ani permits a retropubic position at rest. During micturition, the muscle relaxes, allowing for descent of the bladder neck and emptying of the bladder. During bouts of increased intraabdominal pressure, the levator ani contracts to provide direct support and tensing of the endopelvic fascia, permitting compression of the urethra because of the increased pressure and the hammocklike supportive layer (DeLancey, 1994) (Fig. 22-6).

PELVIC FLOOR FUNCTIONAL ANATOMY

Adoption of an upright posture during human evolution placed the viscera above a hole in the bony pelvis. Adaptive changes developed to prevent outward excursion of the pelvic contents resulting from the forces created by gravity and by the contraction of the diaphragm and the abdominal wall muscles. These changes can be considered separately by anatomic division: bony pelvis, pelvic floor muscles, and endopelvic fascia.

Bony Pelvis

The bony pelvis is formed by the sacrum posteriorly and the ileum laterally; these are united anteriorly by cartilage to

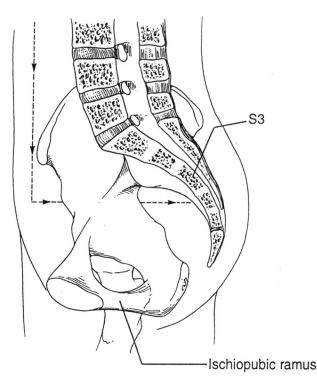

Fig. 22-7. Relationship between the contents of the abdominal and the pelvic cavities in a properly oriented bony pelvis. (From Brubaker LT, Saclarides TJ: *The female pelvic floor: Disorders of function and support,* Philadelphia, 1996, F. A. Davis.)

form the symphysis pubis. Posterolateral projections, the ischial spine, allow for the attachment of the sacrospinous ligaments and are located at its inferior margin.

Natural spinal lordosis and the sacrolumbar curve displace the abdominal contents above the pubic brim, thus decreasing the force vector directly on the opening of the pelvic outlet (Fig. 22-7). The bony pelvis further contributes to the prevention of pelvic organ prolapse by allowing insertion of the pelvic floor muscles and the endopelvic fascia on its solid structure.

Pelvic Floor Muscles

Pelvic floor muscles consist of two groups of muscles, the urogenital and the pelvic diaphragms. The urogenital diaphragm is the most distal structure of the pelvic floor. It consists of the bulbo-cavernosus, the transversalis, and the ischiocavernosus muscles. Its function is to provide stabilization of the perineal body, which is pyramidal and onto which these muscles merge. This, in turn, supports the anal sphincter and the lower vagina. The rectovaginal fascia similarly inserts onto the superior border of the perineal body, and muscular attachments from the levator ani complete its anchorage and stabilization.

The pelvic diaphragm includes the levator ani, obturator, and coccygeus muscles, of which the levator ani is functionally the most important. It is formed from three muscles: the pubo-rectalis acts as a U-shaped sling around the urogenital

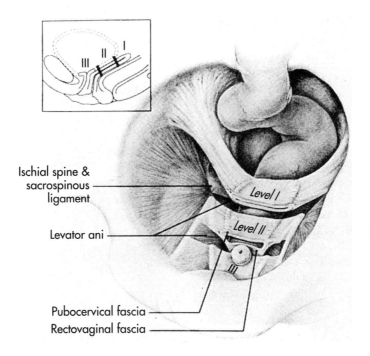

Ischial spine &
sacrospinous
ligament

Levator ani

Pubocervical fascia
Rectovaginal fascia

Fig. 22-8. Level 1 (suspension) and level 2 (attachment). In level 1, paracolpium suspends the vagina from the lateral pelvic walls. Fibers of level 1 extend vertically and posteriorly toward the sacrum. In level 2, the vagina is attached to the arcus tendineus fascia pelvis and to the superior fascia levator ani muscles. (From DeLancey JOL: Anatomic aspects of vaginal eversion after hysterectomy. *Am J Obstet Gynecol* 1992; 166:1717).

hiatus (through which pass the urethra, the vagina, and the anus), and the pubo-coccygeus and the ileo-coccygeus form a posterior plate called the levator plate. Some muscle fibers originating from the pubo-rectalis circle the urethra and vagina (Shafik, 1997). Muscle fibers of the levator ani consist of slow- and fast-twitch fibers. The slow-twitch fibers assure basal tone, whereas the fast-twitch fibers allow voluntary control and reflex contraction in response to rapid increases in intraabdominal pressure (*e.g.*, cough, sneeze).

In the resting state, the sling pubo-rectalis maintains the genital hiatus closed, in proximity to the pubis. The pelvic organs rest above the plate. During micturition, the sling and plate relax, allowing the bladder (or rectum) to evacuate its contents.

Endopelvic Fascia

The endopelvic fascia is a sheathlike connective tissue that supports the supralevator pelvic organs. Its condensations form the round, cardinal, and utero-sacral ligaments. This fascia attaches the pelvic organs to the pelvic sidewall. Between the vagina and the bladder, it is called the pubocervical fascia, and between the vagina and the rectum, it is called the recto-vaginal fascia (Denonvilliers' fascia).

DeLancey (1992) elegantly described the anatomy and function of the endopelvic fascia, which, for the purpose of description, can be divided into three levels (Fig. 22-8). Level 1 is the most proximal and includes the cardinal and utero-sacral complex of ligaments. Its functions are to sup-

port the cervix and the upper vagina and to maintain those structures above the levator plate. The cardinal ligament assures lateral stability, and the utero-sacral preserves posterior stability. When a woman is standing, the uterosacral ligaments are almost vertical in their orientation. Medially, approximately one-third of these ligaments attach on the visceral layer of the vagina, two-thirds attach on the cervix, and they all insert laterally onto the pelvic sidewall.

Level 2 provides lateral attachment to the mid-vagina, on top of which lies the bladder. As stated earlier, the endopelvic fascia is fused to the vaginal mucosa. Anteriorly it forms the pubocervical fascia, and posteriorly it forms the rectovaginal septum (or Denonvilliers' fascia). Laterally, this fascia attaches to the arcus tendineus fasciae pelvis and to the superior fascia of the levator ani. This attachment stretches the vagina transversely between the bladder and the rectum. The arcus tendineus fasciae pelvis is an anteroposterior cordlike structure that inserts anteriorly behind the pubic ramus and posteriorly on the ischial spine, on each side of the pelvis. This structure, also called white line, lies on top of the obturator internus fascia and fuses with the fibers of the obturator fascia, providing the final link to the pelvic sidewall. It is important to realize that this arrangement orients the mid-vagina to a horizontal axis when a woman is erect.

Finally, level 3 provides support to the distal vagina and urethra; it has been described in detail in the section on urethral anatomy. In addition, the levator ani attaches to the vagina directly, by the puborectalis, which at that level takes the name of pubovaginalis. In addition to the fascial attachment previously described, this connection is responsible for the appropriate mobility of the bladder neck and proximal urethra desirable for voiding, but it prevents excessive mobility during bouts of increasing intraabdominal pressure.

MALFORMATIONS

The genital and the urinary tracts develop in close association. In the female fetus, normal development of the mesonephric system precedes, and is partly responsible for inducing, normal development of the müllerian ducts. After fusion of the caudal ends of the müllerian ducts, the downward growth of the müllerian tubercle separates the urogenital sinus into its urinary and vaginal components. A consequence of this interdependence is that abnormalities in one system are commonly associated with abnormalities in the other.

Some important lower urinary tract malformations become manifest during infancy or childhood and are diagnosed by the pediatrician. However, some remain silent into adulthood and are only detected coincidentally as a result of an unrelated imaging study or surgical procedure. Urinary tract malformations of special importance to the gynecologist include unilateral renal agenesis, ureteral duplication, ectopic ureteral orifice, and ureterocele.

Unilateral renal agenesis occurs with an incidence of approximately 1 per 1000 (Magee et al, 1979). Associated genital tract anomalies, usually unicornuated uterus or uterine duplication, develop in 35% to 45% of affected women. Several mechanisms have been proposed, including failed differentiation of the nephrogenic ridge, failed differentiation of the mesonephric duct and ureteral bud, and failed development of the metanephric blastema. The earlier in embryonic development urinary tract aberration occurs, the more severe are associated abnormalities in the genital tract. The diagnosis of unilateral renal agenesis is usually made while the patient is evaluated for symptomatic renal disease or during surgery. When it is identified, a structural evaluation of the genital tract should be conducted. There is no renal functional derangement unless there is compromise of one kidney.

Duplication of the ureter may be partial or total, and it occurs in approximately 1% of the population (Vaughn and Middleton, 1975). Y-shaped partial duplication results when the ureteral bud branches before establishing contact with the metanephric blastema. Two complete ureters result from growth of a duplicated ureteral bud that arises from the mesonephric duct. Ureters usually cross each other within a common vascular sheath so that the ureter draining the upper renal pole enters the bladder more medial and distal to its mate (the Meyer-Weigert rule). It may surface so inferiorly in the bladder that it is sometimes considered an ectopic ureter. The interstitial segment of the distal ureter tends to be shorter and thus is prone to vesicoureteral reflux and resul-

tant upper urinary tract infection. In addition to possible reflux, it is important to recognize this condition clinically so that the duplicate ureter may be avoided during surgery.

An ectopic ureteral orifice may open into the urethra, vestibule, vagina, or uterus (Zornow, 1977). Usually it occurs in a duplicate ureter, with the ectopic ureter draining the superior renal pole as expected by the Meyer-Weigert rule. If the ectopic ureter opens distal to the urethral sphincter or into the genital tract, incontinence results. The usual clinical presentation is constant dribbling of urine with a concurrent normal voiding pattern. In children it may be misinterpreted as enuresis. If the ureter opens into the uterus or the vagina, signs and symptoms of vaginitis may be most prominent. Ipsilateral ureteroureterostomy, or reimplantation into the bladder, is the usual surgical treatment for symptomatic ectopia.

A ureterocele is a cystic dilatation of the distal ureter (Vaughn, 1975). It may be congenital or acquired, and it usually involves the interstitial ureter. It is probably produced by incomplete perforation of the bladder by the ureter that results in a localized increase in hydrostatic pressure. The usual clinical presentation is recurrent urinary tract infection caused by obstruction. Treatment requires surgical resection of the involved segment with reimplantation into the bladder.

PHYSIOLOGY

The lower urinary tract stores urine until conditions are appropriate for the complete expulsion of bladder contents. Its functions are controlled by a complex neurologic system involving central and peripheral components. In infancy, micturition occurs as a reflex and is involuntary. However, with maturation of the cerebral descending pathways, it is brought under voluntary control.

Both components of the lower urinary tract must function reciprocally to accomplish the opposing functions of storing and emptying urine. During storage, the detrusor muscle remains relaxed, through sympathetic inhibition, to accommodate increasing urine volumes while the sphincter, under α-sympathetic stimulation, is contracted to maintain continence. During emptying, the pelvic floor and the urethral sphincter relax to provide a low-resistance conduit through which the urine passes as the detrusor contracts, under parasympathetic stimulation, to expel the bladder contents.

The bladder wall is innervated by sensory fibers that carry sensations of pain, temperature, and proprioception (stretch) to the spinal cord (Bradley et al, 1976). They synapse in the sacral spinal cord micturition center with efferent motor nerves that return to the bladder to complete a reflex arc. Motor neurons supplying the detrusor muscle originate in the sacral spinal segments S2 to S4. In addition, the afferent nerves synapse with other neurons that transmit information about bladder sensation up the cord to the brain stem and the cerebral cortex, where centers coordinating micturition activity are located.

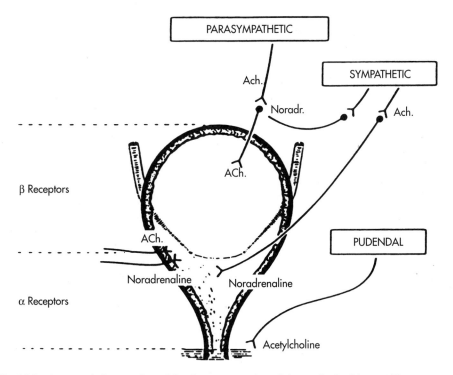

Fig. 22-9. Autonomic innervation of the detrusor muscle and the urethral sphincter. (From vanGeelen H: Drug action on the bladder and urethra. *Int Urogynecol J* 1990; 1:19-24.)

The activity of the efferent neurons controlling detrusor function is modulated by input from bladder afferent nerves and from signals originating in the brain stem and the frontal lobe. The basic micturition reflex consists of detrusor contraction in response to the stretch of bladder filling. Input from higher centers on this reflex is primarily suppressive. Toilet training is a learned response that allows the inhibition of detrusor activity until a socially appropriate time for emptying occurs. Thus the micturition reflex is brought under a degree of voluntary control. After appropriately integrating the information from the bladder with that from higher centers, the sacral micturition center sends signals to the detrusor and the urethral sphincter to initiate a coordinated micturition event. Three characteristics of the event are notable. First, the actions of the detrusor and the sphincter must be coordinated so that the bladder empties through an open outlet. This averts the need to generate excessive intravesical pressures that may create ureteral reflux. Second, detrusor contraction must be sustained until the entire contents are expelled to avoid residual urine retention in the bladder. Third, when the bladder is empty, the bladder and the sphincter must return to the basal states that promote urine storage. Detrusor motor neurons reach the bladder by way of the pelvic nerve. They are parasympathetic and form ganglionic synapses within the wall of the bladder. Postganglionic neurons then carry information to the smooth muscle cells of the detrusor. Release of the neurotransmitter acetylcholine stimulates a detrusor contraction. The role of the sympathetic nervous system in the control of bladder func-

tion is less well established for humans (Gosling et al, 1977). Preganglionic fibers from the thoracolumbar spinal segment synapse in chain ganglia with postganglionic fibers that travel in the hypogastric nerve to the bladder and sphincter. Sympathetic effects are mediated through α- and β-receptors. β-Receptors are predominant in the detrusor, and stimulation of these is thought to inhibit detrusor contractility. α-Receptors are abundant in the sphincter region, and stimulation causes contraction of these muscle fibers. Hence, a picture emerges of autonomic influence on bladder function such that parasympathetic activation initiates bladder emptying, whereas sympathetic activation relaxes the detrusor and stimulates the sphincter to promote the storage function of the bladder (Fig. 22-9).

Despite intense investigative efforts, the mechanism of continence remains incompletely understood. From a simplified point of view, continence is maintained during the bladder storage phase because intraurethral pressure exceeds intravesical pressure at all times. Intravesical pressure remains low during filling because of the relaxed state and high compliance of the detrusor muscle. This allows the bladder to accommodate increasing volumes of urine with only a minimal increase in intravesical pressure. Intraurethral pressure remains high because of a combination of intrinsic and extrinsic factors that contribute to a sphincter-like effect (Hurt, 1988). Intrinsic features of the urethra that determine intraurethral pressure include sympathetically mediated contraction of the smooth muscles of the internal sphincter, contraction of the striated muscles of the external sphincter, tissue turgor that results from blood flow in the paraurethral vascular bed, and mucosal seal that results from the elastic properties of the urethral wall.

Extrinsic structures that support the urethra and bladder comprise an extremely important aspect of the continence mechanism. This is especially true during episodes of increased ambient intraabdominal pressure such as sudden valsalva, coughing, and sneezing. An increase in intraabdominal pressure is transmitted across the wall of the bladder and increases intravesical pressure. As long as the proximal urethra is properly supported and stabilized between the pubic bone and the anterior vaginal wall, the pressure increase is similarly transmitted across its wall, compresses the lumen until it closes, and raises intraurethral pressure to a comparable degree. The pressure relationship between the bladder and the urethra is unchanged, and continence is maintained. If the supports are damaged and the urethra is allowed excessive downward mobility during stress, adequate compression of the urethra will not occur. If intravesical pressure increases sufficiently, leakage will result.

Pharmacology of the Lower Urinary Tract

An understanding of the neurophysiology of the lower urinary tract has allowed the application of various pharmacologic agents to the treatment of urinary tract disorders (Ginsburg and Genadry, 1984). Drugs that facilitate urine storage are helpful in treating incontinence. They may work either by promoting detrusor relaxation or sphincter contraction. Detrusor relaxation may be induced with anticholinergic agents, direct smooth muscle relaxers, calcium-channel blockers, β-receptor agonists, prostaglandin inhibitors, and tricyclic antidepressants. Clinically, the most effective are oxybutynin, propantheline, and imipramine (Fantl et al, 1996). Drugs that promote sphincter closure include α-agonists, β-antagonists, and possibly estrogen. The mechanism of the beneficial effect of estrogen is thought to be increased blood flow to the paravaginal tissues, increased pliability of the mucosal lining, and increased responsiveness of the smooth muscle to adrenergic stimulation.

Pharmacologic treatment of the disorders of bladder emptying makes use of drugs with opposite actions on the bladder and sphincter. Drugs that enhance detrusor contractility include parasympathomimetics, choline esterase inhibitors, and β-antagonists. Agents that decrease sphincter closure include α-antagonists, β-agonists, and skeletal muscle relaxants. These drugs will be more extensively covered in subsequent sections pertaining to medical therapy of urinary tract dysfunction.

URINARY INCONTINENCE: URINARY STORAGE AND EVACUATION ANOMALIES

Urinary incontinence is defined by the International Continence Society as the involuntary loss of urine that is a social and hygienic problem and that is objectively demonstrable (Abrams et al, 1990). Occasional episodes of incontinence are common in women and should not be regarded as ab-

normal. However, incontinence becomes a medical problem when it interferes with a woman's social life or hygiene. Objective demonstration is important because incontinence can often be confused with vaginal discharge or leakage of amniotic fluid in pregnant women.

Classification and Evaluation
Classification

Classification can be based on symptoms, but because these do not correlate specifically to an underlying disease, this is less helpful than a classification based on a diagnosed abnormality. The breakdown of this is shown in Fig. 22-10 in which, broadly speaking, incontinence is shown to be transurethral or extraurethral. The most common cause is genuine stress incontinence or urethral sphincter incompetence. Genuine stress incontinence is defined as the loss of urine that occurs with increased intraabdominal pressure in the absence of a detrusor contraction. It can be caused by hypermobility (loss of posterior support to the urethra and bladder neck) or to urethral sphincter deficiency. For diagnostic purposes, these two conditions are distinctly defined, but in practice, a large degree of overlap exists. Detrusor instability results from uninhibited detrusor contraction. Its cause may be neurologic (e.g., stroke, Parkinson disease) and thus termed detrusor hyper-reflexia, but in most gynecology patients no concomitant neurologic abnormality is detected. Thus it is considered idiopathic. Loss of urethral pressure before detrusor contraction is a common finding with detrusor instability. If it is seen in the absence of detrusor instability, the loss of pressure is termed urethral instability, but this is rare. Urinary retention with overflow, more common in the elderly, may occur in the young. On the other hand, congenital abnormalities of the urethra usually are seen in infants. In some incontinent women, no underlying causes can be detected. If there is an associated mental disorder, these patients may be classified as having psychogenic incontinence. It is important that the term functional incontinence not be used as a "trash can" diagnosis. Another type of functional incontinence relates to comorbidity and environmental issues seen in the elderly. These are transient causes of incontinence and have been elegantly tabulated (Box 22-1) into a mnemonic, DIAPPERS (Resnick and Yalla, 1985). The extraurethral causes of incontinence are either congenital or acquired. Congenital causes are usually diagnosed in childhood; occasionally, they may be seen during the reproductive years (see section on malformations). Fistulas may be iatrogenic and develop after surgery or radiotherapy, or they may result from malignancy. In the developing world, especially in Africa, they are primarily caused by obstetric trauma.

Clinical Evaluation of the Lower Urinary Tract

History. Lower urinary tract dysfunction includes one or more of the following symptoms: incontinence, irritative symptoms (urgency, frequency, painful micturition), and voiding difficulties.

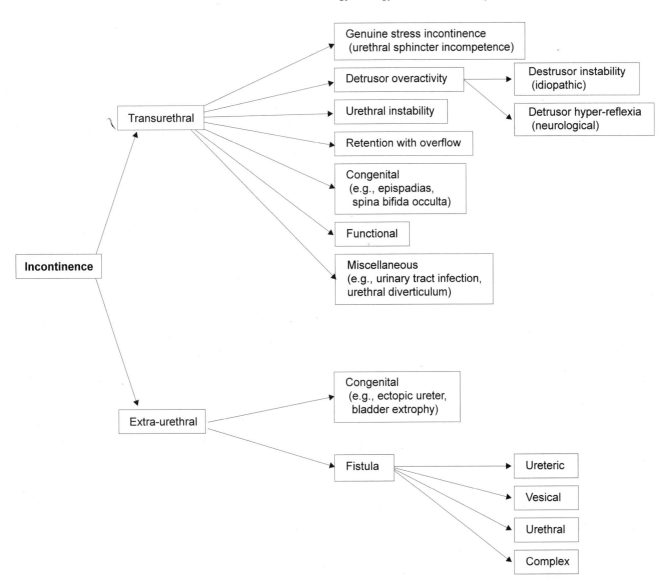

Fig. 22-10. The causes of female urinary incontinence. (Modified from Stanton SL: Classification of incontinence. In Stanton SL, editor: *Clinical gynecologic urology,* St. Louis, 1984, Mosby.)

BOX 22-1
TRANSIENT CAUSES OF INCONTINENCE:
DIAPPERS

D elirium
I nfection
A trophic vaginitis
P harmacologic
P sychological
E ndocrine
R estricted mobility
S tool impaction

Symptoms can be misleading in trying to determine a diagnosis. A careful history is essential because it clarifies the patient's complaint amid coexisting conditions, and it allows the diagnostician to put the investigative findings into context. The reason most women have mixed symptoms is that the primary abnormality induces behavior modification that itself results in symptoms. For example, a woman with incontinence will attempt to reduce her incontinence by keeping her ambient bladder volume at a minimum. This necessitates voiding frequently so frequency becomes a symptom, which often results in urgency. A woman with retention may complain of stress incontinence because when her bladder is full, she may leak urine on coughing. Similarly, a full bladder may be an invitation to colonization by bacteria; she may have recurrent urinary tract infections or symptoms that are primarily irritative.

Stress incontinence is a term used to describe incontinence that occurs involuntarily during physical activity. This activity causes increased intraabdominal pressure, resulting in incontinence. *Urge incontinence*, on the other hand, is a strong and sudden desire to void that results in the involuntary loss of urine. *Dribbling incontinence* is another symptom that may have various underlying causes, ranging from retention with overflow to a fistula or an ectopic ureter.

<table>
</table>

BOX 22-2
CAUSES OF FREQUENCY AND URGENCY

Structural
  Urethral caruncle or diverticulum
Bladder mucosal lesion (*e.g.,* papilloma)
  Small-capacity bladder
  Pelvic mass (*e.g.,* fibroids)
  Radiation cystitis or fibrosis
Infective-inflammatory
  Urinary tract infection
  Urethritis or cystitis
  Chronic retention of urine
  Bladder calculus
  Genital warts
Endocrine
  Diabetes insipidus or mellitus
  Hypothyroidism
  Pregnancy
Lifestyle
  Habit
  Large fluid intake
Miscellaneous
  Idiopathic detrusor instability
  Upper motor neuron lesion
  Diuretic therapy or impaired renal function
  Previous pelvic surgery

BOX 22-3
CAUSES OF VOIDING DYSFUNCTION

Neurologic
  Upper or lower motor neuron lesions
Inflammation
  Urethritis, vulvitis, or vaginitis
Drugs
  Tricyclic antidepressants
  Anticholinergic agents
  α-Adrenergic stimulators
  Ganglion blockers
  Epidural anesthesia
Obstruction
  Urethral stenosis or stricture
  Edema after surgery or parturition
  Fibrosis caused by repeated dilatation or irradiation
  Pelvic mass (*e.g.,* fibroids, retroverted gravid uterus, ovarian cyst, feces)
  Urethral distortion resulting from a large cystocele
Medical
  Diabetic neuropathy
  Hypothyroidism
  Psychosis
Atonic detrusor
  Secondary to overdistension
Functional
  Anxiety, apprehension

Postmicturition dribble is less common in women, but it can occur in the presence of a marked urethrocele or urethral diverticulum. *Nocturnal enuresis* is a term that is applied to bed wetting; however, the patient is awakened by having wet the bed rather than by the desire to void and then has become incontinent. *Giggle incontinence* is found in younger adolescent girls and is often associated with detrusor instability. *Coital incontinence* is usually associated with genuine stress incontinence, but when it occurs with orgasm, it is thought to result from detrusor instability.

Frequency of micturition varies considerably among normal women; some may void only twice a day (cameloid bladder). When voiding occurs more than seven times a day, it is thought to be abnormal. *Nocturia* is a condition of waking up with a strong desire to void. Habitual voiding because the patient wakes up for some other reason is not nocturia. Once per night is normal. Nocturia only becomes significant when it occurs more often. *Urgency* is the strong and sudden desire to void that can be debilitating because the patient thinks of little else. There are many causes of frequency and urgency, and some of them are shown in Box 22-2. When treating a patient with incontinence, it is important to consider the potential for coexisting abnormalities.

Voiding difficulties in women may be accompanied by symptoms of *hesitancy, poor stream, straining to void, incomplete bladder emptying,* or a combination of these.

Again, the causes of voiding dysfunction are numerous and are listed in Box 22-3. Dysuria is a confusing term best avoided because it can refer to painful micturition or difficulty with micturition; instead the actual symptoms should be described. *Hematuria* can result from a number of conditions, from malignancy to infection and should always be promptly investigated. Finally, *backache* is a fairly common nonspecific problem associated with incontinence. Often the cause is musculoskeletal dysfunction, but it can also develop after uterine prolapse. It is sometimes difficult to differentiate between the two. In general, however, backache from the former is worse in the morning whereas backache from the latter gets progressively worse through the day. This back pain should be distinguished from *flank pain,* which, when associated with painful micturition, may be caused by early pyelonephritis.

Physical Examination. As for any surgical or medical condition, a full examination is required. However, for the purposes of lower urinary tract dysfunction, the physician should concentrate on the gynecologic, urologic, and neurologic examinations. Assessment of the patient's mental state is also useful. Testing of the sacral nerve roots S2 to S4 is important because incontinence may have a neurologic origin. The physician has to ascertain whether behavior modification or conservative therapy would be suitable and whether a patient would understand enough and have suffi-

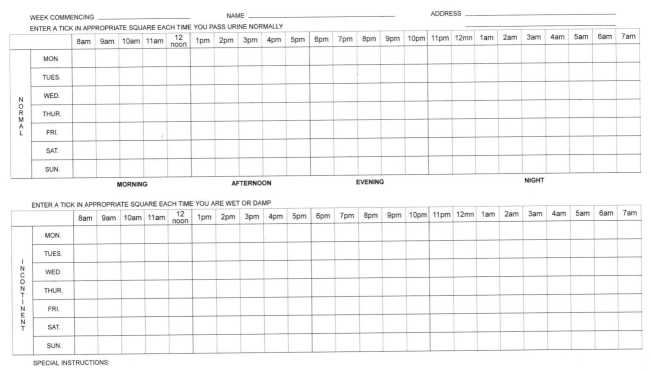

Fig. 22-11. Example of a frequency volume chart or voiding diary (from Kabi Pharmacia).

cient motivation. When considering surgery, the integrity of pelvic floor tissues and the degree of atrophy are important prognostic features. The gynecologic examination should also try to elicit the presence of uterine prolapse. Anterior, vault, or posterior prolapse should be systematically determined. The International Continent Society has developed a standardized and quantified pelvic organ prolapse (POP-Q) tool (see section on disorders of the pelvic floor). It is useful for longitudinal evaluation of a given patient, postoperative assessment of surgical results, and cross-sectional comparison of study populations.

Bimanual gynecologic vaginal examination should be performed to determine concomitant abnormalities and to detect a palpable bladder and localized tenderness. The urethra should be observed while the patient coughs to detect stress incontinence, and it should also be inspected for the presence of a caruncle or of a urethral mucosal prolapse. It should be palpated throughout its entire length for the presence of a diverticulum. The course of the ureter should be palpated for localized tenderness, and the kidneys should be examined for enlargement or tenderness.

Q-Tip Test. The Q-tip test assesses the integrity of the ligamentous support of the proximal urethra and determines the presence of urethral hypermobility (Karram and Bhatia, 1988). A sterile, lubricated cotton swab is placed in the bladder neck, taking care not to insert it beyond the bladder neck and not to insert it too distal because this would yield an erroneous measurement. At rest in the lithotomy position, the urethra (and thus the swab) assumes a 0° angle to the hori-

zontal plane. The patient is then asked to perform a Valsalva maneuver. If the proximal urethra is normally supported, straining displaces the distal end of the swab only slightly. However, with loss of support, straining causes the proximal end of the urethra to descend and the distal end of the swab to move upward to an angle that usually exceeds 30° and often approaches 90°.

Although the Q-tip test is sensitive in detecting hypermobility, pitfalls of the test reside in the large overlap between continent and incontinent patients (Bergman et al, 1987; Montz and Stanton, 1986), making this test nonspecific. However, if patients with stress incontinence have negative findings on the Q-tip test, it should alert the practitioner to the possibility of intrinsic sphincteric deficiency because these patients have been found to have high failure rates with anti-incontinence surgery (Bergman et al, 1989). Realistically, the Q-tip test merely quantifies the descent of the proximal urethra, which is qualitatively visible with the naked eye.

Frequency Volume Charts. Although history taking is essential for obtaining the patient's perception of her problems, this is often at variance with actual events; a frequency volume chart or voiding diary is an important adjunct to the clinical evaluation. Many voiding diaries are available commercially, but they all elicit similar information (Fig. 22-11). Volumes voided give an indication of whether voiding is premature or there is true diuresis; amounts and types of fluid a patient drinks can ascertain it. Documenting changes throughout the day is useful because simple measures can

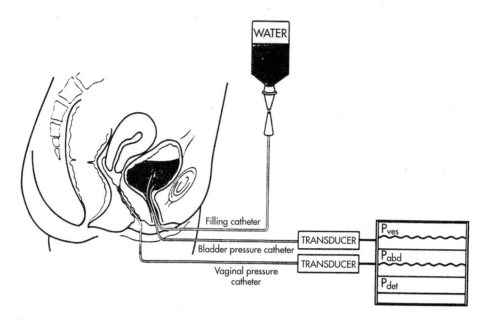

Fig. 22-12. Substracted cystometry. Intravesical and intraabdominal pressures are measured, and true detrusor pressure is electronically derived ($P_{ves} - P_{abd}$). P_{ves}, bladder pressure; P_{abd}, abdominal pressure; P_{det}, detrusor pressure. (From Karram M: *Clinical urogynecology,* St. Louis, 1993, Mosby.)

resolve many difficulties. For example, if the patient drinks large amounts of fluid, especially tea or coffee, late at night, then nocturia is a likely consequence.

Basic Urodynamic Investigations

No matter how careful the physician is in obtaining the history, diagnosis based on the clinical picture alone will commonly be inaccurate (Jarvis et al, 1980; Sand et al, 1988; Shepherd et al, 1982). Even when a computerized questionnaire was used to limit clinician bias, the results (though more predictive than in the previously published studies) displayed an 80% correct classification that is still not acceptable for clinical practice (Versi et al, 1991b).

Cystometry. For patients with incontinence caused by detrusor instability, surgery designed to elevate the bladder neck is usually contraindicated. This is because anatomic repositioning of the bladder neck is not required and because surgery at the level of the bladder neck often results in a worsening of detrusor instability.

The primary objective of any investigation is to exclude detrusor instability, and the mainstay of basic urodynamic investigations is cystometry. Because this requires catheterization, it is important that no patient with a urinary tract infection undergo this procedure. As the term implies, cystometry is the measurement of bladder pressure, and it is a dynamic investigation in that the intravesical pressure is measured not only during filling but also at capacity and during voiding. Because the bladder is an intraabdominal organ, any changes that occur in intraabdominal pressure will be reflected in the intravesical pressure. To account for this, intraabdominal pressures are often measured separately.

This can be done by measuring the pressure inside the rectum or in the upper third of the vagina. The equation

Detrusor pressure =
Intravesical pressure − Intraabdominal pressure

describes three-channel cystometry; the two pressures on the right side of the equation can be measured, and the detrusor pressure on the left side of the equation can be calculated. The standard test for the diagnosis of detrusor instability is three-channel, fluid-filled provocative cystometry (Fig. 22-12). Saline or contrast medium is used because this best approximates urine, and during filling measures are taken to provoke abnormal detrusor contractions. The bladder is filled at a rate faster than the physiologic rate, the fluid tends to be at room temperature, and, while the bladder is filling, the patient is asked to cough intermittently. Any of these measures may elicit a detrusor contraction. During the filling phase, the patient is asked to indicate when she experiences the urge to void. Bladder volume at that moment is noted; the average is between 100 and 300 mL. Some investigators differentiate between a first desire and a strong desire to void. When the patient is unable to tolerate further filling, it means physiologic capacity is reached, and this is usually between 400 and 600 mL. If patients have a low-volume first sensation and bladder capacity, they are deemed to have sensory urgency if no detrusor instability has been noted. If they have a high-volume first sensation and bladder capacity, the diagnosis is a hyposensitive bladder. With a full bladder, the patient is asked to change posture from supine to erect, and this in itself may induce a detrusor contraction. If none of these measures result in a wavelike (systolic or phasic) detrusor contraction and if the pressure increase on filling and on standing is less than 15 cm of water, the patient is deemed to have a stable detrusor, as defined by the International Continence Society Standardization Committee (Abrams et al, 1990). When the patient has a full bladder in the erect or sitting position, she is asked to cough and the presence of stress incontinence is noted. Should this occur in the absence of detrusor contraction, the diagnosis is genuine stress incontinence. After evaluation of the urethral sphincter, the patient is asked to void. During this phase, the detrusor (activity) pressure changes are monitored. Voiding pressure is not helpful because it is highly dependent on urethral resistance. Therefore, if the pelvic floor and the urethra are fully relaxed, a woman may void with little increase in her own detrusor pressure. To determine the strength of detrusor activity, the stop test can be applied. The patient is asked to stop voiding midstream. This results in an instantaneous contraction of the urethral sphincter, but the detrusor muscle does not relax so quickly. An isometric detrusor contraction is noted; the pressure generated by this maneuver is of more interest for the evaluation of detrusor contractility.

Three-channel cystometry requires a urodynamic system that is either computer based or uses amplifiers. Both systems require the use of pressure transducers and a printer or chart recorder. In a bid to simplify and reduce the cost of this test, many investigators have tried to use single-channel (intravesical) cystometry, but, because of the confounding problem of intraabdominal pressure, this technique results in the overdiagnosis of detrusor instability. To avoid messy fluid-filled systems, CO_2 gas cystometry has been used. Unfortunately, carbon dioxide dissolves to form carbonic acid, which is an irritant, and it is thought that this technique also exaggerates the incidence of detrusor instability.

Uroflowmetry. Uroflowmetry measures the rate of urine flow, and the most important diagnostic variable is the peak flow rate. Although peak flow rate declines with age, peak flows in excess of 15 mL per second are accepted as normal. However, before voiding, the bladder must contain more than 200 mL or the detrusor muscle may not be able to develop an adequate contraction. After voiding, the residual should be less than 50 mL; if it is greater than 100 mL, it is regarded as abnormal.

Clearly, uroflowmetry is an essential investigation in a patient with voiding difficulties, but it is also used for preoperative evaluation of a woman about to undergo bladder neck surgery for genuine stress incontinence. A poor preoperative flow rate is a poor prognostic feature for postoperative voiding, irrespective of the cause. Because some women void by abdominal contractions, such a maneuver after surgery for stress incontinence will result in closure of the urethra and in postoperative voiding difficulties.

Pad Testing. Pad tests are important not only for objective verification of urinary incontinence but also for quantification and, hence, definition of the magnitude of the

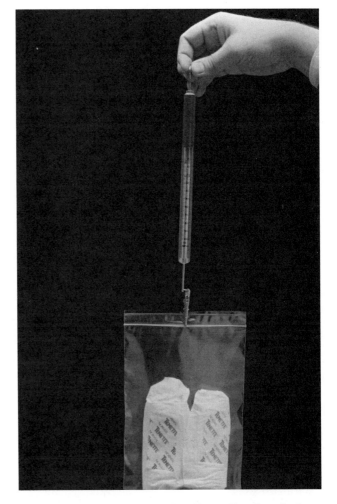

Fig. 22-13. The perineal pad is placed in a self-sealing plastic bag and weighed before and after the test period. Weight increase is a quantification of the degree of incontinence.

problem. However, the degree of incontinence does not always relate to the psychosocial impact. This tends to depend on the patient's background and reaction to the disability.

These tests essentially involve the use of a perineal pad that is weighed before and after the patient has worn it. The difference in weight is interpreted as the weight (volume) of urine that is lost. There are two types of pad tests, those performed in a hospital after a standard exercise regimen and those performed at home (Lose and Versi, 1992). Although the former may be monitored under more controlled conditions, the latter gives a truer description because it is not set in an artificial environment. Cheap and noninvasive, pad tests can be used not only for diagnosis but also to monitor the progress of treatment. Various commercial kits are available, and when these tests are performed in conjunction with a voiding diary, this simple test can yield much useful information about the patient's disability (Fig. 22-13).

Special Urodynamic Investigations

Cystourethroscopy. Cystourethroscopy is useful in the older patient in whom symptoms of frequency and urgency

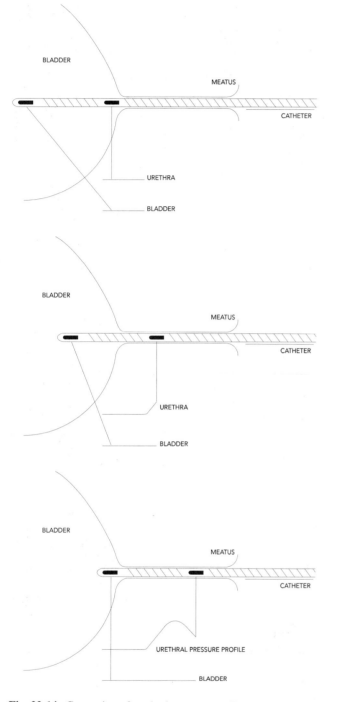

Fig. 22-14. Generation of urethral pressure profile. The catheter is pulled out at a steady rate. As the proximal transducer traverses the urethra, the pressure profile is recorded. Because the bladder sensor is intravesical throughout, no pressure change is registered. (From Versi E, Cardozo LD: Urodynamics. In Studd JWW, editor: *Progress in obstetrics and gynaecology,* vol 8, London, 1990, Churchill Livingstone.)

may be associated with bladder disease. However, in the absence of hematuria in the young patient, its use in the investigation of lower urinary tract dysfunction is not as valuable. If routine urodynamic investigations reveal the possibility of a stricture or a stenosis, such an investigation may be an

appropriate next step. The investigation can be carried out with a flexible cystoscope, and general anesthesia is often not required.

Urethral Pressure Profilometry. Through urethral pressure profilometry, pressure in the urethra can be measured at different points along its course simultaneously with bladder pressure (Enhorning, 1961). It is primarily used for diagnosing urethral sphincter incompetence, but it can be used to diagnose urethral instability, urethral strictures, and diverticula.

The first person to attempt to measure urethral pressures was Victor Bonney (Bonney, 1923), and he used the technique of retrograde sphincterometry. Subsequently, perfusion systems were developed. Although perfusion techniques are simple, their reproducibility has been questioned. Modern techniques use solid-state transducers mounted on catheters (Asmussen and Ulmsten, 1975). The most commonly used catheter uses two transducers mounted approximately 6 cm apart. The catheter is inserted in the bladder through the urethra until both sensors are inside the bladder. While the catheter is withdrawn steadily, the proximal sensor passes through the urethra and obtains a urethral pressure profile at rest (Fig. 22-14). Many measurements can be taken from the resting profile, but specifically they relate to measures of urethral length or maximum urethral closure pressure. If the patient coughs during the procedure, a stress profile can be obtained as well. Clearly, the latter is more important for investigating the integrity of the urethral sphincter. Although the reproducibility of the resting profile is well accepted, the same cannot be said for the stress profile. For this reason, urethral pressure profilometry cannot be used accurately for the diagnosis of genuine stress incontinence (Versi, 1990; Versi et al, 1991b).

Urethral instability can be detected by placing the catheter so that the urethral sensor is at the maximum urethral pressure point. At this point, various fluctuations are seen in urethral pressure; there is a small urethral pulse that is in time with the vascular pulse. There is also a fluctuation in the maximum urethral pressure that usually does not vary by more than one third of the resting value (Versi and Cardozo, 1986). However, in some patients there is sudden and complete loss of urethral pressure that may be associated with incontinence. This often occurs in the patient with detrusor instability before an unstable contraction that mimics the situation during normal micturition. However, in some patients, this loss of urethral pressure occurs in spite of a stable detrusor; therefore, it is diagnosed as urethral instability.

A consistent dip in the urethral pressure profile may indicate a urethral diverticulum, and an aberrant point of abnormally high pressure may be construed as a urethral stricture. Cystourethroscopy or fluoroscopy more easily and directly diagnose these urethral abnormalities. Although urethral pressure profilometry is widely used in urodynamic investigations, diagnostic criteria for genuine stress incontinence have been poorly formulated, which limits the clinical value of this technique.

Electrophysiological Studies. The value of routine electromyography as part of the urodynamic workup for a patient who is neurologically intact but incontinent is also limited. Although this technique is more useful in research, it has a clinical role in the investigation of voiding disorders and concomitant neurologic abnormalities.

Patients with voiding difficulties may have detrusor sphincter dyssynergia. The detrusor muscle contracts, but the urethral sphincter simultaneously contracts instead of relaxing. Voiding dysfunction in neurologically intact young women may be caused by pelvic floor contraction at the time of attempted micturition. Both abnormalities may be detected by electromyography studies.

Imaging Studies

Video-Urodynamics. Video-urodynamic testing is the most useful test for evaluation of the lower urinary tract. Essentially, the investigation involves cystometry using radiographic contrast medium and fluoroscopy so that the bladder and the urethra can be imaged while pressure recordings are made. This form-and-function test can be recorded on videotape and reviewed at a later date for analysis and for teaching purposes.

Video-urodynamic testing is considered the best urodynamic test because it yields a comprehensive array of information about the lower urinary tract. It may be argued that it is unnecessary for the evaluation of uncomplicated incontinence in a neurologically intact patient. However, the technique yields more information than simple cystometry. It is most useful for investigating patients who have undergone previous failed surgery and for those with a voiding dysfunction or a neurologic abnormality.

Ultrasonography. With the improved resolution of ultrasound imaging and the use of vaginal, rectal, and perineal probes, the definition that can be obtained of the lower urinary tract has improved. The main difficulty is that the probe may alter the anatomic configuration of the structure viewed and may influence the findings. Ultrasonography is most useful in the diagnosis of urinary retention. Urethral catheterization to determine a urinary residual has been replaced by simple transabdominal ultrasonography. The bladder is imaged so that all three dimensions can be measured. The product of these dimensions is multiplied by 0.7 to give a bladder volume that is accurate to an error of less than 20%. The ultrasound equipment automatically measures and calculates these indices.

Vaginal probes are able to delineate clearly the bladder neck. When the patient coughs, bladder neck incompetence can be diagnosed (Quinn, 1990). Bladder neck incompetence is of little diagnostic value because many continent women have an open bladder neck at rest and on coughing (Versi, 1991; Versi et al, 1990). For the diagnosis of genuine stress incontinence, it is important to be able to see the urethra open throughout its entire length, but this is not always possible using ultrasonography because of movement during a cough. In addition, if a patient has cough-induced de-

Table 22-1 Genuine Stress Incontinence–Associated Features	
Pelvic floor damage or denervation	Parturition
	Pelvic surgery
Urethral damage	Vaginal (urethral) surgery
	Surgery for incontinence
	Urethral dilatation or urethrotomy
	Recurrent urinary tract infection
	Radiotherapy
Increased intraabdominal pressures	Pregnancy
	Chronic cough (bronchitis)
	Abdominal-pelvic mass
	Fecal impaction
	Ascites
	Obesity

trusor instability, ultrasound imaging sometimes misdiagnoses the condition as urethral sphincter incompetence. There may, however, be a place for ultrasonography in combination with conventional urodynamic pressure studies, but this requires further evaluation. Recently, transvaginal ultrasonography was used to assess the dynamic difference of the genital hiatus in stress-incontinent versus stress-continent patients without prolapse (Boos et al, 1997). At rest and during the Valsalva maneuver, the hiatus in the incontinent group was significantly larger, and there was an added effect of pulling the urogenital hiatus apart at the level of the bladder neck, which probably impacted negatively on the continence mechanism.

Plain Radiology. Micturation cystography is largely outmoded because it is not a dynamic test, and it provides little information in comparison with video-urodynamics. Intravenous urography, though essential for the investigation of the upper urinary tract, has limited value in the investigation of incontinence. This test should be deferred in favor of the more dynamic tests previously mentioned.

Genuine Stress Incontinence
Cause

Genuine stress incontinence is defined as urethral sphincter incompetence. As a result, there is an involuntary loss of urine when intravesical pressure exceeds the maximum urethral closure pressure in the absence of a detrusor contraction (Abrams et al, 1990). Before detrusor contraction, urethral relaxation often occurs. If stress incontinence also occurs during urethral relaxation, it is not because of urethral sphincter incompetence; hence, the rider about excluding detrusor instability is important. Hypermobility causes genuine stress incontinence because of the lack of posterior support during a cough. Intrinsic sphincteric deficiency is the other cause of genuine stress incontinence. It results

---

BOX 22-4
CONSERVATIVE TREATMENT FOR GENUINE
STRESS INCONTINENCE

Pelvic floor exercises
Inferential therapy
Faradism
Vaginal cones
Perineometry
Tampons
Mechanical devices
α-Adrenergic agonists with or without estrogen replacement therapy

---

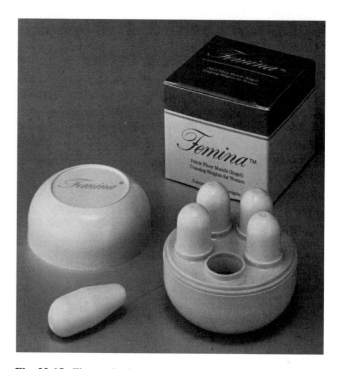

Fig. 22-15. Five vaginal cones. Reproduced from Colgate Medical, Berkshire, UK.

from the lack of urethral coaption, which leaves the urethra gaping, and it can be present with or without hypermobility.

There may be many causes for genuine stress incontinence, and some of these are listed in Table 22-1. Childbirth has definitely been implicated but is not the only cause. Many young nulliparous girls are also incontinent. Thomas et al (1980) found that multiparity was a predisposing factor, whereas Jolleys (1988) noted the association with obstetric trauma. Recent studies on collagen synthesis suggest that deficiencies in the repair process may contribute to the cause of prolapse but perhaps not of genuine stress incontinence (Norton et al, 1992). Electrophysiologic studies have shown that vaginal delivery rather than pregnancy itself can damage the pudendal nerve (Allen et al, 1990), but this does not explain why women experience stress incontinence during pregnancy. It may be that during pregnancy women have transient detrusor instability, whereas after delivery any damage that is caused may be more permanent.

Radical pelvic surgery can cause genuine stress incontinence and voiding dysfunction (Farquharson et al, 1987), possibly because of embarrassment of the nerve supply. On the other hand radiotherapy is more likely to result in detrusor instability and a small-capacity bladder. Few studies suggest that benign gynecologic surgery, in particular hysterectomy, is associated with the development of incontinence (Minaire and Buzelin, 1992). Unfortunately, the data are so flawed with confounding variables that a definitive statement is impossible without additional studies and subgroup analyses (Versi, 1989).

Diagnosis

The diagnosis of genuine stress incontinence can be made with cystometry when stress incontinence is noted in the absence of a detrusor contraction. Stress incontinence can be demonstrated by observing the external urethral meatus or by fluoroscopy. Many practitioners throughout the world use urethral pressure profilometry as a means of making the diagnosis. Although this may be adequate for many patients, results are ambiguous for a large number of them.

Treatment

Conservative Management. Nonsurgical management of genuine stress incontinence has been reviewed elsewhere (Rai and Versi, 1993); the types of treatments are listed in Box 22-4. Pelvic floor exercise is the mainstay of treatment (Kegel, 1948), but electrical therapy can be useful as a trophic stimulus to the muscles and, more significantly, as a biofeedback technique. Contraction of the specific pelvic floor muscles allows the patient to become aware of these muscle groups, which aids pelvic floor retraining (Mantle and Versi, 1991).

Perineometry works in a similar fashion. A vaginal dilator-shaped device is inserted into the vagina, and the patient is asked to contract her pelvic floor. The device measures the strength of the contraction, and the patient receives the biofeedback of pelvic floor activity, thus reinforcing the education process.

Vaginal cones are an interesting innovation (Fig. 22-15). The patient uses a set of five cones, each identical in size but of different weight. The cone of lowest weight is inserted into the vagina by the patient; she is then instructed to hold it in place while walking around. The cones are designed to teach the patient to contract her pelvic floor muscles without contracting her abdominal musculature. Contraction of the latter muscles leads to expulsion of the cone. When the patient has been able to hold a certain weight, she moves to the next weight—weight training for the pelvic floor! Patients find the cones acceptable (Peattie et al, 1988) and easy to use.

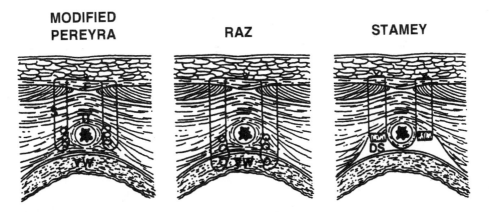

Fig. 22-16. Comparison of the modified Pereyra, Raz, and Stamey operations showing the coronal section of the bladder neck and surrounding tissues. VW, vaginal wall. (From Stanton SL: Surgical management of urethral sphincter incompetence. *Clin Obstet Gynecol* 1990; 33:346.)

The cure rate for these physical treatments is limited, but approximately 70% of patients show significant improvement. The key to successful use of this therapy is patient selection. Women who are highly motivated, young, thin, and fit and who have not undergone incontinence surgery are the most likely to benefit. Other good prognostic features are absence of long-standing incontinence, concomitant prolapse, or chronic cough (Mantle and Versi, 1991).

Medical. In postmenopausal women, α-adrenergic agonists can be used in the conservative management of genuine stress incontinence, and uncontrolled trials have shown subjective improvement (Lose and Lindholm, 1984; Lose et al, 1989; Diernaes et al, 1989). The use of α-adrenergic agonists such as phenylpropanolamine (PPA, 25 to 100 mg twice a day) or pseudoephedrine (15 to 30 mg three times a day) will act at the level of the bladder neck and urethra to stimulate the contraction of smooth muscle (Fantl et al, 1996). However, as seen in a previous section (Anatomy of the Urethra), the female urethra has a very attenuated circular smooth muscle (where the α-adrenergic receptors are localized), in contrast to the male urethra. This limits the effects of α-adrenergic drugs. Combination therapy with estrogen replacement has been shown to potentiate the effects of α-adrenergic drugs (Fantl et al, 1996) and to work in double-blind, placebo-controlled trials (Ahlstöm et al, 1990). These medications are contraindicated in women with hypertension. The side effects of these drugs (anxiety, insomnia, agitation, dyspnea, headache, sweating, and arrhythmia) limit the long-term use of the therapy.

Imipramine has been used for patients with stress incontinence because it has α-adrenergic properties, but valid data supporting its use are few (Fantl et al, 1996). Thus, effective medical treatment for stress incontinence is lacking.

Surgical. More than 100 surgical procedures have been described for the treatment of genuine stress incontinence. Because a full discussion of them is beyond the scope of this chapter, they are described elsewhere (Hurt, 1992). The procedures can be classified into six groups, which are discussed in the next sections.

Before treatment, the general health of the patient must be considered so the most appropriate type of procedure can be planned. Integrity of the local tissues, particularly around the bladder neck, should also be assessed. In postmenopausal women with atrophied tissues, the sutures may tear out. Presurgical treatment with estrogens may be indicated. Voiding function should be assessed before surgery because patients with poor flow rates or high residuals are likely to have more voiding difficulties after surgery, irrespective of the cause of their compromised voiding function.

Vaginal surgery. The vaginal approach with bladder neck buttress sutures (Kelly plication) is one of the most common operations used by gynecologists. However, because the objective 5-year success rate of this procedure is only approximately 50%, many urogynecologists do not favor it (Leach et al, 1997). This operation should be distinguished from anterior colporrhaphy, which involves the placement of bladder base buttress sutures that should remain proximal to the bladder neck, for the reduction of a cystocele caused by a central defect.

Endoscopic needle-suspension techniques. The endoscopic needle-suspension procedures, such as the Pereyra, Stamey, Raz, Muzsnai, and Gittes techniques, all involve the use of a single loop of suture placed on either side of the bladder neck and tied above the rectus sheath (Fig. 22-16) (Griffiths and Versi, 1997). The Pereyra technique makes use of a single loop of suture that has a tendency to cut out. Because the prevesical fascia is not very tough in patients who require this procedure, modifications have been made to improve the anchor of the suture at the level of the bladder neck. The Stamey procedure has a buffer interposed to mitigate against tearing out. The modified Pereyra procedure involves the use of helical sutures through the deep pelvic fascia, whereas the modified Raz procedure goes further to include part of the vaginal wall. The Muzsnai uses two sutures on each side on the vaginal mucosa to add strength to the support, similar to a Burch colposuspension. The Gittes procedure, on the other hand, uses the full thickness of the vaginal wall. As a result, the sutures are exposed to the vaginal environment. However, within 6 weeks of surgery, the vagina reepithelializes over the sutures. Some practitioners are unhappy with this technique because it may result in excessive vaginal discharge in some patients. The overall long-term success rate for these needle-suspension procedures is less than 50% (Leach et al, 1997). It is suggested that they be used for older women and for women whose vaginas have narrowed from multiple previous operations because a retropubic procedure may be more difficult (Hilton and Mayne, 1991; Griffiths and Versi, 1997).

Retropubic procedures. The most commonly performed retropubic procedures are the Marshall-Marchetti-Krantz (MMK) procedure and the Burch colposuspension. Both involve the use of a Pfannenstiel incision and dissection in the space of Retzius. The bladder is dissected medially from the prevesical fascia, and sutures are inserted at the level of the bladder neck. In the MMK procedure, these sutures (one on each side) are then attached to the periosteum of the symphysis pubis. They elevate the bladder neck by elevating the vagina underneath. Some practitioners are concerned about this procedure because of the risk for osteomyelitis of the pubic bone, which is difficult to treat.

Burch colposuspension is more popular because, unlike the MMK procedure, the sutures are not placed in the periosteum of the symphysis pubis but in the iliopectineal ligament on either side, minimizing the risk for osteitis pubis. Because three or four sutures can be used, not only is Burch colposuspension an anti-incontinence procedure, it can reduce a moderate cystocele or at least convert a low symptomatic cystocele to a high asymptomatic cystocele. Long-term follow-up of patients has shown an increased incidence of enterocele and posterior wall prolapse (Wiskind et al, 1991).

The 5-year success rate for retropubic procedures is thought to be approximately 85%. That figure rises to 95% when the procedure is a primary one. The success rate declines with increasing age of the patient, obesity, and previous surgery to reach a plateau of 69% at 10 to 12 years (Stanton and Cardozo, 1979; Alcalay et al, 1995; Borstad, 1997). None of the procedures described must be obstructive to achieve continence. However, there is often an element of postoperative obstruction to voiding. It is important to emphasize that the probability of success is not dependent on the probability of inducing obstruction; patients who have obstruction may not necessarily be continent. In the retropubic procedures, placement of the sutures is crucial. If the sutures are placed too far distant (paraurethral), the patient is likely to have voiding difficulties, but if they are placed too close (by the side of the bladder), the patient is more likely to experience residual incontinence.

Paravaginal repair. First described by White (1909) and more recently popularized by Richardson et al (1976), paravaginal repair has been suggested as an anti-incontinence procedure. Initial results on a large series of patients reported a 95% subjective cure (Richardson, 1981). However, Burch sutures were also placed at the time of surgery. A re-

cent randomized comparative study of Burch and abdominal paravaginal repair for stress urinary incontinence reported a significantly lower subjective and objective cure rate with the paravaginal repair at 1 and 3 years (100% vs. 72% and 100% vs. 61%, respectively) (Colombo et al, 1996). Most pelvic surgeons now use the technique primarily for the correction of cystoceles caused by paravaginal defect. The technique is described in the section covering surgical repair of disorders of the pelvic floor support.

Slings. An ongoing debate concerns whether the sling should be used as first-line surgery for stress urinary incontinence caused by hypermobility. Opponents point out the high complication rate (voiding dysfunction, fistula) cited in the literature and suggest that this procedure be used only when hypermobility of the bladder neck is complicated by intrinsic sphincteric deficiency. Proponents argue that slings are now performed with less tension and, consequently, fewer complications. This controversy will only be resolved when reliable outcome data become available. Other indications for this procedure include medical conditions in which an abdominal approach would result in significant morbidity, and recurrent urinary stress incontinence after failed surgery, though the latter is better addressed by a full urodynamic assessment and surgery planned in light of that assessment.

The purpose of the sling is to restore normal bladder neck support and to compress mechanically the proximal urethra at times of increased intraabdominal pressure. The degree of pull or elevation is crucial to the procedure because it should provide posterior support, permit voiding without obstruction, and some compression with the Valsalva maneuver. Therefore, the success of the sling operation tends to be operator dependent. Many procedures have been described. Slings can be placed either by the vaginal or by the abdominal route, though using the vaginal route increases the danger of infection. The material used can be endogenous (rectus fascia), organic (porcine fascia, cadaveric fascia), or inert (silastic, Marlex, Prolene).

Periurethral injections. The use of injectibles is an easier option for patients with intrinsic sphincteric deficiency in whom a sling procedure would otherwise be indicated. Previously, materials such as Teflon were injected into the periurethral tissues to increase urethral resistance. Complications included urethritis, abscess formation, and even migration of the Teflon particles to the lung and brain. For this reason other materials have been tried. GAX collagen has shown good results. Short-term studies resulted in a 40% cure rate (no residual incontinence) and an additional 30% to 50% of improvement (Smith et al, 1997). Long-term studies resulted in a 48% objective cure (on urodynamic studies) and an additional 9% improvement (Khullar et al, 1997). The probability of remaining dry without additional injections was 71%, 58%, and 46% at 1, 2, and 3 years, respectively (Herschorn et al, 1996). It is thought that the injected material is replaced by endogenous collagen; therefore not only does it appear safe, it is long lasting. These injectables are ideally suited for patients who do not have bladder neck hypermobility.

Artificial sphincters. When all surgical procedures have failed, there is always the option of an artificial sphincter. This is a technique whereby a cuff is placed around the urethra and the control bulb is inserted into the labia majora. By pressing the bulb, it is possible to activate and deactivate the cuff. Most authorities suggest that the cuff should not be activated for several weeks until surgical edema has settled down. Because it is a closed system, if infection has not been introduced at the time of surgery, it is unlikely to develop afterward. It is usual to deactivate the cuff at night to avoid cuff necrosis. Although expensive, artificial sphincters have transformed the lives of many women.

Failures. If all the above procedures fail repetitively, there is still a place for continent urinary diversion or reconstructive surgery. Some patients may not want to subject themselves to yet another operation, or they may not be fit enough to undergo more surgery. For these patients, the conservative option of using diapers and special pants is an option. There have been many advances in absorptive material in the last two decades; it would be advisable to obtain the help of a nurse specializing in palliative care of this sort. Excellent nursing care is essential because excoriation from urine can be a most irritative and debilitating condition.

Mechanical Devices. Tampons and mechanical devices are useful because they provide temporary occlusion of the urethra. These are inserted into the vagina to prevent leakage in patients who experience stress incontinence only during exercise.

Several mechanical devices have been devised to treat urinary incontinence. They can be classified as intraurethral, intravaginal, or external. The urethral plug (Nielsen et al, 1993) and the Reliance (Uromed: Needham, Mass.) (Pigné et al, 1997) are two examples of intraurethral devices. They have been shown to be effective in controlling incontinence, but they have significant side effects (hematuria, bacterial cystitis and intravesical migration).

Intravaginal tampons and simple pessaries have been used with varying success as a way to stabilize the bladder neck. However, pessaries can obstruct the urethra if they are improperly fitted. More recently, specific intravaginal bladder neck support devices have been developed. The Introl (UroMed) (Kando et al, 1997) resembles a pessary with two prongs at one end. These prongs elevate the bladder neck behind the pubic bone. A significant improvement in subjective and objective evaluation of incontinence resulted from its use. Uroflow and bladder imaging ruled out any obstruction or significant residual with it in place. Nevertheless, 26% of the patients reported side effects such as pain, bleeding, irritation, and vaginal laceration. The device requires fitting; it comes in 24 different sizes. A C-shaped vaginal tampon, the Continence Guard (UroMed), was designed to support the bladder neck through the vagina. Objective improvement in incontinence with no effect on residual urine or vaginal pH was reported among patients who used it on a

short-term (Thyssen and Lose, 1996) and a long-term basis (Thyssen and Lose, 1997). Daily change is recommended (every 4 hours during menses) to prevent septic shock syndrome. No signs of erosion, irritation, or change on urodynamic parameters were noted. With this device, an improvement in quality of life was also noted (Sander et al, 1999).

Finally, three external devices have been designed. The FemAssist (Insight Medical, Bolton, Mass.) is the one most studied (Versi et al, 1998; Tincello et al, 1997). It was shown to decrease objective incontinence and to improve quality of life, and it was not associated with urinary tract infection. Because it is held in place by suction, it may cause urethral prolapse and is contraindicated if this condition is already present. A similar device is CapSure (Bard, Covington, Ga.). The Empress (UroMed) effectively blocks off the external urethral meatus by adhering to the surrounding tissue. It also showed a good clinical profile in the control of incontinence (Harris et al, 1994).

Detrusor Instability and Hyperreflexia
Cause

Detrusor instability is defined as the occurrence of spontaneous detrusor contractions during the filling phase when the patient attempts to inhibit micturition (Abrams, 1990). In practice, any detrusor activity can be regarded as abnormal if it occurs inappropriately. It is the second most common cause of urinary incontinence in middle-aged women, and it accounts for approximately 35% of urogynecologic cases. The incidence increases with age, and there appears to be a specific increase after menopause; detrusor instability may well be a condition that is estrogen sensitive (Versi, 1994). If it is secondary to an upper motor neuron lesion (for example, multiple sclerosis), the condition is known as detrusor hyperreflexia. However, in gynecologic practice most cases are idiopathic. Detrusor instability in men is often secondary to outflow obstruction, and it tends to resolve after the obstruction is relieved, though this may take several months (Mundy, 1990). Outflow obstruction in women is rare. The bladder appears to be sexually differentiated in its response to acute obstruction. In women, it tends toward decompensation with the sequel of a hypotonic bladder (see section on overflow incontinence). Some authorities think that insidious obstruction in women, as in men, can result in detrusor instability. After antiincontinence surgery, detrusor instability develops in 18% of women who did not have it before surgery (Cardozo et al, 1979). This may be the bladder's response to outflow obstruction, or perhaps the surgical procedure disrupted neural input at the level of the bladder neck.

Diagnosis

Through cystometry, the condition can be diagnosed during the filling phase if wavelike contractions are seen in association with urgency or if the pressure rise on bladder filling exceeds 15 cm of water (Abrams, 1990). An abnormal detrusor contraction may be provoked when the patient

Table 22-2	Treatment of Detrusor Instability
Psychotherapy	Bladder drill
	Biofeedback
	Hypnotherapy
Drug therapy	Inhibit bladder contractions:
	Anticholinergic agents
	Muscle relaxants
	Calcium-channel blockers
	Tricyclic antidepressants
	Prostaglandin synthetase inhibitors
	Increase outlet resistance:
	α-Adrenergic stimulants
	Local tissue:
	Estrogens
	Reduce urine production:
	Synthetic vasopressin
Denervation	Vaginal denervation
	Sacral neurectomy
Surgery	Bladder transection
	"Clam" ileocystoplasty
	Cystectomy and neobladder construction
	Urinary diversion

changes posture or after a cough. Some urogynecologists regard idiopathic low compliance as a different entity from detrusor instability, but the symptoms and the treatment are similar to those for detrusor instability. Reduction of the filling rate exhibits phasic detrusor instability in many patients with idiopathic low compliance. There are many causes for low compliance, including radical pelvic surgery, radiotherapy, recurrent urinary tract infection, and interstitial cystitis.

Although the clinical presentation varies, frequency, nocturia, urgency, urge incontinence, and enuresis are the symptoms often associated with detrusor instability. Stress incontinence is common among patients with detrusor instability. In young women, incontinence associated with orgasm is thought to be the result of detrusor instability.

Treatment

The main treatment is behavior modification with the help of pharmacologic agents. Although there are legions of other treatments available (Table 22-2), these merely reflect our inadequacy in treating this condition successfully.

Behavior Therapy. There is no evidence that long-term drug therapy is detrimental, but most patients prefer to take medication for only a short time, especially if it has side effects. Thus, the main treatment remains behavior modification in the form of bladder drill (Frewen, 1978). By examining the patient's voiding diary, it is possible to determine the average intervoid time. The patient is then instructed to increase this time interval even at the risk of incontinence. As the intervoid time increases, so does the voided volume, and the result is a reduction in symptoms of detrusor instability. Indeed cystometry carried out after bladder drill shows that

there is either reduction in the degree of instability or resolution of the condition. Such bladder training is more easily accomplished on an inpatient basis; even though it is less successful in the authors' experience, costs dictate that this should be carried out on an ambulatory basis (Frewen, 1982). The key to success lies in the relationship developed between the patient and the trainer, be it a nurse, a physician, or another health care provider. Motivation is crucial, as are constant encouragement and positive feedback (Mantle and Versi, 1991).

Biofeedback. Another successful treatment for detrusor instability is biofeedback (Cardozo et al, 1978; Moore et al, 1992). The patient undergoes catheterization, and her bladder pressure is displayed to her numerically or graphically. She is able to monitor the strength of her own detrusor contractions and is asked to try to inhibit them. Initially patients may not know how they achieve this, but they are able to do so with some practice. Unfortunately, as with other behavior modification techniques, it is time consuming and there is a significant relapse rate; patients must reinforce this kind of feedback intermittently. Similarly, hypnotherapy has been successful, but it requires reinforcement (Freeman and Baxby, 1982).

Electrical Stimulation. Intravaginal electrical stimulation results in the activation of inhibitory nerve fibers in the sympathetic hypogastric nerve and in reflex inhibition of detrusor contractility (Lindstrom et al, 1983). Some clinical reports have suggested that this method is useful for patients with detrusor instability (Fall, 1984). This effect remains in randomized placebo-controlled trials (Brubaker et al, 1997), despite the high placebo response and the fluctuation with time that is seen with detrusor instability.

Medical Therapy. Many different types of drugs have been used for the treatment of detrusor instability, and they can be broadly classified as in Table 22-2. Any drug may have more than one mode of action. All drugs used in the management of these conditions have side effects, particularly anticholinergic side effects. Because there is such a high (up to 60%) placebo response with this condition, it is difficult to be certain about the efficacy of many of the agents used. Oxybutynin chloride is a muscle relaxant, but it has anticholinergic properties. It has a short half-life and so has to be administered (3 or 5 mg) every 6 or 8 hours. There is a high incidence of side effects (Tapp et al, 1990), and it is important to raise the dose until the patient experiences minimal side effects or the dose will be inadequate. Because there is so much patient variation, the dosage regimens have to be adjusted to suit each person. Other useful drugs are emepronium caragenate (300 to 500 mg four times a day) and dicyclomine hydrochloride (20 mg four times a day). To treat nocturnal enuresis and to avoid side effects during the day, imipramine (50 mg at night) or desmopressin (20 μg at night) can be the drugs of choice. When frequency is the only problem, propantheline bromide (15 to 45 mg four times a day) can be effective. Prostaglandin synthetase inhibitors are less favored because of the high rate of side effects. Because no drugs are completely satisfactory and because pharmacologic therapy is inadequate, the new generation of calcium-channel blockers is eagerly awaited.

Although rigorous proof demonstrating the validity of estrogen replacement therapy in postmenopausal women with urgency, frequency, and nocturia is lacking, it is thought that estrogen supplementation may raise the sensory threshold of the bladder (Fantl et al, 1988).

Surgery. If the above measures fail, surgery is an option, though it is one that should not be taken lightly. It is only appropriate to a small number of women who have not responded to conventional conservative therapy, many of whom have a significant neurologic abnormality. These patients should be treated at a tertiary referral center. There are two options: surgery that involves denervation and surgery that requires bladder augmentation.

Denervation. Many denervation procedures have been devised, among them bladder distension, subtrigonal phenol injection, selective sacral nerve blockade, sacral neurectomy, and transvaginal bladder denervation. The postganglionic somata of the parasympathetic nerves supplying the bladder are located in the bladder wall. Bladder distension and phenol injections are likely to disrupt preganglionic and postganglionic fibers. Other procedures designed to denervate the bladder effectively cause preganglionic section. This results in a transient decrease in postganglionic activity and a reduction in detrusor instability. After recovery, however, the situation may be worse than it was before, and it is for this that denervation procedures are less favored.

Bladder transection. Transection of the bladder (either by laparotomy or cystoscopy) above the level of the trigone has been advocated. Because the neuronal supply enters the bladder in conjunction with the inferior vesical artery, circumferential transaction should interrupt the distribution of neuronal supply and leave sensation intact at the trigone (Turner-Warwick and Ashken, 1967). A study has been reported indicating reasonably good results with this technique (Mundy, 1983).

Augmentation. The rationale for augmentation is that by increasing bladder capacity and interposing a segment of bowel, the effect of detrusor activity is dampened. The most common and successful type of bladder augmentation is the "clam" ileocystoplasty (Mundy, 1986). With this technique, the bladder is transected transversely so that it opens like a clam, and a portion of detubularized ileum on its pedicle is sutured onto the defect. This limits the symptoms of detrusor instability, but because these patients often have voiding dysfunction, intermittent self-catheterization often must be used as adjunctive therapy.

Urinary diversion. When all else fails, patients prefer urinary diversion to living as a "bladder cripple" with all the social and medical consequences. Urinary diversion methods can be incontinent (ileal conduit) or continent. The latter involves the creation of an intraabdominal reservoir made from a portion of bowel that is emptied by intermittent catheterization (Mundy, 1993). The simplest form of conti-

nent diversion is the Mitrofanoff procedure; the appendix or a portion of ureter is used as the catheterizable channel with a flap-valve continent mechanism interposed between it and the reservoir.

Mixed Incontinence
Genuine Stress Incontinence and Detrusor Instability

Some women have both detrusor instability and genuine stress incontinence. This poses a particular problem (Karram, 1989). The overall cure rate for surgery in this group is approximately 50%; pharmacologic agents are successful in treating approximately one third of patients. Added to these figures is a small percentage of patients in whom there is significant improvement without cure. The physician has to decide on the predominant condition and tailor therapy toward that. However, when it is difficult to decide, the safer approach is to treat the detrusor instability medically and to resort to surgery only when the residual incontinence is intolerable. Patients need counseling before such surgery, and it must be explained to them that bladder neck surgery may result in a competent sphincter but that detrusor instability may be aggravated by surgery.

Recent data have suggested that retropubic surgery may cure or improve stress incontinence and urge incontinence, if stress incontinence predates urge incontinence. It has been postulated that the passage of urine into the urethra as a consequence of bladder neck funneling may cause the urge sensation and incontinence (Scotti et al, 1998).

Genuine Stress Incontinence and Voiding Dysfunction

Bladder neck surgery in patients who have genuine stress incontinence and voiding dysfunction leads to worse voiding function after surgery. For this reason, pelvic floor exercises with biofeedback should be the first line of therapy. If this fails and surgery is contemplated, the patient should be taught how to conduct clean, intermittent self-catheterization, and surgery should only be performed if the patient accepts that indefinite self-catheterization may be the price for continence.

Detrusor Instability and Voiding Dysfunction

If the voiding difficulty is caused by detrusor dysfunction, bladder drill should be encouraged. If anticholinergic agents are used, the patient may experience retention and require self-catheterization. If the voiding dysfunction is caused by outflow obstruction, relief of the obstruction by urethrotomy may make the incontinence worse.

Overflow Incontinence and Voiding Dysfunction
Cause

Overflow incontinence is defined as "any involuntary loss of urine associated with overdistension of the bladder" (Abrams et al, 1990). Overdistension of the bladder may result from dysfunction of the detrusor muscle or the urethral sphincter.

Many causes have been described, and they may result in either acute or chronic symptoms.

Urinary retention from detrusor dysfunction is the result of hyporeflexia or atony of the detrusor muscle, usually caused by lesions in the lower motor neurons that supply the bladder. Conditions associated with neurogenic urinary retention include cerebrovascular accident, multiple sclerosis, spinal cord injury, cauda equina tumors, diabetic neuropathy, acquired immunodeficiency syndrome peripheral neuropathy, and pelvic nerve damage secondary to radical pelvic surgery (Herbaut, 1993). Detrusor dysfunction also may result from local inflammation, pharmacologic agents, and psychogenic causes.

Urethral obstruction may cause overdistension of the bladder. Compromise of the outflow tract is common in men with prostatic hypertrophy, but it may occur in women because of other causes. Obstruction in women may result from periurethral edema caused by trauma, labor, or vaginal surgery. A severe cystocele or uterine procidentia may cause kinking and obstruction of the proximal urethra. Neurologic conditions may result in failure of the sphincter to relax appropriately during the micturition reflex. Such detrusor-sphincter dyssynergia may occur with upper motor neuron lesions such as cord section or Parkinson disease (Herbaut, 1993).

Diagnosis

Symptoms of overflow incontinence may be difficult to differentiate from those of stress incontinence. Leakage typically occurs with stress; patients may also report dribbling, hesitancy, and prolonged voiding. Physical examination will confirm a distended bladder and may provide evidence of a local cause. Careful neurologic examination of the sacral dermatomes, lower extremity motor function, and perineal reflexes should be performed, and consultation should be sought for any abnormality. Diagnosis is confirmed by identifying an excessive postvoid residual volume by catheterization or ultrasonography. Cystometrography provides information about bladder sensation and bladder capacity. Voiding studies may assist in differentiating obstruction (high bladder pressure with low flow rate) from detrusor hyporeflexia (low bladder pressure with low flow rate). Electromyography permits identification of abnormal urethral or pelvic floor activity. Sometimes, outlet obstruction can be ruled out during routine urodynamic studies with an assessment of the resistance to catheter insertion. Cystoscopy and urethroscopy can be similarly useful.

Treatment

Acute or iatrogenic retention can be treated by catheterization and by leaving a Foley catheter in place for 24 to 48 hours. Patients may be at risk because of increased age, prolonged surgery, too much analgesia, administration of opiates (Tammela et al, 1986), or instrumental delivery. Prevention of long-term damage in these patients should be addressed by monitoring output and using bladder drainage or intermittent catheterization in the early postoperative period to avert residual urine levels greater than 600 mL after voiding (Anderson and Grant, 1991).

Medical therapy to increase detrusor contractility with cholinergic medication has shown disappointing results (Wheeler and Waller, 1992). If the postoperative intravesical instillation of prostaglandin F_2 helps to reduce acute retention (Tammela et al, 1987), its use has not been supported by studies in patients with chronic voiding dysfunction (Andersson et al, 1978). Surgical correction of severe cystocele or urethral dilatation (or urethrotomy) is indicated for outflow obstruction.

Intermittent self-catheterization remains the mainstay of therapy (Lapides et al, 1984). It requires minimal dexterity and coordination, and we have had success in teaching the technique to visually impaired patients. This technique is safe, and it reduces the rate of infection in patients with chronic post-void residual urine (Kass et al, 1981; Maynard and Diokno, 1984). In patients who have spinal cord injury with preservation of the sacral center, the implantation of a nerve root electrical stimulator on S2, S3, and S4 has shown good results (Brindley, 1990).

Genitourinary Fistula

A fistula that bypasses the normal sphincter mechanism may result in total incontinence. Worldwide, most fistulae are caused by obstetric trauma, either from necrosis secondary to prolonged pressure of the fetal head in the birth canal or from delays in surgical intervention. Other causes include surgical trauma, malignancy, and irradiation.

Symptoms of fistula include the continuous loss of urine, vulvar irritation, passage of urine from the vagina, and recurrent infection. Large fistulae are visible on examination, but smaller tracts may be difficult to localize. Urinary dyes, such as oral phenazopyridine (pyridium), may be helpful for visualization. Endoscopic and radiographic studies are necessary to determine whether multiple tracts are present, to delineate the location of the fistula relative to the trigone and the urethral sphincter, and to discover a complex fistula. A common diagnostic tool is the three-swab test, whereby the practitioner places three sponges in the vagina and examines them a few hours later (pyridium or methylene blue may be placed in the bladder to stain the urine). If the sponges are wet or stained, a fistula is strongly suspected. If the deepest sponge is moist but is not stained, a uretero-vaginal fistula is suspected. If it is stained, a vesico-vaginal fistula is suspected.

Genitourinary fistulae are usually treated by surgery, but small lesions may heal spontaneously with long-term drainage. Successful repair requires strict adherence to basic surgical principles. The fistulous tract, including all surrounding scar tissue, must be identified and excised. Wide mobilization of the tissue layers is necessary to assure reconstruction of normal anatomy in layers without tension on the suture lines. Overlapping of suture lines should be minimized. If the blood supply is compromised, a vascular tissue pedicle such as the Martius labial fat pad graft may be interposed between the tissue layers (Elkins, 1990). Catheterization to divert the urinary stream and to prevent distension and stress on the suture lines is necessary during healing.

Urethral Diverticulum

A urethral diverticulum is a saclike herniation of urethral mucosa that develops through a defect in the muscular layer of the urethral wall. The sac cavity is connected to the urethral lumen by one or more small ostia. Reported incidence varies between 1% and 4% (Ginsbur and Genadry, 1984), but the true incidence in women is unknown. Increasing awareness of the condition among clinicians probably increases the frequency with which it is diagnosed. Diverticula usually develop in women between 30 and 50 years of age, and they may occur with higher frequency in black women.

Cause

Occasionally, urethral diverticula are diagnosed in children, which suggests a congenital etiology. They may arise from an inherent weakness in the urethral wall or from persistent mesonephric cell rests (Coddington and Knob, 1983). However, most diverticula are probably acquired lesions. One theory proposes that traumatic injury, such as occurs in childbirth, disrupts the integrity of the urethral wall. However, the condition generally is not associated with increasing parity (Pathak and House, 1970). Other theories have suggested postinflammatory obstruction of the paraurethral glands as a cause. An abscess cavity forms near the obstruction, and subsequent rupture into the lumen of the urethra results in a diverticulum. Inflammation has been proposed as the most common cause (Ginsburg and Genadry, 1984).

Diagnosis

The classic triad of symptoms associated with urethral diverticula consists of dysuria, dyspareunia, and postvoid dribbling. Other symptoms may be related to a urinary tract infection. Included in this group are frequency, urgency, and hematuria. Occasionally, a patient may have a palpable mass lesion. Many patients are asymptomatic, and the diagnosis is based on physical findings.

Diverticula are differentiated from other vaginal cysts primarily by their location. A palpable mass in the anterior vaginal wall suggests a urethral diverticulum. Most diverticula are 1 to 3 cm in diameter and are located in the distal or middle third of the urethra (Andersen, 1967). The ostium almost always occurs on the posterior urethral wall, and the mass is often tender. On palpation of the urethra, pus or urine may be expressed from the meatus.

Diagnosis is confirmed by imaging and endoscopy. Imaging with a voiding cystourethrogram may demonstrate filling of the diverticulum with contrast media. If not, the urethra is filled under positive pressure using a special double-ballooned catheter. Balloons obstruct the external meatus and the urethrovesical junction; contrast media can thereby be forced into even a narrow-necked diverticulum sac. Ultrasonography has been used successfully to delineate these lesions (Keefe et al, 1991). Urethroscopy allows direct visualization of the ostium and occasionally demonstrates more than one opening.

Treatment

Several surgical procedures have been recommended for the treatment of symptomatic urethral diverticula. If a patient has acute infection with cellulitis, simple incision and drainage is appropriate (Ginsburg and Genadry, 1984). If the infection is subacute, excision of the diverticulum sac through a vaginal incision is often performed (Ward et al, 1967). A small probe, a Fogarty balloon catheter, or a dye may be placed in the sac to assist the dissection (Kohorn and Glickman, 1992). Care should be taken not to excise normal urethral tissue with the sac. The defect is closed with a double-breast technique using fine suture material and without tension on the suture lines. Catheter drainage of the bladder is maintained for several days. If the diverticulum is located in the distal urethra, marsupialization can be performed (Spence and Duckett, 1970). An incision is made from the external meatus to the diverticular sac through the vaginal mucosa and urethral wall. Redundant tissue from the wall of the diverticulum is excised. Urethral mucosa is sewn to vaginal mucosa to create a new urethral meatus, but this can result in spraying during micturition. This procedure can also result in iatrogenic incontinence if the incision includes the urethral sphincter mechanism. Other complications of diverticular surgery include urethral strictures, fistula formation, and recurrence of diverticula.

Painful Bladder Syndrome

Painful bladder refers to the syndrome in which patients have irritative symptoms and pain despite negative findings on urine culture. Irritative symptoms include frequency (>7 times/day), urgency and nocturia (>1 time/night), pain with a full bladder, dysuria, and pain on micturition. They can be debilitating and distressing.

Causes of painful bladder syndrome include radiation and post-chemotherapy (cyclophosphamide) cystitis and systemic disease (lupus) affecting the bladder. However, most of the time, the cause is unclear.

Urethral Syndrome

Because it is ill defined, the incidence of urethral syndrome is difficult to assess. Approximately 20% to 30% (Dans and Klaus, 1976) of women who seek treatment for urinary tract symptoms are thought to have urethral syndrome. Although the cause is unknown, current hypotheses include bacterial cystitis (with counts as low as 10 bacteria per milliliter) (Brooks and Mauder, 1977), atypical infection (*Mycoplasma, Chlamydia*), atrophy, allergy, psychosomatic, noxious agents, and trauma.

The diagnosis of urethral syndrome is made by exclusion. A complete history should be taken and physical examination should be performed, particularly to rule out a urethral diverticulum, caruncle, or inflammation. A clean-catch urine specimen for culture is required. If *Chlamydia* infection or vaginitis is suspected, adequate culture should be taken. Voiding dysfunction, with the resultant chronic residual of urine, can cause symptoms similar to those of the urethral syndrome. Hence, a uroflow and a postvoid residual quantification will be useful. If an intravesical abnormality is suspected, cystoscopy is recommended (hematuria or advanced age). Interstitial cystitis, if suspected, should also be ruled out by cystoscopy.

Because the cause of urethral syndrome is undetermined, the treatment is poorly defined. If patient has irritative symptoms, a culture count of 10 bacteria per milliliter of a single organism with evidence of pyuria may be treated with antibiotics (Benness and Hill, 1997). If sterile pyuria is found, an atypical organism may be the cause and empirical treatment with erythromycin or doxycycline may be indicated. If atrophy is detected in postmenopausal women, a vaginal estrogen cream may help. Urethral dilatation has been used with some success in these patients, though the mechanism of its benefits is unclear. It is thought that dilatation and massage against the hard dilator may facilitate drainage of the urethral glands and increase the urethral caliber if a urethral stricture is present.

Interstitial Cystitis

Interstitial cystitis is chronic inflammation of the bladder. Here again, the symptoms may be devastating for patients, especially the pain, nocturia, frequency, and urgency.

Interstitial cystitis was defined for research purposes by the National Institutes of Health (NIH) (Gillenwater and Wein, 1988) as the association of frequency, urgency, nocturia, dysuria, and suprapubic pain. Typical cystoscopic findings in patients with interstitial cystitis are low capacity (<1000 mL under anesthesia), terminal hematuria after cystodistension (80 to 100 mm Hg), petechial hemorrhage (glomerulations), and Hunner's ulcers. A biopsy specimen is necessary not to make the diagnosis but to rule out a neoplastic condition, especially if the patient has an ulcer. Some authors think the NIH criteria are too stringent. A test elaborated by Pearson (the Pearson test) may help in the diagnosis. It consists of the instillation of a dilute solution of potassium chloride into the bladder. Patients without interstitial cystitis should not experience pain; this is in contrast to patients with interstitial cystitis.

Various causes have been postulated. An immunologic cause was suspected, but there was little support for it. More in favor is the hypothesis of a blood-urine barrier defect, with an epithelial leak. Evidence was found suggesting bladder surface proteoglycans or glycoaminoglycans acting as a protective layer between the (irritative) urine and the bladder mucosa (Lilly and Parsons, 1991). Any damage to that barrier would lead to increased permeability and promote irritation of the mucosa by the urine.

Treatment of interstitial cystitis has proven challenging. Antiinflammatory, bladder analgesic, or antihistaminic agents can help as first-line therapy. Antidepressants may be valuable given the possibility that a patient is depressed because of chronic pain and sleep disturbances from nocturia. Two treatments for interstitial cystitis have been shown in randomized controlled trials to be effective: pentosanpolysulfate (Hwang et al, 1997) and bacillus Calmette-Guérin (Peters et al, 1997). Pentosanpolysulfate (Elmiron), a synthetic analogue of glycosaminoglycan, has been used with success in randomized controlled trials. Intravesical instillation of a strain of bacillus Calmette-Guérin was shown in a placebo-controlled trial to improve quality of life, minimum voided volume, and symptoms in patients with interstitial cystitis. Intravesical instillation and subcutaneous injection of heparin, which shares some properties with glycosaminoglycan, has shown good results in uncontrolled trials (Parsons et al, 1994). Intravesical dimethyl sulfoxide (DMSO) has also shown good results, perhaps because of its analgesic properties (Freedman et al, 1989). However, in studies on mice, no positive effect on the bladder was found. In fact, long-term use may prove deleterious (Freedman et al, 1989).

Behavioral therapy in the form of urge suppression techniques, timed toileting, and pelvic muscle exercise may improve symptoms (Chaiken et al, 1993). Surgical therapy such as resection or fulguration of ulcers, cystoplasty, and urinary diversion should be reserved for the most extreme cases.

Sensory Urgency

Sensory urgency is an uncontrolled, strong desire to void, and it may be associated with the fear of pain or incontinence. Urodynamic studies rule out the presence of detrusor instability and reveal low first sensation (<100 mL) and low capacity (<400 mL). Once again the cause is unclear, but the condition may represent undetected detrusor instability. Ambulation urodynamic studies or low-filling cystometrography may help detect instability.

Evaluation should include cystoscopy to rule out an intravesical abnormality (tumor, interstitial cystitis), especially in the elderly. Treatment consists of behavior modification with urge suppression techniques, timed toileting, and biofeedback. Anticholinergic medications such as oxybutinin chloride have also been successful in controlling symptoms.

Urinary Tract Infections

The female urinary tract is more prone to infection than its male counterpart. Shorter urethral length, proximity to the anus, vulvar and vaginal flora, and mechanical massage of the urethra during intercourse may promote the ascension of bacteria to the bladder. Nonetheless, the bladder has an intrinsic ability to prevent infection because of many factors: the dilution of effluent (diuresis), evacuation (micturition), bacteriostatic property of the urine (high urea concentration, low pH), Tamm-Horsfall mucoprotein secreted by the kidney to prevent bacterial adherence (Orskov et al, 1980), and lactobacilli in the vulva from the vagina to prevent colonization with rectal flora.

The incidence of urinary tract infections increases with age at a rate of approximately 1% for each decade of life from age 5 onward (Savage et al, 1967); urinary tract infections become more common with increasing parity. Prevalence rates are found to increase dramatically in the elderly and are reported to be more than 40% in women in their 90s (Blocklehurst et al, 1968). Recurrent urinary tract infections do not necessarily result in pyelonephritis because ascending infections depend on the presence of a vesico-ureteric reflux. In women with normal urinary tracts, this is uncommon.

Most infections are isolated episodes that either resolve spontaneously or are readily treated with antibiotics and that have no recurrence. Half of all women have had a urinary tract infection at least once. Some, however, have a predisposition to relapses despite sterilization of the urine by antibacterial treatment. Disease can recur within 7 to 14 days. When it does recur, it is usually in patients who have stones or who have scarred, damaged, or cystic kidneys. Occasionally disease recurs in patients with diverticula or ureteric stumps. Recurrent infections, however, are usually the result of reinfection. Treatment failure may result from inappropriate therapy, noncompliance, or poor absorption because of vomiting.

Pregnant women are no more likely to harbor asymptomatic bacteriuria than women who are not pregnant. Prevalence rates increase with age and parity, but they may be higher in lower socioeconomic groups. However, women with asymptomatic bacteriuria in early pregnancy have low spontaneous clearance rates and high incidences of acute symptomatic urinary tract infections later in pregnancy. In addition, although pregnant women may not be more susceptible to the acquisition of infection, they do have a greater predisposition to upper urinary tract infection, a more serious condition. Hence patients diagnosed with asymptomatic bacteriuria in early pregnancy should be treated promptly with antibiotics. Interestingly, Bangladeshi women were found to have a significantly lower bacteriuria prevalence rate than white women, 2% versus 6.3% (Versi et al, 1997). Differences in hygiene and clothing may explain this finding. Some Muslim women perform ablutions after defecation and micturition. In addition, Bangladeshi women traditionally dress in loose pants and no undergarments.

Cause

The most common organism causing symptomatic or asymptomatic bacteriuria is *Escherichia coli. Proteus mirabilis* and other coliform organisms are also common pathogens. It is now recognized that coagulase-negative staphylococci are a cause of infection in young women. Less commonly *Klebsiella* species and *Pseudomonas* organisms, along with *Streptococcus faecalis,* can be urinary pathogens, though such pathogens are usually nosocomial rather than primary domiciliary infective agents. Some organisms are difficult to

isolate, and special culture conditions are required for their identification. Examples of this are lactobacilli, corynebacteria, and *Streptococcus milleri.* Similarly, *Chlamydia trachomatis* may be a cause of "sterile" infection.

The best sign of a urinary tract infection is pyuria. It is possible for pyuria to be present even without bacteriuria, as it is in patients with stones or papillary necrosis. Conversely, many patients with bacteriologically proven infection do not have pyuria. Thus, the diagnosis of a urinary tract infection is based on the demonstration of bacteriuria by microbiologic methods. Significant bacteriuria is taken to mean the presence of 100,000 organisms of the same type per milliliter of freshly plated urine. Counts below 10,000/mL, especially if mixed organisms are present, generally indicate contaminated urine rather than an infection. Counts from 10^4 to 10^5 per milliliter are equivocal and require a repeat assessment. If diagnosis is difficult, it is best to obtain an early morning urine sample because stasis during the night results in a greater yield. Samples should be taken before antibiotic therapy is instituted because this will confound the results of culture. If repeated urine samples are contaminated, then recourse to suprapubic aspiration is justifiable (Kunin, 1979). This is rarely necessary if patients are carefully and thoroughly instructed on how to obtain a clean-catch, midstream urine sample. Urethral catheterization for the purpose of obtaining a urine sample for bacteriologic examination is also possible. Although a midstream specimen of urine examined and plated for culture is the standard test for diagnosing urinary tract infection, the dipstick and other chemical methods are usually adequate for screening purposes. Nevertheless, as with all screening techniques, the false-negative rate has to be acceptably low.

Diagnosis

If a patient has recurrent urinary tract infections, an anatomic cause should be sought. Intravenous urography will detect anatomic or functional abnormalities of the upper tracts that may be correctable. Function of the lower urinary tract can be simply assessed by uroflowmetry and postmicturition ultrasonography or catheterization to detect the presence of residual urine. If voiding difficulties are diagnosed (peak flow rate <15 mL/second, residual >100 mL), cystometry is indicated to determine whether the cause is outflow obstruction or poor detrusor contractility. Although it provides greater yield in the elderly, cystoscopy is useful in younger patients with recurrent urinary tract infections.

Treatment

Primary Infection. Before treatment, a midstream urine specimen should be sent for culture and sensitivity, but treatment can be started while waiting for the results. The patient should be encouraged to drink plenty of fluids (4 pints a day). The "best guess" antibiotics are co-trimoxazole (trimethoprim 160 mg + sulpha-methoxazole 800 mg twice a day), ampicillin (500 mg three times a day), and nitrofurantoin (100 mg three times a day). Co-trimoxazole and nitrofurantoin should not be prescribed to pregnant women.

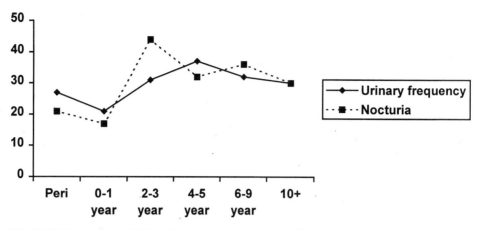

Fig. 22-17. Prevalence of urinary frequency and nocturia in climacteric women according to menopausal age. (From Versi E, Cardozo L, Studd J, et al: Urinary disorders and the menopause. *Menopause*, 1995; 2:93.)

Concomitant treatment with potassium citrate may alleviate symptoms. Antibiotic therapy should be administered for 5 to 7 days, though there is evidence that a 3-day course of therapy may be adequate and that even a single large dose (3 g) of amoxicillin results in a high cure rate in uncomplicated cases (Bailey and Abbott, 1977). Symptoms usually improve in 48 hours. If they do not, the pretreatment urine culture sensitivity should be rechecked.

Recurrent Infection. A patient with recurrent infection should be prescribed a longer antibiotic course of 10 to 15 days. If infection recurs after this, a special examination should be performed. Reinfection, on the other hand, is common and is best treated by explaining prophylaxis to the patient. Again, she should be encouraged to drink 4 pints of fluid every day and to void every 2 to 3 hours. If there is evidence of reflux, she should be encouraged to practice double or triple micturition. If postcoital infection is a problem, she should be encouraged to void immediately after sexual intercourse (Kunin, 1978). Prophylaxis with a single dose of antibiotic after coitus is often helpful. In some patients, long-term, low-dosagee antibiotic prophylaxis may be indicated. The drugs of choice are nitrofurantoin (50 to 100 mg) or trimethoprim (100 mg) at bedtime. Treatment can be continued for as long as 12 months. Drinking cranberry juice helps, as it contains proanthocyanidin, which inhibits adhesion of *E. coli* (Howell et al, 1998).

Although all patients with urinary catheters are prone to infection, those with urethral catheters are twice as likely to have infections as are those with suprapubic catheters. Patients with ileal conduits, neurogenic bladders, or multiple calculi are likely to have frequent infections. They should only undergo treatment when they have symptoms because frequent, multiple antibacterial therapy results in the emergence of polyresistant recalcitrant strains of bacteria that are difficult to treat. In postmenopausal women, evidence suggests that hormone replacement therapy reduces the incidence of urinary tract infections (Raz and Stamm, 1993; Cardozo and Versi, 1993) (see next section).

Menopause and the Lower Urinary Tract

Although symptoms of urinary tract disorders are common at the time of the menopause, it is unknown whether the cause is estrogen deficiency or the aging process. Urge incontinence increases after the age of 50 (Kondo et al, 1992) whereas stress incontinence peaks at approximately 50 years of age and declines thereafter (Jolleys, 1988), perhaps because of a subsequent decrease in overall activity.

Lower urinary tract dysfunction may be manifested as stress or urge incontinence, frequency, urgency, dysuria, recurrent urinary tract infections (more than two a year), or voiding difficulties. We have reported the prevalence of urodynamic diagnoses of urinary disorders in menopausal patients (Versi et al, 1995). Only 59% of the 285 women had normal urodynamics. Genuine stress incontinence was present in 22%, detrusor instability in 10%, voiding dysfunction in 7%, and sensory urgency in 4%. Fifty-three percent reported stress incontinence, 26% reported urge incontinence, and 25% reported post-micturition dribbling. Despite the high prevalence of urinary disorders, there did not appear to be an increased prevalence of symptoms or of urodynamic disease with advancing age. However, the irritative symptoms of frequency and nocturia did increase following menopause (Fig. 22-17).

The lower urinary tract is sensitive to estrogen. The urethral mucosa is lined by estrogen-sensitive epithelium, and hypoestrogenism has been shown to affect the sensory threshold of the urinary tract (Fantl et al, 1988), which increases nocturia. Furthermore, estrogen favors the growth of lactobacilli, which, as discussed in the preceding section, prevents colonization with intestinal flora and decreases the rate of urinary tract infection. With estrogen deprivation, recurrent urinary tract infections are more likely. The effect of progesterone is more debatable. Androgen receptors were found in the lower urinary tract, and their effect was to increase urethral pressure (as does estrogen) in castrated baboons (Bump and Friedman, 1986).

In controlled trials, the use of estrogen in patients with postmenopausal symptoms resulted in reduced stress incontinence when it was used in combination with an α-adrenergic drug. When it was used alone, no difference was detected between placebo- and estrogen-treated groups in most of those trials (Walter et al, 1978; Samsioe et al, 1985; Wilson et al, 1987; Fantl et al, 1988). The only exception was a small study of 12 patients (Walter et al, 1990). Estrogen replacement therapy has been shown to reduce urge incontinence (Walter et al, 1978; Samsioe et al, 1985), irritative symptoms (urgency, frequency) (Salmon et al, 1941; Hilton and Stanton, 1983), and recurrent urinary tract infection (Raz and Stamm, 1993).

DISORDERS OF PELVIC FLOOR SUPPORT
Pathophysiology

The levator ani is the key element for the support of pelvic organs. Its normal function is to close the genital hiatus and to provide a "trampoline" plate for the pelvic organs. Ligaments play a secondary role, providing back-up assistance in case of levator failure (Fig. 22-18).

Several mechanisms play a role in levator failure. Aging leads to neural atrophy with consequent denervation and atrophy of the muscle. Any strain on the pudendal nerve and sacral plexuses can similarly lead to neuropathy. The latter is seen after vaginal delivery and with chronic constipation (Kiff et al, 1984; Lubowski et al, 1988). Mechanical trauma, with tearing of the endopelvic fascial attachment to the arcus tendineus, may result from vaginal delivery, as may torn levator muscles. Collagen itself may be a player in the pathogenesis of prolapse. Intrinsic collagen abnormalities, such as Ehlers-Danlos syndrome, are associated with prolapse. New collagen formed after acute injury is not as strong as native collagen (Norton, 1993). Estrogen receptors are found in fibroblasts, and it is thought that estrogen deficiency may lead to poor collagen formation and remodeling, with ensuing weakness (Holland et al, 1994; Savvas et al, 1993).

Clinical Presentation

Patients with mild degrees of prolapse often are asymptomatic. More extensive prolapse may cause vaginal pressure, introital bulge, and dull pain in the lower back at the end of the day. These symptoms may worsen with prolonged standing, and they may improve on lying down. Prolapse may interfere with sexual intercourse. Advanced stages may culminate in ulcers, which are thought to be caused by friction. Another explanation may be that prolapse exerts traction on the venous plexuses, with decreased venous return causing a stasis ulcer (Coate, 1975). Dryness from exposure to air may predispose a patient to contact trauma; symptoms of this may be exudate or bleeding. Voiding function may be disrupted because the prolapsed bladder can form a kink in the urethra, leading to retention or obstruction. Digitation is a technique patients can use to reduce the prolapse and to

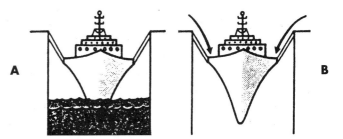

Fig. 22-18. "Boat in dry dock" conception of pelvic floor disorders. **A,** The boat is supported by water (the pelvic floor musculature) and kept in place by its moorings (the pelvic ligaments and fascia). **B,** If the water is removed, the moorings are suddenly placed under great strain. Similarly, pelvic floor tone may place excessive force on the pelvic ligaments and fascia. (From Norton PA: Pelvic floor disorders: The role of ligaments and fascia. *Clin Obstet Gynecol* 1993; 36:926.)

allow micturition (for a cystocele) or defecation (for a rectocele).

Physical Examination

When examining a patient for prolapse, an effort should be made to reproduce the patient's symptoms. The examination should be conducted with the maximal Valsalva maneuver, and the patient may have to change position from supine to semi-supine or even standing to uncover the prolapse.

Pelvic organ prolapse may be graded according to several systems, but two have been popular: the three-grade system and the halfway (0-4) system (Baden et al, 1968). According to the first, prolapse is considered mild (grade 1) if it does not reach the hymenal ring, moderate (grade 2) if it reaches the hymen, and marked (grade 3) if it goes beyond it. The halfway system assesses the position of the lowest part of a urethrocele, cystocele, uterine prolapse, enterocele, and rectocele in relation to a point halfway between the hymen and the apex during maximal strain. Grade 0 indicates no prolapse, grade 1 means it has descended halfway to the hymen, grade 2 means it has reached the hymen, grade 3 means it has descended halfway past the hymen, and grade 4 represents the maximum descent for each site. This last system identifies better than the three-grade system, but only by approximation, the prolapse of each compartment.

In 1994 the International Continence Society elaborated a standardized and quantified pelvic evaluation, the Pelvic Organ Prolapse Quantification (POP-Q) (Bump et al, 1996). The goal was to describe and stage organ prolapse, facilitate intrapatient comparison (treatment outcomes), and permit comparison of populations for research purposes. This system has been relatively easy to teach and is reproducible (Athanasiou et al, 1995; Schussler and Peschers, 1995). All measurements are in centimeters. Anterior, apical, and posterior compartments are evaluated, as is the perineum (Fig. 22-19). The three compartments are measured in reference to the hymen at maximal prolapse (during strain or standing). The anterior compartment is identified by two

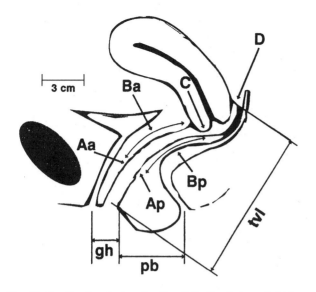

Fig. 22-19. Six sites (points Aa, Ba, C, D, Bp, Ap), genital hiatus (gh), perineal body (pb), and total vaginal length (tvl) used for pelvic organ support quantitation. (From Bump RC, Mattiasson A, Bø K, et al: The standardization of terminology of female pelvic organ prolapse and pelvic floor dysfunction. *Am J Obstet Gynecol* 1996; 175:10.)

landmarks: point Aa (point A of the anterior wall) is located 3 cm proximal to the urethral meatus, and point Ba (point B of the anterior wall) is the most dependent portion of the anterior wall between point Aa and the apex. The posterior compartment is referred to similarly: point Ap (point A of the posterior wall) is 3 cm from the hymen, and point Bp (point B of the posterior wall) is the most dependent edge between point A of the posterior wall and the apex. The apical compartment includes two points: point C identifies the most distal edge of the cervix or vaginal cuff and point D represents the position of the posterior fornix or cul-de-sac of Douglas. This last reference is omitted in patients without a cervix. The length of the vagina during vaginal examination (total vaginal length), the introitus (from the urethral meatus to the posterior hymen, the genital hiatus), and the perineal body (from the posterior hymen to the middle of the anus) are also recorded. The numbers can be listed as a simple line or as a 3 × 3 grid (Fig. 22-20). Each compartment can then be staged (Box 22-5).

The detection of paravaginal defects is unfortunately not included in the POP-Q as currently described. Such an evaluation is better performed with the patient in the supine position, using a Sims' speculum or the lower value of a bivalve speculum. The posterior wall is depressed, and the patient is asked to perform a Valsalva maneuver. If a prolapse is noted, an open Kelly clamp or a sponge forceps is used to support the lateral vaginal fornices and the patient is asked to strain again. The instrument should be oriented toward the sacrum. It should not force open the vagina but support its walls laterally. If the prolapse is reduced, the defect is thought to be caused by a paravaginal defect; if the prolapse persists, the patient has a transverse or a midline

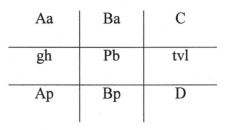

Aa	Ba	C
gh	Pb	tvl
Ap	Bp	D

Fig. 22-20. Three-by-three grid used to express the quantified pelvic organ prolapse (POP-Q) system. Aa, point A of the anterior wall; Ba, point B of the anterior wall; C, cervix or cuff; D, posterior fornix; gh, genital hiatus; pb, perineal body; tvl, total vaginal length; Ap, point A of the posterior wall; and Bp, point B of the posterior wall.

BOX 22-5
PELVIC ORGAN PROLAPSE STAGING

Stage 0:	No prolapse
	Aa, Ba, Ap, Bp are −3 cm and C or D ≤ −(tvl − 2) cm
Stage 1:	Most distal portion of the prolapse −1 cm (above the level of hymen)
Stage 2:	Most distal portion of the prolapse ≥ −1 cm but ≤ +1 cm (≤1 cm above or below the hymen)
Stage 3:	Most distal portion of the prolapse > +1 cm but < +(tvl − 2) cm (beyond the hymen; protrudes no farther than 2 cm less than the total vaginal length
Stage 4:	Complete eversion; most distal portion of the prolapse ≥ +(tvl − 2) cm

Aa, Point A of anterior wall; *Ba*, point B of anterior wall; *Ap*, point A of posterior wall; *Bp*, point B of posterior wall; −, above the hymen; +, beyond the hymen.

---

defect in the pubocervical fascia. A paravaginal defect can be unilateral or bilateral. The distinction between a bilateral or a unilateral defect can be made by closing the instrument, supporting one lateral fornix, and judging the efficacy of that support in reducing the prolapse. A paravaginal defect needs not extend the full length of the vagina. It can be localized and result in a site-specific defect. This can be confirmed at surgery.

Imaging Studies
Fluoroscopy

Physical examination cannot completely delineate defects in pelvic floor support. Fluoroscopic imaging permits better visualization of specific gross anatomic alterations. It involves opacification of the bladder (retrograde filling), vagina (application of thick vaginal paste), rectum (intrarectal application of barium paste), and small intestine (oral barium) with contrast medium. Perineal markers are placed on the perineal body, close to the anus. Imaging is taken while the patient is in three positions: at rest, during a Valsalva maneu-

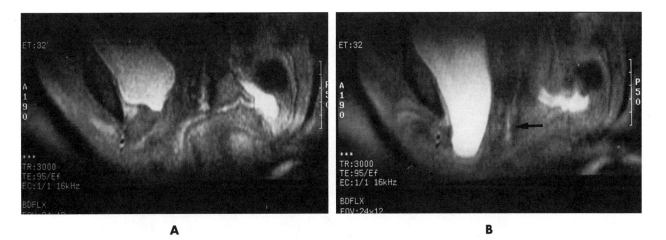

Fig. 22-21. Sagittal T2-weighted (3000/95) image of the pelvic floor in the sitting position at rest (**A**) and with the Valsalva maneuver (**B**). In this patient with known pelvic floor prolapse, there is marked descent of the bladder base, vagina, cervix, and uterus with straining, indicating loss of integrity of the perineal body. The high-signal vaginal canal is marked with an arrow. (From Fielding JR, Versi E, Mulkern RV, et al: MR imaging of the female pelvic floor in the supine and upright position. *J Magn Reson Imaging* 1996; 6:961-963.)

ver and a pelvic contraction (similar to a Kegel exercise), and during micturition and defecation on a special commode. If the patient can evacuate in the erect position, it is especially useful.

Parameters evaluated include urethral mobility and bladder neck opening, cystocele, apical descents (enterocele, vault, and uterine descent), rectocele, and sigmoidocele. In addition, the puborectalis muscle function can be assessed by contraction (Kegel) and relaxation with defecation as a contracted levator imprints posteriorly on the rectum. This study can detect pelvic floor defects that may be missed on examination alone (Altringer et al, 1995). However, the clinical relevance of a defect not otherwise diagnosed is questionable because the relationship between these findings and symptoms has not been well defined.

Magnetic Resonance Imaging

Magnetic resonance imaging (MRI) has been applied to delineate pelvic support anomalies, urethral support system and anatomy, and disorders of the anal sphincter. The landmark used to quantify prolapse in MRI studies is the pubococcygeal line (Yang et al, 1991), and the leading edge of each compartment is measured as the distance in centimeters below it. The bladder and the cervix or vault should not descend more than 1 cm below that line, and the rectum should not descend more than 2.5 cm below it.

Most studies have involved the widely available supine 1.5T MRI. However, because it is preferred that patients be in the erect position for imaging, we have shown that the pelvic floor and the periurethral anatomy can still be assessed using a .5T interventional MRI with the patient in the sitting position (Fielding et al, 1996). MRI is less invasive than fluoroscopy, it does not involve radiation or contrast medium, and it permits visualization of the uterus. However,

it is important to state that pelvic floor MRI is not for routine clinical use but for research in evaluating the pathophysiology of prolapse and incontinence (Fig. 22-21).

Ultrasonography

Ultrasonography was first used as a replacement for catheterization to determine post-void residual urine levels, thus limiting iatrogenic infections. Because it does not involve radiation and the cost is reasonable, its usefulness in urinary and fecal incontinence has been investigated. Its use in genuine stress incontinence was discussed earlier in this chapter (see section on urinary incontinence, imaging studies). Some investigators have used this modality for the evaluation of pelvic floor prolapse, but this is still experimental.

Perineal ultrasonography detects pelvic floor prolapse of all compartments (Creighton et al, 1992) and may be of help in following up patients longitudinally after treatment. In addition, contrast ultrasonography may help in detecting paravaginal defects (Ostrzenski et al, 1997). Neither technique, however, has been compared with clinical pelvic examination, and it is unknown whether they offer more than the POP-Q system and the clinical evaluation of paravaginal defects. As investigational tools, they may permit pathophysiological understanding of prolapse and incontinence.

Management
Behavioral

Behavioral therapy for prolapse consists of pelvic floor exercises to strengthen the levator ani. It includes Kegel exercises, vaginal cones, biofeedback, and electrical stimulation. The mechanism of action is thought to be through hypertrophy of the muscular fibers. However, there is no evidence in the literature that such exercises improve any type of prolapse. Nonetheless, theoretically they prevent additional

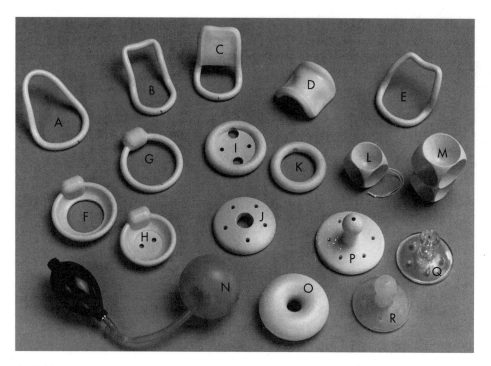

Fig. 22-22. Variety of pessaries. **A** to **C,** Smith-Hodge (with and without support). **D,** Gehrung. **E,** Risser. **F** to **H,** Incontinence Ring (with and without support). **I** and **K,** Ring (with and without support). **J,** Incontinence Dish. **L** and **M,** Cube. **N,** Inflato-ball. **O,** Donut. **P** to **R,** Gellhorn. (From Marlex, Chicago, Ill.)

deterioration of pelvic floor support, just as a stronger levator ani provides better support and decreases the load on ligaments. A stretched or ruptured ligament will not correct itself no matter how much the muscles are exercised.

Mechanical

The mainstay of conservative therapy for prolapse remains the use of mechanical devices such as the pessary. Indications for its use in patients with pelvic organ prolapse include the frail patient for whom surgery and anesthesia may pose a significant risk, the patient reluctant to undergo surgery, the patient who is pregnant, and the patient who desires to be pregnant in the future (surgical repair can be jeopardized by vaginal childbirth). It should not be used in a patient who has poor cognitive functions unless a caretaker can ensure proper follow-up. Hypoestrogenic vaginal mucosa is more prone to erosion; therefore, estrogen cream should be administered before pessary use in any patient with this condition.

Care. A pessary should be removed and cleaned daily (with regular soap and thorough rinsing in water). Most patients are able to remove and replace the pessary themselves, but this is difficult for some. If a caretaker or the physician provides the care, it has been thought that 6 to 8 weeks is the maximum amount of time needed, but it has been our experience that the interval can be extended to 6 months if the vagina is well estrogenized.

Types. Pessaries have been used for a long time, and various forms have been described (Fig. 22-22). Seven types

are the most common, and the first two probably meet the needs of 75% of the patients. The *ring*, with or without diaphragm, is easy to fit. It resembles the contraceptive diaphragm. It offers good support for anterior or apical prolapse. Correctly placed, it lodges behind the symphysis pubis anteriorly and in the posterior fornix (or vault) posteriorly and allows passage of a finger between the pessary and the pubis. The *doughnut* pessary is similar to a ring pessary, but it is much fatter. It enables support for a more advanced stage of prolapse. The *Gellhorn* pessary is used in patients with moderate to severe utero-vaginal prolapse, but it requires good perineal support (perineal body) because it rests on it. The *Gehrung* pessary can also be used to support the anterior wall. When the perineal body is disrupted, the *cube* pessary can be used. The six surfaces of the cube are concave and permit the trapping of vaginal secretions. This results in a very strong odor, and long-term use is limited. The *inflatable* pessary acts similarly to the cube, without the odor. Its application is easy because it is inserted when it is deflated and then it is inflated. It also entails less risk for mucosal erosion. Finally, the *Smith-Hodge* pessary is designed to provide support mainly to the uterus. It is available with a diaphragm over the lower part to offer anterior wall support if that is needed.

Surgical

Surgery is considered the definitive treatment for pelvic organ prolapse. Approaches can be abdominal or vaginal. Morbidity rates are greater with the abdominal route than with the vaginal route, and the recovery is slower. However, long-term success and sexual function seem to be better after the abdominal approach. Laparoscopy is promising, but long-term results compared to with those of traditional open surgery are unknown.

Abdominal Surgery for Cystocele. *Paravaginal repair* is the preferred technique for cystocele due to paravaginal defects. The technique resembles that of a Burch colposuspension, whereby the space of Retzius is dissected until the pelvic floor is reached, demonstrated by visualization of the arcus tendineus fascia pelvis, and the bladder is gently retracted medially. This gentle blunt dissection must be performed carefully because the obturator vessels are located on the lateral wall overlying the fusion of the obturator internus. Once the arcus is reached, the vagina is examined to determine whether it is separated from the arcus or whether the arcus itself is separated from its attachment to the obturator fascia. Placement of interrupted permanent sutures from the endopelvic fascia overlying the lateral vaginal fornix to the arcus tendineus fascia pelvis or the obturator fascia reestablishes the pubocervical fascial attachment to the sidewall. Sutures should start approximately 1 cm from the ischial spines (to avoid the pudendal vessels) and go to the pubic rami if there is a full-length defect. This is done on both sides in patients with bilateral paravaginal defect.

Anterior repair done abdominally has also been described. Once the uterus is removed, the bladder is reflected off the underlying vagina and a triangular wedge of vaginal mucosa is removed, similar to what occurs in vaginal anterior repair. However, this technique does not reduce a midline defect as well as the vaginal approach does because it only reduces the proximal cystocele. There are also concerns that the innervation of the bladder may be more profoundly compromised by this technique.

Abdominal Surgery for Uterine Prolapse. Uterine prolapse can be corrected with or without concurrent hysterectomy using the native support (uterosacral and cardinal ligaments), called *colpexy;* or mesh, called *sacrocolpopexy.* In the former, the vagina or the uterine isthmus (in case of uterine conservation) is attached to the uterosacral ligament. The uterosacral ligaments are identified by traction on the uterus as a cordlike fanning out structure going from the uterus toward the sacrum. A suture is placed proximally and anchored on the vagina or the uterine isthmus. This effectively shortens the uterosacral ligaments, bringing the uterus or vault backward, toward the levator plate, leaving the vaginal axis in a fairly normal orientation.

The technique for vault support is *sacrocolpopexy.* This is easier to perform in the absence of the uterus; nevertheless, it can be performed even if the uterus remains in situ. In brief, the technique involves retroperitoneal suspension of the vaginal apex to the anterior spinal ligament of the sacrum, just below the sacral promontory, by native fascia lata, cadaveric fascia, or synthetic mesh. It is important that the suspensory material be under no tension but that it remains loose, following the hollow of the sacrum, and it is also important that the peritoneum be closed over the bridge, especially when mesh is used, because intestinal loops tend to adhere, and obstruction can result. Complications include bleeding from the sacral perforating vessels, mesh erosion into the vagina, and bowel obstruction.

Abdominal Surgery for Enterocele. *Culdoplasty* is the surgery that corrects for enterocele. Several techniques are described, but two are prevalent. The first one is the Moschcowitz culdoplasty and the second is the Halban culdoplasty. The modified Moschcowitz procedure consists of placing a purse-string suture in the Douglas pouch including the utero-sacral ligaments laterally, posterior vagina and shallow bites of rectal serosa. The Halban technique involves placement of 3-4 parallel sutures starting on the posterior vaginal, picking up Douglas pouch peritoneum and bites of rectal serosa. Either type of culdoplasty is thought to be efficient in obstructing the cul-de-sac and correcting an enterocele but incorporation of the uterosacrals in the former probably results in a sturdier repair. These operations can also be used in the prevention of enterocele, such as at the time of a retro-pubic colposuspension for incontinence.

Vaginal Surgery for Cystocele. Two approaches exist for the correction of cystocele by a vaginal route. The most popular is the *anterior colporrhaphy*, also referred to as the anterior repair. This surgery is most appropriate in cases of midline defect of the endopelvic fascia. The technique involves separating the vaginal mucosa from the bladder, leaving the endo-pelvic fascia on the bladder side. The endopelvic fascia is then plicated, thus reducing the cystocele. Excess of vaginal mucosa is then trimmed and the edges are closed with absorbable suture. A *vaginal para-vaginal repair* is also done in certain centers. The surgery consists of entering the para-vaginal spaces via a standard anterior colporrhaphy incision on the vaginal mucosa. The arcus tendineus is then identified by palpation and sutures, up to 5, are placed into that structure and passed through the pubocervical fascia laterally, and at the level of the superior lateral sulcus of the vagina medially. The sutures are tied to reapproximate the vaginal sulci with the arcus. If any degree of central defect becomes apparent, standard anterior repair is performed. If a patient has just undergone hysterectomy, a transverse defect is present in the pubocervical fascia, and the defect is repaired transversally.

Vaginal Surgery for Uterine Prolapse. *Vaginal hysterectomy* is the preferred surgical cure for uterine prolapse. It is important to isolate the uterosacral ligaments at the beginning of surgery to allow suspension of the vault and to prevent vault prolapse after the hysterectomy. A *Manchester* operation (*Fothergill*) involving cervical amputation can be performed if patients desire uterine conservation. The vaginal mucosa is incised around the cervix, then dissected, and then the bladder is reflected upward. The utero-sacral ligaments are cut as laterally as possible without ureteric injury, and the cut ends sutured anteriorly onto the cervical stump. The vaginal mucosa is sutured over the raw surface of the cervix with a Sturmdorf suture to keep the internal os patent.

Finally, a *LeFort colpocleisis* can reduce advanced uterine prolapse with minimal morbidity. Anterior and posterior rectangular flaps of vaginal mucosa are removed, and the denuded areas are reapproximated with horizontal layers of interrupted absorbable sutures, leaving two small tunnels laterally for drainage.

Vaginal Surgery for Enterocele. Dissection of the enterocele sac from the rectum and adjacent structures (such as the bladder if it is a posthysterectomy enterocele) is the key to repair. The posterior vaginal mucosa is incised longitudinally and reflected laterally to identify the rectocele (if present) and the enterocele. The latter is then opened and carefully dissected from the adjacent structures. A purse string suture is used to close the neck of the sac, and this incorporates the uterosacral ligaments for support. The purse string suture is repeated for added strength, and the redundant sac is excised. After this, any excessive hiatus between the uterosacral ligaments is closed by a *McCall culdoplasty,* which includes bites on the posterior vaginal wall, ipsilateral utero-sacral ligament, peritoneum, contralateral utero-sacral ligament, and contralateral posterior vaginal wall.

Vaginal Surgery for Rectocele. The *posterior colporrhaphy*, or posterior repair, is what gynecologists usually use to repair a rectocele. The posterior vaginal mucosa is dissected longitudinally off the endopelvic fascia overlying the rectum. Placing a finger in the rectum will help identify the defect in this endopelvic Denonvilliers' fascia. The defect is then reapproximated with absorbable sutures, excess vaginal mucosa is excised, and the edges are reapproximated.

ANAL INCONTINENCE
Anatomy

Continence is assured primarily by the integrity of the internal and the external anal sphincters. However, the levator ani (musculus puborectalis) makes an important contribution by creating a sharp anorectal angle, effectively containing stool above the anal canal.

The anal canal is a complex structure consisting of a sensitive mucosa and two anatomic sphincters: the internal smooth muscle and the external striated muscle. Contraction of the internal sphincter is under sympathetic control, which maintains a high basal tone and is responsible for fecal continence. Parasympathetic stimulation permits defecation. The external sphincter is under voluntary control and provides a backup continence mechanism. Sacral segments S1 to S3 supply the innervation of the internal sphincter, whereas the external sphincter's innervation is derived from the pudendal nerve.

The internal sphincter extends from the distal anal canal to the rectum, in continuity with the rectal muscle. The external sphincter has two components, the subcutaneous (the distal ring) and the deep parts that lie beneath and in proximity to the musculus puborectalis (Peschers et al, 1997).

Causes

Anal incontinence may be attributable to diverse causes: functional (diarrhea, overflow resulting from impaction), neurologic (myelomeningocele, dementia, stroke, spinal injuries), trauma to distal muscles (obstetric injuries, anorectal surgery, accidental trauma), aging, chronic or prolonged straining (chronic cough, chronic constipation, vaginal delivery) (Madoof et al, 1992). Chronic or prolonged straining leads to stretch damage of the pudendal nerve and the sacral plexuses.

Diagnosis

Physical examination is important because it can detect a fissure or a disruption of the anal sphincter. It should include a digital rectal examination to rule out neoplasm and impaction. Muscle strength should also be assessed. The musculus puborectalis should contract voluntarily and push the examining finger anteriorly; in this way, anal tone can be evaluated at rest and during contraction.

Until recently, anal function tests were the mainstay for the evaluation of fecal incontinence. They included anal manometry, which measures resting and squeeze pressure, balloon distension, electrical stimulation of the mucosa to assess sensory threshold, and electromyography to identify denervation of the anal sphincter.

Anal endosonography has brought a new perspective on anal disruption as a cause of incontinence. Ultrasonography differentiates between the echogenicity of the mucosa, and the internal and external sphincters and permits the detection of continuity breaks (Law et al, 1991) (Fig. 22-23). In a study that yielded surprising results, Sultan et al (1993) demonstrated that 35% of primipara who delivered vaginally and had apparently intact perineum sustained occult tearing of one or both sphincters. Repair of third- or fourth-degree tears by standard methods resulted in residual defects in 85% of them, as determined by ultrasonography (Sultan et al, 1994a). Disruption of the anal sphincters was corroborated by findings at surgery (Romano et al, 1996; Sultan et al, 1994b) and through electrophysiology (Tjandra et al, 1993). Other imaging studies suggested that structural anatomy is well defined by endoanal MRI (Hussain et al, 1995; Stoker, 1997), yet MRI remains a research tool.

Prevention

Modification of obstetric management may decrease the risk for sphincter tear. Midline episiotomy is strongly associated with sphincteric extension in contrast to mediolateral episiotomy (Woolley, 1995). The same applies to forceps use (Sultan et al, 1994) in contrast to vacuum extraction.

Proper repair along the entire length of the anal canal, including the internal sphincter, may reduce the risk for incontinence. The technique taught to generations of obstetricians, as explained in *Williams Obstetrics* (Cunningham et al, 1993), does not take into account the repair of the inter-

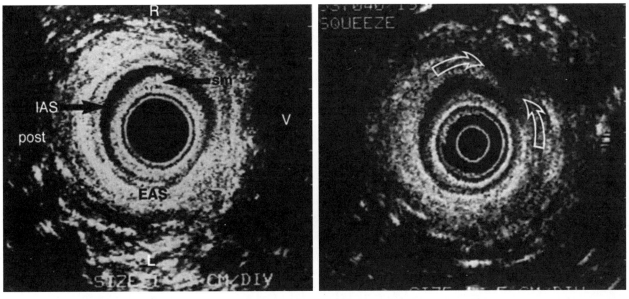

A   **B**

Fig. 22-23. Result of anal endosonography before and after delivery in a primiparous woman with a postpartum defect of the external anal sphincter. **A,** Normal range of the middle portion of the anal canal at 34 weeks of pregnancy. R, right; L, left; IAS, internal anal sphincter; EAS, external anal sphincter; Post, posterior; sm, submucosal (hyperechoic); V, vagina. The probe lies medial to the submucosa. **B,** Anal canal 6 weeks after delivery. Patient had no incontinence of flatus after forceps delivery with an episiotomy. A hyperechoic defect of the external anal sphincter is present between the open arrows. The damage to the anal sphincter was not recognized during repair of the episiotomy (From Sultan AH, Kamm MA, Hudson CN, et al: Anal sphincter disruption during vaginal delivery. *N Engl J Med* 1993; 329:1905. © 1993 Massachusetts Medical Society. Used with permission.)

nal sphincter, and it only reapproximates the subcuticular portion of the external sphincter. This teaching diverges greatly from that in the colorectal literature.

Management

Dietary manipulation can help. The prevention of constipation prevents further impaction. High-fiber diets increase stool consistency and make it easier for the sphincters to maintain continence.

Biofeedback has two roles. It strengthens the levator ani and the external sphincter muscle and it improves the sensation to rectal filling, allowing patients to avert incontinence by regular bowel emptying.

Surgery is the best option for disrupted anal sphincter, especially if pudendal nerve terminal motor latencies are adequate (<2 msec) (Sangwan et al, 1996). The most effective repair technique does not involve debridement of the fibrous tissue and end-to-end anastomosis, but it does involve an overlapping technique using the fibrotic edges for anchorage. If the sphincter is denervated, a neosphincter can be reconstructed using a gracilis muscle flap. Colostomy is a last recourse if other therapeutic modalities have failed.

REFERENCES

Abrams P, Blaivas JG, Stanton SL, et al: The standardization of terminology of lower urinary tract function. *Br J Obstet Gynaecol* 1990; 97(suppl 6):1-16.

Ahlstrom, K, Sandahl B, Sjoberg B, et al: Effect of combined treatment with phenylpropanolamine and estriol compared with estriol treatment alone, in postmenopausal women with stress urinary incontinence. *Gynecol Obstet Invest* 1990; 30:37-43.

Alcalay M, Monga A, Stanton SL: Burch colposuspension: A 10-20 year follow up. *Br J Obstet Gynaecol* 1995; 102:740-745.

Allen RE, Hosker GL, Smith ARB, et al: Pelvic floor damage and childbirth: A neurophysiological study. *Br J Obstet Gynaecol* 1990; 97:770-779.

Altringer W, Saclarides T, Dominguez J, et al: Four contrast defecography: pelvic "flooroscopy." *Dis Colon Rectum* 1995; 38:695-699.

Andersen MJF: The incidence of diverticula in the female urethra. *J Urol* 1967; 98:96-98.

Anderson J, Grant J: Post operative retention of urine: A prospective urodynamic study. *BMJ* 1991; 302:894-896.

Andersson KE, Hendriksson L, Ulmsten U: Effects of prostaglandin E_2 applied locally on intravesical and intraurethral pressures in women. *Eur Urol* 1978; 4:366-369.

Asmussen M, Ulmsten U: Simultaneous urethro-cystometry and urethral pressure profile measurement with a new technique. *Acta Obstet Gynaecol Scand* 1975: 54:385-388.

Athanasiou S, Hill S, Gleeson C, et al: Validation of the ICS proposed pelvic organ prolapse descriptive system. *Neurourol Urodynam* 1995; 14:414-415.

Baden WP, Walker TA, Lindsey JH: The vaginal profile. *Tex Med* 1968;64:56-58.

Bailey RR, Abbott GD: Treatment of a urinary tract infection with a single dose of amoxicillin. *Nephrologie* 1977; 18:316-318.

Benness C, Hill S: Frequency, urgency and painful bladder syndromes: In Cardozo L, editor: *Urogynecology*, New York, 1997, Churchill Livingstone.

Bergman A, Koonings PP, Ballard CA: Negative Q-tip test as a risk factor for failed anti-incontinence surgery. *J Reprod Med* 1989; 34:157-160.

Bergman A, McCarthy TA, Ballard CA, et al: Role of the Q-tip test in evaluating stress urinary incontinence. *J Reprod Med* 1987; 32:273-275.

Bonney V: On diurnal incontinence of urine in women. *J Obstet Gynaecol Br Emp* 1923; 30:358-365.

Boos KPW, Hextall A, Toozs-Hobson P, et al: The dynamic of urinary incontinence. *Int Urogynecol J* 1997; 8(suppl):S61.

Bornstad E: Long-term results after Burch colposuspension: An 11-14 years follow up. *Int Urogynecol J* 1997; 8(suppl): S28.

Bradley WE, Rockswold GL, Timm GW, et al: Neurology of micturition. *J Urol* 1976; 115:481-486.

Brindley GS: Control of the bladder and urethral sphincters by surgically implanted electrical stimulation. In Chisholm GD, Fair WB, editors: Scientific foundations of urology, Chicago, 1990, Year Book Medical.

Brocklehurst JC: Urinary incontinence in the community–an analysis of a MORI poll. *BMJ* 1993; 306:832-834.

Brocklehurst JC, Dillane JB, Griffiths L, et al: The prevalence and symptomatology of urinary infection it an aged population. *Gerontol Clin (Basel)* 1968; 10:242-253.

Brooks D, Mauder A: Pathogenesis of the urethral syndrome in women and its diagnosis in general practice. *Lancet* 1977; 2:893.

Brubaker L, Benson JT, Bent A, et al: Transvaginal electrical stimulation for female urinary incontinence. *Am J Obstet Gynecol* 1997; 177:536-540.

Brubaker LT, Sadarides TJ, eds: *The female pelvic floor: Disorders of function and support.* Philadelphia: 1996, FA Davis.

Bump RC, Friedman CI: Intraluminal urethral pressure measurements in the female baboon: Effect of hormonal manipulation. *J Urol* 1986; 136:508-511.

Bump RC, Mattiasson A, Bø K, et al: The standardization of terminology of female pelvic organ prolapse and pelvic floor dysfunction. *Am J Obstet Gynecol* 1996; 175:10-17.

Cardozo LD, Abrams PH, Stanton SL, et al: Idiopathic bladder instability treated by biofeedback. *Br J Urol* 1978; 50:521-523.

Cardozo LD, Stanton SL, Williams JE: Detrusor instability following surgery for genuine stress incontinence. *Br J Urol* 1979: 51:204-207.

Cardozo L, Versi E: Estrogens and the lower urinary tract. In Asch RH, Studd JWW, editors: *Annual progress in reproductive medicine*, Carnforth, U.K., 1993, Parthenon Publishing Group.

Chaiken DC, Blaivas JG, Blaivas ST: Behavioral therapy for the treatment of refractory interstitial cystitis. *J Urol* 1993; 149:1445-1448.

Coate J: *Principle of gynaecology*, ed. 4, London, 1975, Butterworth.

Coddington CC, Knob DR: Urethral diverticulum: A review. *Obstet Gynecol Surv* 1983; 38:357-364.

Colombo M, Milani R, Vitobello D, et al: A randomized comparison of Burch colposuspension and abdominal paravaginal defect repair for female stress urinary incontinence. *Am J Obstet Gynecol* 1996; 175:78-84.

Creighton SM, Pearce JM, Stanton SL: Perineal video-ultrasonography in the assessment of vaginal prolapse: early observations. *Br J Obstet Gynaecol* 1992; 99:310-313.

Crelin ES: Normal and abnormal development of ureter. *Urology* 1978; 112:2-7.

Cunningham FG, MacDonald PC, Gant NF, et al, editors: *Williams Obstetrics*, ed 19, Stamford, Conn., 1993, Appleton & Lange.

Dans PE, Klaus B: Dysuria in women. *Johns Hopkins Med J* 1976; 138:13-18.

Diernaes E, Rix P, Sorensen T, et al: Norfenefrine in the treatment of female urinary stress incontinence assessed by one-hour pad weighing test. *Urol Int* 1989; 44: 28-31.

DeLancey JOL: Anatomic aspects of vaginal eversion after hysterectomy. *Am J Obstet Gynecol* 1992; 166:1717-1728.

DeLancey JOL: Anatomy and embryology of the lower urinary tract. *Obstet Gynecol Clin North Am* 1989; 16: 717-731.

DeLancey JOL: Anatomy of the female bladder and urethra. In Ostergard DR, Bent AE, editors: *Urogynecology and urodynamics: Theory and practice*, ed. 4, Baltimore, 1996, Williams & Wilkins.

DeLancey JOL: Anatomy and physiology of urinary continence. *Clin Obstet Gynecol* 1990; 33:298-307.

DeLancey JOL: Structural support of the urethra as it relates to stress urinary incontinence: The hammock hypothesis. *Am J Obstet Gynecol* 1994; 170:1713-1720.

DeMartino C, Zamboni L: A morphologic study of the mesonephros of the human embryo. *J Ultrastruct Res* 1966; 16:399-427.

Denis P, Bercoff E, Bizien MF, et al: Étude de la prévalence de l'incontinence fécale chez l'adulte. *Gastroenterol Clin Biol* 1992; 16: 334-350.

Dixon JS, Gosling JA: The role of the pelvic floor in female urinary incontinence. *Int Urogynecol J* 1990; 1:212-217.

Drutz HP: Neurophysiology and neuropharmacology of the lower urinary tract. *Int Urogynecol J* 1990; 1:91-99.

Ek A, Alm P, Andersson KE, et al: Adrenergic and cholinergic nerves of the human urethra and urinary bladder: a histochemical study. *Acta Physiol Scand* 1977; 99:345-352.

Elkins TE, DeLancey JOL, McGuire EJ: The use of modified Martius graft as an adjunctive technique in vesicovaginal and rectovaginal fistula repair. *Obstet Gynecol* 1990; 75:727-733.

Enhorning G: Simultaneous recording of the intravesical and intraurethral pressures. *Acta Obstet Gynecol Scand* 1961; 276 (suppl): 1-68.

Fall M: Does electrostimulation cure urinary incontinence? *J Urol* 1984; 131:664-667.

Fantl JA, Newman DK, Colling J, et al: Urinary incontinence in adults: Acute and chronic management, Clinical practice guidelines, No 2, 1996 update, US Public Health Service, AHCPR Pub No 96-0682, Rockville, Md., 1996.

Fantl JA, Wyman JF, Anderson RL, et al: Postmenopausal urinary incontinence: Comparison between non-estrogen-supplemented and estrogen-supplemented women. *Obstet Gynecol* 1988; 71:823-828.

Farquharson DM, Shingleton HM, Orr JW, et al: The short-term effect of radical hysterectomy on urethral and bladder function. *Br J Obstet Gynaecol* 1987; 94:351-357.

Fielding JR, Versi E, Mulkern RV, et al: MR imaging of the female pelvic floor in the supine and upright position. *J Magn Reson Imaging* 1996; 6:961-963.

Freeman RM, Baxby K: Hypnotherapy for incontinence caused by the unstable detrusor. *BMJ* 1982; 1:1831.

Frewen WK: An objective assessment of the unstable bladder of psychosomatic origin. *Br J Urol* 1978; 50:246.

Frewen WK : A reassessment of bladder training in detrusor dysfunction in the female. *Br J Urol* 1982; 54:372.

Friedman AI, Wein AJ, Whitmore K, et al: In vitro effects of intravesical dimethylsulfoxide. *Neurourol Urodynamic* 1989; 8:277.

Gillenwater JY, Wein AJ: Summary of the National Institute of Arthritis, Diabetes, Digestive and Kidney Diseases Workshop on Interstitial Cystitis, National Institutes of Health, Bethesda, Md., August 28-29, 1987. *J Urol* 1988; 140:203-206.

Ginsburg DS, Genadry R: Suburethral diverticulum in the female. *Obstet Gynecol Surv* 1984; 39:1-7.

Gosling JA, Dixon JS, Critchler HO, et al: A comparative study of the human external sphincter and periurethral levator ani muscles. *Br J Urol* 1981; 53:35-41.

Gosling JA, Dixon JS, London RG: The autonomic innervation of the human male and female bladder neck and proximal urethra. *J Urol* 1977; 118:302-305.

Griffiths DJ, Versi E: Needle urethropexies. *Operative Tech Gynecol Surg* 1997; 2:35-43.

Grobstein C: Inductive interaction in the development of the mouse metanephros. *J Exp Zool* 1955; 130:319-335.

Harris T, Glearson D, Diokno A, et al: External urethral barrier for urinary stress incontinence: A multi-centered trial. *Neurourol Urodyn* 1994; 13:381-382.

Herbaut AG: Neurogenic urinary retention. *Int Urogynecol J* 1993; 4:221-228.

Herschorn S, Steele DJ, Radomski SB: Follow up of intraurethral collagen for female stress urinary incontinence. *J Urol* 1996; 156:1305-1309.

Herschorn S, Steele D, Radomski S: Intraurethral collagen for female stress incontinence. *Neurourol Urodyn* 1993; 12:437-439.

Hilton P, Mayne CJ: The Stamey endoscopic bladder neck suspension: A clinical and urodynamic investigation, including actuarial follow up over four years. *Br J Obstet Gynaecol* 1991; 98:1141-1149.

Hilton P, Stanton SL: The use of intravaginal oestrogen on urethral function in women with stress incontinence. *Br J Obstet Gynaecol* 1983; 90:940-944.

Hofmeister EJ: Pelvic anatomy of the ureter in relation to surgery performed through the vagina. *Clin Obstet Gynecol* 1982; 25:821-830.

Holland EF, Studd JW, Mansell JP, et al: Changes in collagen composition and cross-links in bone and skin of osteoporotic postmenopausal women treated with percutaneous estradiol implants. *Obstet Gynecol* 1994; 83:180-183.

Howell AB, Voisa N, DerMarderosian A, Foo LY: Inhibition of the adherence of P-limbriated *Escherichia coli* to uroepithelial cell surfaces by proanthrocyanidin extracts from cranberries (letter). *N Engl J Med* 1998; 339:1085-1086.

Huffman JW: The detailed anatomy of the paraurethral ducts in the adult human female. *Am J Obstet Gynecol* 1948; 55:86-100.

Hurt WG: Histology of the urinary bladder and urethra in the female. *AUGS Quart Rep* 1988; 6.

Hurt WG: Urogynecology surgery: The master's techniques. In Sanz LE, editor: *Principles and techniques in gynecologic surgery,* New York, 1992, Raven Press.

Hussain SM, Stocker J, Laméris JS: Anal sphincter complex: Endoanal MR imaging of normal anatomy. *Radiology* 1995; 197:671-677.

Hwang P, Auclair B, Beechinor D, et al: Efficacy of pentosan polysulfate in the treatment of interstitial cystitis: A meta-analysis. *Urology* 1997; 50:39-43.

Jarvis GJ, Hall S, Stamp S, et al: An assessment of urodynamic examination in incontinent women. *Br J Obstet Gynaecol* 1980; 87:893-896.

Jolleys JV: Reported prevalence of urinary incontinence in women in general practice. *BMJ* 1988; 296: 1300-1302.

Karram MM: Urodynamics: Cystometry. In Walters MD, Karram MM, eds.: *Clinical Urogynecology.* St. Louis: Mosby, 1993.

Karram MM, Bhatia NN: Management of coexistent stress and urge urinary incontinence. *Obstet Gynecol* 1989; 73:4-7.

Karram MM, Bhatia NN: The Q-Tip test: Standardization of the technique and its interpretation in women with urinary incontinence. *Obstet Gynecol* 1988; 71:807-811.

Kass EJ, Koff SA, Diokno AC, et al: The significance of bacilluria in children on long-term intermittent catheterization. *J Urol* 1981; 126:223.

Keefe B, Warshauer DM, Tucker MS, et al: Diverticula of the female urethra: Diagnosis by endovaginal and transperineal sonography. *AJR Am J Roentgenol* 1991; 156:1195-1197.

Kegel AH: Progressive resistance exercise in the functional restoration of the perineal muscles. *Am J Obstet Gynecol* 1948; 56:238-248.

Kelleher CJ, Khullar V, Cardozo ED: Psychoneuroticism and quality of life impairment in healthy incontinent women. *Neurourol Urodyn* 1993; 12:393-394.

Khullar V, Cardozo LD, Abbott D, et al: Gax collagen in the treatment of urinary incontinence in elderly women: A two year follow up. *Br J Obstet Gyneacol* 1997; 104:96-99.

Kiff ES, Barnes PRH, Swash M: Evidence of pudendal neuropathy in patients with perineal descent and chronic straining at stool. *Gut* 1984; 25:1279-1282.

Kohorn EI, Glickman MG: Technical aids in investigation and management of urethral diverticula in the female. *Urology* 1992; 40:322-325.

Kondo A, Saito M, Yamada Y, et al: Prevalence of handwashing urinary incontinence in healthy subjects in relations to stress and urge incontinence. *Neurourol Urodyn* 1992; 11:519-523.

Kondo A, Yokoyama E, Koshiba K, et al: Bladder neck support prosthesis: A non-operative treatment for stress or mixed urinary incontinence. *J Urol* 1997; 157:824-827.

Kunin CM: *Detection, prevention and management of urinary tract infections,* ed 3, Philadelphia, 1979, Lea and Febiger.

Kunin CM: Sexual intercourse and urinary infection. *N Engl J Med* 1978; 278:336-338.

Lapides J, Diokno AC, Silber SJ, et al: Clean intermittent self-catheterization in the treatment of urinary tract disease. *Br J Urol* 1984; 56:379.

Law PJ, Kamm MA, Bartram CI: Anal endosonography in the detection of fecal incontinence. *Br J Surg* 1991; 78:312-314.

Leach GE, Dmochowski RR, Appell RA, et al: Female stress urinary incontinence clinical guidelines panel summary report on surgical management of female stress urinary incontinence: The American Urological Association. *J Urol* 1997; 158:875-880.

Lilly JD, Parsons CL: Bladder surface glycosaminoglycans: A human epithelial permeability barrier. *Surg Gynecol Obstet* 1990; 171:493-496.

Lindstrom S, Fall M, Carlsson, et al: The neurophysiological basis of bladder inhibition in response to electrical stimulation. *J Urol* 1983; 129:405-410.

Lose G, Diernaes E, Rix P: Does medical therapy cure female stress incontinence? *Urol Int* 1989; 44:25-27.

Lose G, Lindholm P: Clinical and urodynamic effects of norfenedrine in women with stress incontinence. *Urol Int* 1984; 39:298-302.

Lose G, Versi E: Pad-weighing tests in the diagnosis and quantification of urinary incontinence. *Int Urogynecol J* 1992; 3:324-328.

Lubowski DZ, Swash M, Nicholls RJ, et al: Increase in pudendal nerve terminal motor latency with defaecation straining. *Br J Surg* 1988; 75:1095-1097.

Madoof RD, Williams JG, Caushaj PF: Fecal incontinence. *N Engl J Med* 1992; 326:1002-1007.

Magee MC, Lucey DT, Fried EA: A new embryologic classification for urogynecologic malformations: The syndromes of mesonephric duct induced müllerian deformities. *J Urol* 1979; 121:265-267.

Mantle J, Versi E: Physiotherapy for stress urinary incontinence: A national survey. *BMJ* 1991; 302:753-755.

Maynard FM, Diokno AC: Urinary infection and complications during clean intermittent catheterization following spinal cord injury. *J Urol* 1984; 132:943.

Minaire P, Buzelin JM: Epidemiology of urinary incontinence. In Stag A, editor: *Urinary incontinence,* Edinburgh, 1992, Churchill Livingstone.

Minaire P, Jacquelin B: La prévalence de l' incontinence urinaire féminine en médecine générale. *J Gynecol Obstet Biol Rep* 1992; 26:731-738.

Molander U, Milson I, Ekelund P, et al: An epidemiological study of urinary incontinence and related urogenital symptoms in elderly women. *Maturitas* 1990; 12:51-60.

Montz FJ, Stanton SL: Q-tip test in female urinary incontinence. *Obstet Gynecol* 1986; 67:258-260.

Moore KM, Richmond DH, Sutherst JR, et al: One-shot biofeedback in relation to psychoneurotic status and treatment response in detrusor instability. *Neurourol Urodyn* 1992; 11:365-366.

Mundy AR: The etiology of detrusor instability. In Drife Jo, Hilton P, Stanton SL, editors: *Micturition,* London, 1990, Springer-Verlag.

Mundy AR: Long-term results of bladder transection for urge incontinence. *Br J Urol* 1983; 55:642.

Mundy AR: The surgical approach to the treatment of incontinence due to drug resistant detrusor instability with particular reference to "clam" ileocystoplaty. *World J Urol* 1986; 4:45.

Mundy AR, ed.: *Urodynamic and reconstructive surgery of the lower urinary tract.* Edinburgh: 1993, Churchill Livingstone.

Nielsen KK, Walter S, Maegaard E, et al: The urethral plug II: An alternative treatment in women with genuine stress incontinence. *Br J Urol* 1993; 72:428-432.

Norton P, Boyd C, Deak S: Collagen synthesis in women with genital prolapse or stress urinary incontinence. *Neurourol Urodyn* 1992; 11: 300-301.

Norton PA: Pelvic floor disorders: The role of fascia and ligaments. *Clin Obstet Gynecol* 1993; 4:926-928.

Oelrich TM: The striated urogenital sphincter muscle in the female. *Anat Rec* 1983; 205: 223-232.

Orskov I, Ferencz A, Orskov F: Tamm-Horsfall protein or uromucoid is the normal urinary slime that traps type I fimbriated *Escherichia coli* [letter]. *Lancet* 1980; 1:887.

Ostrezenski A, Osborne NG, Ostrzenska K: Method for diagnosing paravaginal defects using contrast ultrasonographic technique. *J Ultrasound Med* 1997; 16:673-677.

Parsons CL, Housley T, Schimidt JD, et al: Treatment of interstitial cystitis with intravesical heparin. *Br J Urol* 1994; 73:504-507.

Pathak U, House M: Diverticulum of the female urethra. *Obstet Gynecol* 1970; 36:789-794.

Peattie AB, Plevnik S, Stanton SL: Vaginal cones: A conservative method of treating genuine stress incontinence. *Br J Obstet Gynaecol* 1988; 95:1049-1053.

Peschers U, DeLancey JOL, Fritsch H, et al: Cross-sectional imaging anatomy of the anal sphincters. *Obstet Gynecol* 1997; 90:839-844.

Peters K, Diokno A, Steinert B, et al: The efficacy of intravesical Tice strain bacillus Calmette-Guérin in the treatment of interstitial cystitis: A double-blind, prospective, placebo controlled trial. *J Urol* 1997; 157:2090-2094.

Pigné A, Biker MO, Cotelle-Bernède O, et al: Reliance urinary control insert: Results of a French multicentered study. *Int Urogynecol J* 1997; 8(suppl):S128.

Quinn MJ: Vaginal ultrasound and urinary stress incontinence. In Drife Jo, Hilton P, Stanton SL, editors: *Micturition,* London, 1990, Springer-Verlag.

Rai R, Versi E: Alternatives to surgery for stress incontinence. In Studd EJ, editor: *Progress in obstetrics and gynaecology,* vol 10. Edinburgh: 1993, Churchill Livingstone.

Raz R, Stamm A: A controlled trial of intravaginal estriol in post menopausal women with recurrent urinary tract infections. *N Engl J Med* 1993; 329:753-756.

Resnick NM, Yalla SV. Management of urinary incontinence in the elderly. *N Engl J Med* 1985; 313:800-805.

Richardson AC, Edmonds PB, Williams NL: Treatment of stress urinary incontinence due to paravaginal fascial defect. *Obstet Gynecol* 1981; 57:357-362.

Richardson AC, Lyon JB, Williams NL: A new look at pelvic relaxation. *Am J Obstet Gynecol* 1976; 126:568-573.

Romano G, Rotondano G, Esposito P, et al: External anal sphincter defects: Correlation between pre-operative anal endosonography and intraoperative findings. *Br J Radiol* 1996; 69:6-9.

Rud T, Andersson KE, Asmussen M, et al: Factors maintaining the intraurethral pressure in women. *Invest Urol* 1980; 17:343-347.

Salmon UJ, Walter RI, Geist SH: The use of estrogens in the treatment of dysuria and incontinence in post-menopausal women. *Am J Obstet Gynecol* 1941; 42:845-8/51.

Samsioe G, Jansson I, Mellström D, et al: Occurrence, nature and treatment of urinary incontinence in a 70 year old female population. *Maturitas* 1985; 7:335-342.

Sand PK, Hill RC, Ostergard DR: Incontinence history as a predictor of detrusor instability. *Obstet Gynecol* 1988; 71:257-260.

Sander P, Thyssen H, Lose G, et al: Effect of a vaginal device on quality of life with urinary stress incontinence. *Obstet Gynecol* 1999; 93:407-411.

Sangwon YP, Coller JA, Barrett RC, et al: Unilateral pudendal neuropathy: Impact on outcome of anal sphincter repair. *Dis Colon Rectum* 1996; 39:686-689.

Savage WE, Hajj SN, Kass EH: Demographic and prognostic characteristics of bacteriuria in pregnancy. *Medicine* 1967; 46:385.

Savvas M, Bishop J, Laurent G, et al: Type III collagen content in the skin of postmenopausal women receiving oestradiol and testosterone implants. *Br J Obstet Gynaecol* 1993; 100:154-156.

Schussler B, Peschers U: Standardization of terminology of female genital prolapse according to the new ICS criteria: Inter-examiner reproducibility. *Neurourol Urodyn* 1995; 14:437-438.

Scott FB, Bradley WE, Timm GW: Treatment of urinary incontinence by an implantable prosthetic sphincter. *Urology* 1973; 1:252-259.

Scotti RJ, Angell G, Flora R, et al: Antecedent history as a predictor of surgical cure of urgency symptoms in mixed incontinence. *Obstet Gynecol* 1998; 91:51-54.

Shafik A: Study on the origin of the external anal, urethral, vaginal and prostatic sphincters. *Int Urogynecol J* 1997; 8:126-129.

Shepherd AM, Powell PH, Ball AJ: The place of urodynamic studies in the investigation and treatment of female urinary tract symptoms. *J Obstet Gynaecol* 1982; 3:123-125.

Smith DN, Appell RA, Winters JC, et al: Collagen injection therapy for female intrinsic sphincteric deficiency. *J Urol* 1997; 157:1275-1278.

Spence H, Duckett J: Diverticulum of the female urethra: Clinical aspects and presentation of simple operative technique for cure. *J Urol* 1970; 104:432-437.

Stanton SL: Classification of incontinence. In Stanton SC, editor: *Clinical gynecologic urology,* St. Louis, 1984, CV Mosby.

Stanton SL, Cardozo LD: Results of colposuspension operation for incontinence and prolapse. *Br J Obstet Gynaecol* 1979; 86:693-697.

Stanton SL: Surgical management of urethral sphincter incontinence (Review). *Clin Obstet Gynecol* 1990; 33:346-357.

Stocker J: New imaging techniques in the diagnosis of faecal incontinence. *Int Urogynecol J* 1997; 8(suppl):S40.

Sultan AH, Kamm MA, Hudson CN, et al: Anal-sphincter disruption during vaginal delivery. *N Engl J Med* 1993; 329:1905-1911.

Sultan AH, Kamm MA, Hudson CN, et al: Third degree anal sphincter tears: Risk factors and outcome of primary repair. *BMJ* 1994a; 308:887-891.

Sultan AH, Kamm MA, Talbot IC, et al: Anal endosonography for identifying external sphincter defects confirmed histologically. *Br J Surg* 1994b; 81:463-465.

Tammela T, Kontturi M, Kaar K, et al: Intravesical prostaglandine F$_2$ for promoting bladder emptying after surgery for women with stress incontinence. *Br J Urol* 1987; 60:43-46.

Tammela T, Kontturi M, Lukkarien O: Postoperative urinary retention, I: Incidence and predisposing factors. *Scand J Urol Nephrol* 1986; 20:197-201.

Tanagho EA, Smith DR: Mechanism of urinary incontinence, I: Embryologic, anatomic, and pathologic considerations. *J Urol* 1969; 100:640-646.

Tapp AJS, Cardozo LD, Versi E, et al: The treatment of detrusor instability in postmenopausal women with oxybutynin chloride: A double blind placebo controlled study. *Br J Obstet Gynaecol* 1990; 97:521-526.

Thomas TM, Plymat KR, Blannin J, et al: Prevalence of urinary incontinence. *BMJ* 1980; 281:1243-1245.

Thyssen H, Lose G: Long-term efficacy and safety of a disposable vaginal device (Continence Guard) in the treatment of female stress urinary incontinence. *Int Urogynecol J* 1997; 8:130-133.

Thyssen H, Lose G: New disposable vaginal device (Continence Guard) in the treatment of female stress incontinence: Design, efficacy and short term safety. *Acta Obstet Gynecol Scand* 1996; 75:170-173.

Tincello DG, Bolderson J, Richmond DH: Preliminary experience with a urinary control device in the management of women with genuine stress incontinence. *Br J Urol* 1997; 87:893-896.

Tjandra JJ, Milsom JW, Schroeder T, et al: Endoluminal ultrasound is preferable to electromyography in mapping anal sphincteric defects. *Dis Colon Rectum* 1993; 36:689-692.

Turner-Warwick RT, Ashken MH: The functional results of partial, subtotal, and total cystoplasty with special reference to ureterocystoplasty, selective sphincterotomy and caecocystoplasty. *Br J Urol* 1967; 39:3-12.

van Geelen H: Drug action on the bladder and urethra. *Int Urogynecol J* 1990; 1:19-20.

Vaughn ED, Middleton GW: Pertinent genitourinary embryology: Review for the practicing urologist. *Urology* 1975; 6:139-149.

Veilas B, Sedeuilh M, Albarede JL: Urinary incontinence: Epidemiological consideration. *Danish Med Bull* 1989; (suppl 8):3-9.

Versi E: The bladder in menopause: Lower urinary tract dysfunction during the climacteric. *Curr Probl Obstet Gynecol Fert* 1994; 17:193-232.

Versi E: Discriminant analysis of urethral pressure profilometry data for the diagnosis of genuine stress incontinence. *Br J Obstet Gynaecol* 1990; 97:251-259.

Versi E: Effect of hysterectomy on bowel function [letter]. *BMJ* 1989; 299:680.

Versi E: The significance of an open bladder neck in women. *Br J Urol* 1991; 61:42-43.

Versi E, Cardozo LD: Urethral instability: Diagnosis based on variations in the maximum urethral pressure in normal climacteric women. *Neurourol Urodyn* 1986; 5:535-542.

Versi E, Cardozo LD: Urodynamics. In Studd JWW, editor: *Progress in obstetrics and gynaecology,* vol 8. Edinburgh: 1990, Churchill Livingstone.

Versi E, Cardozo L, Anand D, et al: Symptoms analysis for the diagnosis of genuine stress incontinence. *Br J Obstet Gynaecol* 1991a; 98:815-819.

Versi E, Cardozo L, Cooper DJ: Urethral pressures: Analysis of transmission pressure ratios. *Br J Urol* 1991b; 68:266-270.

Versi E, Cardozo LD, Studd J: Distal urethral compensatory mechanisms in women with an incompetent bladder neck who remain continent. *Neurourol Urodyn* 1990; 9:579-590.

Versi E, Cardozo LD, Studd JW et al: Internal urinary sphincter in maintenance of female continence. *Br Med J (Clin Res Ed)* 1986; 292:166-167.

Versi E, Cardozo L, Studd J, et al: Urinary disorders and the menopause. *Menopause* 1995; 2:89-95.

Versi E, Chia P, Griffiths DJ, et al: Bacteriuria in pregnancy: A comparison of Bangladeshi and Caucasian women. *Int Urogyncol J* 1997; 8:8-12.

Versi E, Griffiths DJ, Harvey M-A: Efficacy of an external urethral device in women with genuine stress urinary incontinence. *Int Urogynecol J* 1998; 9:271-274.

Wagner TH, Hu TW: Economic costs of urinary incontinence in 1995. *Urology* 1998; 51:355-361.

Walter S, Kjaergaard B, Lose G, et al: Stress urinary incontinence in postmenopausal women treated with oral estrogen (estriol) and alpha adrenoreceptors-stimulating agent (phenyl-propanolamine): A randomized double blind placebo study. *Int Urogynecol J* 1990; 1: 74-79.

Ward J, Draper J, Tovell H: Diagnosis and treatment of urethral diverticula in the female. *Surg Gynecol Obstet* 1967; 125:1293-1300.

Wheeler JS, Walter JS: Urinary retention in females: A review. *Int Urogynecol J* 1992; 3:137-142.

White GR: Cystocele, a radical cure by suturing lateral sulci of vagina to the white line of pelvic fascia. *JAMA* 1909; 53:1707.

Wilson PD, Faragher B, Butler B, et al: Treatment with oral piperazine oestrone sulphate for genuine stress incontinence in post-menopausal women. *Br J Obstet Gynaecol* 1987; 94:568-574.

Wiskind AK, Creighton SM, Stanton SL: The incidence of genital prolapse following the Burch colposuspension operation. *Neurourol Urodyn* 1991; 10:453-454.

Woodburne RT: Anatomy of the bladder and bladder outlet. *J Urol* 1968; 100:474-487.

Woolley RJ: Benefits and risks of episiotomy: A review of the English-literature since 1980, I: *Obstet Gynecol Surv* 1995; 50:806-835.

Yang A, Mostwin JL, Rosensheim NB, et al: Pelvic floor descent in women: Dynamic evaluation with fast MR imaging and cinematic display. *Radiology* 1991; 179:25-33.

Zornow DH: Embryology of urinary incontinence. *Urology* 1977; 10:293-300.

23

Geriatric Gynecology and Aging

KAREN L. MILLER

EBOO VERSI

NEIL M. RESNICK

KEY ISSUES

1. Symptoms and disease are neither inevitable with age nor untreatable.
2. Effective treatment of elderly women requires that the physician understand the implications of age-related decline in physiologic reserve and the need to address the multiple causes of a single disorder, causes often outside the organ system usually assumed.
3. Appropriate decisions about preventive and therapeutic interventions require assessment of the patient's functional status.
4. Estrogen therapy helps prevent and treat cardiovascular disease, osteoporosis, and possibly multiple other conditions in elderly women.
5. Causes of urinary incontinence often lie outside the urinary tract, and evaluation and therapy must include these areas.
6. Decisions about cancer screening and other preventive care should be based on health, not on chronological age.

GERIATRICS OVERVIEW
Demographics and Epidemiology

Sixty percent of the 32 million Americans older than 65 are women, and the proportion rises with age. In those older than 85, the female-to-male ratio is 2.6 to 1. Those older than age 85 comprise the fastest growing segment of the population in the United States, and their number will triple in the next 15 years. One reason for this growth is that life expectancy in elderly women is increasing and is greater than often appreciated: those who are 65 can expect to live 19 more years; those who are 75, 12 more; and those who

are 85, 7 more. Moreover, 50% to 80% of those years will be spent free of dependency. In fact, even at age 85, only 20% of men and women live in long-term care facilities.

Common conditions in elderly women include urinary incontinence, pelvic organ prolapse, urinary infections, vaginal bleeding, gynecologic malignancies, urogenital atrophy, and vulvar disorders. Less common complaints are sexual difficulties, pelvic pain, pelvic infections, mood changes, and cervical dysplasia. In addition to treating these conditions, gynecologic care of the elderly woman includes preventive medicine with cancer screening and with postmenopausal estrogen therapy to prevent osteoporosis, cardiovascular disease, and possibly other disabilities. Treating elderly women requires that the practitioner have knowledge of these conditions and understanding of the basic principles of geriatric medicine. This chapter will focus on aspects of each topic that are particular to older women. As will be seen, however, the relevant data base is surprisingly sparse.

Biology of Aging
Relevant Anatomic and Physiologic Changes

Anatomic changes with aging result from "wear and tear," cessation of ovarian function, and disuse. Estrogen levels decline after menopause, but little is known about subsequent changes. Less appreciated is the fact that estrogen levels and tissue effects (vagina, bone) may vary widely in elderly women, largely as the result of varying peripheral conversion of androstenedione by adipose tissue. Declines in estrogen and androgen production contribute to the sparseness of pubic hair of the vulva and axillae and to vulvar atrophy. The vagina becomes less elastic, shorter, and narrower. These changes can make the pelvic examination, assessment of uterine size, and detection of small pelvic masses more difficult. The cervix is often flush with the vaginal apex, and only a small cervical os is visible. The squamocolumnar junction recedes into the endocervical canal. The uterus decreases in size and is more likely to be axial than it is in younger women. The rectal vault may be widely dilated, a change not necessarily associated with defecation difficulties. By remaining sexually active or taking estrogen supplementation, women can reduce the impact of many of these age-related changes (Leiblum, 1983).

Homeostenosis

The result of aging is not disease but diminished physiologic reserve. This decline in the reserve of each organ system, often referred to as homeostenosis (Resnick and Marcantonio, 1997), begins in the third decade and is gradual and linear, though the rate and extent varies widely among persons and among each person's organ systems. Several important principles follow from these facts:

Persons become more dissimilar as they age.

An abrupt decline in any system or function is always caused by disease rather than by normal aging.

Normal aging can be attenuated by the modification of risk factors.

"Healthy old age" is not an oxymoron.

In the absence of disease, homeostenosis results in neither symptoms nor restrictions on the basic activities of daily living at any age.

Principles of Geriatric Medicine
Impaired Reserve Leads to Earlier Development of Symptoms

At any age, symptoms reflect an imbalance between disease severity and intrinsic compensatory mechanisms (Fig. 23-1). Because of impaired physiologic reserve in older patients, disease often presents at an earlier stage. For example, significant cognitive dysfunction may be precipitated by only mild thyroid dysfunction, hypoxia, or hypercalcemia. Thus, paradoxically, treatment of the underlying disease may be easier in the older patient because it is less advanced at the time of diagnosis. An important corollary of this principle is that drug side effects can occur even with medications and doses unlikely to produce side effects in younger people. First-generation antihistamines may cause confusion or urinary retention, and mild diuretics may precipitate urinary incontinence. Despite the fact that in older patients symptoms develop at an earlier stage of the disease process, diagnosis is often more difficult owing to the next three principles.

Disease Often Presents Through the Weakest Organ System

Manifestation of a new disease depends on the organ system made most vulnerable by previous changes. Because the most vulnerable organ system (the weakest link) often differs from the one newly diseased, presentation is often atypical. For example, in older patients, acute confusion is one of the most common initial symptoms of infections such as pneumonia, urosepsis, or appendicitis. Because the weakest link is so often the brain, the lower urinary tract, or the mus-

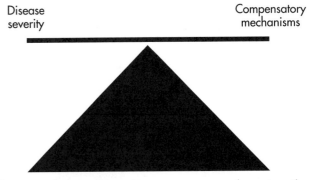

Fig. 23-1. Compensatory mechanisms. Most common symptoms result when the ability to compensate for organ system dysfunction is inadequate. Thus, even mild organ system dysfunction may cause symptoms if compensatory mechanisms are impaired. Because such impairments occur commonly in older patients, evaluation and therapy of most symptoms must extend beyond the organ system usually considered to be the cause. (Modifed from Resnick NM, Marcantonio ER: How should clinical care of the aged differ? *Lancet* 1997; 350:1157-1158. Copyright © 1997, American Medical Association.)

culoskeletal or cardiovascular system, the same symptoms predominate—acute confusion, depression, incontinence, falling, and syncope—no matter what the new disease. Thus, for most common geriatric syndromes, the differential diagnosis is largely the same, regardless of the presenting symptom. The corollary is equally important: dysfunction of the organ system usually associated with a particular symptom is less likely to be the cause of the problem in older patients. Incontinence is less likely to be caused by bladder dysfunction, falling is less likely to be caused by neuropathy, and acute confusion is less likely to be caused by a new brain lesion than in middle-aged patients.

"Abnormal" Findings in the Elderly May Not Equal Disease

Many findings that are abnormal in younger patients are relatively common in older people and may not be responsible for a particular symptom. Examples include bacteriuria, premature ventricular contractions, involuntary bladder contractions, and illness-induced hyperglycemia. Because they may be only incidental, these "abnormalities" can result in misdiagnoses and misdirected therapy.

Etiologies Are Multifactorial; Treatments Should Be Multifaceted

Because comorbid disease and drug use are common in older people, symptoms often have multiple causes rather than one. "Never think of one diagnosis when three will do" is a useful maxim. Postoperative chest pain, cough, tachycardia, and tachypnea are less likely to indicate a pulmonary embolism in an elderly patient than in a younger patient, and they are more likely to result from arthritis in the chest wall, difficulty clearing secretions, and diminished pulmonary reserve. Moreover, even when a single diagnosis is correct,

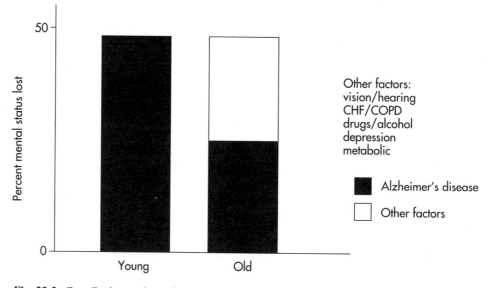

Fig. 23-2. Contributions to loss of mental status in Alzheimer's disease. Young and old patients may appear to be equally affected by Alzheimer's disease, but its extent in older patients is often magnified by comorbidity and drug use. Identification and treatment of these contributing factors improve function in older patients even though the disease itself is not completely treatable. (Modified from from Resnick NM, Marcantonio ER: How should clinical care of the aged differ? *Lancet* 1997; 350:1157-1158. Copyright © by the Lancet Ltd. 1997.)

treatment of a single disorder in an older patient often does not result in cure. In younger patients, incontinence caused by involuntary bladder contractions is often treated effectively with a bladder relaxant. However, an older incontinent patient with the same contractions will not benefit from a bladder relaxant if she also has fecal impaction, takes medications that induce confusion, and has impaired mobility and dexterity because of arthritis. In contrast, disimpaction, discontinuing the offending medications, and treating her arthritis will likely restore continence without the need for a bladder relaxant.

Small Improvements in Diverse Areas May Yield Large Results

Because many homeostatic mechanisms are often compromised concurrently, multiple abnormalities are usually amenable to treatment, and small improvements in each may yield dramatic benefits overall. Even if a primary disease process cannot be cured, therapeutic benefits can be gained through the treatment of concurrent conditions. For instance, cognitive impairment in patients with Alzheimer's disease is often exacerbated by hearing and visual impairment, depression, heart failure, thyroid dysfunction, and electrolyte imbalance (Fig. 23-2). In other words, the patient can often be treated effectively even if the disease cannot be. This is true also of prevention. For instance, though it is impossible to restore normal bone density in older women, fracture may be prevented by implementing interventions that reduce falls—improving balance, strengthening leg muscles, reducing peripheral edema, eliminating nocturia

and urinary urgency, removing environmental hazards, and reassessing medications that induce stiffness, confusion, or orthostasis.

Treatment and Prevention Are Effective

Because older patients are more likely than younger patients to experience adverse consequences of disease, treatment and prevention may be equally or more effective. For example, therapy for hypertension and transient ischemic attacks and immunization against influenza and pneumococcal pneumonia are at least as effective or more so in older patients as in younger ones.

Pharmacology

"Start low and go slow" is the canon of geriatric pharmacology. The elderly experience greater therapeutic effects and greater toxicity from a given medication dose. However, polypharmacy, not patient age or dosage, is the greatest determinant of drug-related complications. The average older American takes 4.5 prescription drugs and 2.1 over-the-counter drugs (Sanders, 1996). Twelve percent borrow prescription medications. Given the diminished compensatory ability of older organs to maintain homeostasis, it is not surprising that the use of multiple medications often leads to impairment. Although the elderly patient may tolerate one medication with mild anticholinergic side effects, the use of more than one may precipitate confusion or urinary retention. In addition to careful monitoring of drug side effects, each practitioner must minimize the number and the complexity of medications.

Important changes in pharmacokinetics (distribution, metabolism, excretion) and pharmacodynamics (drug-receptor interactions) occur with age and are summarized below. Most of these changes necessitate lower doses of medication for elderly patients. Nonetheless, it is important to realize that variability increases with age and that some elderly patients require the same doses used in younger adults. One should first define the goals of therapy and which adverse effects are intolerable, and then increase the dose gradually until encountering one or the other.

Changes in Volume of Distribution

Body composition changes result in diminished lean body mass, greater percentage of adipose tissue, and decreased total body water. Water-soluble drugs, such as aminoglycosides, achieve higher serum levels after the loading dose. Fat-soluble medications such as benzodiazepines, phenothiazines, and anesthetic agents have a longer half-life because they are distributed over a larger area of the body. Serum albumin levels are generally decreased in the elderly, especially in the ill and the malnourished. Consequently, for any given total serum concentration, protein-bound drugs (*e.g.,* warfarin, phenytoin, aminophylline) contain more circulating free ("active") drug with greater effects.

Changes in Clearance: Hepatic and Renal

Liver mass and hepatic blood flow diminish with aging. Although there is usually adequate hepatic reserve, drugs whose clearance is highly dependent on hepatic blood flow, such as lidocaine, often cause problems in the elderly. Synthetic (conjugation) pathways of drug metabolism are less affected by aging than are nonsynthetic (oxidation-reduction, hydrolytic) pathways. Therefore, lorazepam (Ativan) and oxazepam (Serax), which are conjugated in the liver but are not otherwise metabolized, are better sedative-anxiolytic choices for the elderly than are diazepam (Valium), flurazepam (Dalmane), or alprazolam (Xanax), which are oxidated. For the same reason, desipramine and nortriptyline are preferable to imipramine and amitriptyline.

Creatinine clearance declines by approximately 1% per year after age 40, though in one third of persons there is little reduction in the glomerular filtration rate (GFR) (Avorn and Gurwitz, 1997). Because of lower muscle mass in the elderly, reduced GFR is often not reflected by an elevated serum creatinine level. Therefore, in patients older than 70, a lower dose of renally excreted medication should be used initially, unless the risk for subtherapeutic treatment outweighs the risk for overdose. Aged kidneys also have less concentration ability because of diminished tubular secretion and reabsorption; hence, they resorb sodium less quickly and efficiently. Patients are at greater risk for progression to hypovolemia and shock when they are dehydrated, for electrolyte imbalances when they are hydrated intravenously, and for fluid overload when fluids are replaced generously.

EVALUATION OF THE ELDERLY WOMAN
Functional Assessment

Although most elderly persons live independently, many experience some degree of social, physical, and mental impairment. Gynecologic consultants do not have to be experts at geriatric assessment, but *an understanding of the patient's functional level is mandatory.* A simple office interview about a particular medical condition usually fails to detect significant cognitive impairment. It also fails to acquaint the practitioner with how well the patient can care for herself, which is fundamental to her ability to comply with any treatment plan, from obtaining and remembering to take a simple medication to managing her own diet, behavior, or fluid intake.

Function has been divided into three areas: basic, instrumental, and advanced. Information about each is best obtained from questionnaires completed by the patient or caregiver in advance of the office visit. Practitioners can then focus on areas of deficit to pursue their cause and impact. Such instruments also help target the examination. Functional abilities can be assessed with brief screening questions and instruments (Table 23-1, Box 23-1).

Communication with the Elderly

As many as 30% of patients older than 75 suffer from age-related macular degeneration (ARMD), and more than 40% have cataracts (Lichtenstein, 1992). Light reaching the retina can be reduced by two thirds because of yellowing of the lens. Adequate lighting is needed. Before printed material is given to a patient, literacy and ability to see the print should be determined. A font size of 14 (this size) is recommended for handouts given to the elderly, and printed materials should have adequate contrast and low glare. By age 79, approximately 50% of patients have hearing impairment. The most common form is presbycusis, a progressive sensorineural hearing loss in which higher frequencies are more affected. Asking about hearing ability and examining the auditory canals for cerumen early in the consultation is useful, as is the use of amplification devices. The practitioner should speak clearly, enunciate consonants, and increase the volume of speech in the lower frequency range.

Little change in mental acuity occurs with age, but age-associated diseases in some elderly persons can decrease processing speed, memory, or concentration. Increased time may be needed to register important information and to switch from one topic to another. Memory for short, logically associated material is good, but it is less reliable for more complex and logically unassociated material. Unfamiliar words such as medical jargon are often not well retained. Information should be imparted in a clear, simple manner and should be limited to relevant issues and reinforced in writing. Alerting the patient to changes of subject and emphasizing the message with gestures, pauses, deep breaths, touch, and questions enhances retention. Repetition also helps, as does reducing distractions (persons entering or

Table 23-1   Procedure for Functional Assessment Screening in the Elderly

Target Area	Assessment Procedure	Abnormal Result	Suggested Intervention
Vision	Test each eye with Jaeger card while patient wears corrective lenses (if applicable).	Inability to read greater than 20/40.	Refer to ophthalmologist or optometrist.
Hearing	Whisper a short, easily answered question such as "What is your name?" in each ear while the examiner's face is out of direct view.	Inability to answer question.	Examine auditory canals for cerumen and clean if necessary. Repeat test; if still abnormal in either ear, refer to audiometry and possible prosthesis.
Arm	Proximal: "Touch the back of your head with both hands." Distal: "Pick up the spoon."	Inability to do task.	Examine the arm fully (muscle, joint, and nerve), paying attention to pain, weakness, limited range of motion. Consider referral for physical therapy.
Leg	Observe the patient after instructing as follows: "Rise from your chair, walk 10 feet, return, and sit down."	Inability to walk or transfer out of chair.	Perform full neurologic and musculoskeletal evaluation, paying attention to strength, pain, range of motion, balance, and traditional assessment of gait. Consider referral for physical therapy.
Continence of urine	Ask, "Do you ever lose your urine and get wet?"	"Yes."	Ascertain frequency and amount. Search for remediable causes, including local irritations, polyuric states, and medications. Consider urologic referral.
Nutrition	Ask, "Without trying, have you lost 10 pounds or more in the last 6 months?" Weigh the patient. Measure height.	"Yes," or weight is below acceptable range for height.	Perform appropriate medical evaulation.
Mental status	Instruct as follows: "I am going to name three objects (pencil, truck, book). I will ask you to repeat their names now and then again a few minutes from now."	Inability to recall all three objects after 1 minute.	Administer Folstein Mini-Mental Status Examination. If score is less than 24, search for causes of cognitive impairment. Ascertain onset, duration, and fluctuation of overt symptoms. Review medications. Asess consciousness and affect. Do appropriate laboratory tests.
Depression	Ask, "Do you often feel sad or depressed?" or "How are your spirits?"	"Yes" or "Not very good, I guess."	Administer Geriatric Depression Scale. If positive (score above 5), check for antihypertensive, psychotropic, or other pertinent medications. Consider appropriate pharmacologic or psychiatric treatment.
ADL-IADL*	Ask, "Can you get out of bed yourself?" "Can you dress yourself?" "Can you make your own meals?" "Can you do your own shopping?"	"No" to any question.	Corroborate responses with patient's appearance; question family members if accuracy is uncertain. Determine reasons for the inability (motivation compared with physical limitation). Institute appropriate medical, social, or environmental interventions.
Home environment	Ask, "Do you have trouble with stairs inside or outside of your home?" Ask about potential hazards inside the home with bathtubs, rugs, or lighting.	"Yes."	Evaluate home safety and institute appropriate countermeasures.
Social support	Ask, "Who would be able to help you in case of illness or emergency?"	—	List identified persons in the medical record. Become familiar with community resources for the elderly.

Modified from Lachs MS, Feinstein AR, Cooney LM Jr, et al: A simple procedure for general screening for functional disability in elderly patients. *Ann Intern Med* 1990; 112:699-706.

*Activities of daily living–instrumental activities of daily living.

BOX 23-1

Activities of Daily Living

(Everything you do first thing in the morning—self-care)
Transferring
Ambulation
Toileting
Maintaining continence (fecal and urinary)
Bathing
Dressing
Feeding

Instrumental Activities of Daily Living

(Homemaker's duties—require both physical and cognitive
   ability)
Use of transportation
Shopping
Food preparation
Financial transactions
Telephone use
Medications—procurement and administration
Housework
Laundry

BOX 23-2
COMMUNICATING WITH THE ELDERLY

Determine ability to hear and see.
Use written material with adequate font size.
Keep information simple.
Relate new information to something familiar.
Minimize distractions.
Repeat important information.

From Creditor MC: Hazards of hospitalization of the elderly. *Ann Intern Med* 1993; 118:219-223.

BOX 23-3
GERIATRIC GYNECOLOGY HISTORY

Accompanied by
Age, parity
Gynecologic surgery (especially hysterectomy, oopho-
   rectomy)
Urologic surgery (bladder repair)
Age at menopause; hormones used since menopause
Chief symptom, current concerns
History of present illness
Medical history
Gynecologic history (Papanicolaou smears, mammograms,
   cancers)
Review of systems (urologic, gastrointestinal, sexual)
Medications
Allergies
Medical problem list
Surgical history
Functional status: Activities of daily living, instrumental
   activities of daily living
Living situation, support persons, phone numbers
Social history, habits

---

exiting the examination room, television or radio, and pagers) (Box 23-2).

History

Old people have lived long lives. The elderly patient has accumulated a complex medical history and is often unsure how much of it is relevant. The practitioner should allow adequate time when scheduling older patients to avoid frustration on both sides. Several techniques can increase efficiency. History can be obtained by mailing a questionnaire to the patient in advance. The patient should be asked to list all current medications on this form or to bring in all medication bottles, which the nurse can transcribe. Assistants should be trained to inquire about over-the-counter and borrowed medications as well. Full medical history can be obtained over two or three visits. Because the elderly are more likely to have multiple problems, asking about current concerns and then ranking them, rather than merely focusing on

a chief symptom, ensures that the patient's most urgent concerns will be addressed. It is wise to note in the record the name, telephone numbers, and relationship to the patient of anyone who accompanies the patient during the visit.

Noting the pertinent gynecologic history before taking the history of the present illness accelerates the clinic visit by allowing an assessment and a plan to be reached more efficiently (Box 23-3). If the patient has undergone a hysterectomy, it should be clarified whether the cervix was left in situ. Current gynecologic concern(s) can then be elicited. A streamlined medical history consists of a list of medications, a determination of whether the patient has had breast or gynecologic cancer, and brief screening questions about continence, sexual function, activities of daily living, and current home situation. This provides most of the information needed to address gynecologic problems; the list of medications alerts the physician to concurrent medical conditions. For information on urinary problems, additional history must be obtained (vide infra). Dementia is often masked by the conversational style of medical interviews. A low threshold must be maintained to screen patients—particularly women older than 75 who are contemplating surgery or who take potentially dangerous medications such as warfarin—for dementia either with a focused interview or with an instrument such as the Folstein Mini-Mental State Examination (Folstein, 1975).

Pelvic Examination

Annual pelvic examinations are indicated for all healthy women and most debilitated ones. The value of a pelvic examination goes far beyond that of a Papanicolaou smear.

Table 23-2 Physical Examination in the Elderly

Physical Limitation	Recommendation
Short stature	Short gowns to avoid falls
Dorsal kyphosis	2 or 3 pillows to support head
Cardiopulmonary compromise	Elevate back of table
Lower extremity arthritis	Assistants to hold legs
Tender, edematous feet	Assistants to hold legs
Weak upper extremities	Stand at end of table initially, then sit and elevate legs

Whether out of modesty, fear, or competing priorities, elderly women often do not discuss genital problems unless an examination is performed. These are commonly symptomatic vulvar conditions or neoplasms, atrophic vaginitis, pelvic relaxation, and bowel, bladder or sexual dysfunction. In frail elderly women, the examination may be even more important than in the healthy ambulatory population to detect and manage conditions such as vulvar rashes, pressure ulcerations, and fecal impaction.

Differences in the examination of the elderly patient have more to do with physical conditions outside the pelvis than within it (Table 23-2). Alternative positions such as the lateral recumbent position may be required because of physical constraints. If an undressed elderly patient is required to wait for the physician for any length of time, she should be seated comfortably and offered extra blankets because of greater difficulty maintaining body temperature.

The pelvic examination is similar to what it is in the younger patient. During inspection of the vulva, the practitioner should note the observation of lesions, the presence or absence of labia minora, labial agglutination, and subtle fissures, and any color changes. Loss of the labia minora is usually the result of a dermatologic condition (lichen sclerosis, lichen simplex chronicus) rather than simple atrophy. Perianal skin should also be inspected for changes. Introital and vaginal tenderness are often greater, and vaginal stenosis that precludes the insertion of more than a small finger or a small speculum is common in the very elderly. A topical anesthetic can be applied to a tender introitus before speculum insertion. Of course, a speculum appropriately sized for the patient is of the utmost importance in reducing discomfort and visualizing the cervix and vagina. Options include (1) Pederson specula; (2) very narrow specula of normal Pederson length; (3) pediatric specula; (4) medium specula; and (5) large Graves specula. Lubrication reduces discomfort, and the quality of the Papanicolaou smear is not compromised if the cervix is swabbed free of lubricant. Atrophy of the cervix may make visualization difficult, but the cervix can usually be localized by palpation and then inspected.

The uterus and the adnexa are less likely to be palpable or tender than they are in younger women. A palpable adnexum requires additional evaluation. Confounding gastrointestinal lesions such as hard stool, diverticulosis, and colon cancer are more common in the elderly. If hard stool is thought to be the cause of a mass, reexamination after laxative or enema administration is advised before imaging. A large uterus is rare in the geriatric population. If it occurs, the most common cause is still benign leiomyomata (Grover, 1995). Initial palpation of a uterus larger than the size at 8 weeks' pregnancy should prompt subsequent examination, imaging, or endometrial evaluation.

As it is during a pediatric examination, rectal palpation can be used to evaluate the uterus and the adnexa if a patient has a closed or an extremely tender vagina. Rectal examination also evaluates tone, perineal body thickness, rectocele and enterocele, and voluntary pelvic floor muscle contraction. Testing for occult blood during a rectal examination is controversial because of the lack of sensitivity in indicating important colorectal lesions, the increase in false-positive results from the use of antiinflammatory drugs and aspirin, and the high prevalence of benign lesions and neoplasms. However, most primary care providers continue to perform this test, in part because the prevalence of colon cancer increases markedly with age and in part because patients are often not compliant in obtaining and sending stool samples from home. If this is to be done, a new glove should always be used because elderly vaginal tissue is easily traumatized by the speculum alone and by Papanicolaou smears. Specific examination techniques for urinary incontinence and pelvic organ prolapse are covered in Chapter 22. It should be mentioned that the elderly patient, particularly one with dementia, often cannot perform a strong Valsalva maneuver for prolapse evaluation. Having the patient cough or stand erect for the examination may help.

For the patient with dementia, patient and reassuring explanation on the part of the practitioner and those familiar to the patient usually leads to a successful examination. It is inadvisable and virtually impossible to examine an adult who cannot cooperate. Ativan 0.25 to 0.5 mg given 1 hour before an examination usually provides adequate relaxation; occasionally 1 mg is required. Sonographic and radiologic imaging instead of a pelvic examination may provide specific information about pelvic masses, but they do not screen for vulvar, vaginal, and support problems.

HORMONE REPLACEMENT THERAPY IN THE ELDERLY

On average, women live 30 years after the cessation of ovarian function. Many of the health risks of prolonged estrogen deprivation are well known; others are just being discovered. Data suggest that the elderly achieve the same health benefits from postmenopausal estrogen replacement therapy (ERT) as perimenopausal women. Even more important than prolonging life, ERT reduces disability in old age. In this chapter, estrogen and estrogen-progestin therapy will be considered simultaneously, unless otherwise specified, because the addition of a progestin has little impact on the risks and benefits of postmenopausal estrogens other than eliminating the risk for endometrial cancer, a topic addressed in Chapter 21.

Differences in the Elderly

Estrogen use does not usually make elderly women feel better, and it can make them feel worse. They have almost no vasomotor symptoms to alleviate, and vaginal atrophy is usually asymptomatic if the woman is no longer sexually active or has maintained frequent sexual activity. Moreover, there are scant data regarding the preventive benefits or the risks of ERT when it is first initiated in women older than 70. Nonetheless, there are ample reasons to consider ERT strongly for this population.

Cardiovascular Disease

Although randomized trials of estrogen therapy are still lacking, observational data show that ERT benefits elderly patients with clinical and preclinical cardiovascular disease (CVD). The Leisure World Study (Henderson, 1991) followed up almost 9000 retirees (average age, 73) for 7 years, of whom 5000 had used estrogen for at least 1 year. Women who had taken postmenopausal estrogen had a 20% lower all-cause mortality rate than did lifetime nonusers, largely because of the reduction in cardiovascular deaths. Among current users who had taken it for 15 years or more, the all-cause mortality rate was 33% lower and the rate of fatal myocardial infarction was 50% lower. Other studies report a similar 35% to 50% reduction in CVD mortality rates in elderly women (Grodstein, 1996; Bush, 1987; Ettinger, 1996). Estrogen use also has been more beneficial for women with angiographic evidence of moderate or severe coronary artery disease but not for those without such evidence. The 10-year survival rate for estrogen users with critical stenosis was 97%, but it was 60% in nonusers (Sullivan, 1990).

The Cardiovascular Health Study (Manolio, 1993) found that women aged 65 to 74 and those older than 74 experienced equal benefits from ERT and a reduction in cardiovascular risk factors (low-density lipoprotein, insulin, fibrinogen, glucose) and subclinical disease. Current use of estrogen was more beneficial than past use, and past use was more beneficial than no use. In the Nurses' Health Study, the current use of estrogen protected against CVD, but past use and longer duration of use were not important (Grodstein, 1996). Benefit was attenuated within 3 years of discontinuation. The finding that current use rather than past use of estrogen is more protective against cardiovascular disease suggests that ERT will also benefit the very elderly, though no studies have been conducted on this population. Thus, despite the lack of randomized or intervention trials, the evidence suggests that ERT is beneficial in preventing coronary artery disease in elderly women.

Cerebrovascular Disease

The effect of ERT on cerebrovascular disease is uncertain. Some studies reveal a benefit (Ettinger, 1996; Finucane, 1993; Falkeborn, 1993; Hendersen, 1991), others show no effect (Grady, 1992; Boysen, 1988), but none suggest harm.

Osteoporosis

Although estrogen appears to be effective in the prevention and treatment of osteoporosis in the elderly, definitive data are lacking, and it may be less efficacious in preventing hip fractures than vertebral fractures. The antiresorptive effect of estrogen does not diminish with age, at least not before patients are 80. After 1 year of therapy, bone mineral density (BMD) increased 5% to 12% in women 60 to 70 years of age, and there were smaller but continued increases in the subsequent 2 years (Grey, 1994; Lindsay and Tohme, 1990). The Framingham Study (Felson, 1993) found an unimpressive 3.2% higher BMD in women 75 and older after 7 or more years of estrogen therapy than in those who had never taken estrogen (Felson, 1993). However, most of these women had discontinued ERT 10 to 20 years before BMD measurement. A recent study (Schneider, 1997) corroborated a high BMD in older women on estrogen. However, it found no difference in BMD at any site in women who started ERT at menopause and have continued it for 20 years and in women who started ERT after age 60 and have continued it for 9 years.

Although most earlier studies of hip fracture in the elderly show either a nonsignificant reduction among ERT users (Kanis, 1992; Paganini-Hill, 1991; Kiel, 1987) or no reduction (Grisso, 1994; Naessén, 1990; Ettinger, 1985), the most recent and the largest study (Cauley, 1995) suggests that estrogen does provide effective protection against hip fracture. In fact, among the 9700 women older than 64 who were studied, the largest benefit was observed in those older than 75. Previous studies included fewer elderly women and failed to differentiate current from past users of estrogen. Besides improved bone density, estrogen may have effects on neuromuscular strength, postural stability, agility, cognitive function, and prevention of falls, but data are conflicting (Naessén, 1997; Hammar, 1996; Seeley, 1995; Goebel, 1995). Estrogen reduces the incidence of spinal, wrist, and other osteoporotic fractures in elderly women with efficacy equal to that in younger women (Cauley, 1995; Lufkin, 1992; Ettinger, 1985).

Vision

Estrogen replacement therapy may ameliorate age-related macular degeneration (ARMD) and cataract formation. ARMD, which occurs in 40% of those older than 80 and is the leading cause of legal blindness in the elderly (Ernest, 1997), is less common in women using ERT (Smith, 1997; Eye Disease Study Group, 1992). Cataracts, which occur in one of every 7 people older than 40, are 50% more likely in older women than in older men. Lens clarity appears to be higher in older women who have taken ERT for at least 4 years than it is in women who have not and in men (Benitez del Castillo, 1997). The mechanisms are unknown, but estrogen may protect lenses against the damaging effects of transforming growth factor-β (Hales, 1997). Future studies will evaluate the impact of ERT on visual impairment.

Colon Cancer

Several studies suggest a 20% to 50% decrease in the incidence of and mortality from colon cancer with ERT (Calle, 1995; Newcomb, 1995; Troisi 1997; Grodstein, 1998). Current and long-term use seem to be more beneficial. Although one third or more of the subjects studied are elderly, the specific risks for older women are not well delineated. One study found a 65% ERT-related reduction in colon cancer incidence in women 60 to 69 years of age, but the 23% reduction in those older than 70 was not statistically significant (Newcomb, 1995).

Alzheimer's Disease

Alzheimer's disease is the leading cause of dementia before and after age 65, and it has a 3-to-1 female-to-male prevalence. Estrogens may foster the survival of neurons and limit the amount of amyloid-β deposition, but clinical results to date are conflicting, and there is still insufficient evidence to recommend widespread estrogen use in the elderly for the prevention or amelioration of Alzheimer disease (Yaffe, 1998). However, given the devastating nature of this disease, the lack of other good preventive strategies, and the general health benefits of ERT, strong consideration should be given to using it in patients who have the three strongest risk factors for Alzheimer's disease: age older than 65, female sex, and family history of Alzheimer disease.

Osteoarthritis

One large study suggests that postmenopausal ERT may protect against osteoarthritis in elderly women. In this cross-sectional study, white women 65 years and older had a 40% lower incidence of osteoarthritis of the hip and a 50% lower risk for moderate to severe manifestations of the disease. Current and prolonged use increased the benefits (Nevitt, 1996).

Urinary Incontinence and Infections

Estrogens are beneficial for disorders associated with urogenital atrophy. Their use for urinary incontinence and urinary tract infection (UTI) is discussed below.

Menopausal Symptomatology

Atrophic vaginitis can cause postmenopausal bleeding and vulvar and vaginal discomfort. However, most vaginal atrophy is asymptomatic. Dyspareunia is the most common symptom of vaginal atrophy. An older woman often experiences dyspareunia with her new partner after prolonged abstinence because of the illness and death of her husband. ERT is the treatment of choice. It can be administered intravaginally or systemically, and after 3 to 6 months the results are excellent. Careful distinction should be made between vaginal and vulvar discomfort. Vulvar irritation may respond to estrogen creams, but vulvar burning and pruritus are usually caused by a condition other than estrogen deficiency. The therapeutic agent may be the cream itself rather than the estrogen.

Breast Cancer

It is assumed that older women on ERT have the same risk for breast cancer that younger women have, but data are still limited and an age-related increased risk has been reported in some but not all studies (Brinton, 1986; Palmer, 1991). Recent studies show that breast cancer risk is greater in women currently on ERT than in those who were on it in the past (Collaborative Group on Hormonal Factors in Breast Cancer, 1997; Colditz, 1995). Therefore, even elderly women who expect to take estrogen for only a few years must consider the increased risk for breast cancer.

Initiation

It is incumbent on all primary care providers and gynecologic consultants to ensure that each cognitively intact woman, regardless of age or length of time since menopause, be offered the option of ERT. Medical knowledge and opinion have changed in the last 15 years, since the youngest of today's geriatric patients went through menopause. Many elderly women were not given ERT because of medical "contraindications," such as diabetes mellitus, hypertension, smoking, cardiovascular disease, and hypercholesterolemia. These conditions are now generally considered *indications* for ERT. Newer data emphasize the greater benefits (and possible risks) of current rather than past use. Estrogen is probably beneficial at any age for the prevention or treatment of osteoporosis, for the prevention or adjunctive treatment of cardiovascular disease in women with risk factors, and possibly for the other conditions listed above (Table 23-3).

Because of the expense and inconvenience involved, most physicians do not routinely examine the endometrium before they initiate ERT. The progesterone challenge test is an inexpensive way to test the endometrium for estrogen stimulation (a risk factor for endometrial cancer in this age group) before the initiation of ERT (Fig. 23-3). Although not extensively studied, the progesterone challenge test—with a sensitivity of 76% to 100% and a specificity of 96% to 100%—is probably a useful method for finding endometrial growths or abnormalities (Madia, 1993; El-Maraghy, 1994). In the absence of withdrawal bleeding from a progestin, it can be assumed that the endometrium is not stimulated by estrogen and that any bleeding that occurs after ERT is started is not caused by preexisting neoplasia. Therefore, irregular bleeding with ERT can be ignored more confidently for the first 6 to 12 months. It must be kept in mind that a false-negative progestin challenge test could result from a stenotic cervix or possibly from anaplastic endometrial cancer not stimulated by estrogen.

Doses, Side Effects, and Difficulties

Adverse symptoms are more common in elderly women who have not been exposed to estrogen for a decade or more. There is a high discontinuation rate of ERT that may

Table 23-3 Estrogen and Raloxifene Therapy in the Elderly		
Benefit	**Estrogen**	**Raloxifene**
Osteoporosis	Certain	Highly probable*
Cardiovascular disease	Highly probable	Possible*
Atrophic vaginitis	Certain	No effect; may worsen*
Urge urinary incontinence	Probable	Unlikely
Colon cancer	Possible	Unknown
Osteoarthritis	Possible	Unknown
Alzheimer's disease	Possible	Unknown
Cataracts	Possible*	Unknown
Macular degeneration	Possible	Unknown
Stress urinary incontinence	Possible	Unlikely
Cerebrovascular disease	Unclear	Unknown
Risk	**Estrogen**	**Raloxifene**
Breast cancer	Highly probable increase	Likely reduces risk*
Venous thrombo-embolism	Slight increase	Slight increase*
Endometrial cancer	None with progestins	None*

*Data from younger postmenopausal women.

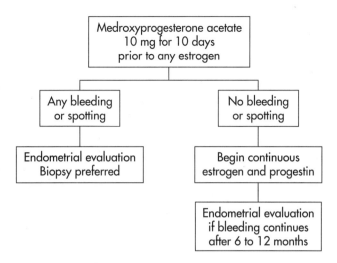

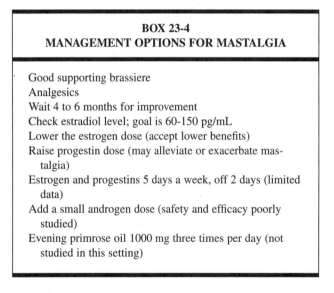

Fig. 23-3. Initiation of estrogen replacement therapy in the elderly woman with the progesterone challenge test.

**BOX 23-4
MANAGEMENT OPTIONS FOR MASTALGIA**

Good supporting brassiere
Analgesics
Wait 4 to 6 months for improvement
Check estradiol level; goal is 60-150 pg/mL
Lower the estrogen dose (accept lower benefits)
Raise progestin dose (may alleviate or exacerbate mastalgia)
Estrogen and progestins 5 days a week, off 2 days (limited data)
Add a small androgen dose (safety and efficacy poorly studied)
Evening primrose oil 1000 mg three times per day (not studied in this setting)

---

be even higher in the elderly. When multiple medical problems arise, estrogen is one of the first medications to be omitted.

Clinical experience suggests that elderly women achieve higher estrogen levels with a given dose than do younger women, but few data are available (Hartmann, 1994). Estrogen absorption and metabolism vary substantially between patients. Dose is usually limited by mastalgia. ERT is usually initiated with a standard dose (conjugated equine estrogen [CEE] 0.625 mg daily or equivalent) and decreased if necessary (Box 23-4). Mastalgia can often be circumvented by starting with a very low dose (CEE 0.3 mg) every other day for 1 month, then administering the same dose daily for 1 month, and then increasing to the standard daily dose. Recent studies have shown adequate skeletal protection using the lower estrogen doses and 1500 mg daily calcium intake (Genant, 1997; Evans, 1996; Naessén, 1997). However, it is premature to use this regimen uniformly because many women lose excess bone mass in spite of ERT. Estradiol levels of 60 pg/mL or more indicate adequate skeletal protection (Notelovitz, 1997). For patients taking less than the standard dose, measuring serum estradiol levels may serve as a guide to increase the dose or to use additional antiresorptive agents when the side effects of standard doses are intolerable. Minimum doses for cardiovascular benefits are unknown.

Bleeding is the side effect that usually leads to the discontinuation of ERT. Physical impairment among patients and lack of familiarity with current menstrual "technology" impede the management of bleeding. Many elderly women have never used tampons or inserted anything into the vagina; some are not aware of self-stick menstrual pads. Patients with weakened and arthritic hands have more difficulty using these products. Most elderly women choose continuous progestin and estrogen and are less likely to bleed on this regimen than are women who are recently menopausal. Nevertheless, as many as 20% of women continue to have bothersome bleeding and spotting after 1 year. Management options are the same as in younger women. One usually begins with an increase in the progestin dose.

When treatment is for urogenital symptoms rather than for preventive health benefits, the local application of topical estrogens may be used. Relief of atrophic vaginitis can be obtained from as little as 2 grams 3 times a week (Nathan, 1996) or from continuous low-dose estradiol delivered with a soft silastic ring such as the Estring (Pharmacia & Upjohn: Bridgewater, N.J.), which stays in the vagina for 3 months. Women who use vaginal estrogens should still be protected from continuous endometrial proliferation. Although not studied in this context, one approach is to give progestins for 12 days every 3 months. This prevents endometrial hyperplasia in most patients (Ettinger, 1994) (Hirvonen, 1994) and tests for estrogen stimulation (Madia, 1993; El-Maraghy, 1994). Because the efficacy of quarterly progestins for long-term uterine protection is uncertain (Williams, 1994; Boerrigter, 1996), the patient who has withdrawal bleeding should be put on a more standard progestin regimen (bimonthly, monthly, or continuous).

Androgens

Of interest for the geriatric patient are the theories linking dehydroepiandrosterone (DHEA) deficiency and problems of aging, including immunosenescence, increased mortality rates, increased incidence of several cancers, loss of sleep, decreased feelings of well-being, osteoporosis, cognitive deficit, and atherosclerosis (Watson, 1996). Epidemiologic studies have demonstrated an association of low levels of DHEA with increased cardiovascular disease in men, whereas no such relationship has been definitively identified in women. Low levels of DHEA and DHEA sulfate have been found in patients with breast cancer. An association between DHEA and cognition has been suggested in one study that noted decreased levels among patients with Alzheimer's disease, but this finding was not replicated. Elderly women in nursing homes who had higher DHEA levels performed better on tests of long-term memory. DHEA has been shown in vitro to enhance T-cell function and to improve insulin sensitivity. In spite of these promising concepts, it will be many years before adequate data are available to evaluate the safety and efficacy of androgen supplementation in women. Beneficial effects are unclear, and side effects are unknown. A large portion of orally ingested DHEA is metabolized into testosterone. Current preparations are sold over the counter in health food stores and are not regulated by the Food and Drug Administration (FDA). This means that dosages, bioavailabilities, and additives are not controlled (Barnhart, 1997). At this time, DHEA supplementation should be used only in an investigative setting.

Selective Estrogen Receptor Modulators

Selective estrogen receptor modulators (SERMs) are estrogens that are modified to yield the beneficial effects of estrogen without stimulating the breasts or the endometrium. Tamoxifen and clomiphene have been used for many years. Recently, the FDA approved raloxifene for the prevention of osteoporosis but not for treatment. Tamoxifen use for ˜ years reduces the incidence of breast cancer in women at ˙isk, and preliminary data suggest a similar effect with ˙e. No data on raloxifene use in elderly women are ˙le. Raloxifene has no benefit for vasomotor ˙s and does not cause vaginal bleeding, which well fits the needs of most elderly women. However, SERMs may not incorporate the full benefits of estrogen for CVD or osteoporosis, and other possible estrogen-associated benefits are unknown (see Table 23-3). Tamoxifen has been associated with ocular toxicity. Additional clinical trials will delineate the best use of raloxifene and future SERMs.

AGE-RELATED ASPECTS OF GYNECOLOGIC CONDITIONS
Osteoporosis

Osteoporosis is a devastating problem, primarily of elderly women, that causes loss of life and creates functional dependence. One fourth of women age 70 and nearly half of women age 80 have vertebral fractures. One of three 90-year-old women has had a hip fracture, which results in long-term institutionalization in as many as 25% and death in as many as 20% (Fox, 1998). *Newer data support the aggressive detection and treatment of osteoporosis in elderly women because slowing bone loss, even if it is not begun until old age, reduces the risk for fracture.*

Definition

Osteoporosis is defined by the World Health Organization as BMD more than 2.5 standard deviations below the peak bone mass in young controls. This low BMD coupled with fractures defines severe osteoporosis. Osteopenia includes BMD between 1 and 2.5 SD below peak bone mass. Using these definitions, almost 90% of American women older than 70 have osteopenia or osteoporosis.

Pathophysiological Differences in the Elderly

With aging there is a decrease in calcium absorption and typically of intake and an increase in parathyroid hormone. Vitamin D levels are lower, even in sunny regions, because of less sun exposure, less efficient skin synthesis, and less intestinal absorption. Vitamin D is also less effective in promoting intestinal calcium absorption (Greenspan and Resnick, 1997). Bone loss continues at least into the ninth decade, and it accelerates with age at the hip (average, 0.7% to 1.0% after age 80). There is also a reduction in the connectivity of the trabecular plates, which not only become perforated and disconnected but continue to thin (Greenspan and Resnick, 1997).

Hip fracture in the elderly is influenced by many factors other than bone density and architecture, notably the risk for falling. Although more than one-third of elderly women fall annually, fewer than 5% of falls result in fracture. Falling to the side carries a greater likelihood of fracture. Patient characteristics that increase fracture risk are a maternal history of hip fracture, previous hyperthyroidism, inability to rise from a chair, poor depth perception, poor contrast vision, poor visual acuity, urinary incontinence, UTIs, dementia, and use of anticonvulsants or long-acting benzodiazepines (Cummings, 1995; Greenspan and Resnick, 1997).

Evaluation

Recent (but not perimenopausal) BMD is helpful in assessing fracture risk in the elderly (Black, 1996a). As in younger postmenopausal women, a decision to measure BMD can be made based on current and projected therapy. If a woman is taking estrogen, bone density need not be measured. If she is not willing to take antiresorptive therapy, densitometry need not be pursued. If, however, she does not take estrogen, requires a reduced estrogen dose, is trying to make a decision about ERT, or is at high risk for osteoporosis, densitometry is indicated. Women with the risk factors of low body weight (<58 kg), current smoking, or a first-degree relative with or personal history of low-trauma fracture should be particularly targeted (Eastell, 1998). Vertebral bone density can be misleading and falsely reassuring because it is increased in anteroposterior measurements by nonspecific calcifications from osteoarthritis, sclerosis, aortic calcifications, and osteophytes. Hip and lateral spine measurements are more useful for women older than 65. Given the increasing variety of efficacious therapies available for the prevention and the treatment of osteoporosis in older women, patients should be screened and treated more aggressively than they were in the past. Studies are ongoing about the combination of estrogen and other antiresorptive agents. If additive benefits are shown, even elderly women taking estrogen therapy should be screened.

If a patient has bone loss or fracture, secondary causes of osteoporosis should be excluded, many of which are more common in the elderly. Older patients with skeletal discomfort should be evaluated by radiography to rule out a fracture or a bony lesion. Persistent groin or labial pain with weight bearing should first be evaluated by plain radiography. However, these can be negative even in the presence of a hip or a pubic ramus fracture, and bone imaging may be necessary to reveal the correct diagnosis.

Treatment

Calcium and Vitamin D. The high intake of calcium slows bone loss in the elderly. Combined calcium and vitamin D supplementation reduces hip and other fractures in healthy elderly women and in elderly women at risk (Eastell, 1998; Dawson-Hughes, 1997; Dawson-Hughes, 1996; Chapuy, 1992; Tilyard, 1992). It is recommended that elderly women taking estrogen ingest 1000 mg calcium daily and those not using estrogen consume 1500 mg daily. Some authors recommend even higher intakes, up to 2000 mg daily (Devine, 1997). Calcium carbonate supplements should be given in divided doses with meals to improve absorption in the elderly, who may suffer from achlorhydria. Calcium citrate can be used as an alternative. Problems with calcium supplementation include exacerbation of constipation, abdominal bloating, and gaseousness, and reduced compliance with medication regimens. Because calcium interferes with zinc absorption, a multivitamin containing zinc should be encouraged. (Greenspan and Resnick, 1997). Elderly women should probably consume 800 IU vitamin D daily (Utiger, 1998).

Antiresorptive Pharmaceuticals. Other than estrogens, bisphosphonates are the most powerful agents to improve BMD and to prevent fractures, even in elderly women (Karpf, 1997; Black, 1996b). Vertebral, hip, and wrist fractures are decreased by 50% or more with 3 years of use. Alendronate has a dose-response relationship, with progressive increases in BMD to at least 10 mg daily. The 5-mg dose is often tolerated when 10 mg is not, and it is roughly two thirds as effective. Etidronate reduces vertebral fractures, but a reduction in hip fractures has not yet been demonstrated. It should be considered for women with osteoporosis who cannot take estrogens or other bisphosphonates. Androgens, including DHEA, increase bone density (Labrie, 1997), but potential adverse effects limit their use. Estrogens and selective estrogen receptor modulators are discussed above.

Exercise and Risk Reduction for Falls. Elderly women should discontinue or substitute medications (including nonprescription) that have adverse effects on cognition, balance, or orthostasis (King and Tinetti, 1996). Common offenders include long-acting benzodiazepines (*e.g.,* flurazepam, diazepam), tricyclic antidepressants (*e.g.,* amitriptyline, imipramine), antipsychotics (*e.g.,* haloperidol), antihypertensives, and agents with anticholinergic side effects. Visual impairment should be corrected. Peripheral edema, which adds at least 3 kg to leg weight, should be reduced or eliminated. Elevating the legs in the evening and wearing pressure-gradient stockings are useful for reducing peripheral edema. Usually the cause of this type of edema is not congestive heart failure, and diuretic therapy in the absence of congestive heart failure can increase the risk for a fall. Environmental dangers such as throw rugs, extension cords, poorly illuminated stairways, and absent hand rails should be corrected. Exercise prevents or reduces the bone loss seen in nonexercisers (Taunton, 1997), though significant BMD increases are rarely seen in elderly women even with weight-bearing exercise. However, strength, conditioning, and balance exercises reduce the risk for falls by improving strength, cognitive processing, and balance (Chandler and Hadley, 1996). For patients with gait disorders, physical therapy should be considered.

Lower Urinary Tract Dysfunction

Urinary incontinence afflicts 15% to 30% of community-dwelling elderly, 33% or more of those in acute-care settings, and 50% of those in nursing homes. Incontinence is underreported by patients and undertreated by physicians, but it is usually treatable and often curable at all ages, even in the frail elderly (Ouslander and Schnelle, 1995; Resnick, 1996a). The approach, though, must differ significantly from that used for younger patients and must focus on diverse physical and environmental areas.

Lower Urinary Tract Changes with Aging

The aging lower urinary tract undergoes many changes that predispose the patient to, but do not cause, incontinence (Resnick, 1996a). Bladder contractility and capacity and the

---

BOX 23-5
CAUSES OF TRANSIENT INCONTINENCE

D elirium
I nfection—urinary (symptomatic)
A trophic vaginitis-urethritis
P harmaceuticals
P sychological—especially severe depression (rare)
E xcess urine output (*e.g.*, congestive heart failure, hyperglycemia)
R estricted mobility
S tool impaction

Modified from Resnick NM: Urinary incontinence in the elderly. *Med Grand Rounds* 1984; 3:281-290.

---

ability to postpone voiding appear to decline in both sexes. Maximum urethral closure pressure and length decline with age in women. The prevalence of involuntary detrusor contractions increases, even in continent elderly persons. The postvoiding residual volume (PVR) probably increases, but to no more than 50 to 100 mL. In addition, the elderly often excrete most of their fluid intake at night, even in the absence of venous insufficiency, renal disease, or heart failure. This, coupled with an age-associated increase in sleep disorders, leads to one to two episodes of nocturia in most healthy elderly persons. Estrogen deficiency may affect the sensory threshold of the urinary tract in elderly patients, causing a decreased volume and time to first sensation. Thinning of the urethral mucosa, submucous vascularity, and connective tissue from estrogen deficiency contributes to the lower urethral closure pressure often found in elderly women (Cardozo and Versi, 1993). Although there are no studies showing that estrogen deficiency contributes to pelvic organ prolapse, the decrease in vaginal connective tissue, principally collagen, is thought to be contributory and is a result of estrogen deficiency (Harvey and Versi, 1998).

Causes of Transient Incontinence

In addition to lower urinary tract function, continence depends on adequate mentation, mobility, motivation, and manual dexterity. Because conditions affecting each of these domains are common in the elderly, geriatric incontinence is rarely attributable to a single cause. Moreover, many of these conditions—particularly those outside the lower urinary tract—respond readily to therapy. Because incontinence often abates once they are addressed, they are considered causes of "transient incontinence." It is important to emphasize that transient incontinence may persist if it is left untreated, and it should be considered even when incontinence is long-standing. After transient and functional causes have been addressed and the search for a serious abnormality reveals none, the lower urinary tract should be evaluated as it is for younger patients.

The causes of transient incontinence can be recalled using the mnemonic DIAPPERS (Box 23-5) (Resnick, 1996a). In patients with *delirium*, incontinence abates after the underlying cause of confusion is identified and treated. Symptomatic urinary tract *infection* causes transient incontinence, but asymptomatic infection (present in 10% to 30% of elderly) does not. Because illness can manifest itself atypically in older persons, incontinence occasionally is the only atypical symptom of a UTI. Thus, if otherwise asymptomatic bacteriuria is found on the initial evaluation, it should be treated and the result recorded in the patient's record to prevent future futile therapy. *Atrophic urethritis* or *vaginitis* often exacerbates incontinence and causes urgency. Occasionally it causes stress incontinence.

Pharmaceuticals are the most common causes of geriatric incontinence, precipitating leakage by a variety of mechanisms (Table 23-4). The most problematic agents are those that contribute to urinary retention because of an underactive detrusor or those that relax the urethral sphincter (α-blockers) and result in stress incontinence. Many of these agents are also used in the treatment of incontinence, which underscores the fact that most medications are "double-edged swords" for the elderly. Attempts should be made to discontinue anticholinergic agents or to substitute agents with fewer anticholinergic side effects. The risk for angiotensin-converting enzyme (ACE) inhibitor-induced cough increases with age and may worsen stress incontinence. *Psychological* causes of incontinence, usually severe depression or lifelong neurosis, are rare in the elderly. *Excess urine output* commonly contributes to geriatric incontinence. It arises from the decreased concentrating ability of the kidneys, excessive fluid intake, diuretics, metabolic abnormalities, drugs (calcium-channel blockers, nonsteroidal anti-inflammatory drugs), disorders associated with fluid overload, and obstructive sleep apnea (present in up to 24% of elderly). *Restricted mobility* can result from numerous treatable conditions. If causes are not correctable, a urinal or a bedside commode may improve or resolve incontinence. Finally, *stool impaction* is implicated as a cause of urinary incontinence in as many as 10% of elderly patients. The mechanism may involve the stimulation of opioid receptors. Patients present with urge or overflow incontinence, and fecal incontinence typically develops. Disimpaction restores continence.

Causes of Established Incontinence

It is important to consider first the serious medical conditions that must not be missed in the evaluation of established incontinence (Box 23-6). These include neurologic lesions of the brain and spinal cord, bladder cancer, pelvic masses, and bladder stones. Multiple sclerosis is uncommon in the elderly. "Functional" incontinence often is cited as a distinct type of geriatric incontinence, and it is attributed to deficits of cognition and mobility. However, incontinence is not inevitable with either dementia or immobility (Resnick, 1996a), and causes of transient incontinence are more com-

Table 23-4 Commonly Used Medications That May Affect Continence

Type of Medication	Examples	Potential Effects on Continence
Sedatives-hypnotics	Long-acting benzodiazepines (*e.g.,* diazepam, flurazepam)	Sedation, delirium, immobility
Alcohol		Polyuria, frequency, urgency, sedation, delirium, immobility
Anticholinergics	Dicyclomine, disopyramide, antihistamines	Urinary retention, overflow incontinence, delirium, impaction
Antipsychotics	Thioridazine, haloperidol	Anticholinergic actions, sedation, rigidity, immobility
Antidepressants	Amitriptyline, desipramine	Anticholinergic actions, sedation
Anti-Parkinsonians	Trihexyphenidyl, benztropine mesylate (not L-dopa–selegiline)	Anticholinergic actions, sedation
Narcotic analgesics	Opiates	Urinary retention, fecal impaction, sedation, delirium
α-Adrenergic antagonists	Prazosin, terazosin	Urethral relaxation may precipitate stress incontinence in women
α-Adrenergic agonists	Nasal decongestants	Urinary retention in women
Calcium-channel blockers	All	Urinary retention; nocturnal diuresis owing to fluid retention*
Potent diuretics	Furosemide, bumetanide	Polyuria, frequency, urgency
Angiotensin converting enzyme inhibitors	Captopril, enalapril, lisinopril	Drug-induced cough can precipitate stress incontinence in women and in some men who have undergone prostatectomy
Vincristine		Urinary retention

Modified with permission from Resnick NM: Geriatric medicine. In Isselbacher KJ, Braunwald E, Wilson JD, et al, editors: *Harrison's principles of internal medicine,* ed 13, New York, 1994, McGraw-Hill, p. 34.

*Dihydropyridine class of calcium-channel blockers, such as nifedipine, nicardipine, israpidine, felodipine, and nimodipine.

BOX 23-6
SERIOUS CAUSES OF INCONTINENCE

Tumors of the central nervous system
Other causes of cord compression
Bladder cancer
Pelvic masses
Bladder stones
Multiple sclerosis
Parkinson's disease

---

mon in these patients. In fact, often the cause is related to the lower urinary tract. Therefore, use of this term should be limited.

Detrusor instability or "overactive bladder," for which the classic symptom is urge incontinence, is more common in the elderly. In older adults, it may exist in the presence of a normally contractile or hypocontractile detrusor muscle (Resnick, 1996a). The latter condition, detrusor hyperactivity with impaired contractility (DHIC), is the usual type of overactive bladder in the elderly. The patient experiences urgency and urge incontinence, but the detrusor contraction is not sustained, usually resulting in a high PVR. However,

residuals may be normal if she strains or voids repeatedly in succession. DHIC is easily misdiagnosed on cystometric testing as stress incontinence or urethral instability owing to the low amplitude of detrusor contractions. Diagnosis can be established by exacting use of the cough stress test and single-channel cystometry (Resnick, 1996b) or by careful multichannel cystometry with or without fluoroscopy. Although generally feasible, anticholinergic therapy may worsen or induce urinary retention, particularly if patients do not have concurrent stress incontinence.

Stress incontinence in elderly women is usually associated with disorders of pelvic floor support, as it is in younger women. However, intrinsic sphincter deficiency appears to be more common in elderly women, though it is mild and results from urethral atrophy superimposed on the age-related decrease in urethral pressure (Resnick, 1996a). Patients with intrinsic sphincter deficiency often can remain continent if bladder volume is kept at a lower level (below 200 mL).

Outlet obstruction is as rare in elderly women as it is in younger ones. When it does occur, its cause may be a large protruding cystocele, a milder cystocele (to the level of the hymen) together with reduced bladder contractility, or obstruction after bladder neck suspension. Rarely is a neoplasm or a bladder calculus the cause.

Detrusor underactivity is usually idiopathic. When it causes incontinence, detrusor underactivity is associated with overflow incontinence; it accounts for less than 10% of geriatric incontinence (Resnick, 1996a). Because of the age-related decline in urethral sphincter strength, the PVR in women with overflow incontinence often is lower than it is in younger women. The mild degree of bladder weakness that occurs in elderly persons can complicate the treatment of other causes.

Diagnostic Approach

Only after the exclusion of serious conditions is the pursuit of a diagnosis of urinary incontinence and its treatment elective. Because the evaluation generally requires a comprehensive approach, it may be conducted over several visits to ease the burden on the patient and to obviate further evaluation in those who respond to simple measures.

History

In addition to urologic baseline history taken in younger women, anticholinergic contraindications (narrow-angle glaucoma), medication use (including nonprescribed agents), cognition, mobility, and manual dexterity should be noted. Sexual function is usually queried in younger women but often overlooked in the elderly. Fecal incontinence should be queried because it often accompanies urinary incontinence, it may affect management, and patients are less likely to volunteer this information. Although history alone is not an accurate predictor of urodynamic diagnosis, the diagnosis is usually clear once the clinical evaluation is complete if several caveats are kept in mind (see below) (Resnick, 1996a).

Physical Examination

In addition to the standard pelvic examination for signs of incontinence, one should check for reversible causes of incontinence and for neurologic disease. The rectal examination assesses fecal impaction, pelvic masses, and sacral reflexes. Many neurologically impaired elderly patients are unable to contract the pelvic floor muscles or the anal sphincter at will, but if they can it is evidence against a spinal cord lesion. If a woman cannot perform a pelvic floor contraction, this should also be assessed rectally, and she should be asked to use her muscles to avoid passing flatus. The absence of the anal wink is not necessarily abnormal in the elderly, nor does its presence exclude an underactive detrusor (owing to diabetic neuropathy, for instance) (Resnick, 1996a).

Voiding Record, Stress Testing, Postvoid Residual Volume Measurement

Literacy, visual acuity, and writing ability should be determined when the voiding diary is requested. The patient's ability to keep a voiding diary provides clues about her ability to follow through with bladder training and other instructions. False-negative cough stress test results occur when the patient fails to cough vigorously or to relax the perineal muscles, the bladder is not full, or a large cystocele kinks the urethra. The PVR can be spuriously low owing to

straining or repeated voiding. It may be spuriously elevated because of failure to relax the urethral sphincter, failure to trigger a detrusor contraction adequately, prolonged interval between voiding and catheterization, or diuresis (caused by caffeine intake) (Elbadawi, 1997). If the PVR is high, it should be remeasured at a subsequent visit. Provided these caveats are addressed, the lower measurement is considered more indicative of the patient's voiding ability.

Empiric Diagnostic Categorization

Initial management is usually possible without further testing (Fig. 23-4). In a woman with a cystocele, placement of a pessary may be sufficient. If the postvoid residual is high, reevaluation of the PVR or a pressure-flow study differentiates mechanical obstruction from detrusor underactivity. The diagnosis can then be clinically categorized as stress incontinence, mixed incontinence, or detrusor overactivity, keeping in mind that detrusor hyperactivity with impaired contractility is a subset of overactive bladder that often, but not always, has an elevated PVR. Therapy is based on the clinical diagnosis, with referral to a specialist or multichannel urodynamics as needed, depending on the expertise of the practitioner.

Therapy

It cannot be overemphasized that successful treatment of established incontinence in the elderly is usually multifactorial and must address conditions outside the urinary tract. Improvement rather than cure may significantly enhance quality of life. Behavioral therapy is the initial mainstay of treatment. Even though physicians are aware of the need to avoid medications in the elderly, they often assume that elderly women are not as capable of learning conservative interventions as younger women. Multiple studies have documented the efficacy of pelvic floor exercises and bladder training in reducing incontinence and improving quality of life for elderly women (Bo, 1997; Wyman, 1997; Fonda, 1995; Burns, 1993).

Detrusor Overactivity

Cognitively intact elderly patients are treated for urge incontinence, as are younger patients, with behavioral modification and pharmacologic treatment but with less emphasis on the latter. Fluid management and adjustment of voiding frequency are particularly important.

Cognitively impaired persons respond well to "prompted voiding." Asked every 2 hours whether they must void, such patients are escorted to the toilet if their response is affirmative. Positive verbal reinforcement is used, and negative comments are avoided. Drugs augment behavioral intervention but do not supplant it in these patients. In one study, oxybutynin added substantially to the clinical effectiveness of prompted voiding in less than 25% of nursing home residents (Ouslander, 1995).

Medications to suppress bladder contractions are often discontinued because of lack of efficacy or side effects.

Address transient causes (DIAPPERS), exclude serious associated conditions, then:

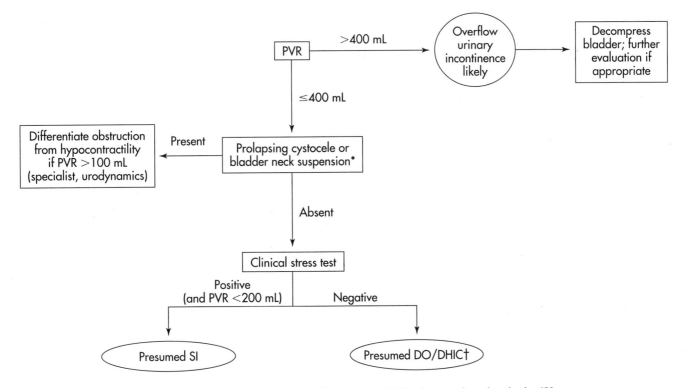

Fig. 23-4. Approach to urinary incontinence in elderly women. *Other than anterior colporrhaphy. †Use bladder relaxants with caution if postvoid residual volume is 50 to 150 mL; avoid them if postvoid residual volume is more than 150 mL. (Modified from Resnick NM: Clinical crossroads: An 89-year-old woman with urinary incontinence. *JAMA* 1996; 276:1832-1840. Copyright © 1997, American Medical Association.)

Treatment with electrical stimulation has not been adequately investigated and is underused in the elderly, but its advantage would be the avoidance of medication. Cost reimbursement and patient compliance are common obstacles.

There are few data on drug efficacy or toxicity in the elderly. Available studies show similar efficacy for most drugs, except flavoxate, which fares poorly in controlled trials (Resnick, 1996a). Thus, the choice of drug should be based on medical factors unrelated to bladder function, such as the avoidance of anticholinergic agents in patients with constipation or cognitive deficits. Combining low doses of two agents with complementary actions, such as oxybutynin and desipramine, occasionally maximizes benefits and minimizes side effects. Tolterodine is a recently approved anticholinergic agent that has shown a lower incidence of xerostomia than oxybutynin in controlled clinical trials. Medications should generally be started in low doses (2.5 mg oxybutynin, 10 mg imipramine, 1 mg tolterodine).

Detrusor Hyperactivity With Impaired Contractility. Management of detrusor hyperactivity with impaired contractility is aimed at limiting the consequences of detrusor overactivity without inducing retention. Timed voiding and judicious use of anticholinergic agents can be helpful. For patients whose incontinence defies other remedies, inducing urinary retention and using intermittent catheterization may be a solution.

Stress Incontinence

Besides behavioral training, mechanical supports and barriers are regaining popularity as conservative therapy; several newer devices and pessaries are available. Estrogen therapy plus an α-adrenergic agonist, such as phenylpropanolamine (50 to 100 mg/day in divided doses), may help patients increase the proximal urethral pressure (Resnick, 1996a). Caution must be used, but α-agonists are often tolerated even by patients with uncomplicated hypertension.

Surgery for stress incontinence is as efficacious for elderly patients as for younger ones, provided that the correct preoperative diagnosis has been established and access is adequate for vaginal procedures. Glutaraldehyde cross-linked collagen injections are minimally invasive and are 50% to 80% efficacious in elderly patients. Improvement, however, is more common than cure (Stanton and Monga, 1997; Khullar, 1997; Herschorn, 1996; Monga, 1995; Faerber, 1996). Endoscopic bladder neck suspensions and retropubic colposuspensions in elderly patients have produced good results in most studies (Nitti, 1993; Griffith-Jones and Abrams, 1990; Golomb, 1994; Peattie and Stanton, 1989; Gillan and Stanton, 1984). Long-term results of needle-suspension procedures have been disappointing in young patients (Leach, 1997), possibly because of suture failure after high-impact activity. Whether they are more durable in the elderly has not been determined. In published series (Carr, 1997; Couillard, 1994), pubovaginal slings have the same efficacy and complication rate in the elderly as in younger patients. Caution is advised for patients with incipient voiding dysfunction. Morbidity and mortality rates are low after incontinence surgery in the elderly. In 66,000 women older than 65 who underwent inpatient continence procedures, the overall mortality rate was 0.33%. Although mortality increased linearly with age, it was still only 2% in those older than 85 (Sultana, 1997).

Underactive Detrusor

Management of detrusor underactivity is directed at reducing the residual volume, eliminating hydronephrosis (if present), and preventing urosepsis (Resnick, 1996a). The first step is to use indwelling or intermittent catheterization to decompress the bladder for at least 7 to 14 days and for as long as 1 month while reversing the factors that contribute to impaired detrusor function (*e.g.,* fecal impaction and medications). If after decompression the detrusor is acontractile, the patient should be started on intermittent catheterization or an indwelling urethral catheter.

Urinary Tract Infection

Whether symptomatic or asymptomatic, urinary infections traditionally have been defined by a culture of 10^5 colony-forming units per milliliter (cfu/mL) of one or more organisms in the urine. However, this definition now applies only to asymptomatic bacteriuria (ASB). Symptomatic UTI is confirmed by a single organism with greater than 10^2 cfu/mL. Unique aspects of these infectious disorders in the elderly are their dramatic increase in prevalence, a change in pathogens, a tendency to colonize upper tracts, and the special concerns about medications in the elderly regarding allergies, adverse reactions, drug interactions, and modification for renal insufficiency. In addition, UTIs can present with any of the common geriatric syndromes—incontinence, falling, altered sensorium, syncope, or depression. *Escherichia coli* is the most common UTI or ASB isolate in the elderly (60% to 80%), as it is at all ages, but other organisms increase in relative frequency, among them *Proteus mirabilis, Klebsiella pneumonia, Enterococcus faecalis,* coagulase-negative staphylococci, and group B streptococci (Childs and Egan, 1996). Estrogen deficiency and the resultant increase in vaginal pH contribute to the prevalence and the altered microbial spectrum of UTI-ASB.

Asymptomatic Bacteriuria

The prevalence of ASB increases with age, from approximately 5% or less in young ambulatory women, to 20% to 30% in women older than 70, and to as much as 50% in women older than 80. Higher residual urine volume, estrogen deficiency, and immune system alterations may play a role (Nicolle, 1997). Functional status and the number and severity of medical diagnoses have an even greater impact than age alone (Nicolle, 1997). Not surprisingly, institutionalized patients have the highest prevalence of ASB (Childs

and Egan, 1996). Conversion between positive and negative ASB states is common, especially in the institutionalized elderly. In an elderly ambulatory population, 5% of women initially negative for bacteriuria were positive 6 months later, and approximately one-third of those initially positive for ASB showed spontaneous clearance in 6 months (Nicolle, 1997).

Although it may be difficult for physicians to avoid treating a patient with a positive urine culture, *it is recommended that no antibiotic therapy be given for ASB* unless the patient is also immunocompromised or an invasive procedure is planned. Such treatment does reduce the incidence of subsequent positive urine cultures in the elderly, but it does not reduce UTI symptoms, morbidity, or mortality, and it increases the prevalence of more virulent organisms (Abrutyn, 1996; Nordenstam, 1986; Nicolle, 1987). The common concurrence in the elderly of ASB and urinary incontinence, lethargy, fatigue, or depression promotes misguided treatment. If the symptom is unchanged by effective antibiotic therapy (documented with a follow-up dipstick or culture), future futile treatments can and should be avoided.

Symptomatic Urinary Tract Infection

Urinary tract infection is a major source of morbidity, mortality, and health care expenditures in the elderly. In a rural outpatient clinic, 60% of antibiotic prescriptions given to elderly women were for UTI (Leistevuo, 1997). It is one of the two most common antecedents of acute confusion in elderly residents of long-term care facilities (Culp, 1997). Risk factors for UTI are similar to those for ASB, which itself is a risk factor for UTI in the elderly (Nicolle, 1997). Urinary tract infections account for 60% of nosocomial hospital-acquired infections in elderly patients (Beaujean, 1997). The risk increases with each year of age, even for geriatric patients. Dehydration and urinary catheters are also contributing factors.

Diagnostic issues in healthy elderly patients do not differ from those in younger ones. Institutionalized patients, however, should be cultured more often rather than administered empiric therapy because of more unusual and resistant organisms. In asymptomatic elderly patients, a negative urine dipstick effectively rules out bacteriuria (Monane, 1995), but because UTI may be caused by a lower concentration of organisms, only a culture can definitively rule out infection. Especially in very old and frail elderly, a high suspicion for UTI must be maintained if there is an onset of any new symptom or illness. In a study of elderly patients with bacteremic UTI, symptoms were confusion (30%), cough (27%), dyspnea (28%), and new urinary symptoms (20%) (Barkham, 1996). Only 63% of those older than 70 were febrile.

Relapse rates were 44% to 60% after short-term therapy (Nicolle, 1988), in part because of colonization of the upper urinary tracts. Infective organisms were localized to the kidneys in more than 50% of ambulatory elderly patients and in more than 66% of those receiving acute or chronic care

(Nicolle, 1987). Although short-term therapy is a reasonable initial approach in healthy, ambulatory women, antibiotics should be prescribed for 10 to 14 days in functionally impaired or ill patients. If symptoms resolve, follow-up cultures are contraindicated because of the high prevalence of ASB.

Antibiotic prescription should be undertaken with the same caution given every medication in the elderly. The likelihood of decreased renal function should be assessed clinically, with dose adjustments made accordingly. The slender 80-year-old whose creatinine clearance was 1.1 last year (presume a decrease in GFR of one-third to one-half) should be prescribed single-strength trimethoprim-sulfamethoxazole (80 mg/400 mg) twice daily rather than double strength to avoid hyperkalemia. The potential for interactions with other drugs should be evaluated. Although rare, the risk for serious adverse reactions to nitrofurantoin (acute pulmonary reactions, interstitial pneumonitis, allergy) (Holmberg, 1980) and probably to trimethoprim-sulfamethoxazole (Stevens-Johnson syndrome, toxic epidermal necrolysis, aplastic anemia, agranulocytosis) increase with age and with peripheral neuropathy. Because of cost, efficacy, and antimicrobial spectrum, generic trimethoprim-sulfamethoxazole is one of the best choices for initial therapy in the elderly (Bjornson, 1997), keeping in mind that resistant *E. coli* and other organisms are relatively common in this age group. (Arstila, 1997). Fluoroquinolones are widely prescribed because of their broad spectrum of antimicrobial activity and their excellent tissue penetration. They are eliminated predominantly by renal excretion. Dosing recommendations for individual quinolones based on age and estimated renal clearance should be reviewed when these are prescribed (Bergan, 1995).

Pelvic Organ Prolapse

Characteristics of pelvic organ prolapse depend more on individual genetic and environmental factors than on age. Nonetheless, some generalizations are worth consideration. Elderly women have more vulnerable epithelium and in most cases a longer duration of estrogen deficiency, leading to greater vaginal atrophy, friability, and tenderness. At the same time, their pelvic tissues are less supple. Apical vaginal agglutination and atrophy of introital muscular support may contribute to difficulties with pessary use. Other barriers to nonoperative prolapse management and pessary use may be less manual dexterity, less familiarity with vaginal insertion, and less flexibility to reach the vagina than younger women. A high postvoid residual in an elderly woman with a cystocele has a much greater chance than in a younger woman of resulting from impaired detrusor contractility rather than from obstruction. Finally, providers often fail to query sexual function and concerns in elderly women.

Elderly patients with genital prolapse are evaluated as their younger counterparts are. Many remain asymptomatic and consequently do not require treatment. No good correlation has been documented between symptomatology and severity of prolapse. Details of the examination are presented in Chapter 22. If the leading edge is protruding through the hymen, the resultant erosion, urinary retention, or ureteric obstruction may necessitate correction. Although elevated urinary residuals caused by detrusor underactivity do not lead to renal damage, obstruction of ureters or of the urethra do endanger the kidneys.

Many elderly women with genital prolapse choose not to undergo surgery and instead elect the use of a pessary. This is addressed in Chapter 22, but a few points must be made that are specific to the elderly. The use of a vaginal pessary in the absence of estrogen treatment is problematic because erosion and the ensuing infection and discharge are common. Thus, estrogen use is advised and is best administered locally (with or without systemic estrogen). Elderly patients may be unwilling or unable to remove the pessary on a daily basis. Fortunately, this is not necessary because the pessary can be removed, cleaned, and, after inspection of the vagina, replaced by the clinician every 3 to 6 months. The patient should be advised to return sooner if there is any discharge. If significant erosion is noted, treatment with estrogen cream and an antiseptic preparation in the absence of a pessary is indicated until the area has healed.

Should surgery be considered, thought should be given to the type of anesthesia (vide infra). Certain procedures, such as colpocleisis, can be performed under local anesthesia (Miklos, 1995). The abdominal approach is thought by many pelvic floor surgeons to be the preferred route for reconstruction. However, in the elderly, the advantages of the "better" result must be balanced against the disadvantage of greater morbidity and slower postoperative recovery. Consequently, vaginal surgery may be preferred.

Sexuality

Sexual interest and capacity persist at least into the ninth decade (Rockstein and Sussman, 1979; Bretschneider and McCoy, 1988). However, many studies document the decline in sexual desire and activity (Roughan, 1993). Endocrine, anatomic, and physiologic changes play a role in the reduced frequency of sexual activity in older women, but illness and lack of an available partner are the major determinants of this decline (Roughan, 1993; Purifoy, 1992). After age 79, there are 39 men for every 100 women (US Bureau of the Census, 1990). A decline in sexual interest is often adaptive on the part of a woman with no partner or a partner who is impotent, and she may sublimate by focusing on offspring and friends as sources of intimacy and enjoyment (Purifoy, 1992; Malatesta, 1988).

Changes with Aging

Studies by Masters and Johnson remain the definitive source regarding the physiologic changes that take place in the sexual response cycle as a person ages (Roughan, 1993). All phases of arousal take longer. For instance, lubrication time may increase from 15 to 40 seconds to 5 minutes. Major changes are decreased congestion of the labia minora, decreased separation of the labia majora, decreased vaginal lubrication and blood flow, decreased orgasmic platform contraction, reduced number of orgasms, and occasional painful spastic contractions of the uterus. There is overall loss of genital and breast tactile sensitivity. In addition, the breasts become less vasocongested, and nipple erection is less likely to occur. Effects of estrogen deprivation include a thinner, flattened vaginal epithelium (leading to dyspareunia and postcoital bleeding), fewer *Lactobacilli* (causing a greater susceptibility to vaginal and urinary infections), decreased vaginal elasticity and lubrication, and reduced vaginal blood flow in response to erotic stimuli (Roughan, 1993). Vaginal function appears to be better preserved, and dyspareunia is less common in estrogen-deficient women who remain sexually active than in those who resume sexually activity after a long period of inactivity (Leiblum, 1983).

Evaluation

In addition to asking a patient about the duration and impact of a problem, the physician should inquire about measures used to solve it, her belief concerning its cause, and her feelings about it (Brandt, 1987). Although validated questionnaires of sexual function exist for men, no such validated instruments exist for elderly women (Kaiser, 1996).

Examination of the elderly woman for sexual dysfunction is essentially the same as it is in younger women. There is a greater likelihood of vulvar abnormalities, with the probable exception of vulvar vestibulitis, though data are lacking. Vaginal depth and suppleness should be evaluated. Tenderness in specific areas, such as the levator ani muscles or the cul-de-sac of Douglas, and whether this reproduces the dyspareunia should be noted, as should pelvic organ prolapse.

Conditions and Treatments

As the number and severity of medical illnesses increase with aging, sexual function is often affected. In contrast to the plethora of conditions that may cause erectile dysfunction in men, few disorders are known to specifically inhibit sexual function in women. Gynecologic conditions treated with radical surgery or radiation may cause vulvar and vaginal problems. Vaginal narrowing after prolapse surgery interferes with intercourse, but it is not common and it responds well to estrogen and dilation (Holley, 1996). Hysterectomy and urinary continence procedures have little impact on sexual functioning (Roughan, 1993; Berglund, 1996). Neurologic injury or disease can impair sensation or sexual function. Even without a direct effect on sexual capacity, most chronic illnesses affect sexual function and enjoyment through general debility, anxiety, depression, or pain. Drugs may also impair sexual function; both the condition being treated and the medication itself may have negative effects on sexual expression.

Common treatable conditions that impair sexual function are atrophic vaginitis, vaginal stenosis, urinary incontinence, and pelvic organ prolapse. Maximum improvements from local or systemic estrogen are seen in 12 to 18 months (Roughan, 1993). One fourth of elderly women experience incontinence during intercourse (Hilton, 1988). One third of women with incontinence and prolapse report that they interfere with sexual activity (Weber, 1995). Careful evaluation of the type of incontinence (stress, urge, overflow) is necessary for effective treatment. In addition, male partners are often not bothered if the condition is explained. Prolapse can be managed by conservative means or by surgery, or it can be managed by having the patient change position for intercourse. Pessaries usually impede vaginal intercourse, but they are not an absolute contraindication. Reduction of the prolapse with a pessary may facilitate other forms of sexual expression.

Approximately 50% of all persons older than 65 have arthritic or rheumatic disorders that cause sexual problems in half of them (Brandt and Potts, 1987). Pain is the most troublesome symptom. In addition to their direct effects on joints, several types of arthritis have systemic features, such as the fatigue of rheumatoid arthritis (RA) and systemic lupus (SLE). Sjögren syndrome, which is often associated with RA and SLE, is also associated with diminished vaginal secretions. Corticosteroids can cause decreased libido and sexual responsiveness. Treatment should start with effective communication between partners so that the patient can let the partner know exactly what does and does not hurt. Otherwise, a frown, a wince, or a move away may be interpreted as sexual rejection. Sexual activity can be planned at a time when the affected partner is most energetic and pain free. Physical therapy and local measures (heat, ice) can be used, as can analgesics or muscle relaxants. Narcotics, however, should be avoided because of their adverse effect on libido. Physician advice on a variety of positions and alternative activities may give the couple the information and license they need to explore new ways of sexual expression.

Only one third of women receive any sexual information after myocardial infarction (Kaiser, 1996). Patients should be encouraged to maintain their normal habits of affectionate touching, holding, and hugging during the recovery period to reduce depression and alienation (Bonner and Gendel, 1987). If a patient can undergo a stress test without pain, dyspnea, or arrhythmia, it is likely that sexual activity may be resumed. No position is safer than another for intercourse; a side-by-side position may minimize incisional discomfort after bypass surgery. Stroke causes sexual dysfunction because of physical disability, changes in libido, spousal rejection, and fear of another stroke (Roughan, 1993; Jain, 1987). Decreased libido has been reported to be particularly common in women with right-sided paralysis. Partners should be taught to touch the unaffected side and, when the patient has hemianopsia, to make sure that the spouse can see him or her. Emptying the bowel and bladder before intercourse may prevent incontinence.

Twenty percent to 30% of couples continue to engage in regular sexual activity when one partner has dementia

(Ballard, 1997; Wright, 1991). Although dementia occurs in 10% of persons older than 65, limited knowledge is available about its impact on sexual activity. Women may be affected as patients or as spouses. Indifference and anhedonia are common in Alzheimer's's disease. Although it is a commonly cited sexual disturbance, sexual disinhibition is found in only a low percentage (3% to 4%) of patients with Alzheimer's's disease. (Derouesné, 1996).

Other conditions relatively common in elderly women that may affect sexual functioning include hypothyroidism, Parkinson's disease, drug abuse or misuse, elder abuse or neglect, depression, diabetes mellitus, and breast cancer. The thyroid-stimulating hormone level should be checked during evaluation for decreased desire or performance. Parkinson's disease may cause personality changes; it can be associated with depression, psychosis, dementia, and muscle rigidity leading to sexual dysfunction. Sometimes treatment with levodopa leads to an increase in libido (Mayeux, 1987). Drug or alcohol addiction may be long-standing or it may occur in elderly persons as a response to the late-life stresses of retirement or bereavement. Overuse or underuse of medications may be intentional or inadvertent, controlled by either the patient or the caregivers (Gottheil, 1987). An estimated 500,000 to 1 million elderly persons in the United States are victims of abuse, a situation that often goes undetected (Kallman, 1987). Treatment of depression is confounded by the frequency with which antidepressants cause sexual dysfunction, a phenomenon that affects elderly and younger patients. Surprisingly little is known about the effect of diabetes on female sexual function at any age. Decreased libido and anorgasmia are slightly more common in women with type II diabetes, and lubrication is decreased. However, there is no evidence that peripheral or autonomic neuropathies affect female sexual response (Roughan, 1993). Loss of a breast to mastectomy is known to result in reduced or absent sexual relations in many couples (Steinberg, 1985); in addition, the pain after radiation therapy may limit activity.

In addition to the relationship issues that cause sexual difficulties in persons of all ages, several concerns are pertinent to the aging couple. Men and women may be unaware that with aging, more direct stimulation is needed to achieve excitement, and they are probably unaccustomed to talking about sexual needs (Roughan, 1993). Male erectile dysfunction with age and illness occurs in more than half of men 75 and older (Meston, 1997). This can lead to a sense of failure on the part of either partner and to withdrawal from all sexual expression. Ill health may lead to a fear of causing pain or to a situation in which one person is the caregiver and the other is infantilized (Roughan, 1993). Guilt and grief limit the willingness of many widows to become sexually involved with a new partner (Schneider, 1996).

Sexuality does not disappear when persons lose autonomy. It is viewed with frank hostility in many institutions for the elderly. Men and women are separated, and signs of sexual interest (*e.g.,* masturbation) are suppressed, often with medication. Sexual "incidents" that involve patients with dementia are often used to argue for the prohibition of sexual activity by all residents (Roughan, 1993). Needs and biases of staff and relatives often take precedence over those of residents. Physicians should avoid viewing sexual behavior in institutionalized elderly as aberrant, but solutions to this complex situation are not simple.

Physicians may be discouraged by their perceived lack of ability to provide helpful solutions to women with major social impediments to sexual expression— being single, widowed, or institutionalized. The benefit of attentive and respectful listening to the sexual concerns of an older woman should not be underestimated. Many women have no other person with whom they can discuss such intimate problems.

Vulvovaginal Disorders

Vulvar neoplasms and dermatologic conditions are relatively more common in elderly women; sexually transmitted infectious diseases and certain vulvar pain syndromes are less so. However, the diagnosis and management are essentially the same in all age groups; this topic is appropriately addressed in Chapter 4. In the elderly, it is best to avoid medications as much as possible. Pruritic or dysesthetic vulvar conditions, whether the diagnosis is nonspecific or specific (lichen sclerosis, lichen simplex chronicus), often respond well to simple petroleum jelly or solid vegetable oil when applied twice daily for several weeks.

PERIOPERATIVE CARE

The goal of perioperative care of elderly women is not the successful completion of an operation. *Outcome must be judged by whether the patient has been restored to full functional capacity and whether her quality of life has been improved.* To achieve these goals, the gynecologist must first take the time and effort to understand the patient's current status including her functional capacity, living situation, specific gynecologic symptoms, and personal goals and values.

Although most surgeons are capable of keeping patients alive until hospital discharge, few have the time or the knowledge to provide geriatric patients with the comprehensive care that will avert prolonged disability and promote rapid recovery. Surgeons should consult liberally with geriatricians, nutritionists, physical therapists, and occupational therapists. Proactive nursing participation for preoperative, intraoperative, and postoperative care should be solicited. Nurses should be educated about the importance of early ambulation, the atypical and subtle symptoms of illness, and the management of delirium. A comprehensive review article by Lusis (1996) outlines nursing interventions to promote functional recovery.

It is usually not difficult to obtain informed consent for surgery from either the patient or her representative. However, the elderly suffer several threats to personal autonomy owing to the increased prevalence of dementia, depression, and physical frailty, which can result in greater social and

Table 23-5   Estimated Energy Requirements for Various Activities*

1 MET	Can you take care of yourself?
	Eat, dress, or use the toilet?
	Walk indoors around the house?
	Walk a block or two on level ground at 2-3 mph or 3.2 to 4.8 km/h?
	Do light work around the house like dusting or washing dishes?
4 METS	Climb a flight of stairs or walk up a hill?
	Walk on level ground at 4 mph or 6.4 km/h?
	Run a short distance?
	Do heavy work around the house like scrubbing floors or lifting or moving heavy furniture?
	Participate in moderate recreational activities like golf, bowling, dancing, doubles tennis, or throwing a baseball or football?
10 METS	Participate in strenuous sports like swimming, singles tennis, football, basketball, or skiing?

Modified from American College of Cardiology/American Heart Association Task Force on Practice Guidelines (Committee for Perioperative Cardiovascular Evaluation for Noncardiac Surgery): Guidelines for perioperative cardiovascular evaluation for noncardiac surgery. Reprinted with permission from the American College of Cardiology (Journal of the American College of Cardiology 1996; 27:910-948).

MET, metabolic equivalent.

*Modified from the Duke Activity Status Index (Hlatky MA, Boineau RE, Higginbotham MB, et al: A brief self-administered questionnairre to determine functional capacity. Am J Cardiol 1989; 64:651-654.) and AHA Exercise Standards (Fletcher GF, Balady G, Froelicher VF, et al: Exercise standards: a statement for healchcare professionals from the American Heart Association Writing Group. Circulation 1995; 91:580-615).

economic dependency. Physician judgments are the accepted criteria for determining capacity to consent (Marson, 1997), and decisions are generally straightforward. When there is doubt, a health care proxy is often available to speak for the patient. In the absence of a proxy, there is still no problem if involved family members and friends concur with the decision. If not, the patient's competence must be determined.

Competence, a legal concept, has four requirements. The patient must be able to express choices; understand relevant information; appreciate her disease, its consequences, and the potential outcomes of treatment; and reason and deliberate (Appelbaum and Grisso, 1988). To test a patient's understanding, she should be asked to paraphrase the information presented to her rather than just repeat it. Any physician may testify to a patient's competence; a psychiatrist is not required. Unfortunately, if a patient has mild dementia, no good criteria exist to establish a patient's capability to consent to a procedure, and physicians agree on such a patient's capacity only half the time (Marson, 1997).

Preoperative Evaluation
Risk Assessment

Preoperative medical evaluation enables accurate risk assessment and optimization of medical conditions. Organ

system reserve, number and severity of illnesses, and magnitude of surgery influence risk. Age contributes little to surgical risk, especially before the age of 80. The number of comorbid conditions, especially cardiac disease, is the primary determinant of increased mortality rates from surgery (Tiret, 1986; ACA/AHA, 1996). Reduced functional status also worsens outcome (Mayer-Oakes, 1991; Inouye, 1998). Gynecologic surgery generally falls into low-risk (<1% mortality rate) and intermediate-risk (<5% mortality rate) categories. Age greater than 85 years was associated with increased readmission rates (8% within 30 days) and mortality rates (1.6% within 30 days) in a study of women older than 64 who underwent surgery for incontinence (Sultana, 1997). Because these numbers include patients with and without comorbid conditions, individual risks may be higher or lower.

The surgeon's task is to determine both the presence of disease and the amount of reserve of the cardiac, pulmonary, gastrointestinal, renal, and central nervous (cognitive) systems. In addition, the high incidence of malnutrition and deconditioning in older persons requires that the history include questions about food intake (Who prepares meals? Does the patient have difficulty swallowing?), weight loss, and level of activity.

Cardiac Function

Cardiac disease is the predominant cause of major perioperative morbidity and mortality. The elderly are at increased risk for cardiac morbidity not only because of the increased prevalence of disease but also because the number and resilience of cardiac myocytes and sinoatrial cells diminish with age (ACA/AHA, 1996). In addition, arterial impedance and ventricular stiffness increase, disease is often asymptomatic, and cardiac symptoms may be atypical (Josephson and Lakatta, 1990). A thorough history of cardiac disease and risk factors must be obtained, and functional capacity should be estimated (Table 23-5). Perioperative cardiac risk is increased if a patient is unable to meet a metabolic equivalent demand (ACA/AHA, 1996). Any decrease in functional capacity or possible cardiac symptoms should prompt consideration of a preoperative cardiac stress test to reveal subclinical disease. If a patient is unable to perform vigorous activities, pharmacologic stress testing should be considered, particularly if the planned surgery is extensive or abdominal. Detection of subclinical disease offers the opportunity for preoperative cardiac optimization by either short-term (medication) or long-term (risk-reduction) interventions.

Pulmonary Function

If pneumonia is included, pulmonary complications are the second most common cause of mortality in elderly patients undergoing surgery (McLeskey and Janis, 1990). The aging respiratory system maintains less vital capacity and has more air trapping, a relative obstructive pattern. In addition, pulmonary defenses are impaired in several ways, including a diminished cough reflex and a reduced antibody response

(Tockman, 1990). Functional residual capacity, already diminished by aging, is further reduced by the patient's lying in the supine position and is made worse by general anesthesia and an abdominal incision. These conditions, along with the age-associated increase in closing volume (air trapping), predispose elderly patients to atelectasis with the attendant risks of hypoxemia and infection. A predicted postoperative forced expiratory volume in 1 second of 0.8 L or greater implies a reasonable risk for surgery (Pompei, 1997). The usefulness of routine preoperative pulmonary function tests in the elderly is uncertain. However, as with cardiac evaluation, either an indication of impairment or an inability to "stress" the pulmonary system with exercise is an indication for testing.

Renal and Gastrointestinal Function

Renal changes and the importance of estimation of renal function are discussed in the section on pharmacology. Diminished function increases the risk for postoperative renal failure. Reduced large bowel motility can lead to constipation in the elderly, but the intestinal tract has such a large functional reserve that most patients remain asymptomatic from other age-related changes.

Cognitive Function

Dementia occurs in at least 3% of women 65 years of age and in more than 30% of those older than 85. Preoperative assessment of cognitive function is an important part of establishing the ability to give informed consent. Formal, brief assessment with an instrument such as the Folstein Mini-Mental State Examination (Folstein, 1975) should be conducted before surgery in all patients older than 70 because dementia is underrecognized and underreported by physicians. The finding of dementia or depression (also common in the elderly) should prompt multidisciplinary interventions before and after surgery to minimize the risk for delirium and to enhance rapid recovery (Table 23-6).

Other Medical Conditions

Other conditions common in the elderly include diabetes mellitus, thyroid disease, and the presence of foreign bodies such as artificial joints, steel rods, and pacemakers. During an office visit, an assessment should be made of the best positioning of arthritic extremities during surgery to provide joint protection and adequate exposure. Age is a risk factor for thromboembolic disease, but the general recommendations for thromboembolism prophylaxis apply to all age groups.

Operative Care

The elderly bruise their extremities easily because of decreased subcutaneous connective tissue; the same is probably true of internal tissues. Disability is minimized and recovery time is quicker with vaginal surgery than with abdominal surgery. Regional anesthesia offers some advantages over general anesthesia in the immediate recovery

Table 23-6   Potential Interventions to Reduce Postoperative Delirium

Preoperative
  Psychiatric consultation to address fears, strengthen confidence, reduce anxieties, improve coping
  Education of patient and spouse about postoperative care and interventions for delirium
  Education of patient about common but transient memory loss, impaired concentration, hallucinations
Postoperative
  Familiar items in room (*e.g.,* photographs)
  Orientation of patient with physical contact at each nursing encounter
  Frequent eye contact, touch, and verbal orientation of patient by family
  Avoidance of sleep disruption
  Clock and calendar with today's date
  Maximum sensory input (glasses, hearing aid, dentures, adequate light, touch)
  Early medical evaluation for any alteration in status
  Frequent evaluation by a geriatrician with additional care for confusion

From Cole MG, Primeau F, McCusker J: Effectiveness of interventions to prevent delirium in hospitalized patients: A systematic review. *Can Med Assoc J* 1996; 155:1263-1268.

period. However, the anesthesiologists's competence in managing elderly patients is more important than the type of anesthesia used. Outcomes are equivalent with well-administered general or regional anesthesia.

Four interventions before and during surgery will help avoid complications:

Preoperative dehydration must be avoided (Josephone and Lakatta, 1990). A patient should be given intravenous fluids long before the start of surgery unless hers is the first procedure of the day. To maintain cardiac output, the older heart is more dependent on preload than the younger one. It is less able to increase heart rate when needed and relies instead on inotropy.

Hypothermia should be avoided (Miller, 1997). The elderly are particularly vulnerable to heat loss and its potential for cardiac dysrhythmias or impaired ventricular function. Aluminized and forced-air body coverings are useful. Preoperative patient warming, warm operating room temperature, and warming of skin preparation solutions, intravenous solutions, and inspired gases may also be helpful.

Careful attention should be given to fluid balance and composition. The elderly kidney is less able to accommodate rapid fluid and electrolyte shifts. Hypovolemia should be treated with normal saline rather than with lactated Ringer's solution because low renal perfusion aggravates the aged kidney's impaired ability to excrete an alkaline load (the lactate) (Zawanda, 1990).

Elderly skin and joints are fragile and need appropriate attention. Bony surfaces should be padded. Joints should not be excessively flexed or extended. If arthritis of the hip is a significant problem, the patient should be positioned before the induction of general anesthesia to prevent damage.

Postoperative Management
Bed Rest

The bed is a dangerous place for the elderly. Most of the physiologic impairments brought on by aging worsen in the supine position. With bed rest, deconditioning occurs rapidly, plasma volume diminishes, baroreceptors become less sensitive (with a resultant increased risk for syncope and falls), closing lung volume increases and fewer alveoli ventilate, arterial oxygen tension reduces, and skeletal demineralization accelerates (Creditor, 1993). Barriers to ambulation also contribute to sensory deprivation and to the increase in urinary incontinence seen in elderly hospital patients. The physician should remove "tethering" tubes and lines as quickly as possible and should encourage the patient to sit upright and move around despite medical "accessories." With a proactive approach, the physician and the health care team can limit the functional decline and medical complications that so often lead to loss of independence and to institutionalization after hospital admission.

Delirium

To reduce the incidence and severity of delirium, familiar persons should be with the patient as much as possible (Table 23-6). Any report of "sundowning" requires that a medical evaluation be completed before treatment is initiated to review potential causes, such as hypoxia, metabolic derangement, infection, central nervous system events, myocardial ischemia, fecal impaction, urinary retention, sensory deprivation, and medication side effects. Anticholinergic medications often cause confusion in the elderly. Therefore, diphenhydramine and similar agents should not be given for sedation or sleep. After medical evaluation, patients with delirium should first be treated nonpharmacologically with frequent verbal and physical contact, additional assistance from family members, and nearness to the nursing station. Soft lights, familiar photographs, a quiet room, and background music may help. A patient who is awake at 2 AM may be a nuisance to the nursing staff, but this is not an indication for sedation. Agitation can be controlled by lorazepam 0.25 mg or haloperidol 0.25 mg, with slowly increased doses. Lorazepam may cause disinhibition and lead to worse behavior in a demented patient. Akathisia (restlessness, pacing, agitation) may occur as a side effect of haloperidol (Pompei, 1997).

Pain Management

Adequate pain control is an important part of early ambulation and deep breathing. This is accomplished in much the same manner as it is with younger patients (Egbert, 1996). However, all analgesics have a greater potential for therapeutic and toxic effects in the elderly. Intrathecal and epidural opioids are usually well tolerated, but they carry a greater risk for respiratory depression and urinary retention than they do in younger patients. Self-administered intravenous narcotics are preferable to intermittent intramuscular injections because of the greater risk for respiratory depression with the latter. Patients with dementia should be given regularly scheduled medications. Meperidine should be avoided because its active metabolite, normeperidine, may accumulate as a result of reduced renal function. Morphine, hydromorphone, and oxymorphone can be given rectally for patients with poor tolerance for parenteral and oral narcotics. The potency is similar to that for the oral route. Nonsteroidal anti-inflammatory drugs (NSAIDs) should be used on a scheduled parenteral, rectal, or oral basis to spare narcotics, enhance analgesia, and decrease inflammatory mediators, with appropriate dose reductions for impaired renal function. NSAIDs should be avoided in frail, elderly patients with dehydration, preexisting renal disease, cirrhosis, or congestive heart failure because of the higher risk for acute renal failure. Propoxyphene (Darvon) should not be used because it is no more potent than acetaminophen, but it can induce or exacerbate confusion. Delirious patients can and do remember pain. If delirium is diagnosed, efforts should be continued to provide pain relief by changing rather than discontinuing analgesics.

Infections

The atypical presentation of infectious disease with common geriatric syndromes (confusion, falling, incontinence) is discussed earlier in this chapter. In addition, it should be noted that fever, leukocytosis, and pain are commonly diminished or absent in the elderly. Because the baseline temperature of an elderly person is often 1°F to 2°F below normal, a temperature of 99°F (37.2°C) or higher may be significant.

Discharge Planning

Although the postoperative discharge needs of younger patients are determined best during recovery, services required for elderly patients often can be anticipated before surgery or early in the postoperative course. Medicare pays for home-health care nursing only if skilled services are required. These include dressing changes, wound assessments, catheter care, and administration of intravaginal medications. Nurses may go into the home to set up medications and check compliance if the patient is visually impaired. Home nurses can also monitor the effects of new medications such as warfarin or antihypertensives, particularly when it requires undue effort on the part of the patient (transportation difficulties, hearing or visual impairments) to come to a physician's office.

If home-care nursing is justified, Medicare will pay for a home health aide to bathe the patient and provide personal care. An aide may take care of light housekeeping if a patient is placed on certain medical restrictions, such as no lifting during the postoperative recovery. Medicare may reimburse physical and occupational therapists for adjunct treatment, such as for arthritis or immobility, that contributes to incontinence.

Often the physician is uncertain of the patient's situation or need, and there may be no family member available for assistance. Medicare sometimes authorizes one home health nurse visit for assessment. Alternatively, the Area Agency on Aging (AAA) Outreach Service can be contacted. Each state, county or district has a federally funded and mandated AAA. An outreach representative can go into the home and assess needs. The representative may then be able to obtain a Medicaid-funded home health aide.

CANCER SCREENING

Cancer is the second leading cause of death. Less widely appreciated is the fact that 55% of all cancers occur in the 13% of the population older than 65. Although absolute cancer incidence rates rise in the middle years and decline in the later years, the age-specific incidence rates rise progressively throughout life. Cancer incidence declines after the age of 95, but at this advanced age, clinical diagnoses significantly underestimate the incidence of cancer and the prevalence of cancer deaths (Stanta, 1997).

Cancer Mortality

Leading causes of cancer deaths in women aged 55 to 74 years of age are lung, breast, and colon. After age 74, lung cancer loses some of its "lead," death rates from colon cancer rise dramatically, and rates of breast cancer mortality continue to rise. The result is that mortality rates are similar for each of these cancers in this age group (Landis, 1998). Among women 85 and older, however, colorectal cancer is by far the leading cause of death from cancer (US Bureau of the Census, 1997). After breast cancer, endometrial cancer is the most common gynecologic malignancy in older women, followed by ovarian and cervical cancer (Termrungruanglert, 1997). Compared to women 40 to 65 years of age, the risk for one of these malignancies to develop in a woman older than 65 is twice as high for uterine cancer, three times as high for ovarian cancer, and one-tenth higher for cervical cancer. The prognosis is worse for elderly women with these cancers largely because of delayed detection and more advanced stages. Mortality rates in women older than 65 are 300% higher for endometrial cnacer and 50% higher for ovarian and cervical cancer than in younger women (Termrungruanglert, 1997). Of these six cancers, mortality rates can be reduced if patients are screened for three of them: breast, colorectal, and cervical.

Age Limits of Screening

Age cutoffs for screening are controversial, largely because of the omission of elderly women from screening trials. Few data are available about the specific usefulness of diagnostic tests in elderly patients, the precise risk with testing, or the efficacy of or risk with treatment. Guidelines must be ex-

Table 23-7   Cancer Screening Recommendations in Healthy Elderly Women

Papanicolaou smears
  Every 1 to 3 years*
  Every 5 years in women who have undergone hysterectomy*
Mammograms
  Annually
Home fecal occult blood
  Annually†
Sigmoidoscopy
  Every 5 years†

*See text.
†Alternative screening methods include colonoscopy every 10 years or air-contrast barium enema every 5 to 10 years.

trapolated from data about younger patients and disease processes.

Health Status

Justification for cancer screening is strongly influenced by a patient's current health and functional status. Average life expectancies suggest that most women should be screened beyond age 85 (Table 23-7). Screening for cancer should be discontinued if the patient is debilitated to the extent that either she or her family member(s) decides that early diseases should not be aggressively treated. This is not to say that symptoms should not be investigated. In an elderly patient who is debilitated or has dementia, screening mammography or Papanicolaou smears may be omitted, but the cause of vaginal bleeding should still be investigated through examination, biopsy, or ultrasonography to plan a future course of action, including supportive care.

Quality of Life

Cancer screening programs are devised to prevent cancer by the detection of precancerous conditions or to find cancer in its early, curable stages. It is difficult to justify *not* screening the elderly for conditions more common or more lethal in this age group. For instance, elderly women are more likely to die *of* breast cancer than *with* it. And even if an elderly woman with breast cancer adds only a few months to her life because of mammography screening, she may avoid months or years of debilitating disease during her remaining "golden" years by finding and treating cancer in the early stages. Moreover, several studies have shown that the elderly withstand well-managed cancer surgery, chemotherapy, and radiation almost as well as younger women. A decision analysis about breast cancer screening showed that only if the operative mortality rate reached a level between 27% and 62% were the risks of screening as high as the benefits (Mandelblatt, 1992). Robinson and Behgé (1997) provide a thorough discussion of individual decisions based on quality of life issues in their review article.

Breast Cancer Screening (Mammography)

Breast cancer is the most common cancer in elderly women, and it carries the third highest mortality rate. Approximately 48% of newly diagnosed breast cancers occur in women 65 and older, but nearly 57% of the breast cancer deaths occur in these same women (Caplan, 1997). Older women are more likely to be estrogen-receptor positive, but when they are matched for it and for disease stage and comorbidity, breast cancer appears to be no less aggressive in elderly women than in younger women (Rosen, 1985; McKenna, 1994; Smart, 1997).

Some strides have been made in the diagnosis and treatment of elderly white women with breast cancer, but they have not been as demonstrable in elderly black women. Mortality rates declined by 1.6% per year from 1989 to 1992 in white women aged 60 to 79 (and in those younger than 60), but not in those older than 80. There has been no decline in mortality rates for black women of any age (Chevarly and White, 1997). Approximately 27% of women older than 65 have never had a mammogram. (Caplan, 1997). Elderly and socioeconomically disadvantaged women undergo less mammography and clinical breast examination screening.

Screening and aggressive treatment of elderly women are indicated and justified on the bases of increased life expectancy, response to therapy approximately equal to that of younger women (McKenna, 1994; Kennedy, 1989) and improved quality of life in those treated for early-stage as opposed to late-stage disease (Feussner, 1997). Annual mammography and clinical breast examination are recommended until worsened health status dictates otherwise. If a patient has a life expectancy of at least 3 years, screening is justified (Robinson and Beghé, 1997). In particular, elderly women taking estrogen therapy should be encouraged to undergo annual mammography because of the probable increased risk for breast cancer and the often decreased sensitivity of mammography because of denser breast tissue.

Colorectal Cancer Screening

Seventy-three percent of all cases of colorectal cancer in women occur in those older than 65 (Feussner, 1997). The annual incidence increases with age; there are up to 400 cases per 100,000 women age 85 and older. Mortality rates have decreased 32% for women in the past 20 years, reflecting decreasing incidence and improved survival (Cancer Facts & Figs, 1997). The adenomatous polyp is the precursor of most, if not all, colorectal cancers (Cohen, 1996). It develops in one third of the population at age 60 (Geul, 1997). Increasing evidence indicates that endoscopic polypectomy prevents colorectal cancer (Geul, 1997; Cancer Facts & Figs, 1997).

Despite our ability to detect and remove colorectal cancer precursors, the optimum screening method remains controversial because none is simple, cheap, sensitive, and risk free. Screening strategies involve digital rectal examinations (DRE), serial fecal occult blood tests (FOBT) obtained at home, and sigmoidoscopy, colonoscopy, and barium enema. DRE has not been shown to reduce mortality rates from colon cancer, nor has office FOBT. Several studies show a small but significant reduction in mortality rates with annual home FOBT screening. Because of the marked increase in colorectal cancer incidence with age, the positive predictive value of the FOBT improves in older cohorts (10 colonoscopies per cancer detected) (Robinson and Beghé, 1997). Flexible sigmoidoscopy screening lowers colon cancer mortality rates more effectively than FOBT. The American Cancer Society recommends annual FOBTs and flexible sigmoidoscopy every 5 years after the age of 50, or colonoscopy every 10 years, or double-contrast barium enema every 5 to 10 years for persons at average risk. Because of the prolonged interval between the appearance of polyps and the development of cancer, benefit would decline as life expectancy falls below 10 years, and it would probably be gone with less than 5 years of life remaining (Robinson and Beghé, 1997).

Cervical Cancer Screening

Twenty-five percent of cervical cancers and 41% of the deaths from this disease occur in women 65 and older (Cervical Cancer, 1996). Elderly women have poorer survival rates with cervical cancer, in part because of the less frequent screening and the more advanced disease stage at the time of diagnosis. For reasons that are unclear, older age is also a risk factor; one theory proposes that more carcinomas in the elderly are not associated with the human papillomavirus and are more biologically aggressive (Adami, 1994).

Epidemiologic data indicate that women who are at low risk but who have a uterus or a cervix in situ can reduce their screening intervals. The American College of Obstetrics and Gynecology and the American Cancer Society recommend that after three normal annual Papinicolaou smears, women can be screened every 3 years. Other organizations recommend discontinuing cervical cytology altogether in recently screened women older than 65 (Feussner, 1997). To consider with confidence that a younger patient is at low risk, a thorough sexual history and an abbreviated medical history must be elicited. This includes age at first intercourse, number of lifetime sex partners, exposure to additional sex partners through male partners, sexually transmitted diseases, smoking history, other substance abuse, and immunosuppression (e.g., chronic steroids for pulmonary or rheumatoid disease). In the elderly, there are no data evaluating the importance of sexual history or other history to the development of cervical cancer. It is plausible that a less active squamocolumnar junction affords some protection from viral and other influences, but this is unknown. Alternatively, if the theory is correct that more cervical cancers in the elderly are biologically aggressive, the screening interval should not be extended.

It is clear from the increased lethality of cervical cancer in the elderly that current screening practices are inadequate in this population. Annual Papanicolaou smears probably should be taken for the healthy elderly woman who has a cervix in situ because of the uncertainty of her sexual history, the uncertainty of its importance, her potential exposure to viruses if she is sexually active, the inevitable degree of noncompliance, and the possibility of more biologically aggressive cancers with advanced age. It should be kept in mind, however, that the greatest reduction in cervical cancer in the elderly would be achieved by targeting populations who have not been screened in more than 3 years (Wain, 1992; Robinson and Beghé, 1997).

Papanicolaou smears are not useful in women who have had total hysterectomy (*corpus* and *cervix uteri*) for benign disease (Pearce, 1996). ACOG recommends "periodic" vaginal cuff Papanicolaou smears in women with any risk factors for cervical cancer or with any endometrial, vaginal, or vulvar neoplasia (ACOG, 1995). Data regarding the usefulness of vaginal cytologic smears in the elderly are lacking. Even in those who have had remote hysterectomies for neoplastic disease, it seems unlikely that a related neoplasia would be detected. However, it is difficult to determine in some elderly women that the cervix has been removed. Because of this and because of frequent uncertainty about the indication for hysterectomy, such as for cervical dysplasia, and the general benefits of pelvic examination, it is reasonable to continue obtaining Papanicolaou smears every 5 years even in healthy women who report that they have undergone hysterectomy.

REFERENCES

Abrutyn EA, Berlin J, Mossey J, et al: Does treatment of asymptomatic bacteriuria in older ambulatory women reduce subsequent symptoms of urinary tract infection? *J Am Geriatr Soc* 1996; 44:293-295.

ACOG committee opinion #152, Committee on Gynecologic Practice, Washington, DC, March 1995, American College of Obstetrics and Gynecology.

Adami H-O, Ponten J, Sparen P, et al: Survival trend after invasive cervical cancer diagnosis in Sweden before and after cytologic screening. *Cancer* 1994; 73:140-147.

American College of Cardiology/American Heart Association Task Force on Practice Guidelines (Committee for Perioperative Cardiovascular Evaluation for Noncardiac Surgery): Guidelines for perioperative cardiovascular evaluation for noncardiac surgery. *J Am Coll Cardiol* 1996; 27:910-948.

Appelbaum PS, Grisso T: Assessing patients' capacities to consent to treatment. *N Engl J Med* 1988; 319:1635-1638.

Arstila T, Huovinen S, Lager K, et al: Positive correlation between the age of patients and the degree of antimicrobial resistance among urinary strains of *Escherichia coli*. *J Infect* 1994; 29:9-16.

Avorn J, Gurwitz JH: Principles of pharmacology. In Cassel CK, Cohen HJ, Larson EB, et al, editors: *Geriatric medicine*, ed 3, New York, 1997, Springer-Verlag.

Ballard CG, Solis M, Gahir M, et al: Sexual relationships in married dementia sufferers. *Int J Geriatr Psychiatry* 1997; 12:447-451.

Barkham TMS, Martin FC, Eykyn SJ: Delay in the diagnosis of bacteraemic urinary tract infection in elderly patients. *Age Ageing* 1996; 25:130-132.

Barnhart KT: Is there evidence to replace DHEA sulfate in aging men and women? *Menopausal Med* 1997; 5:6-12.

Beaujean DJMA, Blok HEM, Vandenbroucke-Grauls CMJE, et al: Surveillance of nosocomial infections in geriatric patients. *J Hosp Infect* 1997; 36:275-284.

Benitez del Castillo JM, del Rio T, Garcia-Sanchez J: Effects of estrogen use on lens transmittance in postmenopausal women. *Ophthalmology* 1997; 104:970-973.

Bergan T: Quinolones in the elderly. *Drugs* 1995; 49(suppl 2):112-114.

Berglund A, Eisemann M, Lalos A, et al: Social adjustment and spouse relationships among women with stress incontinence before and after surgical treatment. *Soc Sci Med* 1996; 42:1537-1544.

Bjornson DC, Rovers JP, Burian JA, et al: Pharmacoepidemiology of urinary tract infections in Iowa Medicaid patients in urban long-term care facilities. *Ann Pharmacother* 1997; 31:837-841.

Black DM: Screening and treatment in the elderly to reduce osteoporotic fracture risk. *Br J Obstet Gynaecol* 1996a; 103(suppl 13):2-8.

Black DM, Cummings SR, Karpf DB, et al: Randomised trial of effect of alendronate on risk of fracture in women with existing vertebral fractures. *Lancet* 1996b; 348:1535-1541.

Bo K: Physiotherapy in the treatment of urinary incontinence in elderly women. *Tidsskr Nor Laegeforen* 1997; 117:2623-2626.

Boerrigter PJ, van de Weijer PHM, Baak JPA, et al: Endometrial response in estrogen replacement therapy quarterly combined with a progestogen. *Maturitas* 1996; 24:63-71.

Bonner EJ, Gendel ES: Sexual counseling for the elderly patient after myocardial infarction. *Med Aspects Hum Sexuality* 1987; 21:100-108. [Supplement].

Boysen G, Nyboe J, Appleyard M, et al: Stroke incidence and risk factors for stroke in Copenhagen, Denmark. *Stroke* 1988; 19:1345-1353.

Brandt KD, Potts MK: Arthritis in the elderly: Assessment and management of sexual problems. *Med Aspects Hum Sexuality* 1987; 21(suppl):57-67.

Bretschneider JG, McCoy NL: Sexual interest and behavior in healthy 80 to 102 year olds. *Arch Sex Behav* 1988; 17:109-129.

Brinton LA, Hoover R, Fraumeni JF Jr: Menopausal oestrogens and breast cancer risk: An expanded case-control study. *Br J Cancer* 1986; 54:825-832.

Burns PA, Pranikoff K, Nochajski TH, et al: A comparison of effectiveness of biofeedback and pelvic muscle exercise treatment of stress incontinence in older community-dwelling women. *J Gerontol* 1993; 48:M167-M174.

Bush TL, Barrett-Connor E, Cowan LD, et al: Cardiovascular mortality and noncontraceptive use of estrogen in women: Results from the Lipid Research Clinics Program Follow-up Study. *Circulation* 1987; 75:1102-1109.

Calle EE, Miracle-McMahill HL, Thun MJ, et al: Estrogen replacement therapy and risk of fatal colon cancer in a prospective cohort of postmenopausal women. *J Natl Cancer Inst* 1995; 87:517-523.

Cancer Facts and Figures—1997. American Cancer Society.

Caplan LS: Disparities in breast cancer screening: Is it ethical? *Public Health Rev* 1997; 25:31-41.

Cardozo L, Versi E: Oestrogens and the lower urinary tract. In Asch RH, Studd JWW, editors: *Progress in reproductive medicine, vol 1*, New York, 1993, Parthenon.

Carr LK, Walsh PJ, Abraham VE, Webster GD: Favorable outcome of pubovaginal slings for geriatric women with stress incontinence. *J Urol* 1997; 157:125-128.

Cauley JA, Seeley DG, Ensrud K, et al: Estrogen replacement therapy and fractures in older women: Study of Osteoporotic Fractures Research Group. *Ann Intern Med* 1995; 122:9-16.

Chandler JM, Hadley EC: Exercise to improve physiologic and functional performance in old age. *Clin Geriatr Med* 1996; 12:761-784.

Chapuy M-C, Arlot ME, Duboeuf F, et al: Vitamin D_3 and calcium to prevent hip fractures in elderly women. *N Engl J Med* 1992; 327:1637-1642.

Chevarley F, White E: Recent trends in breast cancer mortality among white and black women. *Am J Public Health* 1997; 87:775-781.

Childs SJ, Egan RJ: Bacteriuria and urinary infections in the elderly. *Urol Clin North Am* 1996; 23:43-54.

Cohen LB: Colorectal cancer: A primary care approach to screening. *Geriatrics* 1996; 51:45-50.

Colditz GA, Hankinson SE, Hunter DJ, et al: The use of estrogens and progestins and the risk of breast cancer in postmenopausal women. *N Engl J Med* 1995; 332:1589-1593.

Cole MG, Primeau F, McCusker J: Effectiveness of interventions to prevent delirium in hospitalized patients: A systematic review. *Can Med Assoc J* 1996; 155:1263-1268.

Collaborative Group on Hormonal Factors in Breast Cancer: Breast cancer and hormone replacement therapy: Collaborative reanalysis of data from 51 epidemiological studies of 52 705 women with breast cancer and 108 411 women without breast cancer. *Lancet* 1997; 350:1047-1059.

Couillard DR, Deckard-Janatpour KA, Stone AR: The vaginal wall sling: A compressive suspension procedure for recurrent incontinence in elderly patients. *Urology* 1994; 43:203-208.

Creditor MC: Hazards of hospitalization of the elderly. *Ann Intern Med* 1993; 118:219-223.

Culp K, Tripp-Reimer T, Wadl K, et al: Screening for acute confusion in elderly long-term care residents. *J Neurosci Nurs* 1997; 29:86-88,95-100.

Cummings SR, Nevitt MC, Browner WS, et al: Risk factors for hip fracture in white women: Study of Osteoporotic Fractures Research Group. *N Engl J Med* 1995; 332:767-773.

Dawson-Hughes B: Calcium and vitamin D nutritional needs of elderly women. *J Nutr* 1996(April); 126(4):1165S-1167S.

Dawson-Hughes B, Harris SS, Krall EA, et al: Effect of calcium and vitamin D supplementation on bone density in men and women 65 years of age or older. *N Engl J Med* 1997; 337:670-676.

Derouesné C, Guigot J, Chermat V, et al: Sexual behavioral changes in Alzheimer's disease. *Alzheimer's Dis Assoc Disord* 1996; 10:86-92.

Eastell R: Treatment of postmenopausal osteoporosis. *N Engl J Med* 1998; 338:736-746.

Egbert AE: Postoperative pain management in the frail elderly. *Clin Geriatr Med* 1996; 12:583-599.

Elbadawi A, Subbarao VY, Resnick NM: Structural basis of geriatric voiding dysfunction, VI: Validation and update of diagnostic criteria in 71 detrusor biopsies. *J Urol* 1997; 150:1802-1813.

El-Maraghy MA, El-Badawy N, Wafa GA, et al: Progesterone challenge test in postmenopausal women at high risk. *Maturitas* 1994; 19:53-57.

Elward K, Larson EB: Benefits of exercise for older adults. *Clin Geriatr Med* 1992; 8:35-50.

Ernest JT: Changes and diseases of the aging eye. In Cassel CK, Cohen HJ, Larson EB, et al, editors: *Geriatric Medicine*, ed 3; New York, 1997, Springer-Verlag.

Ettinger B, Friedman GD, Bush T, et al: Reduced mortality associated with long-term postmenopausal estrogen therapy. *Obstet Gynecol* 1996; 87:6-12.

Ettinger B, Genant HK, Cann CE: Long-term estrogen replacement therapy prevents bone loss and fractures. *Ann Int Med* 1985; 102:319-324.

Ettinger B, Selby J, Citron JT, et al: Cyclic hormone replacement therapy using quarterly progestin. *Obstet Gynecol* 1994; 83:693-700.

Evans SF, Davie MWJ: Low and conventional dose transdermal oestradiol are equally effective at preventing bone loss in spine and femur at all postmenopausal ages. *Clin Endocrinol* 1996; 44:79-84.

The Eye Disease Case-Control Study Group: Risk factors for neovascular age-related macular degeneration. *Arch Ophthalmol* 1992; 110:1701-1708.

Faerber GJ: Endoscopic collagen injection therapy in elderly women with type I stress urinary incontinence. *J Urol* 1996; 155:512-514.

Fahs MC, Mandelblatt J, Schechter C, et al: Cost effectiveness of cervical cancer screening for the elderly. *Ann Intern Med* 1992; 117:520-527.

Falkeborn M, Persson I, Terént A, et al: Hormone replacement therapy and the risk of stroke. *Arch Intern Med* 1993; 153:1201-1209.

Felson DT, Zhang Y, Hannan MT, et al: The effect of postmenopausal estrogen therapy on bone density in elderly women. *N Engl J Med* 1993; 329:1141-1146.

Feussner JR, Oddone EZ, Wong JG: Screening for cancer. In Cassel CK, Cohen HJ, Larson EB, et al, editors: *Geriatric Medicine*, ed 3; New York, 1997, Springer-Verlag.

Finucane FF, Madans JH, Bush TL, et al: Decreased risk of stroke among postmenopausal hormone users. *Arch Intern Med* 1993; 153:73-79.

Folstein MF, Folstein SE, McHugh PR: "Mini-Mental State:" A practical method for grading the cognitive state of patients for the clinician. *J Psychiatr Res* 1975; 12:189-198.

Fonda D, Woodward M, D'Astoli M, et al: Sustained improvement of subjective quality of life in older community-dwelling people after treatment of urinary incontinence. *Age Ageing* 1995; 24:283-286.

Fox KM, Hawkes WG, Hebel JR, et al: Mobility after hip fracture predicts health outcomes. *J Am Geriatr Soc* 1998; 46:169-173.

Genant HK, Lucas J, Weiss S, et al: Low-dose esterified estrogen therapy: Effects on bone, plasma estradiol concentrations, endometrium, and lipid levels. *Arch Intern Med* 1997; 157:2609-2615.

Geul KW, Bosman FT, van Blankenstein M, et al: Prevention of colorectal cancer: Costs and effectiveness of sigmoidoscopy. *Scand J Gastroenterol Suppl* 1997; 223:79-87.

Gillan G, Stanton SL: Long-term follow-up of surgery for urinary incontinence in elderly women. *Br J Urol* 1984; 56:478-481.

Goebel JA, Birge SJ, Price SC, et al: Estrogen replacement therapy and postural stability in the elderly. *Am J Otol* 1995; 16:470-474.

Golomb J, Goldwasser B, Mashiach S: Raz endoscopic bladder-neck suspension in women younger than 65 years compared with elderly women: A 3-year experience. *Urology* 1994; 43:40-43.

Gottheil E: Drug use, misuse and abuse by the elderly. *Med Aspects Hum Sexuality* 1987 (suppl); 21:29-37.

Grady D, Rubin SM, Petitti DB, et al: Hormone therapy to prevent disease and prolong life in post-menopausal women. *Ann Intern Med* 1992; 117:1016-1041.

Greenspan SL, Resnick NM: Geriatric endocrinology. In Greenspan FS, Strewler GJ, editors: *Basic and Clinical Endocrinology*, ed 5, Stamford, Conn., 1997, Appleton and Lange.

Grey AB, Cundy TF, Reid IR: Continuous combined oestrogen/progestin therapy is well tolerated and increases bone density at the hip and spine in post-menopausal osteoporosis. *Clin Endocrinol* 1994; 40:671-677.

Griffiths DJ, Harrison G, Moore K, et al: Variability of post-void residual urine volumes in the elderly. *Urol Res* 1996; 24:23-26.

Griffiths-Jones M, Abrams P: The Stamey endoscopic bladder-neck suspension in the elderly. *Br J Urol* 1990; 65:170-172.

Grisso JA, Kelsey JL, Strom BL, et al: Risk factors for hip fracture in black women. *N Engl J Med* 1994; 330:1555-1559.

Grodstein F, Martinez ME, Platz EA, et al: Postmenopausal hormone use and risk for colorectal cancer and adenoma. *Ann Intern Med* 1998, 128:705-711.

Grodstein F, Stampfer MJ, Manson JE, et al: Postmenopausal estrogen and progestin use and the risk of cardiovascular disease. *N Engl J Med* 1996; 335:453-461. [Erratum, *N Engl J Med* 1996; 335:1406.]

Grover SR, Quinn MA: Is there any value in bimanual pelvic examination as a screening test? *Med J Aust* 1995; 162:408-410.

Hales AM, Chamberlain CG, Murphy CR, et al: Estrogen protects against cataract induced by transforming growth factor-beta. *J Exp Med* 1997; 185:273-280.

Hammar ML, Lindgren R, Berg GE, et al: Effects of hormone replacement therapy on the postural balance among postmenopausal women. *Obstet Gynecol* 1996; 88:955-960.

Harding GK, Nicolle LE, Ronald AR, et al: How long should catheter-acquired urinary tract infection in women be treated? A randomized controlled study. *Ann Intern Med* 1991; 114:713-719.

Hartmann BW, Kirchengast S, Albrecht A, et al: Absorption of orally supplied natural estrogens correlated with age and somatometric parameters. *Gynecol Endocrinol* 1994; 8:101-107.

Harvey M-A, Versi E: The climacteric bladder. In Lentz G, editor: *Urogynecology: diagnosis and treatment of female urinary incontinence, Current Topics in Obstetrics and Gynecology.* London: 1998, Edward Arnold.

Henderson BE, Paganini-Hill A, Ross RK: Decreased mortality in users of estrogen replacement therapy. *Arch Intern Med* 1991; 151:75-78.

Herschorn S, Steele DJ, Radomski SB: Followup of intraurethral collagen for female stress urinary incontinence. *J Urol* 1996; 156:1305-1309.

Hilton P: Urinary incontinence during intercourse: A common but rarely volunteered symptom. *Br J Obstet Gynaecol* 1988; 95:377-381.

Hirvonen E, Salmi T, Puolakka J, et al: Can progestin be limited to every third month only in postmenopausal women taking estrogen? *Maturitas* 1995; 21:39-44.

Holley RL, Varner RE, Gleason BP, et al: Sexual function after sacrospinous ligament fixation for vaginal vault prolapse. *J Reprod Med* 1996; 41:355-358.

Holmberg L, Boman G, Böttiger LE: Adverse reactions to nitrofurantoin. *Am J Med* 1980; 69:733-738.

Inouye SK, Peduzzi PN, Robinson JT, et al: Importance of functional measures in predicting mortality among older hospitalized patients. *JAMA* 1998; 279:1183-1193.

Jain H, Shamoian CA, Mobarak A: Sexual disorders in the elderly. *Medical Aspects of Human Sexuality* 1987(suppl); 21:14-25.

Josephson RA, Lakatta EG: Cardiovascular changes in the elderly. In Katlic MR, editor: *Geriatric surgery: Comprehensive care of the elderly patient*, Baltimore, 1990, Urban and Schwarzenberg.

Kaiser FE: Sexuality in the elderly. *Urol Clin North Am* 1996; 23:99-109.

Kallman H: Detecting abuse in the elderly. *Medl Aspects Hum Sexuality* 1987(suppl); 21:89-99.

Kanis JA, Johnell O, Gullberg B, et al: Evidence for efficacy of drugs affecting bone metabolism in preventing hip fractures. *BMJ* 1992; 305:1124-1128.

Karpf DB, Shapiro DR, Seeman E, et al: Prevention of nonvertebral fractures by alendronate. *JAMA* 1997; 277:1159-1164.

Keil DP, Felson DT, Anderson JJ, et al: Hip fracture and the use of estrogens in postmenopausal women. *N Engl J Med* 1987; 317:1169-1174.

Kennedy AW, Flagg JS, Webster KD: Gynecologic cancer in the very elderly. *Gynecol Oncol* 1989; 32:49-54.

Khullar V, Cardozo LD, Abbott K, Anders K: GAX collagen in the treatment of urinary incontinence in elderly women: A two year follow up. *Br J Obstet Gynaecol* 1997; 104:96-99.

King MB, Tinetti ME: A multifactorial approach to reducing serious falls. *Clin Geriatr Med* 1996; 12:745-759.

Labrie F, Diamond P, Cusan L, et al: Effect of 12-month dehydroepiandrosterone replacement therapy on bone, vagina, and endometrium in postmenopausal women. *J Clin Endocrin Metabol* 1997; 82:3498-3505.

Landis SH, Murray T, Bolden, S, et al: Cancer statistics, 1998. *Ca Cancer J Clin* 1998: 48:6-30.

Leach GE, Dmochowski RR, Appell RA, et al: Female Stress Urinary Incontinence Clinical Guidelines Panel summary report on surgical management of female stress urinary incontinence: The American Urological Association. *J Urol* 1997; 158: 875-880.

Leiblum S, Bachmann G, Kemmann E, et al: Vaginal atrophy in the postmenopausal woman: The importance of sexual activity and hormones. *JAMA* 1983; 249:2195-2198.

Leistevuo T, Isoaho R, Klaukka T, et al: Prescription of antimicrobial agents to elderly people in relation to the type of infection. *Age Ageing* 1997; 26:345-351.

Lichtenstein MJ: Hearing and visual impairments. *Clin Geriatr Med* 1992; 8:173-182.

Lindsay R, Tohme JF: Estrogen treatment of patients with established postmenopausal osteoporosis. *Obstet Gynecol* 1990; 76:290-295.

Lips P, Graafmans WC, Ooms ME, et al: Vitamin D supplementation and fracture incidence in elderly persons. *Ann Intern Med* 1996; 124:400-406.

Lufkin EG, Wahner HW, O'Fallon WM, et al: Treatment of postmenopausal osteoporosis with transdermal estrogen. *Ann Intern Med* 1992; 117:1-9.

Lusis SA: The challenges of nursing elderly surgical patients. *AORN J* 1996; 64:954-962.

Macia M, Novo A, Ces J, et al: Progesterone challenge test for the assessment of endometrial pathology in asymptomatic menopausal women. *Int J Gynecol Obstet* 1993; 40:145-149.

Malatesta VS, Chambless DL, Pollack M, et al: Widowhood, sexuality and aging: A life span analysis. *J Sex Marital Therapy* 1988; 14:49-61.

Mandelblatt JS, Wheat ME, Monane M, et al: Breast cancer screening for elderly women with and without comorbid conditions: A decision analysis model. *Ann Intern Med* 1992; 116:722-730.

Manolio TA, Furberg CD, Shemanski L, et al: Associations of postmenopausal estrogen use with cardiovascular disease and its risk factors in older women. *Circulation* 1993; 88:2163-2171.

Marson DC, McInturff B, Hawkins L, et al: Consistency of physician judgments of capacity to consent in mild Alzheimer's's disease. *J Am Geriatr Soc* 1997; 45:453-457.

Mayer-Oakes SA, Oye RK, Leake B: Predictors of mortality in older patients following medical intensive care: The importance of functional status. *J Am Geriatr Soc* 1991; 39:862-868.

Mayeux R: The psychiatric and sexual complications of Parkinson's disease. *Med Aspects Hum Sexuality* 1987(suppl); 21:68-72.

McKenna RJ Sr: Clinical aspects of cancer in the elderly: Treatment decisions, treatment choices, follow-up. *Cancer* 1994; 74:2107-2117.

McLeskey CH, Janis KM: Perioperative risk and preoperative preparation of the geriatric surgical patient. In Katlic MR, editor: *Geriatric surgery: Comprehensive care of the elderly patient*, Baltimore, 1990, Urban and Schwarzenberg.

Meston CM: Aging and sexuality. *West J Med* 1997; 167:285-290.

Miklos JR, Sze EHM, Karram MM: Vaginal correction of pelvic organ relaxation using local anesthesia. *Obstet Gynecol* 1995; 86:922-924.

Miller KL: Operating on the elderly woman—what are her special needs? *Curr Opin Obstet Gynecol* 1997; 9:300-305.

Monane M, Gurwitz JH, Lipsitz LA, et al: Epidemiologic and diagnostic aspects of bacteriuria: A longitudinal study in older women. *J Am Geriatr Soc* 1995; 43:618-622.

Monga AK, Robinson D, Stanton SL: Periurethral collagen injections for genuine stress incontinence: A 2-year follow-up. *Br J Urol* 1995; 76:156-60.

Naessén T, Lindmark B, Larsen HC: Better postural balance in elderly women receiving estrogens. *Am J Obstet Gynecol* 1997: 177:412-416.

Naessén T, Persson I, Adami H, et al: Hormone replacement therapy and the risk for first hip fracture. *Ann Intern Med* 1990; 113:95-103.

Nathan, L:Vulvovaginal disorders in the elderly woman. *Clin Obstet Gynecol* 1996; 39:933-945.

Nevitt MC, Cummings SR, Lane NE, et al: Association of estrogen replacement therapy with the risk of osteoarthritis of the hip in elderly white women: Study of Osteoporotic Fractures Research Group. *Arch Intern Med* 1996; 156:2073-80.

Newcomb PA, Storer BE: Postmenopausal hormone use and risk of large-bowel cancer. *J Natl Cancer Inst* 1995; 87:1067-1071.

Nicolle LE: Asymptomatic bacteriuria in the elderly. *Infect Dis Clin North Am* 1997; 11:647-662.

Nicolle LE, Mayhew WJ, Bryan L: Prospective randomized comparison of therapy and no therapy for asymptomatic bacteriuria in institutionalized elderly women. *Am J Med* 1987; 83:27-33.

Nicolle LE, Muir P, Harding GM: Localization of urinary tract infection in elderly, institutionalized women with asymptomatic bacteriuria. *J Infect Dis* 1988; 157:65-70.

Nitta V, Bregg K, Sussman E, et al: The Raz bladder neck suspension in patients 65 years old and older. *J Urol* 1993; 149:802-807.

National Institutes of Health: Cervical cancer. *NIH Consensus Statement* 1996; 14:1-38.

Nordenstam GR, Brandberg CA, Oden AS, et al: Bacteriuria and mortality in an elderly population. *N Engl J Med* 1986; 314:1152-1156.

Notelovitz M: Estrogen therapy and osteoporosis: Principles and practice. *Am J Med Sci* 1997: 313:2-12.

Ouslander JG, Schnelle JF: Incontinence in the nursing home. *Ann Intern Med* 1995; 122:438-449.

Ouslander JG, Schnelle JF, Uman G, et al: Does oxybutynin add to the effectiveness of prompted voiding for urinary incontinence among nursing home residents? A placebo-controlled trial. *J Am Geriatr Soc* 1995; 43:610-617.

Paganini-Hill A, Chao A, Ross RK, et al: Exercise and other factors in the prevention of hip fracture: The Leisure World Study. *Epidemiology* 1991; 2:16-25.

Palmer JR, Rosenberg L, Clarke EA, et al: Breast cancer risk after estrogen replacement therapy: Results from the Toronto Breast Cancer Study. *Am J Epidemiol* 1991; 134:1386-1395.

Pearce KF, Haefner HK, Sarwar SF, et al: Cytopathological findings on vaginal Papanicolaou smears after hysterectomy for benign gynecologic disease. *N Engl J Med* 1996; 335:1559-1562.

Peattie A, Stanton SL: The Stamey operation for correction of genuine stress incontinence in the elderly woman. *Br J Obstet Gynaecol* 1989; 96:983-986.

Pompei P: Preoperative assessment and perioperative care. In Cassel CK, Cohen HJ, Larson EB, et al, editors: *Geriatric Medicine*, ed 3; New York, 1997, Springer-Verlag.

Purifoy FE, Grodsky A, Leonard M, et al: The relationship of sexual daydreaming to sexual activity, sexual drive, and sexual attitudes for women across the life-span. *Arch Sex Behav* 1992; 21:369-385.

Resnick NM: Geriatric incontinence. *Urol Clin North Am* 1996a; 23:55-74.

Resnick NM, Brandeis GH, Baumann MM, et al: Misdiagnosis of urinary incontinence in nursing home women. *Neuroruol Urodynam* 1996b; 15:599-618.

Resnick NM, Marcantonio ER: How should clinical care of the aged differ? *Lancet* 1997; 350:1157-1158.

Robinson B, Beghé C: Cancer screening in the older patient. *Clin Geriatr Med* 1997; 13:97-118.

Rockstein M, Sussman M. *Biology of aging,* Belmont, Calif., 1979, Wadsworth.

Rosen PP, Lesser ML, Kinne DW: Breast cancer at the extremes of age: A comparison of patients younger than 35 years and older than 75 years. *J Surg Oncol* 1985; 28:90-96.

Roughan PA, Kaiser FE, Morley JE: Sexuality and the older woman. *Clin Geriatr Med* 1993; 9:87-106.

Sanders AB: Pharmacology and aging. In Sanders AB, editor: *Emergency care of the elderly person,* St. Louis, 1996, Beverly Cracom.

Schneider DL, Barrett-Connor EL, Morton DJ: Timing of postmenopausal estrogen for optimal bone mineral density. *JAMA* 1997; 277:543-547.

Schneider DS, Sledge PA, Shuchter SR, et al: Dating and remarriage over the first two years of widowhood. *Ann Clin Psychiatry* 1996; 8:51-57.

Seeley DG, Cauley JA, Grady D, et al: Is postmenopausal estrogen therapy associated with neuromuscular function or falling in elderly women? Study of Osteoporotic Fractures Research Group. *Arch Intern Med* 1995; 155:293-299.

Smart CR, Byrne C, Smith RA, et al: Twenty-year follow-up of the breast cancers diagnosed during the Breast Cancer Detection Demonstration Project. *CA Cancer J Clin* 1997; 47:134-149.

Smith W, Mitchell P, Wang JJ: Gender, oestrogen, hormone replacement and age-related macular degeneration: results from the Blue Mountains Eye Study. *Aust N Z J Ophthalmol* 1997; 25(suppl 1):S13-S15.

Stanta G, Campagner L, Cavallieri F, et al: Cancer of the oldest old: What we have learned from autopsy studies. *Clin Geriatr Med* 1997; 13:55-68.

Stanton SL, Monga AK: Incontinence in elderly women: Is periurethral collagen an advance? *Br J Obstet Gynaecol* 1997; 104:154-157.

Steinberg MD, Julian MA, Wise L: Psychological outcome of lumpectomy versus mastectomy in the treatment of breast cancer. *Am J Psychiatry* 1985; 142:34-39.

Sullivan JM, Zwaag RV, Hughes JP, et al: Estrogen replacement and coronary artery disease: Effect on survival in postmenopausal women. *Arch Intern Med* 1990; 150:2557-2562.

Sultana CJ, Campbell JW, Pisanelly WS, et al: Morbidity and mortality of incontinence surgery in elderly women: An analysis of medicare data. *Am J Obstet Gynecol* 1997; 176:344-348.

Taunton JE, Martin AD, Rhodes EC, et al: Exercise for the older woman: Choosing the right prescription. *Br J Sports Med* 1997; 31:5-10.

Termrungruanglert W, Kudelka AP, Edwards CL, et al: Gynecologic cancer in the elderly. *Clin Geriatr Med* 1997; 13:363-379.

Tilyard MW, Spears GFS, Com B, et al: Treatment of postmenopausal osteoporosis with calcitriol or calcium. *N Engl J Med* 1997; 326:357-362.

Tiret L, Desmonts JM, Hatton F, et al: Complications associated with anaesthesia—a prospective survey in France. *Can Anaesth Soc J* 1986; 33:336-344.

Tockman MS: Aging of the respiratory system. In Katlic MR, editor: *Geriatric surgery: Comprehensive care of the elderly patient,* Baltimore, 1990, Urban and Schwarzenberg.

Troisi R, Schairer C, Chow WH, et al: A prospective study of menopausal hormones and risk of colorectal cancer (United States). *Cancer Causes Control* 1997; 8:130-138.

Utiger RD: The need for more vitamin D [editorial]. *N Engl J Med* 1998; 338:828-829.

Wain GV, Farnsworth A, Hacker NF: The Papanicolaou smear histories of 237 patients with cervical cancer. *Med J Aust* 1992; 157:14-16.

Watson RR, Huls A, Araghinikuam M, et al: Dehydroepiandrosterone and diseases of aging. *Drugs Aging;* 1996; 9:274-291.

Weber AM, Walters MD, Schover LR, et al: sexual function in women with uterovaginal prolapse and urinary incontinence. *Obstet Gynecol* 1995; 85:483-487.

Williams DB, Voigt BJ, Fu YS, et al: Assessment of less than monthly progestin therapy in postmenopausal women given estrogen replacement. *Obstet Gynecol* 1994; 84:787-793.

Wright LK: The impact of Alzheimer's disease on the marital relationship. *Gerontologist* 1991; 31:224-237.

Wyman JF, Fantl JA, McClish DK, et al: Quality of life following bladder training in older women with urinary incontinence. *Int Urogynecol J* 1997; 8:223-229.

Yaffe K, Sawaya G, Lieberburg I, et al: Estrogen therapy in postmenopausal women: Effects on cognitive function and dementia. *JAMA* 1998; 279:688-695.

Zawada ET, Horning JR, Salem AG: Renal, fluid, electrolyte, and acid-base problems during surgery in the elderly. In Katlic MR, editor: *Geriatric surgery: Comprehensive care of the elderly patient,* Baltimore, 1990, Urban and Schwarzenberg.

Index

Italic numbers indicate illustrations; numbers followed by b indicate boxes; numbers followed by t indicate tables.